Textbook of

ORTHOPAEDICS

AF869019

Accession Number
9299
Order Number 136091
Price £25-22
Class No. WE100
Date 30-8-06

A Thought from the Student

God created the doctor and his patient. Together they created many hospitals and Medical Institutions. A happy world is what it would have been, had it not been the emergencies in between.

Let this book come in 'handy' when it matters the most.

Dr K Sarawana

Textbook of ORTHOPAEDICS

Third Edition

John Ebnezar

MMBS, D'Ortho, DNB (Ortho), MNAMS (Ortho), DAc, DMT
Consulting Orthopaedic and Spine Surgeon and
Holistic Orthopaedic Expert

Formerly

Assistant Professor of Orthopaedics
Devaraj Urs Medical College
Kolar, Karnataka

Senior Specialist in Orthopaedics
Department of Orthopaedics
Victoria Hospital
Bangalore Medical College

Presently

Chairman
The Physically Handicapped and
Paraplegic Charitable Trust of Karnataka ®

President
The Karnataka Orthopaedic Academy ®

Director
Bangalore Holistic Orthopaedic Centre, Bangalore

Medical Director
Parimala Hospital and Research Centre, Bangalore

Chairman
Ebnezar Institute of Orthopaedics, Bangalore

Anshan
Tunbridge Wells
UK

JAYPEE BROTHERS
MEDICAL PUBLISHERS (P) LTD
New Delhi

First published in the UK by

Anshan Ltd
in 2006
6 Newlands Road
Tunbridge Wells
Kent TN4 9AT, UK

Tel/Fax: +44 (0)1892 557767
E-mail: info@anshan.co.uk
www.anshan.co.uk

Copyright © 2006 by (author)

The right of (authors to be identified as the author of this work has been asserted in accordance with the Copyright, Designs and Patents act 1988.

ISBN 1 904798 683

British Library Cataloguing in Publication Data
A catalogue record for this book is available from the British Library

All rights reserved. No part of this publication may be reproduced, stored in a retrieval system, or transmitted in any form or by any means, electronic, mechanical, photocopying, recording and/or otherwise without the prior written permission of the publishers. This book may not be lent, resold, hired out or otherwise disposed of by way of trade in any form, binding or cover other than that in which it is published, without the prior consent of the publishers.

Printed in India by Replika Press Pvt. Ltd.

Many of the designations used by manufacturers and sellers to distinguish their products are claimed as trademarks. Where those designations appear in this book and where the publisher was aware of a trademark claim, the designations have been printed in initial capital letters.

to

My mother (Late) Sampath Kumari
who taught me that life is more than self and there
is more joy in giving and sharing than taking

My wife Dr Parimala, my lovely children Rakesh and Priyanka
who are an epitome of love, sacrifice, encouragement and inspiration

All my teachers
who made me what I am today
&
All my students past and present

Foreword

I sincerely admire the efforts of Dr John Ebnezar. It is an excellent book for the undergraduates and postgraduate students (their teachers too!). I like the style of his writing.

My heartiest congratulations on his solo herculean efforts.

With best wishes

GS Kulkarni
MS, MS (Ortho), FICS
Professor of Orthopaedics and Director
Orthopaedics Hospital and Post Graduate Institute of Orthopaedics
Swasthiyog Pratishthan, Miraj
(Recognised for MS (Ortho), D (Ortho), Courses by
Shivaji University and Medical Council of India,
Delhi and Recognised for Dip NB (Ortho), MNAMS
by National Board of Examinations, Delhi
Editor, Clinical Orthopaedics India
Secretary ASAMI-India (Ilizarov Association)
Chief Research Director, Sandhata Medical Research Society, Miraj

Foreword

I am very glad that Dr John Ebnezar has written an excellent book on Orthopaedics.

The book is extremely informative and is most up-to-date. It is very stylishly written and is neatly designed. It has so many unique features which is hitherto unprecedented in the history of textbook writing.

What makes this book stand out from the rest is that, it never provides the reader with a single dull moment and makes the reading very interesting and thought provoking. It keeps the reader engrossed and the students will find it very gripping and absorbing.

I am sure students will enjoy reading this book and will find it very useful in their preparation for the examination.

I wish him all the success.

Dr N Ramesh
Former Head of the Department and Prof of Orthopaedics
Bowring and Lady Curzon Hospital
Bangalore Medical College
Bangalore
Karnataka, India

Foreword

Dr John Ebnezar has been my assistant and has worked with me for over two years. Knowing him it is hardly surprising that he has written a textbook on Orthopaedics for such is his keeness and interest in teaching the students. He enjoys teaching and is tremendously popular among the students.

The book is very comprehensive, simple and is neatly written. Never before any book on Orthopaedics has come out with so many innovations and this kindles and sustains the interest in the readers. A good book is one which apart from evincing interest in the readers about the subject, makes them desirous to know more and more about it. This book does that and I am sure students will enjoy reading it and the roller coaster experience it provides. The practical approach and suggestions will help the students in their preparations for the examination.

This is the first ever textbook written by an Orthopaedic Surgeon from Karnataka and I am happy that it comes from my assistant. It is indeed befitting that I write a foreword for his book.

I wish him all the best.

Dr YA Somasundara
Former Senior Professor and Head of the
Department of Orthopaedics
Bangalore Medical College
Bangalore
Karnataka, India

Preface to the Third Edition

It is almost a decade when my *Textbook of Orthopaedics* hit the market. Ever since I have been deluged with an unprecedented love, support and encouragement from teachers and students from all over the country. More than my effort, it is this universal liking that has made this book what it is today. It has broken all the conventional barriers and is galloping triumphantly into the third edition. With each passing year, this book has grown from strength to strength. It is both heartening and humbling to hear encomiums from senior professors to undergraduates. Postgraduate students in orthopaedics find this book invaluable. In short, this book has catered to the needs of all and sundry in orthopaedics. In this edition, I have made sincere attempts to live up to the expectations bestowed upon me by scores of people. I am placing the third edition of this book in your hands with the following changes:

Highlights

- The book has been made in multicolour.
- The book has been thoroughly overhauled
- Each and every chapter has been thoroughly updated
- I have inserted about 1,100 mind-boggling colour diagrams in this edition
- I have inserted a number of colour clinical photographs wherever required
- About 50 new X-rays have been added
- Breaking away from the conventional practice I have introduced lots of innovative and thought provoking diagrams which are an idea of my own. Hope students will like it.
- Eight new chapters have been added and the notable ones among them are:
  1. Soft tissue injuries
  2. Fractures in special situations
  3. Hand injuries
  4. Injuries to the foot
  5. Approach to orthopaedic disorders
  6. Deformities and their management
  7. Treatment of orthopaedic disorders
  8. Sports injuries
- Even the Appendices have been thoroughly revised
- Due to the sheer number of diagrams the book has slightly overgrown its size. However, it is an apparent bulk and not the real bulk as diagrams add to the quality of the book.

My book has been widely appreciated for columns like quick facts, vital facts, flow charts, points to ponder, mnemonics, etc. and many students have told me that they just read these just before the exams. These columns give them the gist of the entire chapters in a jiffy and it is a great boon to them. Copying is the best complement and I now see so many new books coming out in the market in orthopaedics are copying this method of mine thereby stamping their approval of my beliefs and thoughts. To make these features more attractive, I have added the following new exciting subcolumns:

1. Lots of interesting captions like 'Did you know'?, 'myths', etc. have been incorporated, wherever required apart from the usual attractions of the second edition.

2. A new column, 'What is new?', has been added. Change is the way of life. Orthopaedics as a science is evolving everyday. Hence, to keep the students abreast of the latest developments, I have provided what is new in each chapter itself.

- Section on Clinical Examination Methods in Orthopaedics is being offered as a free supplement with this edition.

Nobody is infallible. I am grateful to all those who wrote to me pinpointing certain mistakes in the previous edition. I have corrected these and incorporated the meaningful suggestions. I will be glad to have your feedback on this edition too and help me in my endeavor to maintain high standards. Hope my efforts will be well appreciated by the teachers and student community at large. I will be highly obliged if you can send me your comments, criticisms and suggestions. I will be too happy to make the changes if there are any lacunae.

John Ebnezar

Preface to the First Edition

While I was a final year MBBS student, I fell in love with Orthopaedics lock *stock* and *barrel.* The subject fascinated me so much that I was drawn towards it like a magnet. I always wanted to do something to the subject I loved most. This book is a small effort on my part in this regard.

Students often questioned me during my undergraduate teaching sessions as to which book they should read for Orthopaedics. Whenever I suggested the standard books written for them, they said they found them too inadequate and that the bigger books were too much for them. So they were in a *situation of either too little or too much.* I then asked them as to what sort of book they need? They said that, they wanted a book which is comprehensive and at the same time examination oriented. I learnt that my notes were actively being circulated among the students and after each examination, students came back to me and told that they had done extraordinarily well after reading my notes. This surprised me as I had always taught them more than required. I was a firm believer of the fact that by pruning the subject one cannot do justice to it. Examination should be a part of the learning process and not vice versa. I then decided to write a book for them which was adequate, neither less nor more. Little did I realise then that I was embarking on a journey which was arduous and tumultous. I slogged for three long years to bring out this book. Hope students find my effort informative and useful.

Despite being meticulous, I am sure there will be plenty of mistakes in the book. I request the students to point them out unhesitatingly so that I can improve upon. This book will be a useful handbook for postgraduate students also.

Now about the highlights of this book:

To make the book more educative and also to present an enjoyable reading, I have tried certain innovative methods which hitherto has not been attempted in textbook writing. I am confident that it will be received well.

- Autobiographical anatomy: I have noticed that majority of students skip anatomy for reasons of monotony. To assure that they read anatomy, I planned to make it different. So I decided to let the structures talk about themselves. I hope this self-talking anatomy appeals.
- Good illustrative diagrams
- Differential shading of the tables and columns to highlight the facts in their order of importance.
- Quick short summaries during each chapter to make the student focus their attention towards the important and salient features of the topic concerned.
- Useful mnemonics wherever feasible to enable the students to remember and recall easily.
- Diagrams have been put in tabulated columns with suitable description to make it more useful and attractive.
- Orthopaedics is a part of life and not vice versa. The philosophies of life applies to it also. Hence, an attempt is made to view orthopaedics in a philosophical angle.
- Anecdotes, jokes and a word of caution wherever found neessary.
- Good flow charts to convey the ideas effectively.
- Though examination is not everything, but still it is an inescapable inevitability in any student life. On their request, a list of examination short cases and relevant points have been given at the end of the book. It will be of use if only the subject has been studied properly. It will be complementary and not a substitute for good reading.

- X-rays are put in the end of chapters so that students can browse through it, especially during examinations.
- The chapter on instruments is prepared with great care to maximally benefit the students.
- History of orthopaedics is given equal weightage as much as the recent advances. I firmly believe that it is to the solid foundation laid down by our forefathers we owe our present-day success. It is our duty to remember and know their contributions and build upon it.
- Chapter on low backache is written to educate the students about their back. It is a common problem which every student needs to know irrespective of the subject of interest in future. Hence, an attempt is made to present it more realistically.
- More importantly, I have used the services of my students rather than professionals and I hope they have done a commendable job, as they know the requirements and pulse of the students better.

John Ebnezar

Acknowledgements

Bringing out the third edition of the Textbook of Orthopaedics turned out to be a marathon effort. My belief that it would be a smooth sailing considering the experience of the previous two editions went topsy-turvy. I ended working harder for this venture. A mammoth effort like this cannot be stage managed by a single person hence I would like to recall with gratitude the role played by these good samararitans in making my dream a reality.

First and foremost, I would like to offer my reverence to my beloved mother late Smt Sampath Kumari who unfortunately could not live to see the book getting completed. A disciplinarian and idealistic mother to the core. I owe my very existence and success to her. I thank my wife Dr Parimala, my son Rakesh who is now in his first year medical school at Mysore Medical College and my beautiful and lovely daughter Priyanka for the unstinted and unflappable love, warmth, encouragement and support.

I thank all my teachers who shaped my personality and career right from primary school to my post-graduation in orthopaedics. I thank all the colleagues of Victoria Hospital, Bangalore Medical College for their cooperation. I thank my artist friend Mr Linus for creating such beautiful diagrams as desired by me. His creativity in imagining and translating my thoughts into pictures and producing the right impressions are worthy of praise. But for his skill, the book would not have been what it is today. I thankfully acknowledge with fond memories the role played by students Dr KR Raghavi and Dr Raghvendra in this endeavour of mine. I also thank my Junior Reasearch Assistant Dr Yogita in lending me a helping hand. I also thank all the staff of my hospital for helping me.

A lot of credit should go to Shri Jitendar Pal Vij (Chairman and Managing Director), M/s Jaypee Brothers Medical Publishers (P) Ltd, and his entire team for the hard work, cooperation, unstinted faith, support and commitment in bringing out this book. My special thanks to Mr Tarun Duneja, General Manager (Publishing), Mr Mandal (Regional Manager), Mr Venugopal (Asssistant Branch Manager) and all the Bangalore Branch staff and Mr PS Ghuman (Senior Production Manager), Mr KK Raman (Editor), Mr Sukhdev Prasad (DTP Operator), Mr Manoj Pahuja (Graphic Designer) and Ms Bano for their hard work and dedication.

I thank all the teachers and students for patronizing and supporting my book. Finally, I thank the God Almighty for all the blessings and the gift of life.

Contents

Section 1— Traumatology

General Principles

Section 2— Regional Traumatology

Injuries to the Upper Limb

Injuries to the Lower Limb

Injuries to the Axial Skeleton

Nerve Injuries

Section 3— Non- Traumatic Orthopaedic Disorders

General Principles

Regional Orthopaedics

Section 4— Hand Disorders and Low Backache

Section 5— General Orthopaedics

Section 6— Miscellaneous

Appendices

SECTION ONE

TRAUMATOLOGY

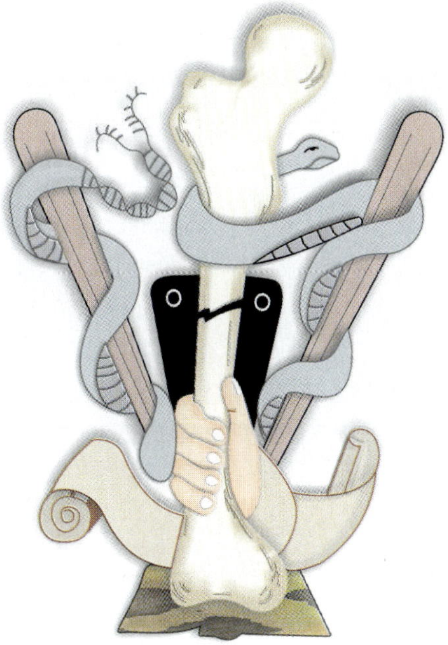

1 Introduction

Orthopaedics has come a long way since the days of Nicholas Andry, a French physician, who is credited for coining the term, orthopaedics from two words, *Ortho = straight* and *Paedics = child* in 1741.

What was a primitive branch then restricted to correcting deformities in children, has developed into a full-fledged speciality with diverse scope ranging from simple treatment, as done by traditional bonesetters to highly advanced joint, spine and hand surgeries.

The development of orthopaedics as a speciality was pedestrian till 18th century. The discovery of anaesthesia and aseptic surgical techniques opened up new avenues of treatment like open reduction, debridement, etc. The discovery of X-rays by Roentgen and the introduction of the usage of Plaster of Paris by Albert Mathysen in 1852 revolutionised the diagnosis and management of orthopaedic disorders. Thus, orthopaedics started breaking through the deadlocks of a crude branch to that of a science.

But what really set the ball rolling was the sudden surge of orthopaedic cases firstly by the two World Wars and of late by the road traffic accidents which is on the rise, both in the developed and developing countries.

Polytrauma, multiple fractures and high-velocity injuries severely exposed the limitations of the conventional treatment in orthopaedics, as the fracture patterns were bizarre and complicated. Thus newer modalities of treatment like improved methods of internal fixation, the AO systems, the interlocking nail system, Ilizarov's method, etc. were introduced into orthopaedic management. Suddenly orthopaedics was being considered a highly specialised branch with vast scope.

Needless to say many pioneers both at the international and national level have contributed enormously for the development of this branch to the present what is today. We salute them for their contribution. A fitting tribute to them is to carry on the good work done by them and to raise the level of this branch to such dizzy heights so that the sufferings of mankind due to orthopaedic disorders is mitigated.

There is a strong notion among the students that orthopaedics is all about trauma. Nothing can be farther from the truth. Though trauma contributes to a major chunk of orthopaedic-related conditions yet it is not the sole contributor. Like any other system in the body, bones and joints are affected by a plethora of disease conditions ranging from congenital disorders, infections, tumours, etc. Degenerative disorders that seem to ravage the musculoskeletal system in old age completes the cup of misery. Needless to say one needs to be equipped both with knowledge and skill to gear up oneself to face the orthopaedic challenges being hurled at surgeons in double quick time of late.

Through this book, I endeavour to arm my students with the all important knowledge so essential to understand and unravel the mysteries surrounding orthopaedic-related conditions. Based on this knowledge, the necessary skills can be acquired through various stages of practical exposures. It always helps to know the common orthopaedic terminologies, tests, surgical procedures, etc. for better and easy understanding. Hence glossary is presented first. It is imperative to know about the fundamentals of bones and joints before undertaking the arduous journey of problems afflicting the musculoskeletal system. Thus basics of this system is talked about next. The ensuing chapters deal extensively first with the traumatic conditions and related problems, followed by non-traumatic conditions.

Finally, the tools required to acquire the all necessary skills are mentioned in the final chapters on instruments and implants. I fervently urge my students to be a stickler for basics and sophistication automatically follows. It pays to know, at the beginning itself, that the reverse is not true.

GLOSSARY

IMPORTANT CLASSIFICATIONS IN ORTHOPAEDICS

Spine

- Allen's—for cervical spine injuries.
- Anderson and D'olonzo's—for odontoid process fractures.
- McAffee's—for thoracolumbar fractures.

Upper Limbs

- Neer's—for proximal humeral fractures.
- Gartland's—for supracondylar fracture of the humerus (extension type).
- Bado's—for Monteggia fractures in adults.
- John Wein's—for Monteggia fractures in children.
- Stimson's—for posterior dislocation of the elbow joint.
- Shorbe's—for side swipe injuries of the elbow.
- Colton's—for olecranon fractures.
- Frykmann's—for Colles' and Smith's fractures
- Mason's—for radial head fractures.

Pelvis Fractures

- Key and Conwell's.
- Tile's.

Lower Limbs

Hip Joint

- Garden's—for fracture neck of femur (intracapsular).
- Pauwell—for intracapsular fracture neck of femur.
- Perlington—for intracapsular fracture neck of femur.
- Delbet's—for fracture neck of femur in children.
- Seinsheimer's—for subtrochanteric fracture of femur.
- Thompson Epstein—for fracture dislocation of the hip.
- Fielding's—for subtrochanteric fracture of the femur.
- Judet—for central dislocation of the hip.
- Neer—for supracondylar fracture of the femur.

Knee and Proximal Tibia

- Smillie's—for meniscal injury.
- Hohl and Moore's—for fracture of the proximal tibia.
- Elli's—for fracture of shaft of tibia and fibula.

Ankle

- Lauge Hansen—for ankle injuries.
- Dennis Weber—for ankle injuries.

Foot

- Essex-Lopresti—for calcaneal fractures.

Peripheral Nerve Injuries

- Sunderland.
- Seddon.

Epiphyseal Injuries

- Salter and Harris.

Miscellaneous

- Gustilo and Anderson's—for open or compound fractures.

IMPORTANT RADIOLOGICAL APPEARANCES

Hip Joint

- Trethovan' sign—seen in slipped capital femoral epiphysis.
- Risser's sign—seen in iliac bone epiphysis.
- Shenton's line—for hip dislocations and displaced hip fractures.
- Hilgenreiner's line—for CDH.
- Perkin's line—for CDH.
- Sagging rope sign—for Perthes' disease.
- Tear drop sign—for Perthes' disease.
- Garden's criteria—for fracture neck of femur.
- Salter extrusion angle—Perthes' disease.

Knee Joint

- Insaal and Blumensaat's lines—for patella alta.

Ankle Joint

- Hawkin's sign—avascular necrosis talus.
- Böhler's angle—for calcaneum.
- Crucial angle of Gissane—for calcaneum.

Shoulder

- Goldie's sign—for periarthritis or frozen shoulder.
- Maloney's line—for shoulder joint, similar to the Shenton's line.

Elbow Joint

- Crescent sign—absence of the normal radiolucent gap of the elbow on the lateral view.
- Tear drop sign—seen in the lateral view of the elbow.
- Anterior humeral line—a line drawn along the anterior border of the distal humeral shaft.
- Fish tail sign—the sharp anterior border of the proximal fragment in supracondylar fracture of the humerus.
- Coronoid line—a line directed proximally along the anterior border of the coronoid process of the ulna.
- Bauman's angle—angle between the horizontal line of the elbow and the line drawn through the lateral epiphysis and the long axis of the forearm.
- MacLaughlin's line—a straight line drawn along the centre of the shaft of the radius cuts the capitulum in the centre irrespective of the position of the elbow.

Hand

- Kaplan's lesion—presence of a sesamoid bone within the metacarpophalangeal joint of the finger (commonly index).
- Scapholunate angle—for carpal injuries.

Spine

- Aneurysmal sign—Pott's spine (anterior type).
- Scottish terrier sign—for spondylolysis due to fracture in pars.

Infection

- Sequestrum—seen in chronic osteomyelitis.
- Cloacae and involucrum—chronic osteomyelitis.
- Spina ventosa—tubercular dactylitis.
- Protrusio acetabuli, Mortal Pestle appearance—TB hip.
- Concertina collapse—TB spine.

Metabolic Disorders

- Champagne glass appearance—rickets.
- Moth-eaten appearance—renal rickets.
- Looser's or Milkman's line—osteomalacia.
- Pin head stippling—primary hyperthyroidism.
- Ground glass and biconcave vertebrae—osteoporosis.
- White line of Frankel—scurvy.
- Scurvy line—scurvy.
- Wimberger's line—scurvy.
- Pelkan spur—scurvy.

Developmental Disorders

- Shepherd's crook deformity—fibrous dysplasia.
- Ribbon ribs—von Recklinghausen's disease.
- Marble bone—osteopetrosis.
- Quadrilateral ilium—achondroplasia.

Congenital Disorders

- von Rosen's line—CDH.
- Kite's index—CTEV.
- Hourglass tibia—congenital pseudarthrosis of tibia.

Bone Tumours

- Soap-bubble appearance—seen in giant cell tumour.
- Onion peel—seen in Ewing's sarcoma.
- Sunrise sign—seen in osteogenic sarcoma.
- Codman's triangle—seen in osteogenic sarcoma.
- Nidus—osteoid osteoma.
- Fluffy, cotton wool, bread crumb or popcorn—chondrosarcoma.
- Pedicle sign—multiple myeloma.

IMPORTANT FRACTURES WITH EPONYMS

Spine

- Hangman's fracture—fracture pedicle lamina of C_2 vertebra.
- Jefferson's fracture—fracture of C_1 vertebra.

- Whiplash injury—ligament injury of the neck.
- Chance fracture—horizontal avulsion fracture of lumbar spine.

Upper Limbs

- Essex-Lopresti fracture—fracture head of the radius with dislocation of the inferior radioulnar joint.
- Night stick fracture—fracture of the shaft of the ulna.
- Galeazzi fracture—fracture distal radius with subluxation or dislocation of the inferior radioulnar joint.
- Fracture of necessity—other name for Galeazzi.
- Reverse Monteggia fracture—other name for Galeazzi.
- Colles' fracture—fracture distal end of radius.
- Smith's fracture—fracture distal end of radius with palmar displacement.
- Chauffeur's fracture—fracture of the radial styloid process.
- Bennett's fracture—intra-articular fracture of the base of the first metacarpal bone.
- Rolando's fracture—extra-articular fracture of the base of the first metacarpal bone.
- Jersey finger—avulsion of flexor digitorum profundus from its insertion on distal phalanx.
- Baseball thumb—avulsion of ulnar collateral ligament.
- Mallet finger or baseball finger—avulsion of the extensor tendon from base of the distal phalanx.
- Barton's fracture—rim fracture of the distal end of the radius.

Pelvis

- Malgaigne's fracture—disruption of the pelvic ring with injury to the pubic symphysis and sacroiliac joint on the same side.

Lower Limbs

- Dash board fracture—fracture patella.
- Bumper's fracture—comminuted lateral condyle fracture tibia.
- Pott's fracture—bimalleolar fracture.
- Cotton's fracture—trimalleolar fracture.
- Aviator's fracture—fracture neck of the talus.
- Jone's fracture—fracture base of the fifth metatarsal bone.
- March fracture—stress fracture of the second metatarsal bone.

IMPORTANT CLINICAL TESTS IN ORTHOPAEDICS

Neck

- Adson's test—for thoracic outlet syndrome.

Shoulder Joint

Tests for anterior dislocation of shoulder:
- Bryant's test.
- Callaway's test.
- Dugas test.
- Hamilton ruler test.
- Regiment badge test—for axillary nerve injury.

Elbow Joint

- Cozen's test—for tennis elbow.
- Gunstock deformity—malunited supracondylar fracture humerus.
- S-shaped deformity—seen in supracondylar fracture humerus.

Forearm

- Volkmann's test—for Volkmann's ischaemia of the forearm.

Wrist Joint

- Wrist drop—for radial nerve injury.
- Thumb and finger drops—for radial nerve injury.
- Finkelstein's test—for de Quervain's disease.

Hand

- Police tip deformity—for Erb's palsy.
- Claw hand—for ulnar nerve injury.
- Benediction test—for median nerve injury.
- Ape thumb deformity—for median nerve injury.
- Pointing index—for median nerve injury.
- Kanaval sign—for ulnar nerve bursitis.
- Froment's sign—for ulnar nerve injury.
- Tinel's sign—for peripheral nerve injury recovery.

Spine

- Anvil test—percussion by the fist thumping to elicit spine tenderness.

- Straight leg raising test (SLRT)—passive straight leg raising test in disc prolapse.
- Fazerstazan test—SLRT with dorsiflexion of the foot.
- Laségue test—hip flexed, knee flexed and the leg is slowly straightened.
- Buckling sign—after doing SLRT knee is suddenly flexed.
- Sicard's test—after doing SLRT great toe is dorsiflexed.
- Well leg raise test—SLRT of the normal leg.
- Bilateral SLRT—SLRT of both the legs.
- Femoral nerve stretch test—reverse SLRT for high disc prolapse.
- Coin test—for TB spine.

Sacroiliac Joint

- Pump handle test.
- Gaenslon's test.

Hip Joint

- Barlow's test—test for CDH in the newborn.
- Ortolani's test—test for CDH in infant between 3 and 9 months.
- Galeazzi's test—knee flexion test for CDH.
- Thomas test—for fixed flexion deformity of the hip.
- Trendelenburg's test—test for abductor mechanism of the hip.
- Ober's test—test for iliotibial band contracture as in polio.

Pelvis

- Destot's sign—pelvic fracture.
- Roux's sign—pelvic fracture.
- Earle's sign—pelvic fracture.

Knee Joint

- Lachman's test—anterior drawer test at 30 degree knee flexion in acute injuries.
- Drawer's test—for anterior cruciate ligament (ACL) tear.
- McMurray's test—test for meniscal injuries.
- Ludloff's test—for avulsion of the lesser trochanter.
- Apley's compression test—for meniscal injuries.
- Apley's distraction test—for knee collateral ligament injuries.
- O'donoghue's triad—injury to the medial meniscus, medial collateral and anterior cruciate ligaments.
- Pivot shift test—for ACL tear.

IMPORTANT ORTHOPAEDIC SURGERIES BY NAMES

Upper Limbs

Shoulder Joint

- Putti-Platt's—Overlapping and tightening of subscapularis tendon for recurrent dislocation of shoulder.
- Bankart's—detached anterior structures attached to glenoid rim by sutures.
- Bristow's—transplantation of coracoid process to anterior rim of the glenoid cavity in recurrent dislocation of shoulder.
- Staple capsulorrhaphy of Destot's and Roux—same as Bankart's but staples used instead of sutures.
- Magnusan and Stack—lateral advancement of subscapularis tendon.
- Eden Hybinette—anterior bone graft over glenoid and scapular neck.
- MacLaughlin—for posterior dislocation of the shoulder.

Elbow Joint

- French osteotomy—lateral closed wedge osteotomy for cubitus varus.
- King's osteotomy—medial open wedge osteotomy for cubitus varus.
- Max page—releasing of structures from medial epicondyle of humerus for VIC.

Wrist Joint

- Fernandez—dorsal wedge osteotomy for Colles.
- Campbell—lateral wedge osteotomy for Colles.

Lower Limbs

Hip Joint

- Souter—release of structures arising from anterior superior iliac spine (ASIS) for polio.

- Yount—sectioning of iliotibial band.
- Meyer—muscle pedicle (quadratus femoris) graft for posterior wall comminution in fracture neck of femur.
- Girdlestone—surgical excision of the hip joint.

Knee Joint

- Wilson—for flexion deformity of the knee.
- Hauser—for recurrent dislocation of the patella.
- Campbell—for recurrent dislocation of patella.

Foot

- Triple arthrodesis—fusion of the subtalar, talonavicular and calcaneocuboid joints.
- Lambrinudi—for severe equinus deformity of the foot.
- Dwyer—lateral closed osteotomy for varus foot deformity.
- Evan—resection of calcaneocuboid joint for CTEV.
- Garceau—transfer of tibialis anterior to middle cuneiform for CTEV.
- Turco—one-stage release of posteromedial structures in mild CTEV.
- MacKay—one-stage release of posteromedial and posterolateral structures in severe CTEV.
- Grice-Green—subtalar fusion.
- Jones'—surgical correction of foot deformity.
- Keller's—surgical correction of halux valgus deformity.
- Steindler's—release of plantar fascia short plantar muscles and long plantar ligament in cavus foot deformity.

TERMINOLOGIES ASSOCIATED WITH FRACTURES

- Fracture—a break in the continuity of the bone.
- Simple fracture—fracture that does not have an open wound in the skin.
- Compound or open—fracture in which there is an open wound at the skin or soft parts that leads into the fracture.
- Comminuted—fracture with multiple fragments.
- Avulsion fracture—small fracture near a joint that usually has a ligament or tendon attached to it.
- Impacted fracture—fracture whose ends are driven into each other.
- Displaced fracture—fracture whose ends are separated.
- Undisplaced fracture—fracture whose ends are not separated.
- Greenstick fracture—incomplete fracture due to break in one cortex of the bone in children.
- Pathologic fracture—fracture that occurs due to bone weakness due to a local or generalised bone disorder.
- Intra-articular fracture—fracture that involves the joint surface of a bone.
- Fatigue or stress fracture—fracture due to repeated minor stresses.
- Torus or buckle fracture—fracture caused by compression of the cortex most commonly in the distal region.
- Epiphyseal fracture—fracture of the growth plate usually in the long bones.
- Occult or hidden fracture—as clinical condition that suggests a fracture. Radiographs 2 to 3 weeks later may show the fracture line or a new bone formation.
- Nonunion—complete failure of fracture union.
- Malunion—union of a fractured bone in a position other than anatomical.
- Cross-union—side-to-side union of fracture.

IMPORTANT ORTHOPAEDIC TERMINOLOGIES

Joint

- Ankylosis—restriction of joint motion.
- Arthrodesis—surgical fusion of a joint.
- Arthroplasty—surgery to restore motion and function to a joint.
- Arthrotomy—opening of a joint.
- Effusion—escape of fluid into a joint cavity.
- Dislocation—complete disruption in the continuity of a joint.
- Subluxation—partial disruption in the continuity of the joint.
- Fracture dislocation—dislocation that occurs in conjunction with a fracture of the bone if incomplete it is called fracture subluxation.
- Osteoarthritis—degeneration of a joint.
- Osteophytes—new bone growth due to degeneration of the joint.
- Arthrocentesis—joint aspiration.
- Arthroscopy—inspection of a joint through an arthroscope.
- Strain—muscle tear.
- Sprain—ligament tear.

- Genu—pertains to knee.
- Cubitus—pertains to the elbow.

Movements

- Flexion—forward bending of the joint.
- Extension—backward bending of a joint.
- Abduction—movement away from the midline.
- Adduction—movement towards the midline.
- Pronation—to rotate the forearm in such a way that the palm looks downwards when the arm is in the anatomical position.
- Supination—to rotate the forearm in such a way that the palm looks forwards when the arm is in the anatomical position.
- Eversion—turning outward of the foot.
- Inversion—turning inward of the foot.

Spine

- Spondylitis—inflammatory condition of the spine.
- Spondylosis—degenerative condition of the spine.
- Spondylolysis—defect in the pars interarticularis of the vertebra.
- Spondylolisthesis—slipping of one vertebra over the other.
- Kyphosis—curvature of the spine with posterior convexity.
- Lordosis—curvature of the spine with anterior convexity.
- Scoliosis—abnormal lateral curvature of the spine.
- Radicular pain—shooting pain due to a spinal nerve involvement.
- Sciatica—shooting pain along the course of the sciatic nerve.
- Laminotomy—opening made in the lamina.
- Hemilaminectomy—partial removal of the lamina.
- Laminectomy—complete removal of the lamina.
- Fenestration—opening made in ligamentum flavum between two laminae.

Foot and Ankle

- Equinus—plantar flexion of the foot.
- Calcaneus—dorsiflexion of the foot.
- Planus—flat foot.
- Cavus—hollow foot.
- Talipes—talus (ankle) + pes (foot).
- Pes—foot.
- Hallux—great toe.

Tendons and Nerves

- Tenotomy—cutting a tendon.
- Tenodesis—attaching a tendon to another tendon or bone.
- Tenolysis—freeing a tendon from adhesions.
- Tendon transfer—transferring a tendon from one site to the other.
- Neurolysis—freeing a nerve from adhesions.
- Neurorrhaphy—repairing a sectioned nerve.
- Neurectomy—sectioning a nerve.

IMPORTANT OSTEOTOMIES IN ORTHOPAEDICS

Upper Limbs

- French—for cubitus varus deformity.
- King's—for cubitus varus deformity.

Hip Joint

- McMurray—for nonunion fracture neck femur.
- Shanz—for nonunion fracture neck femur.
- Pauwel—for nonunion fracture neck femur.
- Salter—for CDH.
- Pemberton—for CDH.
- Steel—for CDH.
- Chiari—for CDH.
- Derotation osteotomy—for CDH.
- Innominate osteotomy—for Perthes.

Knee

- High tibial osteotomy (HTO) for genu varum deformity in osteoarthritis.

Spine

- Spinal osteotomy—for ankylosing spondylitis.

Foot

- Dwyer's—for varus deformity of the heel.

2

Know Your Skeletal System

Section 1

BRIEF ANATOMY

THE BONE SPEAKS

I am a specialised connective tissue. By providing a rigid skeleton I give the all important shape to the human beings. I am proud to be entrusted the job of protecting vital structures like brain, lungs and heart. I am the largest storehouse of the all important mineral, i.e. calcium in the body. I am also concerned with haemopoiesis. I give attachment to the muscles and enable them to act on the joints by acting as a lever for their action. I am made up of 30 per cent organic material (mainly type I collagen) and 70 per cent mineral (calcium hydroxyapatite).

Remember the functions of bone

- Protection of vital organs.
- Support to the body.
- Haemopoiesis.
- Movement.
- Mineral storage.

How I start Developing?

My development begins with the condensation of the mesenchyme in the embryo. There are certain exceptions like the vault of the skull (membranous ossification), the clavicle (mixed ossification) and the mandible (Meckel's cartilage). From this condensation I rapidly form a cartilaginous model. Between the cartilaginous bone and plates, I form small clefts for the future joints. During this period of 12 weeks, I am particularly vulnerable to teratogenic influences.

As early as the fifth week of intrauterine life, I develop a primary centre of ossification which gradually replaces this cartilage model to bone by a process of endochondral ossification. During the late fetal stages or early few years of life, I develop secondary centres of ossification.

Growth plate which keeps the primary and secondary centres of ossification separated from each other till skeletal maturity, helps me grow longitudinally and I increase my width from the growth of the thickened periosteum. In addition, I keep remodelling myself from the fetal stage to the adult stage. Only the rate varies (50% during the first two years of life and 5% per year thereafter till adulthood).

Remember

- Bone development starts as a condensation of mesenchyme.
- Later a cartilaginous model develops.
- There are two types of ossification—endochondral and membranous.
- There are three types of bone cells.

About Osteon

Now let me tell you how exactly I am made up of internally. I am made up of many units called *"osteon"*. I have three types of cells, osteoblasts which form the bone, osteoclasts which remove the bone and are concerned with remodelling, osteocytes which are the resting cells. These cells are present in the lamellae, which surround concentrically the Volkmann's canal (which has the nutrient vessel) and each lamellae is interconnected by the canaliculi through which the nutrients pass. Osteoblasts lay down uncalcified matrix which is subsequently calcified as true bone. These various osteons amalgamate to form large haversian systems, loosely woven in the medullary bone and densely packed in the cortical shell (Fig. 2.1).

Now having known my intrinsic structure, you will be interested to know that I have two major portions, *medulla* and the *cortex*.

About Medulla

Medulla is my softer counterpart and has the dual role of structure and storage. It stores more than 95 per cent of body's calcium and is a storehouse for other minerals too. The other important component of the medulla is the marrow between the medullary bone lattice. This is the source from where the RBCs and WBCs originate. Initially

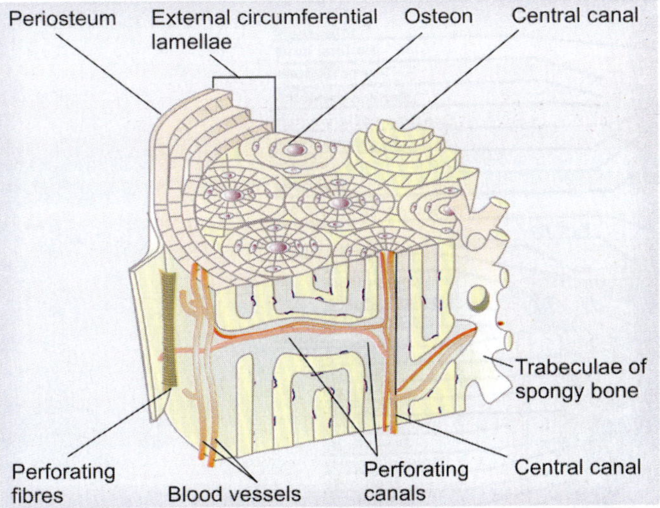

Fig. 2.1: Bone cross section showing its internal structure

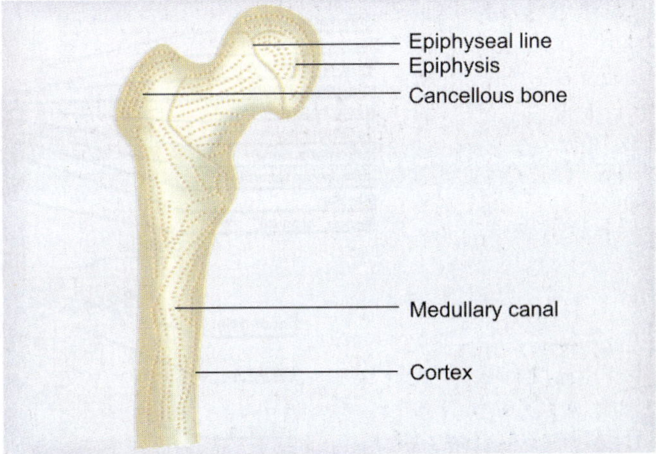

Fig. 2.2: Showing general structure of a long bone

present throughout, it confines itself to the metaphyseal regions of the long bones and in some flat bones like pelvis, rib, etc. as age advances and is replaced by a *fatty white marrow.*

The medulla plays the structural role by its trabecular organisation along maximal lines of stress and clearly identifies itself into *compression* and *traction trabeculae.*

About Cortex

Cortex gives me the remarkable strength which you all admire particularly during compression. Its periosteal cover allows remodelling throughout life. It also gives attachments to ligaments, tendons and muscles through the Sharpey's fibres.

Remember about medulla

- Softer portion.
- Stores 95 per cent of body calcium.
- Marrow is the other important component.
- Also plays a structural role.

About General Structure

Now let me explain to you my general structure. I have an epiphysis and epiphyseal plate (which disappears with growth), metaphysis and diaphysis (Fig. 2.2).

Epiphysis This is an expanded portion at the end, develops usually under pressure and forms a support for the joint surface. It is easily affected by developmental problems like epiphyseal dysplasias, trauma, overuse, degeneration and damaged blood supply. The end result is distorted joints due to avascular necrosis and degenerative changes.

Growth plate (physis) Though mechanically weak it helps longitudinal growth. It responds to growth and sex hormones. It is affected by conditions like osteomyelitis, tumour, slipped epiphysis resulting in short stature or deformed growth or growth arrest.

Metaphysis This is concerned with remodelling of bone. It is the cancellous portion and heals readily. It gives attachment to ligament and tendons. It is vulnerable to develop osteomyelitis, dysplasias and tumours resulting in distorted growth and altered bone shapes.

Diaphysis This is a significant compact cortical bone which is strong in compression and which gives origin to muscles. It forms the shafts of the bones. Healing is slow when compared to metaphysis. In remodelling it can remodel angulation but not rotation. It may develop fractures, dysplasias, infection and rarely tumours.

Remember: Parts of a bone

- Epiphysis
- Physis (growth plate)
- Metaphysis
- Diaphysis

ORGANISATION OF THE BONES

We are 206 in number and are grouped into two subdivisions namely:

1. Axial skeleton—80 bones (Table 2.1).
2. Appendicular skeleton—126 bones (Table 2.2).

Axial skeleton forms the upright axis of the body and the *appendicular skeleton* forms the appendages and girdles that attach them to the axial skeleton (Fig. 2.3).

Out of this 206, some of us are short and some are long. We have different shapes. The shape and size depend upon the functions attributed to us.

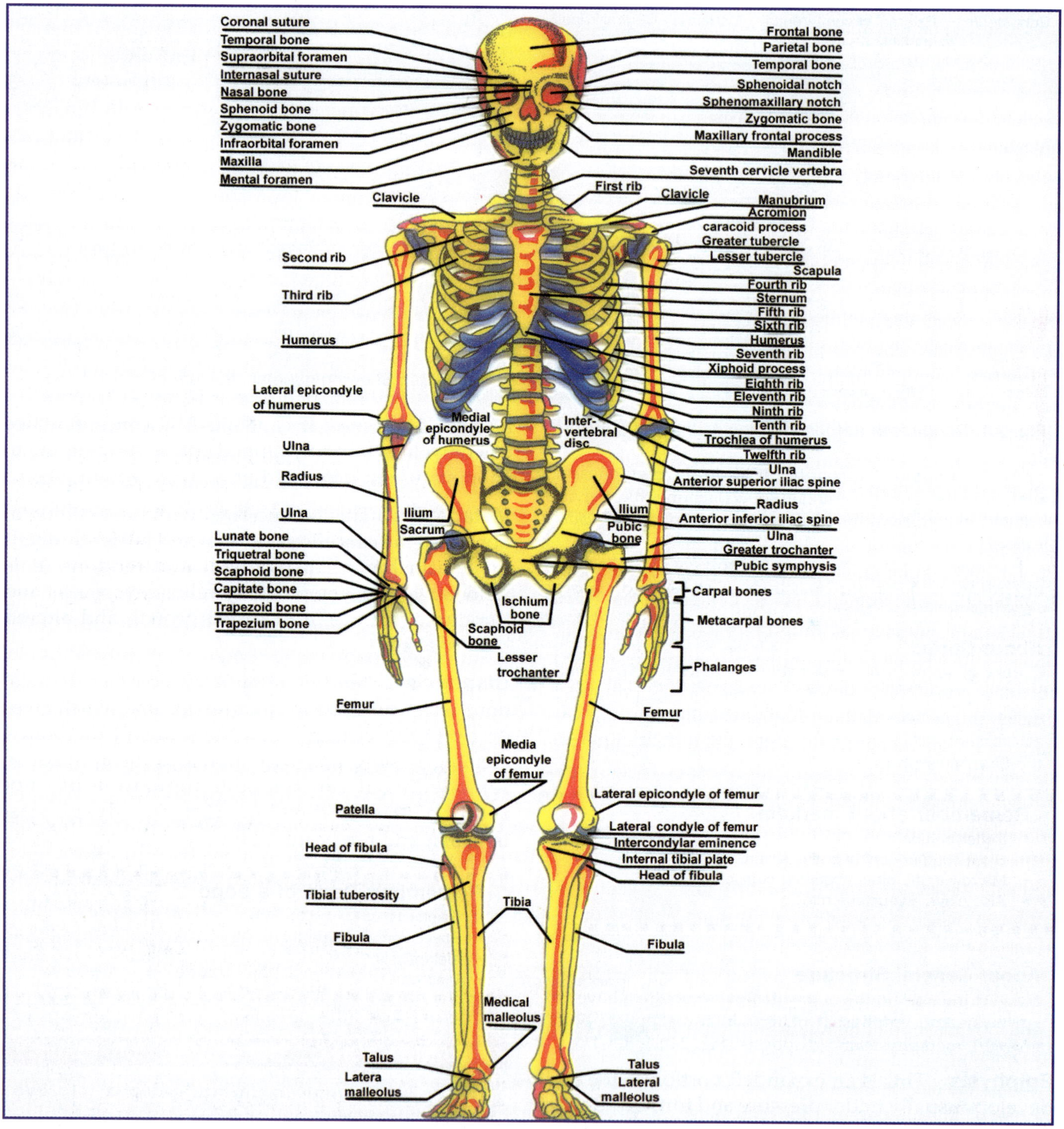

Fig. 2.3: Organisation of bones: Axial and appendicular skeleton

TYPES OF BONES (Figs 2.4A to C)

Long bones (Fig. 2.4C) These serve as levers for the muscle action, e.g. femur, tibia, etc.

Short bones These are generally cube-shaped and are found in areas where limited movements are required. Their primary role is to provide strength (Fig. 2.5).

Table 2.1: Bones in the axial skeleton

Skull		
• Cranium	8	
• Face	14	
Vertebral column		
• Cervical vertebrae	7	
• Thoracic vertebrae	12	
• Lumbar vertebrae	5	
• Sacrum	1	(5 fused bones)
• Coccyx	1	(3-5 fused bones)
Sternum	1	
Ribs	24	(12 pairs)
Hyoid	1	
Ear ossicles		
• Malleus	2	
• Incus	2	
• Stapes	2	
Total	**80**	

Table 2.2: Bones of the appendicular skeleton

Shoulder girdle	
• Clavicle	2
• Scapula	2
Upper extremities	
• Humerus	2
• Ulna	2
• Radius	2
• Carpals	16
• Metacarpals	10
• Phalanges	28
Hip girdle	
• Os coxa	2
Lower extremity	
• Femur	2
• Fibula	2
• Tibia	2
• Patella	2
• Tarsals	14
• Metatarsals	10
• Phalanges	28
Total	**126**

Flat bones (Fig. 2.4A) These consist of parallel layers of compact bone separated by a thin layer of cancellous bone tissue, e.g. scapula, skull, etc.

Irregular bones (Fig. 2.4B) These have a peculiar and irregular shape and are unique in their appearance and functions, e.g. pelvic bones.

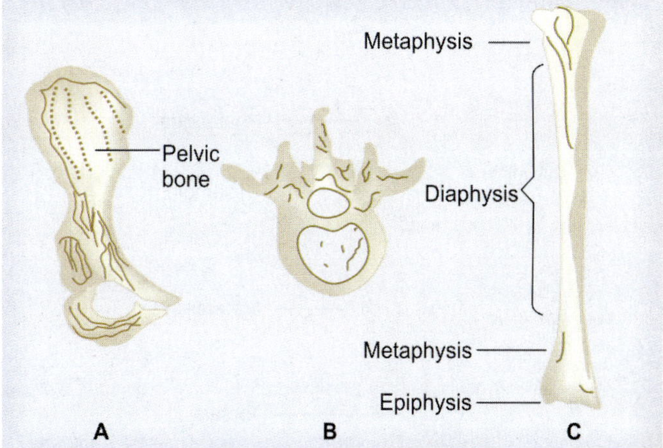

Figs 2.4A to C: Showing types of bones (A) flat bone, (B) irregular bone, and (C) long bone

Sesamoid bones These are small, rounded or triangular bones which develop within the substance of a tendon or fascia. Their name is derived from their resemblance to "sesame seeds", e.g. patella (largest and most definitive of the sesamoid bones).

Remember

Types of bones

- Long bones
- Short bones
- Flat bones
- Irregular bones
- Sesamoid bones

The above bones are arranged in two groups

- Axial—80 bones
- Appendicular—126 bones

Thus, my duty is to serve you to the best of my ability, so that you lead a healthy skeletal life. Much depends on you in keeping me in a proper shape. You need to take good nutritious diet rich in calcium and vitamins to keep me healthy. Proper exercises, protection against injuries and infection enhance my efficiency in serving you, but there are certain inherent problems in me in which you can do precious little. Congenital problems, hormonal problems, metabolic problems, tumour conditions, etc. are some of these.

Though the above problems are troublesome I develop them infrequently. But the problem which poses a serious threat to my integrity are injuries due to trauma. As a child, you are more playful and more prone to fall and this breaks me quite often. As an adult, you are more prone for road traffic accidents (RTAs) and this subjects me to a plethora of different varieties of forces causing many complex, grotesque and bizarre breaks. Though you pride in the fast-paced life of yours, I grieve at my misfortune and at my vulnerability to these vast array of incriminating forces which overcome me putting you out of action for months.

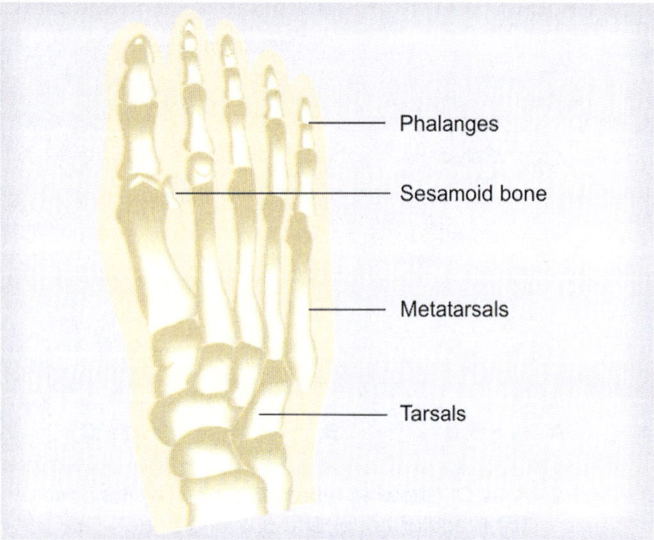

Fig. 2.5: Foot is an assembly of short bones of various sizes

> As you age, my faithful friends, proteins and minerals gradually desert me. I cannot provide you the same strength as earlier. In this phase, I am easily overcome by even trivial forces (pathological fractures). I am sad that I cannot provide you the same privileges as before but I hope you can realise that I am not being unfaithful to you, but I am made helpless by situations beyond anybody's control.

ABOUT JOINTS

A joint exists where two or more skeletal components— whether bone or cartilage, come together to meet. Without joints in between the bones your whole body would be rigid and immobile. It is the existence of the joint that makes movement of the body parts possible. Joints are classified into three major groups:

Fibrous joint or synarthrosis These are immovable joints, e.g. sutures of the skull. In these there are three varieties.

Syndesmosis This is characterised by a dense fibrous membrane that binds the articular bone surfaces very closely and tightly to each other, e.g. distal tibiofibular joint.

Sutures True sutures are found in the skull. Here the adjoining bone margins are united into rigid, jagged interlocking processes, e.g. sagittal suture of the skull.

Gomphosis Here a conical peg or projection that fits into a socket, e.g. teeth and sockets of jaw bones.

Cartilaginous joints or amphorthosis These are slightly movable joints with either hyaline or fibrocartilage in between. Two varieties are described.

Synchondroses Here hyaline cartilage is posed in between, e.g. articulations between rib and sternum.

Symphysis Here fibrocartilage is interposed in between and are usually found in the midline of the body, e.g. pubic symphysis.

SYNOVIAL JOINTS OR DIARTHROSIS

These form the majority of the joints in the body. They have between the bones, a synovial or joint cavity. They form the most mobile joints in the body and hence are more prone for injuries.

It consists of a fibrous joint capsule which helps to hold the articulating bones together. The synovial membrane lines the joint space and secretes the synovial fluid. This fluid serves to lubricate the joints and provides nourishment for the articular cartilage. The articular cartilage is formed by the hyaline cartilage which is a unique type of connective tissue formed by specialised cells called chondrocytes.

TYPES OF SYNOVIAL JOINTS (Figs 2.6A to G)

Uniaxial joints These permit movement in only one plane and one axis. In this there are two types:

Hinge joints Here movement takes place around a horizontal axis, e.g. elbow joint.

Pivot joints Here movement takes place around a vertical axis which permits rotation, e.g. atlantoaxial joint.

Biaxial joints Here movement occurs in two planes and two axes that are at right angles to each other. Two types are described:

Saddle joint Here the articular surface is concave in one direction and convex in the other while the articular surface of the opposing bone is exactly the opposite, e.g. carpometacarpal joint at the base of the thumb.

Condyloid joint In this an oval condyle fits into an elliptic socket or cavity, e.g. radiocarpal joints.

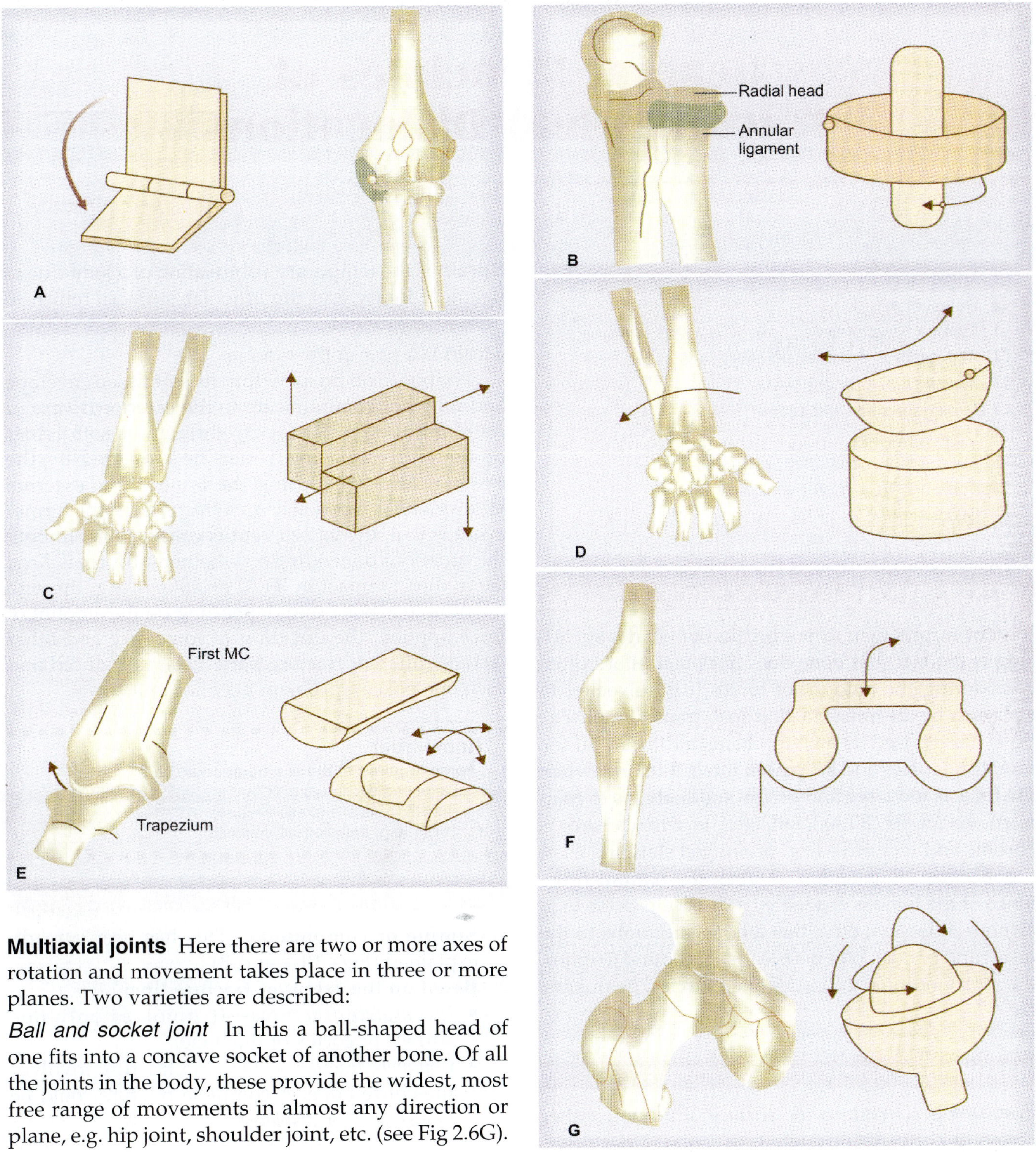

Figs 2.6A to G: Showing different types of joints: (A) Hinge joint, (B) Pivot joint, (C) Plane joint, (D) Ellipsoid joint, (E) Saddle joint, (F) Bicondylar joint, (G) Ball and socket joint

Multiaxial joints Here there are two or more axes of rotation and movement takes place in three or more planes. Two varieties are described:

Ball and socket joint In this a ball-shaped head of one fits into a concave socket of another bone. Of all the joints in the body, these provide the widest, most free range of movements in almost any direction or plane, e.g. hip joint, shoulder joint, etc. (see Fig 2.6G).

Gliding joints These are numerous and gliding movements occur in all planes, e.g. joints between the carpal and tarsal bones and all the joints between the articular processes of the vertebrae (see Fig. 2.6C).

3 General Principles of Fractures and Dislocations

INTRODUCTION

It is not surprising if a bone breaks but what is surprising is the fact that bone does not break more often considering the amount of forces it is subjected to everyday by the muscle action, load transmission, etc. Bone has devised its own mechanism to ward off the unnatural forces and keep itself intact. But only when the force is too large and occurs suddenly [as in road traffic accidents (RTAs), fall, etc.], or when a force is chronic and repetitive (e.g. prolonged standing as in a policeman, nurse, etc.) or when the natural resistance of the bone is eroded by a disease process (e.g. tumour, infection, etc.), that a bone succumbs to the insult and breaks. When it breaks, it is bound to injure the surrounding soft tissues like muscles, ligaments, etc.

DEFINITIONS

Fracture is a break in the surface of a bone, either across its cortex or through its articular surface.

Dislocation is a complete and persistent displacement of a joint in which at least part of the supporting joint capsule and some of its ligaments are disrupted.

Subluxation is a partial dislocation of a joint.

Sprain is the temporary subluxation of a joint due to ligament injury and the articular surfaces return to normal alignment.

Strain is a tear in the muscle.

The bone can break within its soft tissue envelope and may not communicate to the exterior *(simple* or *closed fractures)* or it may rip through its soft tissues or the soft tissue itself may be damaged by the external forces, exposing the bone to the external atmosphere *(compound or open fractures)*. If the former event is bad, the latter event is catastrophic. In both the situations depending on whether the force is *direct* (as in direct impact in RTA) or *indirect* (e.g. through the muscle action), and depending on the amount of force applied, the direction of force, age and other factors, different fracture patterns are produced and each one poses a problem peculiar to its own.

> **Remember**
>
> **Force required to break a bone could be**
> - Large and sudden (e.g. RTA).
> - Repetitive (e.g. a stress fracture).
> - Trivial (e.g. pathological fractures).

TYPES OF FRACTURES

1. **Simple or compound**— This has been already explained (Figs 3.1A and B).
2. **Based on the extent of fracture line:**
   - *Incomplete fractures*—It involves only one surface or cortex of the bone.
   - *Complete fracture*—Here the fracture involves the entire bone. A complete fracture could be *undisplaced* or *displaced.*

> **Causes for displacement**
> - Muscle forces.
> - Gravity.
> - Obliquity of the fracture line.
> - Improper handling of the fracture.

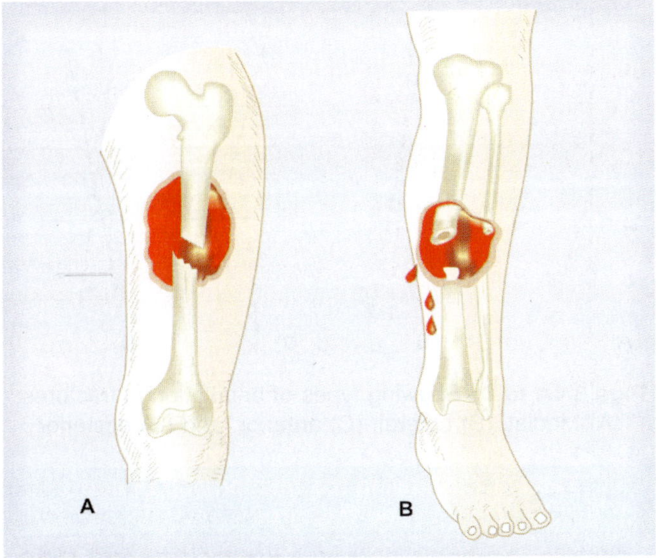

Figs 3.1A and B: Showing simple and compound fractures

3. **Based on fracture patterns (orthopaedic trauma association classification—Figs 3.2A to E)**
   - *Linear fractures* These could be *transverse, oblique* or *spiral*. Any fracture which forms an angle less than 30° with the horizontal line, is called transverse. Angle equal to or more than 30° is termed oblique.
   - *Comminuted fractures* Here the fracture fragments are more than two in number. They are further subclassified into $\leq$ *50% comminution* or more than *50% comminution*. *Butterfly-shaped fractures* are also included in this group.
   - *Segmental fractures* A fracture can break into segments and the segment could be two-level, three-level, a longitudinal split or comminuted.
   - *Bone loss* This could be a < 50 per cent bone loss or more than 50 per cent bone loss or a complete bone loss.

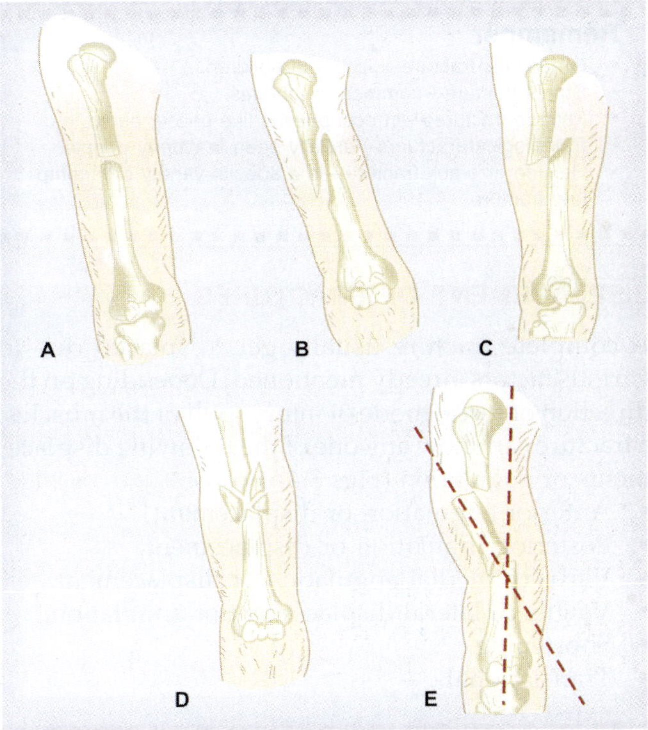

Figs 3.2A to E: Types of fractures based on fracture patterns: (A) transverse, (B) spiral, (C) oblique, (D) comminuted, and (E) segmental fractures

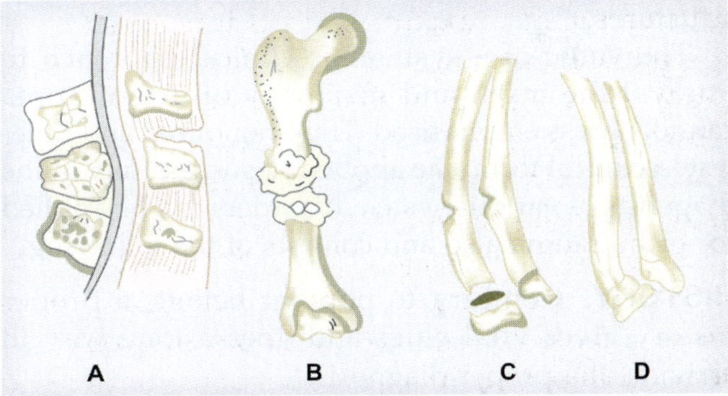

Figs 3.3A to D: Showing atypical fractures: (A) compression, (B) pathological, (C) greenstick, and (D) torus fractures

Atypical Fractures (*Figs 3.3A to D*)

a. *Greenstick fractures* It is seen exclusively in children. Here the bone is elastic and usually bends due to buckling or breaking of one cortex when a force is applied. This is called a greenstick fracture.
b. *Impacted fractures* Here the fracture fragments are impacted into each other and are not separated and displaced.
c. *Stress or fatigue fracture* It is usually an incomplete fracture commonly seen in athletes and in bones subjected to chronic and repetitive stress (e.g. third metatarsal fracture, fracture tibia, etc.).
d. *Pathological fracture* It occurs in a diseased bone and is usually spontaneous. The force required to bring about a pathological fracture is trivial.
e. *Hairline or crack fracture* It is a very fine break in the bone which is difficult to diagnose clinically. Radiology usually helps or still better is CT scan.
f. *Torus fracture* This is just a buckling of the outer cortex.

Remember
- Greenstick fracture—occurs in children.
- Stress fracture—common in athletes.
- Fatigue fractures—in occupations like police, nurse, etc.
- Pathological fractures—usually seen in elderly people.
- Hairline or crack fracture—is a special variety of incomplete fracture.

DISPLACEMENT OF FRACTURES

A complete fracture usually gets displaced due to various factors already mentioned. Depending on the direction of force, mode of injury, pull of the muscles, a fracture can show any one of the following displacements or angulation (Figs 3.4A to D):
- Anterior angulation or displacement.
- Posterior angulation or displacement.
- Varus or medial angulation or displacement.
- Valgus or lateral displacement or angulation.
- Shortening.
- Translational.

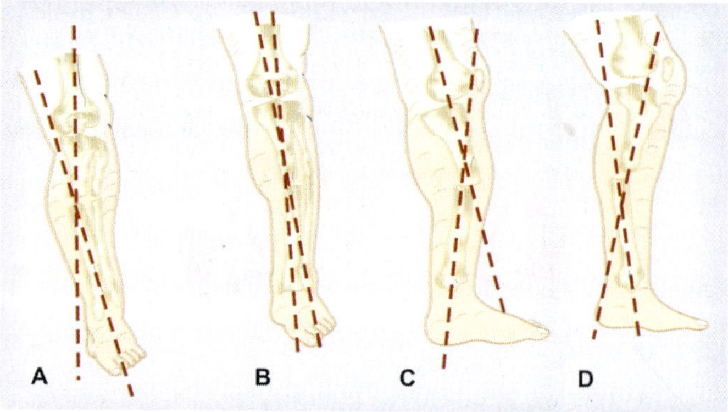

Figs 3.4A to D: Showing types of angulation in fractures: (A) Medial, (B) Lateral, (C) anterior, and (D) posterior

APPROACH TO ORTHOPAEDIC INJURY

Orthopaedic injuries encompass a wide range of problems starting from bone and joint injuries, strains, sprains and damage to associated neurovascular structures.

The value of a systematic clinical approach to unravel the myth and mysteries of orthotrauma cannot be less emphasised. Time-honoured and time-tested clinical formulae applied so successfully in the diagnosis of various system disorders can be applied for orthotrauma also and consists of the following.

HISTORY Contrary to popular beliefs, a proper history gives vital clues and goes a long way in arriving at a proper diagnosis.

Age Certain fractures have predilections for certain age groups (Table 3.1). Hence the practice of first enquiring about the age of the patient is a step in the right direction.

Sex Colles' fracture is more common in females and supracondylar fracture humerus, posterior dislocations of elbow are more common in males.

Table 3.1: Showing the relationship of age and fractures

Age vs	*Fractures and dislocations*
• *Birth*	Brachial plexus injury, fracture, clavicle, fracture humerus, etc.
• *Early childhood*	Supracondylar fracture of humerus. Epiphyseal injuries.
• *Late childhood*	Posterior dislocations of elbow. Slipped capital epiphysis. Monteggia fractures.
• *Adult*	Fracture of long bones. Hip and shoulder dislocations.
• *Elderly*	Colles' fracture. Fracture neck femur.

Note In spite of age predilections, any fracture can be seen in any age group as an aberration.

Mechanism of Injury

This could be different in different age groups as mentioned below in Table 3.2.

Clinical Features

A patient with limb injuries may present with the following complaints.
1. *Pain* This is a very subjective symptom and is invariably the first and the most important complaint. It may be mild, moderate and severe and may be due to tearing of periosteum (which contains the nerve endings), soft tissue injury, nerve injury, etc.
2. *Swelling* It is due to soft tissue injury, medullary, bleeding and reactionary haemorrhage. Swelling is usually more in fractures and less in dislocations.
3. *Deformity* Patients with displaced fractures and dislocations usually present with some deformity.
4. *Inability* to use the affected part is another frequent complaint.

Table 3.2: Showing the relationship of age, types of fractures and mode of injuries

Age	*Common modes of injury*	*Examples*
Children	• Fall on the outstretched hands usually while on play or from a height	Fracture clavicle, Fracture and dislocations of any upper limb bones.
Adults	• Fall from height	• Upper limb injuries, spine injuries, etc.
	• Diving injuries	• Cervical spine injuries.
	• RTA	• Any combination of injuries. • Whiplash injury. • Dashboard injuries like fracture patella, posterior hip dislocation, etc.
	• Sports injuries	• Ankle and shoulder, elbow and knee joint injuries.
	• Assaults	• Long bone fractures (e.g. night stick fracture of ulna).
Elderly	Trivial fall	• Colles' fracture • Fracture neck femur, etc.

Note: High-velocity trauma due to RTA can produce any combination of bone and joint injuries.

Having made a note of the history and presenting complaints, effort is now directed towards eliciting the signs, some of which are general and some are injury specific.

- *Tenderness* This is an important clinical sign in bone and joint injuries and is usually seen after trauma. Importance of tenderness, methods of elicitation and grading is mentioned in the box *(refer p. 20)*.
- *Swelling* The swelling is examined for shape, size, consistency, tenderness, fluctuation, etc.
- *Deformity* This is usually seen in displaced fractures and dislocations. Undisplaced fractures, mild strains and sprains usually show no deformities. Some of the deformities are very characteristic (Figs 3.5A to D) and specific and help in making a spot diagnosis (Table 3.3).
- *Abnormal mobility* between fracture fragments is a sure sign of fracture.
- *Loss of transmitted movements* When one end of the limb is rotated, it automatically gets transmitted to the other end. Due to the break in the continuity this is no longer possible in displaced fractures.

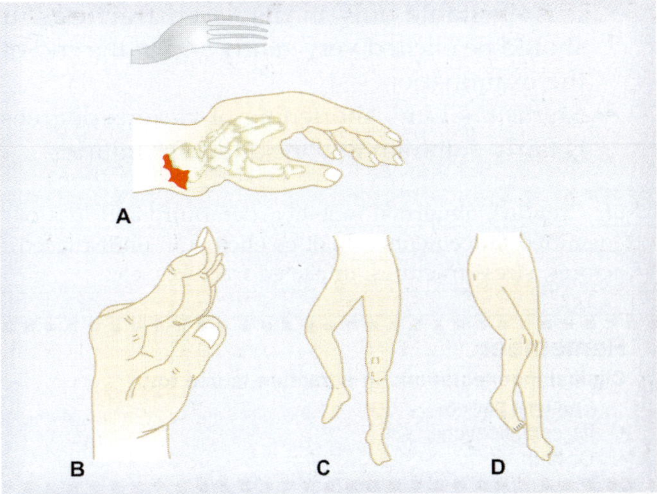

Figs 3.5A to D: Showing some important deformities in orthopaedics: (A) dinner fork deformity, (B) swan neck deformity, (C) anterior dislocation of hip, and (D) posterior dislocation of hip

Table 3.3: Deformity facts

Classical deformities	*Possible diagnosis*
1. Wryneck	Cervical spine injuries.
2. Drooping of shoulder	Clavicle fracture.
3. Flat shoulder	Anterior dislocation of shoulder.
4. S-shaped deformity of humerus	Supracondylar fracture humerus.
5. Dinner fork deformity	Colles' fracture.
6. Boutonniére deformity	Rupture of central extensor slip of finger.
7. Mallet finger	Rupture of distal end of index extensor.
8. Jersey finger	Rupture of distal end of flexor digitorum profundus of index finger.
9. Flexion, adduction and internal rotation	Posterior dislocation of hip
10. Flexion, abduction and external rotation of lower limb	Anterior dislocation of hip
11. Incomplete external rotation of lower limbs	Fracture neck femur (intracapsular).
12. Complete external rotation of lower limbs	Trochanteric fractures, shaft femur, leg bones fractures.
13. S-shaped ankle	Ankle dislocations.

- *Crepitus* This is an abnormal grating sensation produced by the friction between two ragged surfaces of the fracture fragments. Obviously,

Section 1

it is elicitable only in displaced fractures. It should be elicited very gently and in the end of the examination.

- *Shortening* Limb shortening of various degrees is fairly common in bone and joint injuries.

Note Creptius, abnormal mobility, deformity and loss of transmitted movements cannot be elicited in undisplaced fractures, stress fractures, impacted fractures, etc.

Remember

Clinical manifestations in a fracture is due to:
- Fracture per se
- Its complications
- Or both

Interesting Features about the Clinical Signs (Table 3.4)

Various clinical signs are described in fractures. They can be best represented as follows in order of their importance.

Table 3.4: Showing relevance of clinical signs

Clinical signs	
Unfailing signs	• Abnormal mobility • Crepitus
Reliable signs	• Tenderness • Shortening
Important signs	• Bruise • Swelling
Other signs	• Loss of function • Deformity
Late or inconstant signs	• Blisters • Ecchymosis • Swelling due to callus

Remember

***"D"* in fracture**
- Deformity is seen often in displaced fractures.
- Displacement could be anterior, posterior, medial or lateral.
- Distal fragment is the reference point to suggest the type of displacement.
- Dislocation of joints usually presents a deformity.

About crepitus It is defined as an abnormal grating sensation either felt or heard. It could be:
- *Fine* e.g. osteoarthritis
- *Coarse* e.g. fractures
- *Snap* e.g. snapping tendons.

Remember it is unkind to elicit a crepitus in a fracture for fear of hurting the patient.

About tenderness

Remember

Tenderness may be the only evidence of fracture in
- Crack fracture.
- Hairline fracture.
- Stress fracture.
- Fatigue fracture.
- Torus fracture.
- Pathological fracture.

Method of eliciting Proceed from normal area to the affected part for better patient compliance.

Grading
- Grade I—Just a suspect.
- Grade II—Patient winces on pressure.
- Grade III—Patient winces and withdraws.
- Grade IV—Patient will not allow to touch.

This grading of tenderness is superior to the conventional mild, moderate and severe grading.

Clinical manifestations due to neurovascular injuries
Certain fractures are known to cause neurovascular damage quite frequently, e.g. supracondylar fracture of humerus in children. Impending vascular damage is detected by the familiar **five Ps** and nerve injuries are detected by the classical deformities and screening tests (as described in peripheral nerve injuries).

About five Ps

In detecting impending vascular damage in musculo-skeletel trauma
- **P**ain
- **P**allor
- **P**araesthesia
- **P**ulselessness
- **P**aralysis

There are certain bones in the body, the fractures of which are usually missed in the initial examination (see box below). These are known to cause diagnostic difficulties and dilemas.

Missing facts

Do you know the fractures which can give a slip to the clinician:
- Zygoma
- Base of skull
- Odontoid process
- C_7 vertebra
- Ribs
- Radial head
- Impacted fracture neck of femur
- Undisplaced pelvic fracture
- Scaphoid fracture
- Carpal dislocations
- Tarsometatarsal joints
- Talus fracture
- March fracture

Note: Among these, scaphoid tops the list.

INVESTIGATIONS IN ORTHOTRAUMA

Radiography

It is an important diagnostic tool for fractures. Minimum two views, anteroposterior and lateral are required as bone is a cylinder. Sometimes an oblique view and other special views are required depending upon the clinical situations and bone under study.

Vital facts: about Plain X-ray

Radiological clues one should look for on plain X-rays for diagnosis of fractures
- Where is the fracture?
- Situations: Whether it is in the diaphysis, metaphysis, epiphysis and the articular surface.
- Anatomy: Look for the fracture line, whether it is transverse, oblique, spiral, segmental, comminuted, etc.
- Also, look for the alignment, angulation, displacement, rotation, etc.
- Number: How many fragments are seen?
- Bone condition: Identify whether the bone is normal or pathological.
- Joint involvement: Look for the extension of the fracture line into the joint, joint swelling and for evidence of dislocation.
- Soft tissue swelling: The extent of the soft tissue swelling indicates the severity of the injury.

Pitfalls of X-ray
- Presence of a fracture line on an X-ray helps confirm the diagnosis but its absence does not rule out a fracture.
- Hairline fractures tend to get missed (e.g. scaphoid)
- Some dislocations if associated with fractures could be missed (e.g. Monteggia fracture)
- In comminuted fractures the number of fragments could be misleading.
- Beware of artefacts they could mislead you.
- Be careful in interpreting fracture-like appearances, e.g. apophysis
- Avoid interpreting a low quality X-ray.

Role of X-ray

- Helps confirm the clinical diagnosis.
- Helps study the fracture anatomy.
- Helps study the fracture displacement.
- Helps to detect crack and stress fractures.
- Helps to plan the treatment.
- Helps to detect fracture dislocation combinations, e.g. Monteggia.
- Helps to ascertain post-reduction status of fractures.
- Helps in medicolegal study.

Remember the rules in X-rays
- Better no X-ray than one view X-ray.
- X-ray is a shadow. It conceals and distorts. Hence interpret X-rays with caution.
- A joint above and joint below should be included with the fracture under study.
- The fracture should be in the middle of the film.
- Exposure should be adequate and the soft tissue shadow should be delineated properly.
- X-rays should be read by holding the film in an anatomical position.
- Proper protective measures against radiation should be adopted.
- Avoid unnecessary X-rays.
- Check X-rays are to be taken without disturbing the plaster cast.

CT Scan and MRI

These are the most sophisticated investigative methods available now in orthopaedics. Both are noninvasive and are extremely useful in detecting both soft tissue and bony injuries.

Note:
CT scan: This is helpful in detecting fracture of skull, pelvis, spine and identifying loose bodies in the joint.
MRI: This is useful to diagnose any fracture. In addition, it helps to identify soft tissue and ligament injuries. It is certainly the 'Gold Standard' but has its Achilles heel in being expensive.

MANAGEMENT OF FRACTURES

The *goal* of fracture management is to restore the anatomy back to its normal or as near to normal as possible.

The *responsibility* of an orthopaedic surgeon is to ensure that there is no functional disability to the patient following the treatment of fractures.

Management of fracture can be broadly classified and discussed under the following heads:
1. Management of simple fractures.
2. Management of open fractures.
3. Management of complicated fractures.

Management of Simple Fractures

Simple fractures are managed by conservative and operative methods.

Conservative Methods

1. For undisplaced fractures, incomplete fractures, impacted fractures:

a. *Cuff and collar sling* For upper limb fractures.
b. *Strapping* For fracture clavicle, fracture ribs, etc.
c. *Plaster slabs* Plaster of Paris slabs can be used to support the injured limb.
d. *Rest and nonsteroidal anti-inflammatory drugs (NSAIDs)* For impacted fracture neck of femur, etc.

2. *For displaced fractures* Here the aim is to restore back the normal anatomy of the bone by either closed or open reduction.

Management of Fractures by Closed Reduction

This consists of resuscitation, reduction, retention and rehabilitation **(4Rs).**

1. **Resuscitation** Resuscitation is the topmost priority if the patient is in shock following a fracture. ***A to F*** management proposed by MacMurthy is to be followed in all situations of emergencies *(ref. p. 52).*
2. **Reduction** of the fracture fragments if it is displaced. Usually it is done under general anaesthesia after adequate radiographic study.
   Reduction methods are:
   a. *Closed reduction* It is adopted usually for simple fractures. The technique followed is traction and countertraction method. It is a blind technique and needs considerable skill and expertise. It commonly results in malunion.
   b. *Continuous traction* Certain examples where continuous traction can be used for reduction of tractions are Gallow's traction for fracture shaft femur in children, balanced skeletal traction for adult shaft femur fractures, etc.
   c. *Open reduction*. It is done when the above methods fail or if there are specific indications (see box).
3. **Retention** Once the fracture fragments are reduced, it has to be retained in that position till the fracture unites, otherwise it tends to get displaced due to the action of muscles, gravity and inherent factors.
   Retention methods after closed reduction are:
   a. *By plaster of Paris splints* This is the most common splint employed. It could be a slab (encircles half the limb) or a cast (encircles the whole limb) or a functional brace (which permits mobility while the fracture is still under the cast) *(ref. p. 58).*
   b. *By continuous traction* to overcome the muscle forces after closed reduction. The traction could be skin or skeletal traction and is employed as fixed, balanced or combined types of tractions *(ref. p. 63).*
   Use of functional braces This can be used after three weeks, once the fracture becomes sticky *(ref. p. 61).*
4. **Rehabilitation** is by way of physiotherapy and exercises (both active and passive).

Fracture Management by Open Reduction (Operative Management)

As mentioned earlier, open method is indicated once the conservative methods fail and when there are specific indications. These indications could be either absolute, relative or rare as mentioned below:

Indications

Absolute
- Failed closed reduction
- Displaced intra-articular fractures
- Type III and IV epiphyseal injuries
- Major avulsion fractures
- Nonunion
- Replantation of extremities

Relative
- Multiple fractures
- Delayed union
- Loss of reduction
- Pathological fractures
- For better nursing care
- To avoid prolonged bedrest
- Closed methods ineffective in Galeazzi fracture, Monteggia fracture, femoral neck fracture, etc.

Questionable
- Neurovascular injury
- Open fractures
- Cosmetic reasons
- Economic consideration

Methods of Open Reduction After the exposure, the fracture is reduced by direct methods and in the indirect methods the fracture is reduced without exposing by positioning and traction over the fracture tables, skeletal traction, tensioner, lamina spreader, etc.

Principles of open reduction *(known after Lambotte)* Principles of open reduction as suggested by Lambotte includes:

Exposure The fracture is adequately exposed through a proper approach.

Reduction of the fracture fragments under direct vision is carried out.

Temporary stabilisation of the fracture fragments by K-wire is done first.

Definitive stabilisation of the fracture using either plate and screws or intramedullary nail, etc. is done later.

Retention after open reduction After open reduction the fracture fragment invariably needs to be fixed internally by various implants (see box).

The Choice of Implants

K-wire For epiphyseal injuries and for fractures of small bones of hand and feet (diameter of the K-wires varies from 1-3 mm). *Screws* For avulsion fractures and butterfly fragments.

Intramedullary nails For fracture through the narrowest portion of a medullary canal of a long bone.

Plate and screws For proximal and distal third fractures of long bones.

Interlocking nails For segmental fractures comminuted fractures, etc. of long bones.

Hip implants For fracture neck femur. Smith Peterson's nail, Richard's compression screw, multiple cannulated screws, etc. are some of the examples.

Spine implants Steffee plate and screws (VSP's), Luque's rod, Hartshill frame, Harrington's rods, etc.

Steel Wires No 18-20 gauge Useful for tension band wiring for fracture of patella, olecranon, etc.

The rehabilitation process is the same as for closed management of fractures.

Contraindications for open reduction

- Infection
- Small fragments
- Weak and porotic bone
- Soft tissue damage
- Undisplaced or impacted fractures
- Poor general and medical condition

Disadvantages of open reduction

- Closed fracture converted into an open fracture.
- Fracture haematoma is disturbed.
- Scar tissue.
- Anaesthetic problems.
- Foreign body reaction due to metals.

Remember

Success by open reduction depends on

- Proper indications.
- Proper timing.
- Proper surgical approach.
- Proper technique.
- Proper selection of implant.
- Proper surgeon.

Quick facts

About methods of fracture immobilisation

- *External*: Plaster of Paris external fixators
- *Internal*: Fixation with plates and screws, rods, K-wire, etc.
- *Traction*: By skin and skeletal traction

OPEN FRACTURES

Open fracture is a surgical emergency and presents as a problem which is much more difficult than closed fractures. It is defined as a *fracture which communicates with the external atmosphere due to break in the soft tissue cover*. The break in the soft tissues could be from inside to outside or outside to inside.

CLASSIFICATION (Figs 3.6A to E) (GUSTILLO AND ANDERSON'S CLASSIFICATION)

Type I Wound is less than 1 cm in size. It is usually due to a low-velocity trauma.

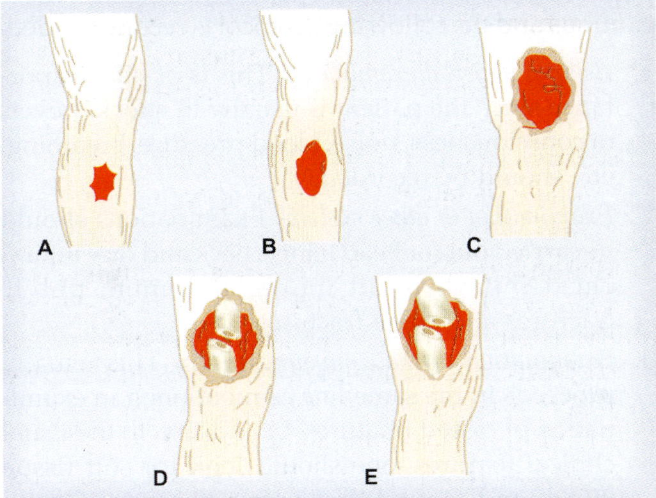

Figs 3.6A to E: Varieties of open fractures: (A) Type I (< 1 cm), (B) Type II (> 2 cm), (C) Type IIIA, (D) Type IIIB, and (E) Type IIIC

Type II Wound is more than 1 cm and less than 10 cm but there is no devitalisation of soft tissue and is associated with very little contamination. These are due to high energy trauma.

Type III Wounds moderate and severe in size (> 10 cm) and the soft tissues are devitalised and contaminated.

Type IIIA Extensive soft tissue injury but with adequate soft tissue to cover the fractured bone.

Type IIIB Extensive soft tissue damage and loss. Bone cannot be covered and is exposed to the atmosphere.

Type IIIC Compound fractures with arterial injuries.

No classification invites so much of debate as for open fractures with only 60% of the surgeons across the globe accepting it. Hence newer modifications are now being suggested like:

a. The modified Gustillo Anderson's classification.
b. The Trafton classification (this combines the Gustillo Anderson's and Tscherne classification).
c. AO classification of soft tissue injury with Alphanumeric classification of fractures.

APPROACH IN COMPOUND FRACTURES

Compound fractures are usually serious injuries and are due to high-velocity trauma.

They may be associated with multisystem and multiskeletal injuries. The approach should be more cautious and the following protocol is recommended.

1. *General physical examination* This is of vital importance since the patient is usually in shock. Levels of consciousness, pulse, blood pressure, breathing, etc. should be recorded.
2. *Examination of other systems* Examinations should be carried out for head injury, neck and face injury, chest injury, blunt injury abdomen, pelvic fractures and spine fractures.
3. *Examination of the compound injury* This usually proceeds in the same line as mentioned in examination of closed fractures. In addition to the usual clinical features, one should look for soft tissue injury and wound, bone loss, absence of bone pieces, distal neurovascular status of the limb, etc.

Note: The term 'open fracture' is more preferable than the old outfashioned term "compound fractures".

Investigations

General investigations Hb percentage, blood group, bleeding time and clotting time, urine examinations, etc. are carried out.

X-ray of the part as for other fractures—look for missing pieces of bone in open fractures.

Management Principles

Aims of treatment

- To convert a contaminated wound into a clean wound and thus help to convert an open fracture into a closed one.
- To establish union in a good position.
- To prevent pyogenic and clostridial infections.

Considerations

1. First to stabilise the general condition of the patient as the patient is usually in shock. This consists of resuscitation, blood transfusion, intravenous fluids, antibiotics, oxygen administration, etc.
2. To keep the wound covered with proper sterile bandages till the patient is ready for surgery.
3. Open fractures are surgical emergencies and surgery is to be done *as soon as the patient is fit.*

Treatment Plan

After stabilising the general condition of the patient, surgical debridement is planned under strict aseptic measures in a major operation theatre.

It is a team work and involves a battery of specialists like the vascular surgeon, plastic surgeon, thoracic surgeon, general surgeon, faciomaxillary surgeon, and of course the orthopaedic surgeon. Once the injuries to the vital organs are managed by these specialists and the general conditions of the patient is stabilised, the fractures are dealt by the orthopaedic surgeon.

Debridement (known as unbriddling) This is the most important step in the management of compound fractures. It consists of the following steps **(4Es)** (Fig. 3.7A):

1. *Exploration of the wound* The wound should be sufficiently explored proximally and distally to have a proper asssessment of the extent of the damage.
2. *Excision of all nonviable structures* A thorough excision of all the nonviable structures is important to prevent infection. The recognition of

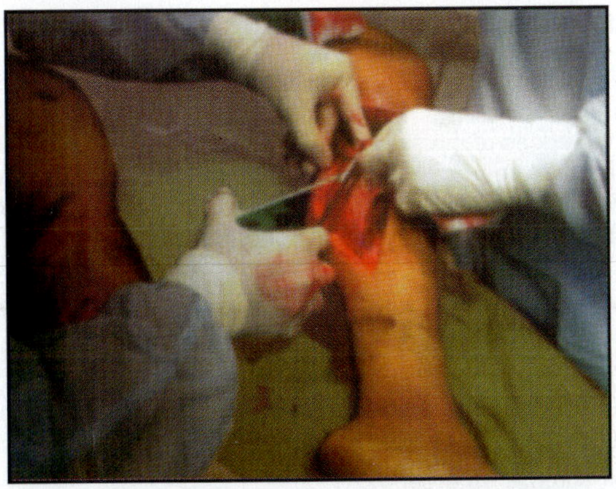

Fig. 3.7A: Showing the technique of debridement

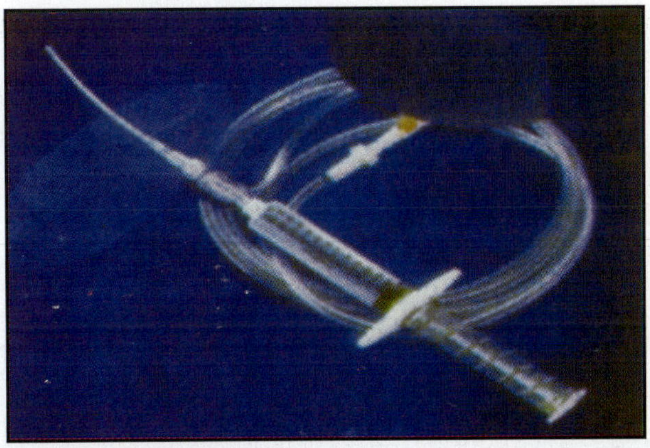

Fig. 3.7B: Irrigation set used in open fractures

nonviable tissue before excision is of paramount importance. The tissues are dealt with as follows:

- *Skin* Here the plan is to excise all the dead skin and yet be conservative.
- *Muscle* Nonviable muscle should be removed but often it is overlooked hence the axiom, *"when in doubt, take it out"*. **5Cs** help in deciding the muscle viability (Table 3.5).

Table 3.5: Showing the criteria to evaluate tissue status

Features	*Viable*	*Nonviable*
Colour	Pink	Pale
Consistency	Firm	Flabby
Capacity to bleed	Preserved	Lost
Circulation	Present	Absent
Contractility	Present	Absent

- *Bones* Small bits of loose bones devoid of soft tissues are removed. Large fragments with their soft tissue attachments are preserved.
- *Nerves and vessels* Primary repair is done if the wound is clean. In contaminated wounds they are dealt with at a later stage.

3. *Evacuation of foreign bodies* like dirt, glass, stones, pebbles, etc. These foreign bodies are a source for infection and may invite a foreign body reaction. Hence, they have to be removed by a thorough irrigation (normal saline is used) (Fig. 3.7B).

About irrigation

- Dilution is the solution of pollution.
- Single most essential step.
- Minimum 10 litres of saline is used.
- Forcible streams are avoided.
- Swirling movements of the irrigation fluid is preferred.
- Irrigation or wound toilet helps to clear the foreign bodies and clots minimising the chances of contamination.

Note:
- Antiseptic additives kill the bacteria.
- Detergent irrigation aims to remove than kill bacteria.

4. *External fixators* are used to fix the fracture fragment after debridement. Plaster of Paris and internal fixation devices have little and controversial role in the fracture management of compound fractures. External fixators help to stabilise fracture fragments, allow daily wound inspection and dressing, permit procedures like skin grafting, etc. to cover the wound, allow soft tissues to heal apart from providing early mobilisation. In open tibial fractures, external fixator can be safely exchanged to internal fixation within 3 weeks with only 5 per cent incidence of deep infection (Fig. 3.8).

Indications for external fixation in open fractures

- Grossly comminuted fractures
- Grossly contaminated wounds
- Side swipe injuries
- Periarticular fractures
- Pelvic fractures
- Pilon fractures
- Tibial plateau fractures
- Acetabular fractures

Primary internal fixation in open fractures

In recent times this concept is undergoing a 'sea change'. The inhibitions regarding the primary internal fixation is fast disappearing. The reasons for this shift in stance is improved methods of wound care, powerful antibiotics, improvements in the investigations and operative techniques, improvements in the external fixation devices, etc.

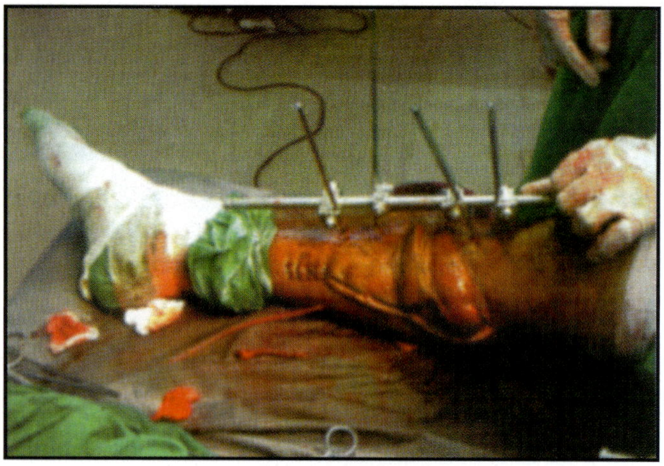

Fig. 3.8: External fixators preferred method of immobilisation in open fractures

Indications for internal fixation in open fractures

- Intra-articular fractures
- Multisystem injuries
- Multiple fractures
- Elderly patients
- Head injuries
- Vascular injuries
- Tibial shaft fractures

Preferred method Interlocking nailing is emerging as a better alternative than plating.

OTHER FORMS OF FRACTURE IMMOBILISATION

1. Pins and plasters—limited use can be tried in type I fractures.
2. Limited internal fixation—in grade I and some grade II, grade IIIC fractures
3. Skeletal traction—overhead olecranon traction for compound supracondylar fracture. Böhler-Braun skeletal traction for open femoral shaft fractures are some of the examples.
4. Plaster of Paris casts practically have no role.

Open facts in open fractures

About fixation methods in open fractures

• External fixators	Liberally used.
• Internal fixators	Sparingly used.
• Skeletal traction	Rarely used.
• Plaster casts	Occasionally used (type I).
• Functional brace	Never used.

Poetic facts

James Learmanth's poem depicts the four major principles of debridement:
On the edges of the skin take a piece, very thin (1); the tenser the fascia, the more you should slasher (2); of muscles much more, until you see fresh gore (3); and the bundles contract at least the impact; hardly any of bone, only bits quite alone (4).

Remember

Problems peculiar to open fracture

- In open fractures soft tissue injury is a dreaded problem than the fracture itself.
- A surgical emergency.
- Three problems:
  1. Infection from the environment.
  2. Problems of soft tissue loss.
  3. Active infection.
- Effective immobilisation rendered difficult.
- Bone repair is delayed. Speed is the watchword in treatment.
- Nonunion, malunion, chronic osteomyelitis are very common.
- Difficulty in using the standard internal fixation methods renders managing the fractures very difficult.

Some interesting treatment guidelines the world over for open fractures

- 17% surgeons cultured wounds on admission.
- 98% gave antibiotics after initial debridement
- 97% used cephalosporins
- Except in grade I debridement was done more than once.
- 14% surgeons discharged patients with oral antibiotics
- Re-operation was done in a few cases

Definitive wound care After resuscitation, debridement and application of external fixators attention is now given to the definitive wound care. This is an extremely important step as the primary objective of treatment in open fracture is to convert an open wound into closed wound. The wound closure could be primary or secondary.

Criteria for Primary Closure

- All necrotic material should be removed.
- Circulation should be normal.
- Nerve supply should be intact.
- The patient's general condition should be stable.
- Wound should be closed without tension.
- No dead space should be left after closure.
- There should be no multisystem injuries.

If all the above criteria are met, the wound is closed by primary suturing. The following alternative measures are considered in the event of the above criteria not being met:

- Split skin graft.
- Pedicle or flap graft.
- Secondary suturing after 2 to 3 weeks.
- Relaxing incisions to mobilise the neighbouring skin.
- Biological dressings (homologous or heterologous skin).
- To leave it open and to follow by regular dressings wound inspection and closure at a later date.

Role of antibiotics It will not replace the wound debridement. Topical antibiotics have very little role. Parenteral administration is recommended. The choice of antibiotics is usually a broad spectrum, bactericidal hypoallergenic agent with adequate serum concentration.

What is new?

Some surgeons have found good results with insertion of antibiotics integrated (2.4 gm of Tobramycin powder) PMMA beads into Type III wounds.

Role of AGGS and ATS The patient has to be protected against tetanus and gas gangrene by effective immunisation against them.

Role of primary amputation in open fractures. This is controversial but can be considered in type IIIC with neural injury and if the warm ischaemia is more than 6 hours.

Remember

In open fractures

- Debridement is the mainstay of treatment
- The procedure is **4 Es**:
  1. **E**xploration of the wound.
  2. **E**xcision of the devitalised tissues.
  3. **E**vacuation of the foreign bodies.
  4. **E**xternal fixators.
- Devitalised tissue recognised by **5 Cs.**
- Wound irrigation is the single most important step.
- Primary aim is to convert an open wound into a closed one.
- Wound closure is to be decided with caution.
- Antibiotics cannot replace wound debridement.
- External fixators have definite role.
- Internal fixators and plasters have limited role.
- Ultimate goal is to restore the patient's limb and function as early as and as full as possible.

APPROACH TO A POLYTRAUMA CASE

This is as mentioned in the approach to a compound fracture. Speed is the watchword in the approach towards a multiple trauma case and should proceed in the following lines:

1. *Initial evaluation* The **ABCDEs** of initial examination of a polytrauma case are as follows: A—airway, B—breathing, C—circulation, D—disability (neurologic examination), E—exposure, F—fracture examination, G—Go back to the beginning for a secondary survey and H—help.
2. *Secondary evaluation* After the initial evaluation and resuscitation, a more systematic and detailed evaluation of the injuries mentioned above are done. Fractures are splinted externally and managed at a later date. But in few cases primary internal fixation is recommended in ipsilateral fractures, multisystem injuries, etc. for faster rehabilitation. Dislocations are promptly reduced.
3. *Fracture examination* This is done systematically as mentioned in the previous discussions.
4. *Investigation* This includes routine blood examinations, radiographs of head, neck, chest, spine and affected parts. CT scan and MRI of injured structures are mandatory.

DISLOCATION

Dislocation is defined as a total loss of contact between the two ends of bones (Figs 3.9A and B). All dislocations are emergencies unlike fractures, for delay in reduction may damage the articular surface which are deprived of nutrition by the synovial fluid. Unlike fractures, all dislocations need prompt reduction and early treatment because the patient will not be relieved of pain due to the persistent capsular stretch. The capsule contains nerve endings which give rise to pain.

Pathology

In a dislocation there could be damage to the capsule, articular cartilage, muscles, ligaments in varying degrees. There could be osteochondral fractures and avulsion injuries.

Types of Dislocation: Congenital or Acquired

Congenital as in CDH and in acquired the following varieties are seen:

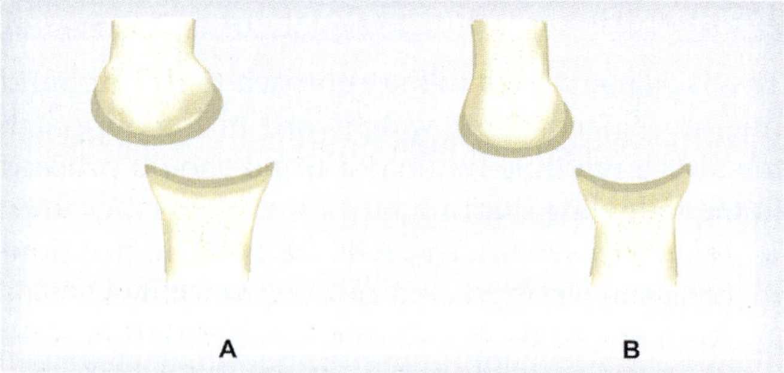

Figs 3.9A and B: Showing (A) subluxation, and (B) dislocation

1. Traumatic common in young adults due to high-velocity trauma.
2. Pathological e.g. TB hip, septic arthritis, etc.
3. Infective e.g. Tomsmith arthritis in infants.
4. Paralytic e.g. poliomyelitis, cerebral palsy, etc.
5. Inflammatory disorders, rheumatoid arthritis, etc.

Clinical Features

Traumatic variety is the most common type of dislocations one encounters in clinical practice (Table 3.6). A patient gives history of trauma usually a road traffic accident (RTA) following which there is pain, swelling deformity and loss of movements. In dislocations of other varieties clinical symptoms and signs pertaining to that particular disease are seen.

Typical deformities in dislocations

- Shoulder—abduction deformity.
- Elbow—flexion deformity.
- Hip: Anterior—flexion abduction and external rotation deformity.
- Posterior—flexion, adduction and internal rotation deformity.
- Knee—flexion deformity.
- Ankle—varus deformity.

Investigations

Radiograph of the affected part should include anteroposterior and lateral views of the joints.

Treatment

Since dislocation is an orthopaedic emergency early closed reduction under general anaesthesia is recommended. The part is immobilised for a period of 3 to 6 weeks to ensure adequate healing. Operative reduction is rarely required and is reserved for compound dislocations and irreducible dislocations.

Table 3.6: Showing common traumatic dislocations

Area involved	*Type of dislocation*
1. *Spine*	Anterior, C_5 over C_6
2. *Upper limb*	
• Acromioclavicular joint	Type I/II/III
• Sternoclavicular joint	Anterior/posterior
• Shoulder joint	Anterior/posterior
• Elbow joint	Posterior
• Isolated dislocation of superior radioulnar joint	Anterior
• Fracture dislocation of superior radioulnar joint	Monteggia fracture
• Fracture head of radius and dislocation of inferior radioulnar joint	Essex-Lopresti fracture
• Wrist dislocations	Perilunar, lunar
• Kaplan's injury	Carpometacarpal joint of the thumb
3. *Lower limb*	
• Hip dislocations	Anterior/posterior/central
• Knee joint	Posterior
• Patella	Lateral dislocations
• Ankle	Anterolateral
• Foot	Intertarsal
— Chopart's	
— Lisfranc's	Tarsometatarsal

Complications

Acute injury to peripheral nerves and vessels can occur, e.g. sciatic nerve palsy in posterior dislocation of hip.

Chronic

Unreduced dislocation which is common in Asian countries due to ignorance, delay in seeking treatment, etc.

Recurrent dislocations due to inadequate and improper healing of soft tissues following initial trauma.

Traumatic osteoarthritis due to damage to the articular cartilage following impaired nutrition by the synovial fluid.

Joint stiffness due to capsular and other soft tissue damage.

Avascular necrosis due to injury to the vessels.

Myositis ossificans More commonly seen than in fractures due to greater periosteal strip.

Remember in dislocation

- It is an orthopaedic emergency.
- Reduction should be quick and prompt.
- Reduction should always be done under general anaesthesia to relax the muscles.
- Swelling is less when compared to fractures.
- Movements are more restricted than in fractures.
- Closed reduction is sufficient most of the times.
- Open reduction is resorted to if specifically indicated.
- Reduction technique should always be very gentle.
- Pain will not subside by splinting unlike fractures.
- Myositis ossificans is a problem more commonly asociated with dislocation.

Subluxation

Subluxation is defined as partial loss of contact between the two ends of the bones. It poses a problem much less serious than dislocation.

Sprain It is a tear in the ligaments. The severity varies from grade I to grade III. Mild sprains are more common and heal by conservative treatment, whereas grade III sprains cause joint instabilities and need to be repaired surgically. Sprains are commonly encountered in knee joints and ankle joints. They are discussed in detail in appropriate sections.

Strain It is a tear in the muscles and is more common in young athletes and usually heals by conservative methods.

These have been dealt with in greater detail in the chapter on Soft Tissue Injuries.

4

Complications of Fractures

INTRODUCTION

Fracture is a disturbing event more so if it develops complications. The complications could be immediate or delayed. Immediate complications are life threatening and delayed complications are more morbid. Some complications develop at the time of injury and are beyond the control of the surgeon. They need to be accurately diagnosed and treated. Whenever a surgeon encounters a case of fracture he should look beyond the fracture and try to detect complications if any. The following are the common complications.

ACUTE RESPIRATORY DISTRESS SYNDROME (SYN: FAT EMBOLISM)

Acute respiratory distress syndrome (ARDS) is defined as a post-traumatic distress syndrome occurring within 72 hours of skeletal trauma. It indicates the presence of fat globules (palmitin and stearine in children and olein in adults) within the lung parenchyma and peripheral circulation after a long bone fracture. It usually manifests within 24 to 48 hours but sometimes may be delayed for several days. It is a dreaded complication often associated with multiple fractures, major bone fractures, pelvic fractures, multisystem injuries like chest and abdomen, head injuries, etc. It is seen in 10 to 45 per cent cases of multiple fractures and is an important cause of morbidity and mortality (11%) in multiple fracture and multisystem injuries.

Historical facts

- Vong Bergman first diagnosed fat embolism syndrome in 1873.

Aetiology

Common aetiological factor is a long bone fracture in young (usually between 20 and 30 years of age) adult or a pelvic fracture in elderly.

Source of fat It could be from two sources:

I. Mechanical theory
   - From bone marrow (accepted).

II. Biochemical theory
   a. *Obstructive theory*
      - From plasma by agglutination of chylomicrons which later acts as an embolus (less accepted).

   b. *Toxic theory*: The free fatty acid destroys the pneumocytes and causes ARDS.

Pathogenesis

Following injury, the bone marrow fat or the platelet agglutination are sucked into the injured vessels and are transported to various sites as emboli giving rise to varied clinical manifestations.

Showing complications of fractures

Acute	Chronic	Complications peculiar to open fractures
• Shock (Hypovolaemic or neurogenic) • **ARDS** • Thromboembolism • Neurovascular injuries 1. Radial nerve palsy in fracture shaft humerus 2. Sciatic nerve palsy in posterior dislocation of hip 3. Supracondylar fractures causing brachial artery injury • Acute Volkmann's ischaemia • Crush syndrome • Deep vein thrombosis	• **Delayed union** • **Nonunion** • **Malunion** • Shortening • Growth disturbances • **Avascular necrosis** • Joint stiffness • Post-traumatic arthritis • **VIC** • **Myositis ossificans**	• Infection • Chronic osteomyelitis • Gas gangrene • Tetanus • Hypovolaemic shock • **Miscellaneous** • Implant failure • Reflex sympathic dystrophy, etc. **The complications emboldened in this table are discussed in detail**

CLASSIFICATION (Sevitt's)

1. *Classical type* In this variety the onset is less than 24 hrs, *tachycardia* is greater than 140/min, *Pyrexia* is greater than 40°C, *tachypnoea, cyanosis,* changing *cerebral signs* vary from confusion, restlessness and coma. *Petechial rashes* (Fig. 4.1) over shoulder, infra- and supraclavicular regions, *retinal petechiae,* and in *conjunctiva of lower lids, if present is pathognomonic.* In this type the blood pressure is maintained throughout.
2. *Fulminating type* Here the sequence of events are very fast and there is no time for the rashes to develop. Patient is comatose within hours and throws repeated seizures. Patient rapidly collapses and death supervenes.
3. *Incomplete type* The manifestation is between the two types. Unexplained tachycardia, fever and rash are its features.

Features of rashes in ARDS

- Seen commonly in classical type.
- Presents across the chest, axilla, root of the neck and conjunctiva.
- Fleeting type.
- Fades rapidly.
- Occurs periodically with attacks of coma.
- Can occur in the retina.
- Diagnosed by fundoscopy.
- Retinal rashes are pathognomonic.

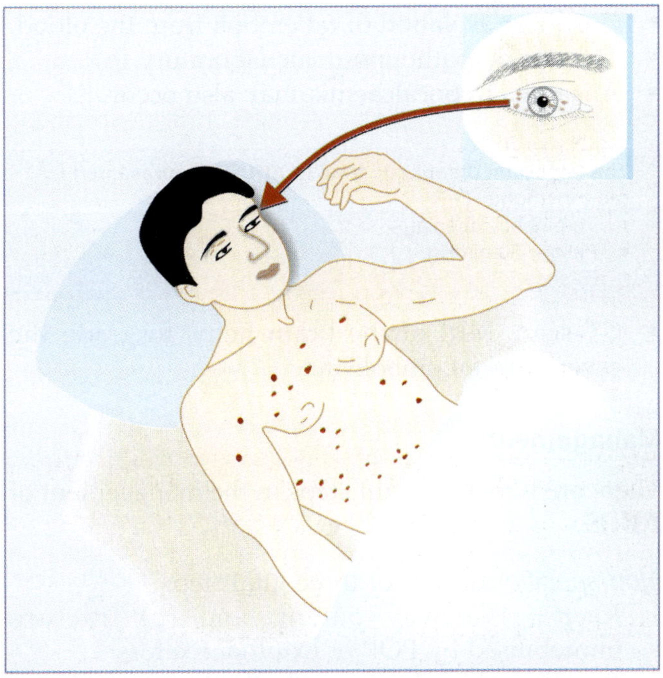

Fig. 4.1: Petechial rashes like these are the hallmark of fat embolism syndrome

Interesting facts

Do you know the Gurd's major and minor criteria for diagnosis of fat embolism syndrome?

Major criteria
- Axillary and subconjunctival petechiae
- $PaO_2 < 60$ mmHg
- CNS depression

Section 1

Minor criteria
- Pulse > 110/min
- Pyrexia > 38.5°C
- Retinal embolism
- Fat in urine
- Reduced platelet count
- Increased ESR
- Fat globules in sputum

Diagnostic criteria: At least one from major criteria and four from minor criteria are required to make a diagnosis of fat embolism syndrome.

Investigations

- *X-ray of the chest* may snow storm appearance and if seen is pathognomonic.
- PaO_2 less than 60 mmHg.
- Platelet count less than 1.5 lakhs.
- ECG shows prominent S-wave.
- Gurd test: Isolation of fat emboli from the blood.
- There is no pathognomonic laboratory test.
- Anaemia, hypocalcaemia may also occur.

The important diagnostic triad in ARDS is represented by the mnemonic TPR
- Thrombocytopenia.
- PaO_2 < 60 mmHg.
- Rashes.

- CT scan, MRI of the brain helps to grade the severity of fat embolism.

Management

There are two important steps in the management of ARDS:

Non-specific consists of three vital steps:
1. ***Keep*** (a) airway patent, and (b) fracture immobilised by POP or external fixators.
2. ***Restore*** (a) blood volume, (b) fluid, and (c) electrolyte balance.
3. ***Avoid*** (a) careless handling of the injured, and (b) unnecessary transportation.

Specific Again three vital steps are described:
1. *Respiratory support* Oxygen administration to restore back PaO_2 or full-fledged ventilatory support.
2. *Drug therapy*
   - *Steroids* are given intravenously. These help gas exchange by decreasing inflammation in the lungs.
   - *Heparin* This acts as a lipolytic and antiplatelet agent.
   - *Low molecular weight dextran* acts by increasing plasma volume.
   - *Intravenous alcohol* is not universally advocated.
   - *Antibiotics* and other treatment.
3. *Definitive fracture treatment* is discussed in appropriate sections. Early fixation of fractures is advocated to prevent worsening of the situation.

Role of antiplatelets in ARDS

- Should be given early
- Given intravenous every 6 to 8 hr in doses of 2,500 IU.
- It improves microcirculatory flow.
- It increases plasma volume.
- Decreases platelet adhesiveness.

What is subclinical fat embolism syndrome?

The presence of only laboratory abnormalities with no obvious clinical symptoms. Remember 4T's to diagnose fat embolism syndrome
- T-tachycardia > 100/min
- T-tachypnoea > 25 breaths/min
- T-temperature elevation > 37.8°C
- T-thrombocytopenia < 2 lakhs

Interesting facts

Do you know the common pulmonary problems in orthopaedics (Mnemonic PAPA-F)
- P—Pulmonary emboli
- A—Atelectasis
- P—Postoperative pneumonia
- A—Atelectasis
- F—Fat emboli

VOLKMANN'S ISCHAEMIA OR COMPARTMENTAL SYNDROMES

DEFINITION Mubarak defined compartmental syndrome as an *elevation of interstitial pressure in a closed osseofascial compartment that results in microvascular compromise* and may cause irreversible damage to the contents of the space.

Sites

1. Anterior and deep posterior compartments of the legs.
2. Volar compartment of the forearm (Fig. 4.2).

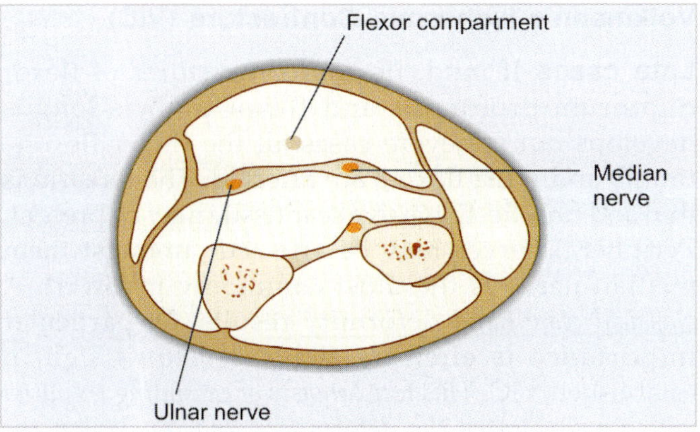

Fig. 4.2: Cross section of the volar compartment of the forearm

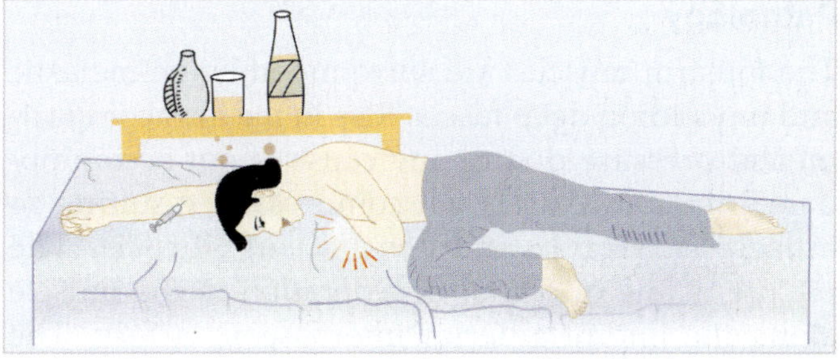

Fig. 4.3: Drug addicts 'beware' lying with your forearm tucked under your body in an inebriated state can lead to compartmental syndrome of the forearm

3. Buttocks, shoulder, hand, foot, arm and lumbar paraspinous muscles are relatively rare sites.

COMPARTMENTAL SYNDROME OF FOREARM

This is one of the most dreaded complications in orthopaedics and ranges from mild ischaemia to severe gangrene. Early recognition and prompt remedial measures are the key to successful countering of this problem. *Needless to say this is an orthopaedic emergency.*

DEFINITION *It is an ischaemic necrosis of structures contained within the volar compartment of the forearm.*

Incidence and Aetiology

It is common in children less than 10 years of age. Supracondylar fracture is the most common cause in children. Crush injuries of the forearm are the most common causes in adults. Occasionally fracture of both bones of forearm dislocation of the elbow, vascular injuries and subfascial haematomas may be the cause. More recently intra-arterial injections in drug addicts who lie on their forearm for prolonged periods in narcotised conditions is mooted to be a cause (Fig 4.3). Improper application of splints is another important cause.

Usually the flexor muscles of the forearm, especially the flexor digitorum profundus and flexor pollicis longus and rarely flexor digitorum superficialis are involved. Volkmann's ischaemic contracture (VIC) is due to the infarction produced by an arterial spasm of the main artery to an extremity with reflex spasm of the collateral circulation. This produces ischaemia of the muscle bellies which results in necrosis and is later replaced by fibrous tissue causing contractures.

Aetiology: According to Matson

1. ↓ Compartment size
   - Closure of fascial defects
   - Tight dressing
   - Localised external pressure
2. ↑ Compartment content
   - Bleeding
   - Vascular injury
   - Bleeding disorders
3. ↑ Capillary permeability
   - Burns
   - Trauma
   - Post exercises
   - Seizures
   - Intra-arterial drugs
   - Exercise
   - Venous obstruction
4. ↑ Capillary pressure
   - Exercise
   - Venous obstruction
5. Muscle hypertrophy
6. Infiltrated infusion
7. Nephrotic syndrome

Pathophysiology

External or internal constrictions → ↑ Arterial spasm or occlusion → Causes muscle ischaemia → ↑ Capillary permeability → ↑ Intramuscular oedema → ↑ Intramuscular pressure → Further arterial compromise → Muscle necrosis → Replaced by collagen → Contractures

Pathology

The forearm muscles are surrounded by an inelastic and unyielding deep fascia. Rise in the intracompartmental pressure due to any cause is not accommodated and the vessels get compressed resulting in muscle ischaemia and consequent fibrosis. The picture is one of *central* degeneration in the muscle along the line of anterior interosseous artery. The greatest damage is at the centre and the muscles commonly affected are flexor digitorum profundus and flexor pollicis longus.

Clinical Features

In the acute stages, the patient gives history of trauma and after an interval of a few hours, severe, poorly localised pain develops in the forearm. The volar aspect of the forearm is swollen, red, warm, tender and tense. Fingers are held in flexion and an attempt to extend the fingers increases the pain (stretch pain) (Fig. 4.4). Peripheral pulses which are present initially, disappear later. Median nerve is more commonly affected than the ulnar nerve.

Note *In VIC the patient complains of pain out of proportion to the injury.*

Impending Volkmann's ischaemia is detected by 6Ps
- **P**ain
- **P**allor
- **P**araesthesia
- **P**aralysis
- **P**ulselessness
- **P**ositive passive stretch test

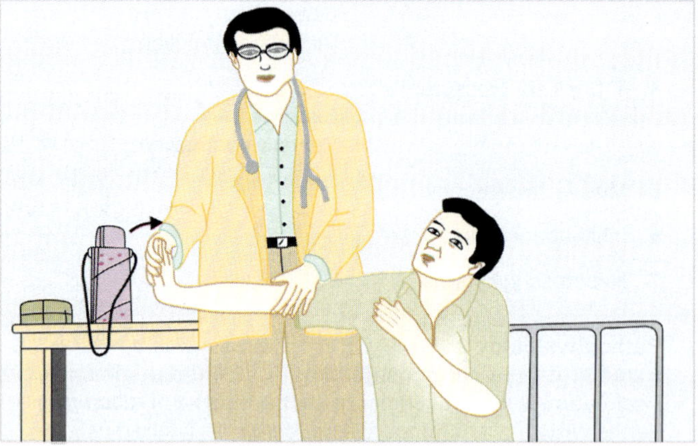

Fig. 4.4: Showing method of performing the passive stretch test

Volkmann's Ischaemic Contracture (VIC)

Late cases If mild, flexion contractures of flexor digitorum profundus and flexor pollicis longus develops but in severe cases all the finger flexors, thumb and wrist flexors are affected. The forearm is thin and fibrotic. Extensive scar tissue may be present. Peripheral nerves may be affected, amongst them median nerve is the most commonly involved. A *classical claw hand* deformity results. Of particular importance is eliciting the *Volkmann's sign* in established VIC. *This test consists of extending the wrist which exaggerates the deformities and on flexion the deformities appear less prominent (Figs 4.5A and B).* Joint contractures and gangrene may also be seen.

In established VIC
Look for
- Claw and deformity.
- Volkmann's sign.
- Extensive scarring of the forearm.
- Joint and soft tissue contractures.
- Neurological deficits.
- Rarely gangrene.

Tsuge's Classification of VIC

Mild	Moderate	Severe
• FDP • FPL involved	• Involvement of FDP+FPL • Superficial finger flexor • Wrist flexors • Thumb flexors	• All flexors. • Few extensors. • Neurologic deficit. • Contracture of joint. • Skin scarred. • Bones deformed.

FDP—flexor digitorum profundus, FPL—flexor pollicis longus.

Management

Acute stage It is a surgical emergency. All encircling tight bandages are removed if present. If there is no improvement, record the pressure within the

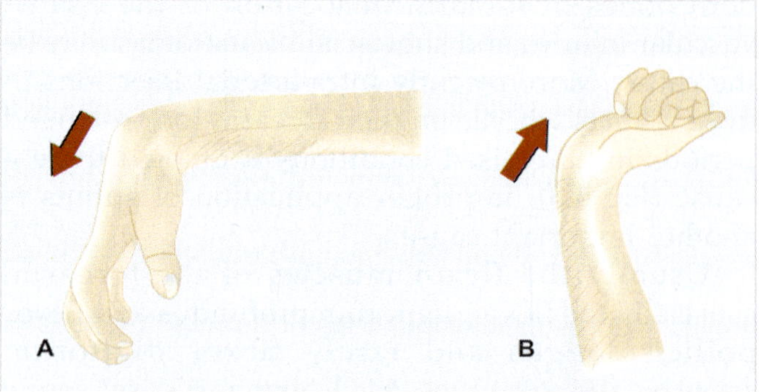

Figs 4.5A and B: (A) Volkmann's ischaemic contracture (VIC) deformity, and (B) Volkmann's sign

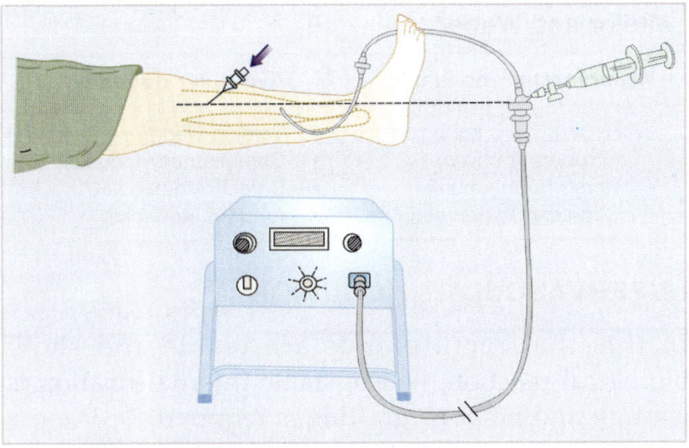

Fig. 4.6: Method of recording the intracompartmental pressure within the leg

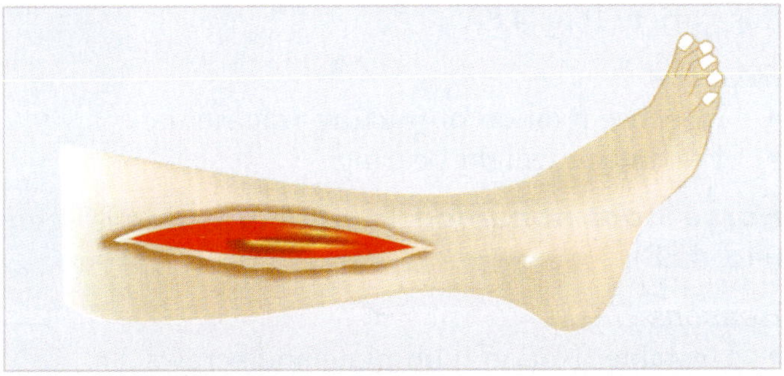

Fig. 4.7: A wide fasciotomy for acute compartmental syndrome

compartment (Fig. 4.6). If it is more than 30 mmHg, an emergency surgical decompression is done by fasciotomy (Fig. 4.7). If the pressure is less than 30 mmHg, continuous monitoring is done.

Methods to Record Intracompartmental Pressure

In any patient with forearm or leg injuries who has a tense compartment and if the patient is unreliable or unresponsive, the intracompartmental pressure should be recorded by using a needle manometer, wick or slick catheter. If the intracompartmental pressure is more than 30 to 40 mmHg or is 10 to 30 mmHg more than the diastolic pressure of the patient, fasciotomy is recommended (see Fig. 4.6).

Established VIC

Here the contractures are well established and the treatment plan depends upon the severity of VIC.

Treatment plan in acute cases

Record ICP → +ve clinical findings → Fasciotomy

Record ICP → If doubtful, record ICP → >30 mmHg → Fasciotomy

If doubtful, record ICP → < 30 mmHg → Monitor IF ICP>30 mmHg → Fasciotomy

Fasciotomy
This is the definitive treatment for acute compartmental syndrome. Here both skin and fascia are divided and left open to be covered by a skin graft later.

Treatment of choice is early decompression

Ischaemia
- more than 4 hours causes myoglobinuria (crush syndrome)
- more than 12 hours—total ischaemia results in contractures

ICP—Intracompartmental pressure

Remember

If 5 Ps help in detection of acute cases, 5 Ps also form clue to the management.

- **P**ressure to be relieved either external or internal.
- **P**ressure to be monitored within the compartment.
- **P**ulse to be recorded continuously.
- **P**assive stretch test indicates the severity.
- **P**utting the fracture back into its position.

Mild type

1. Dynamic splinting.
2. Physiotherapy.
3. Total excision if single muscle is involved.

Moderate type

1. *Max page's muscle sliding operation* This consists of releasing the common flexor origin from the medial epicondyle and passively stretching the fingers. This slides the origin of the muscle down and releases the contractures.
2. *Excision of cicatrix*
3. *Neurolysis* consists of freeing the peripheral nerves from the surrounding fibrous tissue.
4. *Tendon transfers* are done if criteria are met.

Severe type

1. Excision of the scar

2. Seddon's carpectomy—it consists of excising the proximal row of carpal bones thereby shortening the forearm to overcome the effects of contracted muscles.
3. *Arthrodesis* of the wrist in functional position.
4. *Amputation* for very severe cases of VIC with gangrene.

Chronic Compartmental Syndrome

Chronic compartmental syndrome is a pretibial pain induced by exercise seen in the anterior compartment of the leg in athletes. If the compartmental pressure is more than 15 mmHg at rest, more than 30 mmHg during exercise and more than 20 mmHg for 5 minutes after exercise, chronic compartmental syndrome is suspected. Due to the herniation of fat or muscle through the fascial defect, a soft tissue mass is seen in the anterolateral aspect of the lower third of the leg. The patient is instructed to alter or decrease the level of activity, if no relief is forthcoming, surgical decompression is indicated.

NONUNION

The difference between delayed union and nonunion is of degree. In delayed union healing has *not advanced* at the average rate for location and type of fractures but healing can still take place if the limb is immobilised for a longer period. In nonunion there is evidence to show clinically and radiologically that healing has *ceased* and union is improbable and needs surgery. Final status of nonunion is pseudoarthrosis.

DEFINITION (FDA panel) Nonunion is said to be established when a *minimum of nine months* has elapsed since the injury and the fracture shows no radiologically visible progressive signs of healing continuously *for three months*.

CLASSIFICATION OF NONUNION

Two classifications are adopted.

[1]Paley's classification This classification takes into account the amount of bone loss and includes two varieties:

- Type A less than 1 cm bone loss
- Type B greater than 1 cm bone loss

Muller and Weber

Hypervascular nonunion	Avascular nonunion
• Hypertrophic nonunion (Exuberant callus) • Horse hoof nonunion • Oligotrophic nonunion	• Torsion wedge nonunion • Comminuted nonunion • Defect nonunion • Atrophic nonunion

HYPERVASCULAR NONUNION

In this the fracture ends are viable and show biological reaction, hence, stable internal fixation is enough and no bone grafting is required.

Types

Elephant foot nonunion Exuberant callus is seen in this variety (Fig. 4.8A).

Reasons

- Insecure fixation of fracture fragments.
- Premature weight bearing.

Horse hoof nonunion Here poor callus is seen (Fig. 4.8B).

Reasons

- Unstable fixation with plate and screws.

Oligotrophic nonunion Very poor callus is seen in this variety (Fig. 4.8C).

Reasons

This is usually seen in:

- Major displacements, distraction, etc.
- Poor internal fixation.

AVASCULAR NONUNION

In avascular nonunion (Figs 4.9A to D) the fracture ends are not viable due to poor blood supply. No biological reaction is seen, and this needs rigid internal fixation with bone grafting after decortication of nonviable ends.

Types

Torsion wedge nonunion Here the intermediate fragment has healed at one end and not at the other. It is seen in segmental fractures.

Comminuted nonunion is seen in comminuted fractures.

[1]**Dror Paley**. American orthopaedic surgeon.

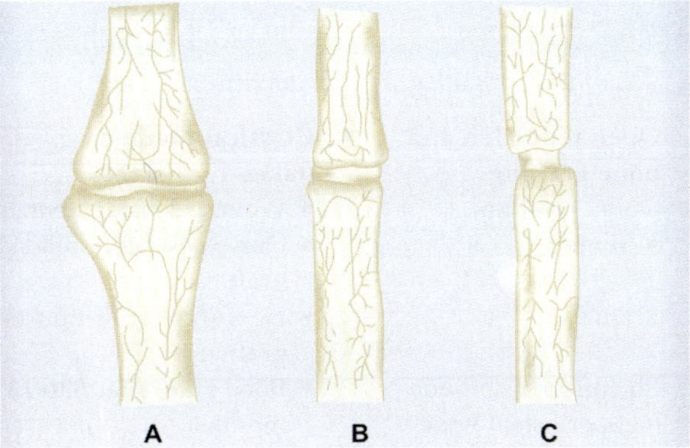

Figs 4.8A to C: Hypervascular nonunion: (A) elephant foot, (B) horse hoof, and (C) oligotrophic

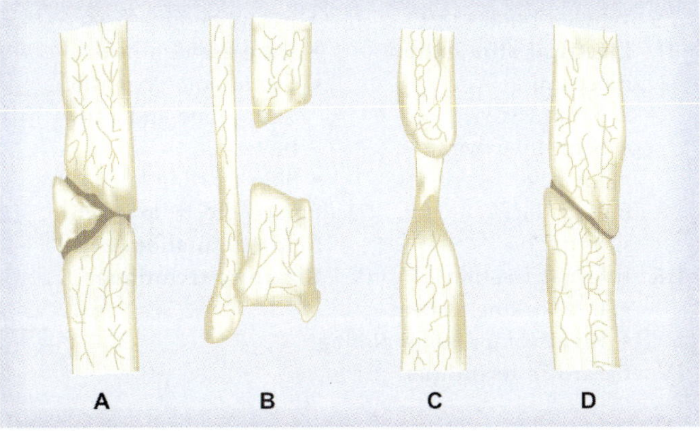

Figs 4.9A to D: Avascular nonunion: (A) comminuted nonunion, (B) gap nonunion, (C) atrophic nonunion, and (D) torsion wedge nonunion

Defect nonunion Here there is loss of fragment, seen in compound fractures, osteomyelitis, etc.

Atrophic nonunion Here the ends are thin and sclerotic with excessive scar tissue in between and the fracture fragments have tapering ends.

CAUSES FOR NONUNION

Nonunion of fractures is a very notorious complication to treat. Infected nonunion challenges the clinical acumen of best of orthosurgeons. There are various causes leading to nonunion and the following are some of those.

Compound fractures There is extensive damage to the soft tissues in open fractures and there could be even loss of small pieces of bone. The former results in impaired blood supply to the fracture fragments jeopardising the chances of union.

Infection This is commonly seen in compound fractures and in postsurgical infections. Hence infections should be kept at a minimum in treatment of fractures.

Segmental fractures In this type of fractures there is a maximum risk of damage to the intraosseous vessels resulting in poor union.

Distraction of fracture fragments This happens when excessive weight is used during skin or skeletal traction.

Soft tissue interposition If soft tissues, like periosteum, muscles, tendons, nerves, vessels, etc. are interposed between the fracture fragments, it obstructs the growth of internal callus and thus jeopardise union.

Ill-advised open reduction Open reduction damages favourable factors for fracture union like fracture haematoma. Periosteal stripping and intramedullary reaming disturbs the vascular supply. All these are detrimental to fracture healing.

Insecure and inadequate fixation of fracture fragments by plate and screws or intramedullary fixation allows micro-movements which prevent union.

Apart from these local factors, the general factors which contribute to poor healing of fractures are anaemia, general debility, cachexia, steroid therapy, osteoporosis, malignancy, etc.

But it can be observed that most of the factors, general or local, responsible for poor fracture healing are preventible if one exercises utmost caution and care during the treatment of fractures.

Clinical Features

This can be discussed under three headings.

History Usually the patient gives history of trauma resulting in fractures, multiple injuries, multisystem or head injuries. There could be history of open fractures, delay or improper or inadequate treatment. It should be noted that in nonunion the history is of a longer duration.

Symptoms The acute symptoms seen in fresh fractures are conspicuously absent in nonunion. There is usually history of no pain or minimal pain. There could be presence of a deformity or loss of function.

Signs The important clinical signs are painless abnormal mobility, no crepitus, shortening, scars and sinuses, deformity, wasting of limb muscles, etc.

Investigations

Radiograph of the part in AP and lateral views (Fig. 4.10). The following points are looked for:

- Gap between the fracture fragments.
- The fragments are rounded and sclerotic.
- The amount of callus formed could be less (avascular nonunion) or more (higher-vascular nonunion).
- Decreased density of bone is due to osteoporosis.

Radiology helps to classify nonunion depending upon the amount of callus.

Management

Principles

1. Nonunion is an absolute indication for surgery and it requires open reduction, rigid internal fixation and bone grafting.
2. There is no role of conservative treatment.
3. Other methods of treatment include electrical stimulation, interlocking nails and Ilizarov's technique (Table 4.1).

Role of Bone Grafting in Nonunion

Bone grafts help in promoting osteogenesis. They also fill in the gap and provide stability.

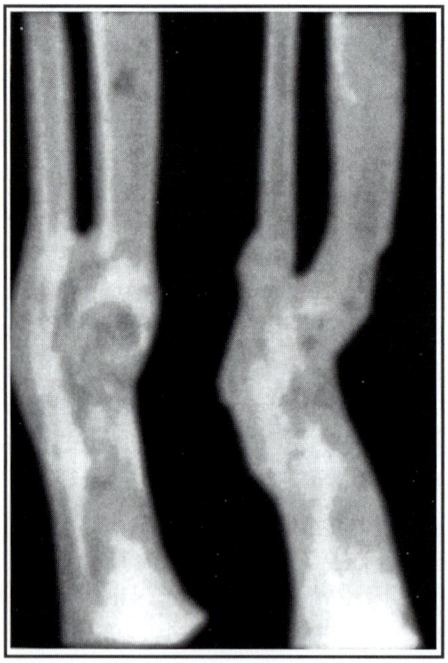

Fig. 4.10: Radiograph showing infected nonunion of tibia and fibula

Table 4.1: Management of nonunion

Uninfected nonunion	*Infected nonunion*
I. Open reduction and bone grafting 1. Onlay grafting • Single • Dual 2. Phemister technique (subperiosteal bone grafting) 3. Cancellous bone grafting 4. Massive sliding graft 5. Whole fibular graft	**I. Classical method (takes 1 yr) stages** • Wound debridement. • One week later split skin graft. • Next week, full-thickness graft. • Bone graft after 6 to 12 months.
II. Electrical stimulation 1. Electrical • Noninvasive • Semi-invasive • Invasive 2. Pulsed EMF stimulation	**II. Active method (takes less time)** • Internal fixation of fractures done first. • Bone grafting next. • Continuous irrigation with saline and antibiotics. • Skin grafting later. **III. Pulsed electromagnetic field stimulation.**
III. Internal fixation • Interlocking system • Rigid compression plating	**IV. Ilizarov's technique.**
IV. Ilizarov's technique	

Types

Cancellous bone graft It is useful in defects less than 2.5 cm. It is very commonly used since it is better tolerated and is rapidly revascularised.

Cortical bone graft provides sufficient fixation and promotes osteogenesis. It has a stabilising property and can be used for nonunion of the shafts of any long bone. When placed on one surface, it is called *single onlay;* when it is placed on both the sides, it is called *the dual onlay;* and when a piece is slided from above to the fracture site, it is called a *sliding graft (Fig. 4.11).*

Phemister bone graft Here the graft is placed subperiosteally. It is simple and blood supply is not disturbed. It is placed posteriorly and is found to be useful in tibia.

Role of Electrical Stimulation in Nonunion

Weak electrical currents of 20 mA delivered to the fracture site by a cathode converts fibrous tissue to

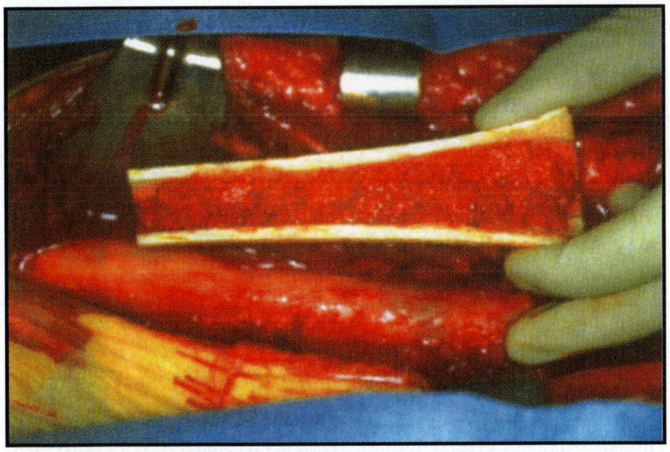

Fig. 4.11: Cortical bone graft

fibrocartilage which gets ossified later by endochondral ossification.

Three types If cathode is placed inside the fracture site, it is called *invasive;* when placed subcutaneously, it is called *semi-invasive;* when incorporated into a plaster cast externally, it is called *noninvasive.*

Pulsed electromagnetic field is the method of delivering the current by electromagnetic field in a pulsed manner. This is also noninvasive.

Union occurs in 85 per cent of cases. Large gap greater than half the diameter of the bone will not unite.

Excision of fibrous tissue followed by bone grafting is done first. Immobilisation by plaster is done to decrease stress.

Union by electrical means is slow and is not always successful.

Role of Ilizarov's Technique in Nonunion

This allows simultaneous correction of all deformities and bone loss. In hypertrophic nonunion gradual compression helps. In avascular nonunion corticotomy, bone transport and compression helps. *Corticotomy* provides some of the same biological benefits as bone graft. Segmental nonunion is also successful. *Ilizarov's* technique provides dramatic results but is technicaly very demanding. It is still the best way to treat cases of infected nonunion.

AVASCULAR NECROSIS

Avascular necrosis (AVN) is a rare but severe complication of certain fractures. It occurs when the blood supply to a segment of bone is affected.

CAUSES

1. Extensive stripping of soft tissues which damage the periosteal blood supply.
2. In certain bones where the blood supply is unique and unidirectional, e.g. talus, scaphoid, neck of femur (Figs 4.12A to C).
3. Other causes like steroid therapy, Caisson's disease, etc. which may cause an embolic block of the blood vessels.

Do you know other causes of AVN other than fractures?
Remember the mnemonic 'SCLERA'
- S—Steroids
- C—Caisson's disease
- L—Lupus erythematosis
- R—Radiation therapy
- A—Alcoholism

Common sites of AVN are head of femur in fracture neck of femur and dislocations of hip, body of the talus in fracture through the neck of talus, proximal pole of scaphoid in fracture through the waist of the scaphoid.

Problems in avascular necrosis The loss of blood supply to a major bone segment impairs healing because the avascular segment cannot participate in the reparative process. This defective healing makes the bone weak and susceptible to external forces. This results in collapse of the bone and late osteoarthritic changes.

Clinical Features

Avascular necrosis of a bone is usually asymptomatic in the early stages. In the later stage, the patient may

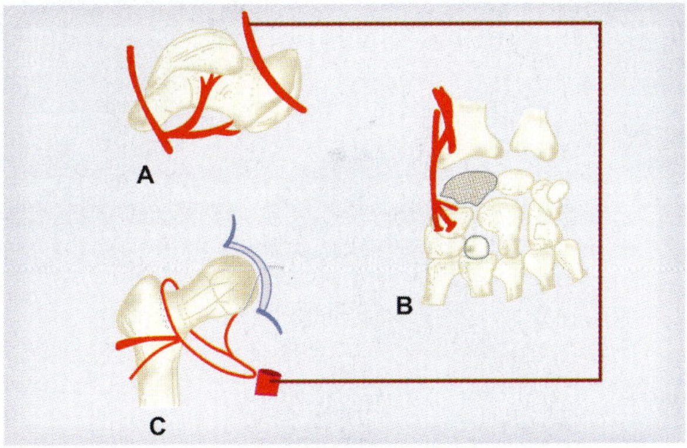

Figs 4.12A to C: Due to the peculiar blood supply avascular necrosis is common in the above three bones: (A) talus, (B) scaphoid, and (C) neck of femur

complain of pain, limp and slight loss of movements. In very advanced cases the patient will show features of osteoarthritis.

Investigations

In the early stages avascular necrosis can be detected by bone scan, radio-isotope study. In the later stages, radiograph shows dense changes in the bone, collapse and osteoarthritic features (Fig. 4.13).

Treatment

Early stages require no treatment. Protective braces may be given to prevent bone collapse. Surgical decompression has a doubtful role. In the late stages total hip replacement is advocated for AVN head of the femur. AVN in scaphoid needs open reduction and bone grafting.

TRAUMATIC MYOSITIS OSSIFICANS

DEFINITION It is a reactive lesion occurring in the soft tissues and at times in the bone periosteum. It is characterised by fibrous, osseous and cartilaginous proliferation of the subperiosteal haematoma. This is later followed by metaplastic changes.

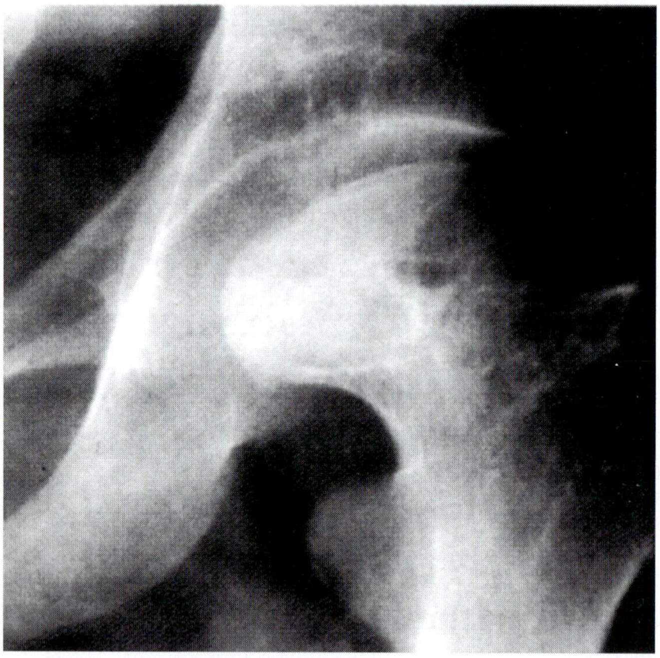

Fig. 4.13: Radiograph showing avascular necrosis of femoral head

CAUSES

Trauma This has a definitive role in the causation of myositis ossificans. Injury to the muscles, ligaments, tendons, periosteum and bones results in bleeding within the soft tissues which in turn may lead to myositis.

Simple blow or repeated minor trauma This could also give rise to myositis due to the repeated and constant soft tissue damage.

Dislocations and avulsion injuries These are more prone to develop myositis than the fractures because of the violent stripping of the periosteum and damage to the muscles.

Ill-advised massage This is by far the most common cause for myositis. Vigorous and improper massage particularly the elbow joint by quacks, etc. explains the frequent occurrence of this problem in patients treated by traditional bonesetters and osteopaths.

Pathology

Muscle is commonly involved, but fascia, tendon and periosteum can also be affected. Basically the process is a peculiar alteration within the ground substance of the connective tissue associated with proliferation of undifferentiated connective tissue.

If the periosteum is involved, the subperiosteal haematoma undergoes proliferation and metaplasia resulting in bone formation. Histological study reveals three zones (Ackermann's zone phenomenon)

- Central highly cellular area.
- Zone of fibroelastic tissue.
- Zone of mature well-oriented bone.

Remember in Myositis ossificans

Muscles commonly involved are:

- Brachialis anticus.
- Quadratus femoris.
- Adductor muscles of the thigh.

Note: All these muscles take origin from a wide area suggesting role of periosteum in its genesis.

CLASSIFICATION (BASED ON ITS LOCATION)

1. Extraosseous.
2. Periosteal—beneath the periosteum.
3. Paraosteal.

Haematoma seems to be a necessary prerequisite in all the three situations.

Clinical Features

In the acute stages, the patient may complain of pain, swelling and loss of movements. On examination there may be tenderness. In the late stages there is no pain and a bony hard lump may be palpated. This may act as a mechanical block to the movements.

Remember

Areas commonly affected

- Elbow joint common in young athletes.
- Ankle joint—(known as footballer's ankle).
- Knee—(known as Pellegrini-Stieda disease).
- Shoulder.
- Hip.
- In head injuries it is more common.

Investigations

Radiography has little role in the *acute stages* but in the late stages a bony growth may be evidently seen (Fig. 4.14).

Treatment

Acute stages Conservative treatment is the method of choice and consists of the following:

- *Immobilisation of the part by splints, etc.*
- *Drugs*—diphosphonate therapy, calcitonin and nonsteroidal anti-inflammatory drugs (NSAIDs).
- *Physiotherapy* Active physiotherapy is encouraged and passive stretching is avoided.
- *Manipulation is done under anaesthesia*. It is a double-edged sword and has to be done very carefully.

Note: Adhesions should snap abruptly and should not be broken gradually.

Chronic stages Surgery is the treatment of choice and consists of soft tissue release and excision of bony spur when it is well formed.

Remember

- The term myositis ossificans is a *misnomer* because skeletal muscle is often not involved and inflammatory changes are rarely seen.
- **Myositis ossificans progressiva** It is a different condition and has nothing to do with the traumatic one. It is a congenital condition affecting all the skeletal muscles

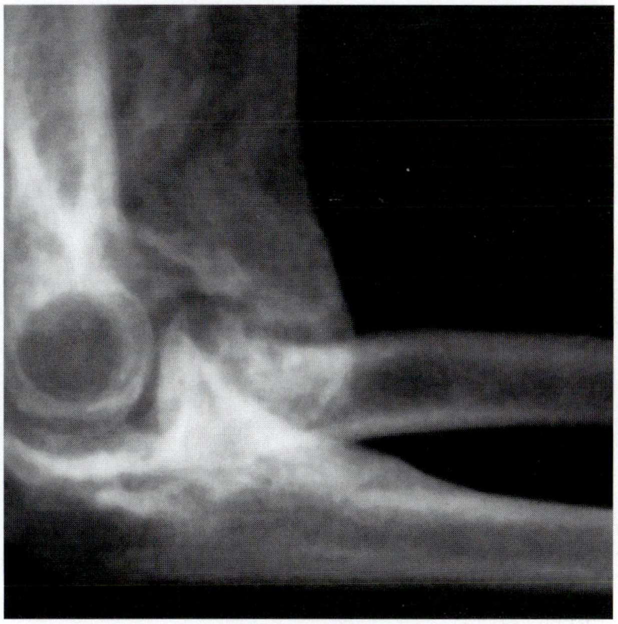

Fig. 4.14: Radiograph showing myositis ossificans (Elbow joint)

MALUNION

When fracture fragments heal in an abnormal position, it is called malunion. It can pose the following problems:

1. It may cause cosmetically unsightly deformity (Fig. 4.15A).
2. It may cause alteration in posture and balance in lower limb fractures.
3. It may cause shortening (Fig. 4.15B).
4. It may interfere with joint function.
5. Altered weight bearing mechanism may lead to premature osteoarthritis of the hip and knee joints.

CAUSES

Treatment methods Malunion is fairly common in fractures treated by closed reduction because it is a blind technique and it is very difficult to assess the accuracy of the reduction.

Improper immobilisation techniques Following reductions if the fracture is not immobilised properly and if immobilised for inadequate length of time, malunion usually results.

Treatment by quacks Due to poor knowledge of fracture anatomy, the osteopaths and the traditional

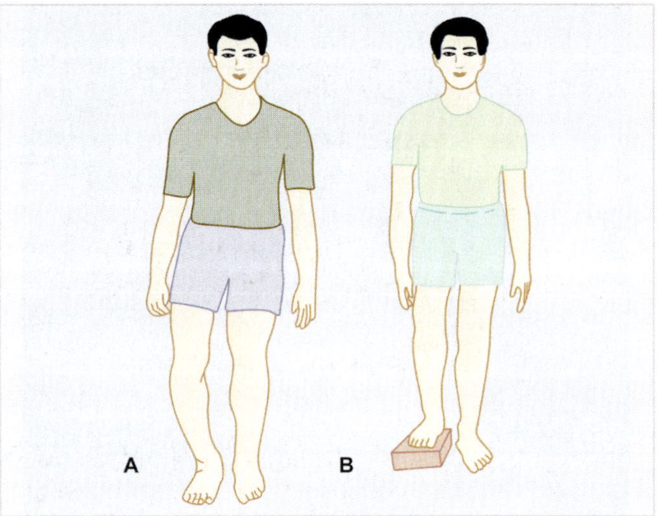

Figs 4.15A and B: Malunion of a long bone like tibia will cause shortening and deformity

bonesetters contribute significantly to the incidence of malunion.

Multiple and multisystem injuries These are life-threatening and assume more importance during treatment and the fractures may go unnoticed by the treating physicians resulting in malunion.

Vital Facts

Postreduction criteria to prevent malunion from developing:

In order to prevent the malunion from developing following closed reductions, certain postreduction criteria should be strictly adhered to like (in order of importance).

- Alignment of fracture fragments to be corrected first.
- Rotation of the fragments corrected next.
- Length of the limb is restored.
- Lastly position of the fragments is adjusted.

CLASSIFICATION

If there is improper correction of any one of the above mentioned criteria, the following types of malunion may be encountered.

1. *Length malunion* This commonly results in shortening of the limb and rarely may give rise to lengthening.
2. *Rotatory malunion* This may cause external or internal rotation deformities.
3. *Angulatory malunion* This may cause varus or valgus deformities.

Of all the factors mentioned above the one factor which is not corrected by remodelling is rotation, while the other three are successfully overcome over the years by remodelling. Hence, all precautions should be taken to correct the rotation element during the initial treatment of fractures.

Types

Significant malunion This impairs both the function and causes a major cosmetic problem.

Insignificant malunion This does not interefere with function but causes only cosmetic problem.

Clinical Features

A patient with malunion of bones may complain of deformity and/ or alteration or rarely loss of function of the affected extremities. There may be shortening and wasting of the involved limbs.

Radiograph of the affected part including the joints above and below are mandatory to assess the malunion (Fig. 4.16).

Treatment

Masterly inactivity if the patient has no functional problems. Cosmesis alone does not form a sufficient indication for surgery unless the patient desires so. But operative treatment is highly justified when malunion affects the function. This can be done by a *corrective osteotomy* at the old fracture site or a *compensatory procedure* may be necessary to restore functions (e.g. Darrach's operation in malunited

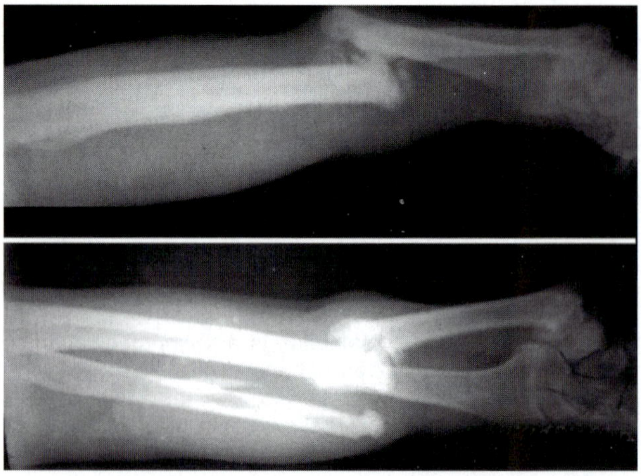

Fig. 4.16: Radiographs showing malunited fractures of both bones of the forearm

Colles). Sometimes pain may be the only predominant symptom necessitating *fusion of the affected joint*.

The optimum time to carry out surgery for malunion is 6 to 12 months after the fracture has occurred.

OTHER IMPORTANT COMPLICATIONS OF FRACTURES

DEEP VEIN THROMBOSIS AND PULMONARY EMBOLISM

Deep vein thrombosis (DVT) is an important complication seen after fractures of spine, pelvis, femur, tibia, etc. The pathogenesis has been described by Virchow's triad of venous stasis, vascular damage and hypercoagulability.

The patient complains of mild-to-severe calf pain, swelling, difficulty in standing or walking and cramps in the calf muscles or foot. The clinical signs include unilateral leg swelling, increased temperature, tenderness, enlarged superficial veins, pitting edema, palpable cord along the involved veins, erythema, etc. (Fig. 4.17).

Homan's sign When forced ankle dorsiflexion produces calf pain, Homan's sign is said to be positive and is pathognomonic of DVT (Fig. 4.18).

Treatment Prophylactic methods consist of early ambulation, foot elevation, elastocrepe bandaging, exercises, etc.

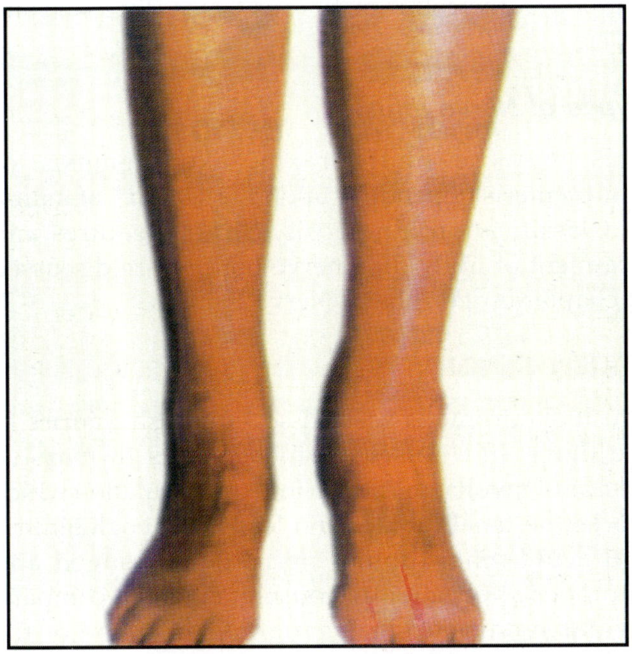

Fig. 4.17: Clinical photograph of deep vein thrombosis

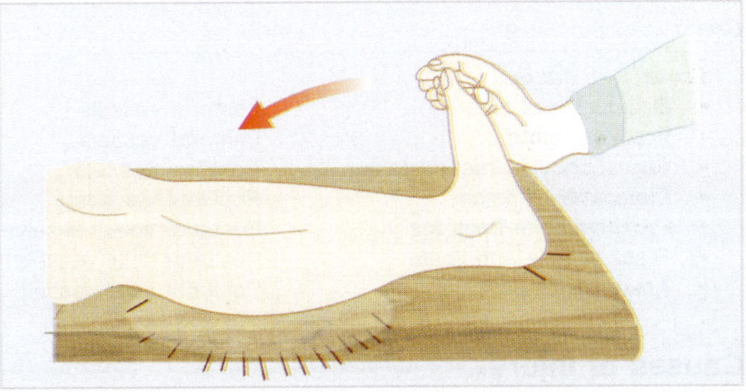

Fig. 4.18: Showing Homan's sign

Anticoagulant therapy This consists of aspirin (600-650 mg), heparin (low dose), low molecular weight dextran, low dose warfarin (2.5-16 mg/day daily orally), etc.

Pulmonary thromboembolism is a serious complication of DVT. The patient with pulmonary embolism complains of unexplained dyspnoea, pleuritic chest pain, hypoxia, tachypnoea, tachycardia, signs of cor pulmonale, etc. Heparin therapy is the treatment of choice.

Chronic venous insufficiency is the common long-term complication of DVT.

Embolic facts

Other important predisposing factors for DVT

- Surgery—orthopaedic/thoracic/abdominal/GU systems.
- Immobilisation due to CCF, MI, stroke, etc.
- Neoplasms
- Oestrogen therapy
- Pregnancy
- Obesity
- Age > 40 years
- TAO, Behçet's disease, etc.
- Hypercoagulable states.
- Total hip and knee replacement, etc.

INJURY TO BLOOD VESSELS

Blood vessels in close proximity to the bones are injured during fractures and dislocations *(see box)*.

Injuries	Blood vessel involved
Upper limb trauma	
• Fracture clavicle	Subclavian vessels
• Proximal humeral fractures	Axillary vessels
• Supracondylar fracture of humerus	Brachial vessels
• Posterior dislocation of elbow	Brachial vessels
• Fracture both bones of the forearm	Anterior interosseous artery

Contd...

Section 1

Contd...

Lower limb trauma	
• Dislocation of hip	Femoral vessels
• Fracture femur	Femoral vessels
• Supracondylar fracture femur	Popliteal vessels
• Dislocation of knee	Popliteal vessels
• Proximal tibial fractures	Posterior tibial vessels
• Fracture tibia and fibula	Posterior tibial vessels
• Ankle injuries	Posterior tibial vessels

Causes of Injury

The blood vessels may be injured in one of the following ways: reflex vasospasm, compression by the fracture fragments or haematoma, incomplete tear, complete tear, partial tear, internal thrombus, tight encircling bandages, etc. (Fig. 4.19).

Effects of Injury

In the initial stages it may range from mild ischaemia to gangrene. In the late stages ischaemic contractures may develop.

Clinical Features

Apart from the usual features, the patient may show impending signs of vascular disaster recognised by 5Ps: pain, pulselessness, paraesthesia, pallor and paralysis. Cold extremities herald the onset of gangrene.

Investigations

Consists of radiograph of the part, Doppler angiogram studies, etc.

Treatment

This consists of prompt reduction of fractures and dislocations and removal of all tight encircling bandages. Thrombectomy, direct end-to-end repair, injection of xylocaine, papaverine, sympathectomy to relieve the vasospasms are some of the commonly recommended methods of treatment. Amputation is considered in irreversible loss of blood supply.

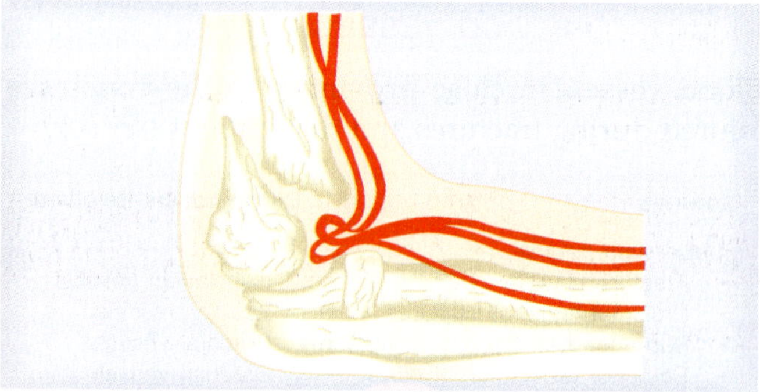

Fig. 4.19: Injury to the brachial vessels can occur in displaced supracondylar fractures of humerus

INJURY TO NERVES

Forty per cent of the bone and joint injuries are associated with peripheral nerve lesions.

Types

Two types are described:

1. *Primary* Here the nerve is injured by the same trauma that resulted in the injury to bone and joint.
2. *Secondary* This is due to involvement of the nerve in infection, scar, callus, etc.

Incidence Radial nerve is the most commonly injured peripheral nerve (45%), followed by ulnar nerve (30%), median nerve (15%), peroneal nerve, lumbosacral plexus (3%) and tibial nerve.

Mechanism of Injury

The nerve may be damaged by the fracture fragments, entrapment between the fragments during fracture reduction, direct injury by the bullets, sharp cutting weapons, etc. In the late stages, the nerve may be trapped in the callus or fibrous tissue (Figs 4.20 and 4.21).

Types of Nerve Injury

This may be neuropraxia, axonotemesis or neurotemesis depending upon the severity of injury.

Classification, diagnosis, clinical features and treatment of individual nerve injuries are discussed in chapter on Peripheral Nerve Injuries.

CRUSH SYNDROME

Crush syndrome is seen in severe crush injuries of the limbs and muscles which results in massive release of myohaemoglobin into the circulation which blocks the renal tubules and leads to myoglobinuria and acute renal tubular necrosis. Prolonged and improper application of tourniquet, acute compartmental syndromes, gas gangrene are some of the other causes of crush syndrome. Treatment is directed

Nerve facts

Trauma	Nerves injured
Upper limb	
• Fracture calvicle	Brachial plexus
• Proximal humeral fracture	Axillary nerve
• Fracture humerus	Radial nerve
• Supracondylar fracture humerus	Radial nerve
• Posterior dislocation of elbow	Median nerve
• Monteggia fracture	Posterior interosseous nerve
• Hook of hamate	Deep branch of ulnar nerve
• Wrist injury	Median nerve
Lower limb	
• Dislocations of hip (posterior)	Sciatic nerve
• Anterior dislocation of hip and shaft femur	Femoral nerve
• Dislocation of knee	Common peroneal nerve
• Proximal tibial fractures and ankle injury	Posterior tibial nerve
• Fracture neck fibula	Lateral popliteal nerve

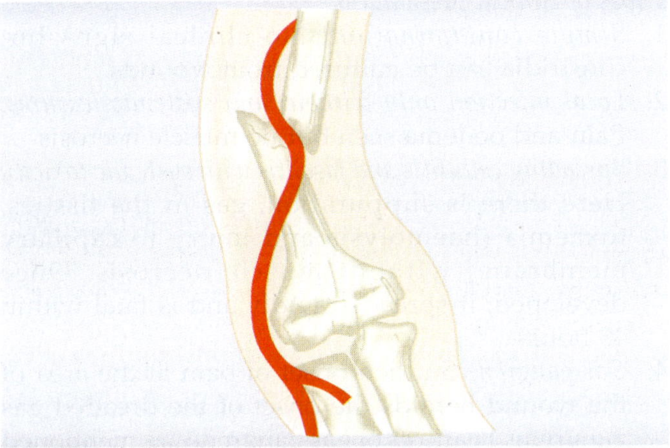

Fig. 4.20: Radial nerve injury can occur in fracture shaft of humerus

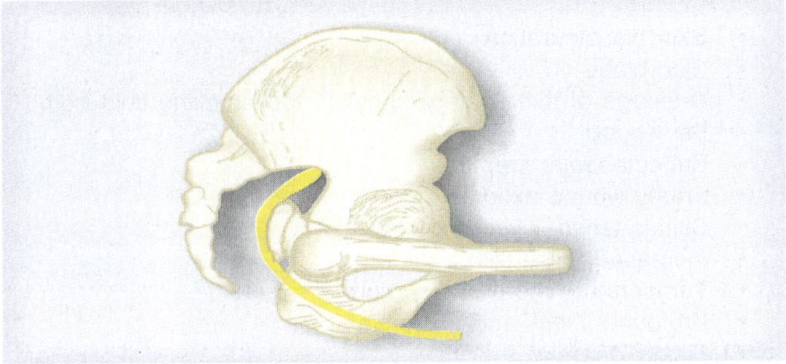

Fig. 4.21: Posterior dislocation of hip joint can damage the sciatic nerve

towards managing acute renal failure in case the patient develops oliguria or anuria.

JOINT STIFFNESS

This is due to improper technique of fracture immobilisation. This can be fairly a troublesome problem. Intra-articular fractures periarticular adhesions of soft tissues, capsules and muscle contractures are some of the other important causes of joint stiffness. Physiotherapy, exercises, manipulation under anaesthesia, surgical excision and lengthening of contractures are some of the important treatment methods.

REFLEX SYMPATHETIC DYSTROPHY

It is an abnormal sympathetic response following fractures. This is commonly encountered in Colles' fracture.

OSTEOMYELITIS

It is common in compound fractures (*see the section on osteomyelitis for details*). The other complications peculiar to open fractures are tetanus, gangrene and hypovolaemic shock.

IMPLANT FAILURE

It can occur due to defective manufacturing or biological reactions within the body.

POST-TRAUMATIC OSTEOARTHRITIS

Post-traumatic osteoarthritis is commonly seen in intra-articular fractures, malunion, etc.

GROWTH ALTERATIONS

Growth alterations are due to epiphyseal injuries in children.

SHORTENING

Shortening of long bones is the other important complication.

COMPLICATIONS PECULIAR TO OPEN FRACTURES

SHOCK

In fractures of major long bones, pelvic fractures, multisystem injuries following road traffic accidents, etc. severe loss of blood may seriously threaten the life of a victim. Delay and apathy in attending a hypovolaemic shock could prove fatal.

Source of haemorrhage This could be external or internal.

a. *External haemorrhage*: This usually happens in compound fractures, pelvic fractures, etc.
b. *Internal haemorrhage*: It is more often seen in blunt injury of abdomen, femur and pelvic fractures, etc.

Note: Internal haemorrhage stealthily snuffs out the life of a victim as it largely goes undetected.

Bloody facts: Do you know the staggering blood loss in fractures?

- Femoral shaft fractures—blood loss could range from 500-2000 ml
- Pelvic fractures—blood loss could range from 1000-2500 ml. It could be much more in multiple fractures.

Clinical features Look for the classical features of shock (see box) apart from the usual features of fractures.

Shocking facts: Look for the classical features

- Sunken eyeballs
- Tongue—pale and dry
- Pale look
- Low BP
- Cold clammy skin
- Cold nose
- Peripheral pulses feeble or absent
- Drowsy or unconscious
- Sweating

Treatment Speed is the watchword in the treatment of shock and includes:

- Resuscitation
- Immediate fluid replacement by:
  a. IV fluids like normal saline, Ringer's lactate, etc.
  b. Haemaccel if blood is not available.
  c. Blood is the best alternative.
- Administration of oxygen, etc.
- Splinting of the fractures.
- Controlling the bleeding points.

GAS GANGRENE

Definition This is an uncommon infection of the superficial and deep fascia following a severe trauma resulting in necrotising fasciitis. The offending organism in most of these situations is *Clostridium* (about 30%). The presence of gas in the tissues implies that due to anaerobic bacterial metabolism, insoluble gases like hydrogen, nitrogen and methane are produced.

Quick Facts: Organisms which can cause gas in the tissues

- *Clostridium welchii* (30%)—Most common
- *C. perfringes*
- *Streptococcus pyogenes*
- Halophilic marine vibrio
- Fungus of rhizopus and *Mucor* species
- *Pseudomonas* and acromonas

Incidence It is about 1.76%

Types of clinical presentation

1. *Simple contamination*: No clinical signs but Clostridia can be cultured from wounds.
2. *Local infection only without any systemic features:* Pain and oedema seen but no muscle necrosis.
3. *Spreading cellulitis and fasciitis with systemic toxicity* Here there is suppuration, gas in the tissues, toxaemia (haemolysis and injury to capillary membrane) without muscle necrosis. Once developed, it spreads rapidly and is fatal within 48 hours.
4. *Gas gangrene* Sudden onset of pain at the area of the wound heralds the onset of the dreaded gas gangrene. Features of gas gangrene are mentioned in the box.

Vital facts: Gas gangrene features

- Skin discolouration
- Skin blebs
- Drainage of thin, watery, greyish, foul-smelling fluid from the wound.
- Subcutaneous crepitus
- Frothy wound exudate
- Skin is tense, white and cool
- Increased pulse rate
- Temperature more or less normal
- Profound shock and toxaemia
- Finally death

Investigation

- Exploration and gram staining of the exudate.
- Plain X-ray of the part.

- CT scan.
- MRI scan.

Prevention Early recognition and excision of all necrotising tissues. The predisposing causes are:

- Penetrating deep wounds of the thigh and buttocks.
- Impaired or loss of blood supply.
- Tight plaster casts.

Treatment Measures

1. *Resuscitative measures*: Include fluid and blood transfusion, respiratory support, etc.
2. *Surgical excision*: Early surgical excision of all necrotising soft tissues.
3. *Antibiotics*: Penicillin G is the drug of choice (20 lac IU/day in adults is the dose).
4. Antitoxin involves administration of AGGS.
5. Hyperbaric oxygen (HBO) Here patients are placed in a chamber at three times the atmospheric pressure. HBO inhibits alpha toxin production by Clostridia. Its role in non-clostridial infection is not clear.

TETANUS

Definition Tetanus is a fatal disease caused by *Clostridium tetani* and can occur in a patient with a superficial wound, deep wound or even in no demonstrable wound.

Pathogenesis *Clostridium tetani*, usually present in faecal matter of humans and animals, enters the body through breaks in the mucosa or skin following a puncture, laceration or abrasion. After an incubation period of 7 to 8 days, it grows and releases two exotoxins, tetanospasmin (acts on the brainstem and spinal cord) and tetanolysin (is cardiotoxic and causes haemolysis), with the clinical effects of the latter over-shadowing the former.

Clinical presentation A full blown tetanus patient presents with the following features:

- Restlessness and headache
- Spasm of the neck and pharyngeal muscles.
- Locked jaw
- In later stages orthotonus, opisthotonus, etc. occur.
- Generalised toxic convulsions can occur. These are triggered easily by external stimuli like light, sound, breeze, etc. Prone for fractures due to fall, etc.
- Death supervenes after 2 weeks to the hapless victim (Mortality rate is 60%).

Treatment A multidisciplinary approach is recommended:

- Respiratory support by oxygen, ventilators, etc.
- Meticulous management of wound is vital.
- Sedation is very important to prevent or control convulsions. Phenobarbitone, secobarbital thiopental sodium, succinyl choline and magnesium sulphate are some of the commonly used agents.
- Good nursing care is required in a dark isolated room.
- Tracheostomy is required if the patient develops pharyngospasm or laryngospasm.
- Pharyngospasm is far more easier to manage than the troublesome laryngospasm.

Prevention This is anytime better and easier than the cumbersome curative methods. The measures recommended are:

- *Active immunisation* This is the best and consists of three doses of tetanus-diphtheria booster. The injection needs to be given once in 10 years for the rest of the life.
- *Passive immunisation* This is done by intravascular administration of 250 IU of tetanus immunoglobulin (TIG).

Pearl: This disease proves that, little things, are so important than the 'hectic damage control' measures so true of life. What can be prevented by little (simple immunisation) cannot be cured by much (the elaborate treatment). A person with a wound who refuses a TT shot is like penny wise and pound foolish who may unfortunately pay through his life.

After the diagnosis is made, human tetanus immunoglobulin is given in the doses of 500–1000 units till a total dosage of 6,000–10,000 is reached.

CRUSH SYNDROME (see page 44)

5

Emergency Care of the Injured

FIRST AID

First aid techniques in managing an injured patient should be learnt first and not last. Proper first aid is a skill which needs to be learnt and developed.

DEFINITION

First aid is the initial care of the injured at the scene of accident.

Anybody can give first aid, but to carry out cardiopulmonary resuscitation measures one should be trained in first aid and should possess a valid certificate issued by a competent body.

First aid executed by a medical person is called *medical aid.*

GOALS OF FIRST AID TREATMENT

Goals of first aid treatment is aptly described by **three Ps**.

- **P**reserve life by carrying out appropriate resuscitative measures.
- **P**revent further injuries by careful handling.
- **P**romote recovery.

INITIAL CARE OF THE INJURED

At the Scene of Accident

- Remove the victim from the accident spot.
- Check his or her vital parameters quickly (pulse, BP, consciousness, etc.).
- Seek the help of bystanders if trained in first aid.
- Ensure that police and ambulance have been informed.
- Remember to carry out first aid according to MacMurthy's A to F regimen *(ref. p. 52).*
- Ensure personal safety.

MODUS OPERANDI IN FIRST AID

AIRWAY

First clear the airway as follows:

- Clear the mouth of clots, dentures, loose teeth, etc (Fig 5.1A).
- Extend the neck slightly as this opens up the pharynx (Fig. 5.1B).
- If the patient is not breathing, begin artificial respiration. First keep a thin cloth over the patient's mouth, blow into the patients mouth keeping his or her nostrils closed (Fig. 5.1C). Blow at the rate of 16 per minute and see for the chest raise. Mouth to nose respiration is carried out if

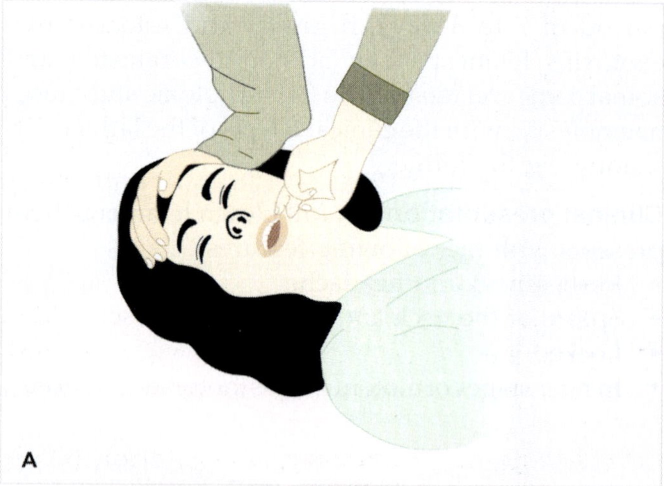

Fig. 5.1A: Technique of artificial respiration. Clear the mouth of debris first

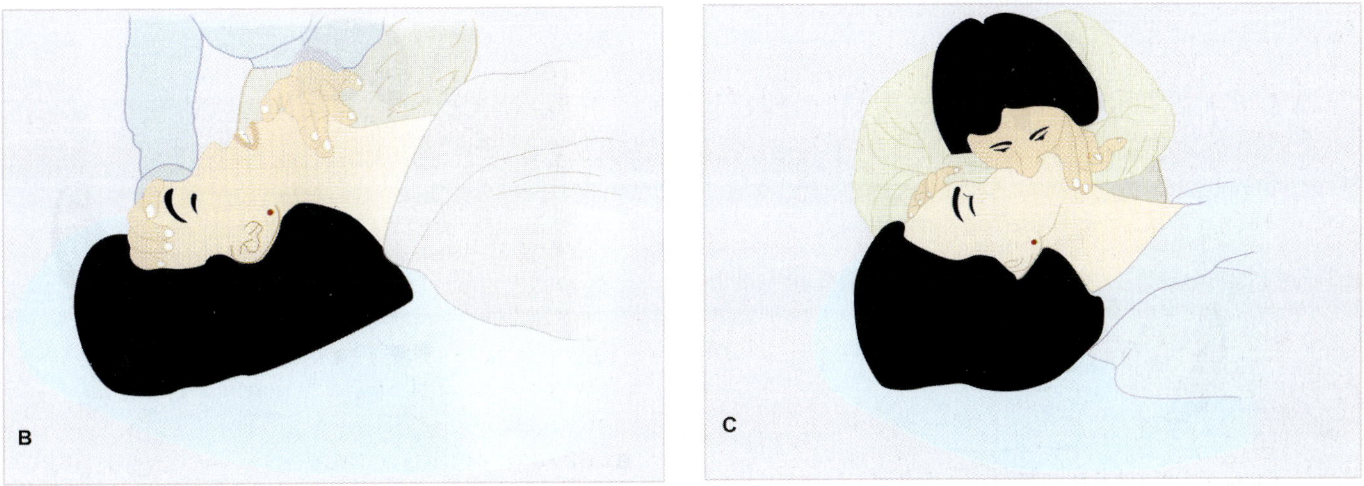

Figs 5.1B and C: (B) Extend the neck (C) Blow into the victim's mouth

there is extensive injury to the mouth. If the patient has suffered extensive facial injuries, put the patient prone, turn the face towards one side and apply pressure over the lower aspect of the chest (Holger-Nelson method).

CARDIA

Examine the radial pulse and the carotid pulse for the function of cardia. If the pulse is absent, initiate cardiac resuscitative measures as follows:

- Ensure that the patient is lying on a hard surface.
- Then pressure is applied with the heel of the palm at the lower end of sternum (Fig. 5.2).
- Optimum pressure should be applied and the depth of each pressure should be 1¼ inch.
- Perform external cardiac massage at the rate of 72 per minute.

  It is preferable to carry out both external cardiac massage and artificial respiration simultaneously by two persons trained in first aid. But if there is no assistance available then cardiopulmonary resuscitation should be carried out by a single person as follows:
  - First artificial respiration is given once and then the same person should quickly change position and carry out external cardiac massage 5 times. So, this 1 : 5 ratio should be maintained throughout.
  - The cardiopulmonary resuscitation (CPR) should be carried out till the patient recovers or at least for half an hour.

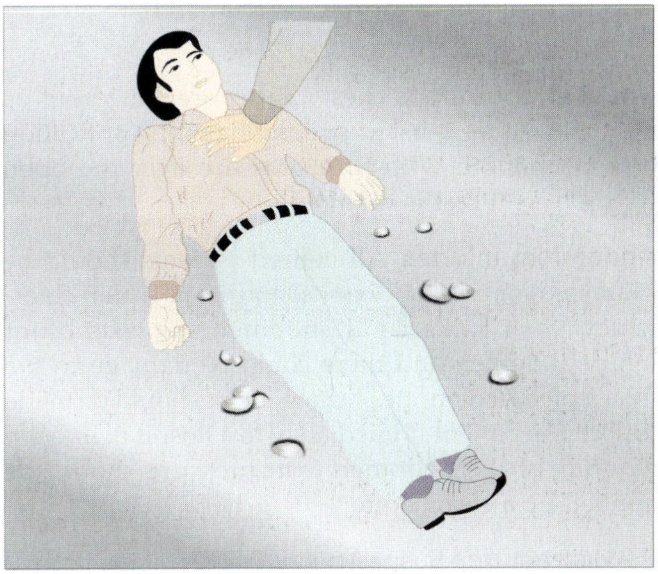

Fig. 5.2: Showing method of external cardiac massage

BLEEDING

It is advisable to arrest the bleeding by elevation or direct application of pressure over the bleeding points (Figs 5.3A and B). *Tourniquet should be avoided and used only as a last resort.*

EXAMINE THE VITAL STRUCTURES

Head injuries Examine the patient for head injuries, cover the skull injuries with a clean cloth, examine pupils and the level of consciousness. Look for neurological deficits.

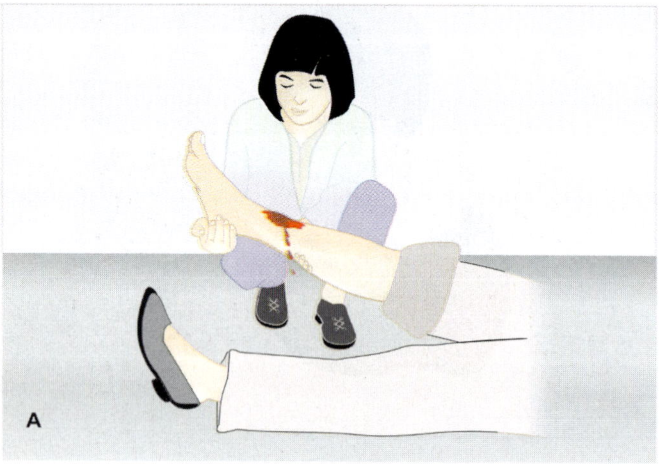

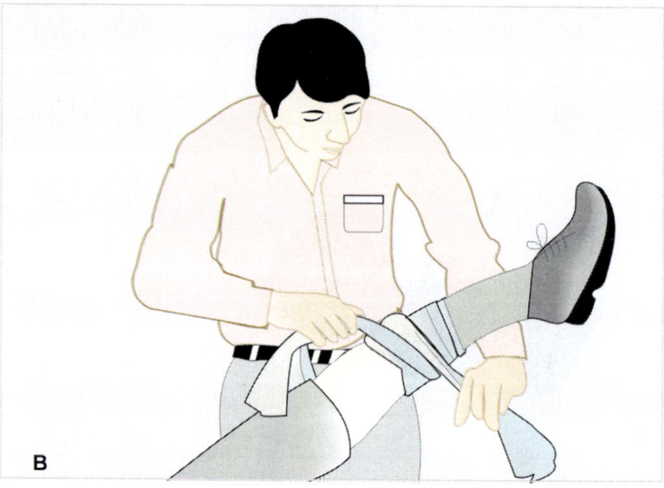

Figs 5.3A and B: Showing methods to control bleeding: (A) Limb elevation, (B) Firm pressure and bandaging at the bleeding site helps control haemorrhage

Chest injuries Open chest injuries are dangerous as they may cause tension pneumothorax. Application of a clean cloth with firm pressure over the open wounds is all that is required.

Abdominal injuries All injured patients should be examined for intra-abdominal injuries as it is an emergency. Board-like rigid abdomen suggests blunt injury abdomen and there could be damage to the liver, spleen, colon, etc. Arrangement should be made to shift the patient immediately to a hospital. In open wounds of the abdomen firm pressure should be applied by a clean cloth.

Pelvic fractures Suspect pelvic fracture if the patient complains of pain during compression test or distraction test which is performed by applying pressure over the iliac bones. Tenderness over the symphysis pubis is also suggestive.

Injuries to the genitourinary system Suprapubic swelling indicates bladder injury, injury to the scrotum or perineal haematoma indicates urethral rupture.

Spine injuries Cervical spine injury should be suspected if the patient is lying still and loathes to turn the neck. Injuries to the thoracic and lumbar spine should be suspected if the patient has developed paraplegia or complains of pain when individual spinous processes are palpated. *Extreme care should be exercised in managing and shifting a patient with spinal injuries.*

Fractures Deformity, pain, swelling, loss of function of a limb are suggestive of fracture.

Fracture needs to be splinted with whatever material is available at the scene of accident (Figs 5.4 to 5.6). They can be managed electively after shifting the patient to the hospital.

Remember

- Fracture is not an emergency.
- Most of them can be managed electively at a later date.
- In A to F management of injured fracture treatment comes last.
- Prepare and improvise splints with available materials at the scene of accident.

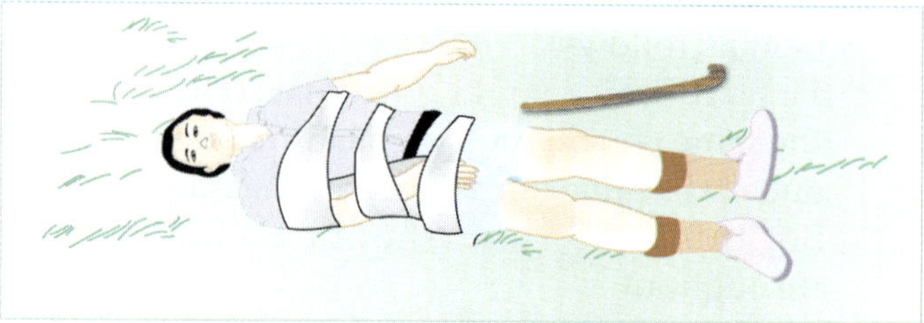

Fig. 5.4: Showing using victim's own body for splinting of fractures

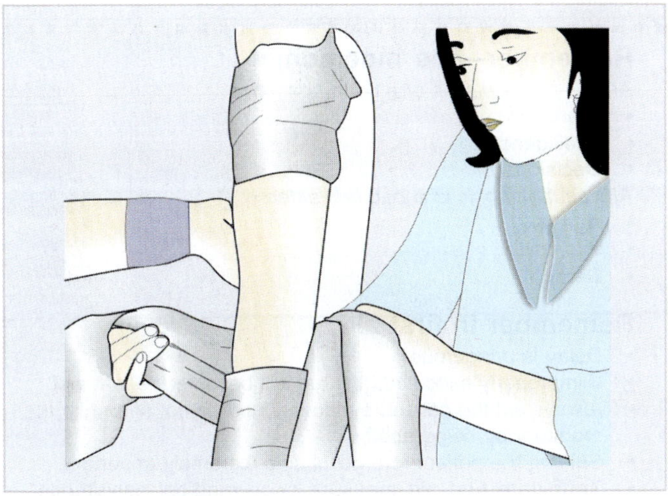

Fig. 5.5A: Showing splinting with a newspaper

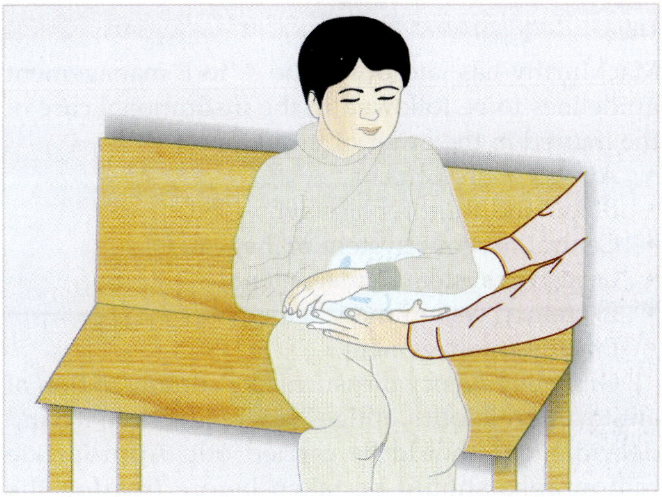

Fig. 5.5B: Showing splinting with a cloth

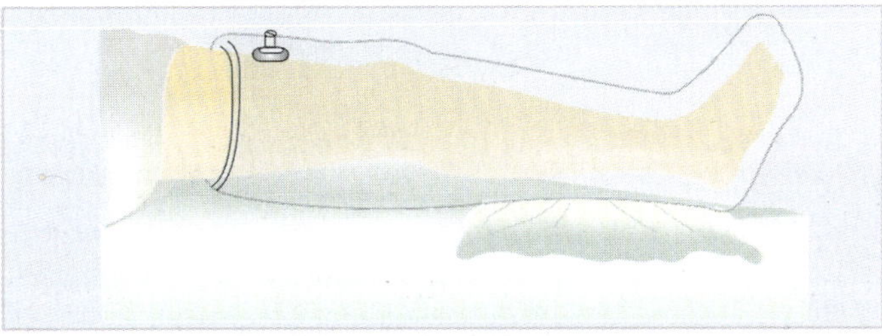

Fig. 5.5C: Showing the modern pneumatic splint

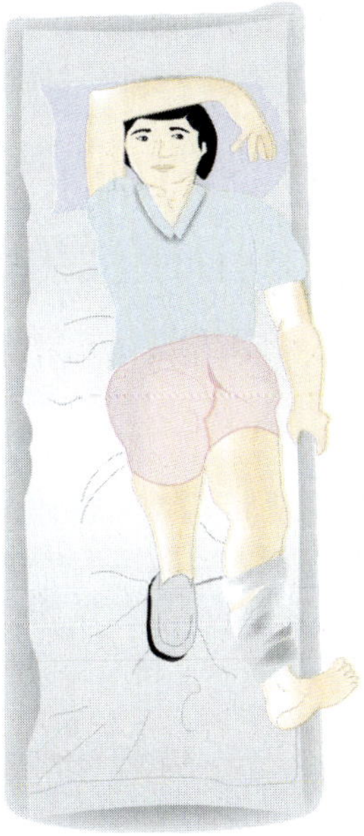

Fig. 5.5D: Splinting with a firm support

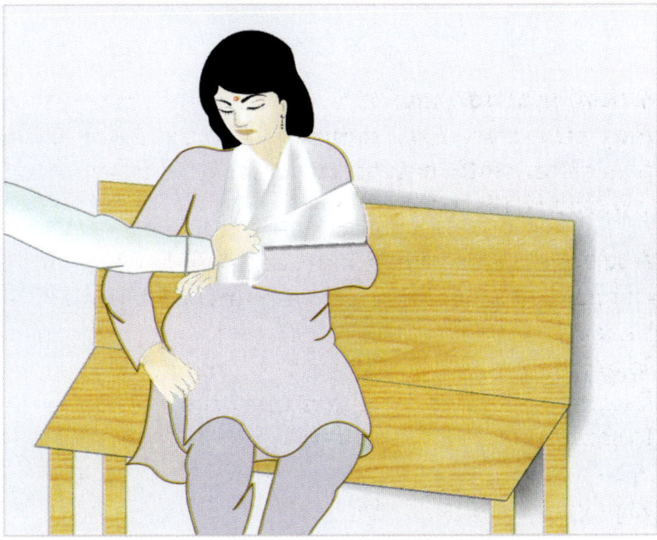

Fig. 5.6: Splinting of the fracture sites with sling and a body bandage

Remember: About fractures in first aid

The management of fractures at the scene of accident.

Five Ss

1. **S**ling for clavicle fractures, shoulder fractures, etc.
2. **S**trap for clavicle and rib fractures.
3. **S**plint, usually improvised. Best would be a Thomas splint or a pneumatic splint.
4. **S**hift the patient with utmost care.
5. **S**eek professional help at the earliest.

Remember the priority in first aid

Three Ss

- **S**hock to be corrected first.
- **S**ystemic injuries to be tackled next.
- **S**pine injuries call for extreme caution.

MANAGEMENT AT THE HOSPITAL

MacMurthy has laid down the A to F management guidelines to be followed in the institutional care of the injured in the order of importance:

- Airway management
- Blood and fluid replacement
- Central nervous system management
- Digestive system management
- Excretory system management
- Fracture management.

Other emergency measures like administration of antitoxin, antibiotics, antigasgangrene serum, wound debridement should be carried out. Appropriate radiographs should be taken before treating the fractures. The treatment of bone and joint injuries are discussed in detail in the relevant chapters.

Remember—the mnemonic

AID as prerequisites of a good first aider

- **A**lertness
- **I**ntelligence
- **D**ecisions

AID as mnemonic of a bad first aider

- **A**pathy
- **I**ndecision
- **D**elay

Remember in first aid

- Delay is dangerous.
- If improperly executed, first aid will become the last aid!
- Always aid the patient to recovery and do not send him to mortuary by being apathetic.
- Shifting the patient to a hospital is extremely important.
- Terminate first aid measure once medical assistance arrives or after shifting the patient to the hospital.

6

Fracture Treatment Methods: Then, Now and Future

"They whose work cannot die, whose influence lives after them, whose disciples perpetuate and multiply their gifts to humanity, are truly immortal." This was how Watson Jones paid tribute to Hugh Oven Thomas.

HISTORY OF FRACTURE TREATMENT: THEN

Our forefathers were no less skilful in treating fractures (Fig. 6.1). The Egyptians were known to be skilled at the management of fractures and many healed specimens have been found. Hippocrates and Celsus described in detail the splintage of fractures by using wooden appliances. But a fascinating account of external splintage was given by Al Zabra, an Arabic surgeon. He used both clay gum mixtures, flour and egg white for casting materials. In 1517, Gersdorf described a method of binding wooden splints using ligatures around the assembled splint and tightening it. Chinese described use of willow board splints for the treatment of tibial shaft fractures and Colles' fracture. The Arabians described a technique of pouring a plaster of Paris mixture around an injured limb. Malgaigne was instrumental in popularising this technique in Europe by the early 19th century. The great disadvantage of all this extensive and heavy forms of immobilisation of limb was the possibility of the fracture disease (Fig. 6.2). In 1873, Sir James Paget described about fracture disease. Thus, he advocated the concept of early mobilisation to prevent this problem.

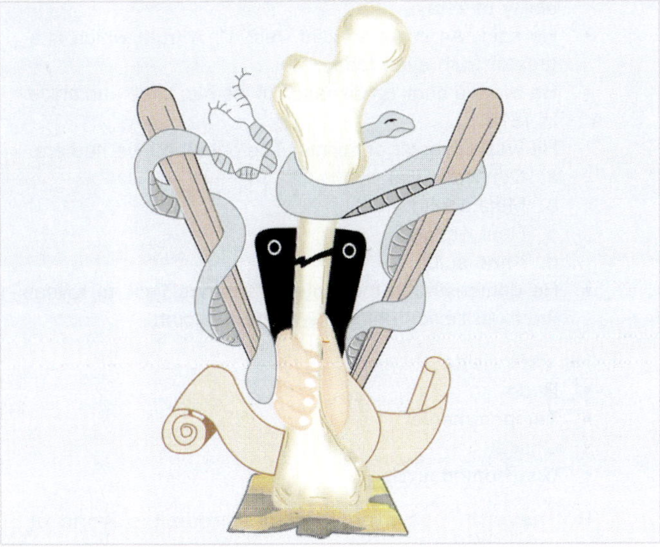

Fig. 6.1: History of orthopaedics

Remember

Hippocrates (Fig. 6.3) and orthopaedics

- Hippocrates was born in Greece in 460 BC.
- He advanced the five concepts of fracture treatment, namely antisepsis, bandaging, reduction, splinting, and traction.
- He dissociated medicine from religion and philosophy.
- He wrote three books on skeletal system.

THE PLASTER BANDAGES

In Holland, in 1852 Antonius Mathysen (1805-1878), a military surgeon, was on the look out of an immobilising bandage that would permit the safe transport of patients with gunshot injuries to specialised treatment centres. He sought a bandage that could be used at once, would become hard in minutes and be adaptable to the extremity. Thus, he

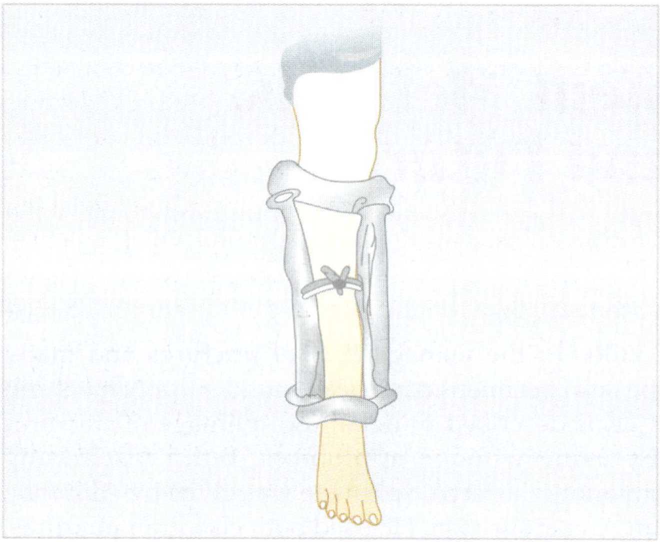

Fig. 6.2: Primitive methods of fracture immobilisation

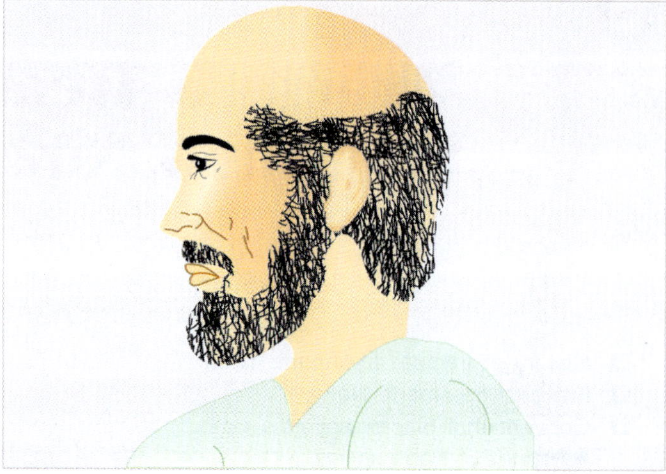

Fig. 6.3: Hippocrates

introduced plaster of Paris (POP) in 1876 at the centennial exhibition in Philadelphia. The use of POP bandages as cast and slabs became popular after his death.

But the most brilliant discovery of a splint was by HO Thomas which came to be known as Thomas splint after his name. It is still used in many centres of the world for treatment of fracture of femur, though it was designed initially to assist in the treatment of TB knee.

TRACTION

Galen (AD 130-200) first described the longitudinal traction to overcome the overriding of fracture fragments. The use of continuous traction in the management of diaphyseal fractures appeared around the middle of the 19th century. In 1800, Albert Hoffa of Wurzburg (the place of Roentgen who discovered X-rays) described the use of tractions for many types of fractures of femur and humerus. Dr Josiah Crosby of New Hampshire gave one of the earliest accounts of the use of continuous skin traction in the treatment of fractures. Professor George Perkins of London described the external splint and advocated a simple straight traction through an upper tibial pin.

Remember

About HO Thomas

- He came from a family of unqualified bonesetters.
- He broke the family tradition by qualifying in medicine in 1857.
- His partnership with his father failed.
- He established his practice individually in the slum of Liverpool.
- He worked there for 32 years taking only six days vacation.
- He died in 1891 at the age of 57.
- He was a great believer of enforced, uninterrupted and prolonged rest in the treatment of fractures.

Interesting Historical Facts

About HO Thomas

I. His brighter side
- Known as the father of British Orthopaedic Surgery
- A genius still unparalled in the field of orthopaedics.
- His diagnosis and management in orthopaedics was spot on even in those dark days despite the unavailability of X-ray.
- He said "An inflamed joint, rest it", A truth which is a greater truth even today.
- He wrote a book on diseases of the hip, knee and ankle in 1875.
- He was a master of splints. The ones he invented are:
  a. Cervical collar
  b. Metatarsal bars
  c. Heel wedge
  d. Knee splint
- He demonstrated the famous 'Thomas Test' to reveal the fixed flexion deformity of the hip joint.

II. His darker side
- Rude
- Temperamental
- Critical
- Unaccomodative

But nevertheless a genius who strode the world of orthopaedics like a colossus.

FUNCTIONAL BRACE

Gooch in 1767 first described the tibial and femoral functional braces. But surprisingly, this concept was pushed into oblivion for over two centuries till Sarmiento revived it. He developed a patellar tendon-bearing cast for the treatment of fractures of tibia after initial standard cast treatment. This heralded the renaissance of functional bracing. In 1970, Mooney described hinged casts for the management of femoral casts.

The widespread use of functional bracing has liberated countless patients from prolonged hospitalisation and permitted early return to function and to gainful employment.

OPEN FRACTURES

Until 150 years ago an open fracture was virtually synonymous with death and generally necessitated an immediate amputation. Ambrose Pare, a French surgeon, first described the technique of ligating the bleeding vessels after amputation. Earlier, it was cauterised. Le Petit in 1718 first described the use of tourniquet to control bleeding from amputation. This brought the mortality from amputation of the lower limbs from 75 to 25 per cent. In 1561, it was Pare again who first described the concept of conserving the limb after an open fracture when he himself sustained an open fracture of tibia due to fall from the horse. The discovery of antisepsis by Pasteur, Koch, etc. brought down the rate of infection due to open fractures drastically.

EARLY FRACTURE SURGERY

In 1770, Malgaigne was the first to describe the earliest technique of internal fixation of fractures by a ligation or a wire suture. The use of screws in bone started first around late 1840s by French surgeons Cucuel and Rigaud. Hansmann of Hampburg in 1886 was the first to describe the plate fixation of bone. Lambotte in 1909 designed a diamond-shaped plate and coined the term osteosynthesis by which he meant stable bone fixation. *He is generally regarded as the father of modern internal fixation.* Lane and Scherman devised their own plates. It was Denis in the year 1940 who by forming an association of Swiss surgeons heralded the modern era of internal fixation.

EXTERNAL FIXATION

Malgaigne in 1840 described the first external fixation device. Later, in 1897 Dr Clayton Parkhill of Colorado devised a new and improved apparatus. In 1902, Lambotte devised a more sophisticated type of external fixator in which the protruding screws were bolted to adjustable clamps linked with a heavy external bar. Pitkin for the first time devised transfixion pins with a bilateral frame as the earlier devices relied upon half pins with a single external linkage device. Ilizarov of Russia in 1952 first described the use of circular external fixator frame. He first showed that external fixator device can also be used for limb lengthening and deformity correction.

INTRAMEDULLARY FIXATION

Dieffenbac of Prussia in 1841 performed early intramedullary nailing with ivory pegs. In 1907, Lambotte emerged as a pioneer in intramedullary fixation for trochanteric fractures. Others who advocated intramedullary nails were Hey Groves of England in 1914, and Rush family.

The person who revolutionised the intramedullary nailing technique was the German military surgeon, Gerhardt Küntscher, who devised a clover leaf nail prior to the World War II. The world was slow to accept Küntscher's design but slowly Sweden in 1943 and America in 1945 absorbed the technique.

In 1958, the Association for the Study of Internal Fixation (ASIF or AO) was born. They suggested many alterations and conducted plenty of educative courses. *They advocated with vigour the concept of rigid fixation and primary bone healing.* Livingston's I beam nail is the earliest example of interlocking nail in the year 1950. At present, interlocking nail has made greater strides.

AO GROUP

Robert Denis of Brussels (1880-1962) is regarded as the father of modern osteosynthesis. He described the interfragmentary compression and the concept of rigid fixation. On 1st March, 1950, a young Swiss surgeon, Dr Maurice Muller, was so much influenced by the work of Denis that he started an association in Sweden in 1958 involving a group of young enthusiastic fracture surgeons. Educating young surgeons from all over the world in their technique was their aim. From 1960 to the present day, they conduct regular annual training sessions.

Thus, it is to our forefathers we owe the tremendous achievements we have made of late in fracture treatment. Needless to say without their sweat and toil we would be way behind.

Remember the pioneers in orthopaedics

- Hippocrates—first described splinting of fracture.
- Galen—traction in orthopaedics.
- Sarmiento—functional cast brace.
- Malgaigne—technique of internal fixation.
- HO Thomas—Thomas splint.
- Lambotte—external fixator.
- Gerhardt Küntscher—intramedullary nail.
- Robert Denis—father of modern osteosynthesis.
- Ilizarov—circular external fixator.
- Mathysen—plaster of Paris.
- And a score of countless unsung heroes.

Remember

About AO or ASIF technique

- Advocated in 1960 by a group of Swiss surgeons.
- Aims at full and rapid recovery of the injured limb by open anatomic reduction and stable internal fixation.
- Healing is by primary intention.
- Eliminates the problem called the fracture disease.

Our Own Heroes in Orthopaedics

Dr BN Sinha and Dr B Mukhopadhya—father of Indian orthopaedics. Known as Sir Robert Jones of India.

Dr KT Dholakia—father of modern Indian orthopaedics.

Dr SM Tuli—who described the famous middle path regime for TB spine.

Dr TK Shanmugasundaram—known for his outstanding work in skeletal tuberculosis.

Dr BB Joshi—who has described the Joshi's external stabilising system (JESS) treatment for congenital talipes equinovarus (CTEV).

Dr Singh—Singh's Index.

Dr GS Kulkarni—known for his work on Ilizarov's treatment.

Dr PS Ramani—eminent neuro and spine surgeon known for his work on IDSS, PLIF and bone bank methodology.

Dr Bakshi—pioneering work on muscle pedicle graft for fracture neck femur.

Dr PC Sethi—well known for his Jaipur foot.

FRACTURE TREATMENT: NOW

The faithful bones support the entire body till its integrity is broken by fractures. Ironically what was known to support, now requires to be supported either externally or internally to regain the lost integrity and revert back to its original role. Before even the orthopaedic surgeons interfere to plan and execute the treatment methodology to restore the bone anatomy, nature has initiated the healing process by immobilising the fracture fragments by its two important mechanisms namely:

1. **Pain** The patient loathes to move his or her injured limbs for fear of pain and thus keeps it immobile.
2. **Muscle spasm** The surrounding muscles go into spasm after the injury and prevent mobility between the fracture fragments.

While pain and muscle spasm keep the fracture fragments immobile, SOS signals are sent by the bone induction agents (e.g. bone morphogenic protein, oxygen gradient, etc.) to the bone cells within the periosteum and endosteum to initiate the fracture healing process. The role of orthopaedic surgeon is to merely assist nature in its mission of putting back the broken bones to normalcy. The ways and means of how he or she can do it is described below.

Remember

- Bones known to support, requires support when broken.
- Pain and muscle spasm are nature's way of immobilising fracture fragments.
- Role of the physician is to merely assist nature to bring about proper fracture healing.
- Remember the adage *Orthosurgeon merely treats the fracture and God (nature) cures it.*

GENERAL PRINCIPLES OF THE METHODS OF FRACTURE TREATMENT

I. Conservative or Non-operative Methods

1. **No treatment** Some fractures need no treatment. Nonsteroidal anti-inflammatory drugs (NSAIDs) and rest suffices, e.g. rib fractures (because of the efficient splinting action of the intercostal muscles).
2. **Strapping** Merely strapping certain fractures to the adjacent normal structures like in undisplaced phalanx fracture of fingers (Fig. 6.4) and toes is sufficient. Other fractures that are treated by strapping are fracture of clavicle, scapula, proximal fumeral fractures, etc.

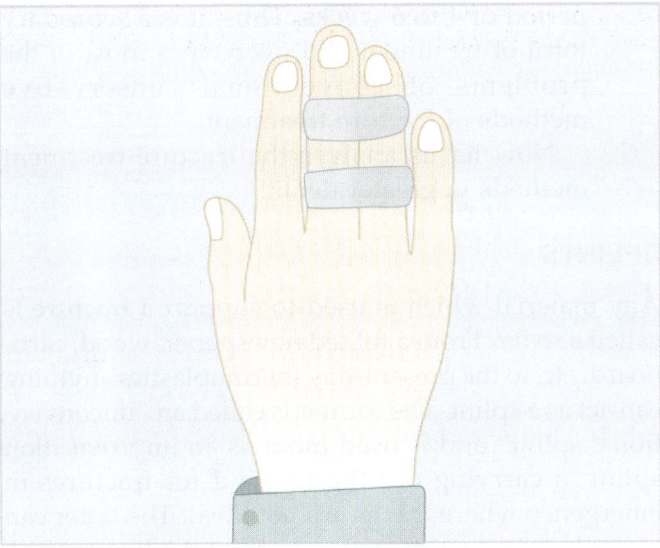

Fig. 6.4: Strapping in a phalanx fracture

3. **Slings** These are used to treat undisplaced upper limb fractures or as first aid measures.
4. **Plaster treatment methods** Two modalities are described.
   a. *Merely support by plaster slabs or splints:* In undisplaced fractures, incomplete fractures, stress fractures, fatigue fractures, support by POP slab often suffices.
   b. *Reduction and support with plaster cast:* Displaced fractures need to be reduced under general anaesthesia before splinting with plaster casts. Reduction can be brought about either by manipulative traction and counter traction methods or by skeletal or skin traction. Principles of closed reduction has already been discussed. Plaster of Paris plays a big role in the conservative management of fractures.
   c. *Spica cast:* This is a plaster cast which encircles a part of the body other than the limb. For example, hip spica, scaphoid cast, etc.
   d. *Traction:* This comparatively plays a less important role and is discussed in detail in a separate section.

Remember

- The cardinal rule of reducing any displaced fracture is to reverse the mechanism of injury preferably under general anaesthesia.

Non-operative Methods

1. **Advantages**
   - Infection chances are nil.
   - Surgical risks are avoided.
   - It is less costly.
2. **Disadvantages**
   - Certain amount of skill is required.
   - Fixation is not rigid.
   - Prolonged immobilisation is required.
   - Malunion is more likely.
   - Fracture disease is a possibility.

II. **Operative treatment of fractures** Operative treatment of fractures becomes mandatory once conservative regimen fails or when there are specific indications (see discussions on open reductions). Once fracture is reduced by operative methods, it invariably needs to be fixed internally by implants. Thus implants act as internal splints. The choice of implants available are as follows:

- *Kirschner's Wire (K-wire)*—useful to fix certain fractures in children and small bone fractures, avulsion fractures, distal radial fractures, etc. in adults.

It pays to know the advantages of K-wire:

- Insertion is stress free.
- Less soft tissue damage.
- It allows early exercises after removal.

Certain important technical facts:

- Diameter ranges from 0.6 to 3.2 mm.
- Length ranges from 160 to 310 mm.
- Pointed at both ends for both antegrade and retrograde insertion.
- The shape of the tips could be—Trocar, diamond, perforated or threaded.

- *Screws*—used mostly to fasten the plates to the bones and rarely used independently to fix avulsion fractures, butterfly fragments, for interfragmentary compression, etc.
- *Intramedullary (IM) nails*—useful for long bone shaft fractures through the narrowest portion of the medullary canal which is usually the middle third. Intramedullary nails are not useful when the fractures are outside this ideal situation and in fractures in children.
- *Plates*—are useful in situation where IM nail is not indicated. Proximal and distal third fractures can be treated by this method. It can also be used in children. However, it has its own set of problems and limitations.

Operative Methods

Advantages
- Anatomic reduction.
- Rigid fixation.
- Early mobilisation.
- Useful in multiple system injuries.
- Useful in multiple fractures.

Disadvantages
- Infection.
- Biologic process hampered.
- More expensive.
- Failure after removal of plate and screws.

III. **Treatment of fractures by external fixators** (Figs 6.5A and B) Open fractures pose a tough problem in the choice of fixation methods. Loss of soft tissues makes application of plaster casts very difficult. At the same time the threat of infection discourages the use of internal fixation devices. It is here that the role of external fixators are clearly defined as it provides both stability and immobilisation of fractures, so essentially required for both the soft tissues and the fracture to heal.

Essentially, all external fixators consist of pins which are passed through the bones above and below the fracture sites and are fastened to the external metallic frames. From the conventional pin fixator to the more recent Ilizarov's circular fixator, the concept of external fixator has a definite place in the treatment of fractures, especially the compound fractures.

IV. **Functional cast bracing** It is a new concept developed by Sarmiento wherein the fracture is mobilised once it becomes sticky after a period of 4 to 6 weeks. Thus, it is a secondary form of treatment and overcomes most of the problems of conventional conservative methods of fracture treatment.

Now let us analyse the fracture treatment methods in greater detail.

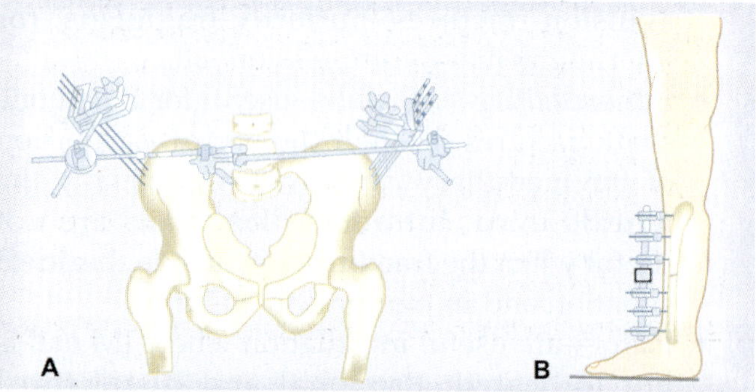

Figs 6.5A and B: Showing treatment of fractures by external fixators: (A) pelvic (B) tibia fracture

SPLINTS

Any material which is used to support a fracture is called a *splint*. From a folded newspaper, wood, cardboard, etc. to the present-day thermoplastics anything can act as a splint. The former is called an "unconventional splint" and is used more as an improvisation splint in carrying out the first aid for fractures in emergency where things are not ideal. The latter can be called "conventional splints" which are more sophisticated and effective. In orthopaedic practice POP splints are the most commonly employed splints.

Remember
- Anything acts as a splint including one's own uninjured part of the body
- Splint is a material used to support fractures.
- *Unconventional splints* are crude, temporary and are used as a first aid measure, e.g. book, paper, umbrella, board wood, etc.
- *Conventional splints* are refined sophisticated and serve both as first aid and definitive measures, e.g. POP splint, Thomas splint, Böhler-Braun splint, etc.

To attain the goal of fracture treatment of restoring anatomy to normal, splints help a long way. They form the mainstay of conservative treatment of fractures.

CONVENTIONAL PLASTER SPLINTS

ALL YOU WANTED TO KNOW ABOUT PLASTER OF PARIS SPLINT

Its History The name plaster of Paris originated from an accident to a house built on deposit of gypsum near the city of Paris. The house was accidentally burnt down. When it rained on the next day, it was noted that the footprints of the people in the mud had set rock hard. Plaster of Paris was first used in orthopaedics by Mathysen, a Dutch surgeon, in 1852. It is made from gypsum which is a naturally occurring mineral. It is commercially available since 1931.

Its chemical formula It is a hemihydrated calcium sulphate. To make plaster of Paris, gypsum is heated to drive off water. When water is added to the resulting powder, original mineral reforms and is set hard.

$$2\,(CaSO_4.\,2\,H_2O) + Heat \leftrightarrow 2(CaSO_4.\,½\,H_2O) + 3H_2O$$

POP Types

Indigenous Prepared from ordinary cotton bandage role smeared with POP powder.

Commercial Plaster of Paris rolls commercially prepared consists of rolls of muslin stiffened by starch, POP powder and an accelerator substance like alum. This commercial preparation sets very fast and gives a neat finish unlike the indigenous ones.

Why is plaster of Paris an ideal splint?

- It is cheap.
- It is easily available.
- It is comfortable.
- It is easy to mould.
- It is quick setting.
- It is strong and light.
- It is easy to remove.
- It is permeable to radiography.
- It is permeable to air and hence underlying skin can breathe.
- It is noninflammable.

Its Various Forms

Plaster of Paris is used in four forms as slab, cast, spica, and functional cast brace.

Slab It is a temporary splint used in the initial stages of fracture treatment and also during first aid. It is useful to immobilise the limbs postoperatively and in infections. It is made up of half by POP and half by bandage roll and hence can accommodate the swelling in the initial stages of fractures.

Slab is prepared according to the required length. There are three methods of applying a slab.

Dry method Here the slab is prepared first and then dipped in water (commonly employed).

Wet method Here the slab is prepared after dipping the POP roll in water. This is rare and requires experience.

Pattern method Here the slabs are fashioned in the desired way before dipping it in water.

Casts (Figs 6.6A to D) Here the POP roll completely encircles the limb. It is used as a definitive form of fracture treatment and also to correct deformities. There are three methods of applying a POP cast.

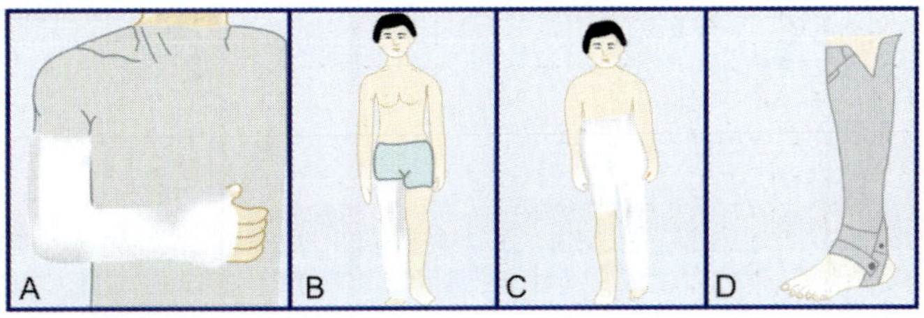

Figs 6.6A to D: Types of plaster applications: (A) above elbow cast, (B) above knee cast, (C) hip spica, (D) functional cast brace

Skin tight cast Here the cast is directly applied over the skin. Dangerous as it may cause pressure sores. It is difficult to remove as hair may be incorporated into the cast and hence it is not recommended.

Bologna cast Here generous amount of cotton padding is applied to the limb before putting the cast. This is the commonly employed method.

Three-tier cast Here stockinette is used first over which cotton padding is done before applying the POP cast. It is an ideal method but is expensive.

Spica This encircles a part of the body, e.g. hip spica for fracture around the hip (Fig. 6.6C), thumb spica for fracture scaphoid.

Functional cast brace (Fig. 6.6D) This is used for fracture tibia after initial immobilisation.

Rules of application of POP casts

1. Choose the correct size, 8 inches for the thigh, 6 inches for the leg, 4 inches for the forearm.
2. A joint above and a joint below should be included. Accordingly, we have an above elbow (Fig. 6.6A) or below elbow POP cast or slab and above knee (Fig. 6.6B) or below knee POP cast or slab. This is done to eliminate movements of the joints on either side of the fractures. However, this is not a hard and fast rule in certain fractures, like a below elbow cast in Colles' fracture, which often suffices.
3. It should be moulded with the palm and not the fingers for fear of indentation.
4. The joints should be immobilised in functional positions.
5. The plaster should just snugly fit and should not be too tight or too loose.
6. Uniform thickness of the plaster is preferred.

Stages of Plastering

First stage Involves application of POP slab or cast (Fig. 6.7).

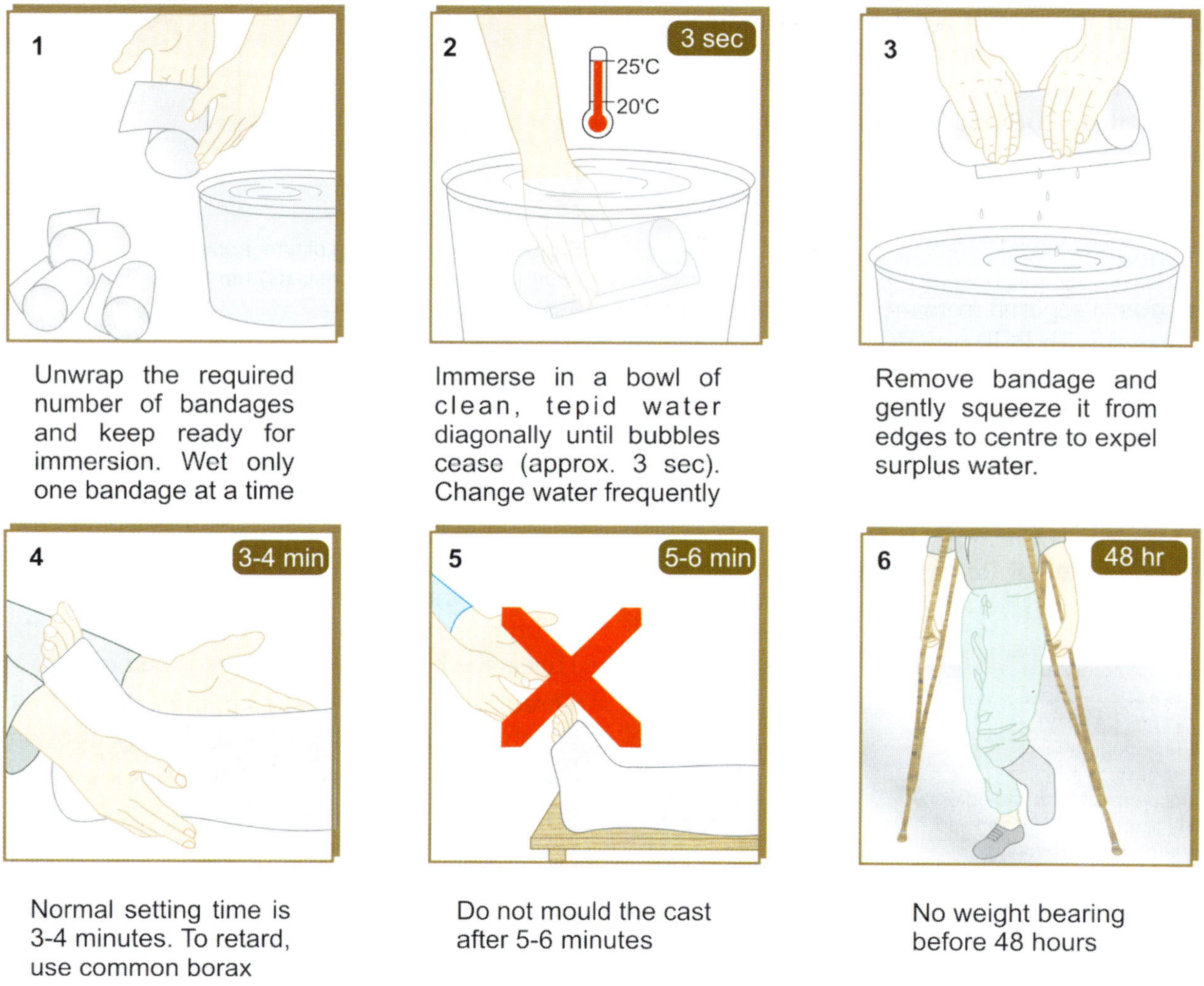

Fig. 6.7: Steps of application of plaster cast

Second stage or cast setting stage This is change of POP to gypsum and is defined as the time taken to form a rigid dressing after contact with water.

Third stage or green stage This is the just set wet cast.

Fourth stage or cast drying By evaporation of excess water when the cast dries. This results in a mature cast with multiple air pockets through which the skin breathes.

Complications of POP

Due to tight fit
- Pain
- Pressure sores
- Compartmental syndromes
- Peripheral nerve injuries
- Cast syndrome (Also called Cast disease).

Due to improper application
- Joint stiffness
- Plaster blisters and sores
- Breakage.

Due to plaster allergy
- Allergic dermatitis.

Unpleasant facts about cast disease

- Muscle atrophy.
- Osteoporosis.
- Joint stiffness.
- Muscle weakness.
- Skin breakdown.
- Compartmental syndrome.
- Blister formation.

Remember about POP

- Used first in the city of Paris.
- The ideal splint.
- Slab for temporary and initial treatment.
- Casts for definitive treatment.
- Spica for hip fracture, etc.
- Functional cast brace for early mobilisation.

FUNCTIONAL CAST BRACE

Introduction If function is allowed during closed method of fracture treatment, it has been observed that, this stimulates osteogenesis, promotes soft tissue healing and prevents development of joint stiffness thus hastening rehabilitation. This concept accepts loss of anatomic reduction to rapid healing. It compliments rather than replacing other forms of treatment. The observation that fracture ribs still unite in spite of continued movements due to the action of intercostal muscles showed that elimination of movements at fracture site is not mandatory for fracture to unite. It was on this concept that Sarmiento devised functional bracing methods.

The mode of action *Here the hydraulic action of muscles is brought into play*. The fracture brace allows movements of the joints and permits the load to be transmitted through the muscles. The muscles which are surrounded by the inelastic deep fascia if encased in a hard plaster cannot be stretched beyond the confines of the cast. On movements and bearing weight, the muscle forces are hence driven inwards towards the fracture and not outwards. This helps the fracture to be held firmly. These hydraulic forces control the fragments and resist overlap and angulation till callus forms (Figs 6.8A and B). Rotation is also resisted by the brace and muscle contraction.

In compound fractures, due to severe disruption of soft tissues, this principle will not work until soft tissues have healed.

Remember

About functional cast brace (Fig. 6.9):

- Fracture ribs indicate that absolute immobility for fracture healing is not required.
- It is a secondary form of fracture treatment.
- Muscle action favours osteogenesis.
- Hydraulic action of muscles stabilises the fracture in a closed compartment.
- Eliminates fracture disease like in AO technique.
- Not useful in compound fractures.
- Popularised by Sarmiento.
- Useful in fracture tibia and fracture femur.

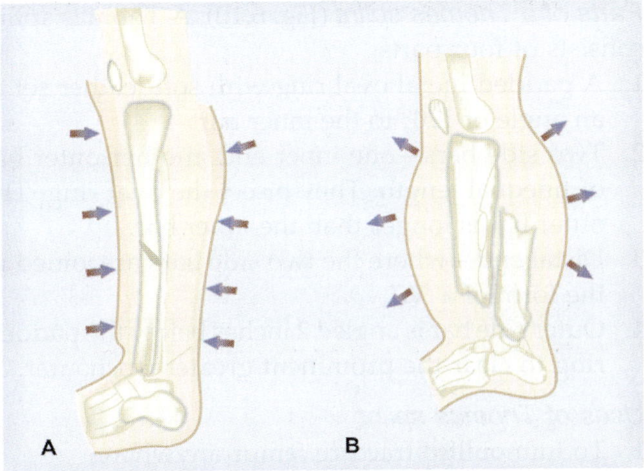

Figs 6.8A and B: Principles of cast bracing: (A) with brace, and (B) without brace

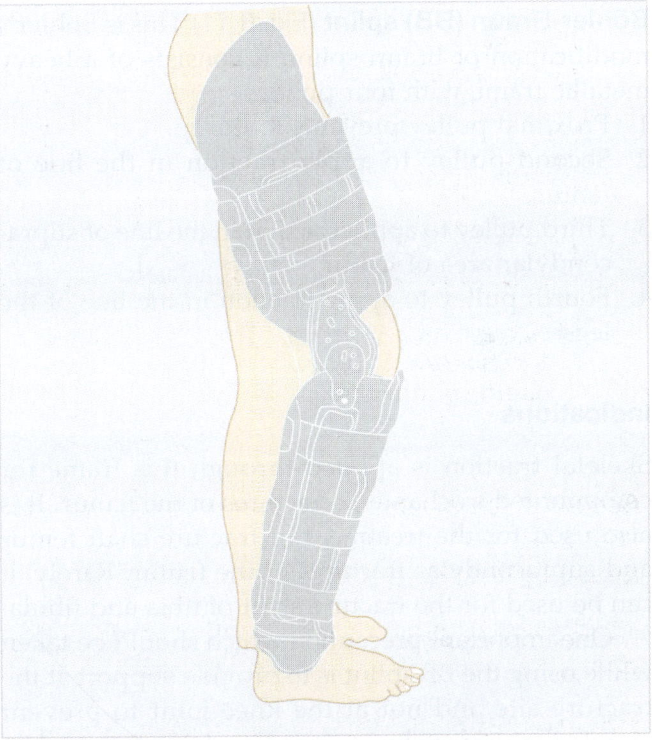

Fig. 6.9: Showing a functional cast brace

IMPORTANT SPLINTS IN ORTHOPAEDICS OTHER THAN POP

Thomas splint This is one of the very commonly used splints in orthopaedics described by HO Thomas in 1876 to assist for ambulatory treatment of TB knee. It is now widely used for the treatment of shaft fractures of femur.

Parts of a Thomas splint (Fig. 6.10) A Thomas splint consists of four parts:

1. A padded metal oval ring with soft leather set at an angle of 120° to the inner bar.
2. Two side bars—one inner and another outer bar of unequal length. They bisect the oval ring. The outer bar is longer than the inner bar.
3. Distal end—where the two side bars are joined in the form of a 'W'.
4. Outer side bar is angled 2 inches below the padded ring to clear the prominent greater trochanter.

Uses of Thomas splint

1. To immobilise fracture femur anywhere.
2. As a first aid measure.
3. For transportation of an injured patient.
4. In the treatment of joint dieases like TB knee, etc.

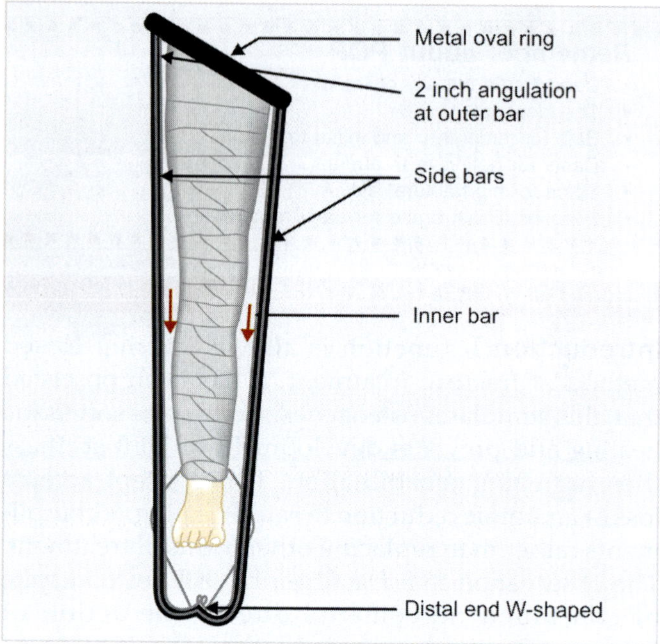

Fig. 6.10: Parts of a Thomas splint and fixed traction method

Böhler-Braun (BB) splint (Fig. 6.11) This is Böhler's modification of Braun splint. It consists of a heavy metallic frame with four pulleys:

1. Proximal pulley prevents footdrop.
2. Second pulley to apply traction in the line of femur.
3. Third pulley to apply traction in the line of supracondylar area of femur.
4. Fourth pulley to apply traction in the line of the legs.

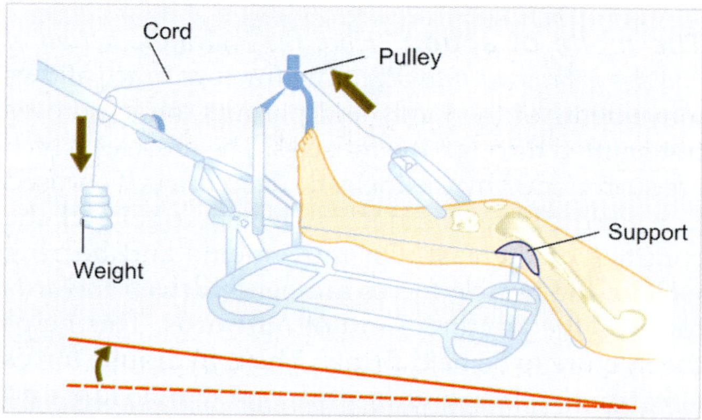

Fig. 6.11: Böhler-Braun splint

Indications

Skeletal traction is applied through this frame for comminuted trochanteric fractures of the femur. It is also used for the treatment of fracture shaft femur and supracondylar fractures of the femur. Rarely, it can be used for the fracture shaft of tibia and fibula.

One important precaution which should be taken while using the BB splint is to provide support at the fracture site and not at the knee joint to prevent angulation, especially in supracondylar fractures of femur.

Problems of BB splint

1. Makes nursing care difficult.
2. It is a heavy and cumbersome frame.
3. It is associated with recumbent problems like bedsores—hypostatic pneumonia, renal calculi, etc.

Care of the splints

1. *Padding* The splint should be well padded at the bony prominences and at the injury sites.
2. *Bandage* This should be tied with optimum pressure.
3. *Exercises* Active exercises of the joints and muscles should be permitted within the splints.
4. *Checking* Daily checking and adjustments of the splints are recommended.
5. *Neurovascular status* Distal neurovascular status should be assessed daily.

Practical points: Other common splints used in orthopaedics

Region	Indications
1. *Cervical spine*	
• SOMI brace	Cervical spine injury
• 4 post collar	Neck immobilisation
2. *Upper limbs*	
• Aeroplane splint	Brachial plexus injury
• Cock-up splint	Radial nerve palsy
• Knuckle-bender splint	Ulnar nerve palsy
• Aluminium splints	Finger injuries
• Volkmann's splint	For VIC
3. *Spine*	
• Milwaukee brace	Scoliosis
• Boston brace	Scoliosis
• Taylor's brace	Dorsolumbar injury
• Anterior spinal hyperextension brace (ASHE)	Dorsolumbar injury
• Lumbar belts and corsets	Backache
4. *Lower limb*	
• Thomas splint and BB splints—mentioned already	
• Footdrop splint.	Footdrop
5. *Miscellaneous*	
• Thomas splint	
• Krammer wire splint	For emergencies

TRACTION IN ORTHOPAEDICS

Traction plays an important role in the management of fractures in orthopaedics.

Uses of Traction

- To reduce a fracture or a dislocation.
- To retain the fracture after reduction.
- To overcome the muscle spasm.
- To control movement of an injured part of the body and to aid in healing.

Methods of Traction

There are four methods of applying traction, namely skin, skeletal, pelvic and spinal.

Skin Traction

Here traction is applied over a large area of skin. Maximum weight that can be applied through skin traction is 15 lbs or 6.7 kg. If the weight used is more than this, the traction will slide down peeling off the skin. When used in fracture, skin traction is applied to the limb distal to the fracture site.

Types of skin traction

Adhesive skin traction Here adhesive material is used for strapping which is applied anteromedial and posterolateral on either side of the lower limbs.

Nonadhesive skin traction Useful in thin and atrophic skin and in patients sensitive to adhesive strap. It is less secure than the former.

Contraindications for skin traction Abrasions, lacerations, impaired circulation, dermatitis, marked shortening, allergy to plaster are some of the important contraindications for skin tractions.

Complications Allergy, excoriations, pressure sores around the malleoli, common peroneal nerve palsy, etc. are some of the known complications in skin tractions.

Remember

Rotation of the limb is difficult to control with skin tractions.

Important Skin Tractions

Buck's extension skin traction This is the commonest type of traction employed for lower limbs. It is used for temporary treatment of fracture neck femur, undisplaced fractures of acetabulum, after reduction of hip dislocation, to correct minor fixed flexion deformity of hip and knee for low backache, etc. (Fig. 6.12).

Dunlop's traction (Fig. 6.13) Used in the upper limbs and is indicated for supracondylar fractures, intercondylar fractures of humerus where elbow flexion causes circulatory embarrassment.

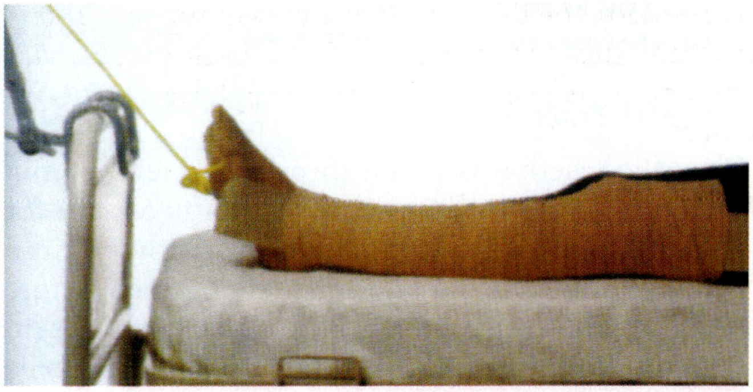

Fig. 6.12: Skin traction (Buck's extension type)

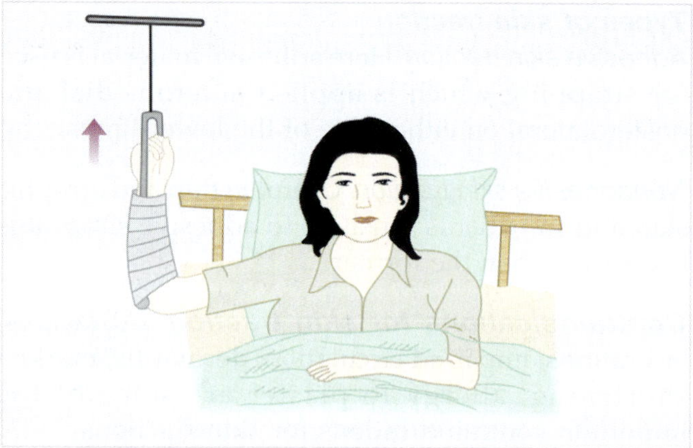

Fig. 6.13: Showing Dunlop's traction

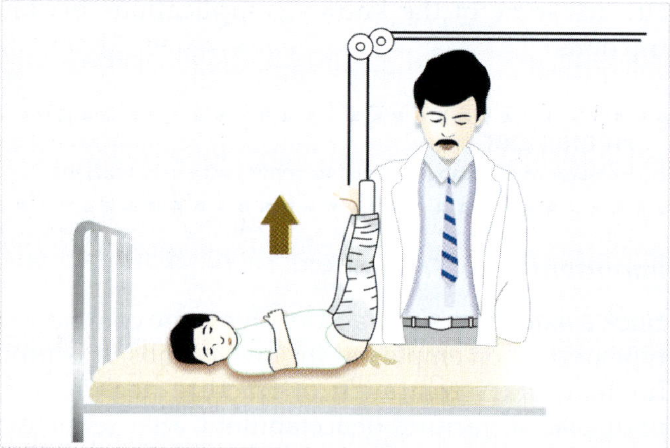

Fig. 6.14: Gallow's traction

Gallow's traction (Fig. 6.14) or Bryant's traction Used for fracture shaft femur in children less than 2 years. If used in children above 2 years, it causes vascular complications.

Did you know?
Buck first used skin traction in a Cecil War.

Skeletal Traction

Here the traction is given through a metal or pin driven through the bone. It is seldom necessary for upper limb fractures but useful in lower limb fractures for reducing and maintaining the fracture reduction. It is reserved for those cases in which skin traction is contraindicated and where the need to be applied weight is more than 5 kg.

Fig. 6.15: Steinmann's pin with Böhler's stirr-up

Know the pins used for skeletal traction

Steinmann's pin It is a rigid stainless steel pin 4 to 6 mm in diameter. Böhler's stirr-up (Fig. 6.15) allows the direction of the traction to be varied without turning the pin in the bone.

Denham pin (Fig. 6.16) This pin is threaded in the centre and engages the bony cortex. It reduces the risk of pin sliding and is useful in cancellous bone like calcaneum and osteoporotic bones.

Fig. 6.16: Denham pin

Traction points Well-known traction in orthopaedics

Tractions	Indications
1. *Head or cervical tractions*	
• Crutchfield or Gardenwells	Cervical spine injuries
• Head halter	Cervical spine injuries
• Halopelvic	Scoliosis
2. *Upper limb tractions*	
• Dunlop's traction	Supracondylar fracture of humerus
• Metacarpal traction	Compound forearm injuries
3. *Lower limb tractions*	
• Gallow's or Bryant's	Fracture shaft femur (<2 years)
• Russel's traction	Trochanteric fracture
• Perkin's traction	Fracture shaft femur in adults
• 90-90° traction	Fracture shaft femur in children
• Agnes Hunt traction	Correction of hip deformity
• Well leg traction	To correct abduction and adduction deformity of hip
• Calcaneal traction	Compound fractures of distal leg and ankle
• Buck's traction	Low backache, etc.
• Pelvic traction	Low backache, etc.

Know the sites and indications for skeletal traction

	Sites of skeletal traction	*Exact point*	*Indications*
1.	*Skull traction*	Outer table of parietal bone of the skull with either Crutchfield or Gardenwells tongs.	• To reduce dislocation or fracture dislocation of cervical spine. • For postoperative treatment of neck. • For cervical spondylosis with severe nerve root compression.
2.	*Upper limbs*		
	Olecranon	$1^{1}/_{4}$ inch distal to the tip of olecranon.	Supracondylar, intercondylar and comminuted fracture lower third of humerus.
	Second and third metacarpals	One inch proximal to the distal end of second and third metacarpal.	Fracture both bones forearm.
3.	*Lower limbs*		
	Greater trochanter	One inch below the most prominent part of the greater trochanter, midway between anterior and posterior surfaces of femur.	Central fracture dislocation of hip.
	Lower end of femur	$1^{1}/_{4}$ inch above the knee joint.	Pelvic fractures, posterior dislocation of hip, trochanteric fractures, shaft fractures, etc.
	Upper end of tibia	3/4th inch below and lateral to the tibial tuberosity.	All of the above indications, supracondylar fractures and intercondylar fractures of the femur.
	Lower end of tibia	Two inches above the level of ankle joint midway between anterior and posterior border.	Tibial plateau fractures. Fracture both bones leg.
	Calcaneum	Two centimetres below and behind the lateral malleolus.	Fractures lower one-third of the leg and ankle injuries.
	Metatarsal bones	Through the base of the metatarsal.	For calcaneal fractures.

Note: Commonest site for skeletal traction is upper end of tibia and common indications for skeletal traction is trochanteric fractures in elderly persons.

K-wire It is of small diameter and is often used in upper limbs.

Know the rules of application

- Skeletal traction should be applied in a major OT under general or local anaesthesia.
- Follow strict aseptic measures.
- Drive the pin from lateral to medial in case of upper tibial traction, to avoid injuring the lateral popliteal nerve.
- Pin should be at right angles to the limb and parallel to the ground.
- Cover the sharp tip on the medial side with a stopper bottle to prevent damage to the normal limb.

Know the complications of skeletal traction

At the time of application

- Anaesthetic problems.
- Vasovagal shock.
- Very rarely death due to vasovagal shock.

During application

- Injury to the nerves (lateral popliteal nerve).
- Injury to the vessels.
- Injury to the muscles, ligaments and tendons.
- Injury to the epiphysis in children (upper tibial epiphysis).
- Pain due to equalisation of intraosseus pressure and atmospheric pressure due to the hole made in the bone.

When pin is in situ

- Infection—due to improper aseptic measures.
- Migration—due to loosening.
- Breakage—thin pin or more weight.
- Bending—same reasons as above.
- Loosening—due to osteoporosis, infection, etc.
- Distraction of fracture fragments—due to excessive weight.

Late effects

- Pin tract infection.
- Chronic osteomyelitis with ring sequestra at the site.
- Genu recurvatum due to damage to the anterior epiphysis of tibia in children.
- Depressed scar.

How to take care of a patient on traction

- Patient on traction need to be looked after as they are unable to take care of themselves.
- Watch for petechial rashes, confusion, etc. which may suggest onset of fat embolism.
- Regular monitoring of temperature, pulse and BP.
- A balanced mixed diet is recommended.
- Use of bed pans is advocated.
- Use of NSAIDs for pain relief.
- Encourage to keep a healthy mental state.
- Proper skin care.

COUNTERTRACTION Traction force will overcome muscle spasm only if another force is acting in the opposite direction as countertraction.

Types

Fixed traction (see Figs 6.10 and 6.17) Here countertraction is achieved through an appliance which obtains a firm purchase on a part of the body. *This can maintain but cannot obtain reduction,* e.g. fixed traction on a Thomas splint for a fracture shaft femur.

Sliding or balanced traction (Fig. 6.18) Here weight of all or part of the body acting under the influence of gravity is utilised to provide countertraction. This can be achieved by raising the foot end of the bed. *Unlike in a fixed traction, both reduction and maintenance of a fracture can be obtained.*

However, the initial traction weight required to obtain a reduction is greater than the traction weight required to maintain the reduction.

Weight Guide Lines
For femoral shaft fracture initial weight required is 10 per cent of patient body weight. For every 1 lb of weight the end of the bed should be raised by one inch. A weight of 10 to 20 kg can be applied through a skeletal traction unlike 6.7 kg in skin traction.

OPERATIVE TREATMENT

IMPLANTS

General Principles

DEFINITION An implant is defined as a material inserted or grafted into intact tissues or body cavity with some specific purpose.

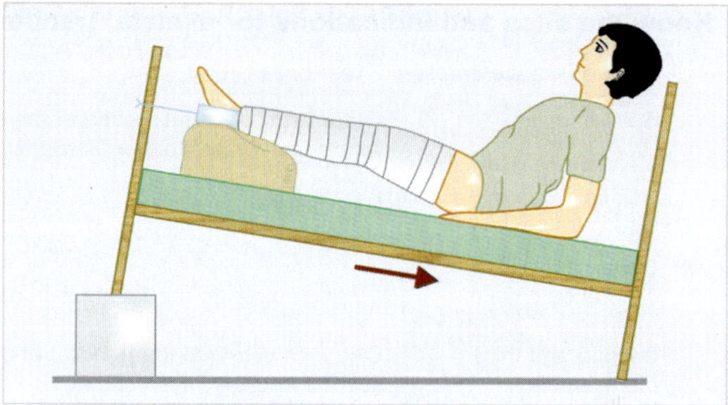

Fig. 6.17: Showing method of fixed traction for fracture shaft femur (also see Fig. 6.10)

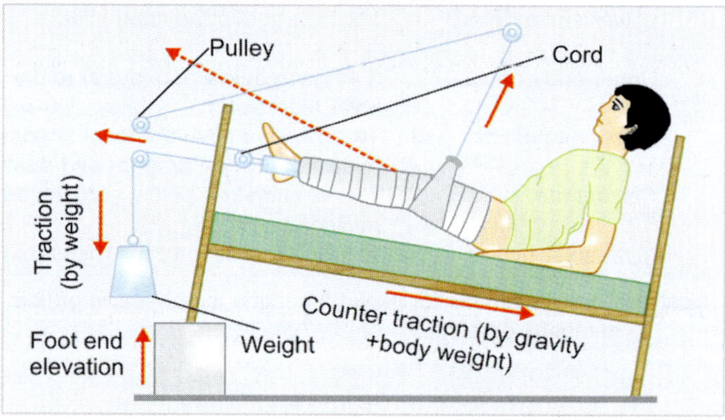

Fig. 6.18: Showing sliding or balanced traction

TYPES OF IMPLANTS

Metallic Generally alloys are used. Three varieties are described.

Iron based (stainless steel) Composition of the alloy is, iron 70 per cent, chromium 20 per cent, nickel 8 per cent, manganese 2 per cent. Commonly used alloy is 18.8S70 stainless steel (18% stands for chromium, 8% for nickel and steel is 70%).

Cobalt based Here the composition is cobalt 60 per cent, chromium 30 per cent, 5 per cent molybdenum, and 5 per cent nickel.

Titanium based This consists of 90 per cent titanium, 6 per cent aluminium and 4 per cent vanadium. Implants made from titanium are very strong and have great corrosion resistance.

Nonmetallic implants usually are made up of plastic materials. Polyethylene, polymethylmethacrylate (PMMA) and silicones are the commonly used nonmetallic implants.

Remember

Characters of ideal implant

- Should be corrosion resistant.
- Should be biocompatible.
- Should have high tensile strength.
- Should have high fatigue limit.

***Three Ps** for implant selection*

- **P**roper material.
- **P**roper design.
- **P**roper size and fixation.

About polymethylmethacrylate (PMMA)

- Called as bone cement
- It has a polymer and a monomer.
- It is not a glue and has no adhesive qualities.
- Called cement because it holds two materials, bone and metal, together by forming an interlocking network between the irregularities.

Note: Corrosion is a chronic reaction that weakens the implants. Addition of chromium and nickel makes the implant corrosion resistant.

VARIETIES OF IMPLANTS

Commonly used implants in orthopaedics are extramedullary and intramedullary fixations.

Extramedullary fixation: This consists of screws, plates K-wires circlage, transfixion, staples and suture anchors.

Screws

Two types of screws are described.

Machine screws (Fig. 6.19) These screws are threaded whole length and may or may not be self-tapping. Used widely with standard bone plates. They are not superior to the ASIF screws because the cutting edge of these screws generates heat at the terminal ends of the screw holes resulting in osteonecrosis and consequent loosening of screws at later date. They are not used of late.

Note: ASIF—Association of the Surgeon of International Fixation (Swiss group).

ASIF screws or AO screws These screws are designed by AO group in which the threads are more horizontal, drill holes are needed as the screws are not self-tapping. Three varieties of ASIF screws are described:

1. *Cortical screws* (Fig. 6.20) These screws are threaded whole length and has a diameter of 2 to 4.5 mm. This functions as a positional screw or a lag screw for interfragmentary compression.
2. *Cancellous screws* (Fig. 6.21) These have larger threads for more purchase in the soft cancellous bone. It is available as 16 mm, 32 mm length and 4 mm to 6.5 mm diameter.
3. *Malleolar screws* These have a sharp pointed tip and may be inserted without predrilling. Used for internal fixation of malleolar fractures.

Other Screws:

a. *Cannulated screws:* These are hollow screws modified over the cancellous and cortical screws. It is used widely for fixation of fracture neck of femur.
b. *Interference screws:* These are special screws without the usual head and is commonly used for bone ligament bone graft reconstruction for torn ACL.

Parts of a screw A screw has a head, neck shaft and tip. The other important aspects of the screws are:

Pitch It is the distance between two threads of a screw.

Lead It is the distance covered by one rotation.

Root diameter It is the minimum cross-sectional area of a screw.

Outer diameter of the screw.

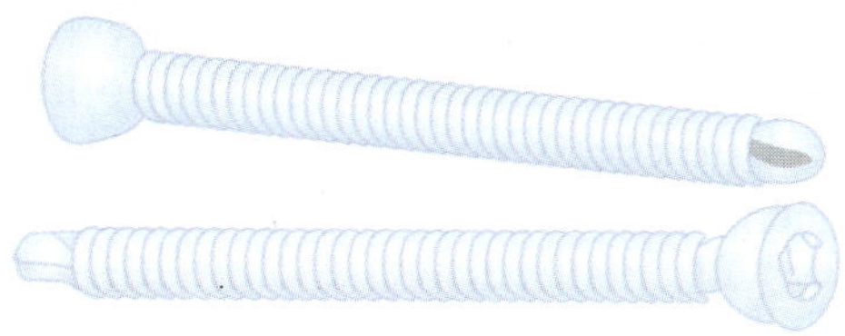

Fig. 6.19: Showing self-tapping machine screws

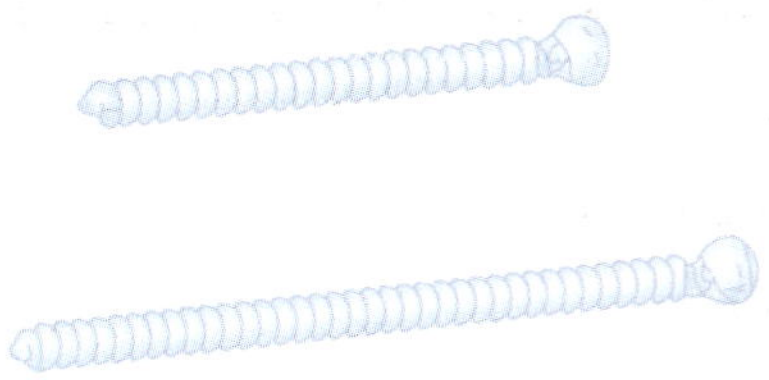

Fig. 6.20: Showing cortical screws—threaded whole length and not self-tapping

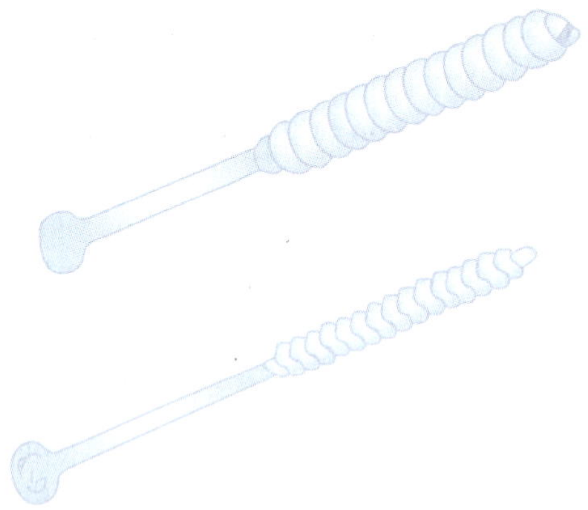

Fig. 6.21: Showing cancellous screw (abov)e and malleolar screw (below)

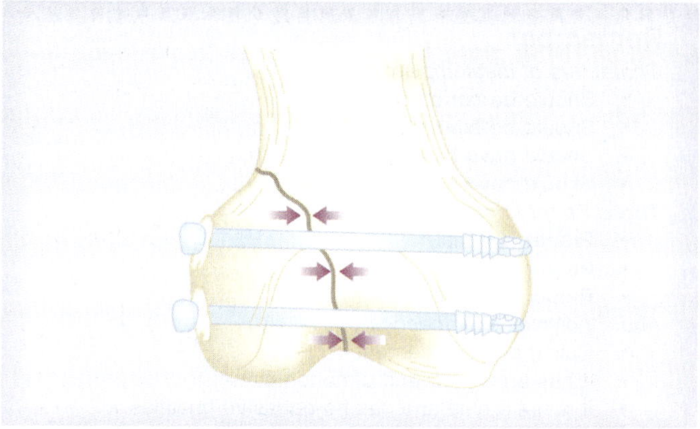

Fig. 6.22: Showing the lag effect produced by cancellous screws

Methods of Providing Compression by Screws

Lag effect To provide compression at the fracture site when cortical screws are used, one has to overdrill the proximal cortex so that the screw will slide down through the hole, pulling the far fragment towards the near fragment.

Cancellous screws provide a lag effect (Fig. 6.22) without over drilling of the proximal cortex since it is half-threaded and pulls the far fragment towards the near fragment.

Remember

The uses of screws

- Used mostly to fasten the plates to the bone.
- Used to fix avulsion fractures, butterfly fractures, etc.
- By overdrilling the cortex, a cortical screw provides interfragmentary compression by producing the lag effect.
- A cancellous screw can produce compression without overdrilling since it is half-threaded.

PLATES

Plates are widely used for internal fixation of diaphyseal fractures. Rigidity and strength depend upon the cross-section and the material used. Ranges from very rigid plates to merely positional plates. There is compensating thickness around the holes.

TYPES OF PLATES

Ordinary Plates

These just function as positional plate to hold the fractures but will not bring about any compression between the fracture sites. They are used in subcutaneous locations or where extreme rigidity is not required. The patients need prolonged immobilisation once this plate is used, e.g. semitubular plate (Fig. 6.23A), Scheurmann plate, etc. for ulna, clavicle, fibula, etc.

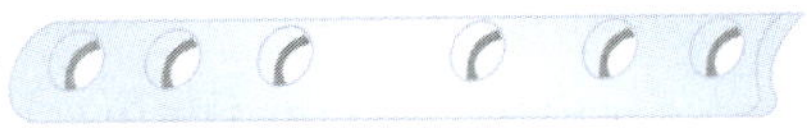

Fig. 6.23A: Showing semitubular plate

Remember about ordinary plates

- Functions merely as a positional plate.
- Useful in subcutaneous situations.
- Needs prolonged immobilisation.
- Hence the role is limited and has given way to compression plating.

AO PLATES

As described earlier, AO techniques aim at early mobilisation of the limb by providing a rigid compression at the fracture site and thereby prevent the possibility of fracture disease. Rigid fixation at the fracture site can be obtained by providing compression at the fracture site. The following are the methods to obtain compression.

METHODS OF PROVIDING COMPRESSION

1. *Static methods* This aims to provide compression by causing lag effect which has been mentioned already.

2. *AO plates with external compression device* Here compression is produced by an external compression device (Muller's device) which is attached to the AO plate. Requires a wider exposure and hence dynamic compression plate (DCP) is preferred.
3. *Dynamic compression* Here no external compression devices are used, on the contrary, the plate holes are designed in such a way that as the screw is being tightened it pulls the fragment in the same direction and brings about compression at the fracture site. This is by far the best method of providing compression at the fracture site.
4. *Tension band principle* There are two forces acting at the fracture site. One is a distraction force seen over the convex surface of the bone and the other is a compression force seen at the concave inner surface. Now if the plate is applied on the compression side, the distraction forces will disturb the fixation and cause implant failure. On the other hand, if the plate is applied on the convex border, it will help convert the distraction force into a compression force and will aid in rigid compression at the fracture site, e.g. tension band wiring for fracture of patella and olecranon, DCP plating for tibia, humerus, etc.

Types

a. *Static tension band*: If the compression is produced by a tension band device only at the time of application, it is static tension band.
b. *Dynamic tension band*: Here in addition to the above compression effect is produced even during physiologic overloading.

TYPES OF ASIF PLATES

a. **AO plates** These are thick plate, with round holes and a slot for the use of compression jig (Fig. 6.23B).
b. **DCP** (Fig. 6.23C) These are heavy duty plates with oval holes.
c. **Special plates** For example, 'T'-plates (Fig. 6.23D), 'L'-plates (Fig. 6.23E), etc. are used for condylar fractures of tibia, proximal humeral fractures, etc.

Flat buttress plate: This is available in the following shapes:

a. 'C' or clover leaf
b. 'H' plate

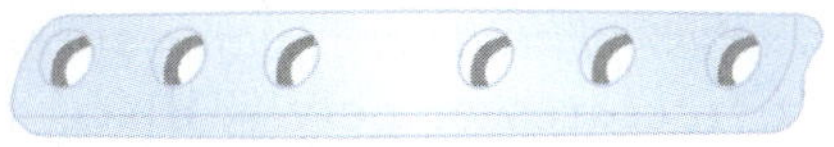

Fig. 6.23B: Showing AO plate

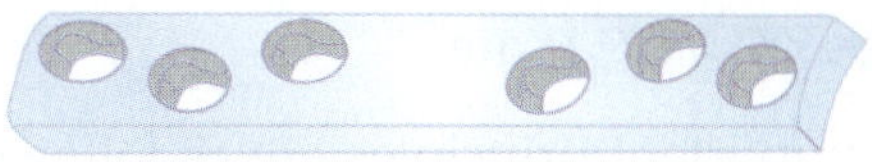

Fig. 6.23C: Showing a dynamic compression plate (DCP)

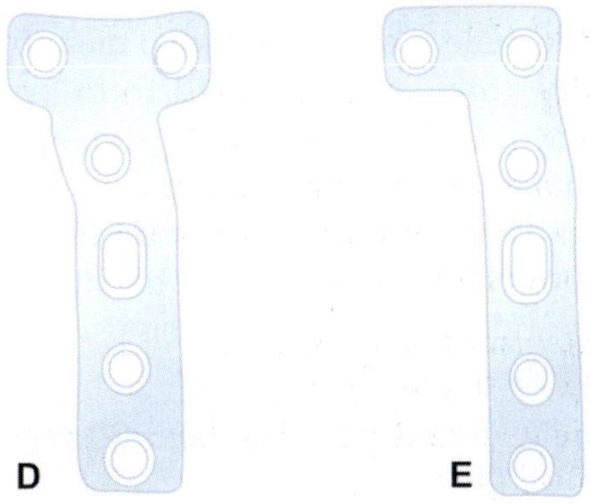

Figs 6.23D and E: Showing (D) special shaped T-plate, and (E) L-plate

c. 'L' plate
d. 'T' plate
e. 'S' or spoon plate.

Indications: It is mainly indicated for buttressing fractures of epiphyseal-metaphyseal junction.

Buttress plate with an antiglide principle

When a lag screw is passed through the buttress plate, it produces both compression and stability and is called the antiglide principle.

- *Wave plate:* Refracture of bone after plate removal is a common pitfall. To prevent this, Weber devised a plate with the cortex not in immediate contact with the plate. Bone graft is used to fill in the gap between the plate and the bone. This is called the wave plate.

d. *Reconstruction plate:* These plates are used to fix difficult fractures of pelvis, distal humerus, calcaneum, etc. as they can be contoured in three planes. Their thickness is in between DCP and buttress plate. In between the holes, they have scallop-like notches at the sides.
Pitfalls: They are less stronger than the DCP plates.

Principles of ASIF Plate

The four important principles are as follows:
1. *Tension band principle* is already mentioned, here the plate is placed on the convex side of an eccentrically loaded bone. This helps to convert the distraction force into compression force.
2. *Neutralisation plate* useful in comminuted fracture. Here the plate is attached to two main fragments. Here the force is transmitted from proximal to distal by passing the fracture site and thus the torsional forces are neutralised.
3. *Buttress plate (Fig. 6.24)* supports thin bone and functions opposite to tension band. The plate is always under compression and is used in fractures around the joints.
4. *Axial compression* for rigid fixation and primary bone healing.

DYNAMIC COMPRESSION PLATES (DCP)

In DC plates screw holes are designed to utilise *spherical gliding principle* with inclined contour of the screwholes and the slope on the under side of the screwhead. As the screw is tightened, its head is guided by the contours of the screwhole in such a way that the head glides towards the centre of the plate until the deepest portion of the hole is reached. Result is that bone fragment into which screw is being driven is displaced at the same time and in the same direction providing rigid compression. It is called dynamic because the bone fragment moves while the screw is being tightened (Fig. 6.25A).

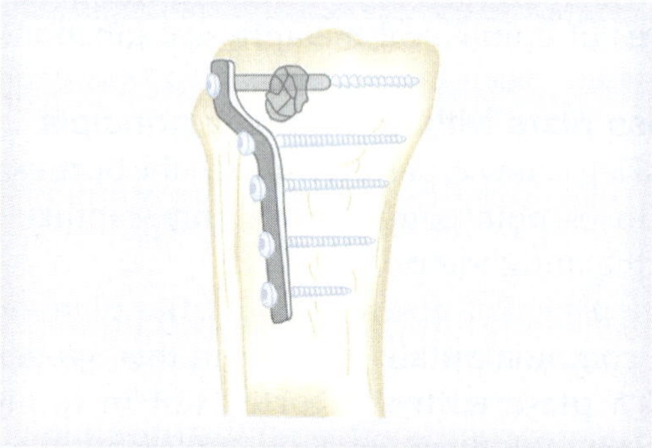

Fig. 6.24: Showing a buttress plate for proximal tibial fractures

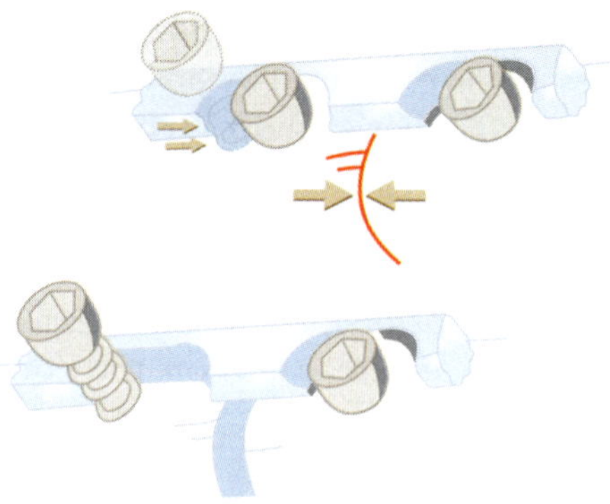

Fig. 6.25A: In DCP, fragment moves as the screw is tightened producing compression

Advantages of DCP

- Less surgical exposure than the conventional surgery.
- Screw and plate fit congruently in any position (Fig. 6.25B).
- Screw may be inserted at any angle.
- All other advantages of rigid fixation.

Remember

About rigid fixation plates
- *Compression at fracture site obtained by*
  — Lag effect.
  — By using external compression device as in AO plating.
  — Self-compression as in DCP.
  — Tension band technique.

Advantages
- Early mobilisation.
- No fracture disease.

Disadvantages
- Heals by primary intention hence callus is not seen on radiographs.
- Poor fracture welding as there is no external callus.
- Excessive compression causes osteonecrosis.
- Refracture is common after removal.
- Requires wide exposure.

Irony. Rigid fixation no doubt permits early mobilisation but this advantage is nullified by the prolonged immobilisation required following implant removal to fill up the screw gaps.
Solution. Interlocking nail emerging as an ideal replacement.

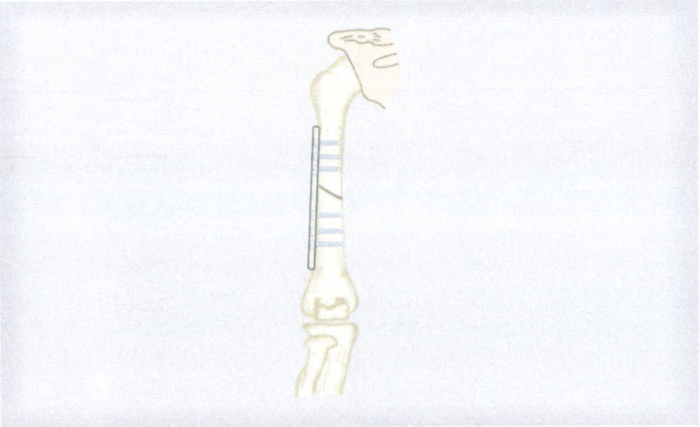

Fig. 6.25B: Fracture shaft humerus fixed with DCP plate and screws

INTRAMEDULLARY NAIL

Salient features about intramedullary nail are as follows:

- Firmly fixes the fracture and permits early mobilisation.
- Useful in diaphyseal fractures at the narrowest portion of the medullary canal.
- Very suitable in young adults.
- Not indicated for children and adolescents as the epiphysis may be damaged while inserting the nail leading to future growth complications.
- The patient should be able to tolerate major surgery.
- Nails should be of suitable length and diameter.
- Suitable instruments, assistants and hospital required.
- Closed technique is better than open.
- Union is peripheral and no endosteal healing due to reamed medullary canal.
- Fat embolism is relatively more common.

Types of IM nails and indications (see the flow chart)

Broadly speaking, there are three varieties of intramedullary nails namely the:

a. Standard or conventional nails e.g. Küntscher's nail (Fig. 6.26)
b. Interlocking nails (ILN) e.g. GK nail, RT nail, etc. (Fig. 6.27)
c. Flexible medullary nails, e.g. Ender's nails.

Flow Chart: Types of intramedullary nails

Intramedullary nails

Standard IM nails or Centromedullary nails

5 designs on cross-section.
1. Clover leaf nail (Küntscher nail)
2. Hansen's nail (diamond shaped)
3. Schneider (double I-beam)
4. Samson's nail (cylindrical rod with flutes)
5. Lottes nail

Indications
- Fracture shaft femur at the level of isthmus in adults
- Fracture tibia (V-nails, K-nails, etc.)
- Fracture shaft of humerus

Interlocking nails

Dynamic → Locked at one end

Static → Locked at both ends

Indications
- Comminuted fractures.
- Segmental fractures
- Nonunion
- Proximal and distal third fractures
- Pathological fractures
- Multiple osteotomies

Example
- Russel-Tailor (RT) nail
- Gross-Kempf (GK) nail

Flexible medullary nails or Condylocephalic nails
- Passed from distal to proximal.
- Fracture fixation is achieved by three point pressure system, e.g. Rush nail and Ender's nail.

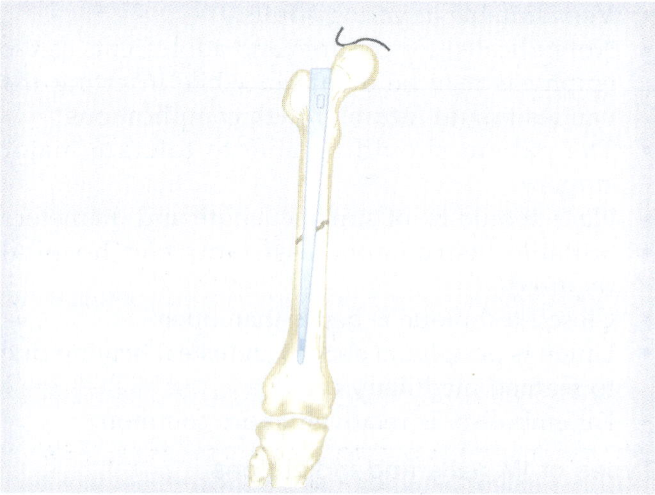

Fig. 6.26: Showing fracture femur fixed with Küntscher's (IM) nail

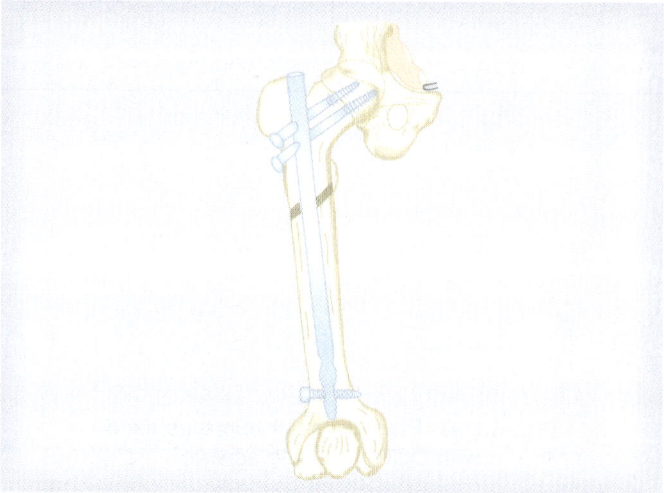

Fig. 6.27: Showing subtrochanteric fracture fixed by an interlocking nail

Presently, the ILN has largely replaced the conventional IM nails.

Requirements of an IM Nail

1. It should be strong and provide a tight fit in the medullary canal.
2. It should provide physiologic stimulus to union.
3. The ends of the nail must be accessible for easy removal.

Mode of Action of Intramedullary Nails

- It is a load-sharing device unlike a plate, which is a load-bearing device.
- It fills the medullary cavity.
- It provides three-point fixation (at the ends of nail and at the point where curve of the nail is in contact with the opposite cortex).
- It resists bending movement but is poor against torsional forces.

Regarding techniques of insertion and complications, see chapter on Instruments.

OTHER IMPORTANT INTERNAL FIXATION METHODS

1. Circlage

This is credited to be the oldest method of internal fixation. It produces an interfragmentary compression effect similar to the interfragmentary screws.

Materials used as Circlage Wires

- 16-gauge 316 L stainless steel wires
- 18-gauge (1 mm) vitallium
- 24-gauge stainless steel wires woven into three strands.

Indications: Circlage wire, like a joker in cards, can be combined successfully with various other fixation methods. This creates a number of permutations and combinations for fixations in orthopaedics.

Here is a list of some important indications:

I. With Steinmann's pin or K-wires
- Fracture patella (Fig. 6.28).
- Fracture malleolus.
- Fracture olecranon (Figs 6.29A and B).

II. With intramedullary nails
- Fracture of femur
- Fracture of tibia, humerus, etc.

III. For fixation of avulsion fractures
- Humerus—Greater and lesser tuberosity
- Femur—Greater trochanter
- Pelvis—Symphysis pubis.
- Tendocalcaneus injury.
- Acromioclavicular injuries.

IV. Spine surgeries
- Sublaminar wiring
- Posterior segmental stabilisation
- Fixation of grafts.

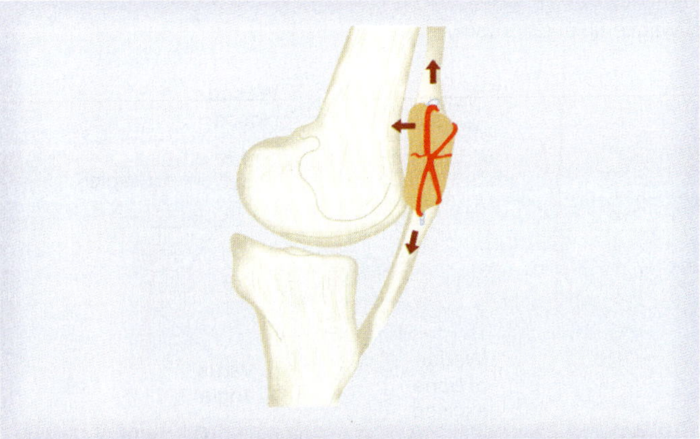

Fig. 6.28: Fracture patella treated with figure of 8 tension band wiring

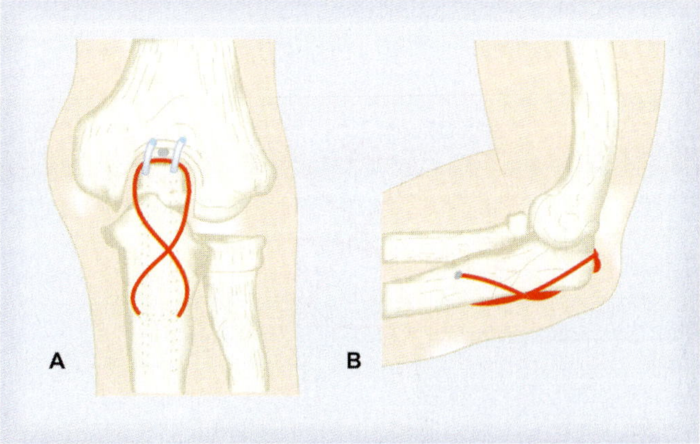

Figs 6.29A and B: Showing tension band wiring (TBW) in fracture olecranon

V. It can be used for primary fracture fixations in selected situations too.

VI. **Miscellaneous**
- For arthrodesis
- For allograft fixation
- For tendon and ligament repairs
- Periprosthetic fractures

Remember

Vital facts about circlage
- It helps provide interfragmentary compression.
- Wires are useful when compression is required and space is limited.
- Like a joker in cards, it can be suited to various fixation methods.
- It creates multiple combinations of internal fixation options.
- This is the oldest method of internal fixation in use since 1775.

2. Transfixion

The first transfixion surgery was done by Volkmann in 1875. It literally means fixation of fracture or bone fragment by penetration or piercing. The most famous transfixion surgeries currently in practice are percutaneous fixations of small bone fractures, distal radial fractures, supracondylar fractures of humerus in children, patellar fractures, olecranon fractures, etc.

Vital Facts about Transfixion

- K-wires or Steinmann's pin is the most common implant used.
- It is the simplest form of fixation.
- It can be used both as percutaneous or open fixation.
- The fixation provided is not stable and needs additional support.
- Loosening, breakage, backing out can occur.

Indications

- Skeletal fractures: This was the initial use.
- For percutaneous fixation of fractures.
- For temporary stabilisation of fractures.
- For stabilising flail and unstable joints.
- As tension band fixation along with circlage for patella, olecranon and malleolar fractures (Fig. 6.30).
- For fixations of small bone fractures of hand, foot, etc. (Figs 6.31 and 6.32).

3. Staples

To arrest the growth of the epiphysis, Blount is credited for popularising the use of staples. They are used in certain special situations.

Staple facts: Indications for staples

- Epiphyseal arrest in children
- Fixation of valgus tibial osteotomy (Figs 6.33A to C).
- For arthrodesis of small joints like:
  a. Wrist
  b. Triple arthrodosis.
  c. Subtalar joint.
- In certain fractures like:
  a. Patellar fractures
  b. Malleolar fractures
  c. Trochanter fractures.

4. Suture Anchors

Earlier to reattach ligaments or tendons to their insertion points in the bone drill holes were made into them. Of late, this procedure is made easy by attaching a sturdy suture to a bone with a screw or

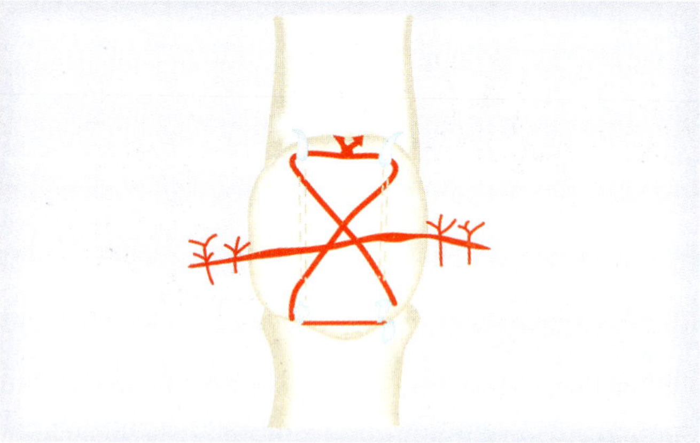

Fig. 6.30: Showing tension band wiring (TBW) for displaced transverse fracture of patella

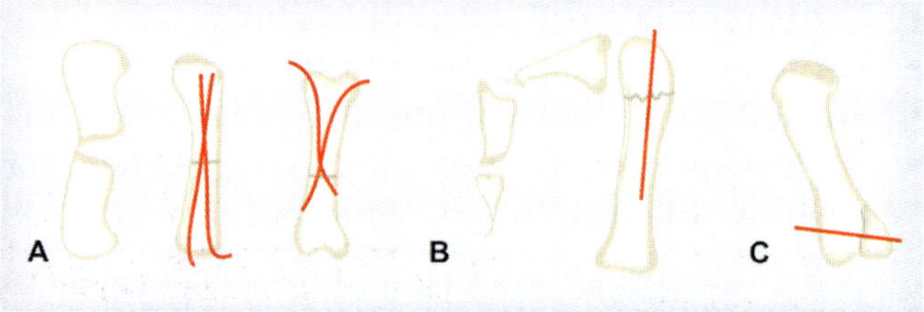

Figs 6.31A to C: Metacarpal fractures treated by closed reduction and percutaneous pinning: (A) unstable fracture fixed with criss-cross K-wires, (B) neck fracture fixed by intramedullary fixation, (C) Bennett's fracture fixed with K-wire

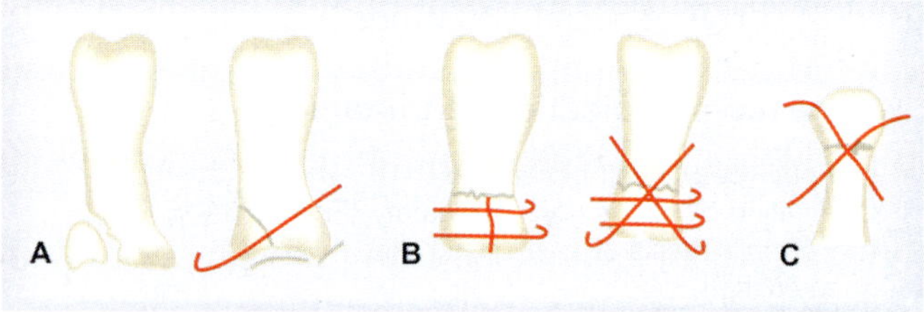

Figs 6.32A to C: Closed reduction and percutaneous fixation of various phalangeal fractures (A) unstable short oblique fractures, (B) comminuted fracture, (C) condylar fracture

spring-like apparatus. These are called the suture anchors. They have a greater pull out strength.

Indications:

- Tendon and ligament surgeries.
- Rotator cuff repairs.
- Shoulder stabilisation procedure.

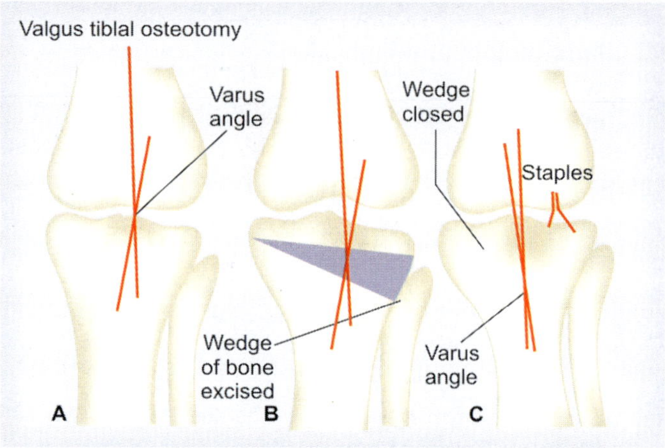

Figs 6.33A to C: Showing fixation of tibial valgus osteotomy with staples

FIXATION TECHNIQUES BY NONCOMPRESSION METHODS

1. Internal splints

Intramedullary rods or nails act as internal splints. They do not rigidly fix the fractures but union is most of the times not a problem. The gliding movements that take place between the fracture fragments allow compression. This concept became popular after the discovery by Küntscher.

2. Biologic fixation

This concept is being mainly applied to plate fixation. Through a limited approach, the fracture is reduced by indirect methods with minimal soft tissue damage. The plate is placed across the comminution without disturbing or manipulating the comminuted fragments. Here no graft is inserted because the comminuted fragments act as vascularised grafts except in situations of bone loss. Here fracture alignment is maintained without compression. This is also known as MIPO (minimally invasive plate osteosynthesis).

Facts about biologic fixations

- Limited exposure.
- Utmost respect for the soft tissue.
- Comminution left undisturbed.
- Limited contact between bone and implant.
- Biocompatible material implants used.

3. Composite Fixation

This refers to fixation of the metalic implants with bone cement. This concept was developed and popularised by Muller. To qualify the fixation as composite, two different fixation materials are used.

Vital facts

Composite fixation is useful in filling defects and fixing it in conditions of tumour, crush injuries, bone loss, etc. Here the gap is filled with cement and the fragments are fixed with nail or plates.

4. Hybrid Fixation

Here, unlike in composite fixation, only one material is used to provide two different fixation methods. An IM device used with an external fixator is an example of hybrid fixation. This method of fixation helps to attain the advantages of two types of fixation. Some of the most common hybrid fixations in common usages are:

- SP nail and plate.
- Jewett nail and plate.
- DHS screw with wide plate device (most common).

5. Bioabsorbable Fixation

Reabsorbable internal fixation devices prevent another surgery, and its attendant complications, for removal of implants. These implants slowly disintegrate and gets absorbed during the course of fracture union (Fig. 6.34).

Materials used The rods and screws are made up of:

- Polyglycolic acid
- Polylactic acid.

Mechanism of action They function as transfixion devices.

Pitfalls:

- Fixation attained is not rigid, hence external immobilisation is required
- Cannot be used for all fractures and hence has limited applications
- Severe synovial reactions are seen due to polyglycolide when used around the knee
- Sinus track formations are fairly common.

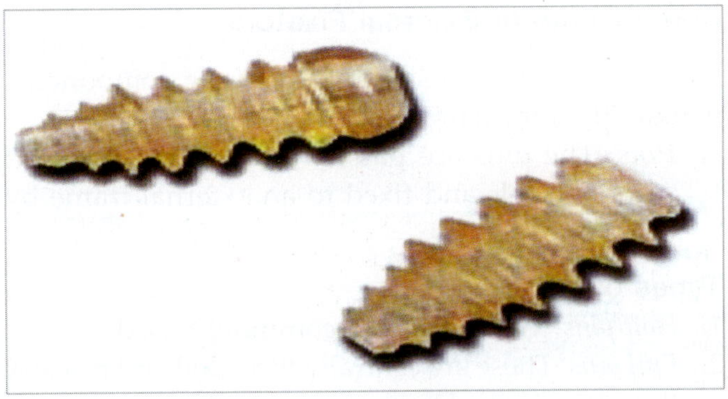

Fig. 6.34: Bioabsorbable screw

Indications It has been used in the following situations with varied success:

- Ankle fractures
- Olecranon fractures
- Osteochondral fractures
- Paediatric fractures
- Radial head fractures
- Repair of soft tissues by arthroscopy.

EXTERNAL FIXATION

Definition An external fixation (EF) is the method of fixing the fractures with a cluster of pins connected to external bars. Lambotte first used it in 1900. From the initial unilateral frames to the subsequent circular frames to the present hybrid fixations, external fixations has come a very long way.

Highlights of External Fixation

1. It provides a stable fixation of fractures and joints.
2. Axial, compression, rotation, distraction, translational and angulatory forces can be applied.
3. It helps in the wound care and reconstructive surgeries.

Indications External fixations has specific indications in the following situations:

1. Open fractures with severe soft tissue injury.
2. To stabilise long bone, periarticular and pelvic injuries in a multiple trauma patient.
3. For fixation of pelvic fractures.
4. For definitive treatment of some fractures of the long bones and pelvis.
5. Circulatory external fixators has its own set of special indications.

Components of External Fixators

External fixators consist of three basic components namely the pin, clamps, external rods.

A. ***Pins:*** The pins are passed through the bones at various levels and fixed to an external frame by the clamps.

Types of Pins

1. *Half pins:* These are very commonly used.
2. *Full pins*: These are centrally threaded and transfix the entire bone. Diameter — 4 to 5 mm.
3. *Thin wires* (1.5 to 2 mm): These are usually used with circular external fixators and it gains its rigidity by tensioning.
4. *Olive wires:* This is a thin wire with a bull protrusion at one end.

Other Varieties

a. *Cortical pins:* Here the thread diameter increases from the tip to the shaft.
b. *Self-drilling pins:* Causes frequent fractures due to osteonecrosis.
c. *Hydroxyapatite coated pins:* These help to prevent pin loosening and migration in porotic bones.

B. ***Clamps:*** These connect the pins to the rods.

Types of Clamps

1. *Simple clamps:* This connects single pin or wires to the rod or ring.
2. *Modules clamps*: These connect several pins as clusters.

Rings: They are extensively used in Ilizarov's and hybrid fixations. They are made up of stainless steel, aluminium and carbon. Types of the rings are:

a. Half rings
b. Full rings
c. 5/8 rings.

C. ***External Rods:*** These connect the cluster of pins through various clamps. They are made up of one of the three materials mentioned above and the cross section varies from circular, square, oval or multiple faced.

Types of External Fixators (Based on Frame Design)

a. *Unilateral frame:* This is the simplest external fixator frame. Four pins, two above and two below the fracture, are passed through the bone and fixed to a frame (Figs 6.35A and B).

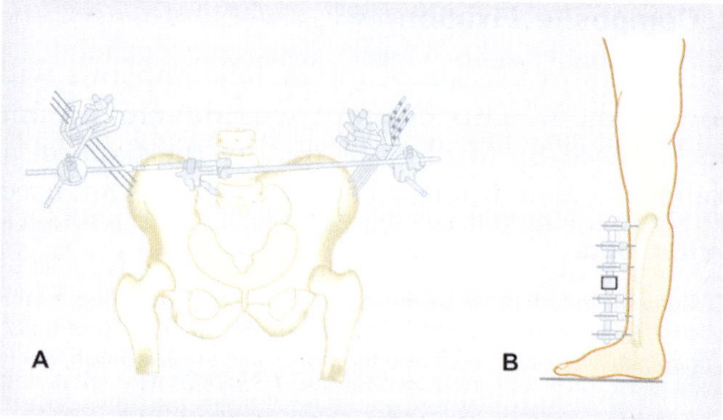

Figs 6.35A and B: Showing treatment of fractures by external fixators (A) pelvic (B) tibia fracture

b. *Bilateral frame:* This improves the frame stiffness and helps in better control of bending and torsional forces.
c. *Ring fixators:* This has been dealt with separately and are multiplanar (Figs 6.36A to C).
d. *Hybrid fixators:* This helps to combine the advantages of uniplanar and multiplanar external fixator devices. They are specially useful in fixing periarticular fractures.

Mode of Action

1. *Compression forces:* These forces help to stabilise certain transverse fractures and also for compression arthrodesis.
2. *Distraction forces:* These make the ligaments, muscles, capsules and other soft tissues taut by ligamentotaxis. These forces help in reduction and also retention of the fracture fragments. This is

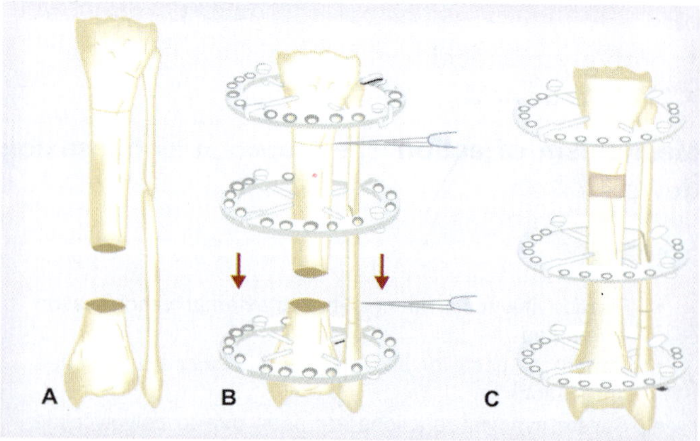

Figs 6.36A to C: Stages of distraction osteogenesis (A) bone gap, (B) corticotomy and distraction and (C) union

commonly used in distal radial, tibial plateau and pilon fractures.

3. *Neutralisation forces:* This provide neutralising forces across the fracture site. These are frequently used in conjunction with some internal fixation. The common application is seen in distal radial comminuted fractures. Here distraction forces are provided to reduce the fractures and later are retained by percutaneous fixation and later the distraction forces are released to provide only the neutralising force across the fractures.
4. *Angular forces:* These are used to bend, rotate and convert the angulations. Used extensively in Ilizarov's technique.

Biotechnical Principles of External Fixation

The mechanical stability of the external fixator is influenced by the following:

1. *Pin size:* Greater the pin size, greater is the stability of fixation.
2. *Pin number:* More number of pins ensure better stability.
3. *Pin placement:* The ideal placement of the pins include very near on either side of the fracture site and farthest away from the fractures. This is known as the "Near Far Construct".
4. *Rod placement:* Rods placed closer to the bone gives better stability. Double stacking the rods also increases the stability.
5. *Clamps:* The rigidity of fixators decreases considerably if the pins are not held firmly by the clamps. Hence periodic tightening of the clamp is a useful and effective practice.

Vital facts: Regarding the case of the external fixators:

- Duration of temporary treatment is 4 weeks
- Duration of definitive treatment is 1 year
- Conversion of external fixators to internal fixators should be planned once the soft tissues heal well
- Up to 10% of external fixators end up in pin tract problems
- Predrilling reduces osteosclerosis
- The tented soft tissues should be released
- Everyday care of the external fixator and pins is a must to prevent complications like infections, loosening, etc.
- Resorption of the bone around the pin for more than 1 mm signifies a significant loosening
- Frequent radiograph (once in 2 weeks) is a must to evaluate the progress of union
- If callus is not seen by 8 weeks, bone grafting should be considered

Complications The following are some of the important complications of external fixation:

1. Pin loosening
2. Pin migration
3. Pin breakage
4. Pin tract infection (10%)
5. Impalement of nerves, muscles, tendons, ligaments, etc.
6. Chronic osteomyelitis (0-4% of cases)
7. Septic arthritis if pin is placed very close to the joint.
8. Soft tissue contractures.

Pin Care Facts:

- Inspect the pins every day
- If there is discharge, dry sterile dressing is advised
- In the event of infections, wash the wound with 50% normal saline and 50% hydrogen peroxide.
- The patient can wash the frame with soap and water for less than five minutes.
- Topical antibiotics should be applied if there is infection
- Loose pins should be replaced.

7

Recent Advances in Fracture Treatment

- ❑ Advances in the existing methods of fracture treatment
  - ■ Improvements in plaster of Paris splints
  - ■ Functional cast brace
  - ■ Improvements in AO technique
  - ■ Improvements in intramedullary nails
  - ■ Interlocking nails
- ❑ Improvements in external fixation
  - ■ Ilizarov's technique
  - ■ Newer external fixators
- ❑ Advances in hip surgery
- ❑ Recent advances in spine surgery
- ❑ Recent Advances in bone grafting method
- ❑ Computers in orthopaedics

ADVANCES IN THE EXISTING METHODS OF FRACTURE TREATMENT

Advances are made in the existing methods of fracture treatment. The notable ones are mentioned here.

IMPROVEMENTS IN PLASTER OF PARIS SPLINTS

Now the days are of ultra short setting plaster casts or slabs made up of a material called polyurethane.

What is New in Plasters?

Fibre Glass Plasters (*Fig. 7.1*)

The more recent 'polyester cast' is composed of a specifically knitted polyester with elasticity, impregnated with polyurethane resin activitated by water.

Advantage Over Conventional Plasters

- Greater comfort.
- *Strength* 20 times stronger and is only 1/3rd the thickness of plaster of Paris.
- *Weight* Much lighter.
- *Shrinkage* Good shrinkage, hence recasting is avoidable.
- *Durability* More durable. Water resistant, smooth and soft edges to prevent scratch skin and snatch clothes.
- *Radiolucency* More radiolucent. Check X-rays are clear.
- *Sanitation* Moisture resistant porous cast, dries easily, prevents bad odour and other skin complications.
- *Colours* Available in different colours like white, green, pink, yellow, blue, black, red, purple, etc.
- *Removal* Easy to remove using conventional cast cutting saw or shear.
- *Dusting* Significantly less dusting and least harmful.

Indications

- Secondary casting of fractures
- Cast braces
- Reconstruction of joints
- Long-term cast
- For immobilisation in injuries

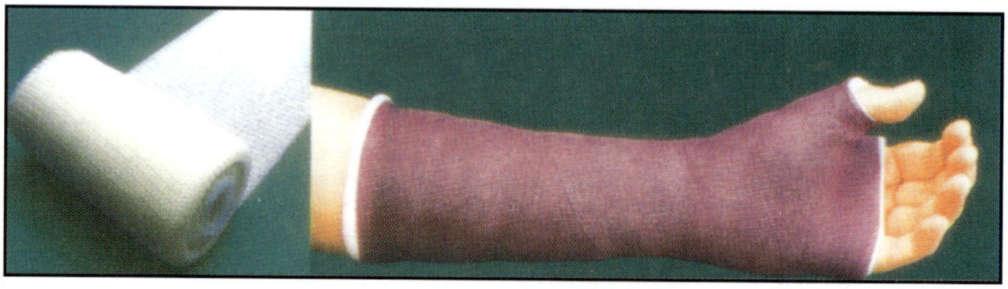

Fig. 7.1: Fibre glass plasters

- To reduce arthritic pain
- To stretch the tight muscles
- To protect an area
- For extra-durability and strength.

FUNCTIONAL CAST BRACE

Earlier application of casts or slabs confined the patient to the bed till the fracture united. Now the concept is to mobilise the patient on the plaster cast by using the functional cast brace, an idea developed by Sarmiento. Discussed at length in the previous section.

IMPROVEMENTS IN AO TECHNIQUE

Introduction of LCDCP (limited contact DCP) is considered as a step in the improvement of rigid fixation by AO technique.

IMPROVEMENTS IN INTRAMEDULLARY NAILS

These are the days of interlocking nails. Earlier intramedullary nails could not be used in proximal and distal third fractures of the long bones because the wider medullary canal in these areas rendered it difficult to control the rotation of the nail. The only alternative left was to use a plate and screw. But the problems associated with plate and screws necessitated the discovery of newer intramedullary nail with the problem of rotation eliminated by locking. Thus, the concept of interlocking nail was born and has made greater strides in the management of difficult fractures of the long bones.

INTERLOCKING NAILS (Figs 7.2A to C)

Standard IM nails designed by Küntscher for shaft fractures leaves two unresolved problems:
— Rotation of the fracture fragments.
— Telescoping at the fracture site.

By locking the nail into the bone by means of self-tapping screw driven through holes located at both the ends, the above two problems are solved. Gross and Kempf locking nail is found to be successful.

Advantages

- It can be used for both simple and compound shaft fracture from subtrochanteric to supracondylar area in the femur and from upper third to supramalleolar area in the tibia.
- It can be used in the treatment of segmental fractures, comminuted fractures, bone loss, etc.
- It can be used for the treatment of nonunion.

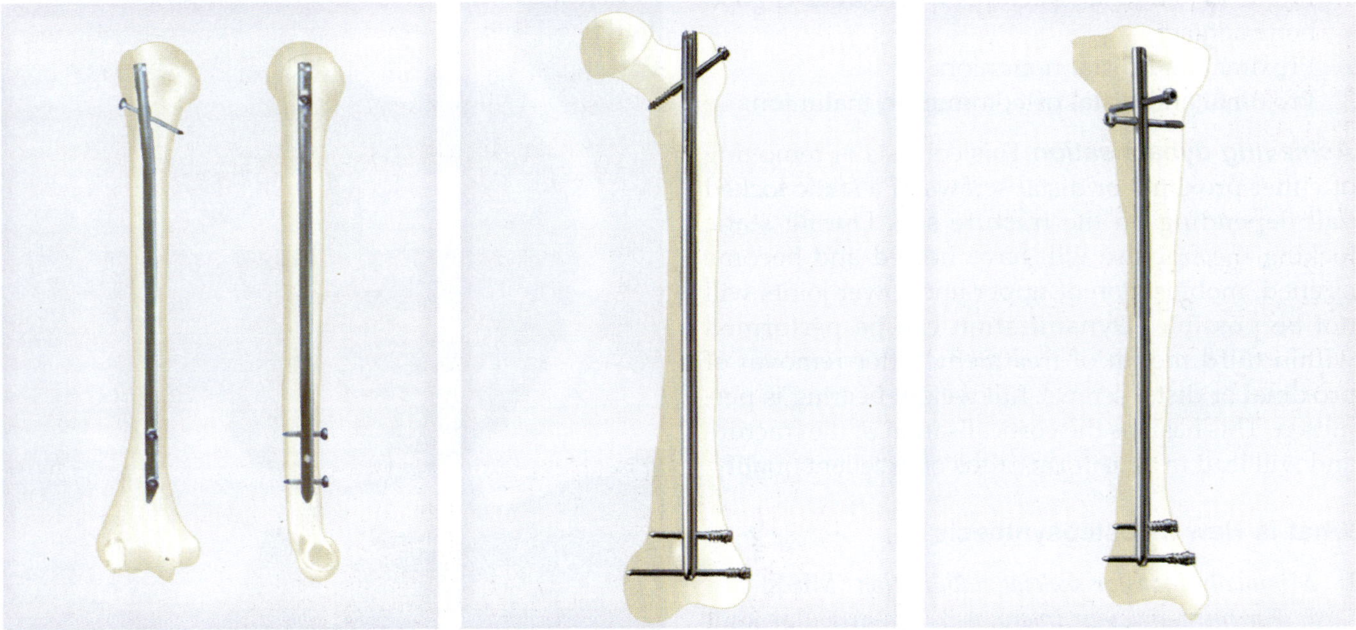

A: Interlocking nail of humerus **B:** Interlocking nail of femur **C:** Interlocking nail of tibia

Figs 7.2A to C: Interlocking nails are a gold standard in the treatment of long bone fractures in adults

- For reconstructive surgery following tumour excision.
- Low blood loss, low risk of infection.
- Short operative time.

Principles

Static locking Here screws are placed both proximal and distal on either sides of the fracture. This neutralises the rotation and restricts telescopy.

Indications

1. Comminuted or butterfly fractures.
2. Spiral fractures.
3. Comminuted fracture with bone loss.
4. Lengthening and shortening osteotomies.
5. Atrophic nonunion.
6. Pathological fractures.

Dynamic locking Here screws are placed either proximal or distal depending on the site of fracture. It neutralises rotation movements but allows certain movements at the fracture site favouring osteogenesis. It allows immediate mobilisation and weight bearing.

Indications

1. Proximal and distal fractures where there is good bone contact.
2. Proximal and distal nonunion.
3. Proximal and distal osteotomies in malunion.

Achieving dynamisation This consists of removing of either proximal or distal screws of a static locked nail depending on the fracture site. During static locking the fracture will have healed and become ossified, mobilisation of upper and lower joints will not be possible. Dynamisation can be performed within third month of treatment. After removal of proximal or distal screws, full weight bearing is permitted. This hastens the corticalisation of the fracture and will lead to a fusiform callus of excellent quality.

What is New in Osteosynthesis?

I. *Minimally invasive skeletal stabilisation (MISS)*
   a. *For intra-articular fractures* Trans-articular joint reconstruction and a retrograde plate osteosynthesis (Mnemonic TARPO).

Remember about interlocking nail

- It is a modification of standard IM nail.
- It extends the indication of IM nail and can be used for a wide range of shaft fractures.
- Low blood loss and low rate of infection.
- Less operative time.
- Technically demanding.
- Requires sophisticated equipment like C-arm (Fig. 7.3).

   Advantages
   - Better visualisation.
   - Quicker fracture healing.
   - Better functional outcome.

   b. *For extra-articular fractures* (Minimally Invasive Percutaneous Plate Osteosynthesis, to remember use Mnemonic MIPPO).
   This technique consists of percutaneous plate fixation through stab incisions (Fig. 7.4).

II. *Less invasive stabilisation system (LISS)* This is another alternative which behaves more like an internal fixator (Fig. 7.5).

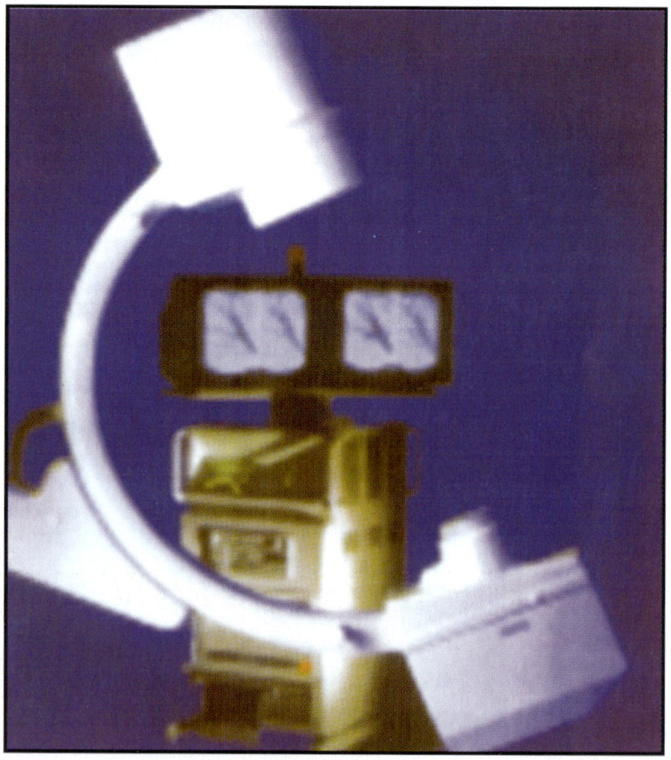

Fig. 7.3: C-arm is a necessary requirement for interlocking nailing and spine surgeries

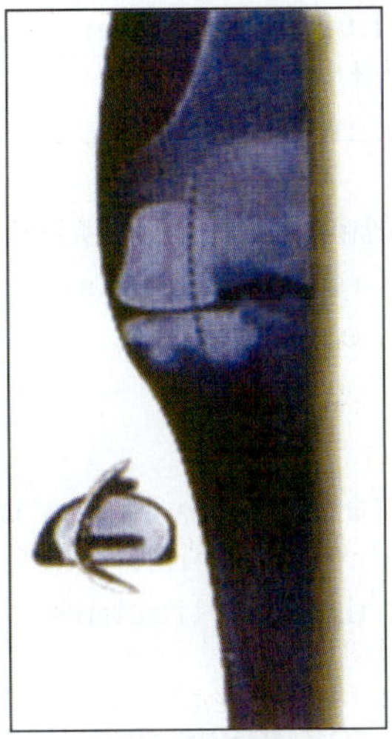

Fig. 7.4: MISS

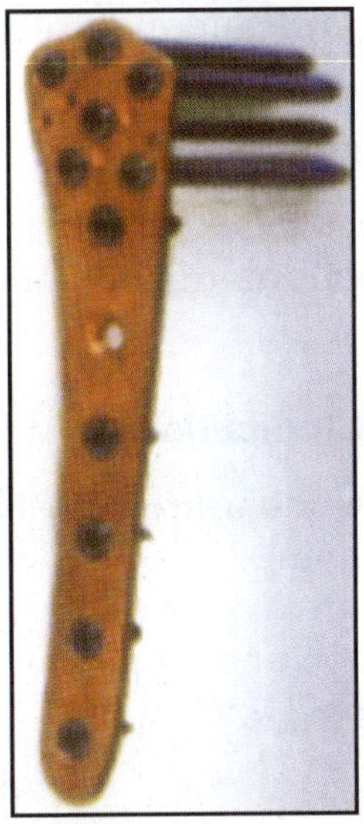

Fig. 7.5: LISS

In a nutshell the newer techniques of osteosynthesis are
- MISS
- TARPO
- MIPPO
- LISS

IMPROVEMENTS IN EXTERNAL FIXATION

ILIZAROV'S TECHNIQUE

Dr GA Ilizarov of Kurgan of Russia had developed a research centre on the role of external fixators in the management of orthopaedic problems. Deviating accidentally from the routine of applying compression, his assistant applied a distraction force much to the discomfiture of Dr Ilizarov. *But he was surprised to see the bone growth in spite of the distraction force*. Little did he realise that he had discovered a new law which was to revolutionise the management of nearly 65 per cent of orthopaedic conditions. He had found an answer to complex orthopaedic problems hitherto unsolvable by conventional orthopaedic procedures.

The use of external fixators in the management of fractures was first described by Hippocrates 2400 years ago. Conventionally, there are two types of external fixators: pin fixator and ring fixator. The ring fixator was developed by Ilizarov in 1951 (Fig. 7.6).

Principles of Ilizarov's Method

An important law of nature which was not known to the biologists was "distraction or pulling apart of living tissue creates a new tissue of its own kind". It was the beginning of a new era of successfully treating unsolved orthopaedic problems. The following are the principles of his method:

Law of tension force When a living tissue is slowly pulled apart at the rate of 1 mm/day, it creates a new tissue. This is called distraction osteogenesis.

Use of a unique ring fixator which is multilevel, multidirectional, multiplane external fixator and hence it is superior to other external fixators.

Corticotomy In this procedure only the cortex of the bone is cut subperiosteally and intramedullary circulation is left intact. Preservation of periosteum and intramedullary circulation produces a better quality of new bone.

About Ring Fixator

Ring fixator is an exceptionally versatile circular external fixator. The system has good range of hard

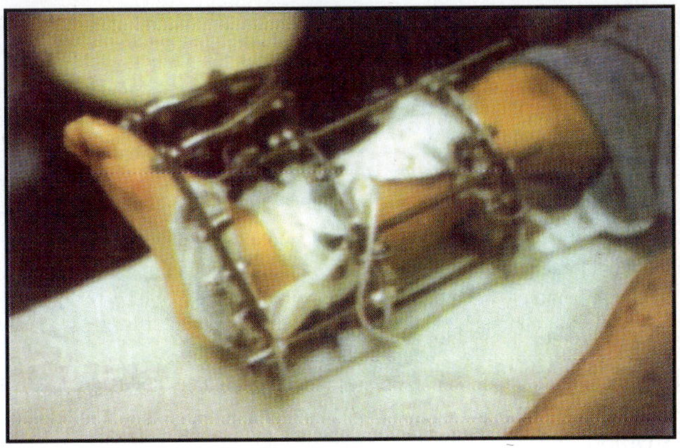

Fig. 7.6: Ilizarov's frame

wires of various sizes and lengths, which can combine to produce a fantastic combination of around 500 types which allows a precise control of bone segments including angulation, rotation, translation, lengthening and compression.

Stages *(Figs 7.7A to C)* Distraction osteogenesis developed by Ilizarov has four stages.

1. Stable fixation of low energy corticotomy to preserve the blood supply.
2. A short latency period before distraction for local bridging of the gap by fibrous tissue.
3. Slow gradual distraction to stimulate ossification during elongation at the rate of 1 mm/day.
4. Newly formed bone extends from each end of the osteotomy in full cross-section parallel to the distraction force. When distraction is discontinued and relative compression is applied, ossification bridges the central gap.

The osteogenic area rapidly remodels to normal macrostructure and microstructure that is indistin–guishable from the host bone histologically and roentgenographically.

Benefits of Ring Fixator System

- Simultaneous correction of multiplane deformities.
- Wide variety of indications treatable with one system.
- Thin tensioned wires allow for stable purchase in small fragments and osteoporotic bones.
- Early patient ambulation.
- Single surgical procedure.

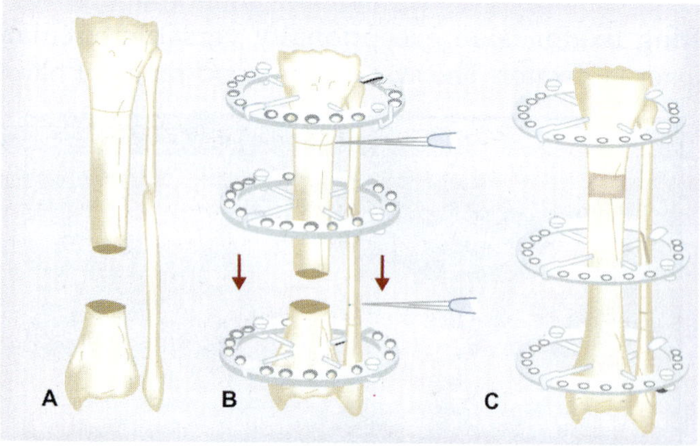

Figs 7.7A to C: Stages of distraction osteogenesis: (A) Bone gap, (B) Corticotomy and distraction, and (C) Union

- Light weight, high strength, radiolucent, composite half rings.
- Relatively simple method, no major surgery required.
- Ilizarov calls this a bloodless surgery as no incision is required, if required it is only 1 to 2 cm.
- Removal of the assembly is very easy.

Indications

Complex fractures Ilizarov is very useful in treating some of the very complex fractures like open fractures, comminuted fractures, intra-articular fractures, etc.

Nonunion Ilizarov gives excellent result in the management of both infected and uninfected nonunion. It simultaneously attends to all the components of nonunion.

Limb lengthening as in achondroplasia and other shortenings.

Deformity corrections due to polio, cerebral palsy, etc.

Other Important Indications

- Congenital pseudoarthrosis of tibia
- Stump lengthening
- TAO
- Tumour excision and lengthening
- Foot deformities.

Complications

- Poor patient compliance.
- Damage to nerves and vessels during insertion.
- Wire tract infection, loosening or breakage.
- Joint contractures.
- Inadvertent injury to the patient or operating room personnel caused by the K-wire.

Remember about Ilizarov

- Makes use of the hitherto unknown principle that distraction stimulates osteogenesis.
- A single frame by arranging it in different combinations can be useful to solve 65 per cent of orthopaedic problems.
- The greatest boon is early ambulation and weight-bearing.
- Low rates of complications.
- Virtually a bloodless surgery.
- Very effective in the treatment of nonunion.
- Cost-effective.

NEWER EXTERNAL FIXATORS

UMEX—Universal Mini External Fixator

This is an indigenous external fixator frame devised and popularised by our very own Indian pioneers. It has the following advantages over the conventional external fixators:

- It is light weight
- It is cheap
- It can be applied to any part of the human skeleton unlike conventional fixators. Hence called universal frame.
- It can be made indigenously.
- Relatively few complications.
- Comparatively less learning curve.
- It can be customized and modulated according to the needs.
- Better patient compliance.

Laser Treatment

Laser treatment for orthopaedic problems like disc prolapse, synovitis, etc. is slowly gaining popularity in the West though it is yet to make a huge impact in our country (Fig. 7.8).

ADVANCES IN HIP SURGERY

Like the spine and the knee, the latest to join the bandwagon of minimally invasive procedure is the hip. Dr G Chana of England has devised minimally invasive surgeries for the hip replacement called the "Minimally Invasive Hip Replacement" (MIH) and 'Minimally Invasive Hip Resurfacing' (MIHR), for trauma and hip diseases. It has the advantages of minimally invasive procedures like:

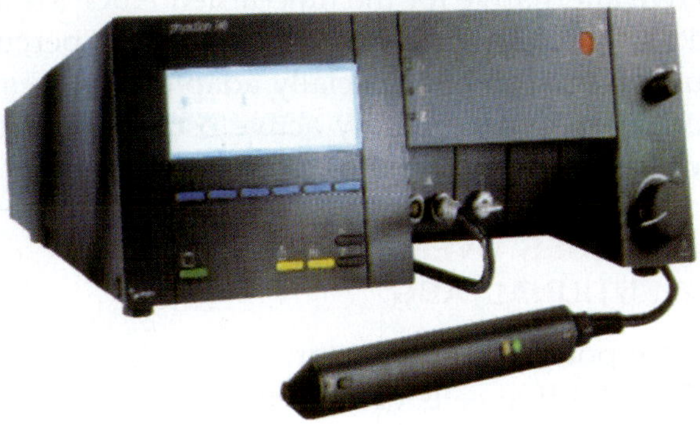

Fig. 7.8: Laser

1. Less blood loss.
2. Minimal exposure.
3. Shorter hospital stay.
4. Reduced hospitalisation cost.
5. Faster mobilisation.
6. Faster ambulations.
7. Minimal scarring.

RECENT ADVANCES IN SPINE SURGERY

Recent advances in spinal surgery paradoxically have resulted in less and less exposure for doing more and more inside the spine. Yes, I am talking about the 'keyhole' procedures which have revolutionised the surgical management of the spine conditions. The notable ones among them are:

1. ***Microscopic lumbar discectomy*** The conventional open method of discectomy resulted in greater morbidity to the patient. With the advent of powerful operating microscope, C-arm and advanced spinal instrumentation, the same procedure can now be done with minimum exposure. This results in widespread benefits to the patients (See box).

Pearls: *Advantages of MLD*

- Less exposure (less than 4 CMS incision required)
- Minimum blood loss
- Early mobilisation (Same day)
- Short hospital stay (2-3 days)
- Relatively inexpensive
- Early return to normal activities and work
- Faster rehabilitation

2. ***Endoscopic lumbar discectomy (ELD)*** (Fig. 7.9) This has the same beneficial effects as MLD and is known to further reduce the tissue trauma and blood loss.
3. ***Minimum invasive spinal surgery (MISS)*** Now through this technique, using an operating endoscope, complex deformities of the spine like the scoliosis, kyphosis, etc. can be corrected at one stage. Earlier these deformity corrective surgeries involved two-stage procedures with extensive blood loss, tissue trauma and big ugly scars. All these undesirable effects are a thing of the past with the advent of MISS.
4. ***VATS (video-assisted thoracoscopic spine surgery)*** This is an endoscopic procedure where anterior thoracic spine pathologies like TB,

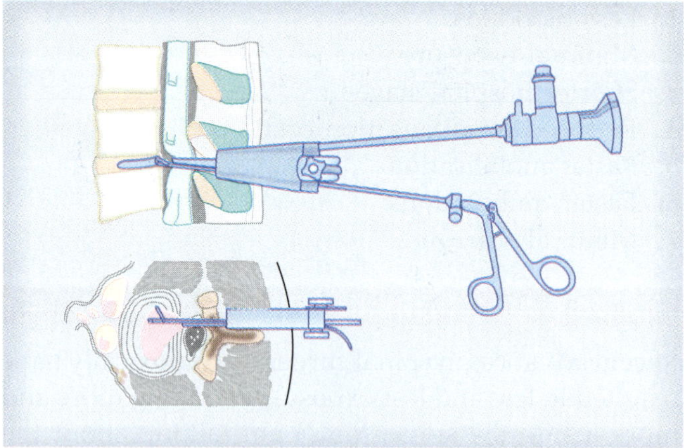

Fig. 7.9: Endoscopic discectomy

trauma, tumour, thoracic kyphosis and scoliosis can be successfully corrected. Here, the patient gets an opportunity to enjoy all the benefits of a MISS and get the above deformity corrected.

Interesting facts:

Remember 'T': in thoracoscopic spine surgery which is indicated in thoracic spine pathologies like:

- T: Tuberculosis
- T: Trauma
- T: Tumours
- T: Thoracic scoliosis
- T: Thoracic kyphosis

Facts you need to now: Get yourself familiar with the following terminology:
MOSS: Moderately open spine surgery
MISS: Minimally invasive spine surgery
MICOSS: Minimally invasive cosmetic spine surgery
VATS: Video-assisted thoracoscopic surgery
MLD: Microscopic lumbar discectomy

5. ***Artificial disc replacement (ADR)*** (Figs 7.10A and B) Of late, damaged discs removed during surgeries are now being replaced by artificial discs. This is known to reduce the postsurgical morbidity and incidences of failed back after surgery.

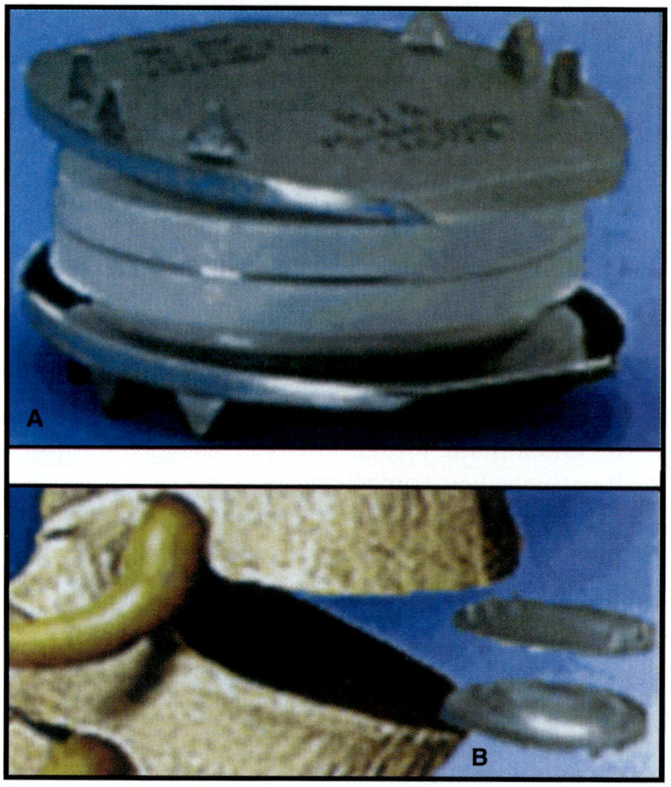

Figs 7.10A and B: Artificial discs

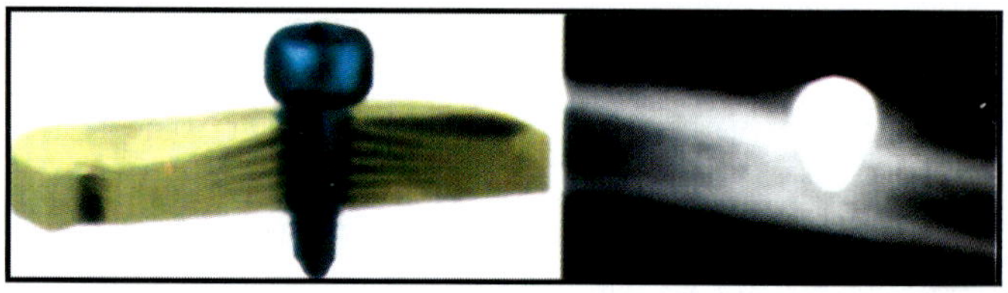

Fig. 7.11: Newer techniques of bone grafting by using differential conical screw

RECENT ADVANCES IN BONE GRAFTING METHOD (Fig. 7.11)

Till recently, autologous bone grafting (ABG) was the 'gold standard' in orthopaedic practice. Adaptive periosteal cambiplasty (APC) is fast emerging as an effective alternative for the time-tested ABG. Mechanical stimulation of healthy tibial shaft by percutaneous application of a specially adapted *"differential conical screw"* yields highly active osteogenic tissue which can be used for autologous bone grafting.

ADVANTAGES OVER THE CONVENTIONAL ABG

- More potent osteoinductor.
- Here the live cells of the cambium layer of the periosteum are activated.
- There is no immune rejection.

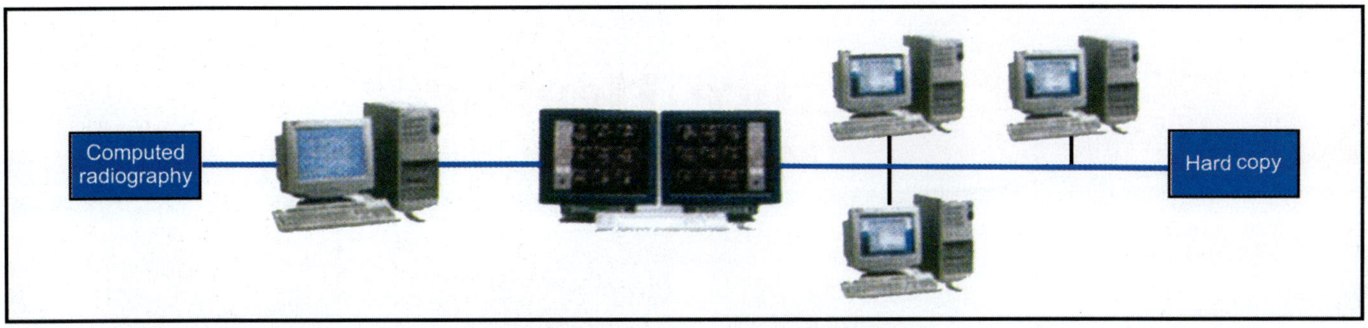

Fig. 7.12: Computers in orthopaedics

- There is minimum artificial injury.
- The healing is faster.

Indications It can be used for the same clinical conditions as ABG but with an enhanced healing response.

COMPUTERS IN ORTHOPAEDICS

Globally computers have made inroads into almost all spheres of human life, so much so that it is hard to imagine life without them. Hence it is no wonder that computers have started knocking the doors of orthopaedic speciality.

In the West and now in our country surgeons are relying more and more on computers for investigations, preoperative planning during operative procedures, especially in arthroplasty, better implant design, etc. Whether all this will improve the quality of orthopaedic services is yet to be ascertained. However, it can be categorically said the future definitely belongs to computer-assisted operations in orthopaedics (Fig. 7.12).

8

Fracture Healing Methods

INTRODUCTION

Bone makes a valiant attempt to get back to its original shape and form after having suffered humiliating fractures due to a myriad of incriminating forces. *Bone is unique in healing itself completely with a tissue that is indistinguishable from the original tissue hence there is no scar left*. The term *bone regeneration* and not *fracture healing* is more appropriate.

Bone is repaired by *callus* which is a new tissue that may develop externally or internally. An *external callus* envelops around the outer aspect of the opposing ends of bone fragments. An *internal callus* forms between the bone ends.

During the first two days at the fracture site and away from the fracture site, in the deep layer of the periosteum the *osteogenic cells* proliferate and lift the fibrous layer of the periosteum away from the bone. *Marrow cells* also proliferate but to a lesser degree. These osteogenic cells differentiate into *osteoblasts* which form the bone trabeculae resembling the embryonic tissue. The osteogenic cells lying away from the fracture site due to *inadequate vascularity* differentiate into chondroblasts and chondrocytes which form the cartilage. The cartilage is finally converted into bone by endochondral ossification.

The internal callus is formed by the mesenchymal cells which convert into pro-osteoblasts and later to osteoblasts laying down new bone. *Remodelling* is an activity of *osteoclasts*, which slowly remove the necrotic bone and create cavities. Osteoblasts line these cavities and lay new bone.

METHODS OF FRACTURE HEALING

A fracture heals by three ways, indirect, direct and distraction histogenesis as described by Ilizarov.

Indirect Fracture Healing

This is the common method of fracture healing where both external and internal callus are formed. Hunter has described six stages in this method of healing (Figs 8.1A to F).

Stage of impact This stage extends from the moment of impact till the complete dissipation of energy causing fractures.

Stage of induction Following fractures, cells possessing osteogenic potential are activated. Other inducing factors are BMP (bone morphogenic protein), fall in oxygen tension and bioelectric effects.

Stage of inflammation In this stage the disruption of blood supply results in necrosis of the bone ends.

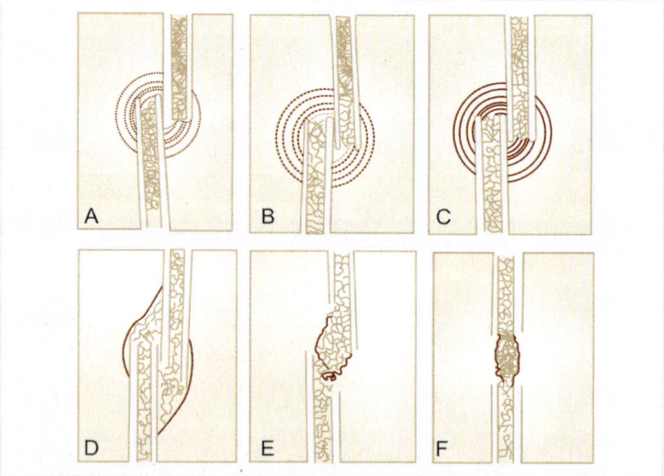

Figs 8.1A to F: Hunter' stages of fracture healing: (A) stage of induction, (B) stage of inflammation, (C) stage of soft callus, (D) stage of hard callus, (E) stage of remodelling, and (F) normal

There is haemorrhage, cellular proliferation and vascular ingrowth.

Stage of soft callus Here the haematoma is organised with fibrous tissue, cartilage and woven bone. Fragments are united with fibrous or cartilaginous tissue or both.

Stage of hard callus Bone fragments are firmly united with bone. If immobilisation is complete, membranous bone healing takes place. If incomplete bone heals by endochondral ossification.

Stage of remodelling Here fibre bone is converted to lamellar bone. Medullary canal is reconstituted and callus diameter begins to decrease in size which takes a few months to several years. However, there will be no remodelling of rotational malalignment.

This method of fracture healing is seen in fractures treated by plaster immobilisation (Fig. 8.2) and other forms of external and some limited internal fixation techniques.

Problems associated with indirect fracture healing

- Less anatomic union.
- Chances of malunion significant.
- Delayed joint mobilisation.
- Possibility of fracture disease.

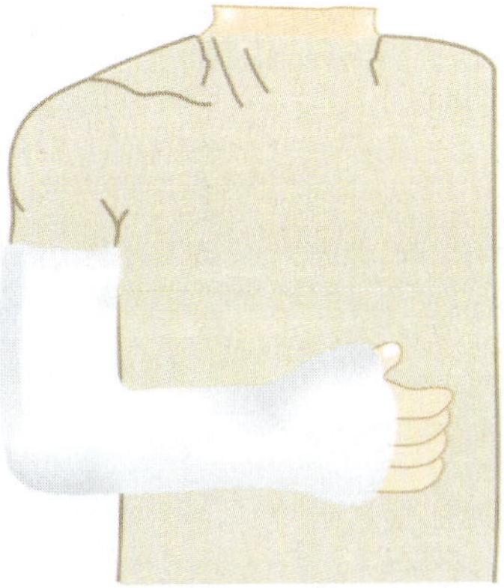

Fig. 8.2: An above elbow cast (Example of indirect fracture healing)

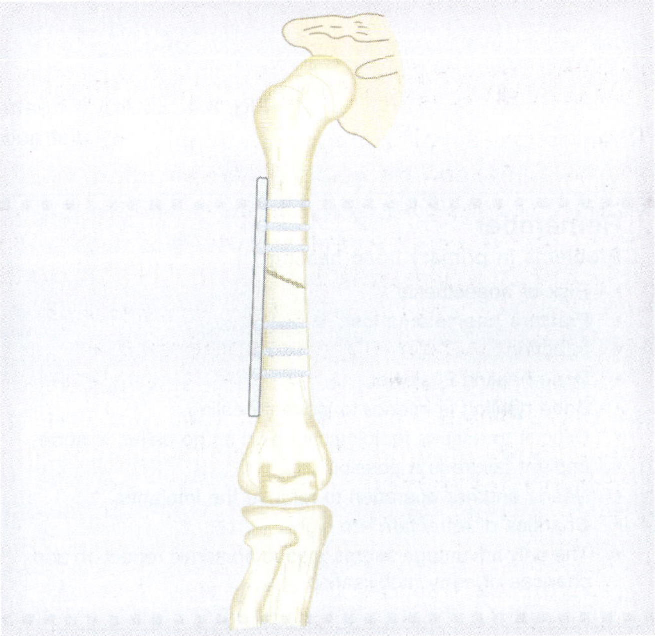

Fig. 8.3: Fracture shaft humerus fixed with DCP plate and screws (Example of direct fracture healing)

Primary Bone Healing (Direct Bone Healing, Healing by Primary Intention)

This type of bone repair is seen when bone fragments are anatomically reduced and rigidly fixed. This cannot be obtained by closed methods of fracture treatment but can be achieved by operative reduction and fixation with special techniques of plate and screws. Here ideally no external callus forms and there is no interposing fibrous tissue or cartilage tissue betwen the fracture sites. The fracture site is bridged by direct haversian remodelling which is almost a direct osteon-to-osteon hookup. The osteoclasts act as cutter heads to remove the bone and are in the forefront promptly followed by osteoblasts behind laying down new bone. This type of bone healing usually occurs in fractures treated by AO techniques developed by Swiss association for osteosynthesis (Fig. 8.3).

Distraction Histogenesis (Fig. 8.4)

Distraction histogenesis is a recent concept described by Ilizarov. Here bone repair is induced by gradual distraction of osteotomies and fracture after an interval of induction say 5 to 7 days. For osteogenesis to occur, the fracture or osteotomy must be stabilised and a slow distraction at the rate of 1 mm per day should be given. For details, see discussion on Ilizarov (p. 81).

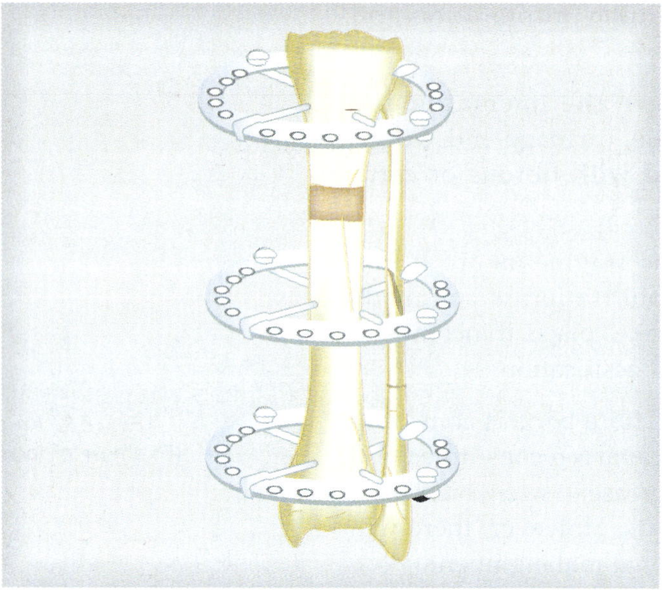

Fig. 8.4: Ilizarov's treatment is an example of healing by distraction histogenesis

Remember

Problems in primary bone healing

- Risk of anaesthesia.
- Fracture haematoma lost.
- Infection.
- Bone healing is slower.
- Bone healing is inferior to indirect healing.
- Difficult to assess radiological union as no callus is seen.
- Implant failure is a possibility.
- Needs another operation to remove the implants.
- Chances of refracture are high.
- The only advantage seems is good anatomic reduction and chances of early mobilisation.

Factors affecting fracture repair

Factors favouring union

- Adequate circulation
- Hormones like growth hormone, parathormone, thyroxine, etc.
- Good nutrition and mineral supplements help passsively
- Bioelectric fixation

Factors detrimental to union

- Poor circulation
- Infection
- Distraction
- Segmental fractures
- Comminution
- Osteoporosis
- Soft tissue interposition
- Inadequate and improper immobilisation, etc.

9 Soft Tissue Injuries

INTRODUCTION

Soft tissue injuries (Fig. 9.1) are not quite 'soft' but 'hard' in terms of management and rehabilitation. The term soft tissue implies skin, subcutaneous tissue, fascia, muscles, ligaments, tendons, synovium, capsules, nerves, etc. Undoubtedly they are more common than bony injuries. Sportspersons are more prone to suffer from soft tissue injuries than the normal population. Unlike in fractures, the soft tissue injury management is essentially conservative and physiotherapy appears to be the mainstay of treatment.

MECHANISM OF INJURY

Direct trauma due to fall, RTA, assault, etc. Contusion, haematomas, lacerations are some of the examples.

Indirect trauma due to avulsion injuries, muscle pull, ligament sprain, etc. More commonly seen in sportspersons.

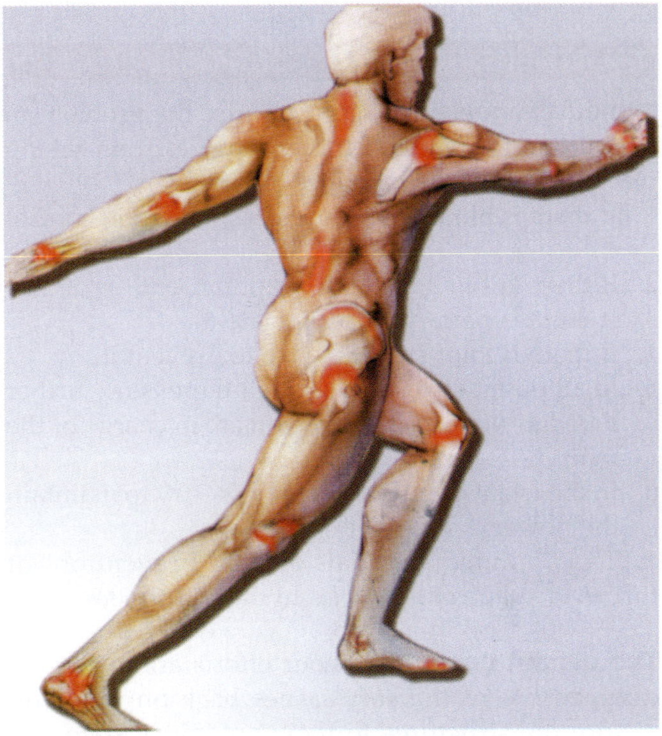

Fig. 9.1: Sites of common soft tissue injuries

APPROACH TO A PATIENT WITH SOFT TISSUE INJURY

The patient's story Listen to what the patient has to say about the problem. Do not be swayed by his story. He may be going overboard. Take his complaints with a 'pinch of salt'. This is the subjective assessment.

Your observation This is your assessment of the problem based on 'his' story. Make an objective assessment of the injury with regard to site, nature, intensity of pain, etc. of the injury. Your evaluation may or may not correlate with 'his' story. Evaluate carefully the functional problem, interpret it analytically and individualise the treatment plan.

Goal setting A surgeon needs to set up goals while treating soft tissue injuries. These could be immediate or long term.

Execution of your plan Having made a careful evaluation of the injury, you have sized up the problem and formulated your modus operandi. Keeping both the short and long-term goals in mind. Unleash your plan of action now to bottle up this genie.

TREATMENT GOALS OF SOFT TISSUE INJURY

Immediate goals This aims to 'nip' the problem in the bud and 'prevent' further damages from taking place. A look at the priorities clarifies this:

1. If there is blood loss—arrest it, prevent it, control it.
2. If there is swelling—try to minimise it.
3. If there is pain—try to alleviate it.
4. If there is joint stiffness—try to prevent it.
5. In all possibility try to see that there is no further damage whatsoever once you are in charge of the injury!
6. In the event of muscle weakness—try to maintain the power.

Thus, immediate goals aim at 'prevention' of further damage and injuries to the soft tissues.

The distant goals Here your efforts are to put the derailed life of the soft tissues back on rails and restore the structures to their pre-injury state. No mean task this and it calls for a sustained and skillful approach. The priorities in this are as under:

1. *Movements* Restore it to as normal as possible.
2. *Mobility* Ensure the affected joints are back to their best.
3. *Strength* The affected muscles need to be given their strength and endurance back.
4. *Kinesthetic/proprioception mechanism* Restore it back to normal.
5. *Daily or functional activities* Restore it back to the original.
6. *Confidence* Boost the patient's morale and also that of the affected part.
7. *Keep away* The swelling, oedema from raising its ugly head again. Once bitten twice shy, hence no more such injuries.
8. *Last but not the least* Ensure that this problem will not surface again by practising effective anti-recurrent methods.
9. *Inculcate* a sense of discipline in practicing regular follow-up and valuing the medical advice. Drive home the advantages of 'home care' programs. Instil in them a thought that, "it pays to be your own doctor in the safe confines of their home!"

CLASSIFICATION OF SOFT TISSUE INJURY

The four broad classification for STI are as follows:

1. Strains
2. Sprains
3. Ruptures
4. Contusions.

Let us now discuss each one in detail.

MUSCLE INJURY STRAINS

Definition Injury to the muscle and tendons is called *strain* (Fig. 9.2).

Reasons

1. Sudden unaccustomed or abrupt action or movements may tear the muscles.
2. Direct trauma can also injure the muscles and tendons.
3. Overstretching of muscles due to indirect trauma, especially in sportspersons.

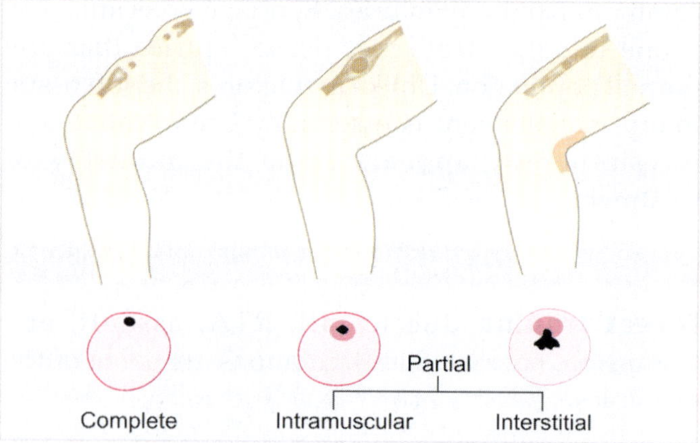

Fig. 9.2: Showing types of muscle strains

Types

1. *Acute strain* This is due to sudden violent force or direct trauma.
2. *Chronic strain* This is due to injury existing since a long period leading to muscle ischaemia and fibrosis.

Pathophysiology

Injury to the muscles leads to pain. As a result, the muscle goes into spasm to limit the movements and reduce pain. But paradoxically, this protective muscle spasm causes pain due to stimulation of pain fibres and thus a vicious cycle sets in (Fig. 9.3). The painful stimuli causes muscle spasm through the peripheral nociceptive stimuli (Fig. 9.4).

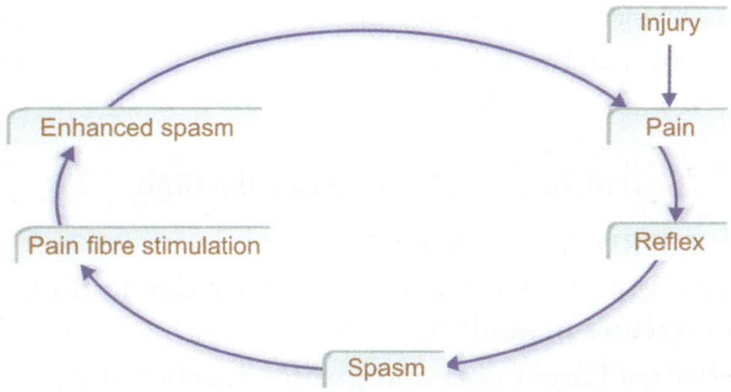

Fig. 9.3: Pain and spasm: the vicious cycle

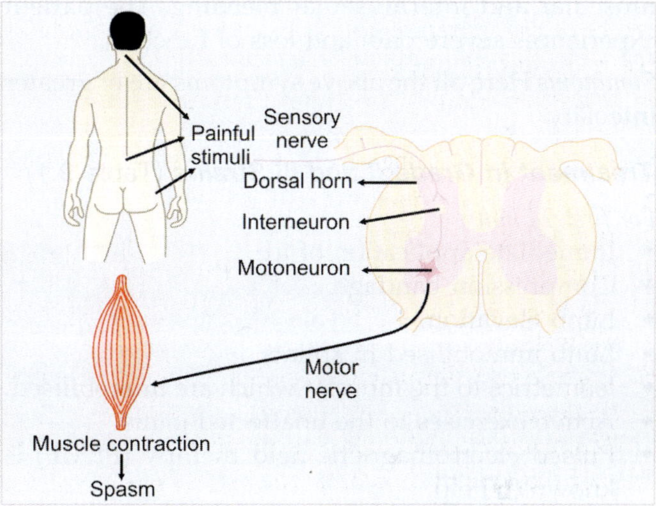

Fig. 9.4: Induction of prolonged muscle contractions (spasm) by peripheral nociceptive stimuli

Severity of Strain

1. FIRST DEGREE STRAIN (MILD CONTUSION)

- This is due to blunt injury and is due to direct trauma of low intensity.
- *Pathology* Few muscle fibres are torn. Bleeding is minimal and the fascia remains intact.

Clinical Features (Fig. 9.5)

- Localised pain and tenderness.
- Pain and spasm prevents muscle stretching.
- Function is not impaired to a greater extent.
- Tenderness over the affected muscles.

Management

- First aid is by cryotherapy (by application of ice) for a period of 20 minutes.
- Gentle active muscle stretch may be permitted after 20 to 60 minutes.
- Compression bandaging with optimum pressure.
- Low dose and low power ultrasound helps.
- Gentle massaging of the surrounding area helps.
- If pain is minimal, the patient can be allowed to do the light work the next day.

2. SECOND DEGREE STRAIN

Cause Here the trauma is more serious.

Pathology

- Greater number of muscle fibres are torn.
- There is more bleeding.
- The fascia is still intact.
- Haematoma is still localised.

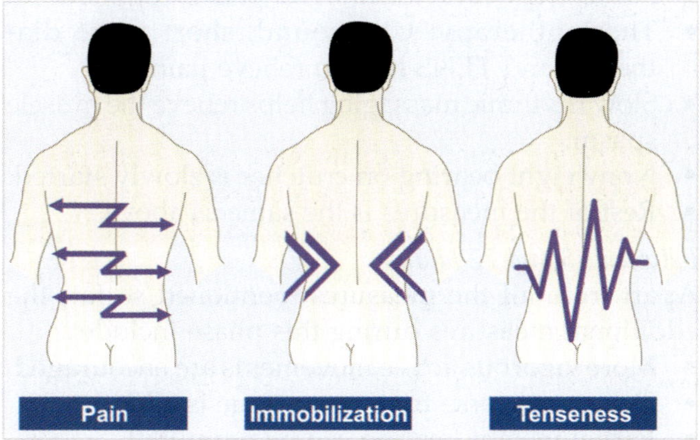

Fig. 9.5: Main symptoms of continuous muscle contractions (muscle spasms) in locomotor system: pain, immobilization and tenseness-tenderness of muscles

Symptoms
- Pain is more severe.
- Tenderness is severe.
- Severe muscle spasm.
- The patient is unable to move the limb.

3. THIRD DEGREE STRAIN

Cause Undoubtedly these injuries are due to trauma of a greater magnitude.

Pathology Larger area and greater number of muscle fibres are involved. More than one muscle group may be involved. The fascia is partially torn. Bleeding is widespread and more. There could be both intramuscular and intermuscular bleeding. The patient experiences severe pain and loss of function.

Symptoms Here all the above symptoms are of greater intensity.

Treatment in Grade II and III Strains (Table 9.1)

For first 24 hours
- Immediate application of ice.
- Compression bandage.
- Limb elevation.
- Limb immobilised in splints.
- Isometrics to the muscles which are immobilised.
- Active exercises to the unaffected joints.
- Pulsed electromagnetic field therapy (PEMF) is known to help.
- No active movements to the affected muscles.

During the next 24 to 48 hours
- The pressure bandage is removed and active muscle exercises are begun.
- Stretching within the limits of pain is commenced.
- Thermotherapy: Ultrasound, short wave diathermy and TENS help to relieve pain.
- Slow rhythmic massaging helps relieve the muscle spasm.
- Nonweight bearing on crutches is slowly started.
- Rest of the measures is the same as above.

Between 48 and 72 hours

Apart from all the measures mentioned so far, the additional measures during this phase include:
- More vigorous active movements are encouraged.
- Deep transverse friction massage is added.
- Partial weight bearing can be permitted.

After 72 hours
- All the above measures are pursued in a more vigorous manner.

Table 9.1: Treatment of muscle strain by conservative methods in a nutshell

Systemic Therapy
Analgesic anti-inflammatory drugs
Antipyretic analgesics
Nonsteroidal anti-inflammatory drugs
Narcotic analgesics
Muscle relaxants
At muscular level
At neuromuscular level
At spinal level
At supraspinal level
Psychotropic drugs
Antidepressants
Neuroleptics
Minor tranquillizers
Others
Calcitonin
Beta-blockers
Local Therapy
Local anaesthetics
Steroids
Transdermal application of analgesic anti-inflammatory drugs (ointments)

- Pressure bandage is totally removed.
- Progressive resisted exercises using the Fowler technique by taking out 10 to 12 repetition maximum (RM), is practised.
- Full weight-bearing should be permitted in injuries of the lower limbs.
- After full movement is regained, the patient is allowed to walk and jog.
- Full functional activity should be regained by 4 to 6 weeks.

4. GRADE FOUR STRAIN

Cause This is usually caused by severe trauma.

Pathology
- Complete tear of the muscle.
- The fascia is torn.
- Considerable bleeding which is intermuscular and diffuse.
- Gross swelling is present.

Clinical Features
- Excruciating pain.
- Severe tenderness is present.
- A snapping sound may be heard by the patient.
- Palpable gap between the muscles felt.
- Severe loss of function.

- Active movements produced by the agonist is absent.
- Active muscle contraction is absent.
- Joint function is not lost.
- Muscle spasm is very severe (Fig. 9.6).

Treatment
- Surgery is advised. This involves opening the ruptured site, evacuating the haematoma and suturing the fascial sheath. Direct muscle repair is avoided.
- Compression bandage is applied and the limb is immobilised for 2 to 3 weeks.
- Active exercises to the unaffected joints.
- Slow rhythmic isometric exercises to the affected muscles.
- Non-weight bearing after 48 hours.
- The use of low frequency current (faradism) to obtain passive contraction are very useful.
- Deep heating modalities like ultrasound, etc. help
- Rest of the measures are same as for Gr II/III injuries.

Note: Mild muscle strain is also called by lay public as muscle pull.

INJURIES TO THE JOINTS

During an injury to a joint, three things could happen:
1. Injury to the ligaments only.
2. Injury to the synovium.
3. Both (According to Bass, 1969).

Ligament Injury

A ligament injury is called "Sprain". Depending on the severity, it could be mild (Grade I), moderate (Grade II) or severe (Grade III).

Anatomy

Ligaments are made of fibrous tissues which are arranged longitudinally. They are tough and elastic. Their vascularity is poor and heal always by scar tissue due to lack of special cells.

Function

Ligaments serve the following functions:
1. *Support* By reinforcing the capsule, they provide support to the joint.
2. *Stability* By holding the bony ends together, it provides stability.

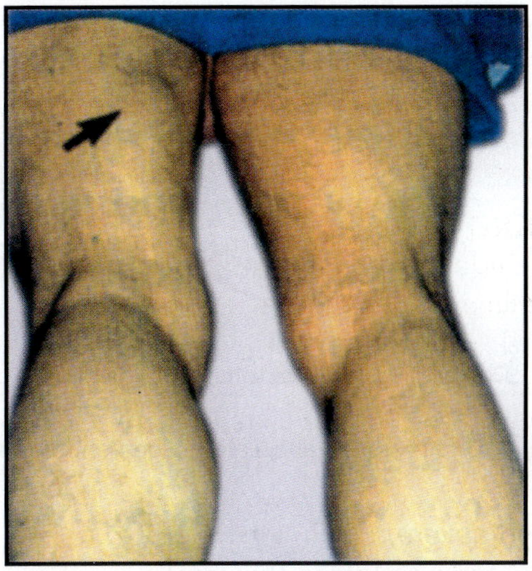

Fig. 9.6: Showing Grade IV muscle strain

3. *Protection* The strength of the ligaments offer protection to the joints along with the muscles.

Problems of Healing

1. Poor vascularity delays the healing.
2. Repair is by scar tissue.
3. Inadequate period of immobilisation results in healing with more fibrous tissue. This will result in excessive laxity making the joint unstable.
4. Intermittent stretching strengthens the ligament while continuous stretch leads to adhesions due to periosteal irritation.

Types of Sprain (Fig. 9.7)

Grade I (minor)
- Slight pain and tenderness at the site of injury.
- Slight swelling and loss of function.
- Stretch test will be positive clinching the diagnosis.

Treatment

First day
- Cryotherapy to alleviate pain.
- Pressure bandage—to prevent swelling.
- Limb elevation—to prevent swelling.
- Active movements of the unaffected joints.

Second day onwards
- Add thermotherapy, stop ice therapy.
- Begin isometric exercises to the affected muscles.
- Weight bearing may be permitted.
- Rest of the measures are same as mentioned above.

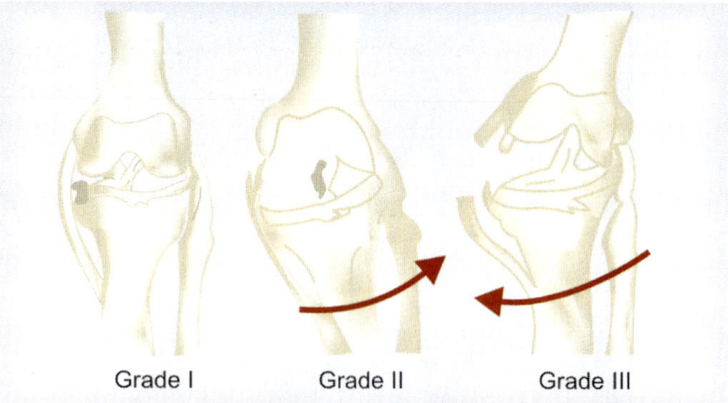

Fig. 9.7: Sprain of medial collateral ligament of the knee

Grade II (severe)

- More force results in this injury.
- The ligament may be partially torn or detached from the attachment.
- Swelling is more severe.
- Pain and tenderness are also more acute.
- Movement is grossly restricted.
- Weight bearing is difficult.
- Function is severely affected.

Treatment

- Cryotherapy.
- Compression bandaging or knee cap and braces (Fig. 9.8).
- Elevation.
- Rest of the measures same as in Grade I.

Grade III (complete rupture)

- Severe violence.
- Gross swelling.
- Pain and tenderness is quite severe.
- Joint is unstable.
- The patient is unable to bear weight.
- Severe loss of function.

Treatment

1. *Conservative*
   - Immediate application of ice.
   - Compression bandaging.
   - Foot end elevation.
   - Isometric exercises to the affected limbs.
   - Active exercises to affected joints.
   - POP cast for 6 to 8 weeks if ligament tear does not cause displacement.
2. *Surgical*
   - If the ligament is torn and displaced, it needs surgical repair and immobilisation with a POP cast for 6 to 8 weeks.
   - Isometric exercises are started after one week.
   - Non-weight-bearing for 3 to 4 weeks.

After Removal of the POP Cast

- *Thermotherapy* Ultrasound, TENS or SWD helps to relieve pain.
- Pressure bandage helps to control the swelling.
- Limb elevation to prevent oedema.

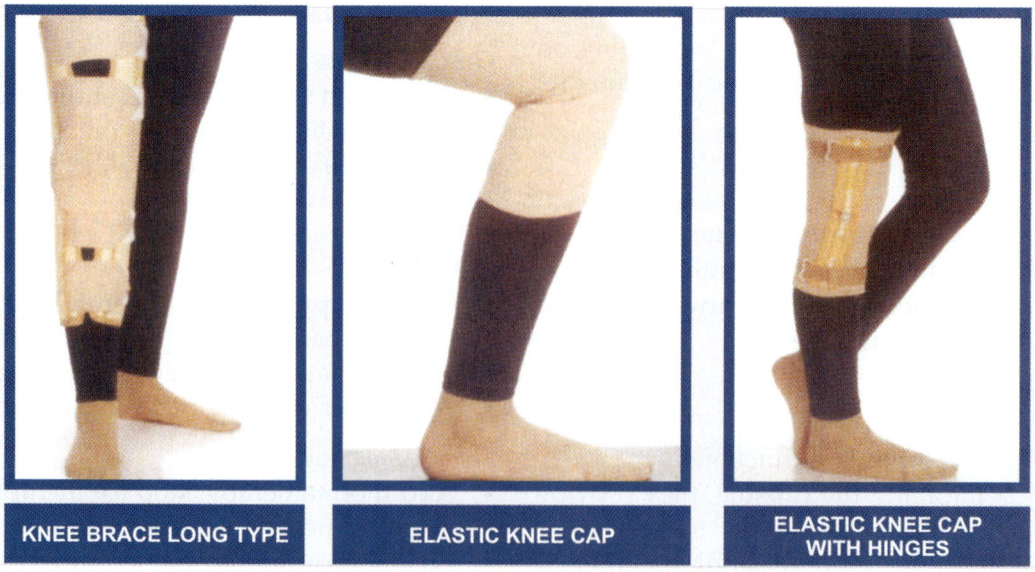

Fig. 9.8: Showing various elastic knee braces to support the knee joint

- Transverse friction massage to relieve spasm.
- Active exercises to the affected joints are begun slowly and progressed gradually.
- Isometrics are done more vigorously.
- Passive ROM exercises.
- Active, active-resisted and self-resisted exercises are prescribed.
- Weight-bearing is slowly encouraged from partial to full after 6 to 8 weeks.
- The patient should be functionally independent by 8 to 12 weeks.

Injury to the Synovium

Relevant Anatomy

Synovium is a lining covering the caspsule of the joint, tendon sheaths, etc. It has a rich blood and nerve supply. It is present throughout the body.

Functions

Synovium produces synovial fluid which serves the following functions:

1. Facilitates frictionless, smooth joint movements.
2. Helps in the nourishment of cartilages.

Causes

Inflammation of synovium is called *synovitis*. It could be due to trauma, arthritis, chondromalacia, rheumatoid arthritis, TB, haemophilia, etc.

Types

1. Acute—due to trauma.
2. Chronic—due to diseases like TB, rheumatoid arthritis, trauma, etc.

Clinical Features in Synovitis

- Swelling of the joint (develops slowly say within 2 to 24 hours).
- The joint is hot and red.
- Pain is present over the injured structure.
- Feeling of tension or pressure due to swelling.
- To accommodate the excess fluid, the joint will assume a flexion attitude (position of ease).
- Muscle atrophy will be quite significant.

In the Event of Synovial Rupture

- The patient feels sudden pain at the back of the knee while getting up from a chair, getting down the stairs, etc.
- The swelling may spread rapidly to the calf muscles. Homan's sign will be positive (see page 43).

Treatment

Aim To prevent muscle atrophy and joint contractures by a graduated exercise regimen.

Methods

During first 24 hours

- Ice therapy.
- Compression bandage.
- Limb elevation.
- Isometric contraction of the affected limb muscles.
- Active movements of the ankle joint.
- Active movements of the unaffected joints.
- Splinting of the affected part.

After 48 hours

- Aspiration of the joint if swelling persists even after 48 hours.
- Sustained isometric contraction of the muscles.
- Small range gradual active movements with adequate support should now be begun.
- Partial weight bearing may be allowed.
- Gradually progressive resistive exercises should be started to achieve full function.

Note: Haemarthrosis vs Synovitis
In haemarthrosis:

1. The swelling is rapid in onset (< 2 hours).
2. Swelling is more generalised.
3. Pain on extreme movements.
4. Joint instability may be present in cases of complete rupture.

Chronic Synovitis

This is due to various diseases affecting the synovium usually of more than three weeks' duration.

Tuberculosis of the joints, rheumatoid arthritis, etc. are some of the examples.

Problems of chronic synovitis

- Firm swelling.
- Muscle atrophy may be gross.

- Joint stiffness may be considerable.
- Lax ligaments create instability.
- Mild pain unlike acute synovitis.

Treatment

- Resistive exercises to the affected limbs.
- Isometric exercises to the affected parts.
- Passive ROM exercises to over come joint stiffness.
- Proper gait training.
- Ultrasound TENS, SWD and other heat modalities to overcome pain and spasm.

Injury to the Bursa

Bursae are thin membranous sac lined with synovial membrane situated at the ends or certain important locations of the bones where tendons, etc. pass over them (Fig. 9.9).

Functions

1. To prevent friction between two structures like tendons and bones that are liable to be rubbed against each other.
2. To prevent wear and tear of muscles and tendons.
3. To protect the structures from pressure and injury.

Types

1. *True bursa* They are normally present in the body at certain important situations like beneath the acromion, elbow, knee, heel, etc.
2. *False bursa* They are also called as adventitious bursa. They develop due to external trauma, pressure, etc.

Causes

The causes of bursitis are as follows:

1. *Trauma* May be due to a single blow or repetitive trauma.
2. *Infection* acute or chronic (e.g. TB).
3. *Metabolic disorders,* e.g. gout, etc.
4. *Abnormal external pressures,* etc. (e.g. hip ischial tuberosity, etc).
5. Inflammatory disorders, e.g. rheumatoid arthritis, etc.
6. Unaccustomed activity, exercise or ill-fitting shoes, etc.
7. Due to excessive pressure, friction, etc. (e.g. olecranon bursitis, student's elbow, etc).

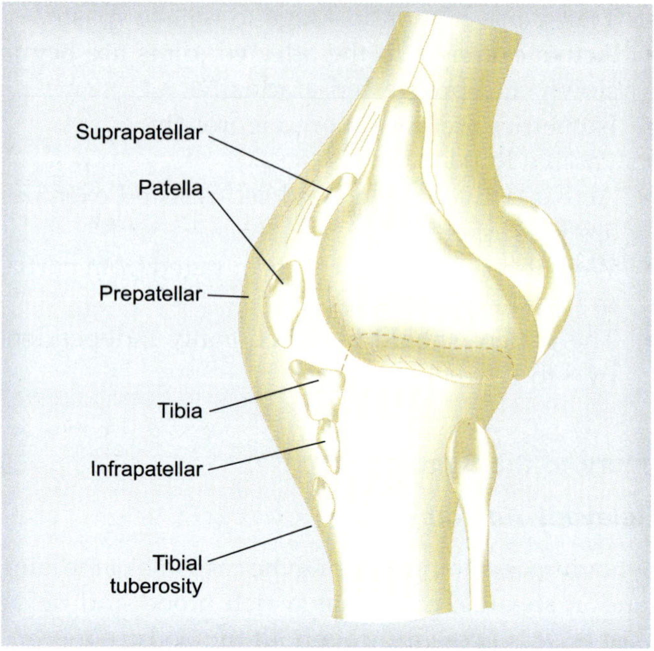

Fig. 9.9: Knee joint has many bursae around it

Common Sites

Upper Limbs

a. Subacromion
b. Olecranon

Lower Limbs

a. Prepatellar
b. Tendo-Achilles
c. Medial side of the great toe
d. Lateral side of the little toe.

Clinical Features

- Pain, more so if it ruptures.
- Swelling is tender and hot.
- Movements of the joint may be painful.
- Tenderness may be present.
- Limp due to gluteal bursitis, etc.

Treatment

1. *In bursitis due to friction*
   - Rest to the part.
   - Thermotherapy: US, SWD, TENS, etc.
   - Cryotherapy in initial stages (first 24 to 48 hours).
   - Restricted weight bearing.
   - Isometric exercises to the affected part.
   - Muscle strengthening exercises.

- Joint mobilisation if there is restriction.
- Injection of hydrocortisone in intractable cases.
- Excision of the bursa, if chronic and troublesome.

2. *Infective bursitis*
   - Appropriate antibiotics
   - Rest of the measures are same as above.
3. *Chronic cases*
   - Appropriate supports like felt pad, footwear modifications, etc.
   - Avoiding repeated frictional movements (e.g. shoulder abduction in subdeltoid bursa).
   - Relaxed passive movements to avoid friction.
   - Active limited ROM exercises with strong isometrics.
   - Progressive resistive exercises.
   - Deep heating like US, SWD, TENS, etc.
   - Deep friction massage.
   - Active exercises to the unaffected joints.
   - Isometrics with limb in elevation helps considerably.

Tenosynovitis

This is due to inflammation of the synovial lining of the tendon sheath. The fibrous sheath is, however, not affected (see Fig. 33.7).

Types

Irritative Due to abnormal or excessive friction. There is pain and crepitus on palpation. The movements are not affected and there are no adhesions. There is watery effusion due to sheath inflammation.

Infective May be due to acute pyogenic infection or chronic infection like TB, etc.

Treatment

Irritative

- Rest to the part by appropriate splints.
- Avoid movements at the joints.
- Bandaging or POP cast.
- Thermotherapy, US, SWD or TENS.
- Deep friction massage.
- Difficult cases, hydrocortisone injection.
- Intractable cases, surgical excision.
- Shoe modifications, etc.

Infective

- Appropriate antibiotics.
- Immobilisation for 2 to 3 months.
- Rest of the measures are the same as mentioned above.

Tenovaginitis

Unlike in tenosynovitis, here the fibrous sheath and not the synovial sheath of the tendon is affected. Though patient may complain of pain, crepitus is conspicuous by its absence, e.g. de Quervain's disease (Fig. 9.10).

Though the exact cause is unknown (Adams 1981), Cyrius (1978) says it may be due to repeated strains. Infection is not known to cause this problem.

Treatment

This is similar to tenosynovitis.

SPECIAL TYPES OF MUSCLE INJURIES

1. **Bruise or Contusion** It is nothing but the Grade I muscle strain. This has already been discussed and is called a superficial haematoma.
2. **Haematomas** These are deep in nature and two types are described:

a. *Intramuscular Haematoma*

- Here blood is contained within the muscle and is bound by an intact muscle sheath.
- Following an injury, bleeding occurs and stops within two hours.
- There is localised swelling.
- If there is further trauma, more bleeding may occur.

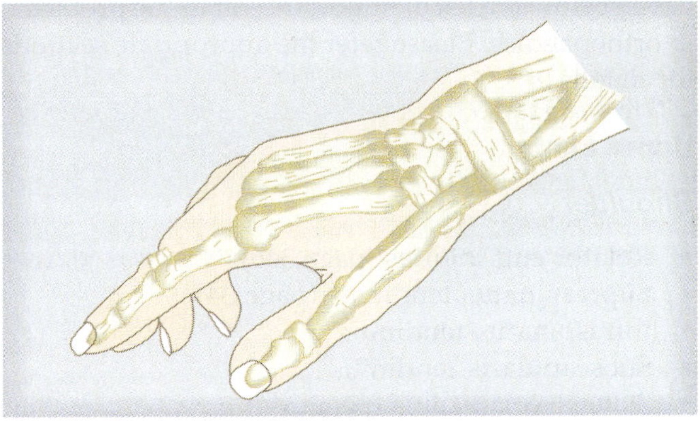

Fig. 9.10: Showing de Quervain's disease, an example of tenovaginitis

Section 1

b. *Intermuscular Haematoma*

- Here the sheath of the muscle is torn resulting in extravasation of blood between the muscle and fascial planes.
- The haematoma is more diffuse.
- Bleeding will be more as the tension does not build up to stop it.
- Due to gravity, it tracks down and may cause discoloration beneath the skin.
- For the first 48 hours it is difficult to differentiate between the above haematomas.

Quick facts

Features of intermuscular haematomas
- Moderate pain
- Swelling reduces drastically by 48 to 72 hours
- Muscle contraction is regained first
- Due to tracking swelling may be seen at a distance away from the site of injury.

Treatment

Aim is to prevent further bleeding.

Methods

- Rest to the part.
- Immobilise the affected part with splint.
- Cryotherapy to relieve pain and spasm.
- Pressure bandage to control the swelling.
- Limb elevation to prevent oedema.

Note In haematomas there is no loss of function. If there is loss of function then it may be a Grade II/III muscle strain.

IMPORTANT SOFT TISSUE PROBLEMS

Given below is a list of important soft tissue problems in orthopaedics. Please refer the appropriate sections for details.

Upper Limb

Shoulder

- Rotator cuff injuries (page 346)
- Supraspinatus tendinitis (page 347)
- Infraspinatus tendinitis
- Subscapularis tendinitis
- Adhesive capsulitis (page 344)
- Tendinitis of the long head of biceps.

Elbow

a. Tennis elbow (page 351)
b. Golfer's elbow (page 353)
c. Student's or miner's elbow (page 354)

Wrist

a. Ganglion (page 356)
b. de Quervain's disease (page 355)
c. Dupuytren's contracture (page 357)
d. Trigger finger (page 356)
e. Carpal tunnel syndrome (page 358)
f. Mallet finger (page 178).

Lower Limbs

Hip and Pelvis

a. Piriformis syndrome
b. Iliotibial tract syndrome
c. Gluteal bursitis
d. Trochanteric bursitis.

Knee and Leg

a. Bursae around the knee (page 386)
b. Collateral ligament injury (page 220)
c. Cruciate ligament injury (page 222)
d. Meniscal injury (page 226)
e. Quadriceps strain (page 235)
f. Hamstrings strain
g. Calf muscle strain
h. Patellar tendinitis
i. Plica syndrome (page 393).

Ankle and Foot

a. Ankle sprain (page 250)
b. Plantar fasciitis (page 400)
c. Calcaneal spur (page 401)
d. Morton's neuroma (page 398)
e. Tendo-Achilles injuries (page 251)
f. Tarsal tunnel syndrome.

For:

- Injuries to tendons, please see the chapter on Injuries of Flexor and Extensor Tendons of the Hand
- Injuries to the nerves, please refer to chapter on Peripheral Nerve Injuries.

10

Fractures in Special Situations

- ❑ Fractures in children
- ❑ Epiphyseal injuries
- ❑ Pathological fractures
- ❑ Fatigue or stress fractures

FRACTURES IN CHILDREN

Fractures in children are different from fractures in adults for the following reasons:

1. Complete fractures are rare due to thick periosteal sleeve and greater elasticity.
2. For the same reasons mentioned above, buckle (Torus fractures) and greenstick fractures are more common.
3. Fracture displacements are relatively less common.
4. Fracture bleeding is also less.
5. Avulsion fractures are more common because bone gives way earlier than the ligaments.
6. Disruptions of the epiphyseal plate are relatively more common because they form the weakest portion of the bone in the children and account for nearly one-third of all childhood fractures.
7. A paediatric fracture unites faster.
8. Differential periosteal activity causes better remodelling which is more likely in (i) the younger the child, (ii) the nearer the fracture to the epiphyseal plate, and (iii) if the deformity is angulated in the plane of the joint movement.
9. All tissues in children not only heal well but rapidly too.
10. Joint stiffness a bugbear in adults, rarely happens in children.

INCIDENCE

- Fracture accounts for 10 to 25 per cent of all injuries in childhood.
- Common between 11 and 14 years of age.
- Boys account for 62 per cent of all cases.
- Fracture distal end of forearm is the most common skeletal injury in children contributing 25 per cent of all fractures in them.

AETIOLOGY

- Falls are the most predominant cause in children.
- Traffic accidents, especially bicycle accidents account for 12 per cent of cases.
- Sporting activities contribute 21 per cent.
- *Birth fractures*—the clavicle is the most commonly injured bone during birth (accounts for 40 to 50% of all birth injuries), followed by brachial plexus injury (usually during instrumental rotation of the vertex), the humerus (injured during breech delivery) and the femur in that order.
- *Pathological fractures*—the conditions leading to pathological fractures could be:
  1. Generalised, e.g. osteogenesis imperfecta, metabolic disorders, etc.
  2. Localised to one limb, e.g. fibrous dysplasia.
  3. Localised to the lesion, e.g. benign cystic condition of the bone, infection, benign and malignant neoplasm, etc.

  Pathological fractures usually result from trivial trauma.
- Child abuse (battered baby syndrome)—80 per cent of child abuse takes place in less than two years of age.
- Stress fractures are not very common. Seen in tibia, neck of femur, etc.

TYPES OF FRACTURES

Greenstick fractures This is a type of incomplete fracture seen exclusively in children. Here one cortex is broken and the other is intact (Fig. 10.1).

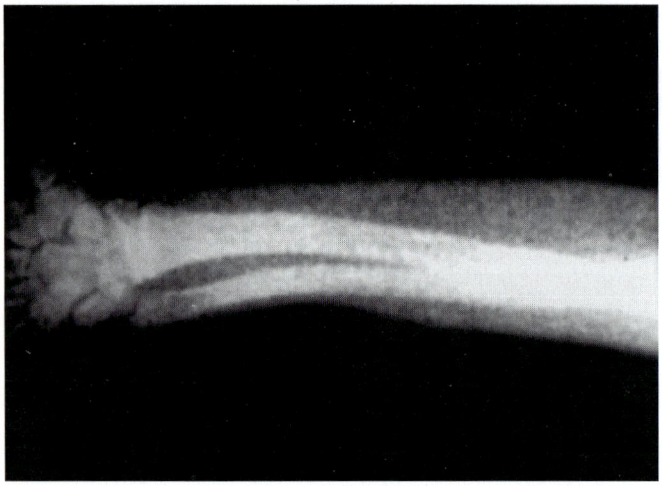

Fig. 10.1: Radiograph showing greenstick fracture of radius and ulna

Buckle fracture (Torus fracture) This is common in metaphyseal region and is due to compressive force. In this fracture cortex is buckled. Common at distal radius.

Treatment Treatment is by plaster cast or Futura type of wrist splint.

Plastic bowing Here bone deforms but does not break. Seen in paired bones. There is a microfracture on the concave side.

Epiphyseal injuries are discussed below.

Patterns of Fractures

- It is simple or compound. The latter variety is rare.
- The fracture in either case could be transverse, oblique, spiral, comminuted or segmental.

EPIPHYSEAL INJURIES

DEFINITION The epiphysis is a specialised growth cartilage of long bones and is most likely to be injured after the age of 10 years.

INCIDENCE

It accounts for nearly 17.9 per cent of all paediatric fractures. Fifteen per cent of these injuries cause growth arrest.

CAUSES

The junction between the metaphysis and the epiphysis is the weakest point of a long bone in children and is, therefore, most vulnerable to shearing forces.

TYPES

[1]Salter and Harris have classified epiphyseal injuries into five types (Fig. 10.2). Rang has added the sixth variety.

Type I Complete separation of epiphysis from the metaphysis without fracture. Common in rickets, scurvy and osteomyelitis.

Type II The fracture involves the physis and a triangle of metaphyseal bone (*Thurston Holland sign*). This is the commonest type of epiphyseal injury accounting for 73 per cent of cases over 10 years of age.

Type III The fracture is intra-articular and extends along the physis and then along the growth plate. This injury is relatively uncommon.

Type IV The fracture is intra-articular and extends through the epiphysis, physis and metaphysis. Perfect reduction is necessary and open reduction is more often necessary to prevent growth arrest.

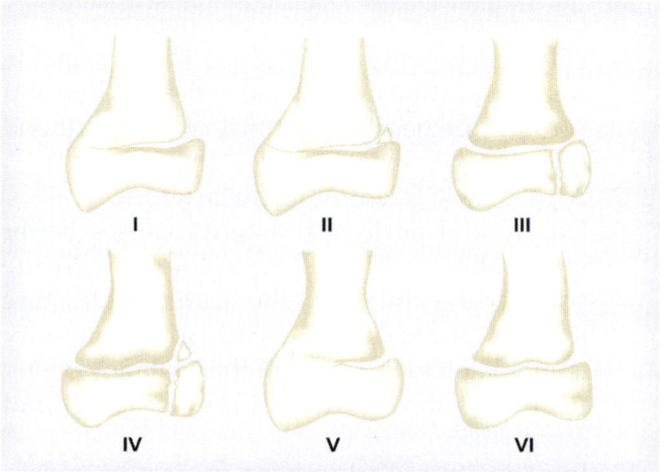

Fig. 10.2: Showing Salter and Harris classification of epiphyseal injuries

[1]**Harris WR, (Toronto) and Robert Salter (Toronto) 1963.** They also described innominate osteotomy for CDH.

Type V Crushing of epiphysis. Growth arrest usually follows.

Type VI There is a peripheral physis lesion and is described by Rang.

Investigations

A routine AP and lateral views of the plain X-ray of the affected limb is enough to make an accurate diagnosis in children.

TREATMENT

Problems of Treatment

- The younger child is fretful and difficult to examine fully.
- Worried parents and a crying child pose problems.
- Many fractures are difficult to see and need X-rays of good quality.
- General anaesthesia required for manipulation.
- Circulatory compromise is relatively common.
- Redisplacement after reduction is common during the first week.
- Wound care should be the same as in adults.
- *Overgrowth after long bone fracture is a very common problem and an overlap of 1 cm should be allowed.*

Remember

The general rules in treatment of fractures in children

- Angulation > 10° is unacceptable.
- Rotation will not be compensated and hence is not acceptable.
- Overlap of the fracture site by 1 to 2 cm is acceptable as there is overgrowth following a long bone fracture.
- Correction occurs at the average rate of 1° per month.

Treatment Options

Type I and II injuries can be managed by closed reduction. Type III and IV injuries usually require open reduction. Angular deformity and shortening are the consequences of premature growth arrest.

I. Conservative Methods

Masterly inactivity NSAIDs, crepe bandage, sling, etc. for undisplaced fractures.

Closed reduction and manipulation This is preferred if the fracture is displaced. Retention is usually by slab, cast and rarely by traction (Figs 10.3A and B).

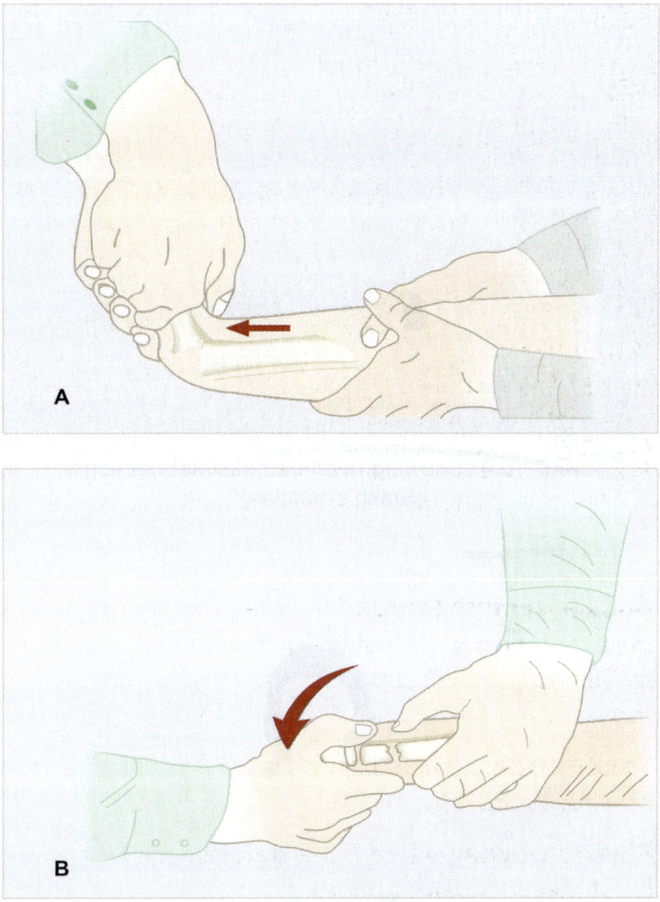

Figs 10.3A and B: Showing methods of closed reduction of a greenstick fracture in children: (A) The opposite intact cortex is broken, (B) The reduction is done

Closed reduction by traction This can also be attempted in certain situations, e.g. Gallow's traction, Dunlop's traction or overhead olecranon skeletal traction in difficult supracondylar fractures of humerus (Figs 10.4 to 10.6).

II. Surgery

Open reduction and internal fixation This is rarely done in children. Indications being failed closed reduction, redisplacement, multiple injuries, neurovascular injuries, delayed union and soft tissue interposition.

Closed reduction and percutaneous fixation Of late, this method of treatment is gaining popularity due to simplicity of technique and reduced complications rate associated with the open techniques.

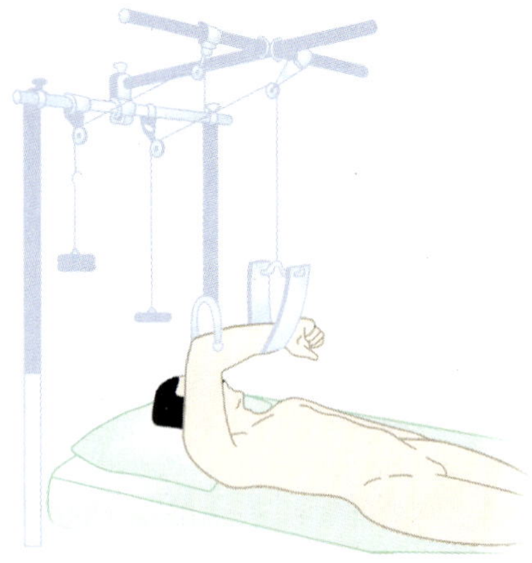

Fig. 10.4: Showing overhead skeletal traction (Smith's traction)

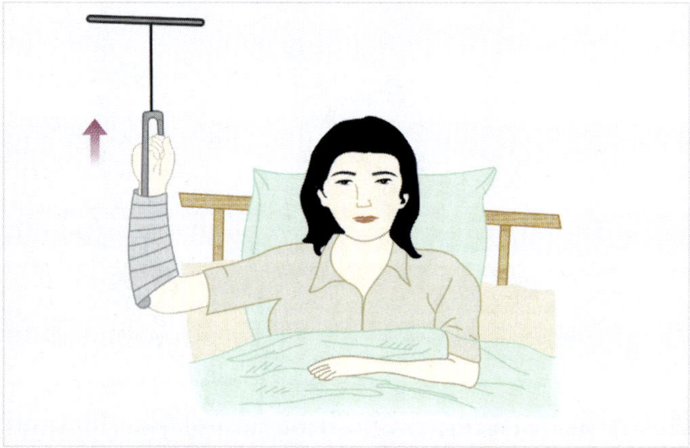

Fig. 10.5: Showing Dunlop's traction

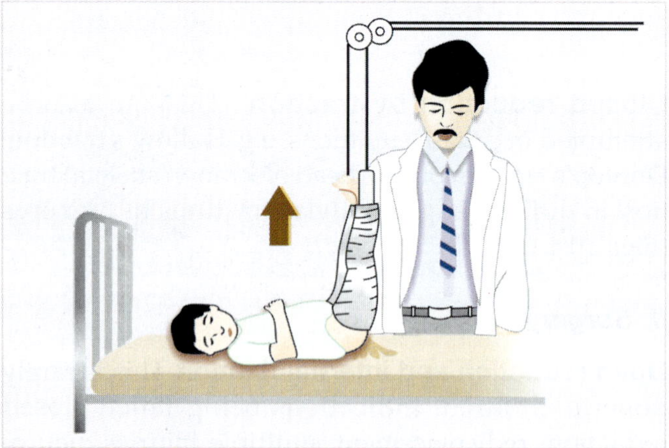

Fig. 10.6: Showing Gallow's traction in children (< 2 years of age)

The most popular example of this technique is closed reduction and percutaneous K-wire fixation of closed displaced supracondylar fracture of humerus in children (Fig. 10.7).

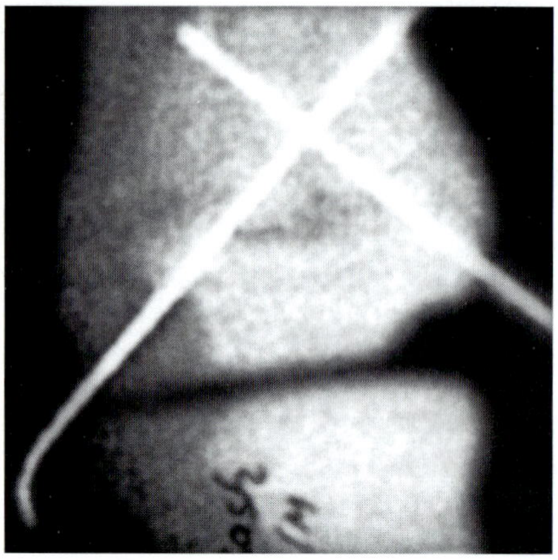

Fig. 10.7: Radiograph showing percutaneous fixation with K-wire of supracondylar fracture of humerus

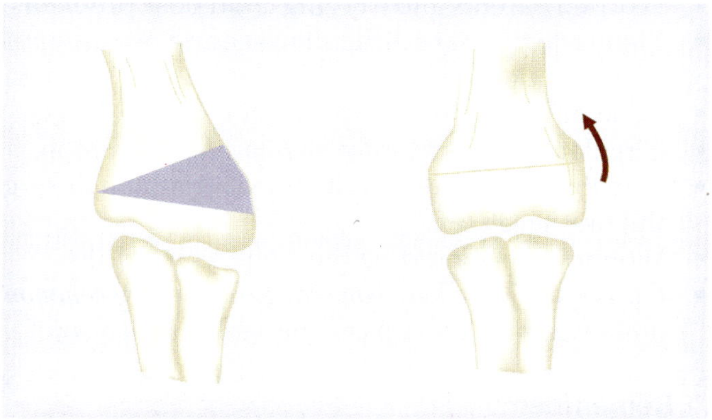

Fig. 10.8: Showing corrective osteotomy in malunited supracondylar fracture of humerus

Corrective osteotomy (Fig. 10.8) This is required in cubitus varus deformity due to malunited supracondylar fracture.

Remember

The principles of treatment in children

Three **Rs**

- **R**ealign the fracture.
- **R**espect the soft tissues.
- **R**emember the child.

COMPLICATIONS

1. Overgrowth—due to stimulation and hypervascularity due to epiphyseal injury.
2. Deformities—due to unequal damage of the epiphyseal plate.

3. Growth disturbances—due to crushing of the growth plate.
4. Growth arrest—due to damage of the growth plate.
5. Shortening —due to crushing of the growth plate.

Important Fractures in Children

1. Monteggia fractures.
2. Supracondylar fractures of humerus.
3. Greenstick fractures and torus fracture.
4. Radial neck fractures.
5. Fracture clavicle.
6. Fracture neck femur.
7. Epiphyseal injuries of ankle and distal end of radius, etc.

Some of these fractures are discussed in detail in appropriate chapters.

Disturbing facts: Do you know the problem fractures in children?

- *Supracondylar fracture of humerus* because of the fear of VIC.
- *Monteggia fracture* here radial head dislocation is often missed.
- *Epiphyseal injuries* leads to growth abnormalities in children.

PATHOLOGICAL FRACTURES

When a fracture occurs through a bone which has already been weakened by a generalised or localised skeletal disorder, it is called a pathological fracture. Unlike traumatic fractures, these fractures take place either spontaneously or due to trivial trauma (Figs 10.9A to E).

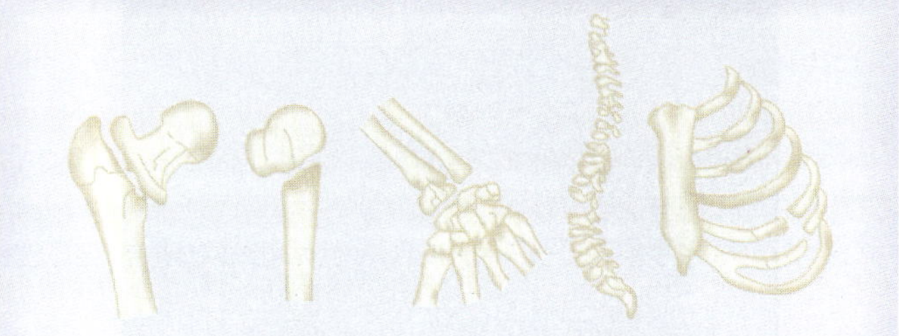

Figs 10.9A to E: Common sites of pathological fractures A—Neck of femur, B—Neck of humerus, C—Distal end of radius, D—Compression fracture of vertebra, E—Fracture of ribs

'Quick glance' at the causes of pathological fractures

1. **Localised diseases**
   a. *Infective disorders*
      - Chronic pyogenic osteomyelitis
      - Tubercular or syphilitic osteomyelitis

   b. *Neoplasms*

      Benign
      - Chondroma
      - Giant cell tumour
      - Haemangioma spine (lung, breast prostate, kidney, etc.)
      - Bone atrophy (e.g. polio, etc.)
      - Tabes dorsalis, etc.

      Malignant
      - Osteogenic sarcoma
      - Ewing's sarcoma
      - Solitary myeloma
      - Metastatic carcinoma
      - Metastatic sarcoma

   c. *Miscellaneous cause*
      - Simple bone cyst
      - Monostotic fibrous dysplasia
      - Eosinophilic granuloma

2. **General affections of bone**
   a. *Congenital disorders*
      - Osteogenesis imperfecta.
      - Fibrous dysplasia
      - Gaucher's disease, etc.

   b. *Generalised rarefaction of bones*
      - Senile osteoporosis
      - Hyperparathyroidism
      - Osteomalacia
      - Nutritional rickets
      - Scurvy

   c. *Miscellaneous*
      - Multiple myeloma
      - Diffuse metastatic carcinoma

   d. *Disseminated tumours*
      - Paget's disease
      - Fibrous dysplasia
      - Gaucher's disease, etc.

CLINICAL FEATURES

The patient usually complains of fracture following a trivial trauma. He or she complains of having suffered pain or discomfort in the region of the affected bone some time before the fracture. The underlying cause for this could be either a generalised disorder or a local skeletal disorder.

Practical point

Common causes for pathological fractures

I. **Local disorders**
   a. *Metastatic carcinoma*
   The primary could be in the lungs, breast, prostate, thyroid or kidney.
   Common sites
   - Vertebral bodies (thoracic/lumbar).
   - Proximal half of femoral shaft.
   - Proximal half of humerus.

   b. *Bone cyst* of a long bone.

II. **Generalised disorders**
   a. *Senile osteoporosis*
   Common sites affected are
   - Thoracic or lumbar vertebral body.
   - Neck or trochanteric region of femur.

   b. *Paget's disease of bone*
   - Shaft of tibia or femur.

Investigations

- *Laboratory investigation* This includes Hbs, TG, DG, ESR, serum Ca, P, alkaline and acid phosphatase, etc.
- X-ray of the affected bones.
- CT scan and MRI are of extreme importance to determine the extent of pathological involvement.
- Bone scan is helpful in determining the spread of disease.

Treatment

Conservative treatment has little role in the treatment of pathological fractures. The treatment recommended is open reduction, rigid internal fixation with or without cement and bone grafting. The aim is to obtain quick union and mobilise the patient early. Pathological fractures due to Paget's disease, osteogenesis imperfecta, etc. unite in the usual time, fractures due to osteomyelitis, bone cyst unite late but fractures due to malignancy, metastasis do not unite at all though union is possible after chemotherapy or radiotherapy.

Do you know the most common causes of pathologic fractures?
- Osteoporosis first
- Metastasis into the bones next

FATIGUE OR STRESS FRACTURES

Definition Fatigue or stress fractures occur mainly in normal bones due to repeated stress or minor trauma to a particular bone usually of the lower limbs.

Clinical Features

Here there is no single specific causative injury as in a traumatic fracture. The onset of pain is gradual or insidious. Activity increases the pain and rest relieves it. On examination, there is significant local tenderness, thickening of bone, local swelling, etc.

Vital facts: Stress fractures

Who are prone for stress fractures? In alphabetical order
- Athletes
- Dancers
- Doctors
- Nurses
- Policemen
- Soldiers
- Sportspersons
- Surgeons
- Unknown group

Radiology

Radiograph of the part at first may not reveal any fractures but may be seen after 3 to 4 weeks. The fracture itself will be hairline, transverse and undisplaced. More striking than the fracture is a zone of callus that surrounds it (Fig. 10.10).

Bone Scan This is of great help in determing the presence of stress fracture (Fig. 10.11).

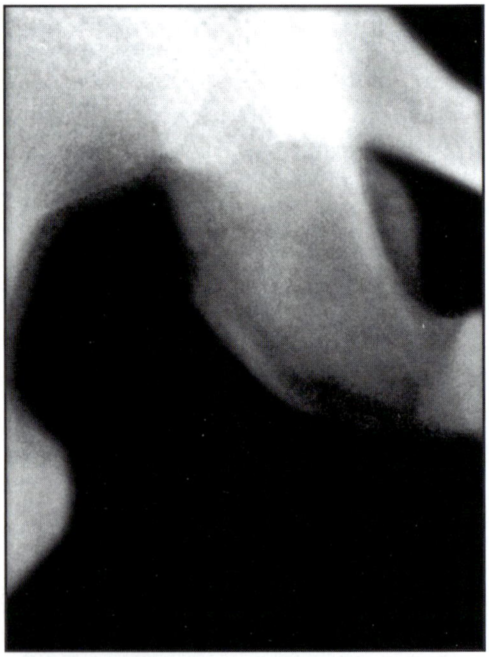

Fig. 10.10: Radiograph showing stress fracture of the ischium

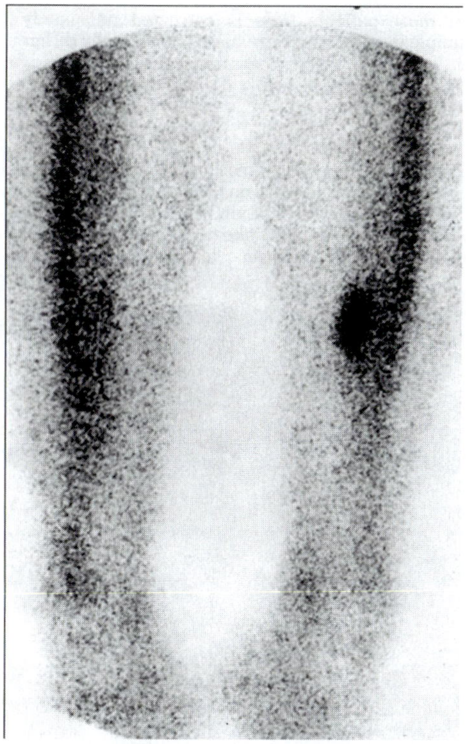

Fig. 10.11: Stress fracture tibia—scintigram

MRI and CT Scan There are the other useful investigations but are expensive.

Treatment

Stress fractures usually heal by rest and support to the affected part.

Practical points: Stress fractures

a. *Common sites*
   - Second and third metatarsal bone—e.g. March fracture (due to repeated marching as in soldiers) (Fig. 10.12).
   - Tibia or fibula—repeated running or dancing.
   - Femur—occasionally.

b. *Radiology*
   - I week—usually no fracture is detected.
   - II/III week—faint hairline fracture, transverse/undisplaced.
   - Zone of callus that surrounds the fracture is more significant than the fracture itself.

c. *Treatment is by rest*

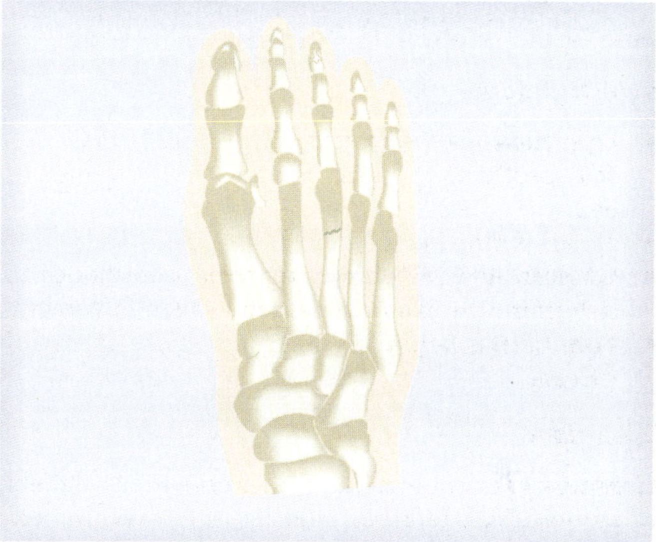

Fig. 10.12: Showing stress fracture of III metatarsal bone

SECTION TWO

REGIONAL TRAUMATOLOGY

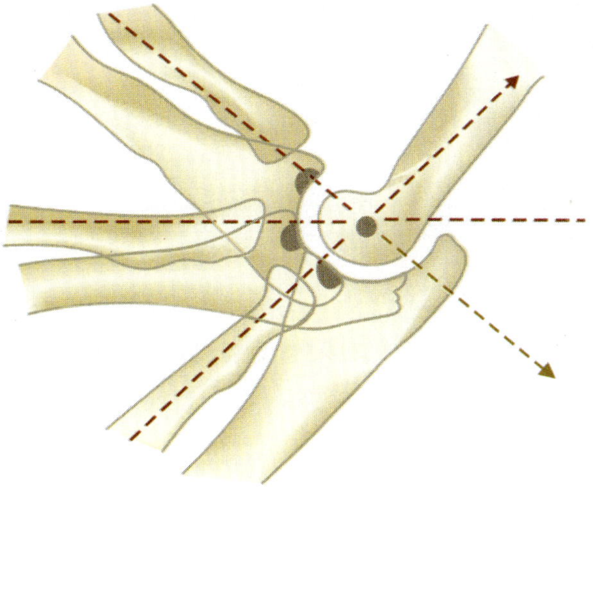

11 Injuries Around the Shoulder

INTRODUCTION

The shoulder joint complex consists of the glenohumeral joint, the acromioclavicular joint and sternoclavicular joint. The injuries concerning all the three joints and the fractures involving the clavicle, scapula and proximal humerus are discussed in this chapter.

FRACTURE CLAVICLE

The term clavicle (Fig. 11.1) is derived from the Latin root *Clavis* meaning *Key*. Clavicle is 'S' shaped and is linked to the music symbol 'clavicula', hence the name.

THE CLAVICLE SPEAKS

- I am the first bone to ossify in the body.
- I ossify from two primary centres.
- I am the only long bone in the body lying horizontal.
- I am the only long bone ossifying from a membrane.
- I am the only link between the appendicular and the axial skeleton.
- I am the most common bone to be fractured in children.
- I invariably end up maluniting after the fracture.

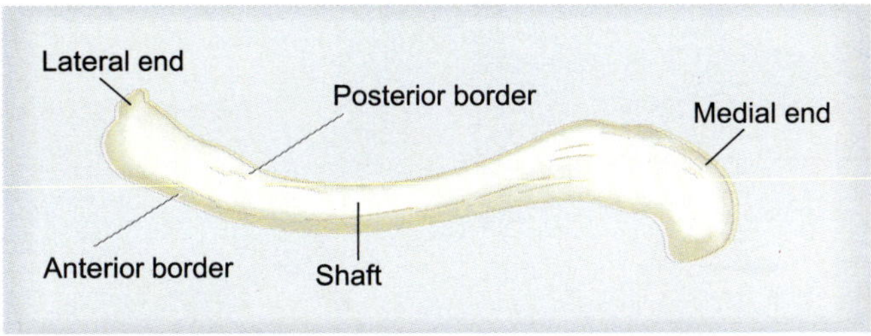

Fig. 11.1: Bony anatomy of the clavicle

FUNCTIONS OF CLAVICLE

1. It increases the arm strength mechanism.
2. It protects the neurovascular bundle consisting of subclavian vessels and brachial plexus.
3. It gives attachments to important muscles around the shoulder.
4. It braces the shoulder back during rest and motion (Strut function).

Mechanism of Injury

Direct Due to fall on the point of the shoulder. This is the most common mode of injury accounting for 91 per cent of the cases (See Fig. 11.7).

Direct trauma over the clavicle due to RTA, etc. accounts for 8 per cent of the cases (Fig. 11.2).

Indirect Fall on the outstretched hands accounts for 1 per cent of the cases.

Sites of Fracture

- Eighty-five per cent of the fracture clavicle occurs at the junction of middle and outer third (Fig. 11.3)
- One per cent at the medial end of the clavicle (5%)
- Lateral end fracture is uncommon (About 10%). (Distal 1/3rd).

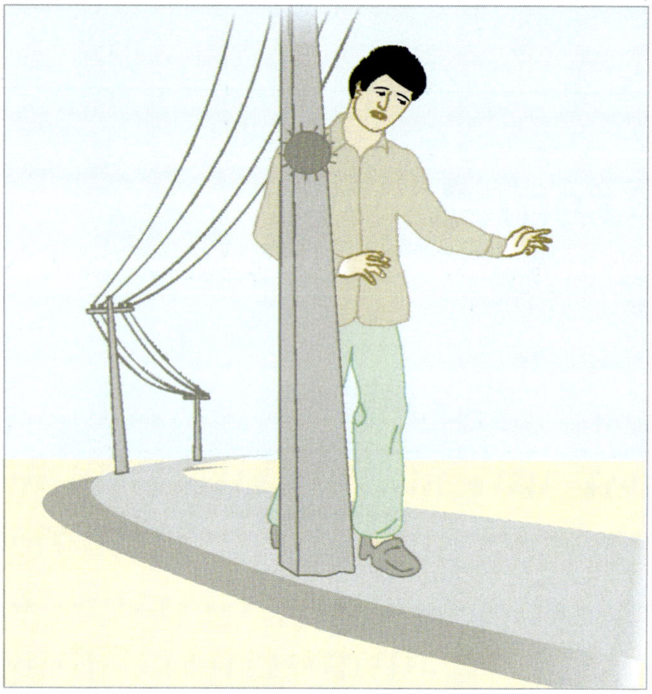

Fig. 11.2: A recklessness like this can break your clavicle bone due to direct injury

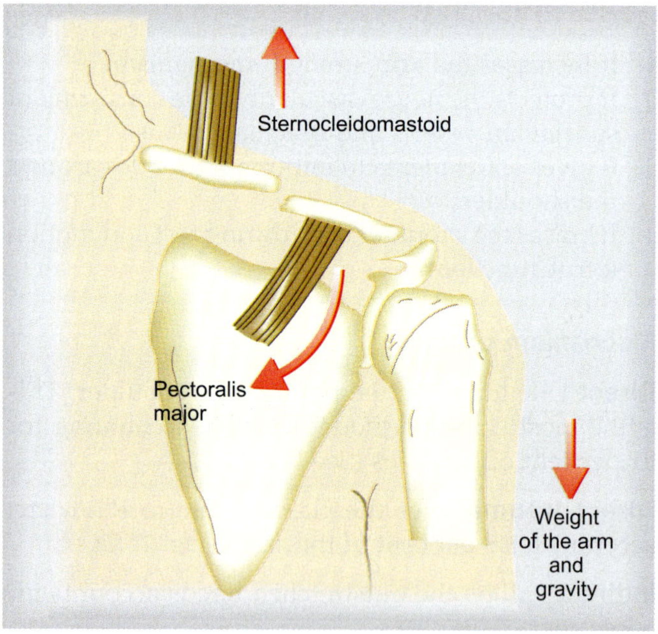

Fig. 11.3: Showing various displacing forces in fracture clavicle

Classification of Fracture Clavicle (Allman's)

Group I are fractures involving middle one-third of the shaft.

Group II are fractures involving the lateral third distal to the attachment of the coracoclavicular ligament. This is further subdivided into two subgroups (Proposed by Neer):

- *Type A* Coracoclavicular ligament intact.
- *Type B* Coracoclavicular ligament ruptured.
- *Type C* Intra-articular extension into ACM joint.

Group III These are medial third fractures.

Clinical Features

The patient presents with pain, swelling, deformity and inability to raise the shoulder. Rarely, the patient may present with pseudoparalysis of the affected arm.

Radiology (Fig. 11.4)

The following views are recommended:

1. Routine AP view of the clavicle.
2. Lordotic view if the fracture is doubtful.
3. Distal clavicle requires special radiography technique.

Principles of Treatment

Before proceeding to the treatment proper one needs to understand the two distracting forces acting on the fracture fragments in clavicle making the treatment difficult (see Fig. 11.2). The medial end of the clavicle is pulled up by the sternocleidomastoid muscle and the lateral end is pulled down by the pectoralis major muscle and gravity acting through the arm.

To counter the above two detrimental forces, the shoulder should be braced up and back and the arm should be supported while treating fracture clavicle.

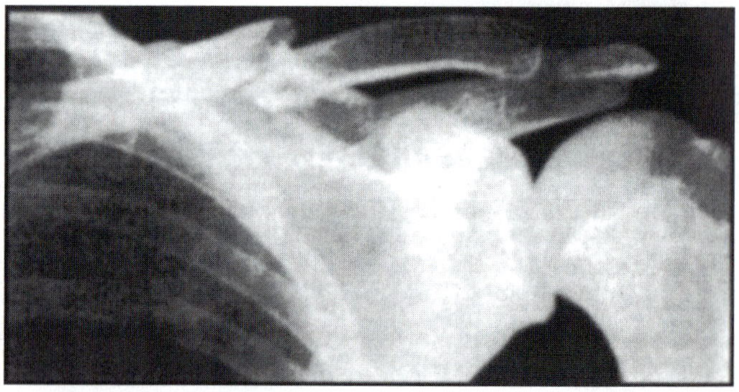

Fig. 11.4: Radiograph showing fracture clavicle of middle third

Conservative Methods

This is the treatment of choice in fracture clavicle and consists of the following methods:

Cuff and collar sling for undisplaced fractures (Fig. 11.5A).

Strapping of the fracture site after reduction of the fracture by elevating the arm and bracing the shoulder upwards and backwards gives good results both in children and adults (Fig. 11.5B).

Sabre method consists of rigid dressing over the fracture. This is no longer used.

Billington Yoke method uses a plaster of Paris over a well-padded figure of '8' dressing.

Figure of '8' This is popularly used and it acts by retracting the shoulder girdle, minimises the overlap and allows more anatomical healing. *It does not immobilise the fracture but acts by serving as a reminder to the patient to hold the shoulder up and back neutralising the forces mentioned above. If they allow the shoulder to slump forward, then the support cuts into the anterior axilla and reminds them to hold the shoulders back* (Fig. 11.5C).

Treatment Plan

Newborn to preambulatory children Treated symptomatically, bind arm to the chest.

Ambulatory stage (2-12 yr) Figure of 8 bandage, tightened after three days and later one week.

Twelve years to maturity Commercially available figure of 8 harness.

Surgery is rarely indicated and consists of open reductions and rigid internal fixation.

Methods of Internal Fixation

- Intramedullary fixation with K-wires
- Rigid plate and screw fixation (Fig. 11.6).

Indications

Open fractures, injury to neurovascular bundle, if the fracture is threatening to penetrate the skin, non-union, fracture near acromioclavicular joint, and displaced epiphysis in children.

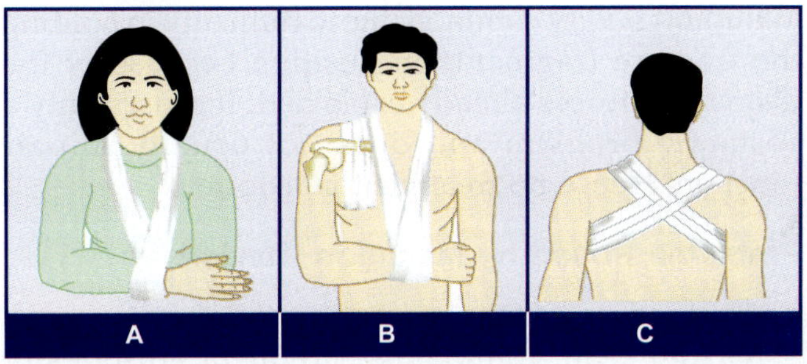

Figs 11.5A to C: Methods of conservative treatment of fractures clavicle: (A) collar and cuff sling, (B) strapping and sling suspension, (C) figure of 8 bandaging

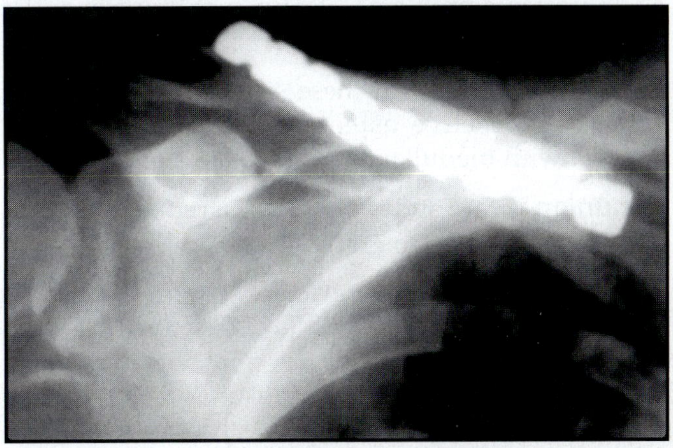

Fig. 11.6: Radiograph showing fracture clavicle plate fixation

More Specific Indications for Open Reduction and Internal Fixation of Fracture Clavicle

- Shortening or distraction of fragments for more than 2 cm.
- More than 100% displacement or fragmentation.
- Bilateral fractures.

Complications of Fracture Clavicle

Neurovascular injury may be immediate due to direct force or delayed due to a very large callus. The structures commonly injured are subclavian vessels and the medial cord of the brachial plexus through which the ulnar nerve is derived. This occurs in fractures of the middle one-third of the clavicle which is the most common.

Did you know?

- The ulnar nerve is the commonest nerve to be injured in fracture clavicle due to its compression between it and the first rib

Malunion is very common due to difficulty in holding the fracture fragments in position because of the distracting forces already explained. It causes only a cosmetic problem and does not usually impair function. Hence no treatment is required.

Problems Posed by Malunion Clavicle

- Cosmetic complaints—mentioned above.
- Orthopaedic complaints—frequent episodes of shoulder fatigue.
- Sleep problems—the patient complains of inability to sleep on the sides.
- Neurologic problems—features of thoracic outlet syndrome.

Remedy If faced with these situations, the patient requires corrective osteotomy and rigid internal fixation with medullary pins or plate and screws.

Nonunion is rare and requires open reduction, internal fixation and bone grafting.

Quick facts: Fracture clavicle

- Most common fracture in children.
- Common mode of injury is direct.
- 80 per cent break at junction of middle and distal third.
- Nearly all fractures are treated closed.
- Open reduction for specific indications.
- Malunion is a rule, but no functional disability.

INJURIES OF THE ACROMIOCLAVICULAR JOINT

Acromioclavicular (ACM) joint is a diarthrodial joint with a fibrocartilaginous disc between the two bones (similar to a meniscus).

THE ACROMIOCLAVICULAR JOINT SPEAKS

- I am essentially a plane joint. I permit gliding rotation between the clavicle and the scapula. My structural integrity depends on the intrinsic capsular element, the superior acromioclavicular ligament and the extrinsic coracoclavicular ligament which forms a hood over the interval between the coracoid process and the acromion

Incidence is 12 per cent and is common in the young. Male : Female ratio is 5:1.

Do you know

- The common name for ACL injury is shoulder separation.
- ACL injuries are 4 to 5 times more common than sternoclavicular injuries

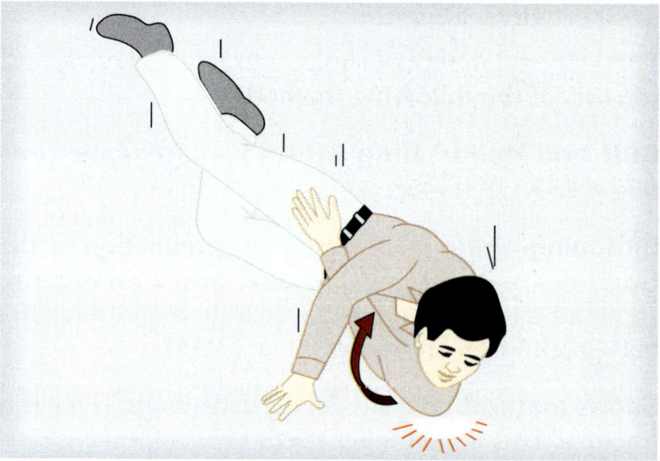

Fig. 11.7: Showing the most common mechanism of injury of ACM joint

Mechanism of Injury

Direct force This is the most common mechanism (Fig. 11.7) of injury as in RTA, assault, athletic events like the tackling, etc.

Indirect force is due to fall on the outstretched hands.

Downward indirect force through the upper extremity This is relatively rare.

Clinical Features

The patient complains of pain, swelling, and difficulty in raising the arm up. The patient supports the affected shoulder by holding the elbow with unaffected hand. On examination, there is tenderness and the lateral end of clavicle is prominently felt (Fig. 11.8).

Classification (Sage and Salvatore's)

Based on injuries to acromioclavicular and coracoclavicular ligaments (Fig. 11.9):

Type I Minor sprain to acromioclavicular ligaments.

Type II Rupture of ACL, sprain of CCL.

Type III Both ACL and CCL ruptured, clavicle is displaced upwards.

Type IV Same as type III , but with upward and posterior displacement of clavicle.

Type V Type III with severe displacement of the clavicle towards base of the neck.

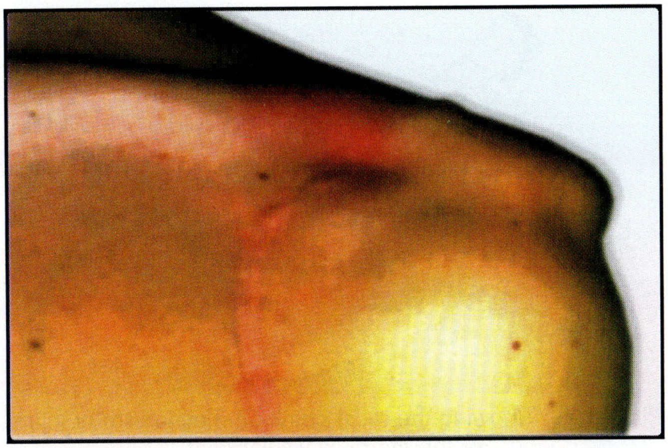

Fig. 11.8: ACM joint injury, the clinical appearance

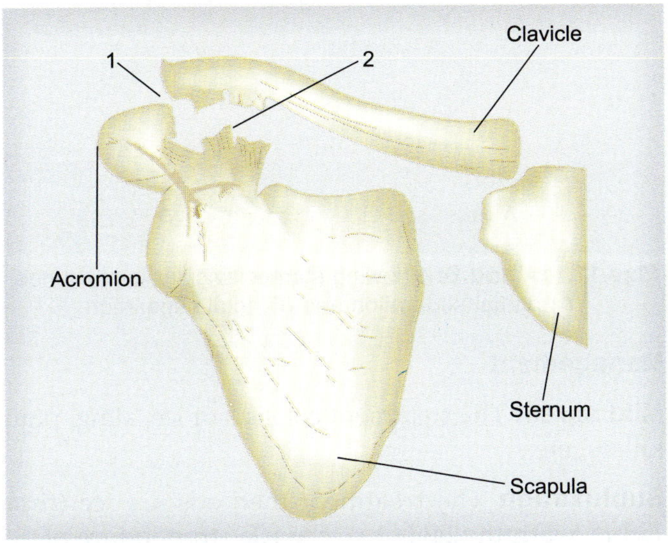

Fig. 11.9: Acromioclavicular joint injury shows: (1) ruptured acromioclavicular ligament (ACL), and (2) ruptured coracoclavicular ligament (CCL)

Type VI Inferior dislocation with clavicle towards base of the neck.

Radiology

The following views are required:

1. AP view with 15° cephalic tilt to prevent overlap of the spine of scapula on routine AP views.
2. Lateral view—axillary view of the shoulder.
3. Stress radiographs—to differentiate from type II and type III by suspending a weight of 10 to 15 lbs around the wrist.

Management

Type I Rest, ice bags, NSAIDS, etc.

Type II Sling for 10 to 14 days, adhesive strapping, elastic strapping, cast or harness. Surgery is required for persisting pain.

Type III Conservative methods like reduction and retention with sling and harness.

Surgical methods include:

1. Acromioclavicular repair.
2. Coracoclavicular repair.
3. Excision of distal end of clavicle for old symptomatic cases.
4. Dynamic muscle transfer by transferring the coracoid process.

Types IV, V, VI Require open reduction, internal fixation, repair and reconstruction.

Complications

1. Associated fracture clavicle.
2. Coracoclavicular ossification.
3. Osteolysis of distal clavicle.
4. Complications after surgery like infection, etc.
5. Complications after non-operative treatment like joint stiffness, periarthritis, etc.

Delayed complications: These include:

- Step-like deformity
- ACM joint arthritis
- Pain during weightlifting.

INJURIES OF STERNOCLAVICULAR JOINT

THE STERNOCLAVICULAR JOINT SPEAKS

- I am a saddle joint and represent the only bone-to-bone connection of the upper limb to the trunk. To absorb the shock transmitted from the arm to the shoulder, I have a fibrocartilaginous disc between clavicle and the manubrii. I derive my structural strength from the interclavicular and costoclavicular ligaments along with the anterior and posterior sternoclavicular ligaments. The intra-articular disc ligaments and the capsular ligaments strengthen me to a great extent.

Mechanism of Injury

This is the least commonly dislocated joint because of the strong ligaments.

Section 2

Direct force rarely causes this injury. For example, collision of an athlete with another person or a post, etc.

Indirect force this is the most common mode of injury. For example loading the upper shoulder while someone lies on the sides (Fig. 11.10).

Incidence is about three per cent and is more common in young males.

Causes

Road traffic accident (RTA) is responsible for 80 per cent of the cases, sports-related injuries account for the remaining 20 per cent.

Classifications (Figs 11.11A and B)

Anatomical classification
- Anterior dislocation (more common)
- Posterior dislocation

Aetiological classification
- *Traumatic*
  - Sprain
  - Acute dislocation
  - Recurrent dislocation
  - Unreduced dislocation.
- *Atraumatic*
  - Voluntary
  - Involuntary
  - Congenital
  - Degenerative
  - Infective.

Clinical Features

The patient complains of pain and swelling. Medial end of the clavicle is prominent in anterior dislocation. Affected shoulder is short. Lateral compression test is positive.

Radiology

1. AP view is often difficult to interpret.
2. Special 90° cephalocaudal views—this helps to see the medial ends of both the clavicles (serendipity view).
3. Tomograms are useful.
4. CT scans and MRI help to study the position of clavicle with respect to sternum and soft tissues respectively.

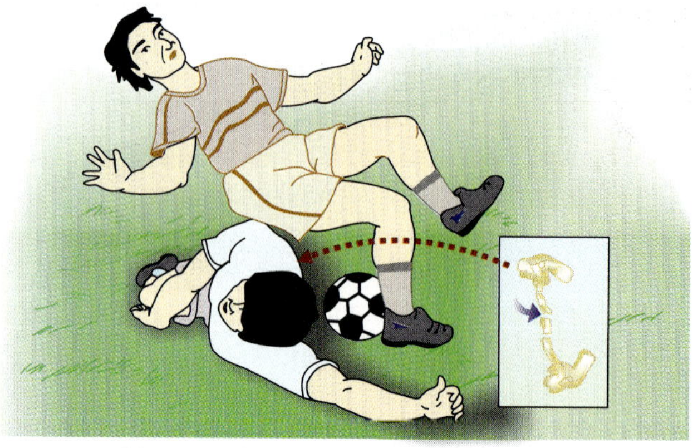

Fig. 11.10: Showing the most common mechanism of injury of the sternoclavicular joint

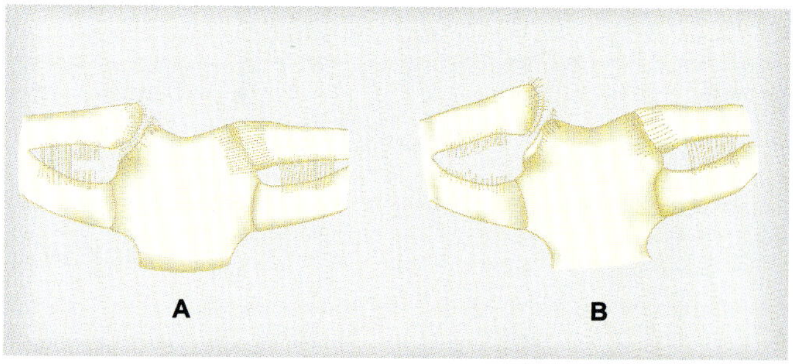

Figs 11.11A and B: Showing sternoclavicular joint injuries: (A) partial separation and (B) total separation

Management

Mild sprain The treatment consists of ice, sling, pain killers, etc.

Subluxation The treatment methods are ice (first 12 hr), warmth (24-48 hr), clavicle strap, figure of '8' and excision of medial end if pain persists.

Dislocation The treatment of choice is closed reduction by firm digital pressure followed by figure of 8, clavicle strap, sling, etc. If it fails, open reduction and internal fixation using K-wire is done.

PROXIMAL HUMERAL FRACTURES

This is common in elderly patients and it accounts for 4 to 5 per cent of all fractures. It is more common in elderly females due to osteoporosis.

Mechanism

- Fall on the outstretched hands is the classical history.
- Blow on the lateral side of the arm is the other mode of injury.

Classification

Four segments are described with respect to proximal humerus. They are the:

1. Anatomical neck (incidence of AVN is high)
2. Greater tuberosity
3. Lesser tuberosity
4. Shaft or surgical neck of the humerus. Incidence of AVN is less.

Neer has proposed a classification for fractures of the proximal humerus based on this 4-segment concept.

Role of Muscle Forces (Fig. 11.12)

1. *Greater tuberosity:* Supraspinatus, external rotators are attached here and displace the fracture segments up.
2. *Lesser tuberosity:* Subscapularis inserted here which generates a deforming force and displaces medially.
3. *Shaft:* It gives attachment to pectoralis major, which causes medial and internal rotation.
4. *Anatomical neck.*

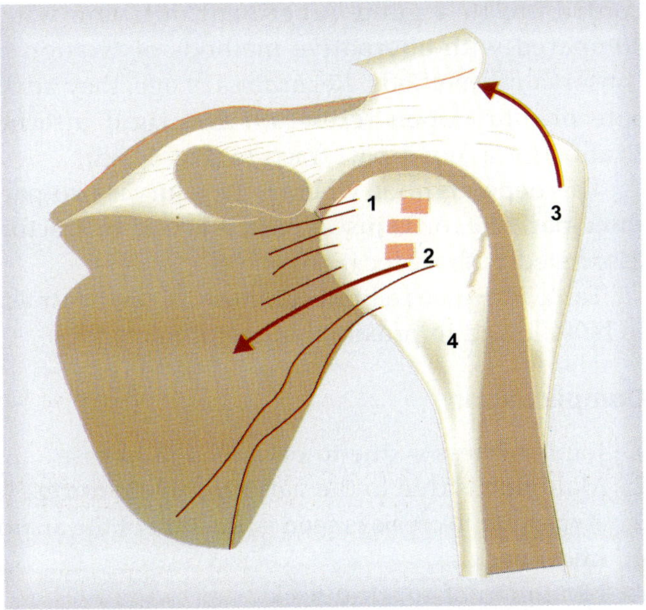

Fig. 11.12: Four segments represented by: (1) anatomical neck, (2) lesser tuberosity being pulled by subscapularis, (3) greater tuberosity pulled by supraspinatus, and (4) surgical neck or shaft

These above muscles pull the fracture fragments in different directions leading to widespread displacements and angulations. When any of the 4 major segments is displaced more than 1 cm or angulated more than 45°, fracture is considered displaced. Eighty per cent of the fracture displacement is minimal and only 20 per cent of the fracture displacement is significant.

There are four major categories of fractures as described by Neer.[1] *Earlier, the number of fracture lines were taken into account to label the proximal humerus fractures as two-part, three-part and four-part fractures. But now the number of "displaced segments" is taken into consideration than the earlier "number of fracture lines".* Thus, for clarity, it can be said that:

A one-part fracture is fracture with minimal displacement.

A two-part fracture is where one segment is displaced in relation to the other.

A three-part fracture is where two segments are displaced in relation to the other two.

A four-part fracture where all four major segments are displaced.

These above fractures when associated either with anterior dislocation or with posterior dislocation of shoulder are called two-part fracture dislocation, three-part fracture dislocation, etc. (Figs 11.13A to D).

Clinical Features

The patient complains of pain, swelling and other features of fractures. Movements of the shoulder joint are grossly restricted.

Radiology and Other Investigations

1. Trauma series consists of AP view and lateral view of shoulder joint in scapular plane (Fig. 11.14).
2. Axillary view of the shoulder.
3. Laminagrams to judge the articular defects.
4. CT scan helps to study the fracture lines with greater accuracy.

[1]**CS Neer** (1970) USA. He also described replacement arthroplasty for glenohumeral osteoarthritis.

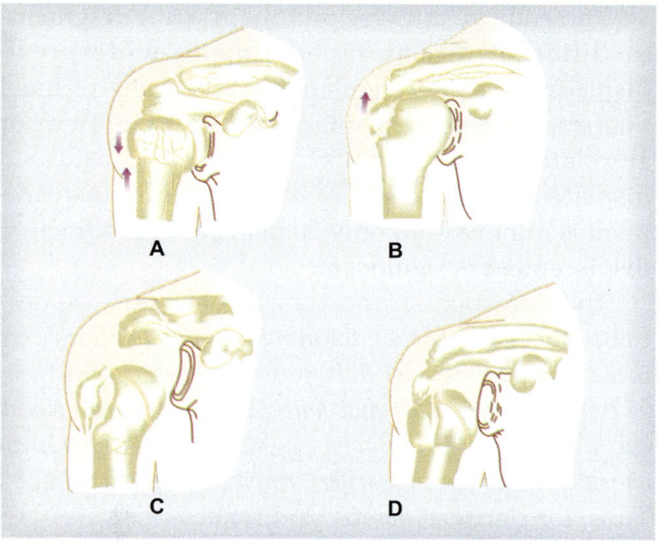

Figs 11.13A to D: Showing (A) 2-part surgical neck, (B) 2-part greater tuberosity, (C) 3-part fracture, (D) 4-part fracture

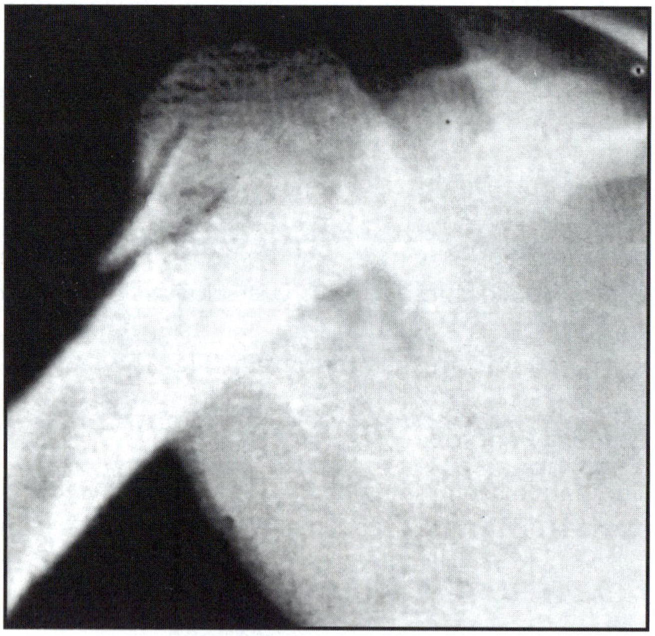

Fig. 11.14: Radiograph showing proximal humeral fracture

Management

Non-operative Treatment

Indications

- Undisplaced fractures
- Surgical neck fractures
- Poor health
- Poor surgical risks
- Very old patients.

Conservative treatment consists of rest, NSAIDs, sling, ice and heat therapy in the initial stages.

Since 80 per cent of the fractures are minimally displaced, early motion of the shoulder is the mainstay of treatment to prevent stiffness of the joint.

Pendulum exercises, elevation, pulley, external and internal rotation and wall climbing exercises are some of the recommended methods, in the later stages.

Treatment facts

- About 80 to 85% of proximal humeral fracture can be treated by conservative methods.

Operative Treatment

Hinterman et al advocate rigid internal fixation of displaced fracture of the proximal humerus in older patients with a blade-plate device and this provides sufficient primary stability to allow early functional treatment.

Restoration of anatomy and biomechanics may contribute to a good functional outcome when compared with alternative methods of fixation or conservative methods. Regardless of age, they advocate primary open reduction and rigid internal fixation for a 3-or 4-part fracture (Fig. 11.15).

This depends upon whether the injury is two-part, three-part, etc. or is just a plain fracture or fracture associated with dislocation.

Table 11.1 gives a brief summary of the treatment to be followed in proximal humeral fractures.

Complications

1. Joint stiffness is due to periarticular fibrosis.
2. Malunion is due to the varying muscle forces.
3. Avascular necrosis is seen in fracture of the anatomical neck.
4. Nonunion of surgical neck.
5. Myositis ossificans due to vigorous massage and treatment.

Mystifying facts

- Did you know that axillary nerve is the most commonly injured nerve in proximal humeral fractures?

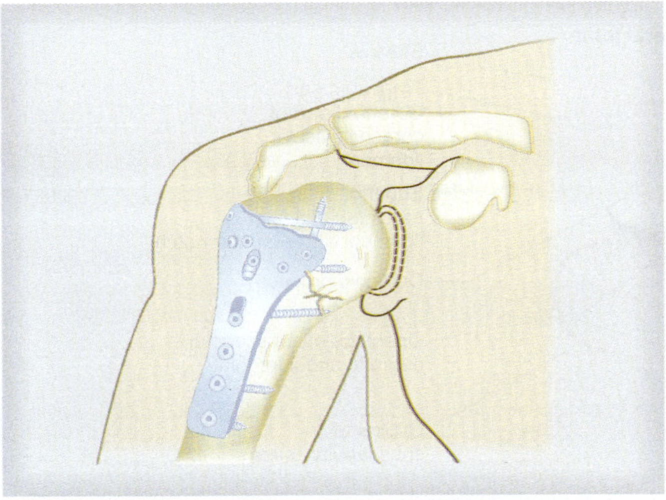

Fig. 11.15: Method of fixation of proximal humeral fracture with T-plate and screws

Table 11.1: Summary of operative treatment followed in proximal humeral fractures

Pattern

1. *Two-part fracture*
   a. *Anterior neck* OR + IF (risk of AVN is high)
   b. Shaft
      • Impacted and angulated → Disimpaction and correction
      • Unimpacted → Closed reduction if reducible. Tension-band wiring if unreducible or T-plate
      • Comminuted → overhead skeletal traction
   c. *Greater tuberosity* If > 1cm displacement, OR + IF
   d. *Lesser tuberosity*: Requires OR+IF
2. *Three-part fracture*
   • Needs open reduction and replacement of the humeral head with Neer's prosthesis or a AO T-plate can be used for fixing the fracture fragment.
3. *Four-part fracture*
   • Invariably require OR + IF
   • When fracture is associated with dislocation:

1. Anterior dislocation with proximal humeral fracture
   a. 2 part → Closed reduction is successful
   b. 3 part → requires OR + IF with T-plate or circlage
   c. 4 part → OR + IF + tuberosity repair

2. Posterior dislocation with proximal humeral fractures
   a. 2 part: Associated with avulsion of lesser tuberosity. Closed reduction sufficient
   b. 3 part: Requires OR + IF
   c. 4 part: Risk of AVN is high and needs early prosthetic replacement (Neer's prosthesis)

What is new?

- Internal fixation with intramedullary locked nail (Polarus Nail) in proximal humeral fracture is fast gaining momentum.

THE GLENOHUMERAL JOINT SPEAKS

I am a multiaxial ball and socket joint. I am proud to be the most mobile joint in the body. Let me introduce my various components (Fig. 11.16) that I am made up of:

a. **Humeral head** It is approximately one-third of a sphere and is oriented at 45° from the long axis of the shaft and retroverted 30°. The indistinct anatomical neck consists two important landmarks, the lesser tuberosity anteromedially and the greater tuberosity superolaterally separated by the bicipital groove.

   The shallow-shaped glenoid cavity is anteverted approximately and inferiorly angulated 5° from the long axis of the scapula.

b. **Labrum** It is a fibrocartilage which is triangular in cross-section and is attached to the outer perimeter of the glenoid. It increases the contact area by 70 per cent and also helps me in my stability.

c. **Ligaments** The fibrous capsule gets attached peripherally to the margins of glenoid cavity and anatomic neck. I have three intrinsic capsular ligament called the glenohumeral ligaments which reinforce me. The coracohumeral ligament assists the capsule in supporting the arm.

d. **Rotator cuff** This is the name given to four inter-related muscles, infraspinatus, supraspinatus, subscapularis, and teres minor. By their co-ordinated activity, they provide me help in the finer adjustments of the humeral head within the glenoid cavity.

e. **Bursae** To provide smooth movements, I am aided by numerous bursae of which subdeltoid or subacromial bursa is the most important. I can carry out various activities like flexion, extension, adduction, abduction, internal and external rotation and circumduction with ease, thanks to the anatomy which the nature has designed for me.

DISLOCATION OF SHOULDER

Shoulder joint is vulnerable for dislocation more often than any other joint in the body. The extreme mobility it enjoys, jeopardises its stability. The shoulder has an "Achilles point" at the inferior part of the capsule providing the joint with a potential weak spot, so much so that 99 per cent of the anterior shoulder dislocation occur here. Ninety-five per cent of the shoulder dislocation is anterior and the remaining five per cent is posterior. An attempt is made here to

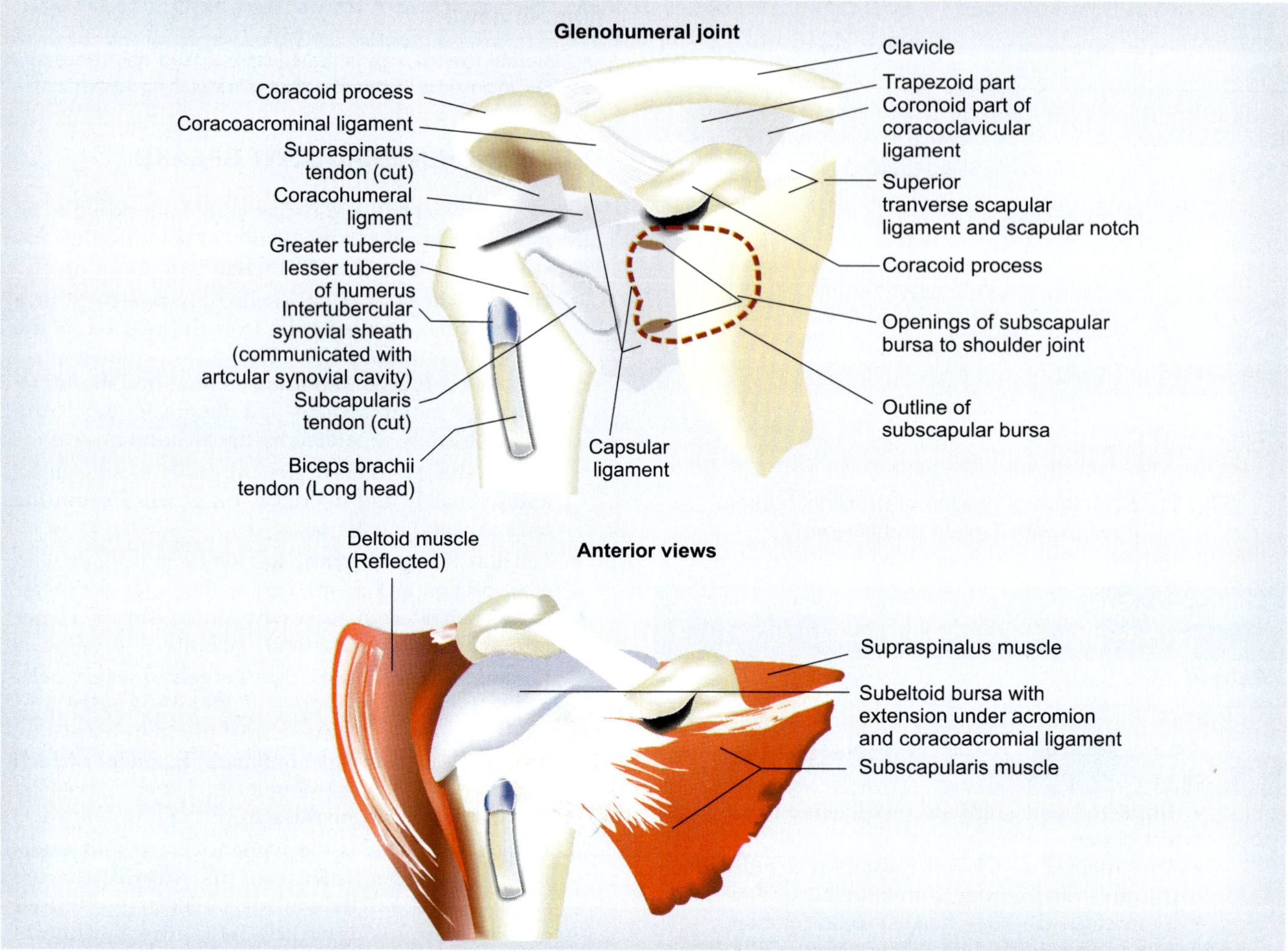

Fig. 11.16: Showing normal anatomy of shoulder joint

present a comparative study of both the dislocations for better understanding and easy remembrance (Table 11.2).

Matsen identifies two groups of dilocations with mnemonics TUBS denoting traumatic group, and AMBRI denoting atraumatic group. These are usually applied to anterior dislocation (Fig. 11.17) but can be applied to posterior dislocation also.

ANTERIOR DISLOCATION OF SHOULDER

As mentioned earlier, this is the most common type of shoulder dislocation.

Mechanism of Injury

It could be due to either direct or indirect forces. The latter is more common.

Varieties

The anterior dislocation of shoulder could be either subcoracoid, subglenoid, subclavicular or intrathoracic. Among these, the most common variety is the subglenoid (Figs 11.18A to E).

Clinical Features

The patient complains of severe pain and inability to use the shoulder joint. Flat shoulder, rounded anterior prominence and the arm held in a position of abduction and external rotation are some of the unmistakable clinical signs. Due to injury to the axillary nerve, there could be loss of sensation on the outer aspect, of the upper arm and is called the 'Regiment Badge' sign (Fig 11.19). Other clinical tests are denoted in the box (see page 122).

Table 11.2: Comparative study between anterior and posterior dislocation of shoulder

		Anterior Dislocation (95%)	Posterior Dislocation (5%)
1.	*Classification* *Traumatic injuries*	1. Sprains 2. Acute subluxation 3. Acute dislocation 4. Recurrent dislocation 5. Unreduced dislocation	1. Sprains 2. Acute subluxation 3. Acute dislocation 4. Recurrent dislocation 5. Unreduced posterior dislocation
	Atraumatic	1. Voluntary or habitual 2. Involuntary 3. Congenital	1. Voluntary 2. Involuntary 3. Congenital
	Based on anatomical location of humeral head	1. Subcoracoid* 2. Subglenoid* 3. Subclavicular 4. Intrathoracic	1. Subacromial 2. Subglenoid 3. Subspinous
2.	*Mechanism of injury*	• *Direct force* Blow from the posterior aspect of the shoulder • *Indirect force*—due to Abduction + External rotation + Extension injury (common)	• *Direct force* Blow from the anterior aspect of the shoulder • *Indirect force*—due to Internal rotation + Adduction + Flexion injury *(common)*
3.	*Clinical features for diagnosis*	• Severe pain • Arm is held in abduction and external rotation • Adduction is restricted • Normal contour of shoulder is lost and there is anterior shoulder fullness	• Severe pain • Arm is in position of adduction and internal rotation (Classical 'sling' position) • Abduction is restricted • Normal contour of shoulder is lost
	Clinical tests for diagnosis	• Posterior aspect is flat • Coracoid process is not identified • Axillary nerve injury may be present	• Posterior shoulder fullness present • Anterior aspect is flat • Coracoid process is more prominent
4.	*X-ray views taken:* 1. Routine X-rays in AP view in internal and external rotations 2. AP view in plane of scapula. 3. Axillary lateral view. 4. True scapula lateral view	• *Bankart's lesions* (Lateral defect anterior). • *Hill-Sachs lesion* (posterolateral defect in the head of the humerus seen in 100% of cases). • *Erosions of rim of glenoid*	• Anterolateral defect • *Vacant glenoid sign* (Fig. 11.22) • *Daylight sign* (complete gap) • *"The trough line"*. Similar to Hill-Sachs lesion and is found on the anteromedial aspect of the head of the humerus
5.	*Transthoracic lateral X-ray* 5. Diagrammatic representation of dislocations *Other investigations* • *Arthrography*: It is more helpful to evaluate rotator cuff tears due to previous dislocations. • *CT scan*: It helps to detect the defect in the head more accurately. • *MRI*: It is very useful to evaluate both soft tissue and bony injuries.	C-shaped rolling line (Fig. 11.21)	V-shaped rolling line (Figs 11.23A and B)

Contd...

Table 11.2: Contd...			
		Anterior Dislocation (95%)	*Posterior Dislocation (5%)*
6.	*Techniques of reduction*	I. Closed reduction: 3 methods 1. *Hippocrate's method* Reduction with foot in the axilla 2. *Stimson's gravity method:* Patient is in prone position with weight attached to the wrist. Gravity helps in reduction 3. *Kocher's method* Most effective and commonly followed method. II. Open reduction: This is indicated in failed closed reduction, soft tissue interposition, greater tuberosity fracture displaced > 1 cm after reduction and large glenoid rim fractures	Reduction under general anaesthesia Distal traction on the injured limb with lateral rotation on the upper arm.
7.	*Complications*	• Recurrent dislocation • Unreduced dislocation • Traumatic osteoarthritis • The risk of developing secondary osteoarthritis following anterior dislocation of shoulder is 10 to 20 times greater than normal people • Axillary nerve damage	• Recurrent dislocation • Unreduced dislocation • Traumatic osteoarthritis

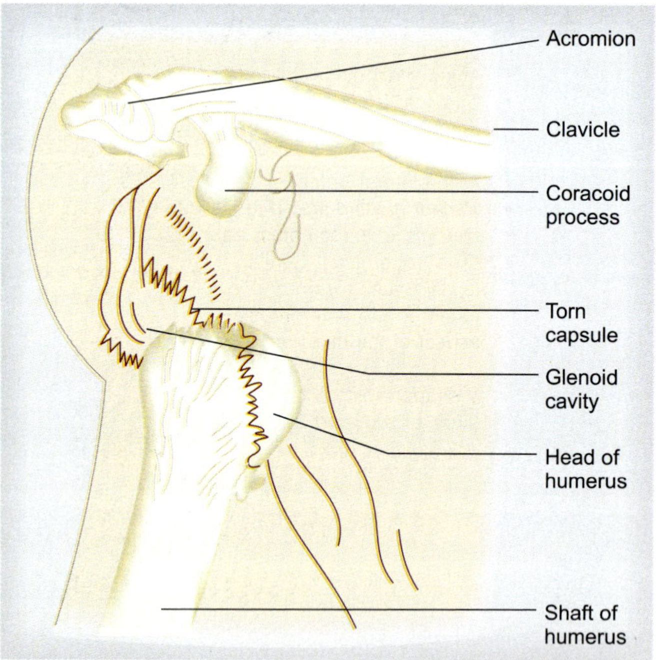

Fig. 11.17: Showing anterior dislocation of shoulder joint

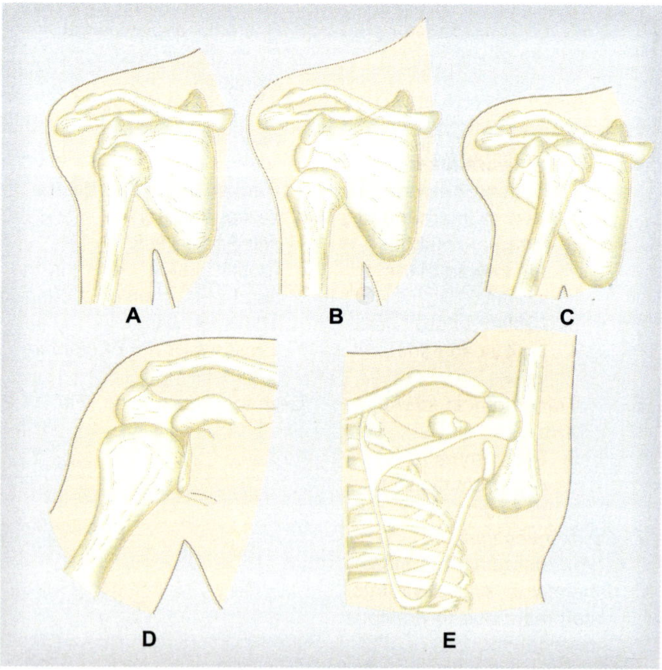

Figs 11.18A to E: Showing various varieties of shoulder dislocation: (A) subcoracoid, (B) subglenoid, (C) infraclavicular, (D) posterior, (E) inferior (luxatio erecta)

Radiology

Various views are required to detect the lesions due to the dislocation (See Table 11.2).

Treatment

Anterior dislocation of the shoulder is an emergency and has to be immediately reduced. There are various

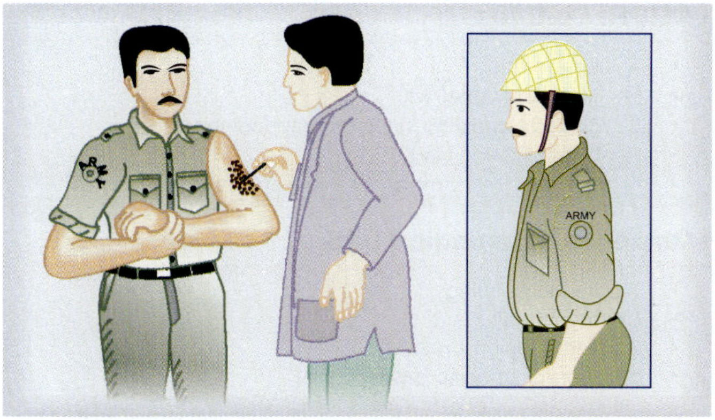

Fig. 11.19: Showing the 'Regiment Badge' sign

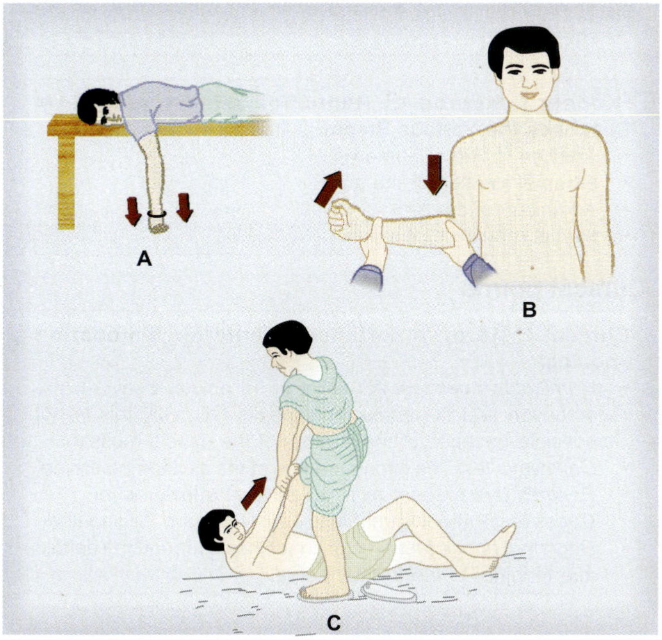

Figs 11.20A to C: Showing different methods of reduction of shoulder joint dislocation: (A) Stimson's gravity method, (B) Kocher's method (most preferred method, (C) Hippocrates method (outdated)

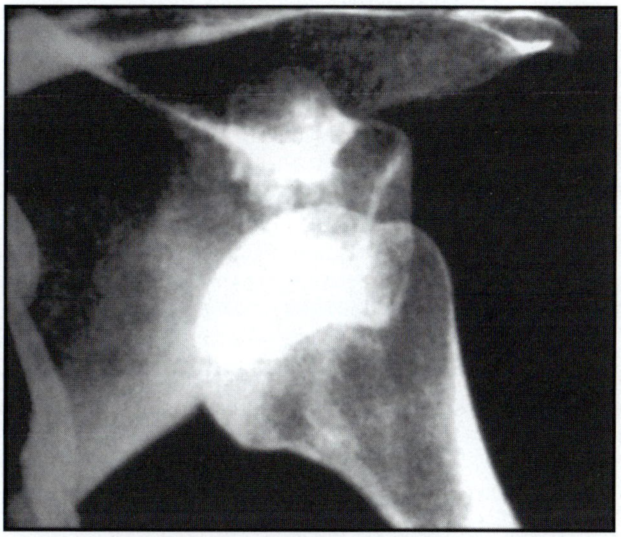

Fig. 11.21: Radiograph showing anterior dislocation of shoulder

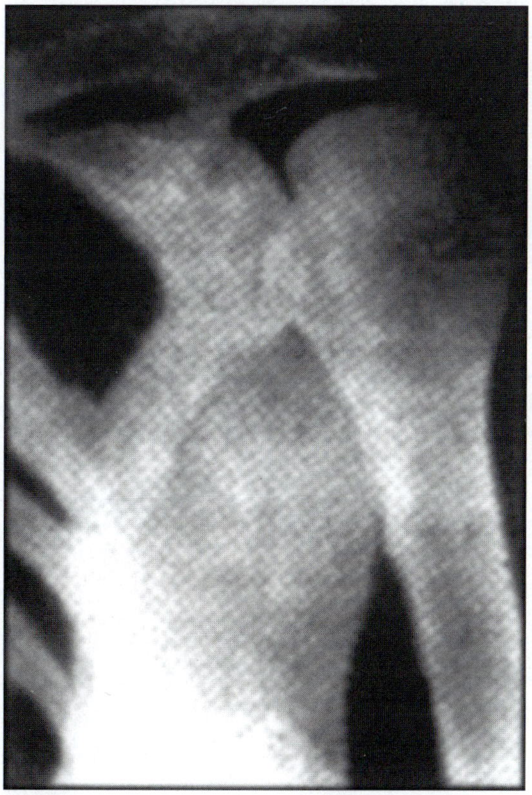

Fig. 11.22: Radiograph showing posterior dislocation of shoulder

methods of reduction (See Table 11.2 and Figs 11.20 A to C) but the most commonly used method is the Kocher's method. The various steps of this method of reduction is denoted in a box (see Fig. 11.24).

Note: Reduction should be gentle and should be done preferably under general anaesthesia.

After Treatment

After the reduction, the arm should be fastened to the chest with a body bandage for a minimum period of three weeks (Fig. 11.25). Failure to do this leads to the development of recurrent dislocation of the shoulder due to the faulty healing of the capsular rent.

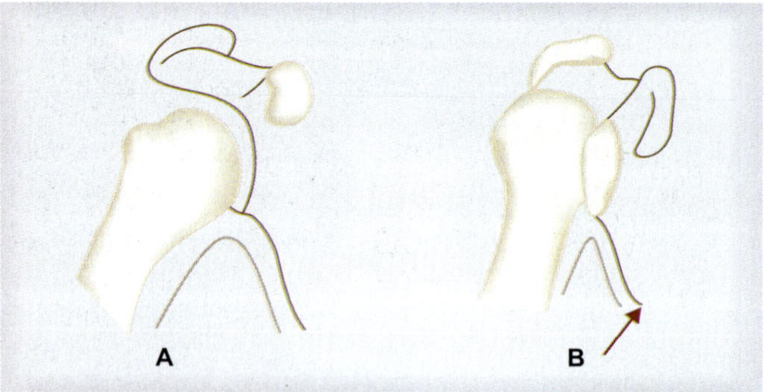

Figs 11.23A and B: Moloney's line (A) Normal, (B) Moloney's akin to Shenton's line in the hip. Seen in posterior dislocation of shoulder

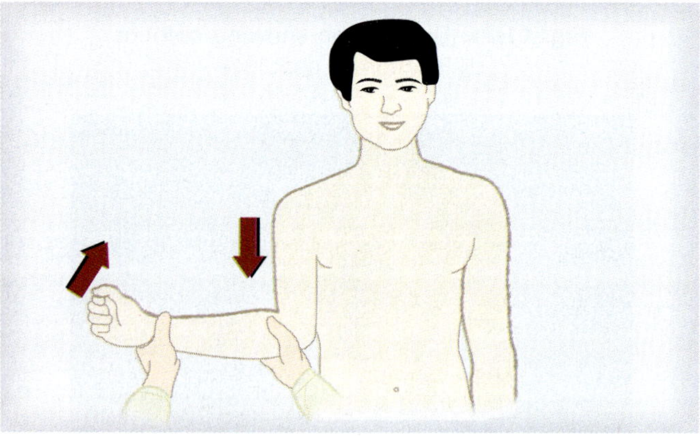

Fig. 11.24: Kocher's method of reduction of anterior dislocation of shoulder. The method consists of four important steps (mnemonic TEAM): T—traction (longitudinal), E—external rotation, A—adduction, M—medial rotation

AMBRI Denotes

- A—Atraumatic
- M—Multidirectional with
- B—Bilateral shoulder findings responding to
- R—Rehabilitation and
- I—If surgery, perform an inferior capsular shift.

Matsen' s Mnemonic TUBS

- Traumatic aetiology
- Unidirectional
- Bankart's lesion present
- Surgery for specific cases

Did you know?

- Hippocrates was the first person to give a detailed description about the anatomy and dislocation of the shoulder.

[2]Kocher's Method of Reduction (Mnemonic TEAM Describes the Various Steps)

- Traction in line of humerus
- External rotation of the arm
- Adduction of the arm
- Medial rotation of the arm

Clinical points

Clinical tests of importance in anterior dislocation shoulder

- *Hamilton's ruler test* A ruler can be placed between the acromion and the lateral epicondyle. Normally this is not possible because of the contour of the deltoid muscle.
- *Callaways test* The circumference of the axilla is increased.
- *Bryant's test* Anterior axillary fold is at a lower level.
- *Dugas test* Patient is unable to touch the opposite shoulder.
- *Regiment badge test* Area of anaesthesia around the deltoid due to injury to the axillary nerve.

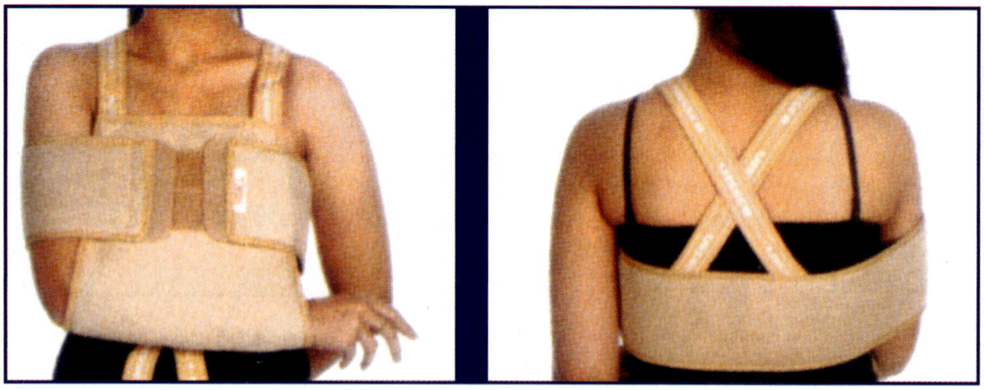

Fig. 11.25: Showing method of shoulder immobilisation after reduction of ADS (failure to do this for at least 3 weeks is the prime cause of RDS)

[2]**Theodor Kocher**, Switzerland. Described the method in 1970.

Quick facts

Anterior dislocation shoulder
- Commonest dislocation.
- Subcoracoid and subglenoid account for 99% of cases.
- Capsular injury in 30% : Labral lesion in 60%.
- Prompt reduction required. Kocher's method is the best.
- Check for axillary nerve injury before reduction.
- Immobilise for three weeks and relative immobilisation for further three weeks.
- Prolonged rehabilitation.
- Avoid provocative positions for 6 weeks.

RECURRENT ANTERIOR DISLOCATION OF THE SHOULDER (RDS)

This is a very common complication of anterior dislocation of shoulder and accounts for greater than 80 per cent of dislocations of the upper extremity. Age at the time of initial dislocation is an important prognostic factor, recurrence rate being 55 per cent in patients 12 to 22 years old, 37 per cent in 23 to 29 years, and 12 per cent in 30 to 40 years old.

Did you know?

- *One* in every three anterior dislocation of shoulder becomes recurrent dislocation of shoulder.

Causes

- Failure to immobilise the shoulder for 3 to 4 weeks after initial dislocation.
- Size and nature of damage at the time of initial dislocation.
- Greater the trauma, lower the incidence.
- Younger the patient, less is the recurrence.

Mechanism of Dislocation

In some individuals, the dislocation can be predictable and can be avoided. In others, the mechanism is unpredictable and thus makes it a very disabling problem. *The usual mechanism of dislocation is external rotation in abducted position* (Figs 11.26A to C).

Pathological Anatomy

No single deformity is responsible for recurrent dislocation of shoulder. Three important reasons have been cited and they have been called the essential lesions.

Triad of Essential Lesion

Hill-Sachs lesion is a posterolateral defect in the head of the humerus. This is produced due to the impact

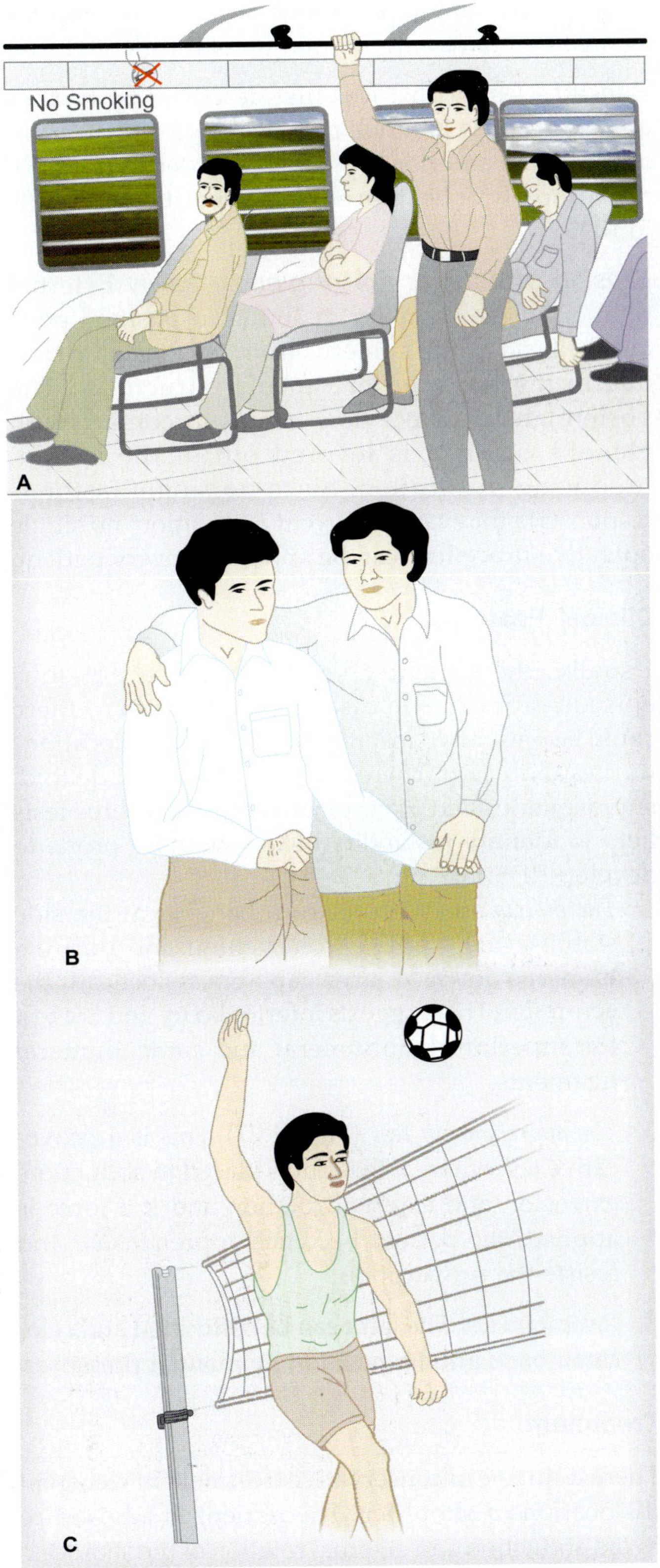

Figs 11.26A to C: Are you a victim of RDS? If so beware of routine innocuous activities like these that will knock out your shoulder joint repeatedly

Section 2

of the posterolateral part of the head of the humerus against the sharp anterior margin of the glenoid rim.

Bankart's lesion This was first described by Perthes as defect in the anterior part of the glenoid labrum and also the anterior capsule. If this defect does not heal properly or heals in elongated position, it results in RDS.

Erosion of anterior rim of glenoid cavity External rotation of the shoulder in abducted position pops out the head of the humerus from the glenoid cavity due to the lax anterior capsular structures. The posterolateral defect now comes in contact with glenoid rim and is levered out of the socket, producing dislocation. Since no single factor is responsible for every recurrent dislocation, no single operative procedure can be applied to every patient.

Clinical Features

Usually, the patient gives history of a previous episode of traumatic dislocation. After that, there could be one or two instances of repeated dislocations during abduction. There could be wasting of deltoid, supraspinatus and infraspinatus muscles. Three tests help to identify instability of the shoulder prone to develop RDS:

1. *The sulcus test* With the arm hanging at the side stabilise the scapula from behind and pull the humerus down. A large gap appears beneath the acromion. This suggests inferior laxity and is a test for superior glenohumeral and coracohumeral ligaments.
2. *The apprehension test* (Fig. 11.27) This is a provocative test where if the arm is placed in abduction, extension and external rotation and if a force is applied, the patient becomes apprehensive and resists the provocation.
3. *Relocation test* The joint can be dislocated and relocated back into its position by manual pressure.

Treatment

There is no role of conservative treatment in recurrent dislocation of shoulder. The patient is advised to avoid abduction and external rotation of the shoulder.

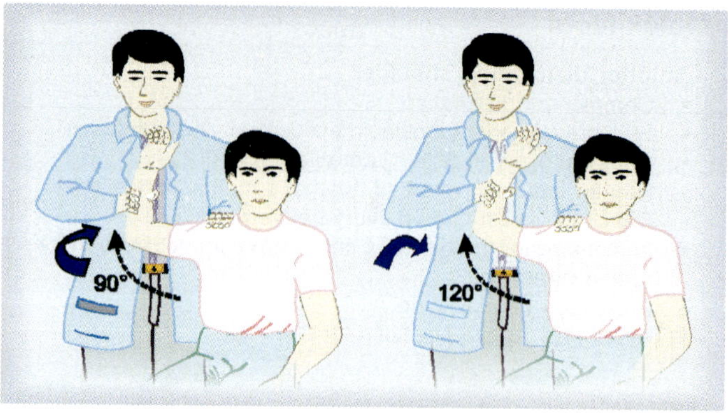

Fig. 11.27: Shoulder apprehension test

However surgery is the treatment of choice and is indicated if the patient has more than three episodes of RDS.

More than 150 operations are devised. Few are mentioned here. All the surgeries aim at correction of the essential lesions and prevent external rotation of the arm.

Name of the Surgery	What is done?
[3] *Bankart's operation* (Fig. 11.28)	Detached anterior structures are attached to the rim of the glenoid cavity with suture
Staple capsulorrhaphy of Destot and Roux	Bankart's lesion attached to labrum with staples
[4] *Putti-Platt's operation*	Subscapularis tendon and capsule is overlapped and tightened
Magnuson and Stack	Subscapularis tendon and capsule is advanced laterally on the humerus.
Eden Hybinette	Bone graft is placed against the anterior aspect of neck of scapula and rim of glenoid cavity
Bristow's	Transplantation of coracoid process with its attachments to the anterior rim of glenoid
MacLaughlin's	Tendon of subscapularis is transplanted into the posterolateral defect

Did you know?

- Bilateral facts about shoulder dislocation. Though anterior dislocation is more common than posterior dislocation, bilateral posterior dislocation is more common than anterior variety. The reason being, the mechanism of injury of adduction and internal rotation of posterior dislocation is common in seizures, which is more prevalent while simultaneous abduction and external rotation for anterior dislocation of shoulder is relatively rare.

[3] **A & B Bankart** (1938). London described pathology and treatment for RDS in 1938.
[4] **Putti Vittoria** (1880-1940) Bologna, Italy and Harry Platt (1886-1986) Manchester, England.

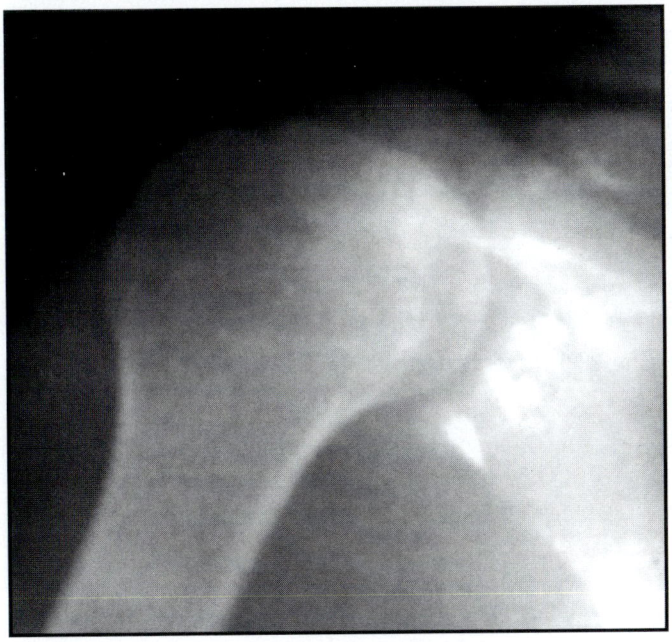

Fig. 11.28: Radiograph showing Bankart's repair

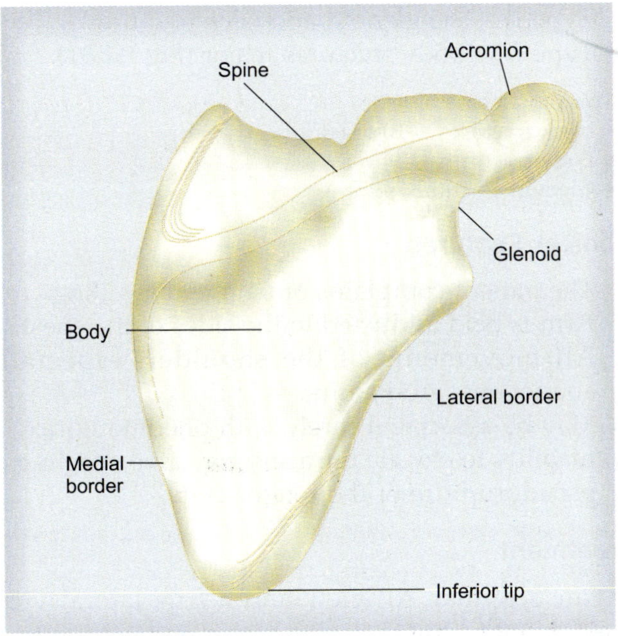

Fig. 11.29: Shows bony anatomical features of scapula

Inferior Dislocation (Luxatio Erecta)

Here the head of the humerus is below the glenoid cavity and the humeral shaft is pointing overhead. It is due to hyperabduction force and is a rare injury. Here shoulder is locked in 100 to 160° of abduction with the forearm behind the head (see Fig. 11.18E).

FRACTURE OF THE SCAPULA

Scapula is a flat bone thickly covered by muscles (Fig. 11.29).

Incidence

It is a rare injury.

- 3 to 5% of all shoulder girdle injuries.
- 0.4 to 1% of all fractures.
- Mean age is 35 to 45 years.

Functions

- Stabilises the upper extremity against the thorax.
- Links the upper extremity to the glenoid.

Mechanism of Injury

- Direct blow—fall of a heavy object on the shoulder blade (Fig. 11.30).
- Axial loading on the outstretched hands.

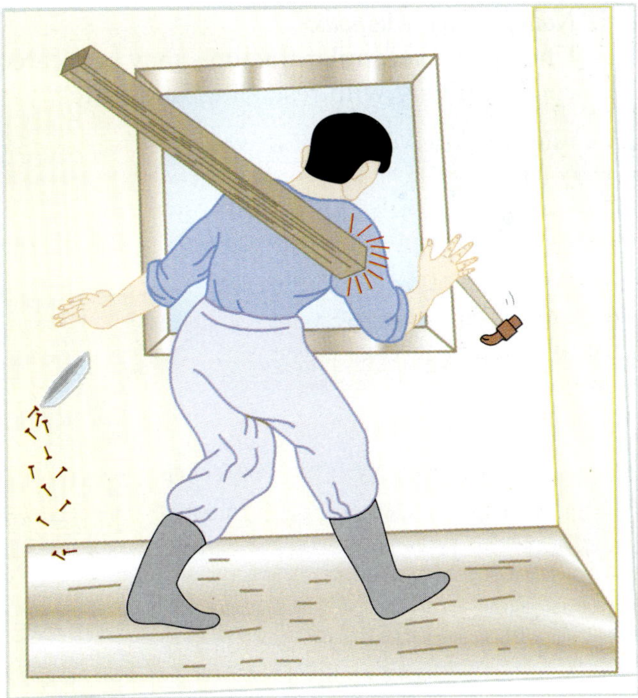

Fig. 11.30: Most common mode of injury causing scapular fracture

Classification (Thompson's)

- Type I—Coracoid, acromion and small fractures of the body.

- Type II—The glenoid and neck fractures.
- Type III—Body fractures major (Fig. 11.31).

Note:
- Neck fractures —10 to 60%
- Body fractures—49 to 89%
- Glenoid fractures—9%

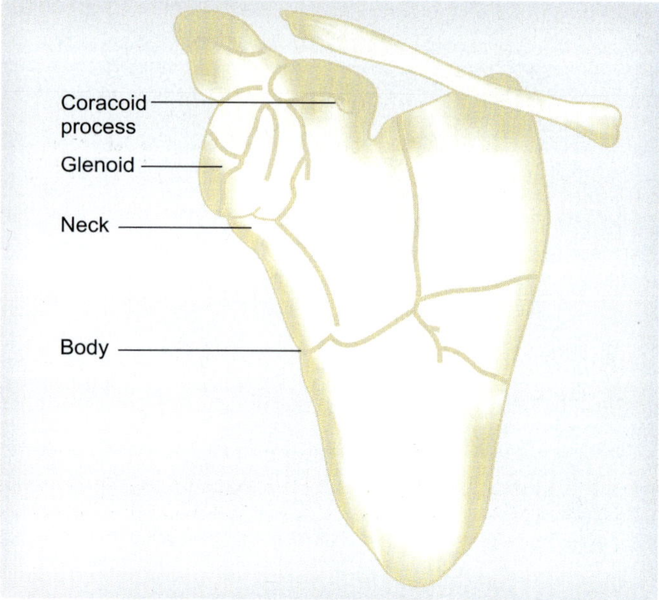

Fig. 11.31: Types of scapular fractures

Clinical Features

- The patient complains of pain and swelling.
- Arm is held adducted to the sides of the chest.
- All movements of the shoulder, especially abductions, are painful.
- May be associated rarely with pneumothorax.
- Inability to elevate the arms may give a feeling of pseudorupture of the rotator cuff.

Treatment

A true scapular AP view and a true lateral view (axillary view) helps to make the diagnosis.

Treatment Methods

I. *Nonoperative Methods:*
Undisplaced scapular fractures may be treated conservatively with rest, sling, strap, etc.

II. *Operative Methods:*
Displaced fractures need open reduction and internal fixation with K-wires, screws, etc.

12

Injuries of the Arm

- Fracture shaft humerus
- Distal humerus fractures

FRACTURE SHAFT HUMERUS

Fracture shaft humerus is more common in adults than in children.

ANATOMIC CONSIDERATIONS

The deformity is influenced by the muscles of the upper arm. If the fracture is between pectoralis major and deltoid, the proximal fragment is adducted by pectoralis major, teres minor and latissimus dorsi, while the distal fragment is pulled upwards by the deltoid (Figs 12.1A and B).

If the fracture is below the insertion of deltoid, the proximal fragment is abducted by the deltoid while the distal fragment is pulled upward by the coracobrachialis, biceps and triceps.

MECHANISM OF INJURY

1. *Direct force* This may produce a transverse or comminuted fracture.
2. *Indirect force* It is due to fall on an outstretched hand and this will produce an oblique or spiral fracture.
3. *Birth injuries* This is the second most common birth fracture after clavicle.

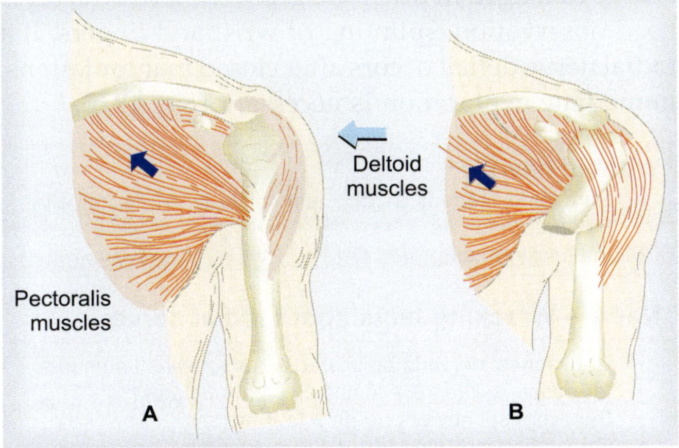

Figs 12.1A and B: Showing deforming muscle forces in fracture humerus: (A) Below the insertion of deltoid, (B) Above the insertion of deltoid

CLINICAL FEATURES

Clinical features show all the signs and symptoms of a fracture. A careful neurologic and vascular assessment is important. Injury to radial nerve is common in fractures at the spiral groove or lower one-third of humerus.

RADIOLOGY (Fig. 12.2)

Radiography of the entire upper arm including both the shoulder joint above and the elbow joint below should be taken. It helps to study the level and pattern of the fracture.

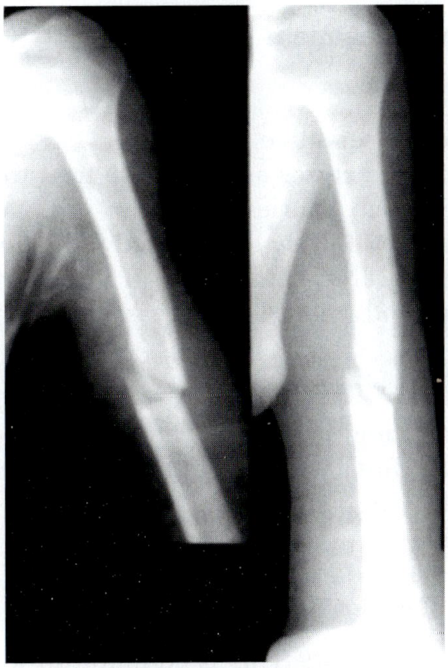

Fig. 12.2: Radiographs showing fracture shaft humerus

Section 2

TREATMENT METHODS

Conservative Methods

This consists of splinting the fracture if it is undisplaced. In displaced fractures, splinting is done after closed reduction preferably under GA (Fig. 12.3).

1. *Simple splint* in birth fractures.
2. *Simple sling* may be sufficient in young children.
3. *Hanging cast* (Fig. 12.4A) is useful in older children and adolescents. Here gravity aids in reduction of the fracture. They are not suitable if the level of fracture corresponds to the upper limit of the cast, because of the deforming effect of the proximal end of the cast. It is indicated in comminuted fractures of the distal third. If the cast is too heavy it may cause distraction and consequent delayed or nonunion.
4. *A plaster U-splint or Co-aptation splint* is sufficient in most of the situations of fractures of the proximal and middle third portions of the humerus (Fig. 12.4B).
5. *Functional cast brace (Sarmiento):* This uses the muscular force to both reduce and retain the fracture (Fig. 12.4C).

Did you know?

- Hanging cast was described by Caldwell and the weight should not exceed two pounds.

Operative Treatment

Indications

1. Failed conservative treatment.
2. Multiple fractures and unstable fractures.
3. Multisystem injuries.
4. Radial nerve palsy after closed reduction.
5. Pathological fractures.
6. Compound fractures with vascular injuries.

Methods

1. DCP plating for fractures at all levels.
2. Intramedullary fixation at middle third fractures.
3. Interlocking nail is being tried recently.
4. Flexible retrograde IM nailing.

COMPLICATIONS

Radial nerve injury This is common in lower one-third fractures and is usually of a high variety. It may also be damaged in the spiral groove. Closed fractures need observation, splinting of wrist and fingers. If a radial nerve deficit occurs after closed manipulations, immediate exploration is necessary (Fig. 12.5).

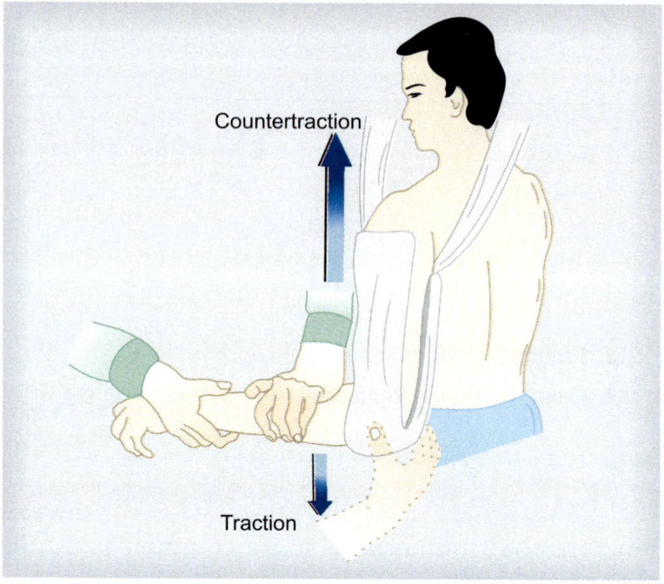

Fig. 12.3: Showing method of reduction and application of U-slab for fracture shaft humerus

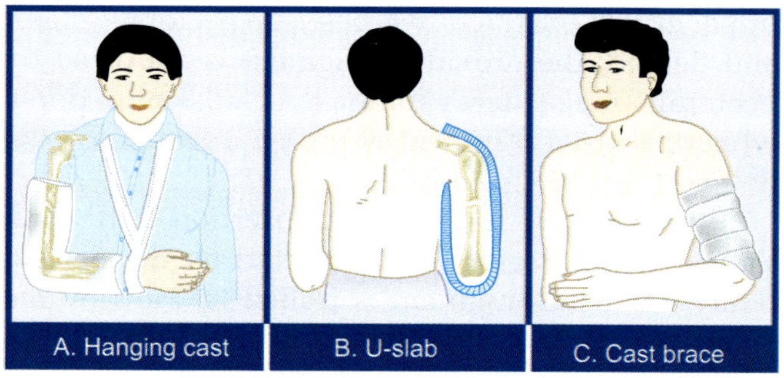

Figs 12.4A to C: Showing different conservative treatment methods in fracture shaft of humerus

What is new?

- Sarmiento brace is a good alternative to IM nailing with 84% success rate.
- Interlocking nail.

Nerve—Wracking facts about radial nerve:

- Commonest nerve to be injured in fracture shaft humerus.
- Incidence is 2 to 18% at middle 1/3rd fractures.
- Recovers spontaneously by 3 to 4 months.
- Exploration indicated beyond 3 to 4 months.
- Radial nerve palsy appearing after closed reduction is an absolute indication for exploration.

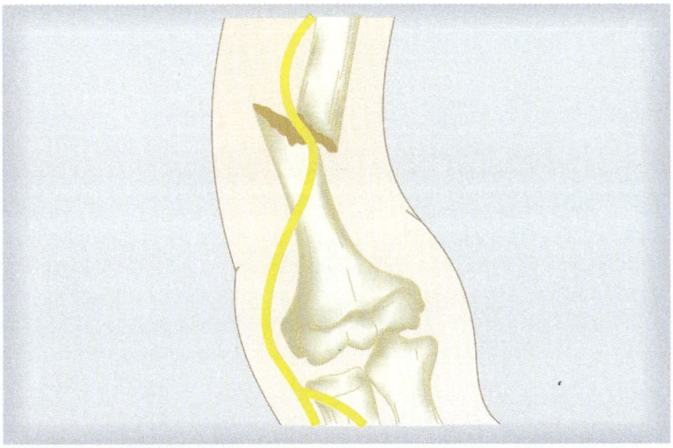

Fig. 12.5: Showing entrapment of radial nerve in between the fracture fragments of the humerus

Vascular injury To the brachial vessels is unusual. It requires repeated assessment and prompt treatment.

Malunion In humeral fractures angular deformity of 20° is acceptable in the middle and distal one-third; while in the proximal one-third, 30° is acceptable. Thick muscles in the upper arm usually conceal the malunion.

Do you know the 'acceptable' levels of malunion?

- Up to 3 cm shortening
- 20° of varus angulation
- 30° of anterior or posterior angulation.

Nonunion is not very common but may be seen due to overweight hanging cast. This requires open reduction, excision of the fibrous tissue, rigid plating and bone grafting.

Operative methods In properly indicated cases, open reduction and rigid internal fixation with DCP plate and screws is the recommended method. Interlocking nail technique is now being more commonly used for comminuted fractures of the humerus (Fig. 12.6).

Interesting Facts

What is Holstein-Lewis fracture?

- It is a spiral fracture of the distal third wherein radial nerve is more often injured.

DISTAL HUMERUS FRACTURES

REGIONAL ANATOMY

The distal most of the lateral column is the capitellum and the distalmost part of the medial column is the non-articular medial epicondyle. The articular segment is formed by the trochlea (medial) and the capitulum (lateral). The trochlea forms the tie-arch between the lateral and the medial columns. This articular segment is tilted 40°forward. In the AP view, the articular surface makes an angle of 4 to 8° valgus to the shaft axis. Anteriorly, there are two fossae, 'radial fossa' and the 'coronoid fossa'; posteriorly, there is 'olecranon fossa' and these receive the head of the radius, coronoid and olecranon process of the ulna respectively.

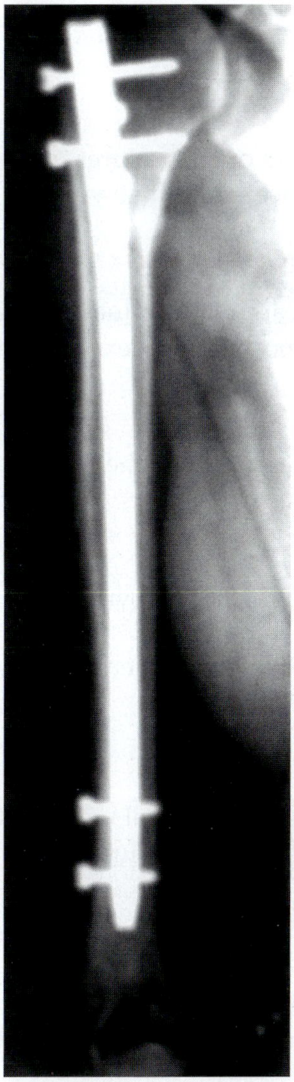

Fig. 12.6: Radiograph showing ILN humerus

INCIDENCE

- Rare fractures
- Comprises 0.5% of all adult fractures

- *Individual incidences:*
  1. Type A — 10%
  2. Type B — < 5%
  3. Type C — 85%
- 41% cases are open fractures.
- Age incidence—About 40 years of age.

MECHANISM OF INJURY

These injuries are mainly due to longitudinal force through the elbow that is flexed beyond 90°.

CLINICAL FEATURES

The patient presents with the following:
- Pain around the elbow
- Gross swelling
- Deformity
- Severe loss of elbow movements
- Crepitus
- Neurovascular impairment may be present in the forearm or hand.

INVESTIGATION

Good quality AP and lateral views of the plain X-ray are enough to make an accurate diagnosis.

CLASSIFICATION (OTA)

1. Type A — Extra-articular
2. Type B — Partially articular
3. Type C — Completely articular (T- or Y-shape)

Three Types of C-variety

a. Simple T- or Y-variety
b. Simple articular fracture with the nonarticular supracondylar area is comminuted.
c. Articular segment is comminuted.

TREATMENT

I. Nonoperative Treatment

Indications

- Frail and debilitated patients.
- Extreme osteoporosis.

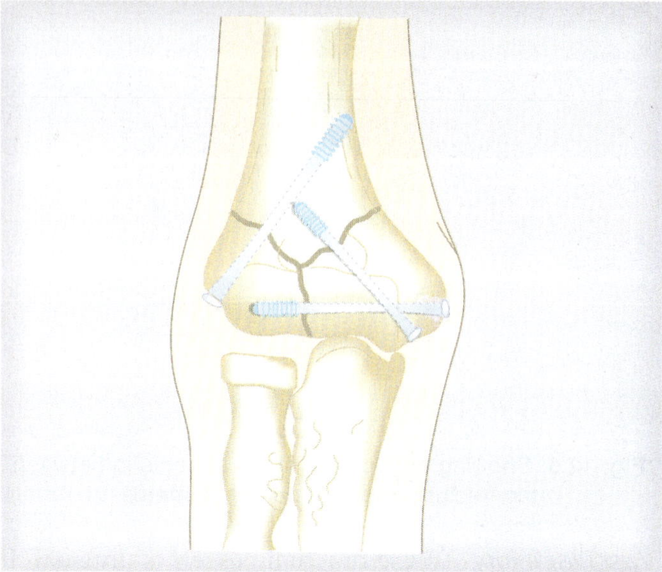

Fig. 12.7: Showing method of internal fixation of Y-intra-articular fracture of the distal humerus

- Local conditions of the skin not conducive for surgery.
- Open degloved or crushed elbow.

Methods

- Overhead skeletal traction through the olecranon
- Initial traction converted to cast, cast brace or hinged brace.

II. Operative Treatment

This is the treatment of choice in unstable distal humeral fractures. This can be accomplished by open reduction and rigid internal fixation with screws or plate and screws. Reconstruction of the lateral and medial columns have to be done and fixed with plate or screws with fixation of the intra-articular segment (Fig. 12.7).

ADVANTAGES

- Reconstructs the distal humerus more accurately.
- Helps in early mobilisation of the elbow.
- Enables early restoration of elbow functions.

13

Injuries Around the Elbow

- Brief anatomy
- Injuries around the elbow
- Supracondylar fracture
- Physeal fractures
- Dislocation of elbow joint
- Side swipe injuries
- Radial head fracture
- Fracture of the olecranon
- Coronoid fractures
- Capitellum fractures

BRIEF ANATOMY

Elbow joint is the most notorious joint in the body for it is associated with many complications following injury or trauma to the elbow.

THE ELBOW JOINT SPEAKS

- I am a compound paracondylar joint as the lower end of humerus articulates with both radius and ulna. Though basically I am a hinge joint allowing only flexion and extension through an arc of 150°, more specifically the humeroulnar component of mine is a modified sellar joint and the humeroradial component is an unmodified ovoid. I have the proximal radioulnar joint which is a modified ovoid joint. All the three components of mine mentioned so far share the same joint capsule. This makes me respond differently to trauma, exercises, masssage, etc. I have a capsule which is reinforced laterally by the radial collateral ligament and medially by the ulnar collateral ligament. The annular ligament holds the head of the radius in its position (Fig. 13.1).
- I flex mainly due to the action of biceps and brachialis supported by brachoradialis, pronator teres and common flexors. I extend due to the action of triceps, aided by anconeus and common extensors. Biceps and supinator help me supinate and pronator teres and quadratus help me pronate. Three important nerves of the upper limb pass through me: (i) the radial nerve crosses laterally, (ii) the ulnar nerve passes beneath the medial epicondyle and enters the forearm through the flexor carpi ulnaris, and (iii) the median nerve crosses me in front.

Interesting Facts

What is patella cubitis
These are accessory bones present in the triceps near its attachment at olecranon.

Vital Facts

- Primary elbow flexor-brachialis and is called the "workhorse" of elbow flexion.
- Primary elbow extensor-triceps.

POSTERIOR ELBOW GEOMETRY

Mnemonic CRMTOL: helps to remember the secondary centres of ossification around the elbow. (All are multiples of two) (Fig. 13.2)

- Capitulum appears at 2 years (6 months to 2 years)
- Radial head (4 years)
- Medial epicondyle (6 years)
- Trochlea (8 years)
- Olecranon (8–10 years)
- Lateral epicondyle (12 years)
- Internal epicondyle appears at 6 years.
- Trochlea appears at 9 years.
- External epicondyle appears at 12 years.

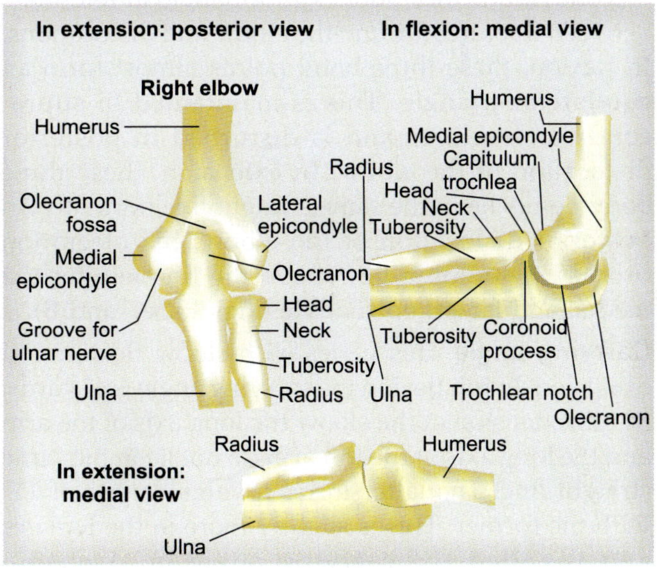

Fig. 13.1: Showing anatomy of elbow joint

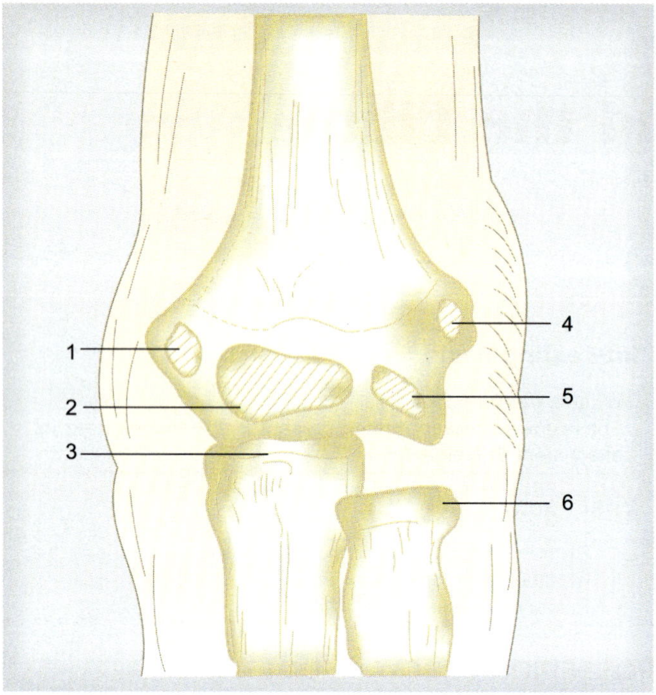

Fig. 13.2: Showing secondary centres of ossification: (1) Medial epicondyle, (2) Trochlea, (3) Olecranon, (4) Lateral epicondyle, (5) Capitulum, (6) Radial head

Note: The importance of these secondary ossification centre is that they are often mistaken as fractures in children.

Triangle Sign

The relation between the three bony points around the elbow namely lateral epicondyle, medial epicondyle and olecranon is important to differentiate between fractures around the elbow and dislocations. In flexion, these three bony points almost form an equilateral triangle. This is maintained in supracondylar fractures and is disturbed in posterior dislocation of the elbow. In extension, these three bony points lie in the same straight line normally. In posterior dislocation of the elbow, the olecranon process of the ulna lies above the line joining the medial and lateral epicondyle (Figs 13.3A and B).

Carrying angle This varies with elbow flexion and extension. In full flexion the carrying angle is 6° varus. In full extension of the elbow the long axis of the arm and the long axis of the forearm do not lie in the same straight line. The latter forms a valgus angle of 11° with the former. This is slightly more in the females and is called the carrying angle in extension (see Fig. 13.2). The carrying angle helps the elbow to

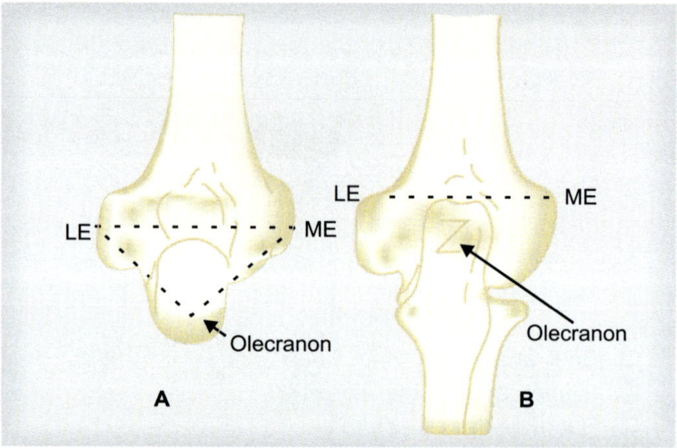

Figs 13.3A and B: Showing the relationship between the three bony points of the elbow in flexion and extension between LE–lateral and olecranon epicondyle, ME–medial epicondyle

clear the pelvis. Increase in this angle results in cubitus valgus deformity (Fig. 13.4) and decrease in the angle forms the cubitus varus deformity. However, the carrying angle disappears with full flexion of the elbow, and it is in this position that the long axis of the forearm and long axis of arm lie parallel to each other.

INJURIES AROUND THE ELBOW

Fall on the outstretched hands is more common in children because they are more playful and hence

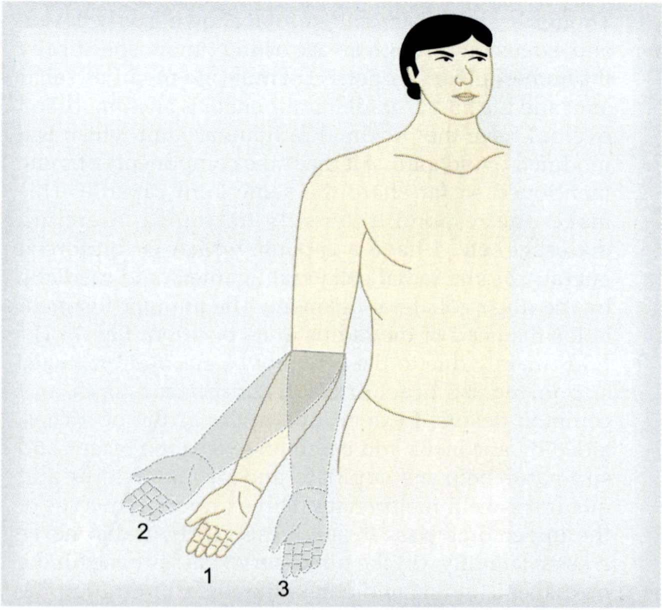

Fig. 13.4: Carrying angle of elbow (1) normal, (2) increased (cubitus valgus), (3) decreased (cubitus varus)

more prone to fall. Thus, upper extremities are vulnerable to fractures. Sixty-five to seventy-five per cent of all fractures sustained by children are seen in upper limbs.

Incidence of injuries around the elbow	Percentage
• Supracondylar fractures	65.4
• Condylar fractures	25.3
• Fracture neck radius	4.7
• Monteggia fractures	2.2
• Olecranon fractures	1.6
• T-condylar fractures	0.8

In children, forearm bone fractures rank first followed by fractures around the elbow region. The incidence of distal humeral fractures are as follows:

• Supracondylar	69
• Lateral condyle	16.8
• Medial condyle	14.1
• T-condylar	1

Classification of Fractures of Distal Humerus in Children

A. *Supracondylar:*
   - Flexion type
   - Extension type.

B. *Physeal fracture:*
   - Involving lateral condylar physis.
   - Involving medial condylar physis.
   - Involving total distal physis.
   - Involving medial epicondylar physis.
   - Involving lateral epicondylar physis.

C. *T-condylar fracture.*

SUPRACONDYLAR FRACTURE

As mentioned earlier, supracondylar fractures of the humerus is very common in children. The reason lies in the bony architecture of the supracondylar area (Fig. 13.5) in children. The mechanism of injury and the predisposing factors exploit this potential weakness in this area and break it more often than any other bone in children.

Do you know?

Supracondylar fracture of humerus is also called Malgaigne's fracture.

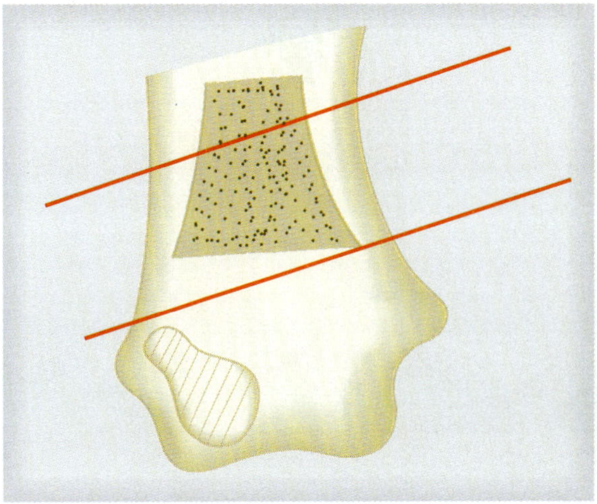

Fig. 13.5: Showing the supracondylar area in children

Vital facts of pathological anatomy

Why common in children < 10 years?
Bony architecture at the supracondylar region is weak and vulnerable because in this region:
- Bone is remodelling.
- It is less cylindrical.
- Metaphysis is just distal to 2 fossae, coronoid and radial.
- Here the cortex is thin.
- Anterior cortex has a defect in the area of coronoid fossa.
- Laxity of ligaments permits hyperextension at the elbow.

Important facts

Predisposing factors for juvenile supracondylar fractures are:
- Ligamentous laxity at the elbow leads to hyperextension.
- Hyperextension converts linear force into bending force. Olecranon concentrates this force to the weak supracondylar area.
- Anterior capsule is taut.
- Bony architecture of a supracondylar area.

Mechanism of Injury

Fall on an outstretched hand with hyperextension at the elbow with abduction or adduction, with hand dorsiflexed (Fig. 13.6).

Quick review of statistics

- *Age*—first decade, 5–8 years, 84% cases < 10 years
- *Sex*—boys 63.6%
- *Sides* (L)—58.6%; (R)—42.4%
- *Open* fracture—2.3%
- *Nerve injury*—7% ————→ Radial nerve—45%; Median nerve—32%; Ulnar nerve—23%
- *VIC*—0.5%
- *Fracture of ipsilateral extremity*—1.2%
- *Flexion type*—2.3%
- *Extension type*—97.7%

Section 2

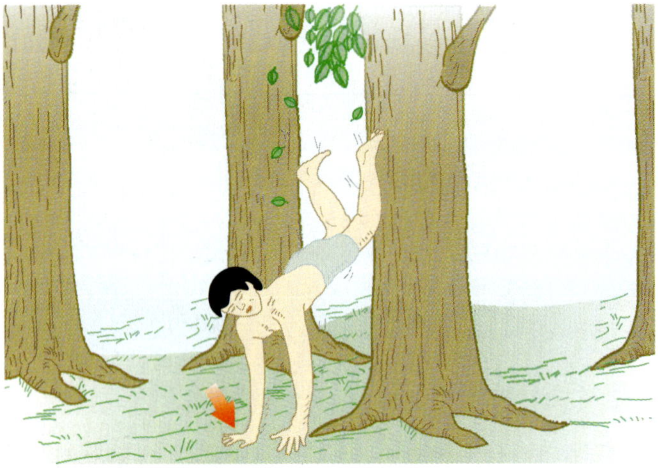

Fig. 13.6: Fall on outstretched hands is a common mechanism of upper limb fractures in children

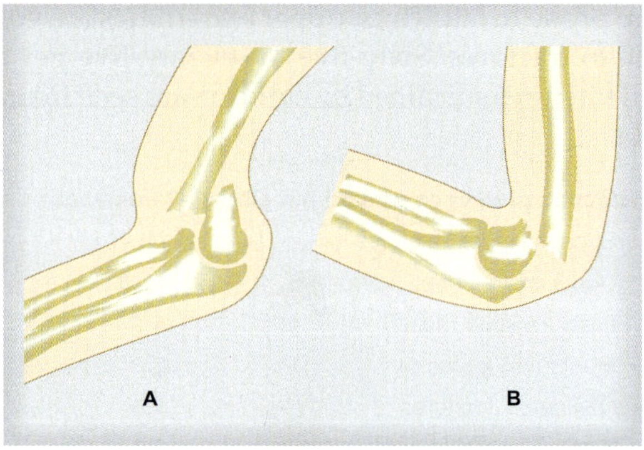

Figs 13.7A and B: Showing types of supracondylar fracture: (A) extension type 97.7%, (B) flexion type 2.3%, and

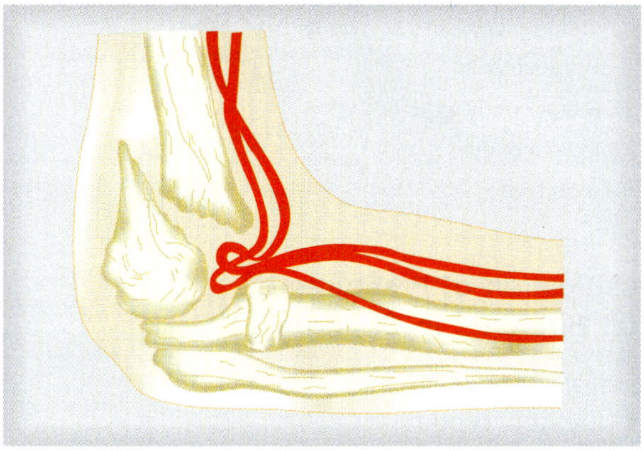

Fig. 13.8: Showing extension type of supracondylar fracture causing neurovascular injuries

Classification

Supracondylar fracture (Figs 13.7A and B) is broadly classified into *extension type* and *flexion type* (Fig. 13.8). In extension type, the fracture line runs *upwards* and *backwards;* and in flexion type, it runs *downwards* and *forwards.*

Extension type of supracondylar fracture is further classified into the following subtypes.

Gartland's Classification (In Children)

- *Type I*—undisplaced
- *Type II*—displaced, but posterior cortex is intact.
- *Type III*—displaced, but no intact posterior cortex and the distal fragment could be either displaced:
  a. Posteromedial or
  b. Posterolateral.

Clinical Features

The patient complains of pain and swelling which is gross, "S"-shaped deformity of the upper arm is obvious and there is loss of both active and passive movements of the elbow. Symptoms relating to vascular and nerve injury may also be seen. The patient may also complain of pseudoparalysis. Tests should be carried out for brachial artery and all the three nerves of the upper limb, namely the radial nerve, the median and ulnar nerves.

The following are the characteristic clinical signs in supracondylar fracture:

- Arm is short, forearm is normal in length.
- Gross swelling, and tenderness.
- Crepitus is present but should not be elicited for fear of increasing the pain and damaging the neighbouring neurovascular structures.
- "S"-shaped deformity.
- Dimple sign due to one of the spikes of proximal fragment penetrating the muscle and tethering the skin.
- Relationship between three bony points is maintained.
- "Soft spots" is an effusion beneath anconeus muscle.
- Movements of the elbow both active and passive are decreased.

Radiology

X-ray of the elbow A proper study of the radiological signs both in AP and lateral view (Fig. 13.9) of the elbow is extremely important not only to study the fracture anatomy but also to check for the adequacy and accuracy of reduction, a failure of which results in malunion later.

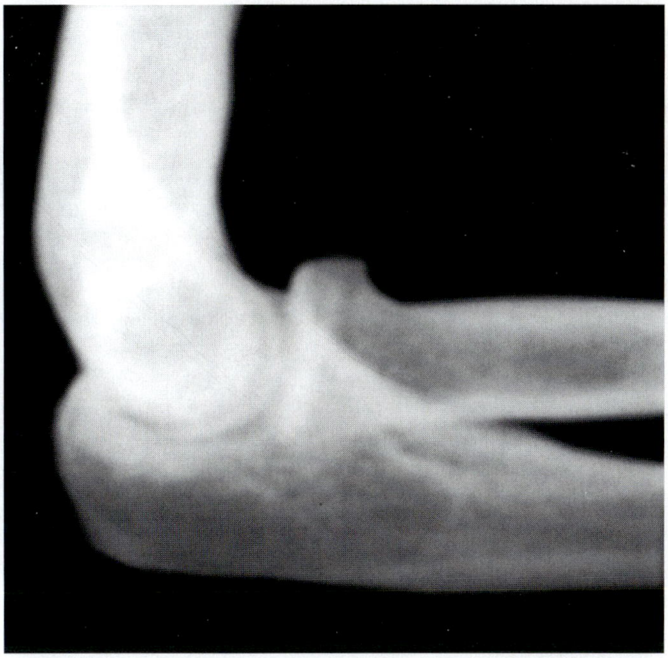

Fig. 13.9: Radiograph showing normal lateral view of elbow

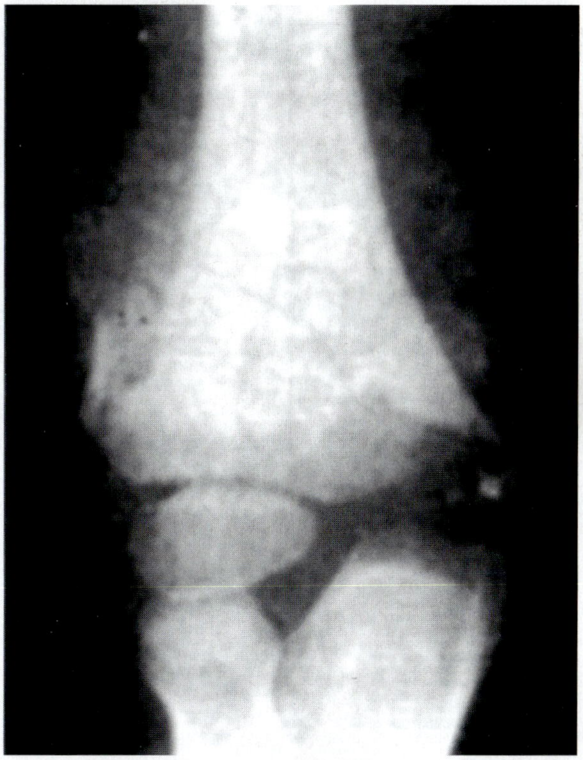

Fig. 13.10A: Radiograph showing extension type of supracondylar fracture: AP view

AP view (Fig. 13.10A) The following are the radiological parameters of importance in this view.

- *Baumann's angle* Angle between the horizontal line of the elbow and the line drawn through the lateral epiphysis and long axis of the arm. Normally it is less than 5° and should always be compared with the other side.
- Angle between the long axis of humerus and the transverse axis of the elbow is normally 90°.
  —Less than 90° suggests cubitus valgus
  —Greater than 90° suggests cubitus varus.

Lateral view (Figs 13.10B and 13.11A to D)

- *Tear drop sign*—it is disturbed in supracondylar fracture, but it is seen in the normal radiograph.
- Normally, there is an angulation of 40° between the long axis of humerus and long axis of lateral epicondyle.
- *Anterior humeral line*—a line drawn along the anterior border or the distal humeral shaft passes through the middle 1/3rd of capitulum. If it passes through anterior 1/3rd, it indicates posterior displacement of the distal fragment.
- *The coronoid line*—a line directed proximally along the anterior border of the coronoid process of the ulna should just barely touch the anterior portion of the lateral condyle. Posterior displacement of

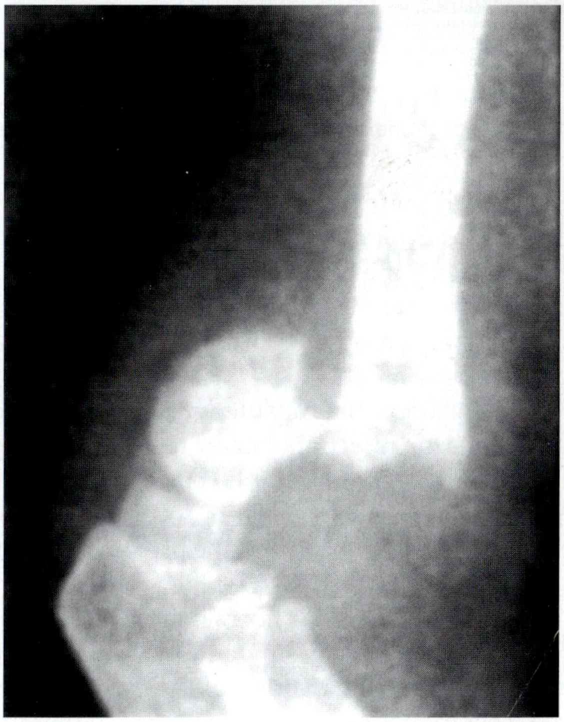

Fig. 13.10B: Radiograph showing extension type of supracondylar fracture: lateral view

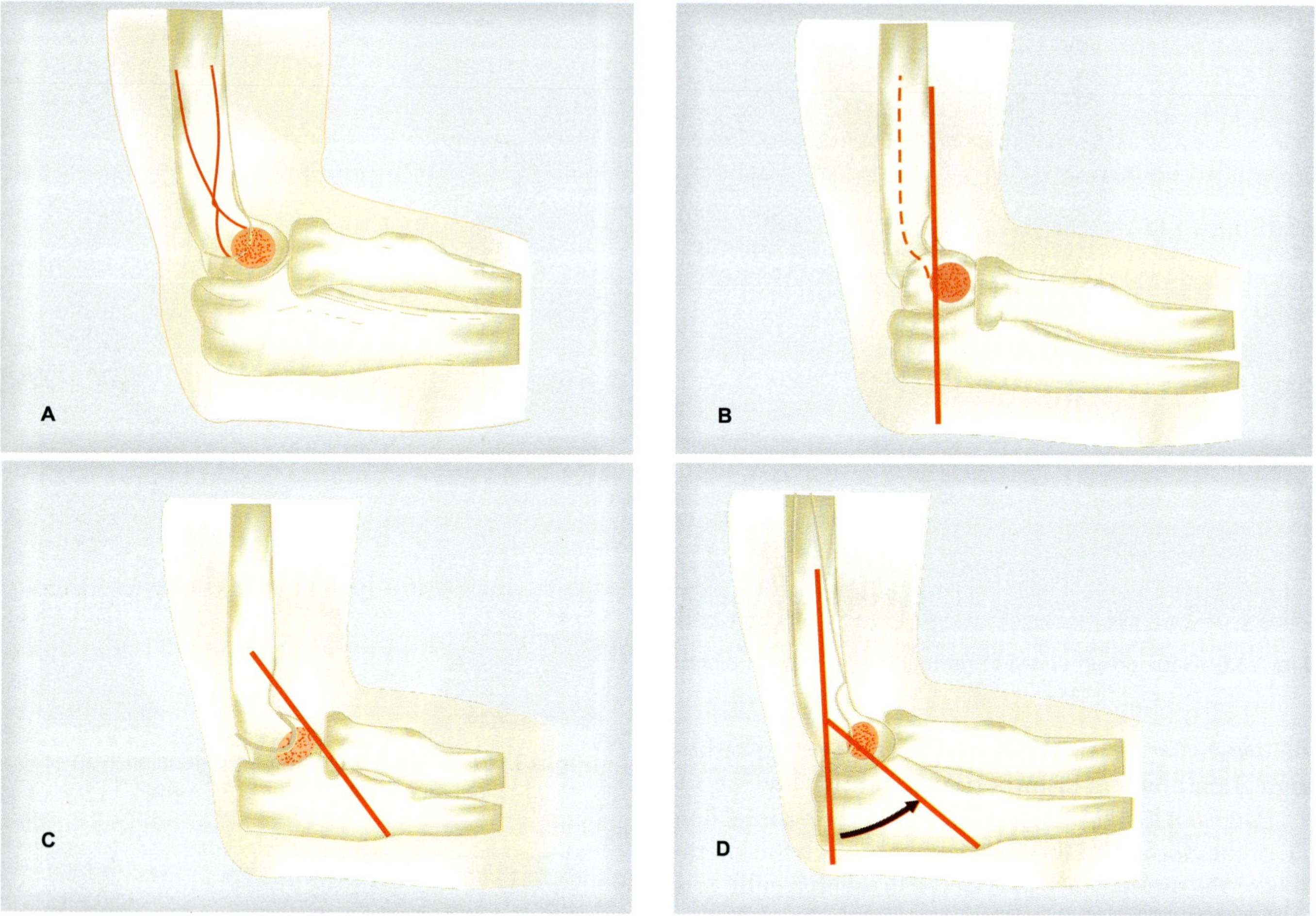

Figs 13.11A to D: Look for these important landmarks on the lateral view of the elbow X-ray: A—Tear drop sign, B—Anterior humeral line, C—Coronoid line, D—Relationship between axis of humerus and that of lateral epicondyle

the lateral condyle will project the ossification centre posterior to this line.

- *Fat pad sign*—the olecranon fossa is deep and thus the fat pad here lies totally contained within the fossa. Not seen on the normal lateral radiograph of the elbow at 90°.

  Distension of the capsule with an effusion due to trauma or infection causes the olecranon pad to be visualised as a radiolucent gap.
- *Fish-tail sign*—due to rotation of the distal fragment, the anterior border of the proximal fragment looks like a sharp spike (See Fig. 13.10B).
- *Crescent sign*—here the normal radiolucent gap of the elbow joint is missing and a crescent-shaped shadow due to the overlap of the capitulum over the olecranon is evident and indicates either varus or valgus tilt of the distal fragment.

Quick facts

Radiological points

1. *Posterior displacement of the distal fragment: indicated by*
   - Loss of tear drop sign.
   - Coronoid line.
   - Fat pad sign.
   - Anterior humeral line.
2. *Coronal tilt of the distal fragment: usually varus tilt rarely valgus indicated on radiography by*
   - Crescent sign.
   - Baumann's angle.
3. *Horizontal rotation of the distal fragment: indicated by fish-tail sign*

Management (Table 13.1)

Conservative management Initially, closed reduction is tried under general anaesthesia by traction and countertraction methods (Figs 13.12A to C). The

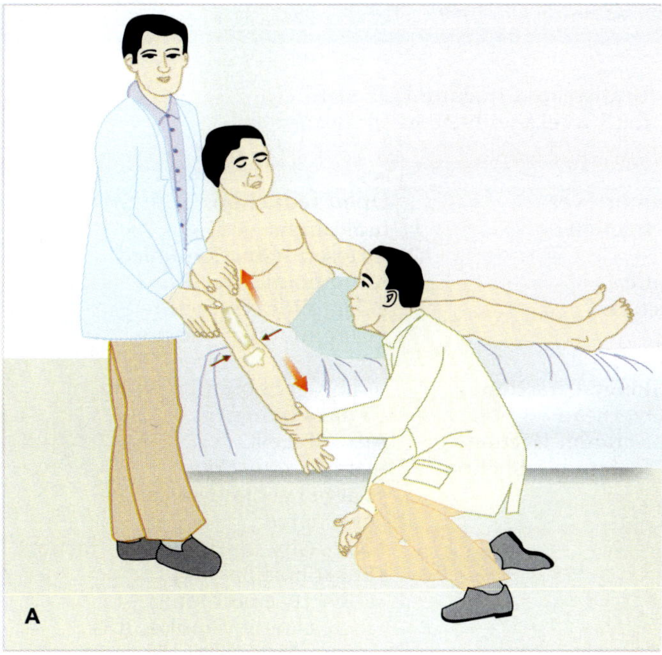

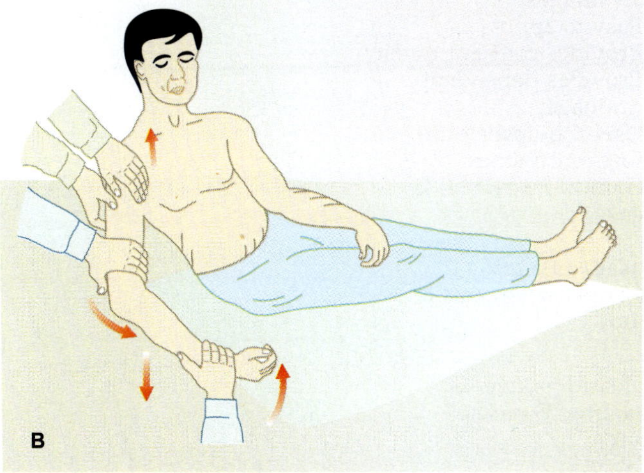

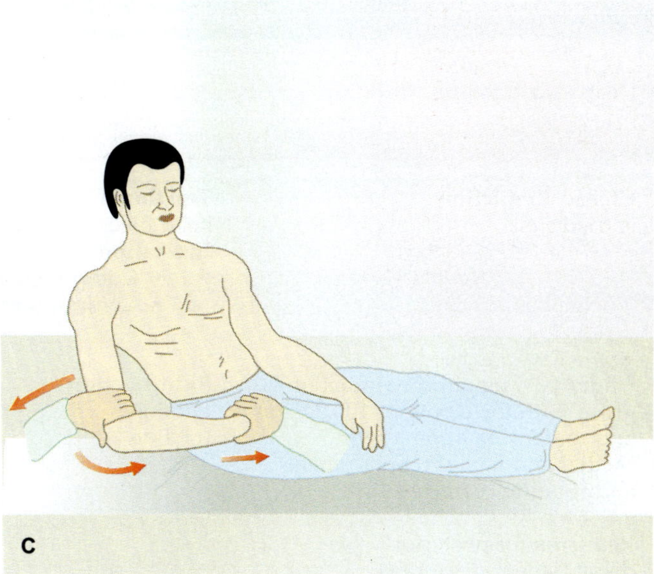

Figs 13.12A to C: Showing the technique of closed reduction of a supracondylar fracture of humerus. A—Longitudinal traction and correction of medial and lateral tilts, B—Correction of posterior tilt, C—Final position

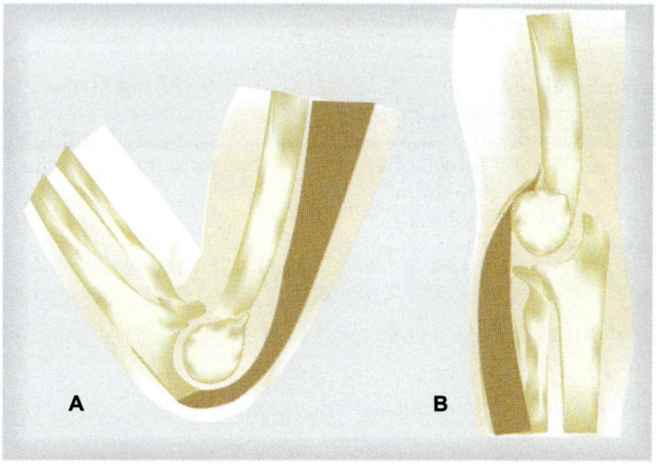

Figs 13.13A and B: Showing methods of immobilisation of supracondy lar fracture of humeros: A—Extension type, B—Flexion type

medial and lateral tilt is corrected first and posterior displacement next. *An immediate check can be made whether the reduction has been successful by noting the long axis of the forearm and arm which should be parallel.* Any deviation from the normal indicates residual uncorrected deformities. Two to three attempts under the same anaesthesia can be made and the elbow is immobilised in hyperflexion, as in this position the triceps acts as an internal splint (Figs 13.13A and B and 13.14) and the forearm is pronated as in this position the medial periosteal hinge closes the cortex laterally. Check radiograph is taken and all the angles so far discussed should be restored to normalcy, failure of which requires to consider alternative methods of treatment like skeletal traction or open reduction and internal fixation.

Table 13.1: Management of supracondylar fracture

- Displaced fracture
- Undisplaced fracture POP slab for 3 weeks with elbow in flexion

Displaced fracture ↓

Closed Reduction is tried first

↓

Under GA, longitudinal traction is given with the elbow in 10° flexion and forearm in supination. Medial and lateral displacement and rotation corrected first

↓

Reduction of posterior displacement done next.

↓

Distal fragment is finally secured to the proximal fragment by supinating the forearm and hyperflexion of the elbow. Take a check X-ray and check for the restoration of the radiological signs both in AP and lateral

- **No Swelling** Elbow immobilised in hyperflexion to neutralise the forces of forearm muscles and to enable the triceps to act as an internal splint.
- **Swelling Gross** Fracture is stabilised by medial and lateral percutaneous pins.

Traction: Dunlop traction or over head olecranon skeletal traction

Indications

- Compound fracture
- Comminuted fracture

↓

- **Skin traction** Dunlop traction
- **Skeletal traction** Overhead olecranon traction (Smith's traction)

↓

Advantages

- Easy to apply
- Provides constant traction
- Provides dependent drainage
- Useful in ipsilateral forearm fracture
- Clinical inspection is easy.

Disadvantages:
Hospitalisation cost is more

Open reduction
Indications: (4 C's)

- Closed reduction failed
- Compound fracture
- Complicated fracture
- Comminuted fracture

↓

Timing: Should be within 5 days of injury

Advantages:

- Direct reduction
- Large haematoma can be evacuated
- Necessity in irreducible fracture
- Short hospital stay

OR + IF is becoming increasingly popular. It is particularly useful in cases needing traction as it reduces the hospital stay.

↓

- Elbow is immobilised at least for 3 weeks.
- Pins or casts are removed after 3 weeks.
- Active exercises are begun.

Modified shoulder spica for 3 to 4 weeks has given good results in some.

Surgery or skeletal traction methods It is indicated if conservative methods fails (Fig. 13.15A and Table 13.1).

Closed reduction and percutaneous fixation In cases where hyperflexion of the elbow cannot be done due to gross swelling in and around the elbow and in grossly unstable fractures, percutaneous fixation of the fragments with K-wires on either side after closed reduction is an acceptable form of treatment and is widely accepted (Fig. 13.15B).

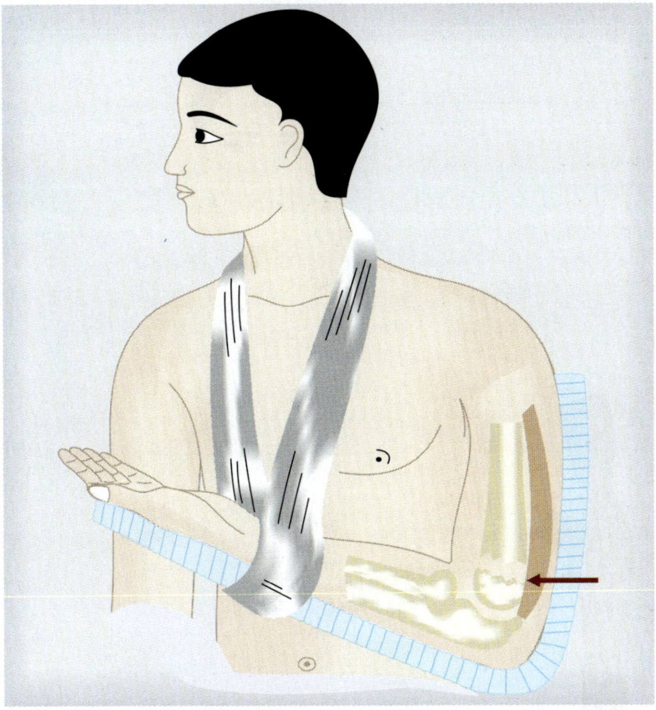

Fig. 13.14: Triceps muscle acts as an internal splint in supracondylar fracture humerus when flexed beyond 90°

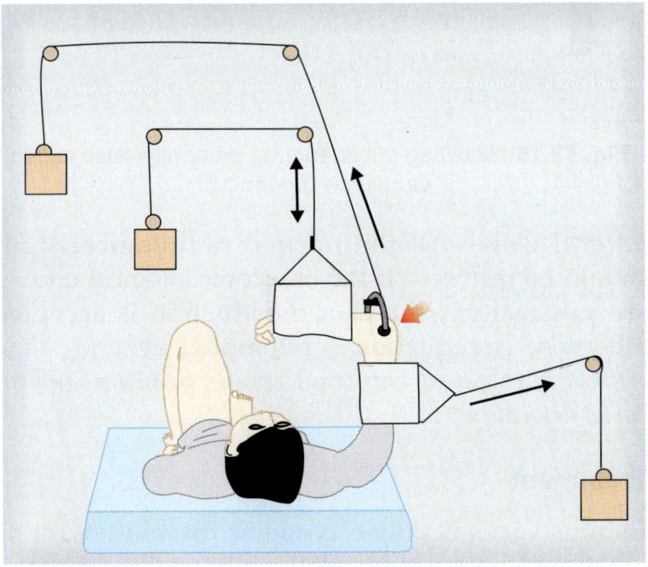

Fig. 13.15A: Showing overhead olecranon traction (Smith's traction)

COMPLICATIONS

These are broadly divided into two categories:

1. Those that cause functional impairment of the extremity and is more serious.
2. Those that produce only a cosmetic sequelae.

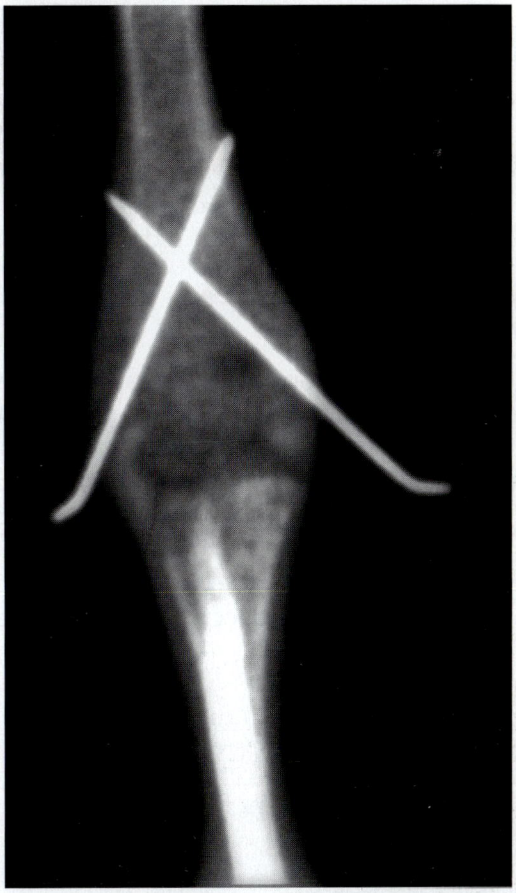

Fig. 13.15B: Radiograph showing percutaneous fixation with K-wire of supracondylar fracture of humerus (*Courtesy:* Dr RB Uppin, Associate Professor Orthopaedics, JN Medical College, Belgaum)

Complications Causing Functional Impairment

Neurological involvement Overall incidence is around 7 per cent.

1. Radial nerve—most commonly affected and is usually injured in posteromedial displacement.
2. Median nerve—injured during posterior displacement.
3. Anterior interosseous nerve injury is seen in posterolateral displacement of the distal fragment.
4. Ulnar nerve—injured in overhead skeletal traction and in flexion type of supracondylar fracture.

Vascular injury The incidence is between 0.5 and 1 per cent. Common with extension type and is usually due to direct injury of brachial artery by the fracture. The other causes are internal thrombus, intimal tear, brachial artery spasm, external compression by proximal fracture fragment of the humerus, fracture hematoma, partial or complete rupture of brachial artery.

Loss of mobility Average loss of flexion is 4° and is usually due to posterior displacement which unites in that position causing mechanical block for flexion.

Myositis ossificans is rare and is seen in manipulative closed reduction and open reduction.

Complications that Produce Cosmetic Abnormalities

Cubitus varus (Gunstock elbow) is called so because the deformity resembles a rifle gunstock (Fig. 13.16). This is the most common complication of supracondylar fracture. Incidence varies from 9 to 58 per cent. The deformity becomes obvious in an extended elbow.

The following are three static deformities of cubitus varus (all with respect to distal fragment):

1. Posterior displacement.
2. Horizontal rotation.
3. Coronal tilt.

Quick facts

Causes of cubitus varus: 4 I's

- Improper persons treating.
- Improper reduction.
- Improper interpretation of radiographs.
- Improper follow-up.

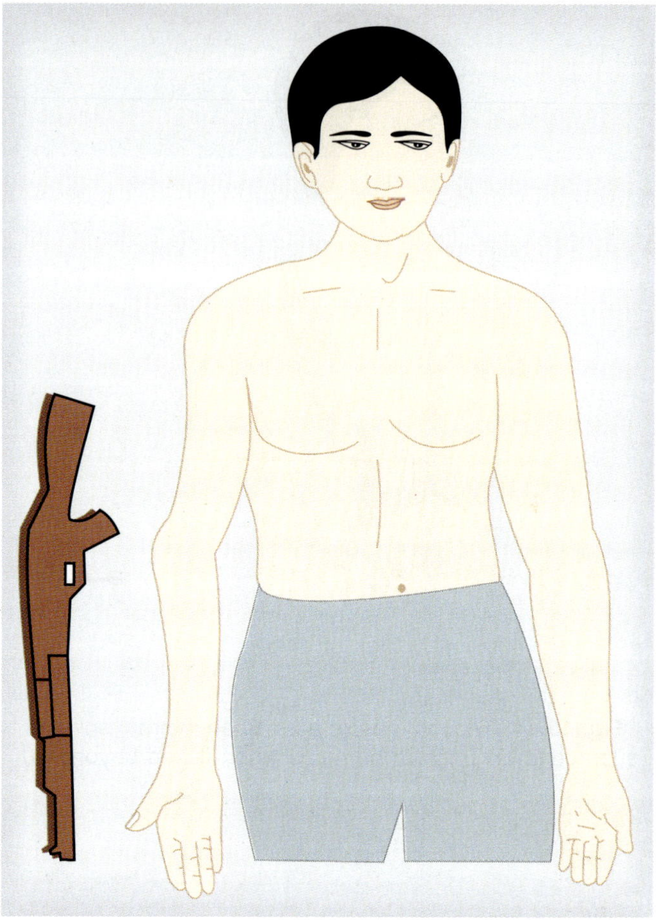

Fig. 13.16: Showing cubitus varus deformity (also called Gunstock deformity)

PATHOMECHANICS

Posterior displacement and horizontal rotation predisposes to coronal tilt. Because the edges of the fracture fragments are thin, there is very little resistance to coronal tilt, if the fragments are horizontally rotated, and also contraction of the biceps produce a medial tilting force.

All these three components should be corrected during the initial reduction of the fracture otherwise, cubitus varus deformity results.

Determination of the quality of fracture reduction after the initial injury can be assessed by the following clinicoradiological tests.

Clinical Tests

Long axes of the forearm and humerus should be parallel when elbow is flexed after reduction.

Radiology

AP view—Baumann's angle should be less than 5°.

Lateral view—All the normal radiological signs should be restored. If the clinicoradiological criteria are satisfactory, the closed reduction is accepted otherwise re-reduction is attempted. *Ignoring these criteria after closed reduction results in future cubitus varus deformity.*

Treatment

Cubitus varus is only a cosmetic disability with no functional impairment of the elbow. Treatment of choice is corrective osteotomy and is deferred till skeletal maturity as cosmesis gains importance at this age and also for the fear of recurrence of deformity if surgery is done before growth stops since there is still potential for growth left.

Osteotomy Methods

1. *Lateral closed-wedge osteotomy (French and modified French)* This operation (Fig. 13.17) is simple and

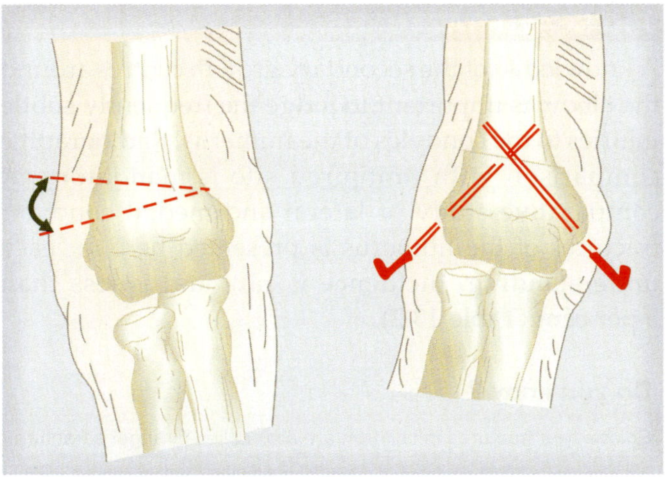

Fig. 13.17: Showing French osteotomy

easy to perform and the posterior triceps splitting approach is used. In this method, osteotomy is done between two screws, the first screw being placed anteriorly in the distal fragment and the second screw is being placed slightly posterior in the distal fragment. After the osteotomy, the distal fragment is rotated such that both the screws become parallel to each other indicating correction of rotational deformity. A wedge of bone is removed from the lateral cortex and the gap is closed and both the screws are secured against each other by a figure of 8 stainless steel wire. This way the cubitus varus is corrected.

Treatment facts of cubitus varus

Cubitus varus (see Fig. 13.16) is a cosmetic problem and not functional

Before skeletal maturity
- Observation.
- Cosmetic considerations are not very important before 18 years.
- If surgically corrected, deformity may recur.

After skeletal maturity
- No further growth left, hence the recurrence chances are nil.
- Deformity is full blown.
- Girls and boys are more cosmetically concerned at this age and hence corrective osteotomy is performed.

2. *Medial open-wedge osteotomy (King's osteotomy)* This is the opposite of lateral closed-wedge osteotomy. In this, a wedge of bone is resected on the medial aspect and the deformity is corrected.
3. *Derotation osteotomy* This technique is not as Popular as the lateral closed- and medial open-wedge osteotomies mentioned above (see Fig. 13.15B).

Cubitus valgus This is rare and may be seen in posterolateral displacement in the extension type of supracondylar fracture. Unlike cubitus varus, it is cosmetically acceptable and the treatment is by medial closed-wedge osteotomy. Tardy ulnar nerve palsy is a distinct possibility in cubitus valgus deformity.

Flexion type of supracondylar fracture This is extremely rare and has an incidence of only 2.5 per cent.

Mechanism of Injury

The common method of injury is direct blow to the posterior aspect of the arm. Angulations seen in lateral radiography are reverse of extension type. This fracture is associated with high incidence of ulnar nerve injury.

Treatment

Closed reduction and immobilisation in above elbow cast in extension is undesirable as it causes elbow stiffness. To overcome this, Sultanpur technique is used (see box). If reduction can be achieved by closed methods, the fracture can be stabilised in flexion with percutaneous pins. If reduction cannot be achieved then open reduction and internal fixation is contemplated.

Quick facts: Sultanpur technique

- Described by Sultanpur of Bahrain.
- A technique which helps to immobilise flexion supracondylar fracture in flexion rather than the conventional extension (Figs 13.18A and B).
- Two-stage casting.
- First, cast is put till distal end of the proximal fragment and is allowed to set.
- Next, the distal fragment is pushed back against this cast.
- Cast is then completed with elbow in flexion.

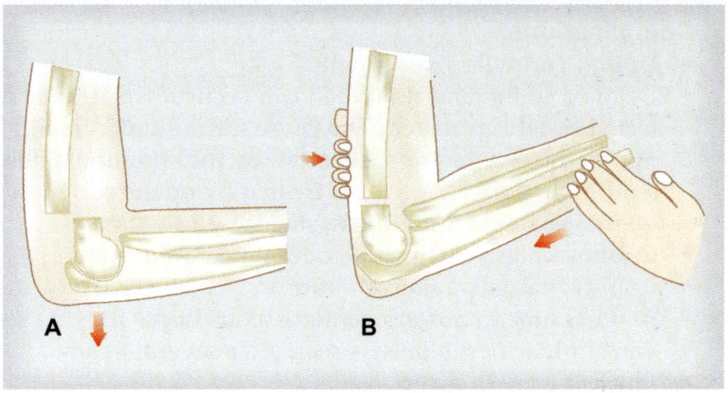

Figs 13.18A and B: Showing Sultanpur technique of reduction

Section 2

Complications

Injury to ulnar nerve is common in this type of fracture. Loss of elbow flexion is another important complication commonly encountered.

Quick facts: Supracondylar fracture of humerus

- The second most common injury next to forearm fractures in children
- Characteristic pathological anatomy
- Extension type accounts for 98 per cent
- Study and restoration of radiological anatomy is very vital
- Closed reduction difficult
- Open reduction in specific indications
- Cubitus varus is the most common complication

PHYSEAL FRACTURES

A knowledge of the secondary growth centres around the elbow is important to judge the frequently subtle injuries to the condyles of the humerus. Radiographic comparison with uninjured site is mandatory. A comparative study of lateral and medial condylar fractures of the humerus is presented here for easy understanding. Incidence is rare and is less than 5 per cent (Table 13.2).

Do you know?

Epicondylar fractures in children are also called Granger's fracture.

Table 13.2: Showing comparison of lateral and medial condyle fracture of humerus

Lateral condyle of humerus (Jupiter fracture)	*Medial condyle of humerus*
Accounts for 16.8 per cent fractures of distal humerus and can be associated with dislocation of elbow and fracture olecranon	Rare in children (1%) Age 8 to 14 years
Classification (2 ways) 1. *Anatomical location* (Figs 13.19A and B) • Type I—fracture line lateral to trochlea through the capitulotrochlear groove. Elbow is stable (high Jupiter fracture). • Type II—fracture line extends into apex of the trochlea, elbow is unstable (low Jupiter fracture). 2. *Stages of displacement* • Undisplaced • Displaced • Displaced and rotated (Fig. 13.20)	**Classification** (2 ways) 1. *Anatomical Location (Milch)* (Figs 13.21A and B) • Type I—fracture line through the apex of trochlea • Type II—fracture line through the capitulotrochlear groove. 2. *Stages of displacement (Kilfoyle's)* • Impacted • Complete • Displaced and rotated (Fig. 13.22).
Clinical features This consists of little distortion of the elbow and less swelling, tenderness and crepitus is positive over the lateral condyle	**Clinical features** Usual signs and symptoms of fracture, tenderness and crepitus is positive over the medial condyle
Radiology Routine AP and lateral views of the elbow help to make a diagnosis	**Radiology** Routine AP and lateral views help to make an accurate diagnosis
Treatment *Stages I and II* Closed reduction and percutaneous pinning *Stage III or If the fracture is > 24-48 hours old:* Open reduction and K-wire fixation	**Treatment** *Stages I and II* Above elbow cast or splint *Stage III* Open reduction and internal fixation
Complications • Lateral condylar overgrowth. • Delayed union and nonunion can occur if fracture is undetected or left untreated. The cause for nonunion could be due to the constant force exerted by the common extensor tendon. In early stages, it is treated by open reduction and internal fixation, and in late stages by osteotomy. • Cubitus valgus—This is a common complication. • Cubitus varus is relatively rare. • Acute injury to posterior interosseous nerve may be seen. • Tardy ulnar nerve palsy—seen after several years. • Physeal growth arrest. • Avascular necrosis—rarely seen. • Myositis ossificans—fairly common.	**Complications** • Missed diagnosis • Nonunion with cubitus varus • Delayed union • Cubitus valgus due to growth stimulation • Ulnar neuropathy

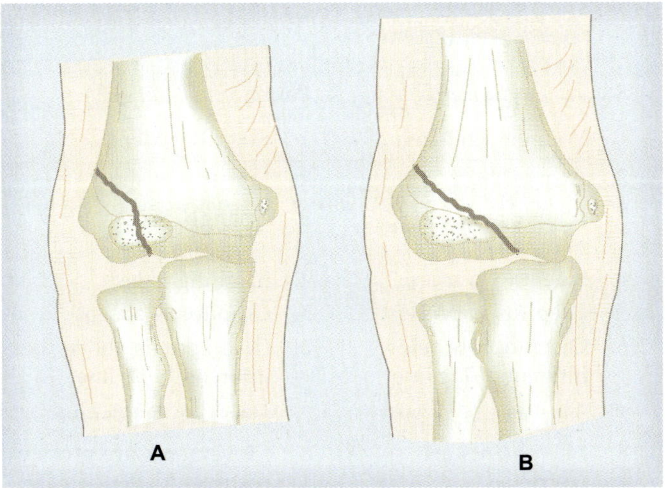

Figs 13.19A and B: Showing lateral condyle fractures. Undisplaced fractures A—Type I, B—Type II

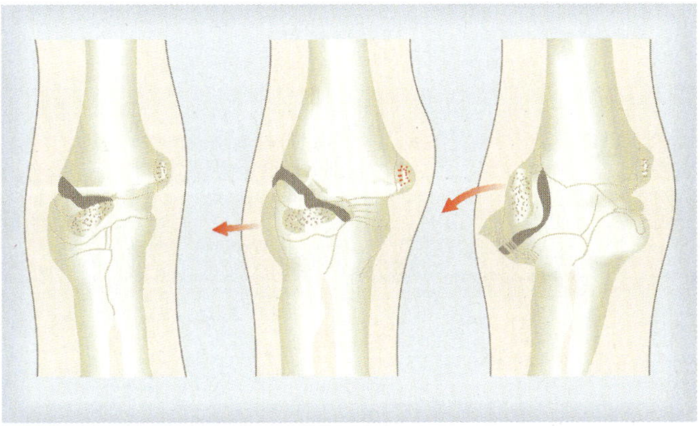

Fig. 13.20: Displaced lateral condyle fractures

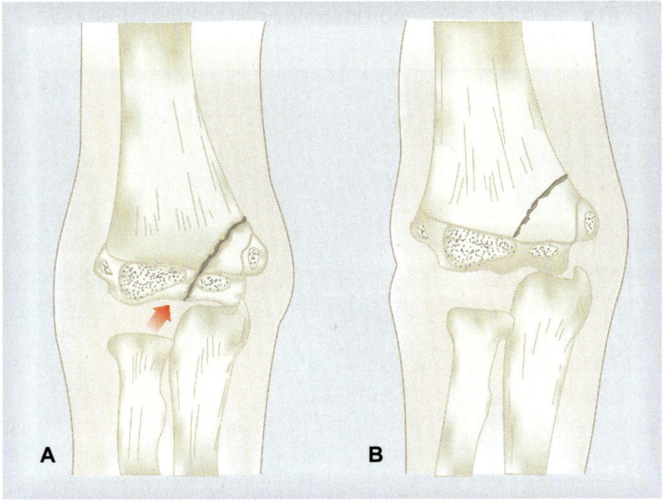

Figs 13.21A and B: Showing types of medial condyle fractures Undisplaced A—Type I, B—Type II

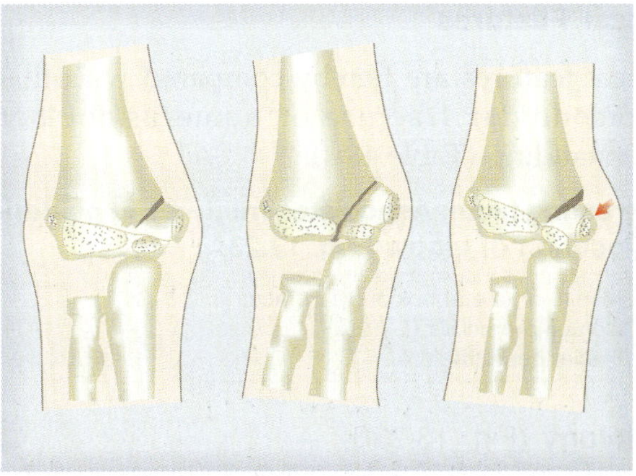

Fig. 13.22: Displaced medial condyle fractures

DISLOCATION OF ELBOW JOINT

It is rare in children below 10 years of age.

- *Incidence*—3 to 6 per cent
- *Males*—71 per cent
- *Nondominant extremity*—62 per cent.

Fifty per cent of all elbow dislocations occur in patients less than 20 years of age.

Mechanism of Injury

This is frequently due to fall on the outstretched hands with elbow slightly flexed. A valgus twist is added to the longitudinal force by the projecting trochlea and thus the dislocation is usually posterolateral. Commonly seen in sporting events and in RTA.

Classification (Stimson)

He described elbow dislocation with respect to the position of radioulnar unit to the distal humerus (Table 13.3).

Table 13.3: Stimson's classification

Proximal radioulnar joint intact	*Proximal radioulnar joint disrupted (divergent dislocation)*
A. *Posterior (90%)*	A. *Anteroposterior*
• Posterolateral	• Radius is anterior
• Posteromedial	• Ulna is posterior
B. *Anterior*	B. *Medial lateral (transverse)*
C. *Medial*	• Radius is lateral
D. *Lateral*	• Ulna is medial

Do you know?

What is "terrible triad" of the elbow? Well it is,

- Posterior dislocation of elbow.
- Radial head fracture.
- Fracture coronoid process of ulna.

Clinical Features

Clinical features are hereby compared with that of supracondylar fracture of humerus for better understanding (Table 13.4).

Interesting facts: Associated fractures in posterior dislocation of elbow (Fig. 13.23A)

- Medial or lateral epicondylar fractures (18–34%)
- Coronoid process (5–10%)
- Radial head fracture.

Radiology (Fig. 13.23B)

AP view Greater superimposition of distal humerus with proximal ulna and olecranon is seen.

Lateral view Coronoid process lies posterior to the condyles of the humerus.

Treatment

Conservative treatment by closed reduction under general anaesthesia is attempted first and reduction by operative methods is reserved for those rare cases of failed closed reduction.

Stimson's principles of closed reduction According to Stimson, the effective methods of overcoming the muscle forces are:

Step I Traction along the long axis of the humerus to overcome contraction of biceps, brachialis and triceps muscles.

Step II Once these forces are neutralised, second force along the long axis of forearm is employed to pull the proximal radius and ulna back into position.

Techniques of reduction

Closed reduction

Open reduction
Indications
1. Inability to obtain closed reduction.
2. Open dislocation.

Pusher's technique (Fig. 13.24A) (method employed in children)
↓
Pushing force is applied to the tip of olecranon with the thumb and with the patient lying prone. This is useful in younger children.

Puller's Technique (Fig. 13.24B) (method employed in adults)
↓
Pulling force applied to the forearm with elbow in 70° of flexion. This is useful in older children and young adolescents.

Table 13.4: Comparitive features between SC fracture humerus and posterior dislocation of elbow

SC fracture humerus	*Posterior dislocation*
1. Younger children	1. Slightly older
2. Arm is short	2. Forearm is short
3. Bony triangle maintained	3. Triangle is disrupted
4. Swelling is more	4. Swelling is less
5. Crepitus is present	5. Crepitus is absent
6. Olecranon is below intercondylar line	6. Olecranon is above the intercondylar line
7. Step sign is negative	7. Step sign is positive
8. Movements are restricted	8. Movements are grossly restricted
9. Radial nerve commonly affected	9. Medial and ulnar nerve injured

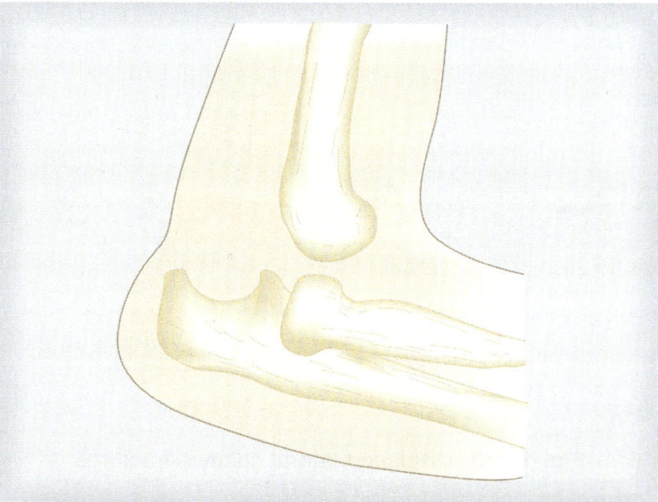

Fig. 13.23A: Showing posterior dislocation of elbow

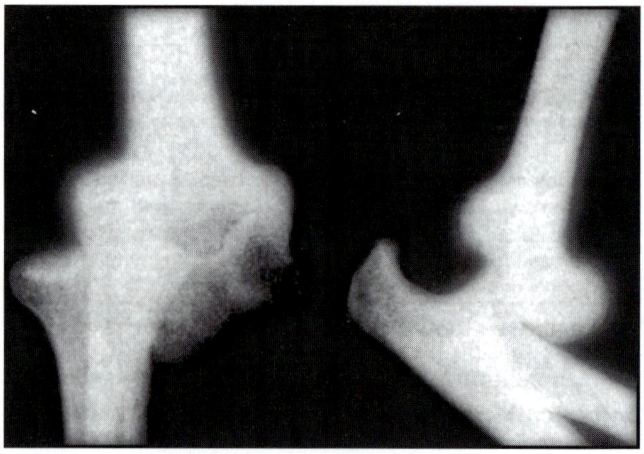

Fig. 13.23B: Radiograph showing posterior dislocation of elbow joint: AP and lateral views

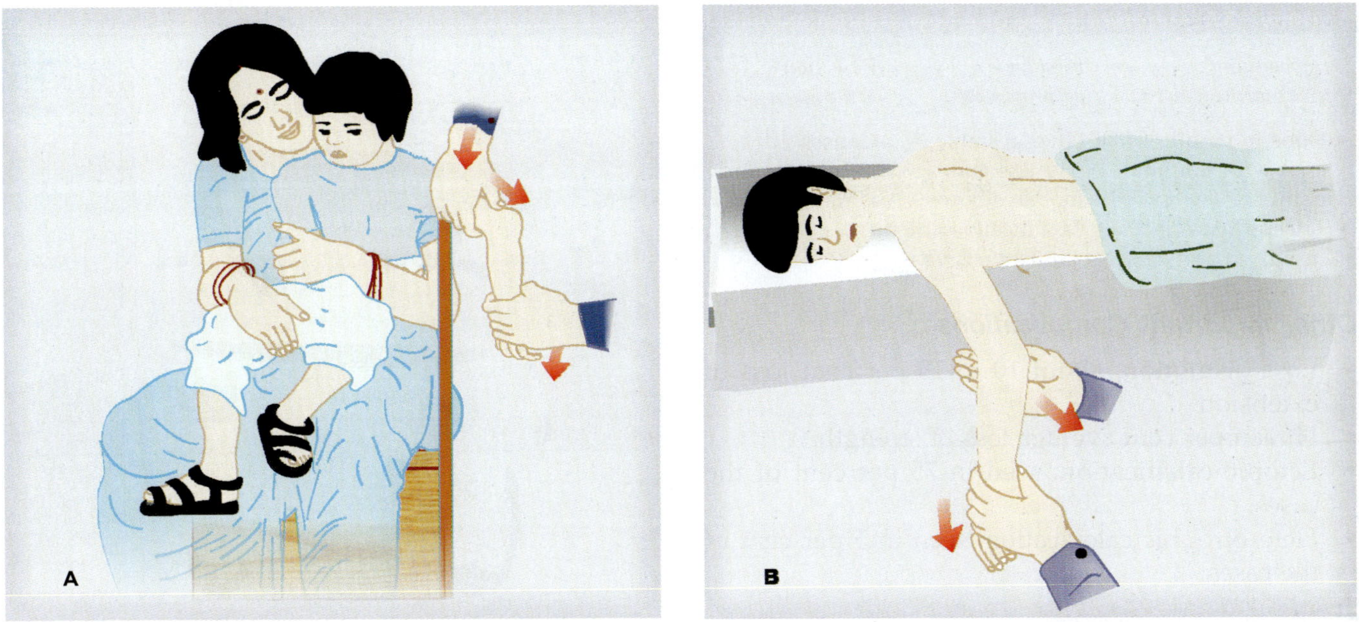

Figs 13.24A and B: Showing methods of reduction of posterior dislocation of elbow joint. A—Pusher's technique (in children) B—Puller's technique (in adults)

An above elbow POP slab is applied with 90° elbow flexion and midpronation for a period of 3 weeks.

Complications

1. *Neurological injuries* In these, the ulnar nerve is very commonly injured, followed by radial and median nerve in that order.
2. *Myositis ossificans* This has an incidence of 5 to 18 per cent and is generally not due to the injury *per se* but due to the manner in which it is treated. *Causes* Delay in initial treatment, use of hyperextension force during reduction, vigorous active physiotherapy and massage are some of the common causes.
3. *Arterial injuries* are rare but brachial artery injury may be seen in open fractures.
4. *Recurrent dislocation* This is relatively rare but can be seen in males and is usually found to be confined to the paediatric age group.

   Pathology Lax ulnar collateral ligament, pocket in the radial collateral ligament and a defect in the posterolateral aspect of the lateral condyle are the common pathological findings.

   Treatment Surgery is the treatment of choice. Soft tissue procedures consist of tightening the radial collateral ligament.

   • *Bony procedures* Here a graft is placed to deepen the semilunar notch of the ulna.
5. *Proximal radioulnar translation* This is an extremely rare complication and is due to very vigorous force used during reduction methods.
6. *Osteochondral fractures* These are relatively uncommon.
7. *Unreduced dislocation* Though rare it is more often seen in Asians due to ignorance, treatment by quacks, etc.

Clinical Features

The patients with unreduced posterior dislocation of the elbow joint have fixed flexion deformity and gross restriction of elbow movements. There may be wasting of the arm and forearm muscles.

Treatment Methods

Children Open reduction and resection of myositis is done in children

If it is less than 3 months' duration, open reduction alone is done.

If the injury is greater than 3 months, open reduction is combined with arthroplasty if necessary.

Adults In adults, open reduction is invariably followed with one of the following arthroplasties (Table 13.5).

Table 13.5: Different types of elbow arthroplasties

Interpositional (fascial) arthroplasty	*Implant arthroplasty*	*Resection arthroplasty*
• Done in mobile joint with minimal pain. • Triceps fascia is used.	• Gives a stable, painless and mobile elbow. • Technically difficult and expensive.	Causes instability and is rarely used.

Other Important Complications

- Loss of motion: about 10 to 15 per cent loss of extension
- Fifteen per cent average loss of strength.
- Ectopic calcification: seen in 75 per cent of the cases.
- Heterotrophic calcification: seen in 5 per cent of the cases.

SIDE SWIPE INJURIES (SYN: TRAFFIC ELBOW, CAR WINDOW ELBOW)

Everybody in the metropolis has heard about traffic jam, but have you heard about traffic elbow? Well, it is a shattered elbow syndrome, a consequence of callous neglect while travelling. Traffic jams are policemen's nightmare, while traffic elbow is orthopaedicians nightmare!

Mechanism of Injury

It is due to the force applied to an elbow projecting from a car window by a passsing vehicle or when it hits a fixed object or when it overturns (Fig. 13.25A).

Shorbe's Classification

Group I—only soft tissue injury.

Group II—only tip of the elbow is injured and there is fracture olecranon.

Group III—fracture of both radius and ulna.

Group IV—variations of comminuted intercondylar fractures of the humerus.

Group V—severely injured, fracture of all bones around the elbow with considerable soft tissue injury. Extensive open wounds are not unusual.

Investigations

Plain X-ray, MRI, CT scan, arteriogram, Doppler study, etc. are some of the important investigation methods.

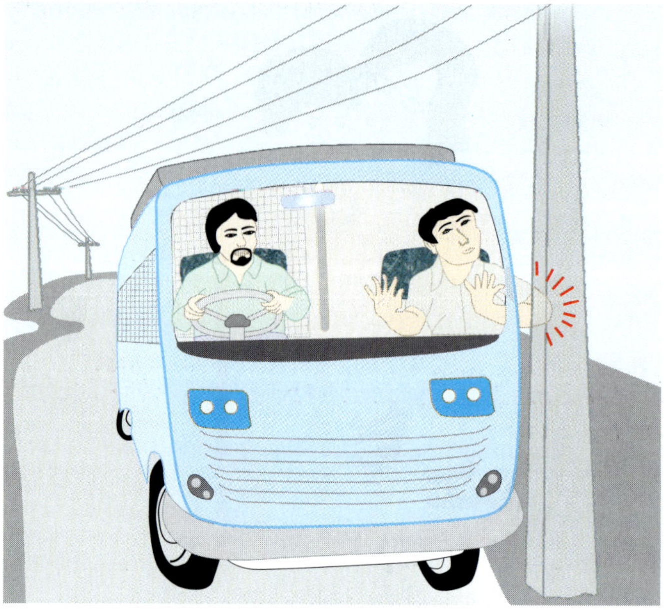

Fig. 13.25A: How many times you are guilty of sitting like this while travelling? Thank God you have not landed up with a "traffic elbow" !

Methods of Treatment

Treatment must be individualised. Various combinations of internal fixation, external fixation and traction should be tried (Fig. 13.25B). Initial debridement must be thorough. Primary nerve repair is indicated if the cut is clean. In crushed injuries, nerve should be repaired secondarily.

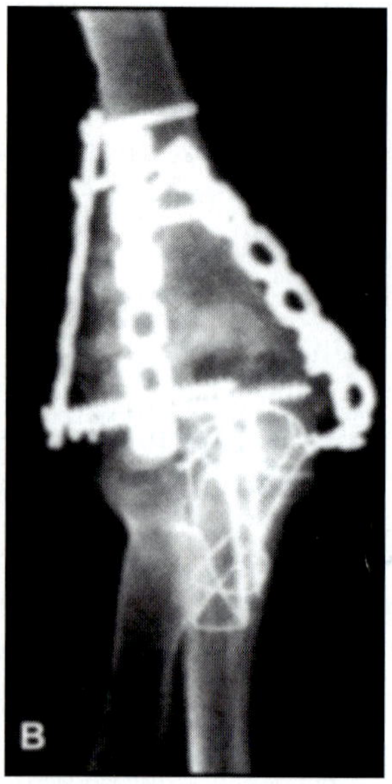

Fig. 13.25B: Radiograph showing reconstruction of fractures due to traffic elbow

Primary amputation This is indicated in the following situations:

1. Irreparable vascular damage and a non-viable extremity.
2. Segmental disruption of all three nerves around the elbow.

But it should be remembered that a pain-free elbow (either stiff or unstable) is better than amputation.

RADIAL HEAD FRACTURE

Radial head fracture is a common injury in adults and is rare in children.

Mechanism of Injury

1. Indirect trauma due to fall on an outstretched hand.
2. Direct trauma due to RTA, assault, etc. in adults.

Mason's Classification (Fig. 13.26)

Type I—undisplaced fracture

Type II—marginal fracture with displacement

Type III—comminuted fractures

Type IV—radial head fracture with posterior dislocation of elbow.

Clinical Features

The patient with radial head fracture complains of pain on the lateral side of the elbow, minimal swelling and restriction of elbow movements and supination, pronation of the forearm. There is tenderness over the radial head and crepitus can be elicited.

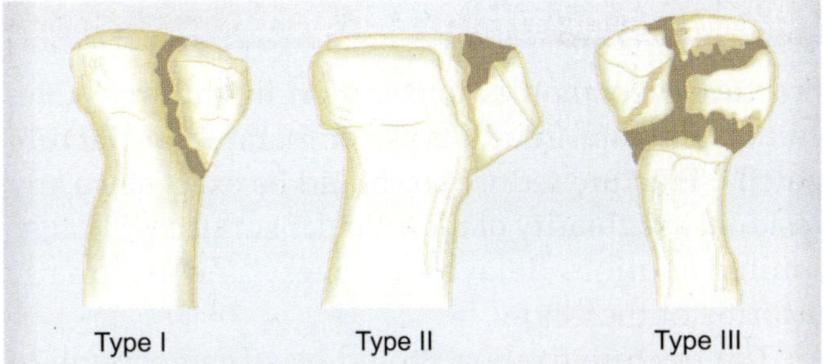

Fig. 13.26: Fracture head of the radius. Type III fracture with posterior dislocation of the elbow is called as type IV

Investigation

Anteroposterior and lateral radiographs of the elbow. Additional oblique radiograph delineates the fracture line better. CT scan helps to delineate the fracture pattern better.

Treatment

This varies according to the type of fractures (Table 13.6).

Radial head replacement is controversial since excision of the head is usually effective in isolated comminuted radial head fracture that too if the medial collateral ligament is intact. However, metal radial head replacement is superior to silicone prosthesis.

Complications

Injury to the posterior interosseous nerve, osteoarthritis and elbow stiffness are the common complications of radial head fractures.

Mystifying facts

Radial head excision does not cause instability (due to the presence of interosseous membrane) or functional impairment (due to the distal radioulnar joint).

Note: In olecranon fracture more than 2 mm separation between fracture fragments is called displaced fracture.

Table 13.6: Methods of treatment for different types of fractures of head of radius

Type I	*Type II*	*Type III*	*Type IV*
Nonoperative means • Aspiration of elbow within first 24 hours decreases pain • Early mobilisation within 24 hours	Excision head of radius (MacLaughlin's criteria for immediate excision) • Angulation > 30° • Depression > 3 mm • Involvement of > 1/3rd of head	• Radial head excision is indicated within first 24 hours • Excised head is replaced with prosthesis	• Prompt reduction of the dislocation is a must • Assess status of the head. If it meets the criteria for excision, do it within 24 hours.

Section 2

FRACTURE OF THE OLECRANON

Fracture olecranon is uncommon in children. Olecranon fracture in adults is comparable to fracture patella. Fracture reduction should be exact since any residual irregularity of the articular surface will cause limited motion, delayed recovery and traumatic arthritis of the elbow.

The fracture fixation should be strong enough to allow gentle active exercises even before radiographs show evidence of complete union.

As separation of the fracture of the patella causes quadriceps insufficiency so does displaced fracture olecranon causes triceps insufficiency.

Mechanism of Injury

1. *Direct* Trauma due to fall on the point of elbow. This is the frequent cause (Fig. 13.27).
2. *Indirect* due to forcible triceps contraction.

Colton's Classification (Figs 13.28A to C) (Modified Schtazker)

1. Undisplaced fracture
2. Displaced fracture
3. Avulsion fracture
4. Transverse/oblique fracture
5. Fracture dislocation (Monteggia group)
6. Comminuted fracture.

Clinical Features

The patient complains of pain, swelling and inability to extend the elbow. Clinically, tenderness and crepitus can be elicited.

Radiology

Radiograph of the elbow Routine anteroposterior and lateral views of the elbow help in confirmation of the diagnosis (Fig. 13.29).

Treatment

Conservative

Indications This is indicated for undisplaced fractures and in fractures with less than 2 mm displacement.

In children, closed reduction is done and the limb is immobilised in an above elbow plaster slab or cast for 3 to 4 weeks and this is often successful.

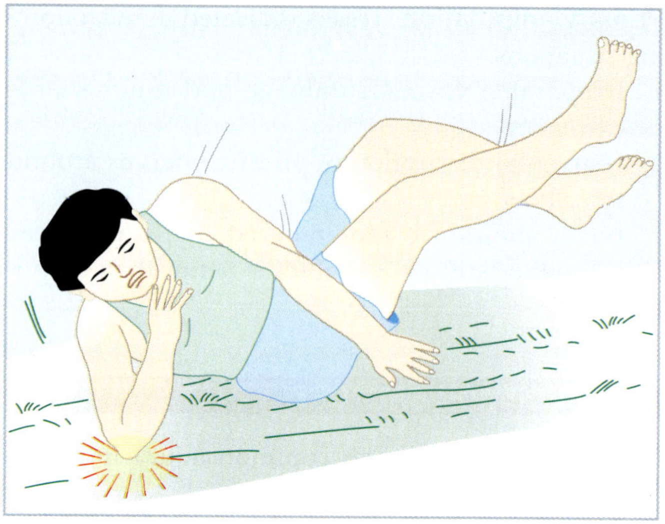

Fig. 13.27: Showing most common mechanism of olecranon fracture

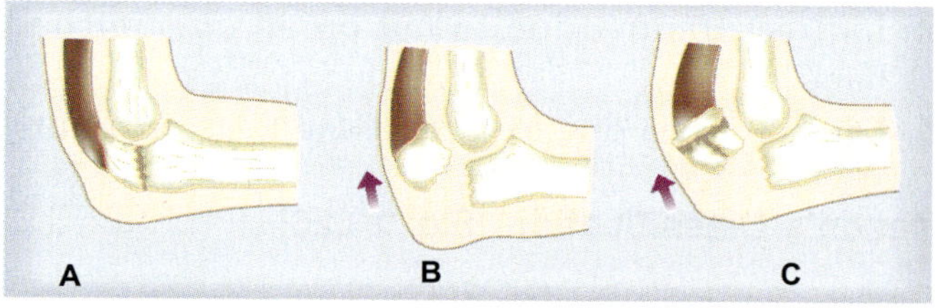

Figs 13.28A to C: Showing undisplaced fractures: (A) Displaced, (B) Comminuted, (C) Fracture of olecranon

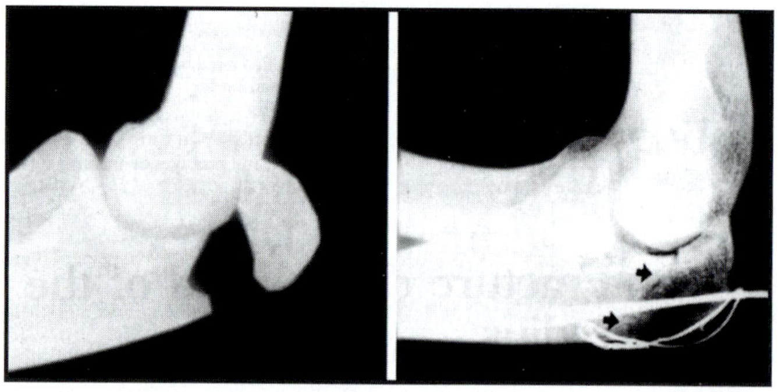

Fig. 13.29: Radiographs showing olecranon fracture

Surgery

In adults, repair of triceps is done for avulsion fractures. There is no place for conservative treatment, because closed reduction needs immobilisation in extension for 6 to 8 weeks, which except in children causes permanent stiffness. Hence, surgery is the treatment of choice in adults.

Three methods of operative treatment

1. **Open reduction and internal fixation with figure of 8 wire loop** (Figs 13.30A and B) This method

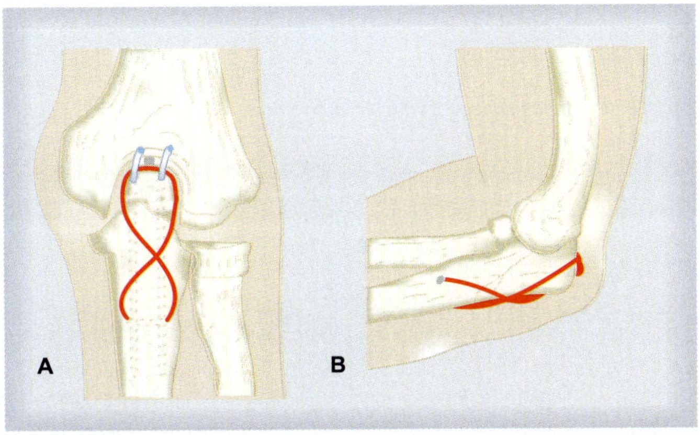

Figs 13.30A and B: Showing tension band wiring (TWB) in fracture olecranon

is used for avulsion and transverse fractures of the olecranon and for fractures which are uncomminuted and proximal to the coronoid fossa.

Disturbing facts

Reoperation rate after tension band wiring in olecranon fracture is as high as 71.7 per cent due to backing out of the K-wire.

2. **Medullary fixation by a single interfragmentary screw** This is indicated in comminuted fracture of olecranon when its distal fragment and the head of the radius are dislocated anteriorly. Rigid fixation is required to prevent recurrence of dislocation.
3. **Excision of the proximal fragments**
   Indications
   - In comminuted fractures
   - In delayed union or nonunion of fractures in upper half.
   - If the patient is greater than 50 years of age and is not involved in heavy work.

This method is useful only if enough of the olecranon is left to form a stable base for the trochlea. Thus, it is not indicated when comminution extends as far as the coronoid.

Complications

Nonunion of the fracture, osteoarthritis of the elbow, triceps insufficiency and restricted movements of the elbow are the common complications of fracture olecranon.

When do you consider olecranon fracture as stable?
If after reduction it does not separate or if the separation does not increase with flexion of elbow to 90°.

Quick facts

Treatment of displaced olecranon fractures in a nutshell:
- Avulsion fracture—TBW/LS
- Transverse fractures—TBW/LS
- Transverse fractures with—Plate and screws with bone grafting
- Oblique fractures—LS/Plate
- Communition—Excision/plate/TBW
- Fracture dislocation—Wire/LS/Plate

TBW—Tension band wiring
LS—Lag screw fixation

CORONOID FRACTURES (Fig. 13.31)

Fractures of the coronoid process of the ulna was earlier thought to be an avulsion fracture involving the brachialis muscle. Of late, this notion has been dispelled as it is found that the insertion of this muscle is more distal.

Interesting facts about coronoid fractures

- Its presence indicates a significant trauma to the elbow
- It also points towards the possibility of acute recurrent dislocations.

Mechanism of Injury This fracture occurs due to the impact of the coronoid process against the trochlea following a fall on an outstretched hand.

Classification of Regan and Morrey

Type I—Avulsion fracture of the tip of the coronoid.

Type II—Fracture involving greater than 50 per cent of the coronoid.

Type III—Fracture involving the base of the coronoid.

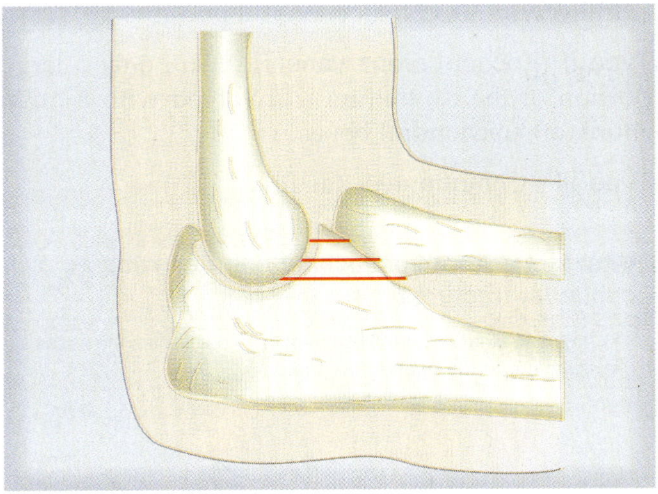

Fig. 13.31: Showing types of coronoid fractures

Section 2

Clinical Features

Isolated fractures of the coronoid process are usually rare and are usually associated with greater elbow trauma. Clinical features like pain, swelling, deformity, movement restriction of the elbow, etc. depends on the extent of damage.

Radiograph This fracture can be easily identified over a true lateral X-ray of the elbow.

Treatment Though small undisplaced fractures can be managed conservatively with an above elbow plaster cast, displaced fractures need open reduction and internal fixation with screw or wires.

CAPITELLUM FRACTURES

Capitellum is the anterior portion of the lateral humeral condyle. This fracture is unique in being intra-articular always.

Mechanism of Injury

Fall on an outstretched hand, with flexion or extension of the elbow, and the resulting shear forces through the radial head slices the capitellum.

Classification Based on the size of the articulating fragment, it is classified into three types (Figs 13.32A and B).

Type I (Hahn-Steinthal variety)—This involves a large portion of the capitellum and a small chunk of trochlea with less of subchondral portion.

Type II (Kocher-Lorenz variety)—Here only a large portion of the capitellum is involved with a huge chunk of subchondral bone.

Type III—Comminuted fracture.

Vital facts: About associated injuries with capitellar fractures

- Injury to ulnar collateral ligament in 69 per cent of the cases
- Fracture of the head of the radius.

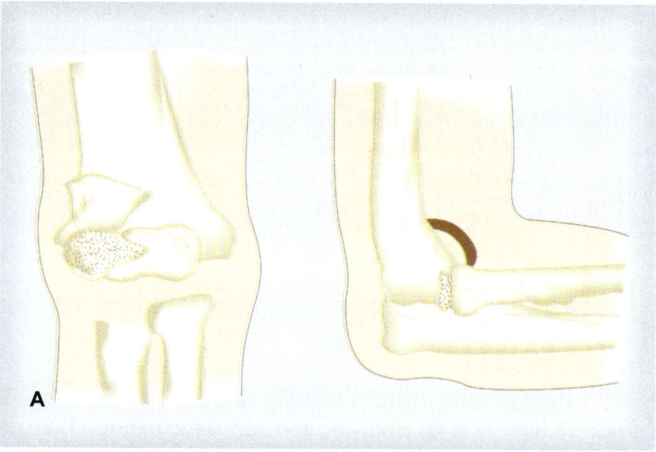

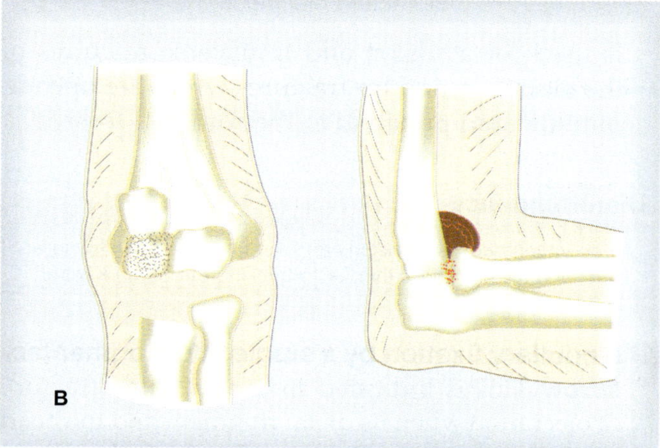

Figs 13.32A and B: Showing types of capitellum fractures. A—Type I, B—Type II

Clinical Features

The patient complains of pain and swelling over the lateral aspect of the elbow. Elbow and forearm movements are also restricted.

Radiograph A true lateral view of the elbow is mandatory to accurately diagnose this fracture. The characteristic finding of this fracture is the presence of "double arc sign" described by McKay over the X-ray.

Treatment Undisplaced fractures can be managed conservatively by an above elbow plaster cast or slab for 3 to 4 weeks.

Displaced fractures need open reduction and internal fixation with minifragment screws.

14 Injuries of the Forearm

INTRODUCTION

Injuries of the forearm present an interesting combination of injuries like fracture both bones of forearm (Fig. 14.1), Monteggia fractures, Galeazzi fractures, Essex-Lopresti fracture, etc. The muscle attachments of the forearm make the treatment of these fractures difficult. The supinator muscle is inserted in the proximal third of the forearm bones and supinates this part of the forearm after the fracture. The middle third gives attachment to the pronator teres muscle and the distal third to the pronator quadratus. When the fracture occurs in the middle third, the forearm is held in the position of midpronation due to the balancing action of supinators and pronator quadratus muscle. In fractures of the distal third, the forearm is pronated due to the action of pronator quadratus. Hence, the treating physician should be aware of the various muscular forces (Fig. 14.2) acting in the forearm to effectively neutralise them and bring about proper union between the fracture fragments. Immobilising the forearm in *supination* in upper third fractures, *midpronation* in middle third fractures and *pronation* in distal third fracture is found to effectively counter the muscular forces which threaten to displace the fracture fragments.

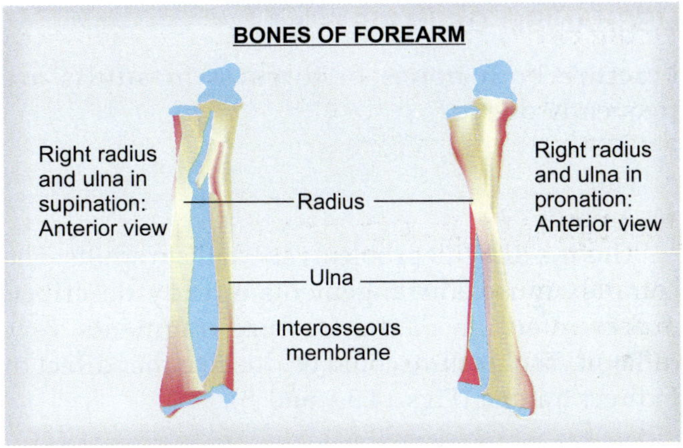

Fig. 14.1: Bones of the forearm

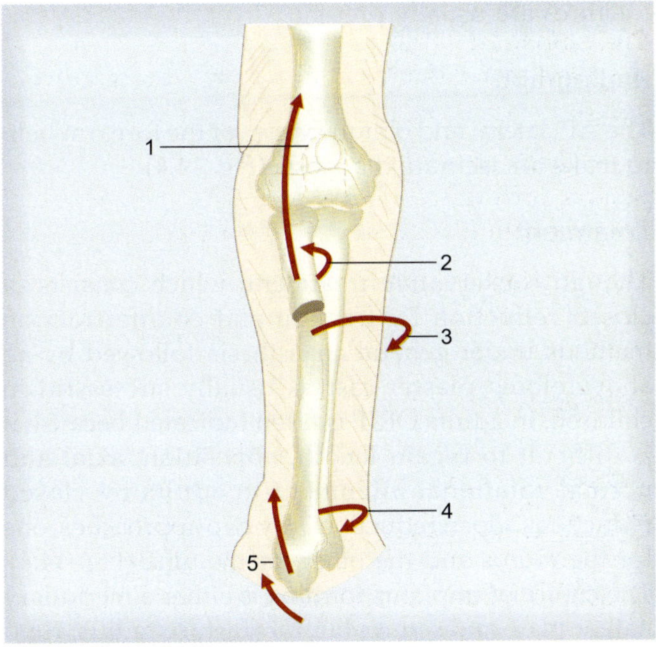

Fig. 14.2: Muscle forces in fracture both bones of forearm: (1) Biceps, (2) Supinator, (3) Pronator teres, (4) Pronator quadratus, (5) Brachoradialis

Monteggia fracture along with Galeazzi fracture forms a rare and interesting combination of injuries where there is fracture of one bone with dislocation of the other. Curiously both are described in the forearm with the former involving the upper and middle forearm, and the latter involving the distal forearm.

FRACTURE BOTH BONES OF THE FOREARM

MECHANISM OF INJURY

Fracture both bones of forearm in adults are frequently due to:

- RTA
- Fall
- Assault

This is a difficult problem especially in adults. The complex muscle arrangements already described makes retention of the fracture fragments very difficult. The fracture could be due to either direct or indirect trauma (Figs 14.3A and B).

Clinical Features

The patient presents with severe pain, swelling and deformity of the forearm. Movements of the forearm are severely restricted and all other features of fractures are usually present.

Radiograph

The AP, lateral and oblique views of the forearm help to make an accurate diagnosis (Fig. 14.4).

Treatment

Though conservative treatment, which consists of closed reduction by traction and countertraction methods under general anaesthesia followed by an above elbow plaster cast, is usually successful in children, in adults ORIF is often indicated because it is difficult to regain length, apposition, axial and normal rotational alignment in adults by closed reductions. Open reduction is by two approaches, one for the radius and the other for the ulna (Fig. 14.4). The choice of implants for ulna is either a medullary nail or plate and screws but for fracture radius, rigid compression plating is usually desired. Cancellous bone grafting is done if the comminution is more than one-third of the circumference of the bone (see Fig. 14.3C).

What is new?

Treatment of fracture both bones of forearm. It is the advent of intramedullary interlocking nailing and is being mainly used in the paediatric group than adults.

Indications

- Segmental fracture
- Open fracture with soft tissues injury and/or bone loss.
- Multiple injuries.
- Failed plating.
- Pathological fractures.

Advantages

- Less exposure.
- Less periosteal stripping.

Complications of Fracture Both Bones of Forearm

1. *Volkmann's ischaemia* Because of the tight fascial compartment, a patient with fracture both bones forearm is more prone to develop acute compartmental syndrome.

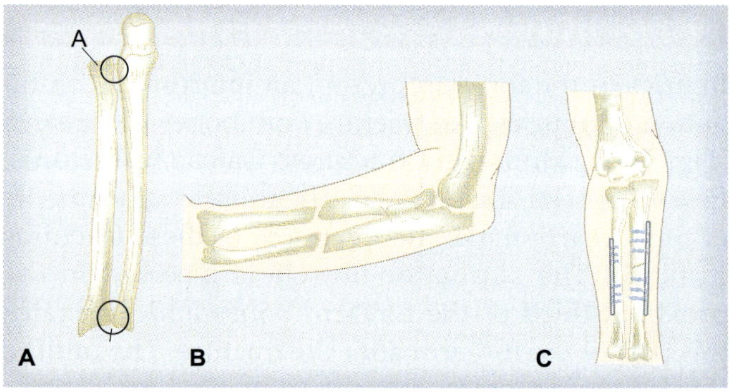

Figs 14.3A to C: Showing (A) normal both bones of the forearm with superior and inferior radioulnar joints, (B) fracture both bones of the forearm, (C) fracture both bones fixed rigidly with plate and screws (preferred method)

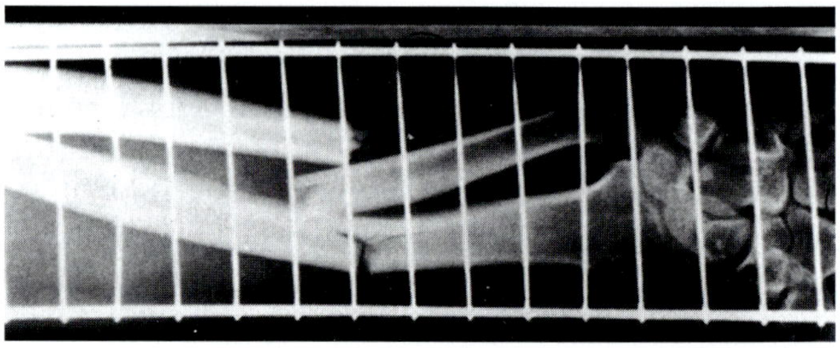

Fig. 14.4: Radiograph showing fracture of radius and ulna

2. *Delayed union and nonunion* This can be encountered due to soft tissue interposition, inadequate immobilisation, etc. It has to be treated by open reduction, rigid internal fixation and cancellous bone grafting.
3. *Malunion* Due to the complex muscular forces it is difficult to retain the position of both bones in perfect alignment after closed reduction. It is in this situation that malunion commonly results. It is treated by corrective osteotomy, plating and bone grafting.
4. *Cross union* This is due to malunion of a radial fracture in a medially deviated position which occupies the interosseous space and blocks pronation and supination. If the cross union takes place in the middle third of the forearm, it can be left alone as the forearm is held in midpronation with less functional damage. Elsewhere it needs corrective osteotomy and rigid internal fixation.

ISOLATED DISTAL ULNAR FRACTURE (ALSO CALLED NIGHT STICK FRACTURE)

This is relatively rare when compared to fracture both bones of the forearm.

It is usually due to direct blow on the subcutaneous border of the ulna (Fig. 14.5). Three types are described:

1. Simple fracture.
2. Comminuted fracture without distal radioulnar joint involvement.
3. Type II with involvement of the distal radioulnar joint.

Interesting facts

Night stick fracture derives its name from the peculiar incident of a burglar getting caught during his misadventure in the night and trying to ward off the policeman's blow with the stick with his forearm (Fig. 14.5).

Treatment

Type II and III varieties are treated by open reduction and rigid internal fixation with plate and screws.

MONTEGGIA FRACTURE (TABLE 14.1)

DEFINITION It is a fracture upper third of ulna with dislocation head of the radius.

This is usually called a "treacherous lesion" because the dislocation is often missed (see box for the reasons).

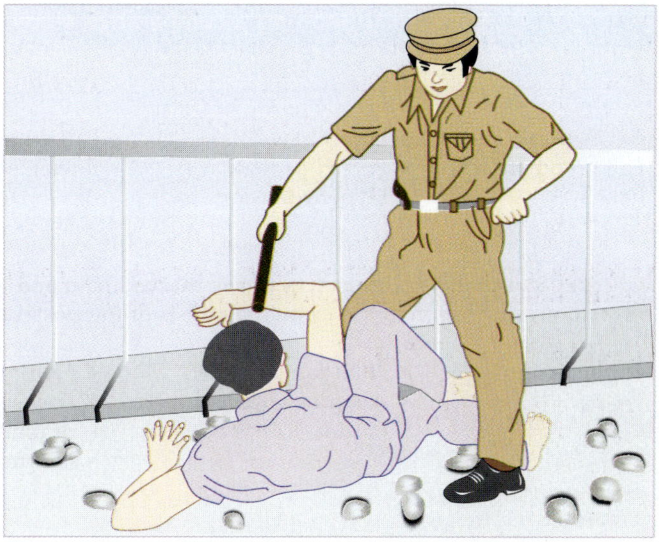

Fig. 14.5: Mechanism of night stick fracture

It was first described by Monteggia in 1881.

Monteggia fractures, Why called as treacherous?
Because dislocation of the head of the radius is often missed.

Reasons

- *Missed by patient*: As he reflexly pulls the elbow after fall and reduces the dislocation unknowingly.
- *Missed by quack* due to ignorance
- *Missed by physician:* Fails to order to include the elbow in radiographs of forearm bone fractures
- *Missed by radiologist:* If he or she fails to utilise the McLaughlin's line

MECHANISM OF INJURY

Monteggia fractures are more common in children and are due to fall on the outstretched hands either in hyperpronation or in hyperextension (Fig. 14.6).

Classification

Bado's classification (Table 14.2) is employed in adults and John Wein's classification (Table 14.3) in children and which takes into consideration the greenstick fractures in them (Figs 14.7A to E).

Monteggia equivalents These are variants of Monteggia fracture dislocations and are a result of pronation injuries. The following types are described:

1. Isolated dislocation of head of the radius.
2. Fracture shaft ulna with fracture neck radius.
3. Fracture shaft ulna with fracture shaft radius (distal).

Section 2

Table 14.1: Showing a comparative study of the various features of Monteggia fractures

	Type I	Type II	Type III	Type IV
Mechanism of injury Fall on outstretched hands	• Direct blow • Forced pronation • Hyperextension	Fall with elbow in flexion of 120°	• Forced supination • Forced pronation • Supination with hyperextension	Same as in type I and if force continues
Clinical Symptoms	All four types have marked pain and tenderness about the elbow. There will be no flexion/extension/ pronation/supination at the elbow. Paralysis of the posterior interosseous nerve may occur.			
Clinical signs	• HOR felt anteriorly • Anterior angulation of ulna	• HOR posterior • Posterior angulation of ulna • Shortening of forearm	HOR is lateral Lateral angulation	HOR is anterior Deformity is at the fracture level
Treatment				
In children	• Closed reduction is tried first • If unsuccessful OR of fracture ulna + CR of HOR is done • If this also fails, OR of fracture ulna with OR of head of the radius with repair or reconstruction of annular ligament using forearm fascia or fascia lata is done	CR tried first. OR if it fails	Closed reduction is successful most of the times	CR is tried first If it fails OR + Rigid IF with plate and screws for radius and ulnar fractures is done.
In adults	• OR + IF of fracture ulna with plate and screws • CR of HOR • If it fails, OR, HOR + IF fracture ulna is done • If fracture > 6 weeks Excision HOR is done	Same as in type I	Same as in type I	Same as in type I

Note: CR → Closed reduction, OR → Open reduction, IF → Internal fixation, and HOR → Head of radius

Table 14.2: Bado's classification (adults)

Type I (60%)	Anterior dislocation of head of the radius with fracture ulna at upper third and with anterior angulation.
Type II (5%)	Posterior dislocation head of the radius and fracture proximal ulna with posterior angulation.
Type III (20%)	Lateral dislocation head of the radius and fracture proximal ulna with lateral angulation.
Type IV (15%)	Fracture radius and ulna in their upper one-third and anterior dislocation of head of the radius with anterior angulation.

Table 14.3: John Wein's classification (children)

It takes into account greenstick fracture in children

1. Anterior bend.
2. Anterior greenstick.
3. Anterior complete
4. Posterior
5. Lateral

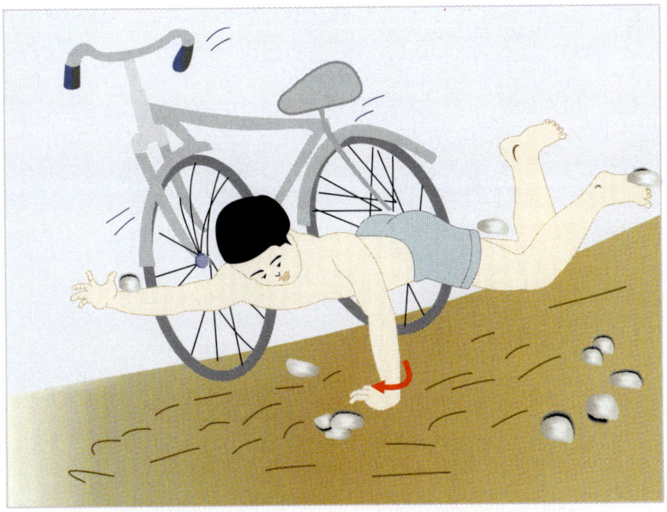

Fig. 14.6: Showing hyperpronation injury leading to fractures like Monteggia

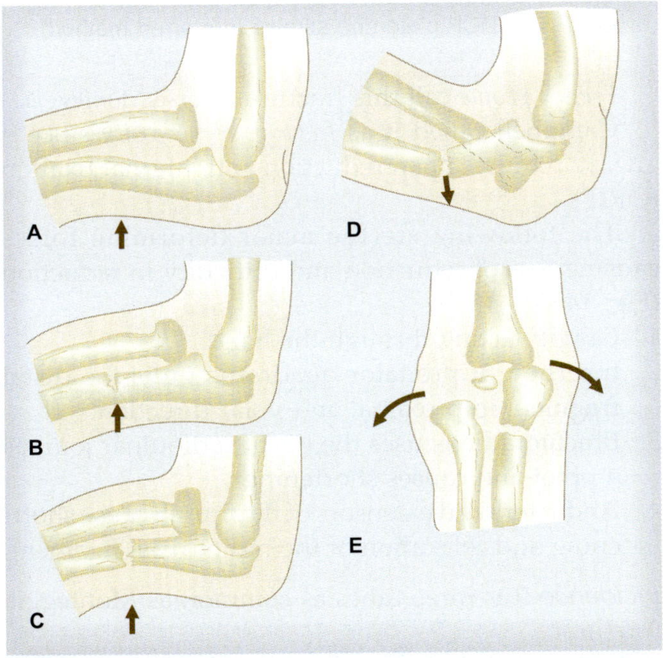

Figs 14.7A to E: Diagrammatic representation of the displacements in Monteggia fracture; **Bado's Types** (Adults) C-type I, D-type II, E-Type III; **John Wein's Types** (Children) A-Anterior bend, B-Anterior greenstick, C-Anterior complete

4. Fracture ulna with fracture radial neck, dislocation of shaft of the radius.

In these cases closed reduction is tried first. If it fails, open reduction and internal fixation is done (Figs 14.8A to C).

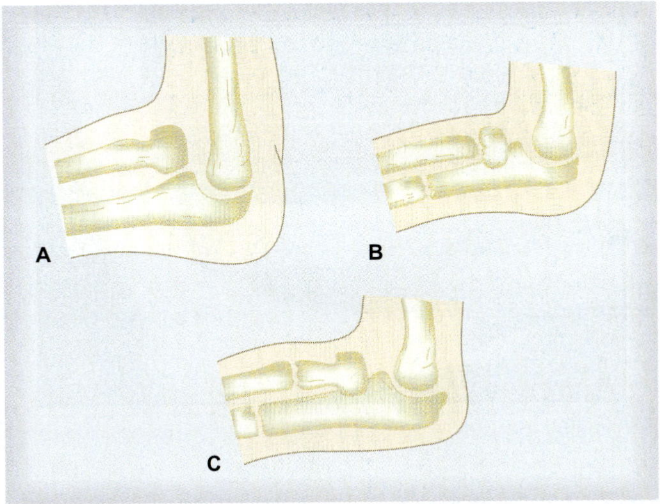

Figs 14.8A to C: Showing types of Monteggia equivalents: (A) isolated anterior dislocation head of the radius, (B) fracture ulna and fracture neck radius, and (C) both fracture ulna (distal) and radius (proximal)

Clinical Features

A patient with Monteggia fracture complains of pain, swelling, deformity and severe loss of forearm movements.

Depending upon the type of Monteggia fractures the head of the radius and the ulnar angulation may be felt anteriorly, posteriorly or laterally.

Radiology (Fig. 14.9A)

In order to avoid missing the diagnosis of dislocation of the head of radius, MacLaughlin's line is employed as described below (Figs 14.9B).

A straight line drawn along the centre of the shaft of the radius cuts the capitulum in the centre irrespective of the position of the elbow.

Treatment

Monteggia fractures can be managed successfully in children by conservative methods and by operative methods in adults (see Table 14.1).

Complications

1. Unreduced dislocation head of radius.
2. Posterior interosseous nerve palsy.
3. Malunion of fracture ulna.
4. Nonunion of fracture ulna.
5. Myositis ossificans.

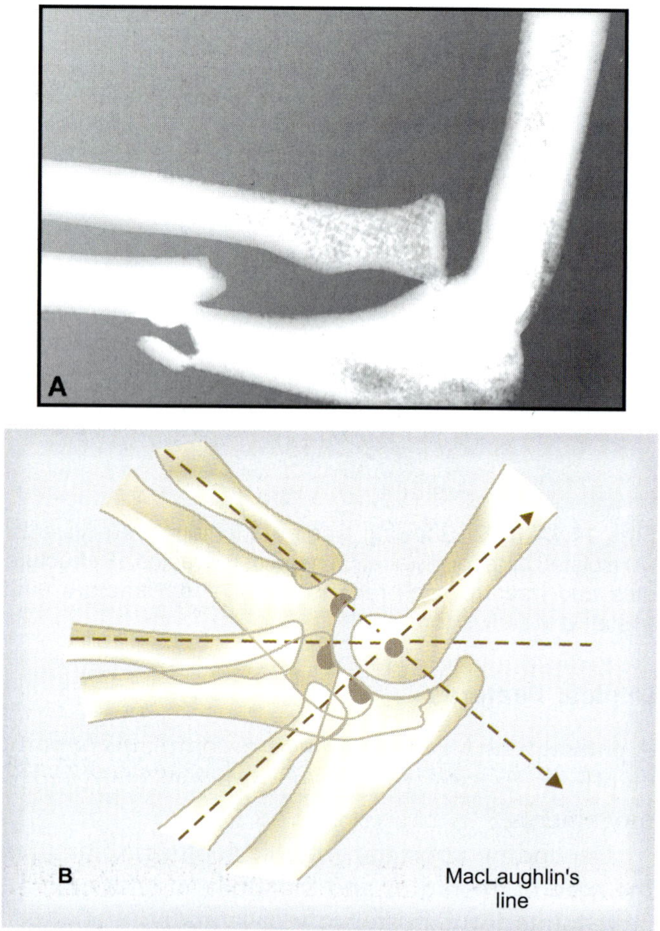

Figs 14.9A and B: (A) Radiograph showing Monteggia fracture, (B) MacLaughlin's line

6. Synostosis between radial head and proximal ulna.
7. Tardy posterior interosseous nerve palsy.
8. Proximal migration of radius.
9. Dislocation of inferior radioulnar joint.
10. Cubitus valgus deformity.

DISTAL SHAFT RADIUS FRACTURE

Also called "Piedmont fracture" (after Piedmont Orthopaedic Society).

GALEAZZI FRACTURE

Definition This is a fracture of radius at the junction of middle and distal third with associated subluxation or dislocation of the distal radioulnar joint. Subluxation of this joint may be present initially or occur during treatment (Figs 14.10A and B).

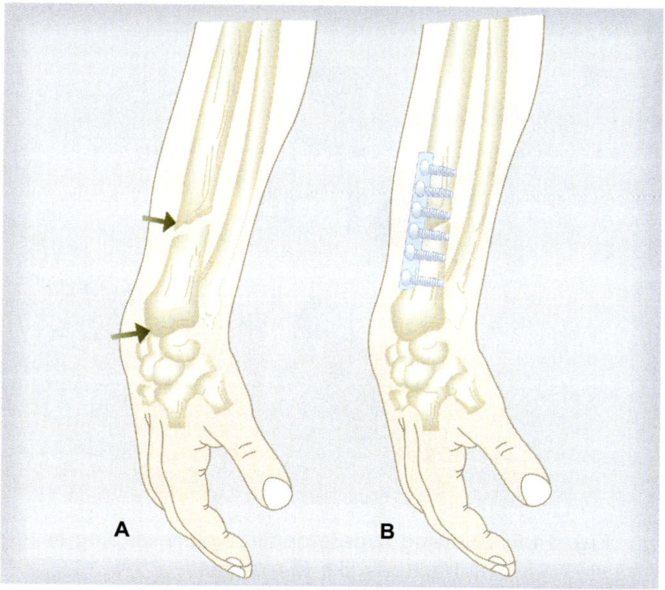

Figs 14.10A and B: Showing (A) Galeazzi fracture, (B) ORIF with DCP plate and screws (preferred method)

French people call this fracture *reverse Monteggia.*

Campbell called it as *fracture of necessity* since it always requires open reduction and internal fixation (ORIF).

The following are the major deforming forces causing loss of reduction and difficulty in reduction (Fig. 14.11).

1. Gravity acting through the hand.
2. Insertion of pronator quadratus pulls the distal fragment in proximal and volar direction.
3. Brachioradialis uses the distal radioulnar joint as a pivot and causes shortening.
4. Abductors and extensors of the thumb cause shortening and relaxation of the radiocarpal ligament.

Incidence It is three times as common as Monteggia fracture.

Mechanism of Injury

1. Fall on an outstretched hand with marked pronation of the forearm.
2. Direct blow on the dorsolateral side of the forearm.

Clinical Features

The patient complains of pain, swelling and deformity of the lower end of the forearm. Pronation and supination are severely restricted. All other features of fractures are present.

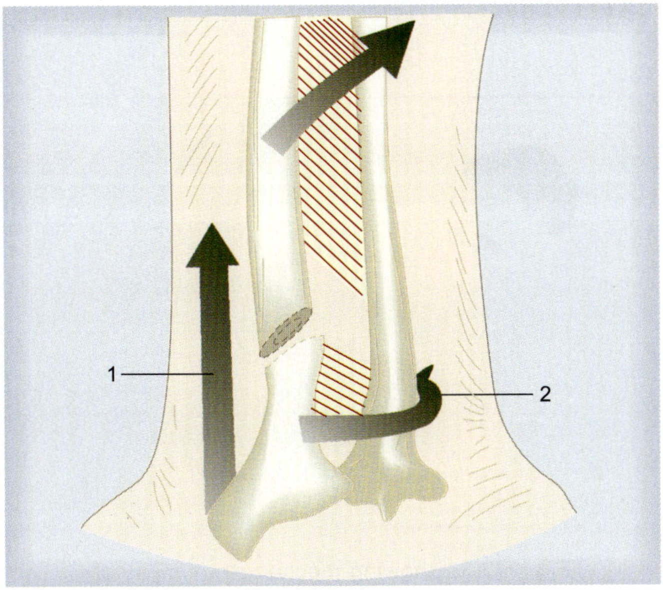

Fig. 14.11: Showing displacing forces in Galeazzi fractures, (1) Brachioradialis, (2) Pronator quadratus

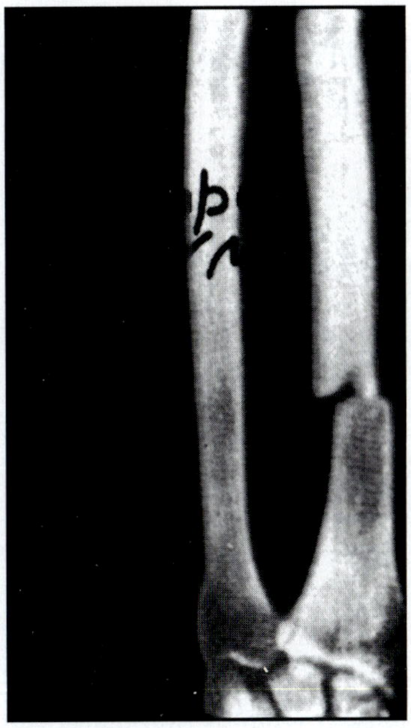

Fig. 14.12: Radiograph showing Galeazzi fracture

Radiology

Important radiological features of Galleazzi fracture are as shown in the box (Fig. 14.12).

AP view	Lateral view
• Fracture radius, transverse or short oblique • Comminution is less • Distal radioulnar joint is dislocated • Radius appears short	• Radius is angulated dorsally • Head of the ulna is prominent dorsally

Treatment

Closed reduction is usually not successful due to the deforming forces of the muscles. Hence, ORIF is the preferred method of treatment. Intramedullary nails and small plates do not provide adequate fixation, long plate (LCDCP plate) and screws are thus used and the dislocated distal radioulnar joint may be fixed with K-wire.

Complications

Nonunion and malunion are notorious complications. Angulation of the fracture and subluxation of the distal radioulnar joint can also occur. Rarely entrapment of extensor carpi ulnaris tendon in distal radioulnar joint is encountered.

ESSEX-LOPRESTI FRACTURE

DEFINITION This is a fracture of the radial head with injury to the distal radioulnar joint.

It is a relatively rare fracture and in order to avoid missing it, radiograph of the wrist joint should be taken in all cases of fracture of head of the radius. If there is disruption of distal radioulnar joint, excision head of the radius is likely to aggravate the proximal migration of the radius. Hence, if fracture radial head needs excision, it has to be replaced by silastic prosthesis.

RADIAL STYLOID FRACTURE (Chauffeur's Fracture)

Radial styloid fracture (Hutchinson's fracture) is similar to the posterior marginal fracture of the radius.

Mechanism

It is usually as a result of the starting crank of an engine being suddenly reversed by a backfire and striking the wrist with a force. It is common in chauffeurs and is an avulsion fracture of the radiocarpal ligament (Fig. 14.13).

Note: These are also seen in motorcycle accidents and fall from heights.

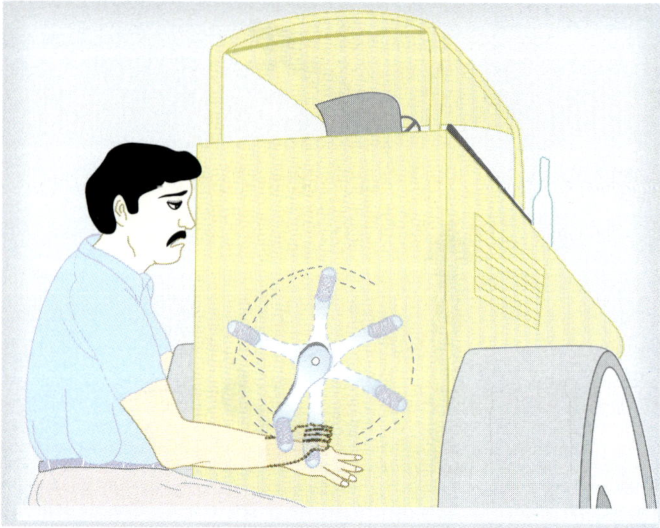

Fig. 14.13: Showing mechanism of injury of Hutchinson's fracture

Clinical Features

The patient complains of pain, swelling and tenderness over the radial styloid process. Movement of the wrist, especially radial deviation, is painful.

Radiology

Radiograph AP view of the wrist shows it as a transverse fracture.

Treatment

This fracture is best treated by closed reduction and above elbow plaster cast. However, unstable fractures need percutaneous fixation with K-wire.

SMITH'S FRACTURE

Definition It is a fracture of distal one-third of radius with palmar displacement. Hence, it is called as *reverse Colles' fracture*. Though it is less common than Colles' it is readily confused with Colles' fracture. It has a clear fracture dorsally with comminution of the palmar surface (Fig. 14.14A).

Did you know?
Smith's fracture occurs about 1/10 as frequent as Colles' fracture. The greatest problem with this fracture is executing the treatment mistaking it to be a Colles' fracture!

Mechanism of Injury

There are three modes of injury like fall on the back of the dorsum of the hand, fall on the forearm in supination and a direct blow to the flexed hand.

Clinical Features

The patient complains of pain, swelling, deformity and loss of wrist functions. The deformity is opposite to that of Colles' fracture and is called the 'garden spade' deformity.

Radiograph

Anteroposterior view of the wrist shows the carpus proximally displaced. There will be anterior displacement of the fragment with palmar angulation of distal radial articular surface. The ulnar styloid process is frequently fractured.

Treatment

The treatment of choice is closed reduction and immobilisation in a long arm cast with forearm in supination and wrist in extension. For unstable fractures, fixation with percutaneous K-wire or open reduction and plate fixation may be required (Fig. 14.14B).

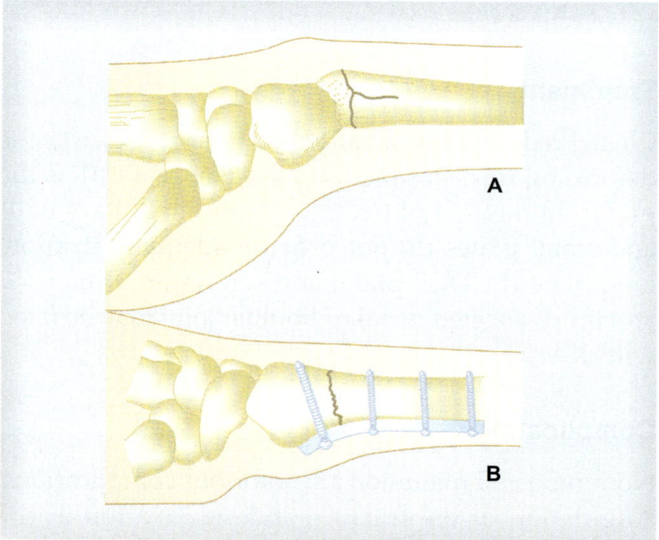

Figs 14.14A and B: Showing (A) Smith's fracture, (B) Method of fixation of Smith's fracture

Complications

1. Misinterpretation of radiographs for Colles'.
2. Other complication of Colles'.

BARTON'S FRACTURE

Rim fractures of the distal radius are called Barton's fracture. Dorsal (Fig. 14.15) or volar (Figs 14.16 and 14.17) rim could be involved and these fractures are invariably intra-articular. A comparative study of these two fractures is presented in Table 14.4.

Table 14.4: Comparison between dorsal Barton's and volar Barton's fracture

Dorsal Barton	*Volar Barton*
• Dorsal rim fracture of distal radius • Variant of Colles'	Palmar rim fracture of distal radius
Mechanism	***Mechanism***
Fall with dorsiflexion and pronation of the distal forearm on a flexed wrist	It is due to palmar tensile stress and dorsal sheer stress and is usually combined with radial styloid fracture
Radiology	***Radiology***
Best seen on the lateral view. Dorsal lip of distal radial articular surface is displaced proximally and posteriorly and may be associated with dorsal subluxation of the wrist	Palmar rim of distal radial articular surface is displaced dorsally
Treatment	***Treatment***
Conservative	*Conservative*
Short arm cast with wrist in neutral position	Reduction is simple, but retention is difficult. Long arm cast is used
Surgery	***Surgery***
Unstable fracture is fixed by percutaneous pins or OR IF with small plate is done. Healing, prognosis, complications are similar to Colles'	If reduction does not remain satisfactorily with wrist in neutral or slight palmar flexion, fixation with K-wire, external fixators and buttress plate, etc. may be used

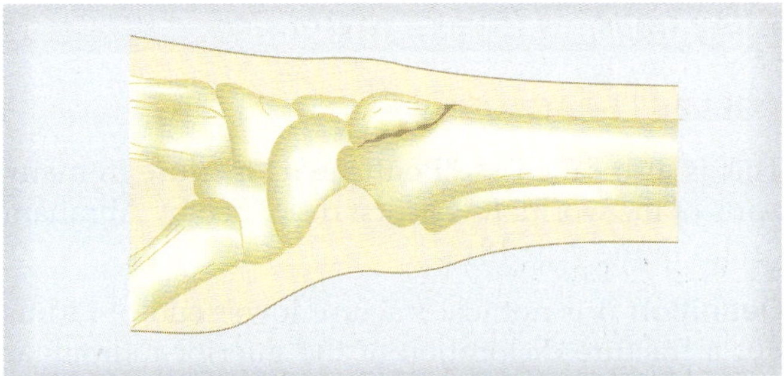

Fig. 14.15: Showing dorsal Barton's fracture

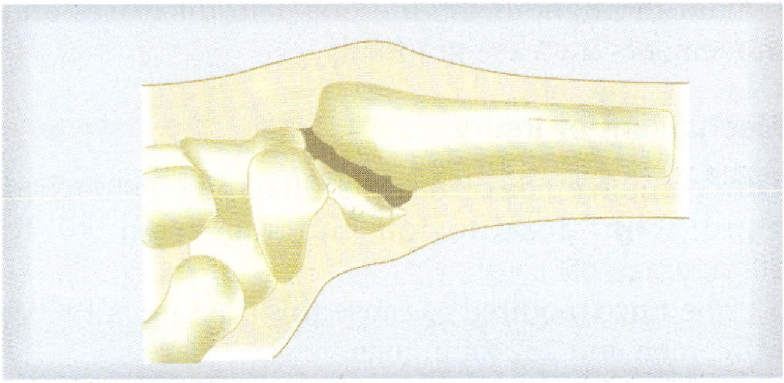

Fig. 14.16: Showing volar Barton's fracture

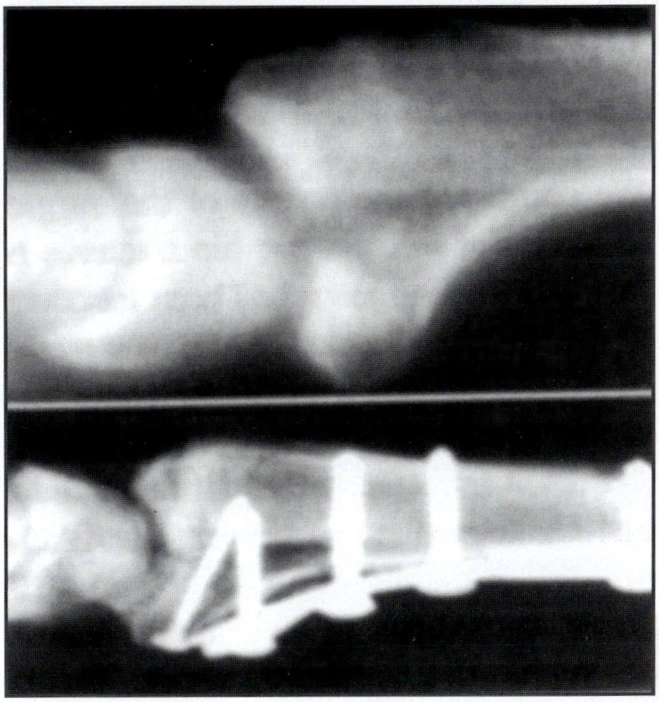

Fig. 14.17: Radiographs showing volar Barton's fracture fixed with plate and screws

Section 2

DISTAL FOREARM FRACTURES

COLLES' FRACTURE

This is also called as **"Poutteau's"** fracture in many parts of the world. It was first described by Abraham Colles in the year 1814.

Definition It is not just fracture lower end of radius but a fracture dislocation of the inferior radioulnar joint. The fracture occurs about 1½" (about 2.5 cm) above the carpal extremity of the radius (Fig. 14.18).

Following this fracture, some deformity will remain throughout the life but pain decreases and movements increase gradually.

Mechanism of Injury

The common mode of injury is fall on an outstretched hand with dorsiflexion ranging from 40 to 90°(average 60°).

The force required to cause this fracture is 192 kg in women and 282 kg in men.

Fracture pattern It is usually sharp on the palmar aspect and comminution on the dorsal surface of the lower end of radius.

Clinical Features

Usually, the patient is an elderly female in her 60s and the history given is a trivial fall on an outstretched hand (Fig. 14.19). The patient complains of pain, swelling, deformity and other usual features of fracture at the lower end of radius. Though *dinner fork* deformity is a classical deformity in a Colles' fracture, however, it is not found in all cases but seen only if there is a dorsal tilt or rotation of the distal fragment (Figs 14.18 and 14.20). However, the styloid process test is more reliable. There are six classical displacement in a Colles' fracture (Table 14.5).

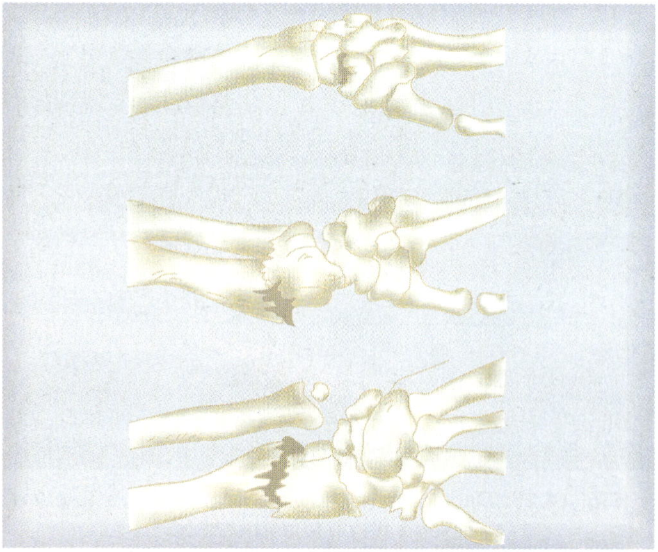

Fig. 14.18: Showing Colles' fracture

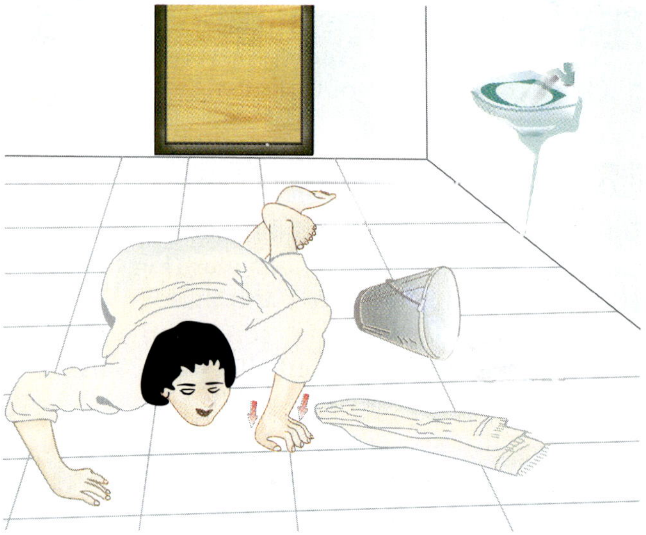

Fig. 14.19: Colles' fracture is usually due to a slip and fall on the outstretched hands in elderly females

> **Did you know?**
> Dinner fork deformity is also called:
> - Silver fork deformity.
> - Spoon-shaped deformity.

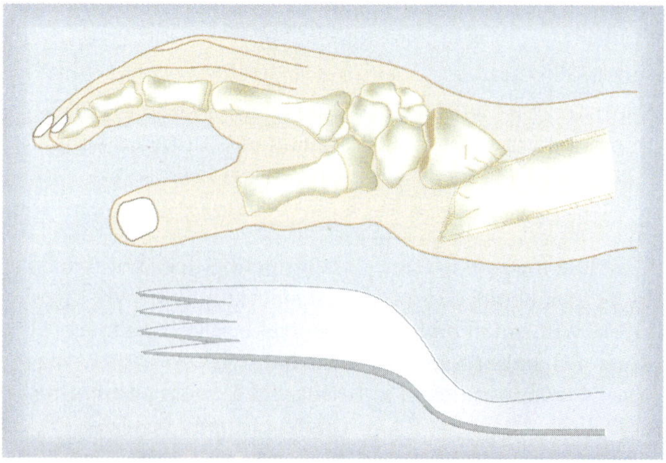

Fig. 14.20: Colles' fracture (A dinner fork deformity)

Table 14.5: Colle's "A Fracture of 6"

6 Displacements	6 Immobilisation methods	6 Complications: *Early complications*	6 Complications: *Late complications*
1. Dorsal displacement	1. Below elbow cast (10-20° palmar flexion, 15-20° ulnar deviation) Colles' cast (see Figs 14.24A and B)	1. Unstable reduction	1. Malunion
2. Dorsal rotation	2. Above elbow cast in supination	2. Median or ulnar nerve stretched	2. Rupture of extensor pollicis tendon
3. Lateral displacement	3. Above elbow cast in pronation	3. Postreduction swelling	3. Sudeck's osteodystrophy
4. Lateral rotation	4. Above elbow cast in midpronation is the best (tension on interosseous membrane is less because brachioradialis muscle is relaxed in this position)	4. Compartmental syndrome	4. Frozen shoulder
5. Impaction	5. Cotton loder's position (wrist fully flexed, useful in markedly displaced fractures)	5. Anaesthesia problems	5. Carpal tunnel syndrome
6. Supination	6. External fixators. Immobilised for 6 weeks	6. Injury to proximal segment of the bone during reduction	6. Nonunion
Principal displacements 1. Dorsal displacement 2. Dorsal angulation			

Styloid process test Normally, the radial styloid process is lower by 1.3 cm when compared to the ulnar styloid process. In Colles' both radial and ulnar styloid processes are at the same level and are found in all displacements of Colles' fracture. *Hence, this is a more reliable sign than dinner fork deformity* (Figs 14.21A and B).

Note: Dinner fork deformity is seen only in *d*orsal displacement and Dorsal tilt in a Colles' fracture (note the *d's*).

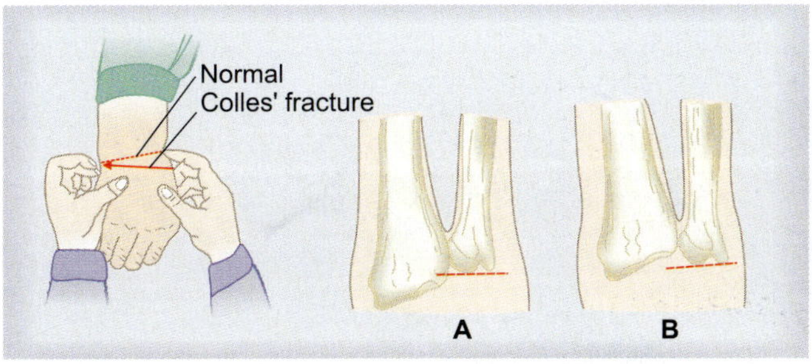

Figs 14.21A and B: Styloid process test: (A) Normal (B) In Colles' fractures

Radiology

Radiographs of the wrist (Figs 14.22A and B) both AP and lateral views of the affected wrist and lower end of the radius are taken. The points noted in the AP view are metaphyseal comminution, fracture line extending into the radiocarpal or inferior radioulnar joint and fracture of the ulnar styloid process (seen in about 60% of the cases). In the lateral view, the points noted are dorsal displacement and dorsal tilt of the distal fragment, sharp palmar surface and dorsal comminution of the lower end of radius, distal radioulnar joint subluxation, etc.

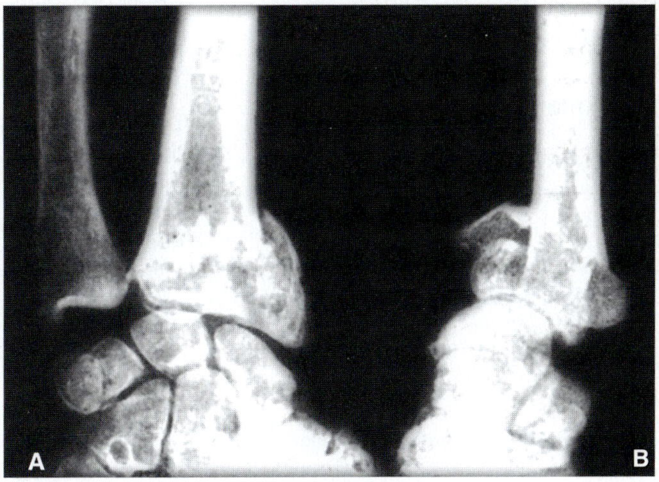

Figs 14.22A and B: Radiographs showing Colles' fracture: (A) AP view, and (B) lateral view

Classification

Contrary to popular belief, Colles' fracture is both intra-articular and extra-articular and not only extra-articular. Frykmann's classification takes into consideration both and also the fracture of ulna (Fig. 14.23).

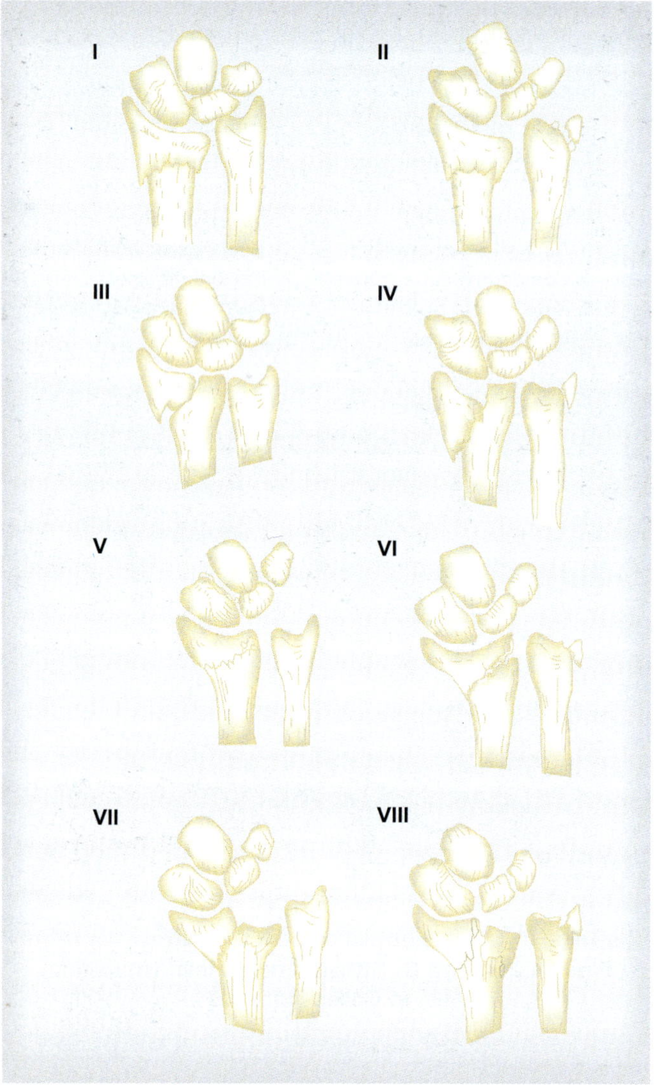

Fig. 14.23: Showing Frykmann's varieties of Colles' fracture

Frykmann's Classification

Fracture line	Distal ulnar fractures Absent	Present
I. Extra-articular	I	II
II. Intra-articular (involving radiocarpal joint only)	III	IV
III. Intra-articular (involving distal RU joint only)	V	VI
IV. Intra-articular (both RC+inferior RU joints)	VII	VIII

RC = radiocarpal, RU = radioulnar

Treatment Methods (Figs 14.24 to 14.26)

Aim The aim of treatment is to restore fully functional hand with no residual deformity. The treatment methods include conservative methods, operative methods and external fixators.

Conservative methods Here fracture reduction is carried out by closed methods under general anaesthesia (GA) or local anaesthesia (LA). The examiner holds the hand of the patient as if to shake hand. With an assistant giving counteraction by holding the forearm or arm of the patient, the examiner gives traction in the line of the forearm. This disimpacts the fracture and the examiner corrects the other displacements of the fracture. At the end of the procedure, styloid process test is carried out to check the accuracy of reduction. If the level of the styloid processes are restored back to normal, it indicates that the reduction has been achieved satisfactorily. Then the limb is immobilised by any one of the methods in the table above (mainly Colles' cast) and a check radiograph is taken. The plaster cast is removed after 6 to 8 weeks and physiotherapy is begun (Figs 14.27A to D).

Colles' cast

It is a below elbow cast in supination and ideally it has to meet the following 4 criteria:

- Firm fit at the dorsum.
- Firm fit at the volar fracture apex.
- Just snuggly fitting at the forearm.
- Metacarpophalangeal joints should be free to move.

What is new?
Sonographically guided closed reduction is an accurate, radiation free, simple tool that is as accurate as the conventional radiographic techniques.

The common causes for failure of reduction are incomplete reduction of the palmar fracture line and dorsal comminution of the lower end of radius.

Vital Facts

Do you know the acceptable limits of Colles' fracture after reduction?

- A dorsal tilt of less than 10 degrees.
- A radial shortening of less than 5 mm.

Operative methods Operative treatment is rarely required for Colles' fracture and may be required in the following situations:

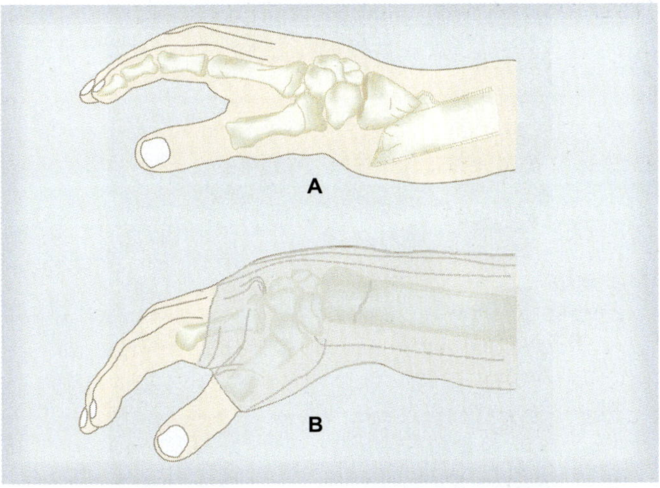

Figs 14.24A and B: Showing (A) A typical Colles' fracture, (B) A typical Colles' cast

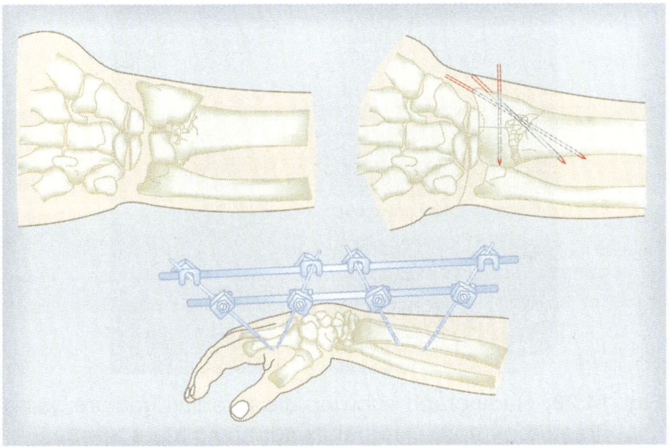

Fig. 14.25: Treatment method of Colles' fracture by external fixation

Indications Extensive comminution, impaction, median nerve entrapment and associated injuries in adults.

Modalities of operative treatment Depending upon the degree of comminution and the intra-articular extensions, one of the following surgical methods is chosen:

1. *Closed reduction and percutaneous pinning with K-wires* Here, after closed reduction by the usual methods, the fracture fragments are held together by percutaneous pinning by one or two K-wires. *Arm control*: This method is known to prevent collapse and gives good results in a few select cases (see Fig. 14.26).

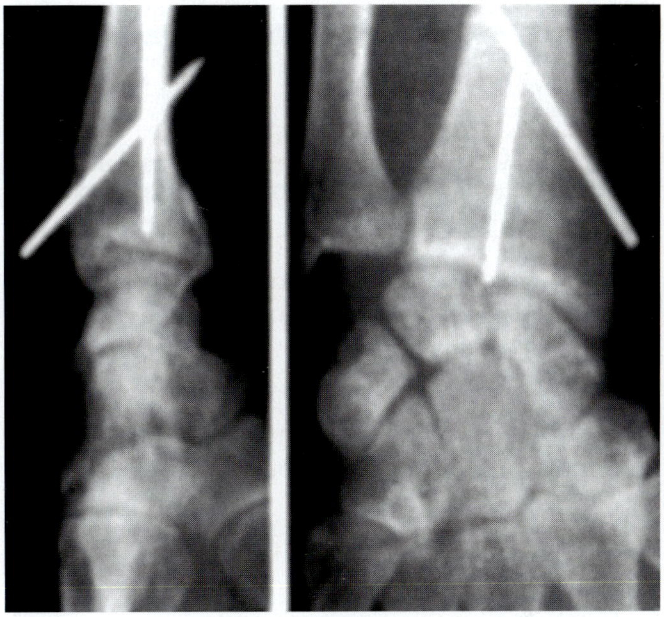

Fig. 14.26: Radiographs showing distal radius fracture percutaneous fixation

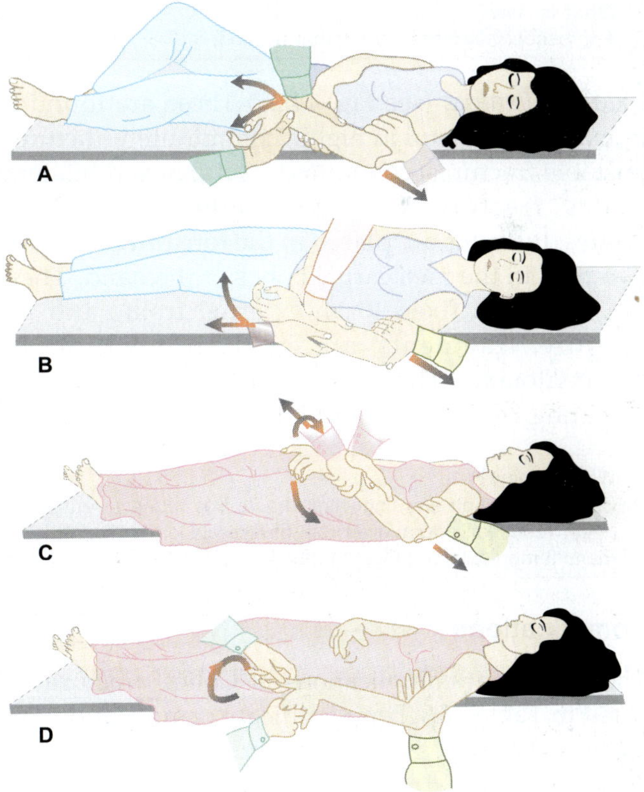

Figs 14.27A to D: Showing the step by step closed reduction methods of Colles' fracture in an elderly woman: (A) Dis-impaction, (B) Correcting anteroposterior displacements, (C) Correcting medial and lateral displacements, (D) Final manipulation

Salient features of percutaneous fixation
- Is becoming popular as it is simple.
- It prevents redisplacement.
- Always needs an external support.
- One of the cortex should not be comminuted.
- Preferably two pins are used (one radial and other dorsal).
- Care should be taken not to injure the radial sensory branch, the tendons, etc.

2. *Open reduction* In certain fractures involving the rim of the distal articular surfaces (Barton's variety), open reduction and plate fixation (Ellis plate) is advocated (Fig. 14.28).

Indications Same as for external fixation and for marginal volar or dorsal Barton's fractures.

Advantages
- Provides buttress.
- Resists compression.
- Load sharing.
- Early mobilisation.

What is new?
Arthroscopically assisted internal fixation.

External fixators (see Fig. 14.25) These are found to be extremely useful in highly comminuted fractures, unstable fractures, compound fractures and bilateral Colles' fracture. Through a lightweight UMEX frames, two pins are placed in the forearm bones and two pins in the metacarpal bones of the hand. These pins are then fixed to an external frame and the fracture fragments are held in position by ligamentotaxis. The frame should be applied after obtaining closed reduction by the usual method.

What is new?
Closed reduction and finger-trap traction is found to ensure better reduction and a lower rate of redisplacement than just manual manipulation (Figs 14.29).

Complications

The important complications of Colles' fracture are listed in Table 14.5. Few significant complications are discussed here.

Malunion This is the most common complication of Colles' fracture. Six important causes are responsible for it.

- *Improper reduction* If the fracture is not reduced properly, in the initial stages it may result in malunion later.

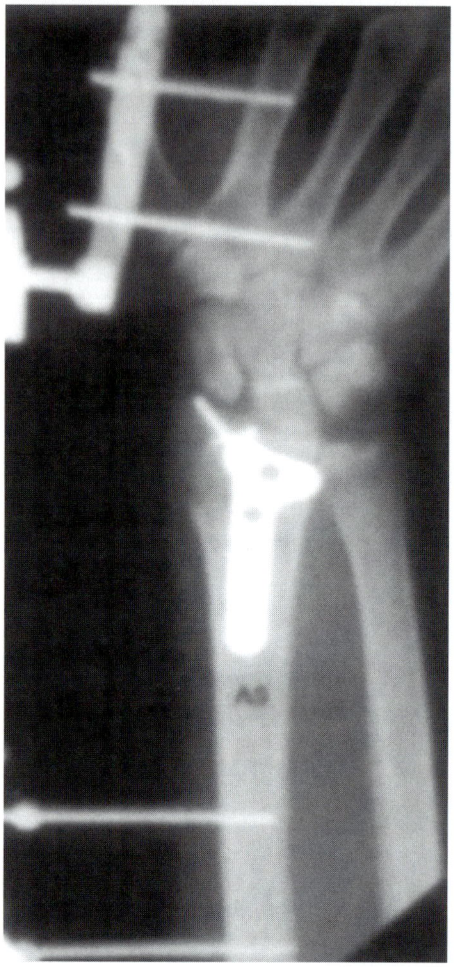

Fig. 14.28: Radiograph showing distal radius fracture being treated by both external fixator and plate screws

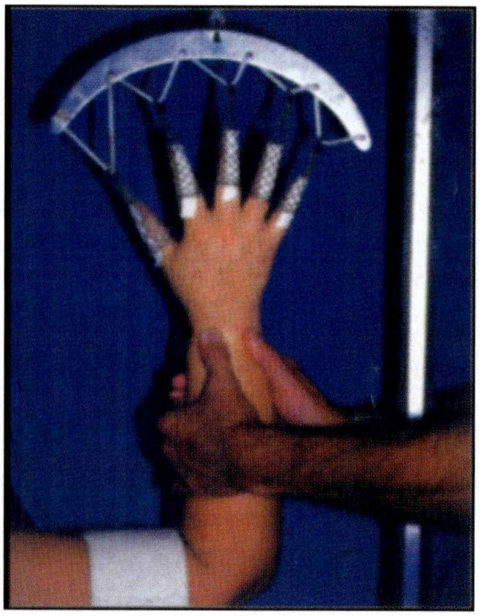

Fig. 14.29: Showing finger-trap traction

Section 2

- *Improper and inadequate immobilisation* This fracture needs to be immobilised at least for a period of six weeks failing which malunion results.
- *Comminuted dorsal surface* Due to extensive comminution, the fracture collapses and recurs again after reduction and casting.
- Osteoporosis may lead to collapse and recurrence.
- *Recurrence* This is due to extensive comminution and osteoporosis.
- *Rupture of the distal radioulnar ligament* This usually goes undetected in the initial stages of treatment and is responsible for the later recurrence.

Treatment

There are six options of treatment in a malunited Colles' fracture:

1. No treatment is required if the patient has no functional abnormality.
2. Remanipulation is attempted if fracture is less than 2 weeks old.
3. Darrach's operation is more often indicated if the patient complains of functional disability.
4. Corrective osteotomy and grafting if the patient wants cosmetic correction and if the patient is young (Fernandes and Campbell).
   Fernandes is a dorsal wedge osteotomy and Campbell is a lateral wedge osteotomy.
5. Arthrodesis (for intra-articular fracture): The patient complains of pain in the wrist joint due to traumatic osteoarthritis following an intra-articular fracture. In these patients arthrodesis of the wrist in functional position is the surgery of choice.
6. Combination of these like Darrach's operation with osteotomy, etc. is also tried in some situations.

Rupture of extensor pollicis tendon This occurs due to the attrition of the tendon as it glides over the sharp fracture surfaces. This usually occurs after 4 to 6 weeks and may be repaired or left alone with no residual disability.

Sudeck's osteodystrophy This is due to abnormal sympathetic response which causes vasodilatation and osteoporosis at the fracture site (Fig. 14.30). The patient complains of pain, swelling, painful wrist movements and red stretched shiny skin. Treatment consists of immobilisation of the affected part with plaster splints, injection of local anaesthetics near the

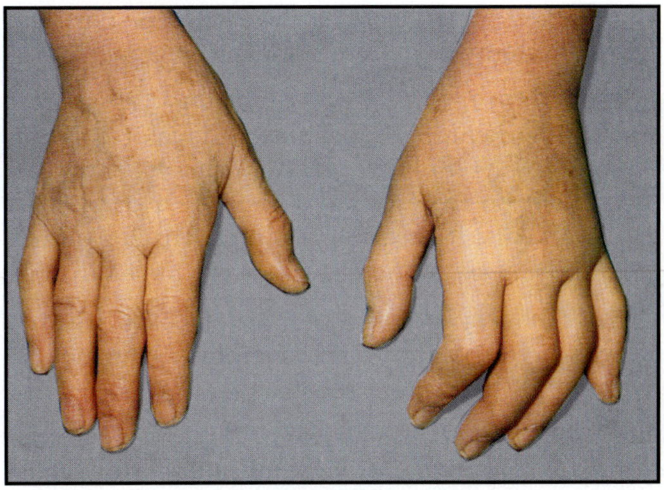

Fig. 14.30: Sudeck's osteodystrophy

Approach to a patient with malunited Colles' fracture

Ask the patient what he or she wants

Desires cosmetic correction	Desires better function	Both cosmesis and function
↓	↓	↓
Young adults Corrective osteotomy: ↓ **Types** 1. *Fernandes osteotomy* 2. *Campbell osteotomy*	*Darrach's* operation* (excision of 2.5 cm of distal ulna including the head leaving behind the periosteum)	A combination of *osteotomy* and *Darrach's* operation*

↓

How does it help?
- Removes the mechanical block and hence ↑ movements
- ↓ Pain which is due to stretching of joint capsule
- Ugly prominence due to persistent dislocation of head of ulna removed

Advantages
- Simple
- No nonunion/malunion
- Improves function

*Darrach's is the most common surgery done for malunited Colles' fracture. It improves the function more than cosmesis, but still it is preferred because Colles' fracture usually occurs in elderly women for whom function is important rather than cosmesis. If cosmesis is the priority, corrective osteotomy done at the radial fracture site gives good results.

sympathetic ganglion in the axilla or cervical sympathectomy in extreme cases.

Frozen hand shoulder syndrome This is a troublesome complication which develops due to unnecessary voluntary shoulder immobilisation by the patient on the affected side for fear of fracture displacements. It is said that the patient has performed a *mental amputation* and kept the limb still.

Carpal tunnel syndrome Malunion of Colles' fracture crowds the carpal tunnel and compresses the median nerve.

Nonunion This is extremely rare in Colles' fracture because of the cancellous nature of the bone which enables the fracture to unite well. However, soft tissue interposition may cause this problem. The treatment consists of open reduction, rigid internal fixation and bone grafting.

Quick facts

Colles' fracture—Why is it called fracture of 6?

- Common at 60 years.
- Force required to cause Colles' fracture are multiples of 6.
- 6 classical displacements.
- 6 methods of fracture immobilisation.
- 6 weeks immobilisation.
- 6 important early and late complications.
- 6 causes for malunion.
- 6 methods of managing malunion.
- 60 per cent cases have fracture ulnar styloid.

15

Injuries to the Wrist

- ❑ Brief anatomy
- ❑ Scaphoid fracture
- ❑ Injuries of the carpometacarpal joints of the thumb
- ❑ Radiocarpal injuries
- ❑ Lunate fractures
- ❑ Triquetral fractures
- ❑ Pisiform fractures
- ❑ Hamate fractures
- ❑ Capitate fractures
- ❑ Trapezoid fracture
- ❑ Trapezium fracture

BRIEF ANATOMY

THE WRIST JOINT SPEAKS

I am not a single joint but made up of radiocarpal, midcarpal and intercarpal joints. The middle finger, the third metacarpal and the capitate are the axial bones of the hand. The midcarpal component of mine allows flexion and extension as this being a hinge joint (Fig. 15.1). My main flexors are flexor carpi ulnaris and radialis aided by finger flexors. I extend mainly by the action of extensor carpi radialis, longus and brevis supported by extensor digitorum and extensor carpi ulnaris. This movement of mine occurs at radiocarpal joint. I adduct mostly at radiocarpal joint by the action of flexor and extensor carpi ulnaris. I abduct entirely at the radiocarpal joint due to the combined action of extensor carpi radialis longus, extensor pollicis brevis, abductor pollicis longus and flexor carpi radialis. My normal range of movement includes flexion 80°, extension 70°, radial deviation 20°, and ulnar deviation 30°. My functional position is 30° dorsiflexion.

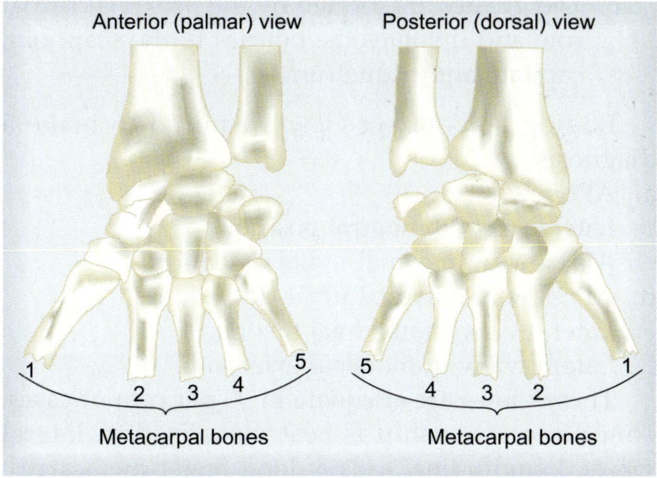

Fig. 15.1: Bony anatomy of the wrist

General Principles of Carpal Injuries

Carpal injuries have an overall incidence of 6 per cent of all skeletal injuries.

Relative incidences

- Scaphoid fracture—60 per cent.
- Dorsal chip radius fracture—10 per cent.
- Post-traumatic carpal instability with or without dislocations—10 per cent.
- Lunate fracture—3 per cent.
- All other carpal bone fractures—7 per cent.

Mechanism of Injury

Carpal injuries usually result from fall on the outstretched hands. Frequenly misdiagnosed, it is known for complications like early avascular necrosis, late carpal instability and arthrosis. Hence, prompt and correct treatment is mandatory. Lack of callus in fractures in this region makes judgement about the progress of union difficult.

Clinical Features

Pain, swelling, tenderness and loss of wrist movements are some of the common complaints of carpal injuries. Careful examination of the entire wrist is mandatory to localise the nature and type of injury.

Investigations

1. **Radiology:** *Plain X-rays of the wrist* preferably the PA view, lateral and oblique views with the wrist in neutral position helps to make an assessment. In the PA view, look for the following:
   a. The dorsal radioulnar articular surfaces.
   b. The lesser arc at the midcarpal joint (This involves the radial styloid, midcarpal and lunatotriquetral space).
   c. The greater arc formed by the proximal carpal row and involves the injuries to the scaphoid, capitate and triquetrum.

   Radiographs of six views required to make a diagnosis:

   a. AP view.
   b Lateral view in neutral position.
   c. AP view in maximal radial deviation.
   d. AP view in maximal ulnar deviation.
   e. Lateral view in maximal flexion.
   f. Lateral view in maximal extension.

   These views are adequate in 90 per cent of cases. Angular relationship is best visualised in lateral views. Longitudinal axes of long finger metacarpal, capitate, lunate and radius all fall in the same line. The following are the important features on radiographs:

   a. *Lateral view—scapholunate angle* It is formed normally between longitudinal axis of lunate and scaphoid and is 30 to 60° (average 47°).
      - Greater than 70° indicates instability.
      - Greater than 80° indicates definite instability of dorsiflexion type.
      - Greater than 20° capitulolunate angle (between the long axis of capitulum and lunate) suggests carpal instability.

   b. *AP view:* There is constant space between the carpal bones in all the movements of wrist. Joint width between scaphoid and lunate is normally 1 to 2 mm. Space of greater than 3 mm is considered abnormal.
2. *Fluoroscopy*: This helps to assess carpal kinematics radiographically.
3. *CT Scan*: This is a very important investigative tool and it detects features not picked by routine plain X-rays.
4. *MRI*: Though less useful, it helps to detect AVN, nonunion, cartilage condition, etc.
5. *Technetium bone scan*: It helps to detect carpal bone fractures 6 to 8 hours after injury and those not seen clearly on X-rays.
6. *Arthrography*: This helps to detect soft tissue and ligament injury.
7. *Ultrasonography*: This helps to detect ganglion, cyst, soft tissue injuries, etc.
8. *Arthroscopy*: It has both diagnostic and therapeutic role in wrist fractures.

Treatment

Principles

- Most carpal injuries need surgical intervention.
- Conservative treatment is reserved for fractures with < 1 mm displacement or < 1-2 mm diastasis.
- If associated with soft tissue injuries, it needs surgical repair.

Methods

- Conservative treatment is by short arm cast immobilisation.
- Percutaneous fixation for displaced fractures is by fixation with K-wires.
- Open reduction and rigid internal fixation for displaced fractures with K-wires or screws.
- External fixation is indicated for difficult, communited and open injuries.

SCAPHOID FRACTURE

Interesting Features

- This bone forms the radial part of the carpus.
- Lies obliquely at 45° to longitudinal axes of 2 rows.
- Articulates with 5 bones (radius, lunate, triquetral, trapezium, capitulum).
- Central indentation is called waist.
- Since it crosses 2 rows of carpus, it is more susceptible to fracture.

Anatomical peculiarities

1. It articulates with distal radius and with four carpal bones. It moves in all the movements of the wrist.
2. It has a precarious blood supply (Fig. 15.2A).
   - Sixty-seven per cent of the scaphoid have arterial foramina throughout its length.
   - Thirteen per cent have predominant blood supply in the distal one-third.

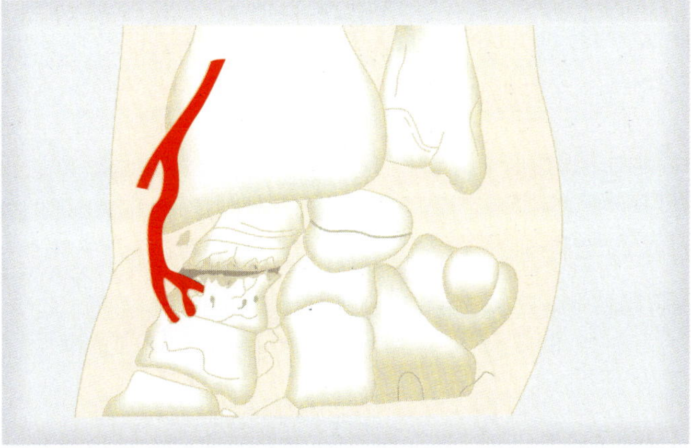

Fig. 15.2A: Blood supply of scaphoid is peculiar (see text)

- In about 20 per cent most of the foramina are in the waist with no foramina in the proximal one-third.

This suggests that one-third of the fractures occurring in the proximal one-third is without adequate blood supply resulting in avascular necrosis in 35 per cent of cases at this level and has poor prognosis.

Aetiology

It is common in young adults though it can be seen in patients of 10 to 70 years of age.

- The common mode of injury is fall on an outstretched hand with hyperextension and slight radial deviation at the wrist.
- It is associated with other fractures of the carpus and forearm bones in about 17 per cent.
- It is the commonest fracture among carpal bones.
- Among the wrist fractures, it is second only to the fracture lower end of radius.

Classification

Cooney, Dobyn's, Linscheid's Classification

- *Stable fracture*
- *Unstable* The following are the criteria to label it as unstable:
  a. Scapholunate angle greater than 70°.
  b. Capitulolunate angle greater than 20°.
  c. Separation of scaphoid and lunate greater than 3 to 4 mm.

Anatomical Classification (Fig. 15.2B)

1. Proximal pole fracture (20%).
2. Waist fracture (70%).

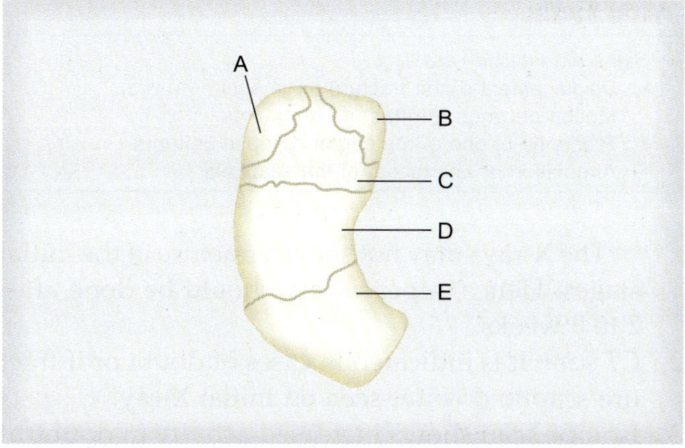

Fig. 15.2B: Showing different levels of scaphoid fracture (A) Fracture of the tuberosity, (B) distal articular fracture, (C) Distal one third fracture, (D) Waist fracture, (E) Fracture of the proximal pole

3. Distal body fracture (10%).
4. Tuberosity fracture.
5. Osteochondral fracture.

Clinical Features

Patient complains of pain and swelling of the wrist. Tenderness in the antomical snuff box is a characteristic finding. The movements of the wrist may be painful.

Investigations

1. **Radiology (Fig. 15.2C)** *Plain X-rays:* The views of the radiographs are (AP, lateral, oblique and ulnar deviation).

   These four views can diagnose scaphoid fracture in 97 per cent of the cases.

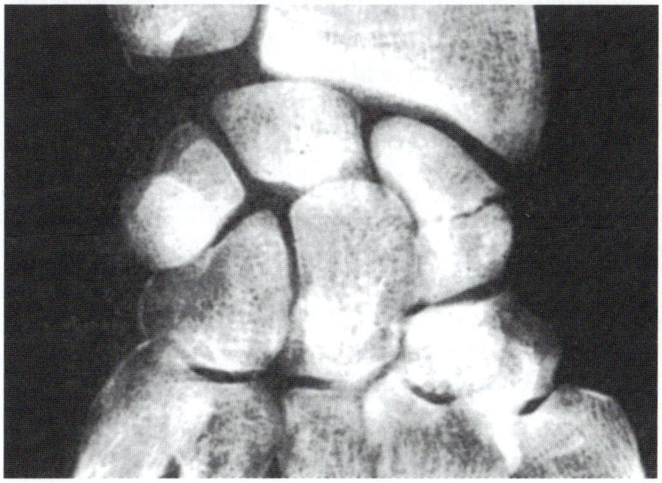

Fig. 15.2C: Radiograph showing fracture scaphoid

Section 2

Vital facts:

Signs of instability are:
- Displacement of the fracture fragments (> 1 mm).
- Motion between the fracture fragments.
- Presence of one of the carpal collapse patterns.
- Angulation or shortening of the scaphoid.

The X-rays may not show a fracture in the initial stages. Hence, repeat X-ray should be done after 2 to 3 weeks.

2. *CT scan:* It is indicated in cases of doubt or if fract ure scaphoid is not seen on initial X-ray.
3. Isotope scan shows increased activity in doubtful cases.
4. *MRI:* This helps to assess the vascularity, especially of the proximal fragment.

Principles of Treatment

- *Common is transverse fracture of the waist.*
- *Injury to the wrist and tenderness in the region of the scaphoid should be treated as if they had a fracture until a fracture has been disapproved by the radiographs at 2nd and 4th week.*

Conservative Methods

This is indicated in undisplaced, <1 mm displacement or <15° angulation.

- *Once a fracture is diagnosed, if undisplaced, Böhler gauntlet type short arm cast from proximal forearm to midpalmar area with proximal phalanx of the thumb is put. Expected rate of union is 95 per cent within 10 weeks of time* (Fig. 15.3).
- *In displaced fracture treatment is by reduction and casting. Union rate is 54 per cent. Closed percutaneous K-wire fixation is also successful if reduction cannot be retained by scaphoid cast.*

Surgical Management

ORIF is the treatment of choice in displaced fractures.

Indications

1. Operative treatment has no place in the management of acute scaphoid fracture except for displaced fractures.
2. In delayed union and nonunion (> 12–16 weeks).
3. Preiser's disease which is an ischaemic necrosis of fracture scaphoid.

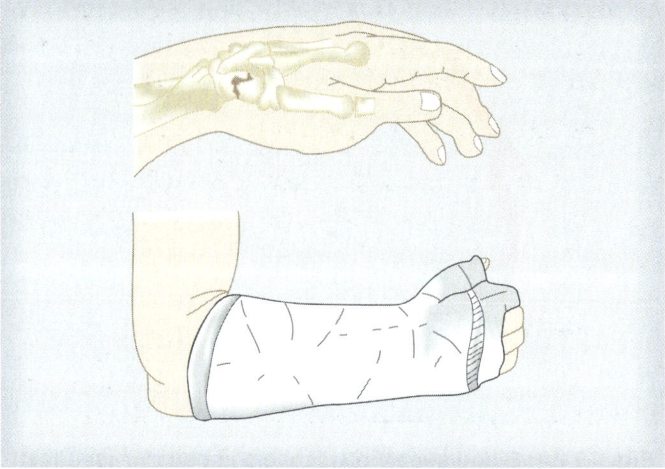

Fig. 15.3: Showing scaphoid fracture being treated by a "scaphoid cast"

Surgical Methods

Closed reduction and percutaneous fixation by three point pressure.

Osteosynthesis It consists of open reduction and internal fixation or bone grafting or both. K-wire and small corticocancellous screws (Herbert screws, headed or headless and Acutrak screws) along with cancellous bone grafts are also used (Fig. 15.4).

Fusion techniques are used if the patient is young, the opposite hand and wrist are normal and if much stressful activity is required.

Note:
1. Open reduction and internal fixation is the most acceptable method.
2. Palmar approach is popular.
3. Herbert screw is preferred for internal fixation.

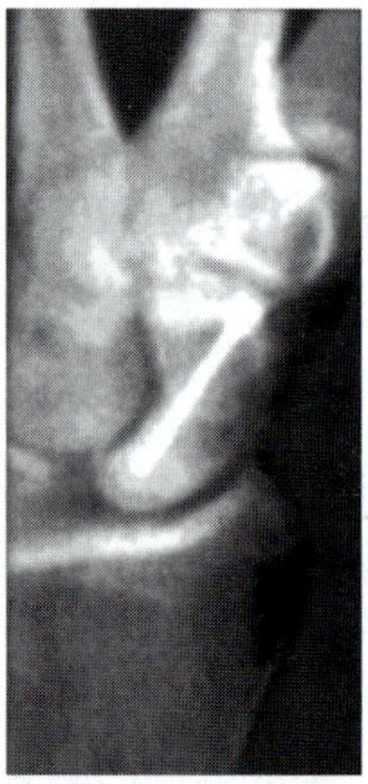

Fig. 15.4: Radiograph showing scaphoid fracture treated by ORIF with Herbert screw

Arthroplasty This is useful for older patients, with significant osteoarthritic changes in the wrist, e.g. radial styloidectomy, silastic implants, etc.

Arthrodesis is less commonly indicated.

Excision of proximal fragments is indicated when fragment is less than ¼'' in size and when bone grafting has failed.

Complications

- Nonunion due to delayed diagnosis, displacement and associated carpal injuries.
- Forty per cent cases are undiagnosed in the initial stages of fracture.
- Incidence of avascular necrosis is as high as 40 per cent.

Quick facts: Scaphoid fracture

- Accounts for 70 per cent of carpal injuries.
- High incidence of AVN.
- Fracture may not be seen on initial radiograph.
- Treat according to symptoms and repeat radiograph at 10 to 14 days.
- If still painful and if still suspicious, cast it.
- If undisplaced, cast it including the thumb.
- If displaced, cast after manipulation.
- Open reduction if gap is more than 2 mm or if still a step remains after reduction, if union is slow or if AVN develops open reduction, internal fixation and bone grafting is done.

What is new?

- Percutaneous cannulated screw fixation for undisplaced fracture scaphoid bone is found to result in faster radiographic union than the conventional plaster cast immobilisation.

INJURIES OF THE CARPOMETACARPAL JOINTS OF THE THUMB

Introduction

Carpometacarpal joints act as a link between the wrist and hand. The joints of the index and middle fingers are stable while that of the thumb and the little fingers are more mobile. Thumb carpometacarpal dislocations are more common and are dealt here. The two important dislocations are Bennett's fracture dislocation and Rolando fracture dislocation.

1. BENNETT'S FRACTURE

Bennett's fracture is a fracture dislocation of the palmar base of the first metacarpal bone of the thumb with either subluxation or dislocation of the first carpometacarpal joint. It was described by Edward Bennett in 1882. It is an intra-articular fracture.

Mechanism of Injury

The common mechanism of injury is an axial blow directed against the partially flexed metacarpal, in most cases during "fist fights."

Characteristics of this Fracture

- Fracture line separates major part of the metacarpal from a small volar lip fragment producing disruption of the carpometacarpal joint.
- It is an avulsion rather than a pure dislocation. It occurs because of strong anterior oblique ligament.
- Size of the volar lip fragment and amount of shaft displacement vary.

Base of the thumb metacarpal is pulled dorsally and medially by the abductor pollicis longus (Fig. 15.5), while the distal attachment of adductor further levers the base into abduction.

Clinical Features

The patient complains of pain, swelling and tenderness over the base of the thumb. Movements of the thumb are severely restricted.

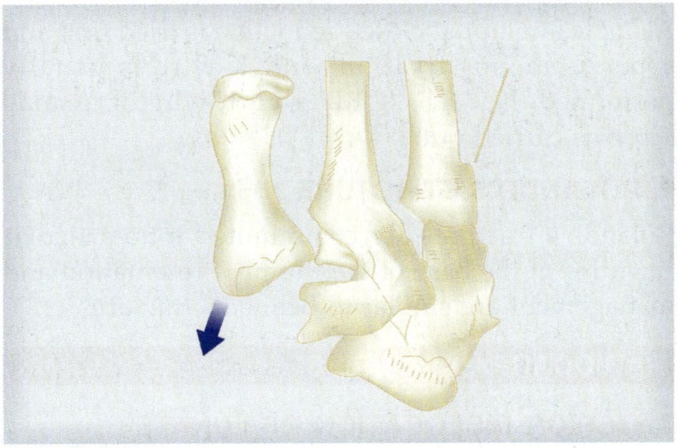

Fig. 15.5: Showing Bennett's fracture. Thick arrow indicates the line of pull of abductor policis longus

Section 2

Flow Chart: Depicting the treatment plan in scaphoid fracture

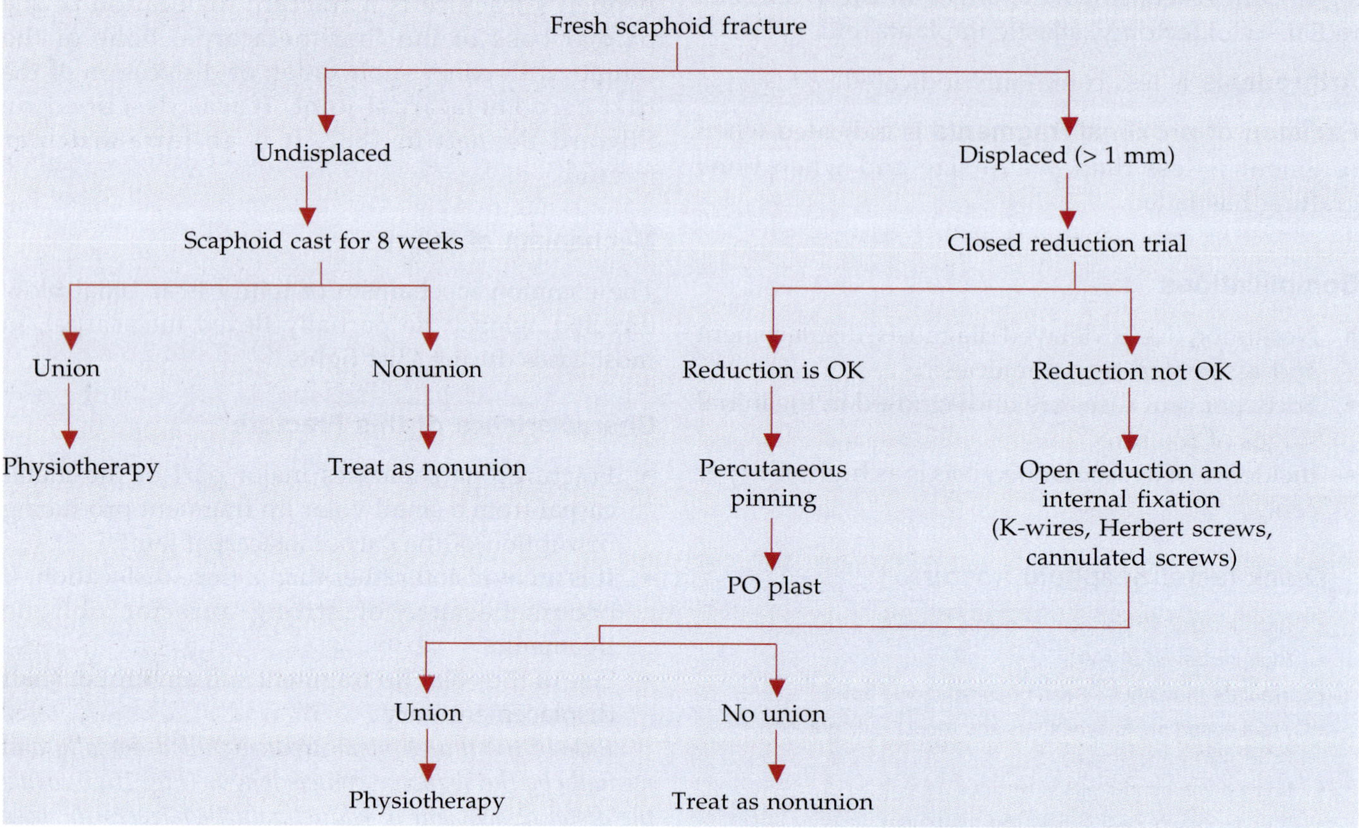

Investigations

Plain X-rays help to make the diagnosis accurately (Fig. 15.6).

Treatment

A single attempt at closed reduction is tried first and a percutaneous fixation with K-wire is usually performed. If it fails, ORIF with K-wire or a small screw is carried out.

2. ROLANDO'S FRACTURE

Rolando's fractures are comminuted intra-articular fractures of the base of the thumb. Presentation and management are similar to Bennett's fracture.

RADIOCARPAL INJURIES

ANTERIOR DISLOCATION OF LUNATE

It is a common carpal dislocation.

Mechanism of injury and clinical features are as described in general principles.

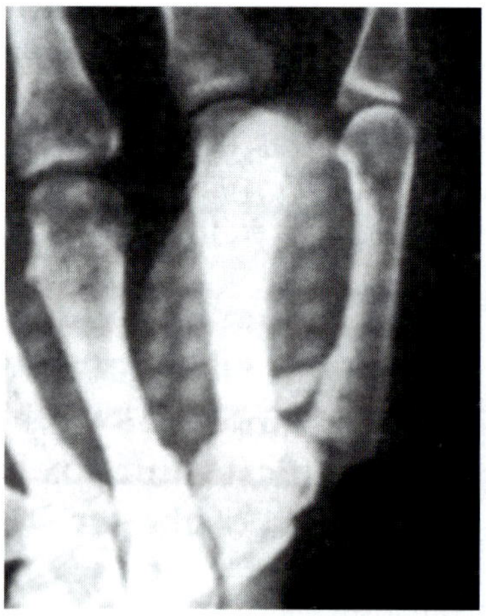

Fig. 15.6: Radiograph showing Bennett's fracture

Radiology

In radiograph of the lateral view normally lunate forms a half-moon shape, which is lost in this dislocation. And in the anteroposterior view the normal rectangular profile is lost.

Problems

- This may cause compression of the median nerve.
- If left untreated it may cause permanent palsy, hence, reduction should be carried out as an emergency procedure.

Treatment

- If seen early, reduction is easy and immobilisation for 3 weeks with wrist in slight flexion usually gives good results.
- If seen after 3 weeks, open reduction is done.
- If lunate cannot be reduced by open reduction, resection of the proximal carpal bones or arthrodesis of the wrist may be necessary.

VOLAR TRANS-SCAPHOID PERILUNAR DISLOCATION

This is a rare injury and is due to fall on dorsum of the flexed wrist.

Mechansim

Mechansim of injury is opposite to the dorsal perilunar dislocation.

Treatment

Treatment is by closed reduction and casting.

DORSAL TRANS-SCAPHOID PERILUNAR DISLOCATION

It is usually diagnosed late. Early closed reduction is the best treatment. When accurate reduction of the scaphoid is not obtained, open reduction and bone grafting or internal fixation is indicated.

Treatment

The following are some of the important principles in treating this injury:

- Less than 3 weeks closed reduction can be tried
- More than 3 weeks OR + IF by K-wires
- More than 2 months arthrodesis or resection of the proximal carpal row is carried out.

LUNATE FRACTURES

These are relatively rare and is due to hyperextension injury of the wrist or may be due to multiple repetitive trauma.

Clinical Presentation

- Pain, swelling and tenderness over the dorsum of the wrist.
- Restricted wrist movements
- Decreased hand grip
- Boggy swelling due to synovitis in the late stages.

Investigation

Plain X-rays are inconclusive. MRI is a better option.

Treatment

This is essentially conservative and consists of application of a below elbow plaster cast.

Complications

Avascular necrosis of lunate, called the Keinbock's disease is known to occur.

TRIQUETRAL FRACTURES

This is the fourth most common carpal bone fractures (after scaphoid, capitate and lunate). It was first described by Destot in 1926.

Mechanism of Injury

- Direct blow
- Fall on an outstretched hand
- Avulsion or chip fractures

Types

These are divided into two types:

1. Body fractures.
2. Peripheral chip or avulsion fractures.

Investigations

Plain X-ray of the wrist (AP, lateral or oblique views) may reveal the fracture. If still in doubt, CT scan is recommended.

Treatment

Body Fractures

- If undisplaced, it is treated by short arm cast for 4 to 6 weeks.
- If displaced (> 1–2 mm), surgery is the treatment of choice namely:

a. Arthroscopic approach and percutaneus pinning
b. Open reduction and internal fixation through K-wires or screws.

Chip or Avulsion Fractures

Symptomatic treatment by orthotics in most of the cases helps and rarely excision may be required in intractable cases.

PISIFORM FRACTURES

There are very rare and account for only 1 to 3 per cent of all carpal bone fractures. This fracture is compared to patella fractures.

Mechanism of Injury

- Due to a direct blow resulting is comminuted fractures.
- Due to an indirect force following an avulsion or pull of the flexor carpi ulnaris tendon. This results in transverse fractures.

Investigations

Pisiform fractures are difficult to visualise on plain X-rays. CT scan is more desirable.

Treatment

Undisplaced fractures are treated by short arm cast for 4 to 6 weeks. Displaced fractures are treated by excision. Open reduction and internal fixation is rarely done in these fractures.

HAMATE FRACTURES

This accounts for 2 to 4 per cent of all carpal fractures.

Mechanism

It could be due to a direct blow or indirect force while trying to grip an object.

Types

Hamate fractures could be either:
a. Body fractures, or
b. Hook fractures.

Clinical Features

Pain in the medial side of the palm and comes on with grip is quite typical of hamate fractures. Few patients may present with ulnar nerve (distal) paraesthesia or palsy. Ruptures of the ring and little fingers are seen in some severe cases.

Investigations

Plain X-ray of the wrist (AP, lateral and oblique views) usually helps in detecting the fracture. CT scan helps in doubtful cases.

Treatment

- Acute fractures are treated by immobilisation with short arm cast for 6 to 10 weeks.
- Nonunions of the hook are usually treated by excision.

CAPITATE FRACTURES

These are rare injuries and account for 1 to 2 per cent of all carpal fractures. It is often associated with carpal-metacarpal dislocations.

Mechanism of Injury

Isolated capitate fractures are rare and are known to occur due to an axial loading injury to the middle finger to which the capitate is attached below. Direct blow is the other mechanism of injury.

Types

Three types are described:
1. Isolated capitate fracture—is rare.
2. Associated with carpal-metacarpal dislocation.
3. Scaphocapitate syndrome: This is more common. This consists of fracture of the waist of the scaphoid and a proximal capitate fracture.

Clinical Features

Pain, swelling and restricted wrist movements are seen.

Investigation

Capitate fractures can be diagnosed by plain X-ray of the wrist. In difficult cases CT scan is advised.

Treatment

Conservative

Undisplaced fractures are treated by a below elbow cast for 4 to 6 weeks.

Surgery: Displaced fractures and scaphocapitate syndrome are treated by open reduction and rigid internal fixation.

TRAPEZOID FRACTURE

These are very uncommon fractures. Dislocations are more common than isolated fractures.

Mechanism of Injury

- Direct blow
- Axial loading injury to the index metacarpal

Treatment

- Undisplaced fractures are treated by below elbow cast for 4 to 6 weeks.
- In displaced fractures (> 1 mm or diastasis > 2 mm) open reduction and rigid internal fixation is advised.

TRAPEZIUM FRACTURE

This accounts for 1 to 5 per cent of wrist fractures. It could be isolated fracture or dislocations.

Mechanism of Injury

- Fall on an outstretched hand
- Direct blow over the dorsum of the hand.

Classifications

Trapezium fractures are divided into:
1. Body fractures
2. Ridge fractures (Palmar)
   a. Type I—fracture base of the trapezoid ridge.
   b. Type II—fracture of the tip of the trapezial ridge.
3. Dislocations: This could be dorsal, palmar or radial and may be associated with fracture of the scaphoid and trapezium.

Clinical Features

The patient complains of pain, swelling and tenderness over the wrist. Resisted flexion produces pain. Plain X-rays though useful are not reliable. CT scan is a better option.

Treatment

- Undisplaced fracture: Thumb spica for 4 to 6 weeks.
- Displaced fracture (> 1 mm or > 2 mm diastasis): Open reduction and rigid internal fixation is advised.
- Dislocation is treated by open reduction and K-wire fixation.

16

Hand Injuries

INCIDENCE

- Hand fractures account for 17.5 per cent of all fractures.
- *Among the hand fractures:*
  a. Phalangeal fractures— 46 per cent
  b. Metacarpal fractures—36 per cent
  c. V Metacarpal bone neck fracture—9.7 per cent
- *Among the phalangeal fractures*
  a. Proximal phalanx—57.4 per cent
  b. Middle phalanx—30.4 per cent
- Single fracture seen in 98.6 per cent of cases
  Multiple fractures—1.4 per cent
- Male : Female = (1.8 : 1)
- Mode of injury:
  a. Sports injuries in 3rd decade
  b. Workplace injuries in the 5th decade.

KNOW ABOUT THE UNIVERSAL HAND SPLINT—THE BURKHALTER SPLINT

Steps of Application

- Fracture reduction of the fingers are done and checked for stability
- Now the hand and forearm are padded
- First a volar slab is applied up to the level of the proximal palmar crease with the wrist in extension
- A second dorsal slab is applied up to the level of the proximal IP joint level with the MP joint in maximum flexion
- This splint neutralises the intrinsics
- Duration of immobilisation: 3 to 4 weeks
- Active movements of the IP joints should be encouraged.

GENERAL PRINCIPLES OF THE TREATMENT OF HAND INJURIES

This includes injuries to the phalanges, metacarpals and carpal bones. The following principles should be followed in treating hand fractures:

1. All stable fractures need closed reduction and splinting.
2. K-wire is the commonly used internal fixation device.
3. While using the K-wire, injury to the tendons, ligaments and extension into the joints should be avoided.
4. Rotational malalignment of the fingers (Fig. 16.1) should be avoided and this can be done by looking at the alignment of the fingers when the fingers are flexed at metacarpophalangeal and interphalangeal joints. The fingers should point towards the scaphoid bone.
5. The safe position for hand immobilisation is 70° flexion at MCP joint 15 to 20° flexion at PIP joint, and 5 to 10° flexion at DIP joint. This is called the intrinsic plus position or the James position (Fig. 16.2).

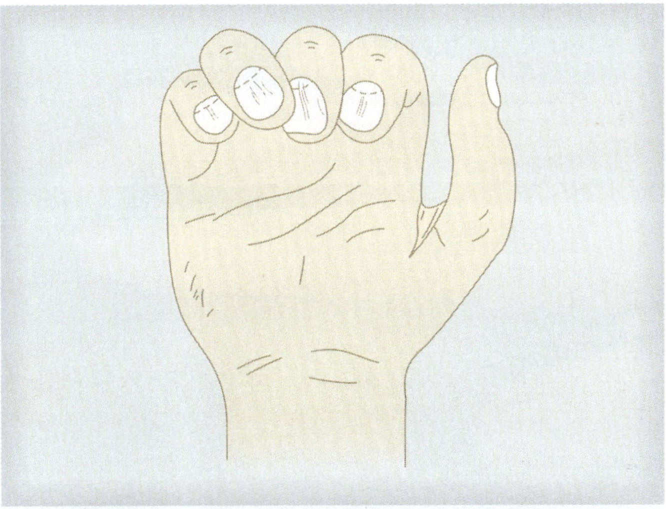

Fig. 16.1: Showing assessment of rotational malalignment of fingers

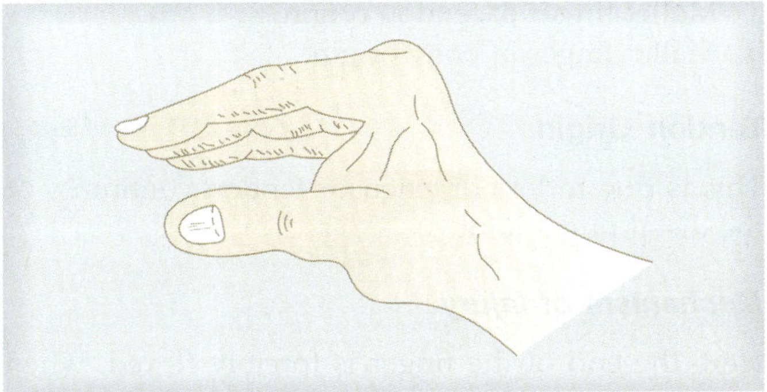

Fig. 16.2: Functional position of the hand (James position)

Indications for Open Reduction in Hand Injuries

a. Intra-articular fractures with a small fragment.
b. Severely displaced fractures.
c. Highly unstable fractures.
d. Multiple fractures.
e. Soft tissue (e.g. tendon) interposition.

After open reduction, internal fixation is usually done by K-wires (Fig. 16.3). Intraosseous tension band circlage wiring, intramedullary fixation, small AO plate and screws are the other but less commonly used fixation methods.

INJURIES TO THE PHALANX

DISTAL PHALANX FRACTURES

- Very commonly injured
- Soft tissue coverage is less
- In nailbed injuries, haematoma can be seen through the nailbed.

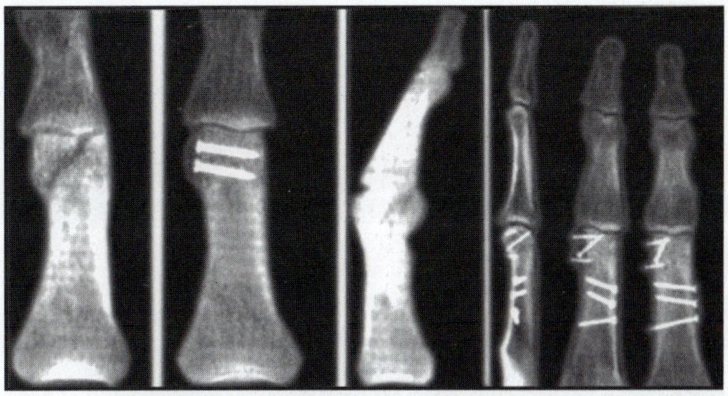

Fig. 16.3: Radiographs showing phalangeal fractures fixed with K-wires

Mechanism of Injury

It is mainly due to direct crush injuries. Indirect forces may result in avulsion injuries.

Classifications

Distal phalangeal fractures are classified into:

- Longitudinal (36%)
- Transverse
- Tuft (63%)
- Basal fractures (18%)
  a. Dorsal
  b. Volar
- Intra-articular complete fractures.

Do you know the difference between dorsal base and Mallet fracture?

- Mallet fingers: < 25 per cent involvement of articular cartilage and hence stable.
- Dorsal basal fractures: > 25 per cent involvement of articular cartilage and hence unstable.

Treatment

Three modalities of treatment are described namely:

I. *Conservative Method:* This is reserved mainly for undisplaced, longitudinal and tuft fractures. The method employed is splinting for 3 to 4 weeks (Fig. 16.4).

II. *Closed Reduction and Percutaneous Fixation:* This is reserved for:
   a. Transverse shaft fractures where external splinting fails to hold the fragments and
   b. Dorsal base fractures with > 25 per cent involvement of articular surfaces. Here the K-wire pinning should be done across the DIP joint.

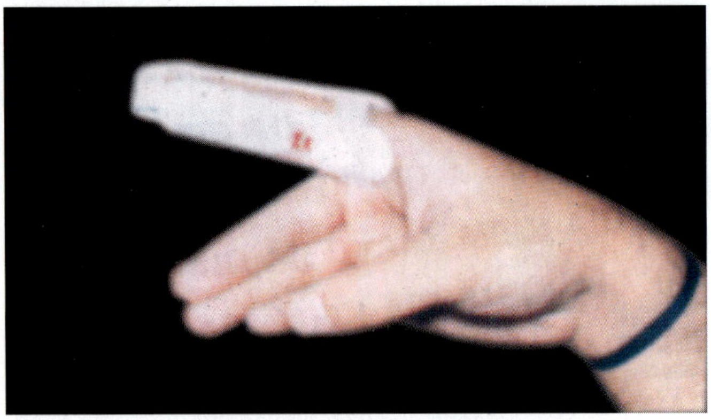

Fig. 16.4: Finger cot splint

III. *Open Reduction and Internal Fixation:*

This is indicated in:

a. Volar base fractures with disruption of the flexor digitorum profundus (FDP) insertion.
b. Dorsal base fractures with 30 to 40 per cent involvement of the articular surface.

DISTAL INTERPHALANGEAL JOINT INJURIES

The following are some of the salient features of these injuries:

- These injuries are usually due to ball catching sports.
- Pure dislocations without tendon ruptures are rare.
- Most of the times DIP joint dislocations are missed initially.
- Dislocation is mainly dorsal.
- Isolated injury to the collateral ligament and volar plate are rare.

Famous DIP Joint Injuries

a. *Mallet finger*: This is the dorsal base extensor tendon avulsion.
b. *Jersey finger*: This is the volar base FDP avulsion.

MALLET FINGER (Syn: Baseball finger, Drop finger, Cricket finger)

Mallet finger (Fig. 16.5) is a common injury usually due to forced flexion of the distal phalanx while the extensor tendons are actively trying to extend the finger. The baseball catcher, football receiver and others are vulnerable to this injury.

Depending upon whether the thin extensor tendon is torn in its substance or pulls off a small piece of bone at its insertion, two types are recognised:

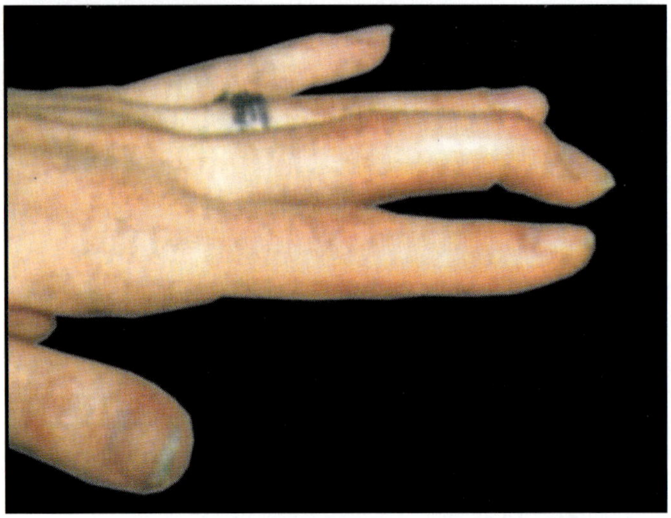

Fig. 16.5: Mallet finger

a. Mallet finger of tendon origin.
b. Mallet finger of bony origin.

Tendon Origin

This is due to loss of extensor tendon continuity at the distal finger joint.

Mechanism of Injury

Here the end of the finger is forcibly flexed, when extensor tendon is taut, e.g. while tucking the bed, catching a ball, striking an object with extended finger, etc. (Figs 16.6A and B).

Several Types

1. *Extensor tendon stretched* In this, degree of drop is less. There is loss of 5 to 20° of extension. There is weak active extension.
2. *Extensor tendon ruptured* from its insertion into distal phalanx. There is 40 to 45° loss of extension. No active extension.
3. A small fragment of distal phalanx is avulsed with the extensor tendon. There is no active extension and it should be treated as tendon injuries rather than fractures.

If the flexion deformity is severe, a secondary hyperextension deformity of PIP joint occurs, because of imbalance of the extensor mechanism.

Radiology: X-ray of the affected finger may show an avulsion fracture of the dorsal lip of the base of the distal phalanx (Fig. 16.7).

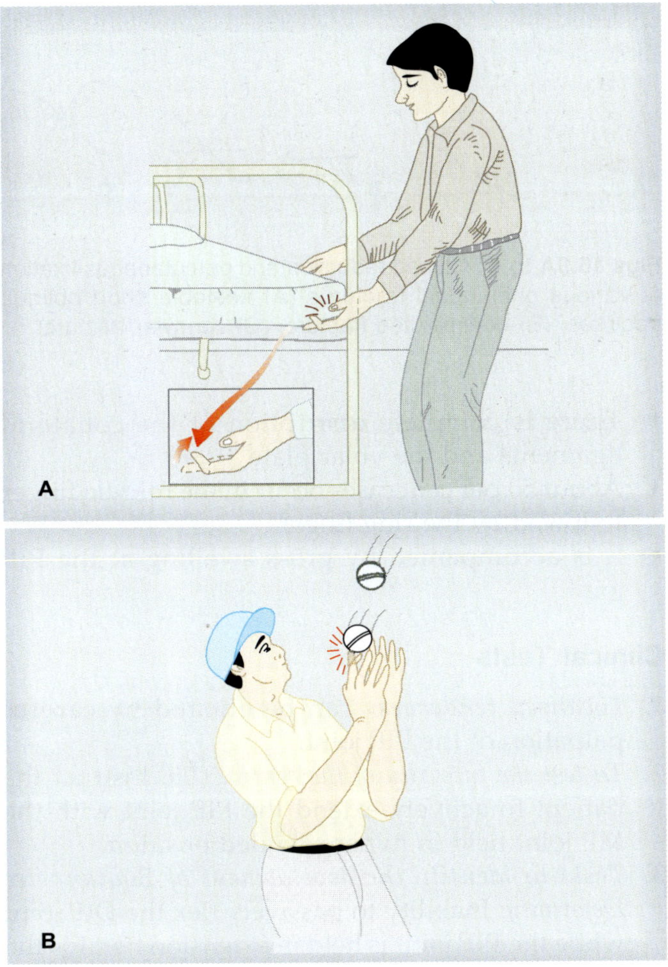

Figs 16.6A and B: Showing common mechanism of injury pertaining to mallet finger

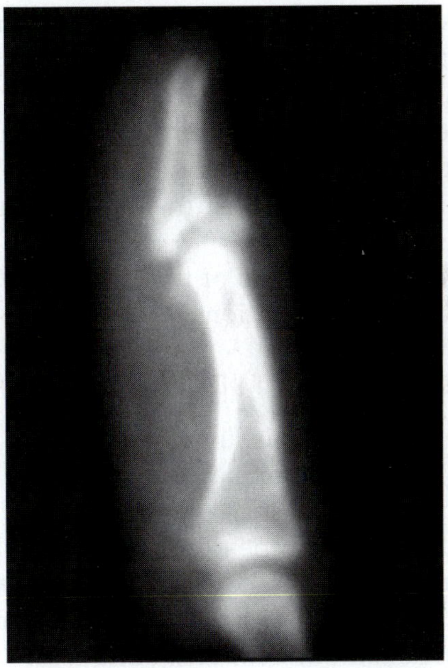

Fig. 16.7: Radiograph showing mallet fracture

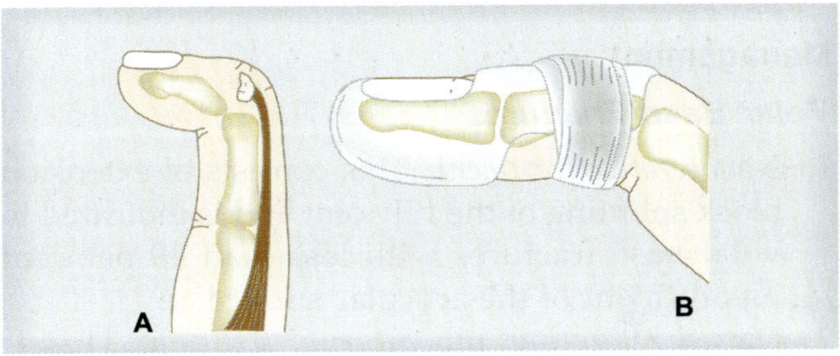

Figs 16.8A and B: Showing (A) mallet finger (B) treatment by a dorsal splint

Facts about Mallet Splints

In these cases, proximal interphalangeal joint of the finger is not immobilised but only the distal joint is immobilised by using:

a. Simple volar unpadded aluminium splint which provides three-point pressure.
b. Dorsal padded aluminium splint.
c. A stack plastic mallet finger splint (Figs 16.8A and B)

Distal joint is put in slight hyperextension. The splint may cause pain and the amount of hyperextension should not cause blanching of the skin over DIP joint.

Splints are useful in cooperative patients, and in uncooperative patients. Smellie's cast is used. About 6 to 10 weeks of continuous immobilisation is required. K-wire fixation is considered in patients like dentist or surgeon who wants to return to work quickly.

Mallet Finger of Bony Origin

This is less common. It is usually fixed with K-wire, if more than one-third of the dorsal articular surface is involved and if remainder of the distal phalanx is subluxated volar-wards.

Lesser Known But Important Thumb Injuries

- *Bowler's Thumb:* It is a traumatic neuropathy of the digital nerve of the thumb due to repeated friction from gripping a ball.
- *Game Keeper's or Baseball Thumb:* This has been explained earlier.

Treatment

1. **Nonoperative measures:** This is reserved for pure dislocations, collateral ligament injuries and mallet finger. Various custom-made dorsal hyperextension splints are used for immobilising the DIP joints.
2. **Closed reduction and percutaneous fixation:** This is reserved for mallet injuries in professionals like

dentists, surgeons, sportspersons, etc. who cannot keep their fingers immobilised for long due to professional commitments.

3. **Open reduction and internal fixation:** This is indicated in the following situations:
   a. Avulsion of the profundus tendon and its reinsertion.
   b. Chronic subluxation of the DIP joint (> 3 wk).
   c. Irreducible dislocations.

FRACTURES OF THE MIDDLE PHALANX

The three important injuries of special interest relating to the middle phalanx are:

1. Isolated fracture of the volar base.
2. Isolated fracture of the dorsal base.
3. Pilon fractures. This consists of extensive metaphyseal comminution with involvement of the entire articular surfaces and bone loss.

All these injuries can pose problems in the management.

Management

Volar Base Fractures

1. *Nonoperative treatment:* This consists of extension block splinting of the PIP joint and is indicated in volar base fractures with less than 40 per cent involvement of the articular surface.
2. *Closed reduction and internal fixation:* This is indicated for both dorsal and volar base fractures of the middle phalanx with less than 40 per cent articular surface involvement (Figs 16.9A and B).
3. *Dynamic traction:* This is a unique method of treatment and is indicated in volar base fractures of more than 40 per cent and in the very difficult Pilon fractures.
4. *Volar plate arthroplasty:* This is indicated in chronic injuries and in volar base fractures greater than 40 per cent.
5. *Open reduction and internal fixations:* This is indicated in single large fragment and in fixing bone graft to the metaphysis.

For dorsal base fractures, extension block pinning after closed reduction is the treatment of choice.

DISLOCATIONS OF THE PIP JOINT

Clinical Features

- These are frequently missed
- Common in ball catching sports

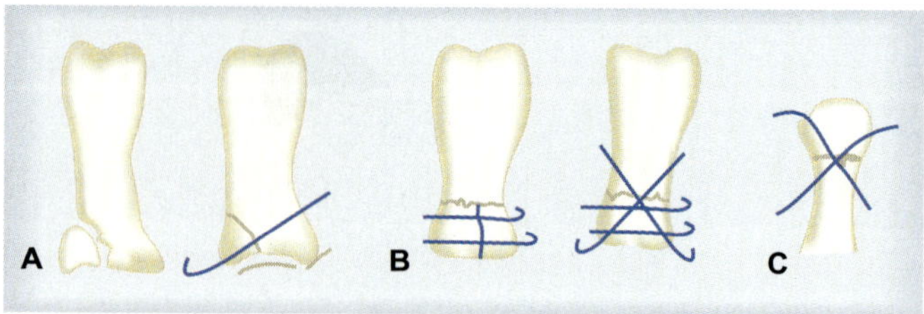

Figs 16.9A to C: Closed reduction and percutaneous fixation of various phalangeal fractures (A) unstable short oblique fractures, (B) comminuted fracture, (C) condylar fracture

- There is complete disruption of the collateral ligaments and the volar plate
- About 50 per cent cases occur in the middle finger followed by the ring finger
- It is accompanied by gross swelling at the PIP joint.

Clinical Tests

1. *Localised tenderness* can be elicited by careful palpation of the PIP joint.
2. *To test the integrity of the central slip*: Instruct the patient to actively extend the PIP joint with the MP joint held in hyperextended position.
3. *Tests to identify the development of Boutannéire Deformity:* Inability to passively flex the DIP joint while the PIP joint is held in extension heralds the onset of the Boutanneire deformity.
4. *Stress tests:* Lateral stress testing is performed with the fingers in complete extension and 30° of flexion. Greater than 20° of opening indicates complete tear of collateral ligaments.

Types of PIP Joint Dislocation

- Dorsal dislocation (most common)
- Pure volar dislocation
- Rotatory volar dislocation
- Complete collateral ligament disruption.

Treatment

Nonoperative Management

This is indicated for closed injuries and for reducible injuries. After reduction:

a. Buddy taping with immediate AROM for rotatory volar dislocation (Fig. 16.10).
b. For collateral ligament injuries buddy taping with immediate AROM.

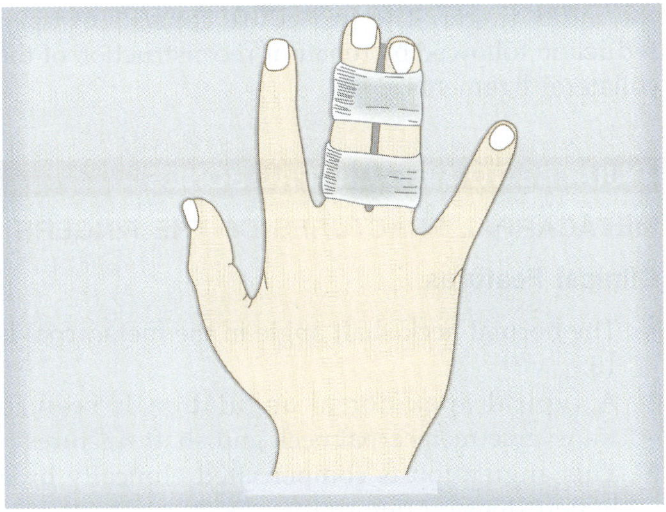

Fig. 16.10: Showing buddy taping

c. For central slip disruption and volar dislocation, 4 to 6 weeks of PIP extension, splinting followed by a 2-week daytime dynamic splinting and a static night splinting. Throughout the period of splintage, DIP joint should be actively exercised (Fig. 16.11).
d. Extension block splinting for 3 to 4 weeks for hyperextension injuries (dorsal dislocation).

Operative Management

Open reduction is indicated for open injuries, irreducible dislocations and injury to the collateral ligament of the index finger.

PROXIMAL AND MIDDLE PHALANX FRACTURES

Clinical Features

- Due to the deforming forces of the intrinsic muscles, transverse and short oblique fractures of the proximal phalanx angulate dorsally.
- The spiral and long oblique fractures shorten and rotate rather than angulate.
- Due to the action of FDS, fractures of the middle phalanx tend to angulate in either direction.

Classifications

- Head fractures—Mainly intra-articular
- Neck and shaft fractures—Extra-articular
- Base—Both extra-articular and intra-articular.

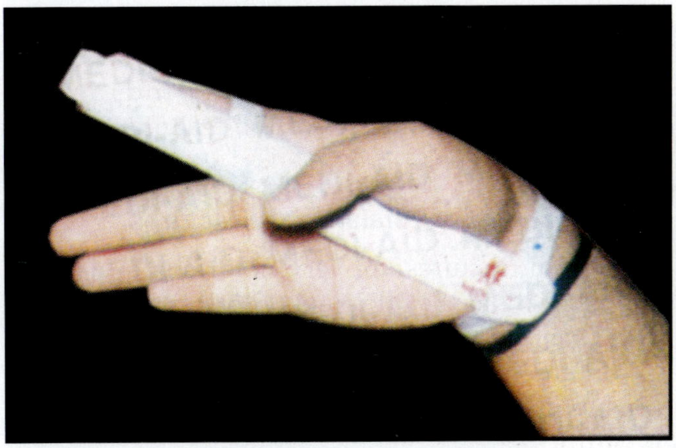

Fig. 16.11: Finger extension splint

All these fractures could be:
1. Minimally displaced but stable.
2. Reducible but stable.
3. Reducible but unstable.
4. Irreducible.

Treatment Methods

Nonoperative Treatment

This is indicated for undisplaced and for reducible but stable extra-articular fractures. The methods employed are Buddy taping for undisplaced fractures and Burkhatter spint for the rest.

Closed Reduction and Internal Fixation (IF)

This is indicated in the following situations:
a. Oblique neck fracture.
b. Reducible and stable intra-articular fracture of the middle phalanx.
c. Reducible and unstable extra-articular fractures (see Fig. 16.9C).

Open Reduction and Internal Fixation

This is indicated in:
a. Open fractures.
b. Multiple fractures.
c. Soft tissue injury.
d. Intra-articular proximal phalanx fractures.

The options for internal fixation after open reduction are:
- Intraosseous wiring
- Composite wiring

- Screws only
- Plate and screw fixation.

The choice of the fixation depends on the experience and familiarity of the technique by the operating surgeon.

Complications of Phalangeal Fractures

Phalangeal fractures are very notorious to develop complications as the PIP joint is very less tolerant joint of the hand:

1. Malunion.
2. Nonunion.
3. Stiffness.
4. Extension lag.

METACARPOPHALANGEAL JOINT DISLOCATIONS

Clinical Features

- Dorsal dislocations are more common than volar
- Small finger collateral ligament injuries are more common followed by the index finger
- Dorsal dislocations are present with hyper-extension deformity and are easy to reduce
- During the dislocations, the volar plate does not get disturbed
- Reduction methods include:
  a. Flex the wrist to relax the flexor tendons.
  b. Apply firm but not excessive longitudinal tractions along the finger.
  c. Now gently flex the joint to achieve reduction.
- Irreducible dislocations are called complex dislocations and is due to the volar plate entrapment. This is more common in index finger. Pathognomonic sign is the presence of sesamoid bones within the joint and puckering of the volar skin.
- Volar dislocations are very unstable but fortunately rare.

Treatment

Nonoperative Treatment

This is indicated in simple dorsal dislocations and collateral ligament ruptures. The fingers are immobilised in Jones position as the digits are buddy taped.

Operative Treatment

This is indicated in complex dorsal dislocations, volar dislocation and radial collateral ligament injury of the index finger. The procedure consists of open reduction followed by repair or reconstruction of the collateral ligaments.

INJURIES TO METACARPAL BONES

METACARPAL FRACTURES OF THE FINGERS

Clinical Features

- The normal neck shaft angle in the metacarpal is 15°
- A typical apex dorsal angulation is seen in transverse metacarpal neck and shaft fractures
- This angulation is compensated clinically by a hyperextension deformity
- Spiral and oblique fractures tend to shorten and rotate than angulate
- Rotational malalignment is not acceptable more than 10°
- Due to the overlapping bone shadows, special X-ray views like the Brewerton view is required. (Reverse oblique views and the Skyline views are other special views)
- Metacarpals are responsible for the formation of the following three arches of the hand:
  a. Transverse arch at the carpometacarpal joints.
  b. Transverse arch at the MP joints.
  c. A longitudinal broad convex dorsal arch.

These arches are maintained by:

1. The interosseous ligaments at the bases.
2. Deep transverse intermetacarpal ligaments distally:
   - Volar aspect of the neck of the metacarpal is the weakest point.
   - Intrinsic muscles are the primary deforming forces which can be neutralised by MP joint flexion.
   - Reduction can be achieved by longitudinal traction and by flexion of the PIP joint.

Treatment Methods

Nonoperative Treatment

This is indicated in the following situations.

a. Undisplaced fractures
b. Stable fractures (These have <50 per cent displacement, < 40° angulation and fracture obliquity of < 60°).

Methods: The hand can be immobilised by:

- Burkhalter splint: This is ideal and is known to give good splints.
- Compression glove for 2 weeks.
- Hand-based cast is also effective and permits the patient to return to the work early.

Closed Reduction and Internal Fixation

This is indicated for fractures that are unstable after reduction and for base fractures. This is mainly used for extra-articular fractures but can also be used for intra-articular fractures that are stable with K-wire fixation alone after reduction.

Open Reduction and Internal Fixation

This is indicated in the following:

- Multiple fractures
- Open fractures
- Irreducible fractures
- Displaced intra-articular fractures.

The choice of the method of internal fixation devices could be:

- Intramedullary fixation through a Steinmann's pin, multiple prebent K-wires, etc. (Figs 16.12A to C).
- Screws only
- Plate and screws
- Intraosseous wiring
- Composite wiring.

The choice of fixation should be the one with which the surgeon is most familiar with.

External Fixations

This is reserved for comminuted intra-articular fractures of the base of the fifth metacarpal bone where internal fixation is not suitable.

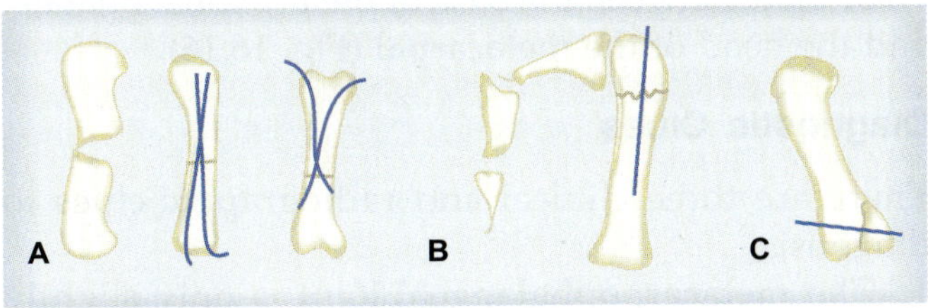

Figs 16.12A to C: Metacarpal fractures treated by closed reduction and percutaneous pinning: (A) Unstable fracture fixed with criss-cross K-wires, (B) Neck fracture fixed by intramedullary fixation, (C) Bennett's fracture fixed with K-wire

Complications of Metacarpal Bone Fractures

- Nonunion
- Avascular necrosis in periarticular fractures.
- Angular malunion
- Rotational malunion
- Intra-articular malunion
- Stiffness of the fingers.

METACARPAL FRACTURE OF THE LITTLE FINGER (BOXER'S FRACTURE)

When a boxer punches the jaw of his opponent with his fist and wins the bout, his ecstasy may be shortlived when he finds his little finger is broken, what he has actually broken is the neck of the fifth metacarpal bone and this is due to a direct impact on the dorsum of the hand (Fig 16.13).

This injury is also seen in assaults, RTAs, fall, etc. These fractures need to be accurately reduced with no rotational malalignment. This can be done by closed reduction and fixation with either plaster cast or percutaneous K-wire fixation.

METACARPAL FRACTURE OF THE THUMB

Clinical Features

- Most of the thumb metacarpal fractures are intra-articular at the carpometacarpal joint
- The volar beak of basal fracture is not palpable
- Special X-ray views consisting of true AP and lateral views are required
- Basal fractures of the thumb are divided into:
  a. Extra-articular fractures: Transverse/oblique
  b. Partial articular fracture (Bennett's)
  c. Total articular fracture (Rolando's).

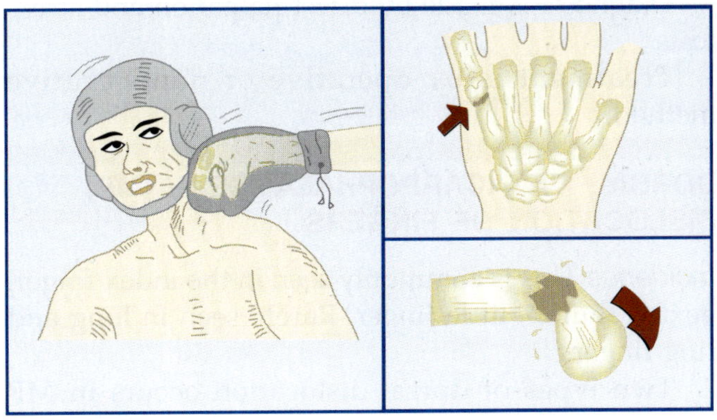

Fig. 16.13: Mechanism of injury in boxer's fracture

Displacing Forces in the Bennett's Fracture

- At the distal fragment, it is the adductor pollicis.
- At the proximal fragment, it is the abductor pollicis longus muscle.

Treatment Methods

Nonoperative Methods

This is indicated in undisplaced fractures and also in extra-articular fractures with less than 20° angulation. Closed reduction and external splinting with a thumb spica is the treatment method of choice.

Closed Reduction and Internal Fixation

This is indicated in:
- Bennett's fracture (Fig. 16.14A)
- Rolando's fracture (Fig. 16.14B)
- Oblique extra-articular fracture.

Open Reduction and Internal Fixation

This is indicated in uncomminuted Rolando's fracture and irreducible Bennett's fracture.

External Fixations

This is indicated in highly comminuted Rolando's fracture where internal fixation is contraindicated.

DISLOCATION OF THE THUMB METACARPOPHALANGEAL JOINT (GAMEKEEPER'S THUMB, SKIER'S THUMB)

Injury to the ulnar collateral ligament of the first metacarpophalangeal (MP) joint is very common but a complete dislocation is rare. It heals with some residual instability (Fig 16.15).

Diagnosis is made by direct palpation and stress tests.

Treatment is by operative or nonoperative methods.

DORSAL METACARPOPHALANGEAL (MP) DISLOCATION OF FINGERS

Incidence This is commonly seen in the index finger, next is thumb, little finger. Rarely seen in long and ring fingers.

Two types of dorsal dislocation occurs in MP joints:

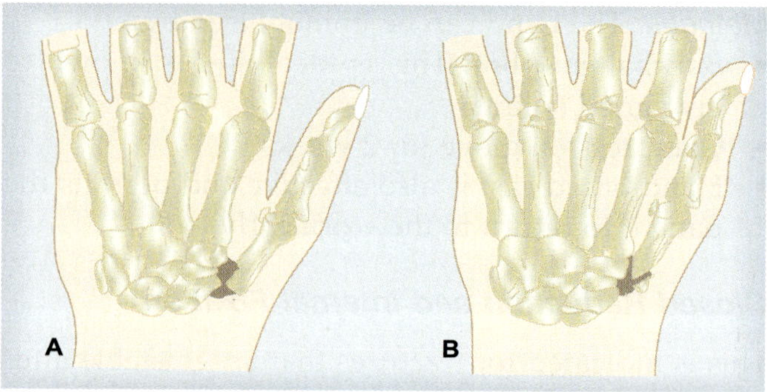

Figs 16.14A and B: Showing (A) Bennett's fracture (B) Rolando's fracture

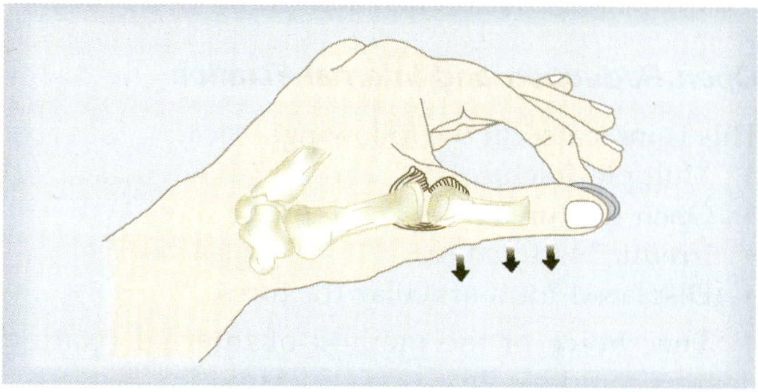

Fig. 16.15: Showing gamekeeper's thumb

Simple This can be reduced by closed methods.

Complex This is irreducible and usually requires open reduction.

Both result from hyperextension injuries and in both the volar plate is torn at its proximal insertion into the metacarpal neck.

Complex (Irreducible) Metacarpophalangeal Dislocation (Kaplan's Lesion)

Kaplan described buttonholing of the metacarpal head into the palm. Here there is an interposition of volar plate between the base of the proximal phalanx and the head of the metacarpal (Fig. 16.16).

Diagnostic Clues

There are three clinical and radiographic clues to diagnosis:

1. The metacarpophalangeal joint is only slightly hyperextended, and the interphalangeal joint is flexed. In the radiographs proximal phalanx and metacarpals are nearly parallel.

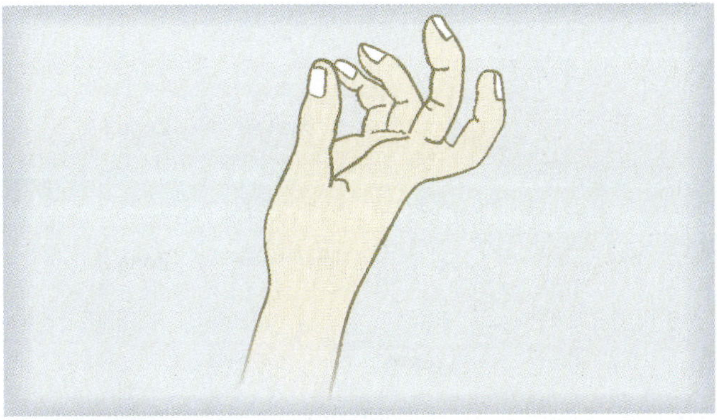

Fig. 16.16: Dislocation of II MP point (Kaplan's lesion)

2. A constant finding is puckering of the volar skin which is more readily seen in thumb than index finger.
3. Pathognomonic radiographic sign is the presence of a sesamoid bone within a widened joint space. This is normally present with volar plate.

Treatment

A single attempt at closed reduction is made; and if this fails, surgical reduction either by the volar (Kaplan's operation) approach or by the dorsal approach is done.

Note: The single most important element preventing reduction in a complex metacarpophalangeal dislocation is interposition of volar plate within the joint.

TENDON INJURIES

Either flexor or extensor tendons of the hand can be injured when the patient sustains hand injuries by a sharp cutting object. Flexor tendons are more commonly injured than the extensors (Fig. 16.17). These tendon injuries are more often missed by the clinician who treats it, if he or she does not explore the hand or the wrist wounds and look for the possibility of tendons being severed. Old healed scars over the hand or wrist with loss of function of the injured tendon confirms the diagnosis.

FLEXOR TENDON INJURIES

Both flexor digitorum superficialis (FDS) or flexor digitorum profundus (FDP) could be injured, singly or together. Flexion of the proximal interphalangeal joint of the fingers is brought about mainly by FDS; and since FDP crosses this joint, it also aids FDS, but FDP is solely responsible for the flexion of distal interphalangeal joint.

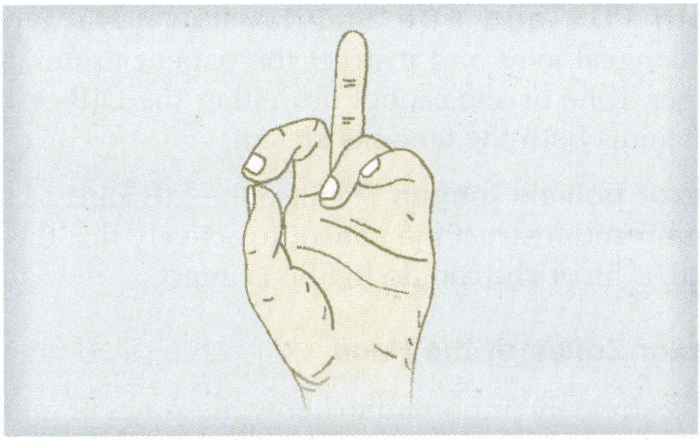

Fig. 16.17: If the flexor tendon is injured, the finger does not flex but remains straight

Tests to Diagnose Flexor Tendon Injuries

Test for Profundus

FDP (Fig. 16.18) Instruct the patient to actively flex the DIP joint while you stabilise the PIP joint. If he or she can flex it, there is no injury to FDP tendon.

Test for Superficialis

FDS (Fig. 16.19) Hold the two adjacent fingers in complete extension. This anchors the FDP tendon in the extended position and prevents it from flexing the PIP joint, if he or she can do it, FDS is intact.

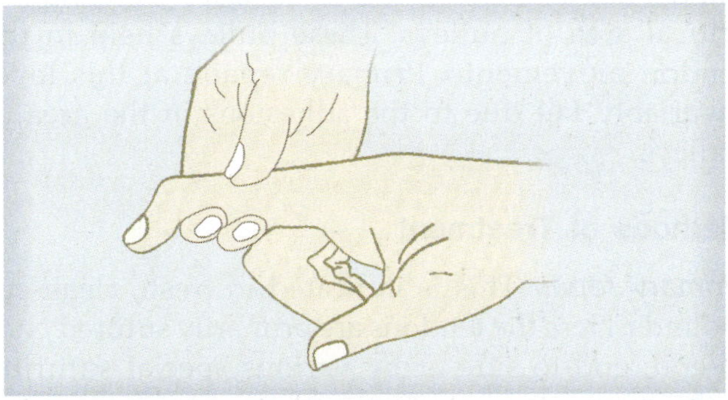

Fig. 16.18: Clinical method of testing FDP

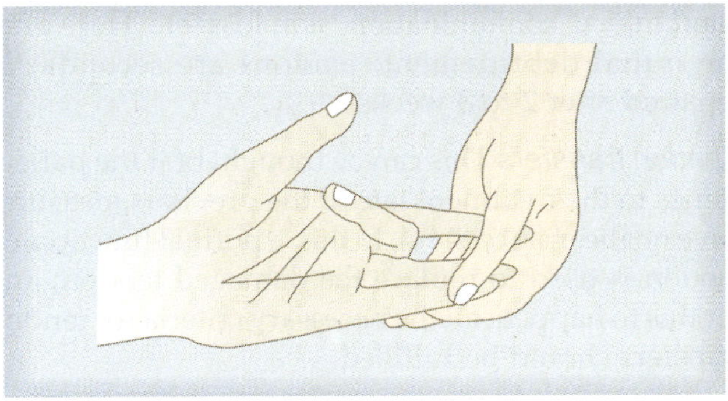

Fig. 16.19: Clinical test to examine FDS

Both FDS and FDP Stabilise the metacarpophalangeal joint and instruct the patient to flex the finger. If he or she cannot flex either the DIP or the PIP joints both the tendons are cut.

Flexor pollicis longus Stabilise the MP joint of the thumb and instruct the patient to actively flex the IP joint, if he or she can do it, FPL is intact.

Flexor Zones of the Hand

It is extremely important to know the zones of injury with regard to flexor tendon injuries of the hand and wrist. There are five zones (Fig. 16.20):

Zone I	This extends from the tip of the finger to the middle of the middle phalanx.
Zone II	This extends from the middle of the middle phalanx to the distal palmar crease.
Zone III	This overlies the palm.
Zone IV	Overlies the transverse carpal ligament of the wrist.
Zone V	Extends from the wrist crease to the level of the musculocutaneous junction of the flexor tendons.

Importance of the Zones

Bunnel has labelled Zone II as *no-man's* land and is a critical area of pulleys. These pulleys help in the tendon movements. Primary repairs at this level invariably fail due to the adhesions in the area of pulleys.

Methods of Treatment

Primary repair This is indicated in fresh, clean-cut wounds. Here the tendons are primarily sutured end-to-end, end-to-side or by various special suturing techniques.

Secondary repair This may be necessary in severe hand injury, contamination, skin loss, etc. Here after the initial debridement, tendons are secondarily repaired after 2 to 3 weeks.

Tendon transfers This can be thought of if the patient comes to the treatment late or the previous measures have not been successful. In this, a normal functioning tendon is used to replace the damaged tendon; and for this to happen, all the necessary criteria for tendon transfers should be fulfilled.

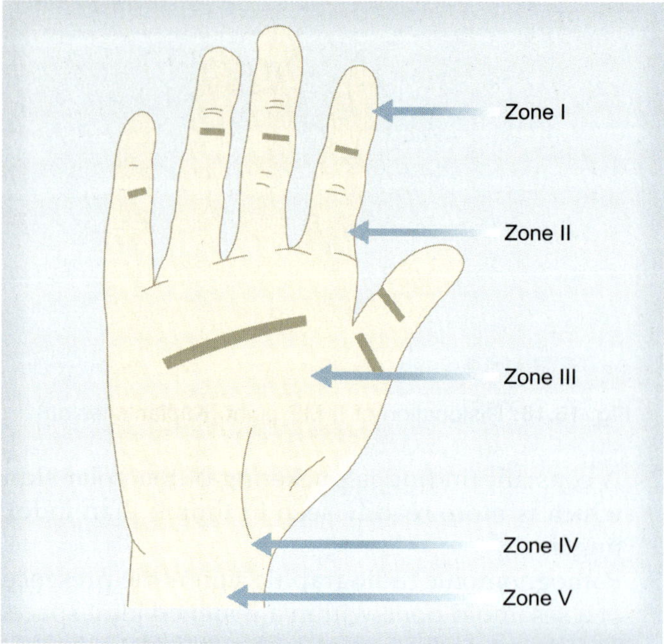

Fig. 16.20: The flexor zones of the hand

Tendon grafting In the event of loss of tendons due to crush injury, tendon grafting can be considered. Donor tendons for grafting in order of preference are the palmaris longus, the plantaris, the long extensors of the toes, etc.

EXTENSOR TENDON INJURIES

Extensor tendons of the hand are less commonly injured than the flexor tendons.

Test

Instruct the patient to extend the metacarpophalangeal joint. If the long extensors are severed, he or she will not be able to do so. But, however, he or she can extend the IP joints due to the action of the intrinsic muscles of the hand.

Treatment

The extensor surface of the hand is also divided into six zones. But unlike in the flexor tendons, extensor tendons can be primarily repaired at almost any level if the injury is clean-cut. In contaminated or crushed injuries, secondary repair after 2 to 3 weeks can be done with good results.

Quick facts

- Flexor tendons are more commonly injured than extensors.
- Primary flexor tendon injury repair is unsuccessful in Zone II.
- It is likely that tendon injuries can be missed during the initial evaluation and treatment of hand injuries.
- Primary repair is done in clean-cut injuries while secondary repair is done in contaminated wounds.
- Extensor tendons can be successfully sutured in any zone

INTERESTING FINGER INJURIES

JERSEY FINGER

It is due to avulsion of flexor digitorum profundus from its insertion on distal phalanx (Fig. 16.21). This is the opposite of 'mallet finger' and the patient is unable to flex the distal interphalangeal joint. It is seen in football and rugby players.

Boutannéire injury This is due to the rupture of central extensor slip which results in dorsal displacement of lateral bands (Fig. 16.22).

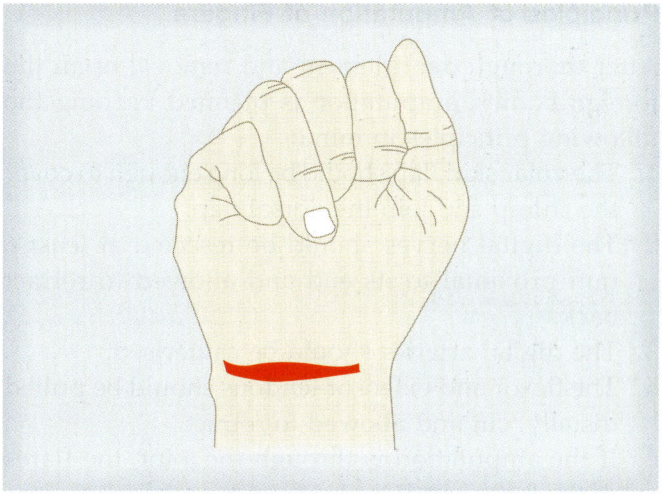

Fig. 16.21: Showing jersey finger

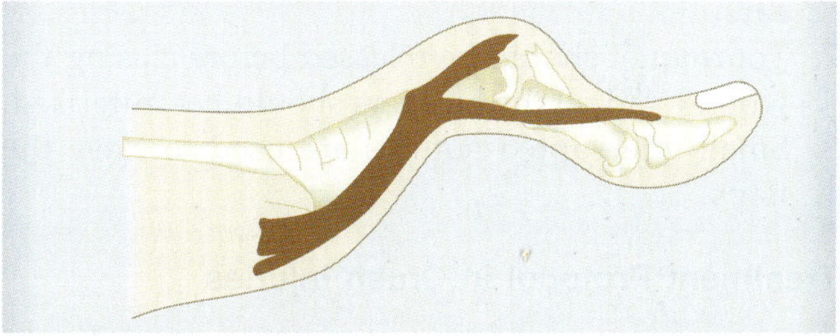

Fig. 16.22: Showing Boutannéire injury

SOFT TISSUE INJURIES OF THE HAND

Subungual haematoma This is due to blunt injury of the fingertips. If it is painful, decompression can be done by puncturing it with a 16-gauge needle.

Nailbed lacerations Before repairing the wound, distal phalangeal fractures should be reduced if any and the original nail if available should be reinserted back.

Fingertip avulsions If the soft tissue defect is more than 1 cm, it should be closed by split or full-thickness grafting.

Frostbite injury In this condition extreme cold causes vasoconstriction which may result in thrombosis of the digital vessels. The treatment consists of rapid rewarming in a water bath at 40 to 45°C.

CRUSH INJURIES OF THE HAND AND AMPUTATIONS

Crush injuries of the hand are very serious injuries seen in industrial accidents, RTAs, fire-cracker injuries, machine tool injuries, etc. Amputation of the fingers or hand is not readily advocated and the following considerations are taken into account before making this painful decision:

1. Is the part injured suffering from absolute or irreversible loss of blood supply? If so, this is the only absolute indication for primary amputation.
2. Are the other fingers normal? If not, delay the amputation of the affected finger.
3. If the finger is left unamputated, will the ultimate function of the hand be good?
4. What is the status of the five tissue areas namely the skin, tendon, nerve, bone and joint? If three or more than three of these five areas require special procedures like grafting, etc. give a serious thought about the possibility of amputation.
5. Is the victim a child? If so exercise caution.
6. If both the flexor tendons and digital nerves are damaged and if the patient is an adult, consider amputation.
7. Is the thumb badly injured? Do everything to salvage the thumb.

Thus, in badly crushed hand injuries, it is advisable to avoid radical amputations and to be as conservative as possible in excising the vital parts of the all important hand.

Principles of Amputation of Fingers

After thorough debridement and removal of all the foreign bodies, amputation is planned keeping the following principles in mind:

1. The volar skin flap should be long enough to cover the stump and join the dorsal flap.
2. The digital nerves should be resected at least 6 mm proximal to its end and allowed to retract back.
3. The digital arteries should be cauterised.
4. The flexor and extensor tendons should be pulled distally, cut and allowed to retract.
5. If the amputation is through the joint, the flares of the bony condyles is excised.
6. No much consideration should be given to the dog ears.
7. Tourniquet should be released before closing the wound and all the bleeders should be cauterised.
8. Small interrupted sutures are used to close the flaps.

Treatment Protocol in Crush Injuries

Whatever treatment protocol is followed, it should aim to fulfil the following objectives:

1. It should promote primary healing.
2. The injured parts should be salvaged.
3. It should aim to prevent infection.

The recommended protocol is as follows:

First aid These measures include covering the wound with a sterile dressing, hand elevation and judicious application of a tourniquet if required.

First examination Here status of the skin is assessed in sterile conditions without probing the deeper structures. After the skin, tests are conducted to assess the damages to bones, tendons and nerves. Each of these structures should be considered as damaged until proved otherwise. Radiograph of the hand and general measures like IV fluids, antibiotics, etc. is then done.

Second examination This is the most important step and is done in a major operation theatre under general anaesthesia or a regional block. After a thorough debridement, all the structures are very carefully inspected again. Skin is examined for viability, bones, nerves, tendons, vessels are inspected for crushing, loss, viability, etc. All the nonviable structures are excised and loose small pieces of bones are removed.

If the wound is clean, all the structures are primarily repaired and the bone is fixed either by K-wire or Joshi's external fixators. If the wound is contaminated, secondary repair of the tendons, nerves, etc. are planned after 2 to 3 weeks. If the wound is badly crushed and nonviable, then primary amputation is considered as discussed above.

Postoperative Considerations

After the surgical procedures mentioned above, the hand is splinted in functional positions—Fig. 16.2 (as discussed earlier) and is kept elevated. Active and passive physiotherapy, wax bath and other rehabilitative measures are planned and appliances given if necessary.

17 Injuries Around the Hip

BRIEF ANATOMY

THE HIP JOINT SPEAKS

- I am an articulation between the femoral head and the acetabulum. I am a ball and socket variety of joint with a high degree of stability and an excellent range of movements exceeded only by my counterpart the shoulder joint. The ball is formed by the head of the femur which has a small fovea in the centre. This gives attachment to the ligamentum teres which carries a small artery to the head. The deep socket of mine is formed by the acetabulum which is lined by a horse shoe-shaped articular cartilage. Its inferior aspect is formed by the acetabular notch which is devoid of hyaline cartilage. The socket is completed by the transverse ligament inferiorly.
- The neck of femur is placed at an angle of 135° to the shaft and it projects 10 to 12° anteriorly to the coronal plane. My inherent strength depends upon the trabecular pattern (Fig. 17.1) which consists of primary and secondary compression and tensile trabeculae. These trabeculae are continuous with the trabeculae of the acetabulum. The degree of movements include flexion 0 to 140°, extension 0 to 15°, adduction 0 to 25° and abduction 0 to 30°.

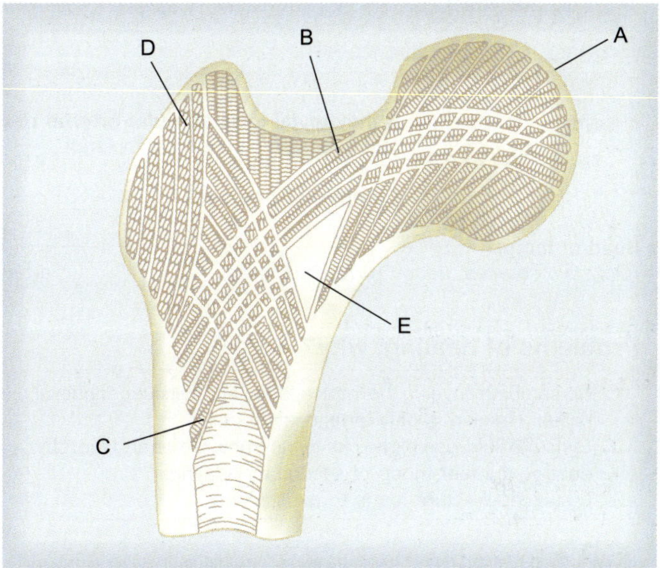

Fig. 17.1: Showing trabecular pattern or proximal femur: (A) primary compressive trabeculae, (B) primary tensile trabeculae, (C) secondary tensile, (D) secondary compressive trabeculae, (E) Ward's triangle

FRACTURE NECK FEMUR

QUOTATION: *"We come to the world under the brim of pelvis and go out of the world through the fracture neck of femur"*

Fracture neck femur could be intracapsular or extracapsular (see Figs 17.12A to C). Intracapsular fracture neck femur is notoriously known as an orthopaedic enigma, since a permanent solution for its treatment still eludes the orthopaedic surgeon. Hence, it is infamously termed as an unsolved problem. Fracture neck of femur does not unite readily and this makes it a difficult problem to tackle (see box for the reasons).

BLOOD SUPPLY OF FEMORAL HEAD

Femoral artery → **Profunda femoris artery**

Medial circumflex artery ← ↓ → **Lateral circumflex artery**

(Along with some contribution from superior and inferior gluteal artery)

→ **EXTRACAPSULAR ARTERIAL RING** ←

Few branches | *Main branches from this ring arise*

↓ **Medullary branches** | ↓ **Ascending cervical arteries** (retinacular vessels)

Small metaphyseal vessels | (Injured early in fracture neck)

Neck of femur (has three sources, hence AVN is rare)

Branches from these divide into *anterior, posterior, medial, and lateral group.* Of these, *lateral group is the most important source*

(Few branches)

↓ At the margin of articular cartilage, these vessels form a

Subsynovial intra-articular arterial ring ← (could be complete or incomplete)

↓ **Epiphyseal branches**

↓ **Head of femur** ← **Artery of ligamentum teres** (branch of obturator or medial circumflex artery (MCA) present in 1/3 cases)

(Only two sources, hence AVN is common)

Problems of healing, why?

1. No cambium layer in the intracapsular area, so no peripheral callus. Healing is only by endosteal callus.
2. Synovial fluid lyse blood clot at the fracture site and thereby destroy another mode of secondary healing.
3. Displaced fracture leads to avascularity.

Clinical Significance of Vascular Anatomy

Avascular necrosis of femoral head and nonunion fracture neck femur are the two very important and common complications of intracapsular fracture neck femur. A thorough knowledge of the vascular anatomy (Fig. 17.2) is a must to understand the reasons behind. Femoral head circulation is through three sources:

1. Intraosseous cervical vessels.
2. Artery of ligamentum teres.
3. Retinacular vessels.

In fracture neck femur, intraosseous cervical vessels are disrupted and blood supply are dependent on artery of ligamentum teres and retinacular vessels only. Artery of ligamentum teres supplies only a small portion of head, hence, avascular necrosis of the head of the femur occurs if retinacular vessels, the only main source, are damaged in fracture neck femur. There are two sources of viability of femoral head after a displaced femoral neck fracture:

1. Residual uninjured vascular supply.
2. Revascularisation of neck of femur from surrounding soft tissue before late segmental collapse.

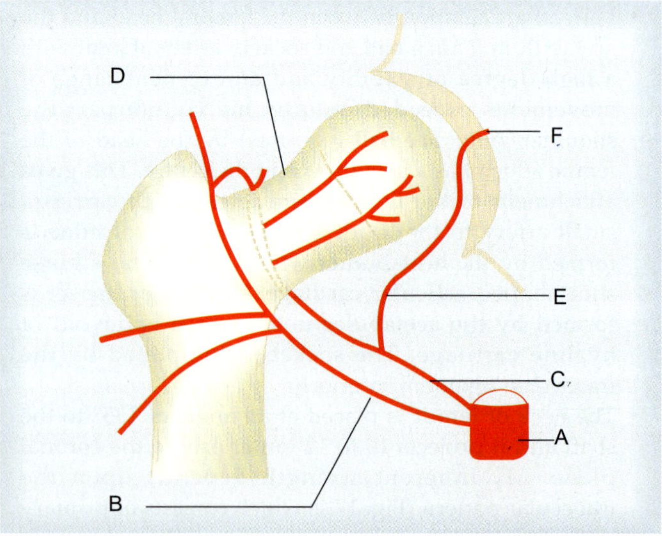

Fig. 17.2: Vascular anatomy of femoral head: (A) profunda femoris artery, (B) lateral circumflex artery, (C) medial circumflex artery, (D) ascending retinacular vessels, (E) obturator branch of medial circumflex artery, (F) artery of the ligamentum teres

"Therefore, the aim of treatment is early anatomical reduction, impaction and rigid internal fixation to protect the existing circulation and to allow revascularisation to take place before late segmental collapse can occur."

Aetiology

1. It is common in older patients with osteoporosis or osteomalacia (12%) and in them usually it is fracture through a pathological bone.
2. It is common in elderly women secondary to senile osteoporosis. It also causes marked comminution of the posterior cortex and thus decreases the quality of reduction.

Mechanism of Injury

- Majority are due to trivial fall, as a result of direct blow over the greater trochanter (Fig. 17.3).
- Second mechanism is mainly due to lateral rotation of the extremity which causes marked posterior comminution of the neck.
- Recent suggested mechanism is cyclical loading due to muscle force and torsion.
- Major trauma in young adults like road traffic accident (RTA), fall, etc.

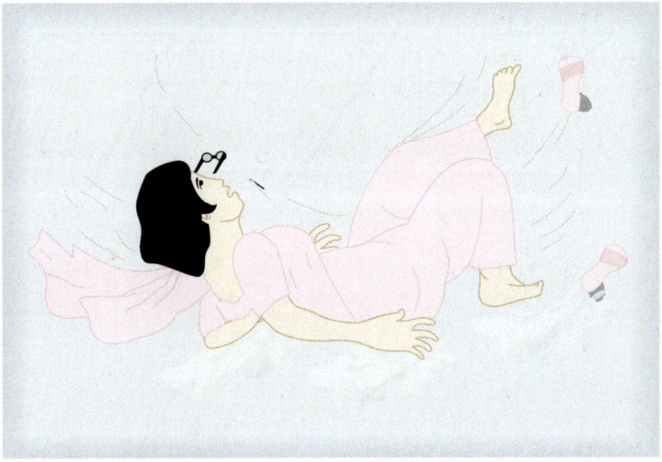

Fig. 17.3: Fracture neck femur is common in elderly females due to trivial fall like a slip and fall in the bathroom

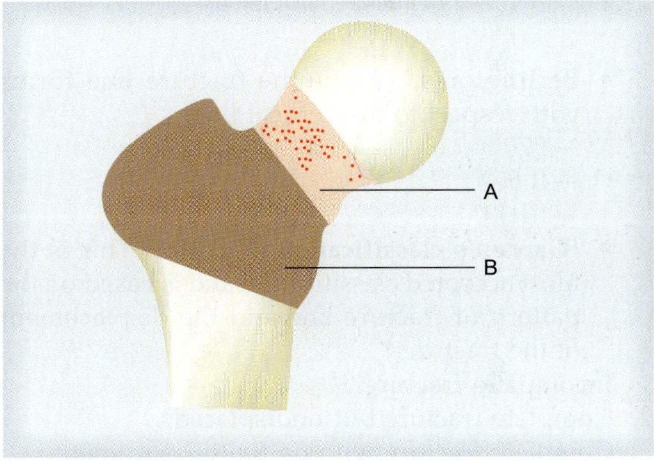

Fig. 17.4: Showing fracture neck femur types (A) intracapsular region, and (B) extracapsular region

Classification

Many classifications are proposed for fracture neck femur. Few important ones are mentioned here.

Broad Classification

1. Intracapsular—from subcapital area to the middle of the neck.
2. Extracapsular—from base of the neck to the pertrochanteric region (Fig. 17.4).

Structural Classification

1. Impacted—here the fragments are telescoped into each other.
2. Undisplaced.
3. Displaced.

Causatively

1. Stress fractures (seen in soldiers, athletes, etc.).
2. Pathologic fractures (seen in osteoporosis, etc.).
3. Postirradiation fractures.

Based on Fracture Character

a. Anatomical location
   1. Subcapital—beneath the neck.
   2. Transcervical—in the middle of the neck.
   3. Basal—at the base of the neck.
      - **Bank's** subclassification
        —Classical subcapital
        —Wedge subcapital (common)
        —Inferior beak appearance.

b. Fracture angle
   - **Pauwel's** (Angle the fracture line forms with respect to horizontal line—Fig. 17.5).
     More the angle more is it likely to be unstable.
     —I 30°
     —II 50°
     —III 70°

Section 2

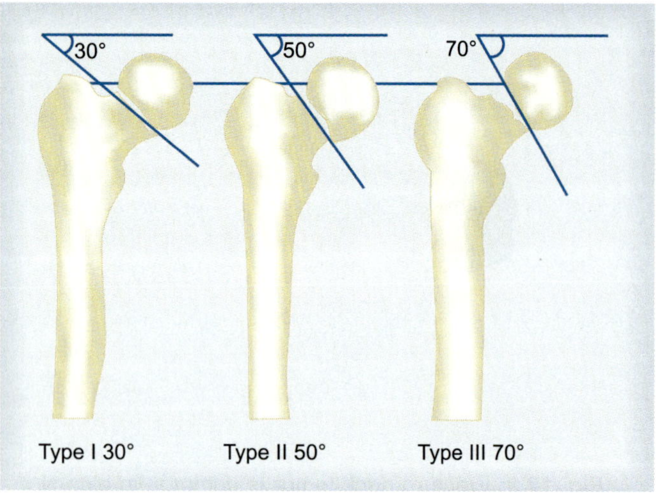

Fig. 17.5: Showing Pauwel's classification of fracture neck femur

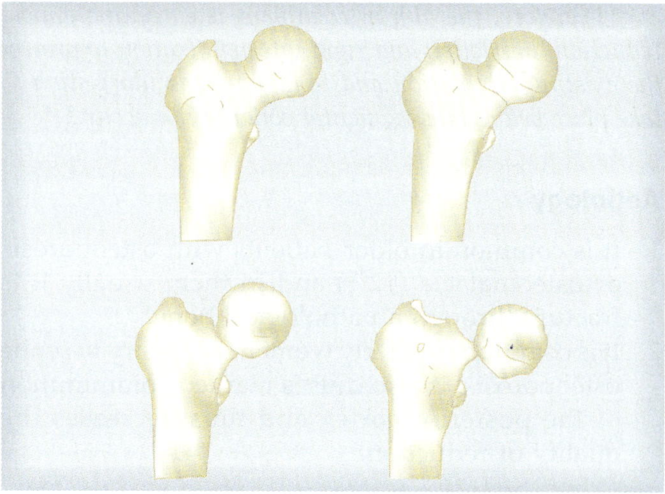

Fig. 17.6: Showing Garden's classification

- **Perlington's** (Angle the fracture line forms with respect to the vertical line)
  —I 70°
  —II 50°
  —III 30°
- [1]**Garden's classification** (Fig. 17.6) This is the most accepted classification and is based on the pattern of fracture line and the displacement of the fracture:

1. Incomplete fracture.
2. Complete fracture but undisplaced.
3. Complete fracture with partial displacement.
4. Complete fracture with total displacement.

Delbet's Classification (Fig. 17.7)—in Children

1. Transepiphyseal—at the junction of the head and neck.
2. Transcervical—through the middle of the neck.
3. Cervicotrochanteric (basal) at the junction of neck and shaft.
4. Intertrochanteric in between the greater and lesser trochanters.
5. Pertrochanteric—at the level of the trochanter.

Note: Garden's and Pauwel's classification in adults and Delbet's classification in children are widely used while the others are mentioned for students information.

Clinical Features

Usually, the patient is an elderly female and gives history of trivial trauma like slip and fall in the bathroom (see Fig. 17.3). The patient complains of pain and restriction of movements of the affected hip. On examination, there is tenderness over the anterior hip joint line. There is minimal shortening and external rotational deformity of the affected limb due to the fracture being intracapsular. The capsule prevents the muscular forces from displacing the fracture fragments grossly. Active straight leg raising is difficult. In impacted fracture neck of femur, the patient complains of groin pain, antalgic gait and restriction of hip movements.

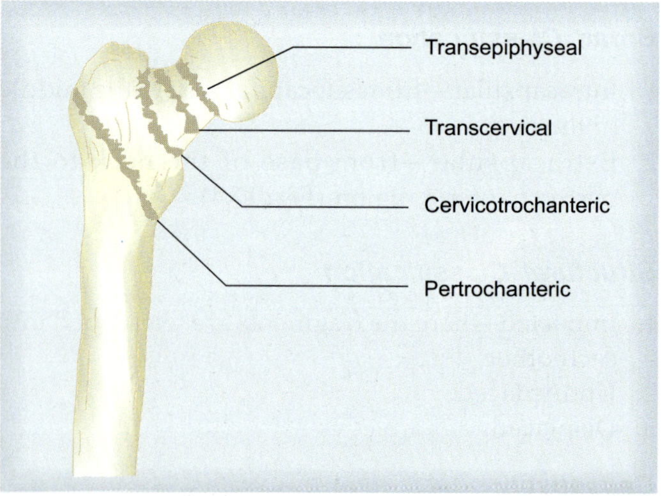

Fig. 17.7: Delbet's classification for fracture neck of femur in children

[1]**RS Garden**. Orthopaedic surgeon, Preston, England, described this classification in 1961.

Investigations

Radiography Consists of routine AP and lateral views of the hip joint. The following points are noted (Fig. 17.8).

- The extent of fracture line whether complete or incomplete.
- The fracture angle.
- Break in the **Shenton's line** (Fig. 17.9).
- Posterior wall comminution of the neck is best seen in the lateral view.
- Prominent lesser trochanter.
- The degree of osteoporosis (Singh's index).

Shenton's line is a line drawn from the superior margin of the obturator foramen to the margin of the neck.

- **Singh's Index** This is a classification system that measures the degree of osteoporosis in the proximal femur based on radiographic evaluation of the trabecular pattern (Fig. 17.10). This helps to decide the choice of implants.

Other Investigations

Radiography has got limited value in assessing the vascular status of the femoral head. The time period required for a radiograph to show avascular changes is 3 to 6 months (Fig. 17.11). Hence, viability and vascularisation of femoral head at the time of surgery is determined by:

- Oxygen tension measurement
- Venography

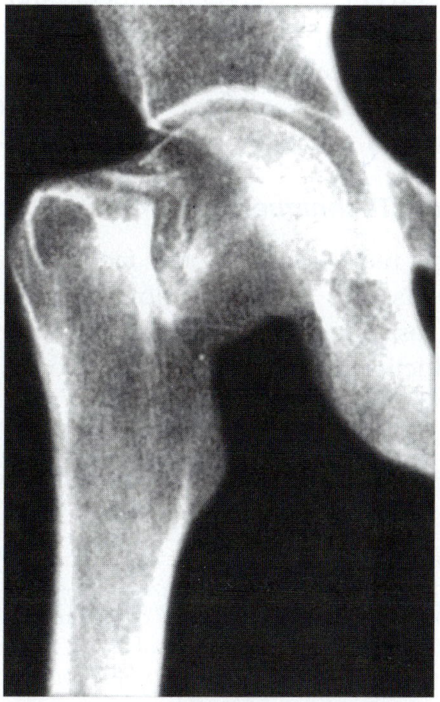

Fig. 17.8: Radiograph showing intracapsular fracture neck femur

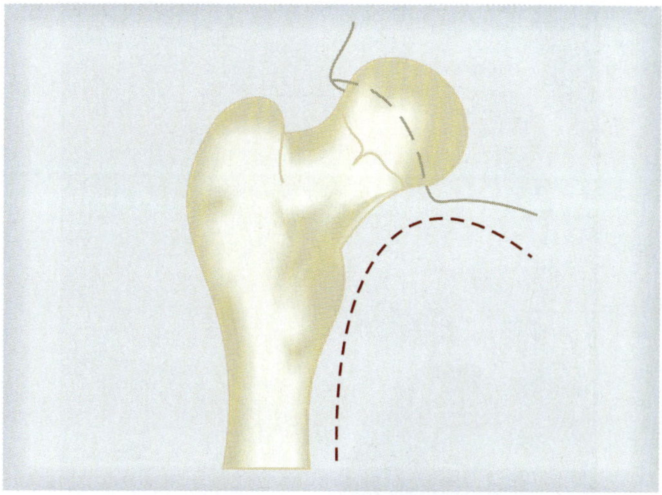

Fig. 17.9: Shenton's line

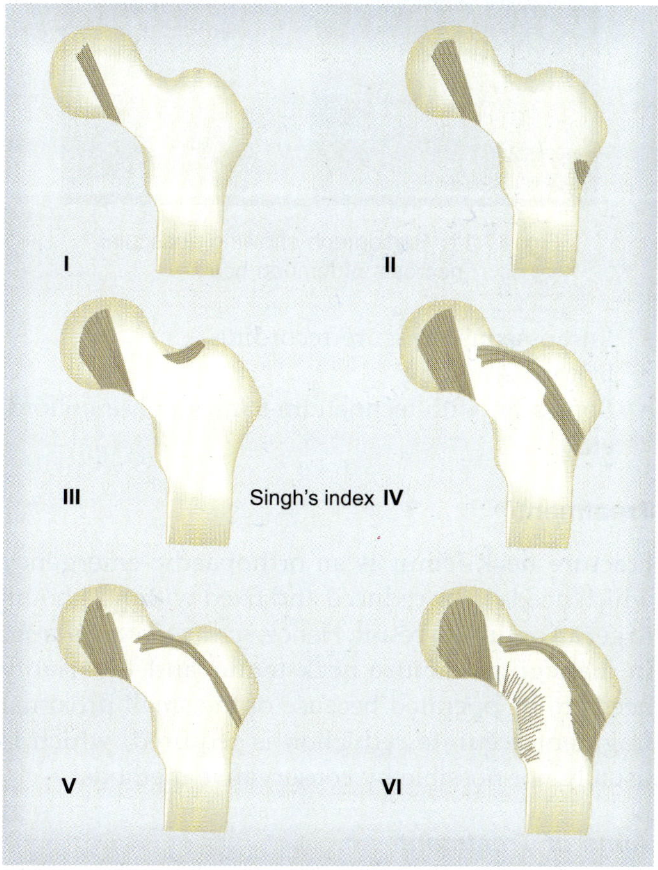

Fig. 17.10: Singh's index

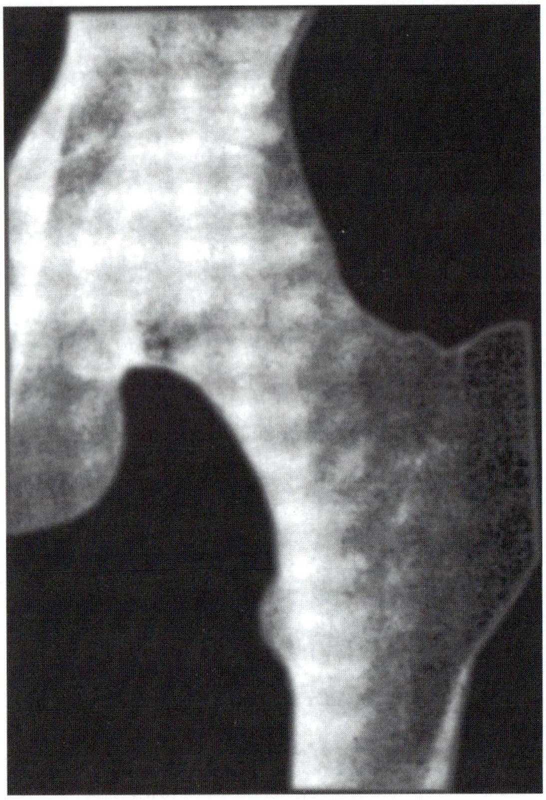

Fig. 17.11: Radiograph showing avascular necrosis of femoral head

- Intraosseous pressure recording
- Isotope scanning
- Bone scan with technetium-99m, sulphur colloid, etc.

Treatment

Fracture neck femur is an orthopaedic emergency which needs to be reduced and fixed within 24 hours to get an optimum result. Hence, *speed is the watchword* in managing fracture neck femur and invariably needs to be operated because of the small proximal fragment accurate reduction is required, which is usually not possible by conservative methods.

Aims of Treatment

- *Early anatomical reduction which helps prevent further vascular damage.*
- *Impaction of the fracture fragments.*
- *Rigid internal fixation: enables revascularisation from the surrounding soft tissues and uninjured bones which helps in early callus formation.*

Broad treatment guidelines

Age group	Undisplaced	Displaced
>70 years	• Dynamic hip screws (DHS)	• Prosthesis • Total hip replacement (THR)
Young adults	• DHS • Cannulated screws (ASNIS)	• DHS • Later osteotomy or prosthesis
Children	• HIP spica • Multiple Moore's pinning	• Multiple Moore's pinning • Osteotomy • Arthrodesis

Treatment Plans as per Garden's Classification

Garden I

a. *Conservative* Hip spica is applied if fracture is several weeks old and if the patient is unfit for surgery.
b. *Surgical* Multiple pins by Moore, Knowles cannulated screws, etc.

Garden II Here the fracture is complete and may get displaced. Hence, it is fixed with either DHS or multiple cannulated AO screws.

Garden III/IV Conservative treatment is rarely indicated except in severely ill patients and mentally ill patients, e.g. hip spica and well leg traction. Surgery is the treatment of choice.

Surgery Goal of surgery is anatomical reduction, impaction and stable internal fixation.

Reduction Techniques

Acceptable reduction is the key factor in decreasing risk of avascular necrosis following fracture neck femur. Closed reduction is tried first failing which open reduction is resorted to. The following are the closed reduction methods:

Closed reduction with hip in extension	*Closed reduction with hip in flexion*
Whitmann's method Extension + internal rotation + abduction movements of the hip	**Lead better method** Flexion of hip, traction along long axis of femur, thigh internally rotated and abducted. Evaluate reduction by *"heel palm test".

Closed reduction with hip in extension	*Closed reduction with hip in flexion*
Massie Forceful internal rotation of the limb	**Smith Peterson** Slight hip flexion + then internal rotation + abduction + extension
Mc Elevenny Extension + external rotation + Internal rotation+ adduction movements	**Flynn** Flexion, traction along the femoral neck
Deyerle Traction with extension + foot is internally rotated + force applied on greater trochanter from anterior to posterior direction	

Note* **What is 'heel palm' test?
It is a clinical test to assess the accuracy of reduction of fracture neck femur. The heel of the affected limb should remain neutral in the palm of the clinician's hand and not lie externally rotated after reduction.

Radiology

Radiographic evaluation of the accuracy of reduction of the fracture neck femur, obtained by any one of the methods employed above is done. It is mandatory before proceeding with internal fixation. The following are some of the parameters:

1. Head and neck always form an "S"-shaped curve. If the radiograph reveals an unbroken "C"-shaped curve the fracture is not reduced.
2. *Garden's criteria* In AP view, normal alignment index between proximal and distal fragments post reduction is 155 to 180°.
   In lateral view, it is 160 to 180°. If the angle is less than 155° or more than 180° in either of the views, then the reduction is not acceptable.
3. *Lateral view* helps to detect the posterior wall comminution. Stability of reduction depends on posterior wall comminution which causes nonunion in 60 per cent of the cases.
4. Slight valgus with 2 to 3 mm separation of the fracture site at the medial calcar is not acceptable. However, varus is not accepted at all.

If two attempts at closed reduction fails, then open reduction is resorted to. Probably, there is no other fracture which needs such an accurate reduction before proceeding for internal fixation. Hence, the reduction should be accurately assessed to get good results.

Techniques of Internal Fixation for the Fracture Neck of Femur

Though there are many choices for internal fixation in fracture neck femur, the principles of preoperative preparation, reduction of the fracture, C-arm or radiographic control, surgical approaches and methods of insertion of fixations are the same.

Procedure The patient is fixed to the fracture table after anaesthesia. Closed reduction of the fracture is done under radiograph or C-arm control. If the reduction is satisfactory, the greater trochanter and upper end of femur is exposed through a lateral incision. Midway between the anterior and posterior cortices of the lateral femur and about 2 cm distal to the edge of the greater trochanter drill a hole and insert a guide pin at an angle of 45° to the shaft and parallel to the ground. Check the positions of the guide-wires by lateral radiographs or C-arm. If satisfactory, insert the cannulated screws or Moore's pins parallel to the guide-wire and if Richard's screw is used through the guide-wire. Confirm the position of all the pins as mentioned above and close the wound in layers. Postoperatively, the patient is mobilised early.

Cardinal Points in Internal Fixation

- Guidepins should be inserted at an angle of 45° to the shaft and parallel to the ground.
- Guidepin should be in the centre and stop short of the head by 1.3 cm.
- The internal fixation screws or pins should be in the midcentre of the neck or below and posterior to prevent damage to the retinacular vessels.
- The guidepin should be inserted slowly and should pass smoothly without any resistance.
- The screws or pins should be 0.6 cm shorter when placed above and 0.6 cm longer when placed below the guidepin.

Complications of Internal Fixation

Infection This is due to poor aseptic measures during surgery. The infection may be superficial or deep and is a troublesome problem to treat.

Nonunion results if the fixation methods are not rigid.

Avascular necrosis This is due to faulty position of the pins in the superior part of the neck which may damage the retinacular vessels leading to avascularity.

Loss of fixation This could occur due to osteoporosis, loosening, etc.

Methods of Internal Fixation

After having accurately reduced the fracture and ascertained the accuracy, the fracture neck femur can be fixed by any one of the methods mentioned below. However, no ideal internal fixation methods are available.

Multiple Pins (Knowles, Moore) For impacted fracture, percutaneously for medically unfit persons, and for fractures in children (Fig. 17.12A).

ASNIS This is a system of cannulated screws that provide improved pullout and bending and torque strengths as compared to Knowles pins. These are the commonly preferred screws for the intracapsular variety.

Fixed angle nail has fallen into disrepute because the nail is rigid and may penetrate the joint (Fig. 17.12B).

Sliding or telescoping nails (dynamic hip screws) It has replaced the fixed angle nail. The nail offers collapsibility which ensures continuous impaction at the fracture site and which lessens the chance of nail penetration through the femoral head. *This is the most commonly employed fixation method for fracture neck femur,* especially the extracapsular variety (Fig. 17.12C).

Meyer's Muscle Pedicle Graft

A mention has to be made about the posterior muscle pedicle grafting technique. Muscle pedicle graft from the gluteus maximus or quadratus femoris (Meyer's technique), is particularly useful in posterior wall comminution. This technique has been popularised by Dr Bakshi of Kolkata.

Other Treatment Options

These include hemireplacement arthroplasty, osteotomy and very rarely THR. However, they are not recommended as the primary modality of treatment in fresh fracture neck of femur. They are indicated in special situations like nonunion, AVN, etc. and are discussed below.

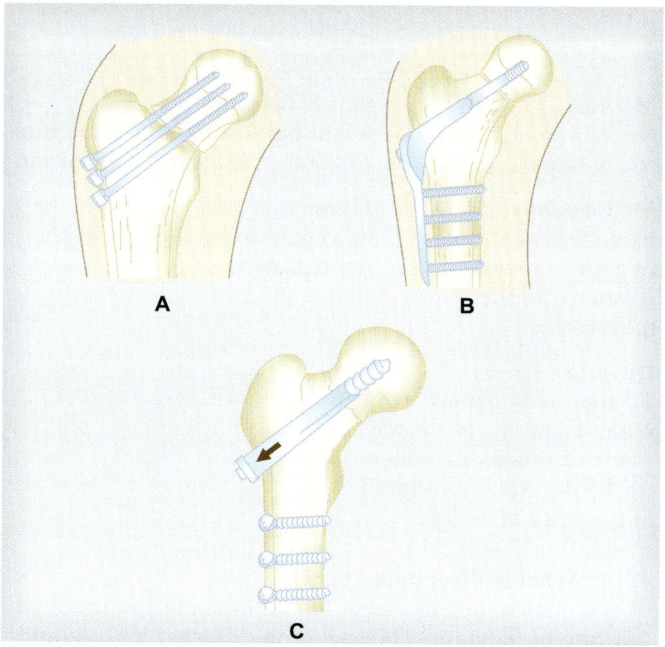

Figs 17.12A and C: Showing methods of internal fixation of intracapsular fracture neck of femur: (A) Multiple pins, (B) Blade plate fixation, (C) Dynamic hip screw

Hemireplacement arthroplasty as a primary treatment in displaced intracapsular fracture neck of femur over 70 years is a better option than internal fixation except in very frail patients where internal fixation seem to do better.

However, after 70 years, in displaced fracture of femoral neck, amongst the treatment options of internal fixation, hemireplacement arthroplasty and THR, THR seems to be the best bet with lower complications.

COMPLICATIONS OF FEMORAL NECK FRACTURE

THROMBOEMBOLISM

Thromboembolism is a leading cause of death within first 7 days. Incidence is 40 per cent.

NONUNION

Only one-third of the fracture neck femur are known to heal with OR + IF. Nonunion rate is 85 to 95 per cent. If there is no evidence of radiological healing taking place between 6 and 12 months at treatment on a radiograph, it is declared as nonunion.

Causes

a. Inaccurate reduction.
b. Poor internal fixation.
c. Lack of cambium layer in the periosteum of the neck.
d. Avascularity of femoral head.
e. Posterior wall comminution.

Clinical Features

The patient is unable to bear the weight on the affected side. Trendelenburg test, telescopic test will be positive. Wasting of the muscles and minimal shortening of the affected lower limb are the other features.

Radiology

Radiographs of the hip reveals ununited fracture neck of femur and there may be avascular changes in the head.

Treatment

Surgery is the treatment of choice. The method chosen takes into account the viability of the head.

- Head viable
  - ↓ Osteotomy (McMurray's displacement osteotomy or (Fig. 17.13A) Shanz angulation osteotomy) + Bone grafting
- Head not viable
  - Acetabular cartilage viable
    - ↓ • Hemireplacement arthroplasty by using a prosthesis
    - • *Bipolar arthroplasty (in young)*
  - Acetabular cartilage not viable
    - ↓ Total hip replacement

OSTEOTOMY

To treat nonunion of fracture neck femur, two types of osteotomies and their modifications have been described and they are as follows:

McMurray's displacement osteotomy (Fig. 17.13A) In this, the osteotomy is made just proximal to the lesser trochanter and the distal fragment is pushed medially and fixed internally.

Shanz angulation osteotomy (Fig. 17.13B) In this, the osteotomy is made through or just distal to the lesser trochanter. A laterally based wedge of bone is removed and the varus angulation is corrected and fixed with plate and screws.

Role of Osteotomy

Displacement or angulation (Figs 17.13C and D) osteotomy helps to convert the shearing force at the fracture site into compression force by changing the line of weight bearing and thereby enhances the chances of fracture union.

Among the two, angulation osteotomy is preferable because the position of greater trochanter is more satisfactory, function of the abductor muscles is re-established more effectively, there is no further shortening and internal fixation is maintained more satisfactorily.

Osteotomy as a treatment for nonunion fracture neck femur has a role only if the head of the femur is viable otherwise hemiarthroplasty is preferable.

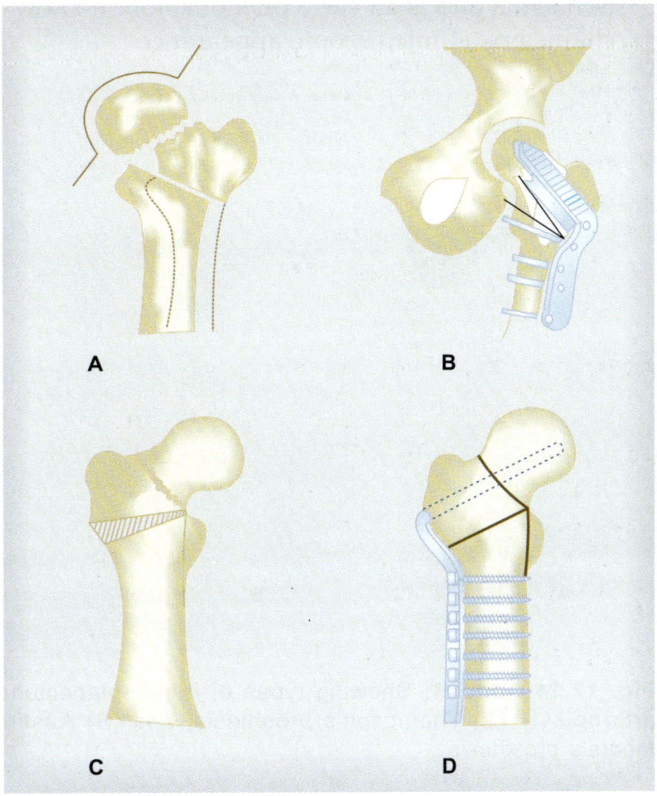

Figs 17.13A to D: Different types of osteotomies (A) McMurray's osteotomy, (B) Shanz angulation osteotomy, (C) Angulation osteotomy, (D) Pauwel's osteotomy

Hemireplacement Arthroplasty

As mentioned earlier, if the head is not viable but the acetabular cartilage is viable, and if the patient is over 60 years of age, hemireplacement arthroplasty is the treatment of choice. However, the choice of prosthesis depends upon the existing calcar femori. If sufficiently present (at least 1 to 3 cm),[2]Austin Moore's prosthesis (Figs 17.14A and B) is the choice and if it is inadequate [3]Thompson prosthesis is preferred *(ref. to section on instruments for details)*. Bipolar hip replacement is another option (Fig. 17.15).

Total Hip Replacement

If both the femoral head and the acetabular cartilage is not viable and if the patient is more than 60 years old total hip replacement is the surgery of choice.

AVASCULAR NECROSIS

It is the next important complication. Two types are described:

1. Due to actual AVN—this is secondary to ischaemia and is an early phenomenon. It shows characteristic microscopic appearance.

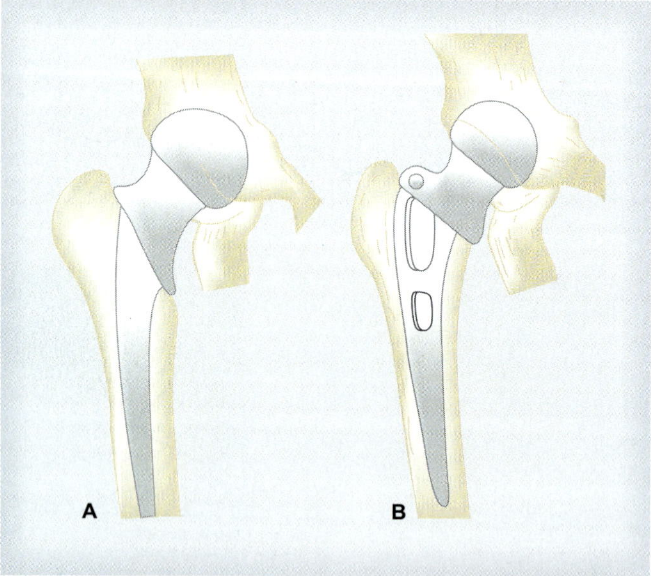

Fig. 17.14A and B: Showing types of hemireplacement arthroplasty (A) Thompson's prosthesis, and (B) Austin Moore's prosthesis

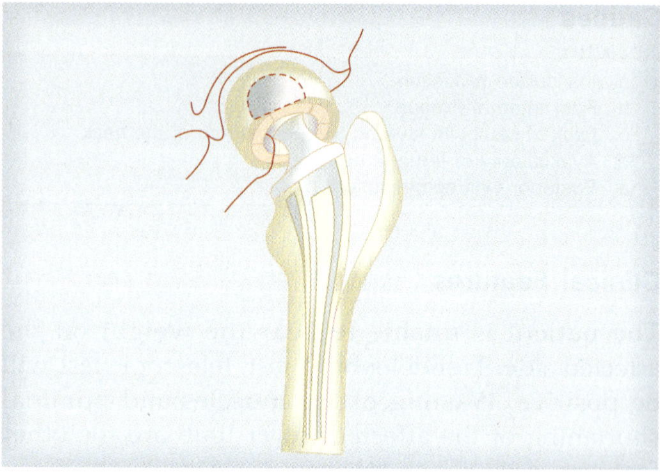

Fig. 17.15: Showing bipolar arthroplasty

2. Late segmental collapse—it is due to collapse of subchondral and articular cartilage that overlies infarcted bone. It occurs late.

Incidence

- Aseptic necrosis—66 to 84 per cent.
- Late segmental collapse—7 to 27 per cent.

In displaced femoral neck fracture, femoral head survival is dependent on vessels of ligamentum teres which is absent in one-third cases and subfoveal artery anastomosis which is variable and incomplete. All vessels within femoral neck and most of the retinacular vessels are disrupted in displaced fracture. Hence, survival of head depends on:

- Uninjured vascular supply
- Revascularisation.

Vascular injury occurs:

a. At the time of fracture commonly.

b. During reduction or internal fixation.

Hence, good anatomical reduction and stable internal fixation is required to preserve the remaining blood supply, which helps in revascularisation.

Investigations

Radiograph shows increased density of the femoral head, and this may take 6 months to 2 years to be seen on radiograph (see Fig. 17.11).

[2]**Austin Moore** (1957), USA. He described (a) Self-locking hip prosthesis. (b) A new low posterior approach for hip (Southern approach).
[3]**Frederick and Thompson** (1955), USA.

Bone scan Early and accurate determination of avascularity can be made, but it is not 100 per cent accurate.

Treatment

1. Symptomatic treatment like bedrest, nonsteroidal anti-inflammatory drugs (NSAIDs), etc.
2. Displacement or angulation osteotomy in early stages.
3. If acetabular cartilage is viable, hemireplacement prosthesis is preferred.
4. Total hip replacement if acetabular cartilage is not viable.

Fracture neck of femur at a glance

- An unsolved problem.
- Fracture of the elderly.
- Majority due to trivial fall.
- Garden's classification widely accepted.
- It is an orthopaedic emergency.
- Speed is the watchword in management.
- Early anatomical reduction, impaction, and rigid internal fixation is the aim of treatment.
- DHS and multiple cannulated cancellous screws is the currently accepted method of fixation.
- Nonunion and AVN are very common.

PROXIMAL FEMUR FRACTURES

SUBTROCHANTERIC FRACTURE (Fig. 17.16)

Subtrochanteric region is defined as an area between the lesser trochanter and a point 5 cm distal to it. Subtrochanteric fracture is a difficult fracture due to problems like malunion, delayed union, nonunion, shortening, angular deformity, rotational malalignment, etc. Two factors responsible for slow union are:

1. Fracture through the cortical bone.
2. Large biomechanical stress at the fracture site results in implant failure.

Mechanism of Injury

It is usually due to direct trauma due to RTA or fall and is common in young individuals.

It can be broadly considered under two headings:

Stable fracture Intact or possible to re-establish bone to bone contact of the medial and posterior femoral cortex anatomically.

Unstable fracture Posteromedial cortex apposition is not obtainable.

Classification

Fielding's Classification

This is based on distance at or below the lesser trochanter (Fig. 17.17).

Type I	Fracture at the level of the lesser trochanter
Type II	Fracture 1" below the lesser trochanter
Type III	Fracture 2" below the lesser trochanter

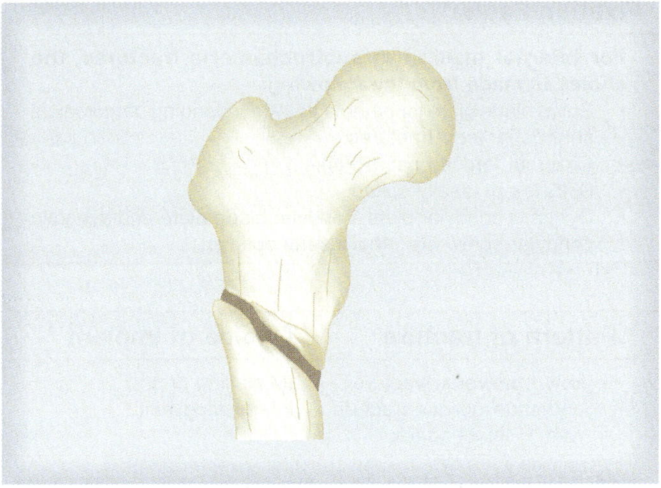

Fig. 17.16: Showing subtrochanteric fracture

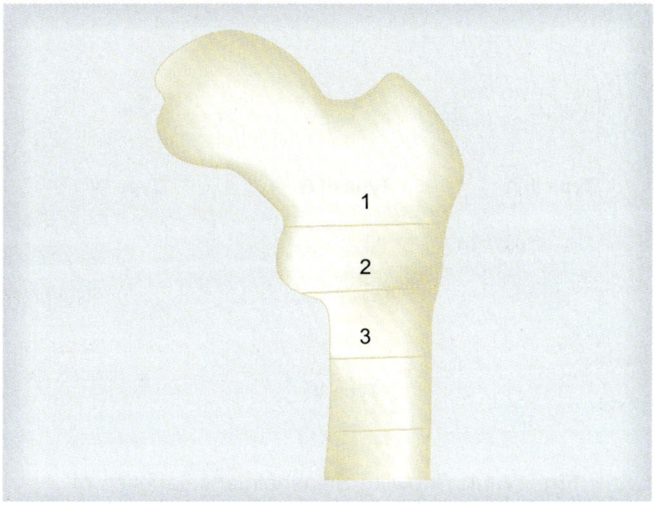

Fig. 17.17: Fielding's classification

Seinsheimer's Classification

This is based on the number of major fragments and the location and shape of fracture lines (Figs 17.18).

Type I	Undisplaced fracture
Type II	2 Part fracture
Type III	3 Part fracture A—Lesser trochanter is the 3rd fragment B—Butterfly fragment is the 3rd part
Type IV	4 Part fracture
Type V	Subtrochanteric comminuted fracture with intertrochanteric extension

Clinical Features

The patient presents with pain, swelling, shortening, external rotation deformity and other usual features of fractures.

Radiology

Radiograph helps to study the level and pattern of fracture and thereby plan the treatment (Fig. 17.19).

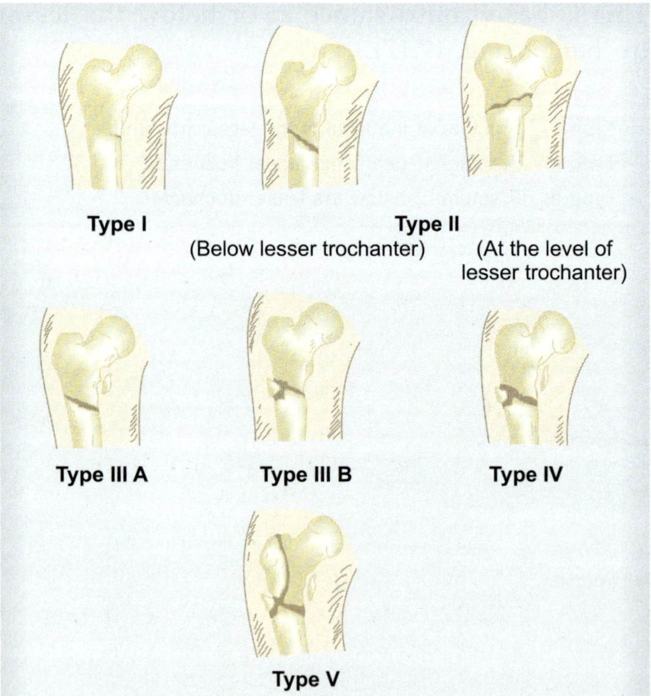

Fig. 17.18: Showing Seinsheimer's varieties of subtrochanteric fractures of femur

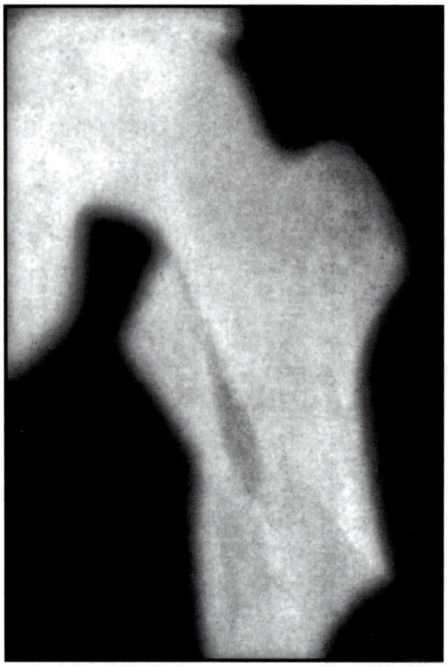

Fig. 17.19: Radiograph showing subtrochanteric fracture femur

Treatment

Conservative methods are advocated if the patient is young. In severely comminuted fractures, modified cast brace with pelvic band is used.

Surgery This is the preferred method of treatment in adults and ORIF is chosen for those fractures which can be made stable by closed or open reduction (Figs 17.20A and B). The choice of implants in different levels of the fracture is shown in the box.

Fixation Facts:

For internal fixation of subtrochanteric fractures, the choice is made from the following:
- Spiral blade plate for pathological or impending pathological subtrochanteric fractures.
- Proximal femoral nail (PFN).
- DHS is not ideally suited.
- Dynamic condylar plate, condylar blade plate and dynamic condylar screw are other useful options.

Pattern of fracture	Choice of implant
1. Low transverse fracture and short oblique fracture with 1" intact cortex	IM Nailing or a interlocking nail

Contd...

Contd...

Pattern of fracture	Choice of implant
2. In fracture above this level without trochanteric extension	Locking nail or Zickel nail
3. In fracture above this level with trochanteric extension	Sliding compression hip screw *Medial stability is obtained by either compression of inter-fragment or medial displacement or valgus reduction* *Fixed nail plate is not recommended. Bone graft is used.*

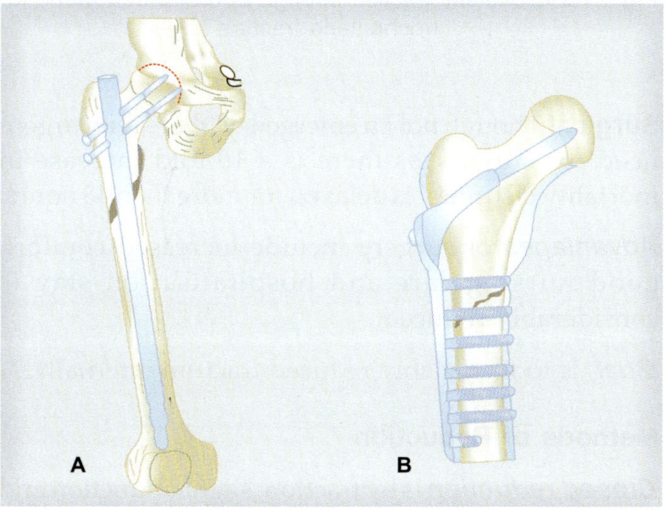

Figs 17.20A and B: Showing different methods of fixation for subtrochanteric fracture: (A) Interlocking nail, (B) Blade plate fixation

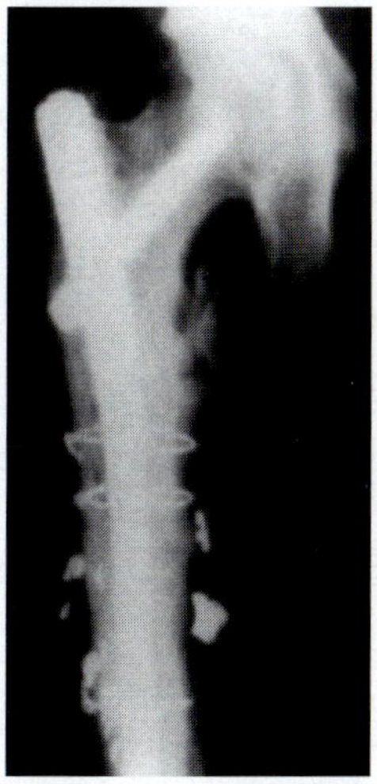

Fig. 17.21: Radiograph showing subtrochanteric fracture fixed with gamma nail

Recent trends in the fixation of pertrochanteric and subtrochanteric fractures: With the gamma nail, stable osteosynthesis of subtrochanteric and pertrochanteric fracture femur is obtained independently of the fracture classification (Fig. 17.21). Patients can be mobilised immediately with this method. However, care must be taken to avoid technical errors.

TROCHANTERIC FRACTURE

Salient Features

- An intertrochanteric fracture occurs along a line between greater trochanter and lesser trochanter with variable comminution.
- Totally extracapsular.
- Internal rotators of the hip remain attached to the distal fragment, short external rotators are attached to proximal head and neck. Hence, limb has to be kept in external rotation after reduction to align the distal fragment with proximal one.
- Cancellous bone, heals well by 8 to 12 weeks.
- Four times more common than intracapsular fracture.

Age Seen in elderly patients 10 to 12 years older than intracapsular fracture neck femur.

Sex More common in females (2.8 : 1).

Mechanism

Direct trauma as in RTA, fall, etc.

Indirect due to muscle pull, etc.

Clinical Features

The patient will have pain, marked shortening of the lower limb, complete external rotation deformity, swelling, ecchymosis and tenderness over the greater trochanter (Fig. 17.22).

Radiology (Fig. 17.23)

A true anteroposterior view in internal rotation and a lateral view help to study the fracture pattern.

Treatment

Conservative treatment There is 10 per cent mortality associated with conservative treatment.

Indications

1. Poor medical and surgical risk patients.
2. Terminally ill patients.
3. Very old patients.

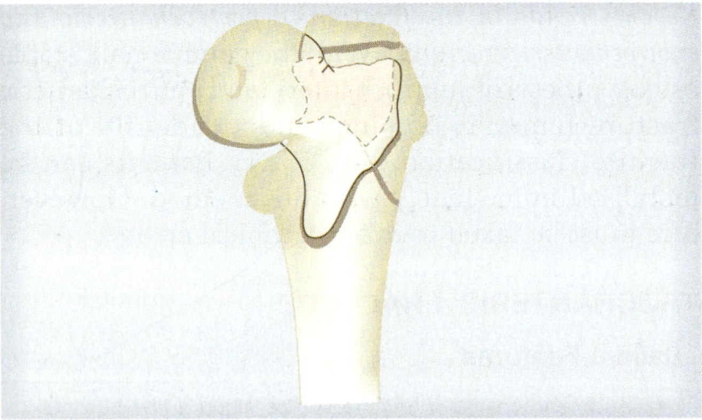

Fig. 17.22: Showing comminuted intertrochanteric fracture

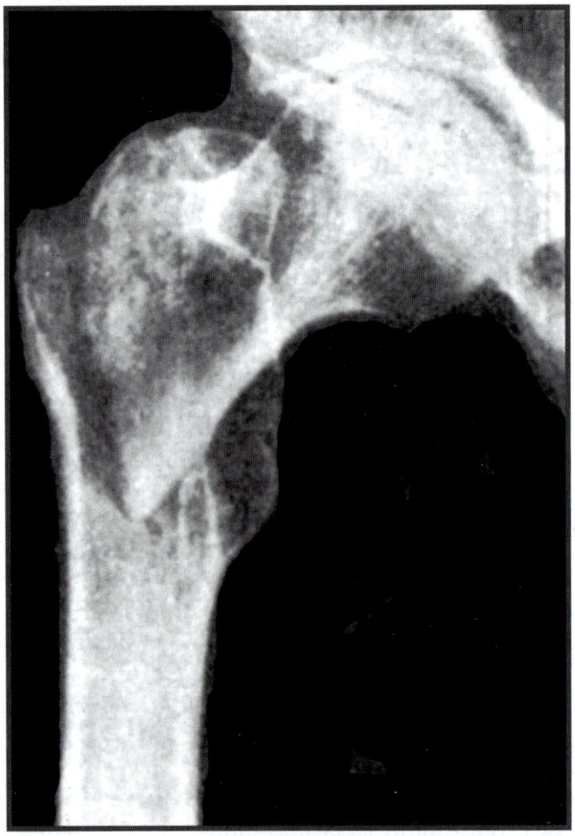

Fig. 17.23: Radiograph showing comminuted trochanteric fracture femur

Methods

1. Simple support with pillows
2. Buck's traction
3. Plaster spica
4. Skeletal traction through distal femur or tibia for 10 to 12 weeks (Fig. 17.24).

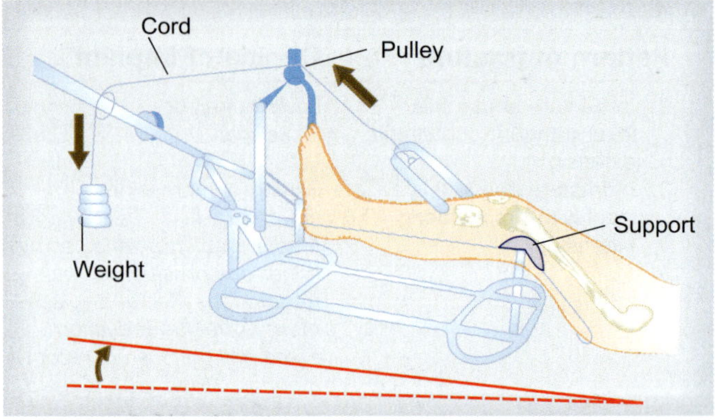

Fig. 17.24: Skeletal traction through Böhler-Braun frame for trochanteric fracture

Surgical Though not an emergency, there is an urgent need for surgery as there is a 10-fold increase in mortality if surgery is delayed for more than 48 hours.

Advantages of surgery include increased comfort, good nursing care and hospitalisation stay is considerably reduced.

Goal is to fix a stably reduced fracture internally.

Methods of Reduction

Closed reduction is by traction, slight abduction and external rotation. If reduction is not obtained, open reduction is done.

Open reduction

Indications

- Failed closed reduction.
- Large spike on proximal fragment with lesser trochanter intact.
- Reverse oblique fracture.

Choice of an Implant

Once stable reduction has been obtained either anatomically or by any one of the non-anatomical means (e.g. by osteotomy, etc.), implants are chosen. For stable fractures, choice of an implant does not matter. For unstable fractures, sliding hip screw (DHS) is most suitable and the 135 to 150° angle side plates are most commonly used. Placement of the DHS screw in the neck should be either central or posteroinferior.

Dynamic hip screw (DHS) allows to secure fixation of the fracture and permits controlled impaction at the fracture site thereby reducing the risk of fixation failure seen in rigid nail-plate like SP nail, etc. (Fig. 17.25A).

Comparison of fracture neck femur and trochanteric fracture

Features	*Fracture neck femur*	*Trochanteric fracture*
1. *Age*	Elderly	More elderly
2. *Incidence*	Common	Four times more common
3. *Blood loss*	Less	More
4. *Mechanism*	Trivial fall	Major trauma
5. *Signs:*		
Shortening	Minimum	Gross
Deformity	Minimum external rotation	Gross external rotation
Site of tenderness	Anterior hip joint line	Over greater trochanter
6. *Conservative treatment*	Not successful	Successful
7. *Surgery*	Absolutely indicated	Indicated for early mobilisation
8. *Complications*		
Nonunion	Very common	Rare (1%)
Malunion	Unheard	Very common

What is new in the treatment of trochanteric fractures?
Proximal femoral nails (PFN) are emerging as an effective internal fixation device.

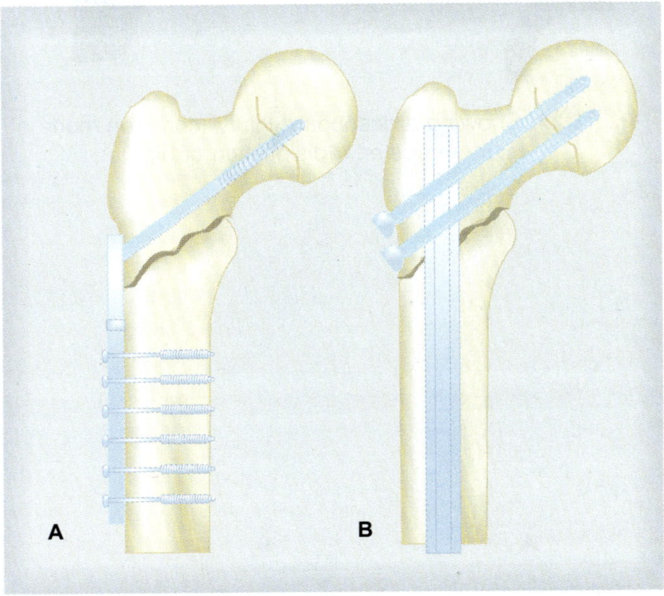

Fig. 17.25: Internal fixation methods for trochanteric fractures (A) DHS, (B) PFN

Complications

Due to the cancellous nature of bone, these fractures unite well unlike fracture neck femur but malunion is quite common. Coxa vara, nonunion is less than 2 per cent (rare) and traumatic osteoarthritis are also seen. These fractures also carry a higher incidence of mortality (more than 10%). Avascular necrosis is very rare (0.8%).

Quick Facts:

In intertrochanteric fracture the success of fracture implant fixation depends upon:

1. Degree of osteoporosis (Singh's index).
2. Fracture pattern.
3. Accurate reduction.
4. Implant designs.
5. Placement of the implant.

Vital Facts:

Treatment of Proximal Femoral Fractures

- Stable trochanteric fractures are fixed with DHS
- Unstable trochanteric fractures cannot be fixed with DHS as it cuts through due to comminution. Hence, the choice of implants in these situations are:
  a. Medoff plate or trochanteric stabilisation plate (TSP, AO).
  b. Condylocephalic nails: These could be proximal femoral nails, Ender's nail or Gamma nail.
  c. 95° condylar blade plate or dynamic condylar screw.
  d. Proximal femoral nails (PFN) (Fig. 17.25B).

In comminuted unstable trochanteric fractures, IM nails are better suited to resist the deforming muscle forces. Hence, proximal femoral nailing is superior to DHS.

Advantages of PFN

- It can be inserted quickly
- Less blood loss
- Early ambulation
- Sliding and limb shortening is less
- It is more successful in reverse oblique fractures.

Features of PFN

- Standard length is 24 cm.
- Long PFN is available in >36 cm length (for low subtrochanteric fractures or two level fractures).
- Proximal wide portion: Here a long screw and hip pin can pass through the head and neck.
- Distal part has a dynamic and static taking holes.

Problems with PFN

- Entry point has to be chosen carefully (preferably pyriformis fossa).
- Excessively curved femur is a central indication.
- Postoperative thigh pain is seen
- It cannot be used if fracture line extends into pyriformis fossa (Here DCS or condylar blade plate is better).

DISLOCATION OF THE HIP JOINT

Dislocation and fracture dislocation of the hip are severe injuries and are due to major forces. These are associated with the disruption of the head-acetabular relations (broken Shenton's line), significant soft tissue damage, etc. If associated with fractures (seen in 50%), small osseous or cartilaginous fragments often remain in the joint space and prevent reduction. These injuries are usually associated with significant injuries elsewhere. *Dislocation and fracture dislocation of the hip are orthopaedic emergencies and are easily missed when there is associated ipsilateral fractures of the femur.*

The dislocations are labelled as anterior, posterior, and central depending upon the relationship of the femoral head to the acetabulum (Figs 17.26A to C). A comparative study of the dislocation is presented (Table 17.1) for easy understanding and better remembrance.

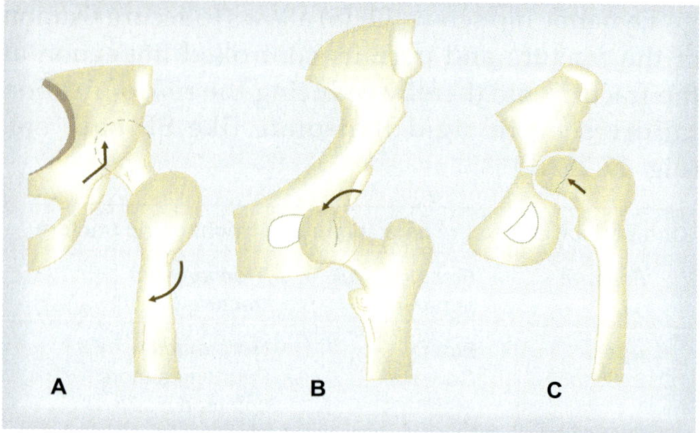

Figs 17.26A to C: Types of hip dislocation (A) Posterior dislocation of hip, (B) anterior dislocation of hip, and (C) central fracture dislocation of hip

POSTERIOR DISLOCATION OF HIP JOINT

It is an interesting observation that if anterior dislocation is common in shoulder joint, it is the posterior dislocation, that is common in the hip joint. Traumatic posterior dislocation is usually a car dashboard injury (Fig. 17.27) or is due to fall of weight on the back of a stooping miner.

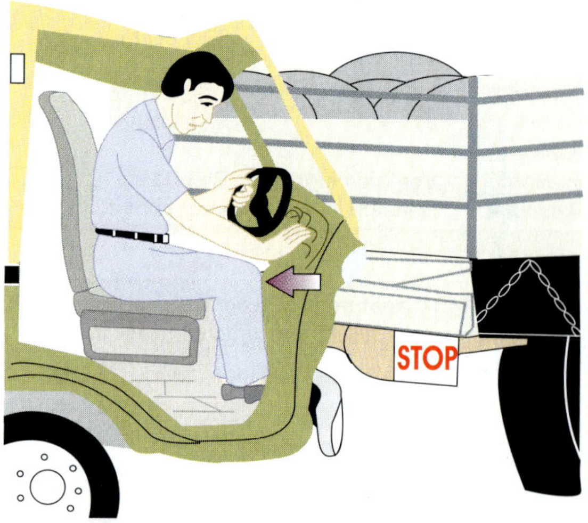

Fig. 17.27: Showing a dashboard injury (common mode of injury in posterior dislocation of hip)

Mechanism of Injury

It is usually due to a backward directed force along the line of femur in a flexed hip. If the femur is more adducted at the time of impact, pure dislocation results and if the femur is slightly abducted, fracture dislocation results.

Clinical Features

There is usually history of trauma and the patient has a flexion, adduction and medial rotation deformity of the affected limb (Figs 17.28A and B). There is marked shortening and gross restriction of all hip movements. Head of the femur is felt as a hard mass in the gluteal region and it moves along with the femur. There could be features of sciatic nerve palsy.

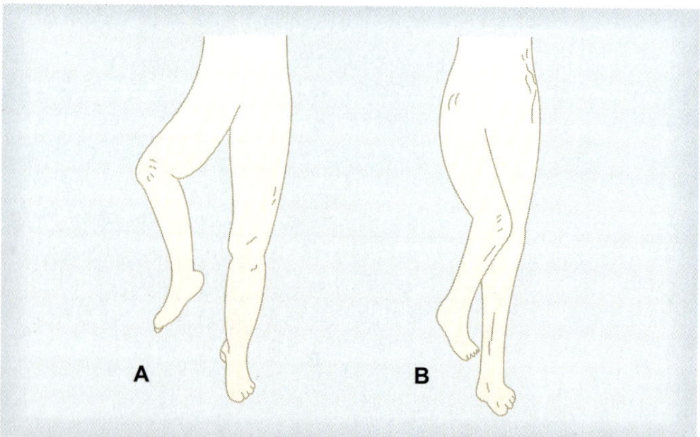

Figs 17.28A and B: Appearance of classical deformities in dislocation hip: (A) anterior, and (B) posterior

Investigations

Radiography of the pelvis showing both the hip joints is usually preferred. Lateral view and oblique views

Table 17.1: Comparative features of dislocations of hip

	Posterior dislocation	*Anterior dislocation*	*Central dislocation*
1. **Incidence**	Common (70%)	10–15%	Rare
2. **Mechanism of injury**	• Dashboard injury as in RTA • Flexed knee + neutral adduction results in simple dislocation. • Flexed knee + slight abduction results in fracture dislocation	• Dashboard injury with thigh abducted • Fall from height • Blow to the back in squatted position	• Due to direct blow over trochanter • Common in patients with epilepsy, convulsions, etc.
3. **Classification**	*Thompson and Epstein* • *Type I* with or without minor fracture • *Type II* with a large single fracture of rim acetabulum • *Type III* comminution of acetabular rim with or without major fragment. • *Type IV* with fracture of femoral head	*Type I* (superior) • *IA* No fracture • *IB* Associated head fracture • *IC* Associated fracture acetabulum *Type II* (inferior) • *IIA* No fracture • *IIB* Associated head fracture • *IIC* Associated fracture acetabulum	*Judet's* Dislocation associated with • Undisplaced fracture • Inner wall fracture of acetabulum • Superior rim fracture of acetabulum • Bursting fracture of acetabulum
4. **Clinical features**	• Limb shortening • Flexion/add/IR deformity • Thigh rests on the contralateral limb • Head felt in the gluteal region. • Vascular sign-ve (Narath). • Movements of hip ↓ • Injury to sciatic nerve	*Superior type* flexion + abd + external rotation deformity *Inferior type* hip is extended and externally rotated • Head felt superiorly or inferiorly • Vascular sign (Narath) +ve • Injury to femoral nerve artery or vein	• No limb shortening • Limb is neutral in position • Bruising over the greater trochanter • Per rectal examination reveals head of femur
5. **Treatment**	*4 Methods of Closed Reduction* 1. *Stimson's gravity method* least traumatic but associated injuries prevent prone positioning 2. *Allis* Traction is given in line of deformity 3. *Bigelow's method* reduction is done by causing the opposite methods of ext/abd/ER 4. *Classical Watson-Jones method* Limb is brought to the neutral position first then longitudinal traction in the line of femur is given.	1. *Stimson's gravity method* 2. *Allis method* 3. *Reverse Bigelow's method* Here position of hip is flexion and adduction 4. *Classical method* is as described for posterior dislocation	Reduction is attempted through skeletal traction on greater trochanter in line of the neck of femur. If it fails, open reduction is indicated.
6. **Complications**	*Early* • Sciatic nerve palsy • Irreducible fracture dislocation • Missed knee injuries • Recurrent dislocations *Late* • Myositis ossificans • Avascular necrosis of bone • Post-traumatic arthritis • Unreduced posterior dislocation	*Early* • Neurovascular injuries • Femoral artery, vein, nerve injury • Irreducibility *Late* • Post-traumatic osteoarthritis • Aseptic necrosis • Recurrent dislocation	*I Early* • Sciatic nerve palsy • Superior gluteal artery injury • Bowel obstruction • Thrombophlebitis • Infection • Recurrent dislocation *II Late* • Post-traumatic arthritis • AVN • Nonunion • Myositis ossificans

of the affected joint gives clue to the fractures of the posterior acetabular rim (Fig. 17.29). CT scan and MRI study of the hip joint is more reliable in assessing the acetabular fractures.

Treatment

In order to prevent early onset of secondary osteoarthritis and also to reduce pain, immediate reduction of the hip has to be carried out under general anaesthesia.

Techniques of Reduction

There are various methods of reduction of the hip joint (Table 17.1), but the most commonly employed method is the "classical method" (*see* Fig. 17.33). In this method the patient is supine and is on the floor

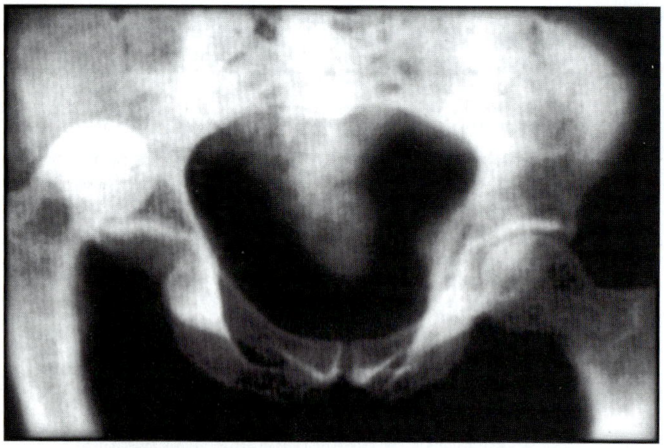

Fig. 17.29: Radiograph showing posterior dislocation of hip

under general anaesthesia. The hip is flexed to 90° and with an assistant stabilising the pelvis, a longitudinal traction is given in the line of femur. If reduction is achieved a loud click sound is heard. Immediately after the reduction tests for the stability of hip joint is done by moving it around in all directions. In fracture dislocations the hip joint redislocates again.

Note: To clinically assess the stability after reduction, flex the hip to 90° and apply a posterior force. If the hip remains reduced, it is considered stable.

After Treatment After reduction, the patient is put on a skin traction or immobilised in a Thomas splint for 3 weeks. Full weight bearing is permitted after 6 weeks.

Indications for open reduction The following are some of the important indications for open reduction:

1. Failure of close reduction: This could be due to obstruction by bony fragments or by soft tissues like acetabular labrum and capsule or locking of fracture surfaces or due to buttonholing of femoral head through the capsule.
2. Instability after reduction is usually due to large posterior chunk of acetabulum.
3. Sciatic nerve palsy, etc.

Complications

Myositis ossificans (2%) It is seen commonly in posterior dislocation with head injury and is unknown in simple posterior dislocation. It may be seen after reduction also. It can be prevented by avoiding repeated manipulation, early immobilisation and by immobilising for 6 weeks in hip spica.

Sciatic nerve injury Incidence of this injury is 10 to 13 per cent. It is 3 times more common in fracture dislocation than simple dislocation (Fig. 17.30). Usually it is a neuropraxia and the peroneal division is commonly affected. It may be due to stretch of the nerve or may be due to impalement between the fracture fragments. If it is associated with acetabular fracture the nerve should be explored. Prognosis is variable.

Traumatic osteoarthritis due to avascular necrosis (35%) For head of the femur major blood supply enters from the capsule and to a lesser extent through the ligamentum teres. If both these sources are damaged, it gradually leads to AVN followed by osteoarthritis of the hip joint. Incidence is about 10 per cent and the treatment has already been discussed *(ref. p. 197)*.

Recurrent dislocation This is due to fracture acetabulum and sometimes due to rent in the capsule and gluteus minimus. This requires exploration and fixing of the acetabular fragments with screws.

Unreduced dislocation This is common in Asian patients due to ignorance and illiteracy. Manupulative reduction is tried first. If it is unsuccessful, operative reduction is attempted. Arthrodesis if acceptable is the best treatment. Total hip replacement is usually not preferred because the patient is usually young. In hips where there is useful range of painless movements corrective osteotomy is done. In painful stiff joints, girdlestone excision is preferred.

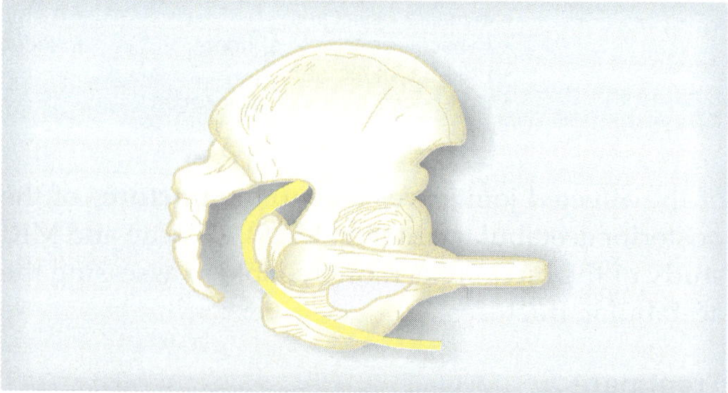

Fig. 17.30: Showing injury to sciatic nerve due to posterior dislocation of hip hoint

Irreducible dislocation (31%) This may be due to bony (acetabular fragments, femoral head, etc.) or soft tissue (acetabular labrum, etc.) obstruction. It may also be due to coma, ipsilateral fracture femur or dislocation of opposite hip. It may require exploration and open reduction.

Hip dislocation with associated acetabular fracture (Figs 17.31 and 17.32).

- It is a severe injury.
- Prompt initial reduction is a must.
- This has to be followed by acetabular fracture reconstruction after 8 to 10 days.
- Failure of reduction and neurologic impairment requires immediate open reduction and internal fixation.
- AVN, secondary OA, heterotropic calcification are the important complications.

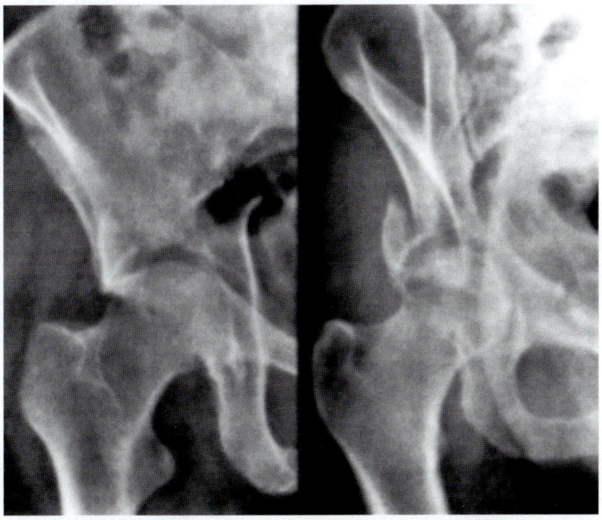

Fig. 17.31: Radiographs showing acetabular fractures

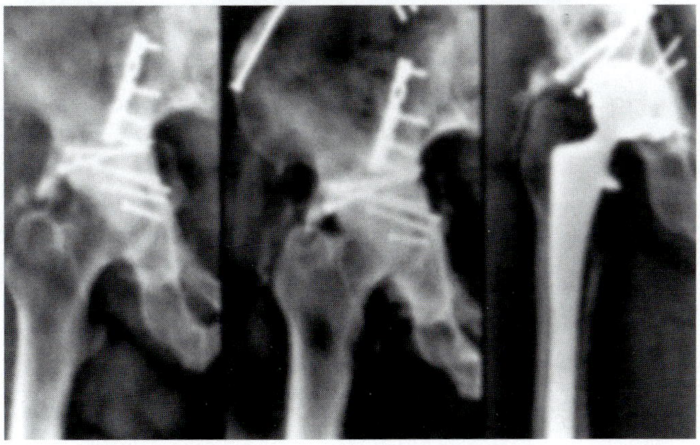

Fig. 17.32: Radiographs showing fixation of acetabular fractures

Differential Diagnosis

Posterior dislocation of hip has to be differentiated from anterior and central dislocations of hip (*see* Table 17.1).

Methods of Reduction of Hip Joint:

Classical Watson Jones method This technique is useful in both anterior and posterior dislocation of the hip. Irrespective of the type of dislocation, the limb is first brought to the neutral position. In this position, the head of the femur lies posterior to the acetabulum even in anterior dislocation. Now with an assistant steadying the pelvis, the head of the femur is reduced into the acetabulum by applying a longitudinal traction in the long axis of the femur. It is simple and effective when compared to Bigelow's method (Fig. 17.33).

The story of a student who was smarter than his teacher— **Jacob Bigelow** when working as a house surgeon in the casualty in one of the hospitals in the UK encountered a case of posterior dislocation of hip. A call was officially sent to the professor. Meanwhile, Bigelow carried out the reduction by his own technique. Expecting a congratulatory note from his professor, he was dismayed when he was severely reprimanded by his professor for having carried out the reduction before he could attend the case! Bigelow promptly redislocated the hip and sent the case back to his professor who could not reduce the dislocation in spite of several attempts! Bigelow was summoned and was asked to reduce the dislocation again which he promptly obliged! This time he received a bouquet and not the brickbat from his professor. *His technique consisted of creating the opposite movements of extension, abduction and external rotation for reducing post dislocation of the hip and vice versa for anterior dislocation.* However, his method is now replaced by a simpler classical Watson Jones method.

Note: Posterior dislocation of hip should be reduced early to prevent post-traumatic osteonecrosis and relieve compression on the sciatic nerve.

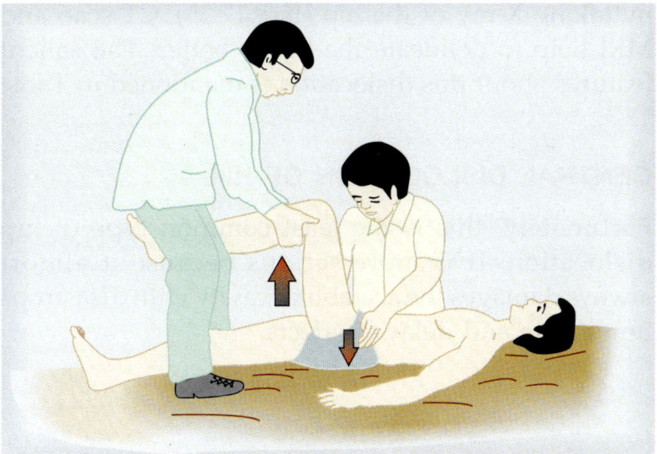

Fig. 17.33: Classical Watson Jones technique for reduction of hip dislocation

Section 2

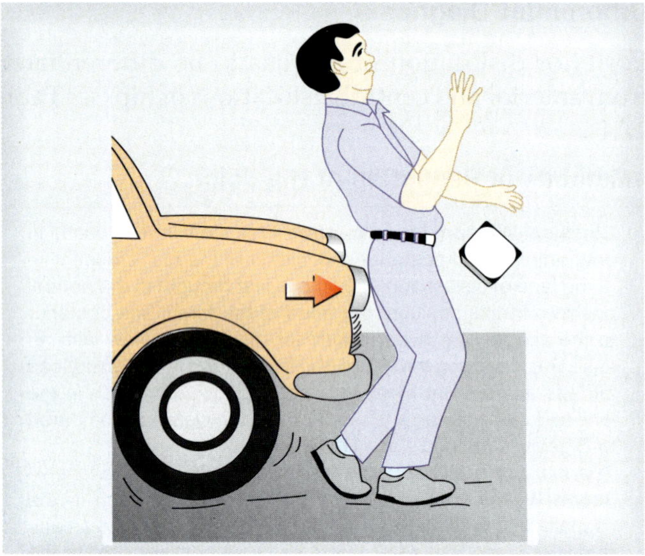

Fig. 17.34: Showing common mechanism of anterior dislocation of hip

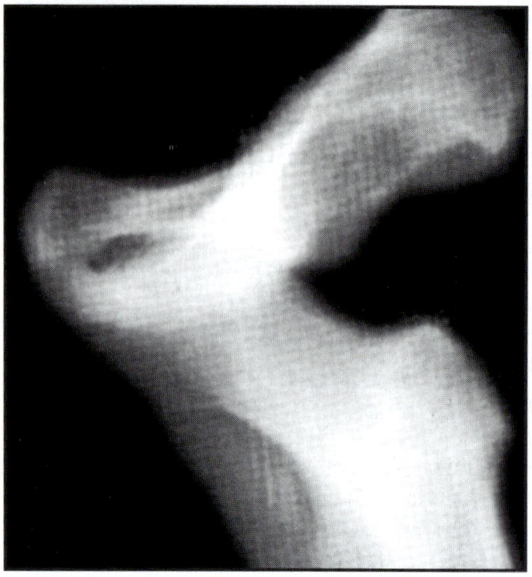

Fig. 17.35: Radiograph showing anterior dislocation of hip

Vital Facts about

Traumatic Hip Dislocation in Adults

In these cases reduction of the dislocation should be prompt to prevent AVN of the head of femur. Though there are various methods to reduce the dislocation, the superiority of one technique over the other has not been shown in literature and the choice must be tailored to the condition of the patient. However, they may be associated with multiple injuries that may limit the options available for initial treatment.

ANTERIOR DISLOCATION OF HIP

This is relatively uncommon and may be due to direct blow from the back (Fig. 17.34). It can be diagnosed by taking X-ray of the hip (Fig. 17.35). CT scan and MRI help to delineate the injury better. The salient features about this dislocation is mentioned in Table 17.1.

CENTRAL DISLOCATION OF HIP

Fortunately, this is the least common type of hip dislocation. It is more serious because it almost always damages the acetabular cavity with disastrous immediate and delayed effects.

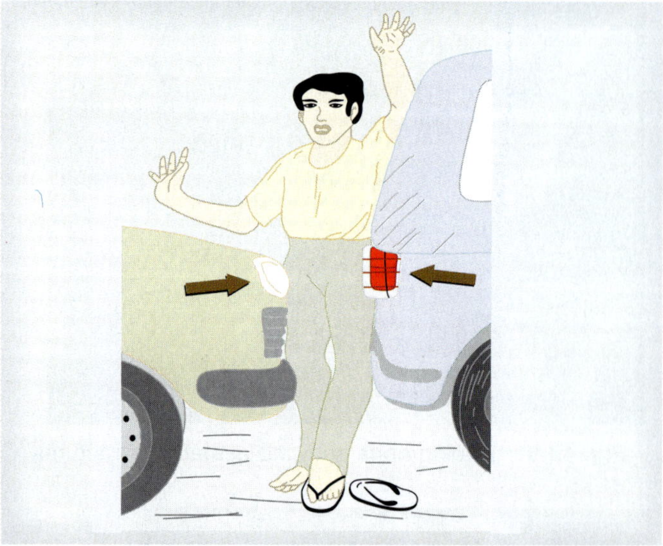

Fig. 17.36: Showing common mechanism of central dislocation of hip joint

It is usually due to direct blow over the trochanter (Fig. 17.36). See Table 17.1 for the features of this dislocation.

18

Fracture Femur

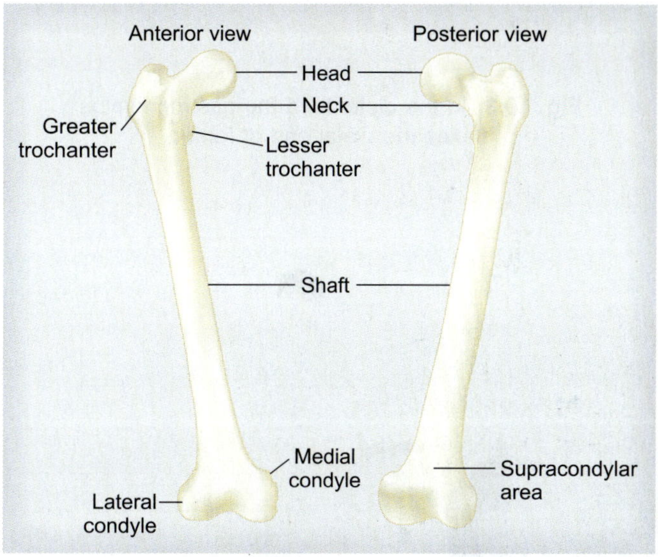

Fig. 18.1: Bony anatomy of femur

SALIENT FEATURES ABOUT FEMUR (Fig. 18.1)

FEMUR: A MUST KNOW FACTS

- It is the longest and the strongest bone in the body.
- It is the heaviest bone.
- A person's height is four times the length of femur.
- It has three parts: proximal end, distal end and shaft.
- The shaft extends from the level of the lesser trochanter to the flare of the condyles.
- The shaft is slightly bowed anteriorly and is narrowest at the midshaft.
- The cross-section is circular.
- Linea aspera is the thick ridge of bone situated mid-posterior.
- Muscle forces (Fig. 18.2) acting on the femur at different sites.

  Proximal third Iliopsoas flex, abductors abduct and external rotators cause abduction and external rotation of proximal fragment, while adductors adduct the distal fragment.

  Middle third There is shortening and adduction.

  Distal third This is flexed due to the action of gastrocnemius muscle (Fig. 18.3).

  The blood supply to the shaft of femur is rich and adequate and thus the fracture in this area usually unites well.

  The above muscular forces should be taken into consideration while planning the treatment for fracture shaft femur.

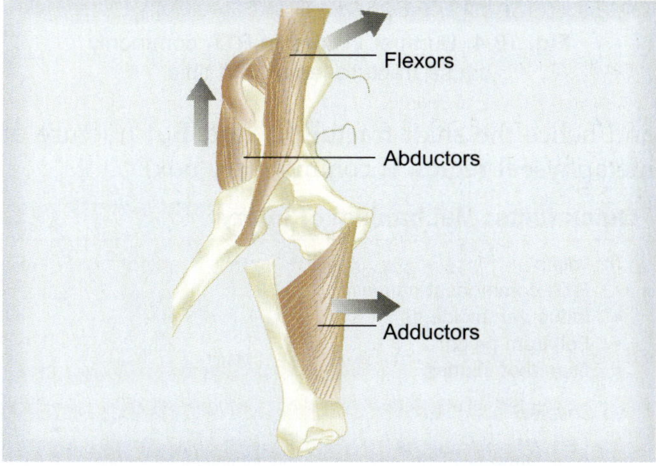

Fig. 18.2: Showing muscle forces acting across the shaft of femur

FRACTURE SHAFT FEMUR

Fracture shaft femur is a serious injury and is usually due to severe violence. It may be associated with severe blood loss (up to 1,500 ml), multiple fractures and multisystem injuries, but heavy musculature, however, provides unlimited blood supply and thus the fracture heals well.

Mechanism of Injury

Usually, it is due to major violence, and is common in young adults because the strong metaphyseal areas transmit the forces to the shaft causing fracture (Fig. 18.4). In old age, the metaphyseal areas are brittle

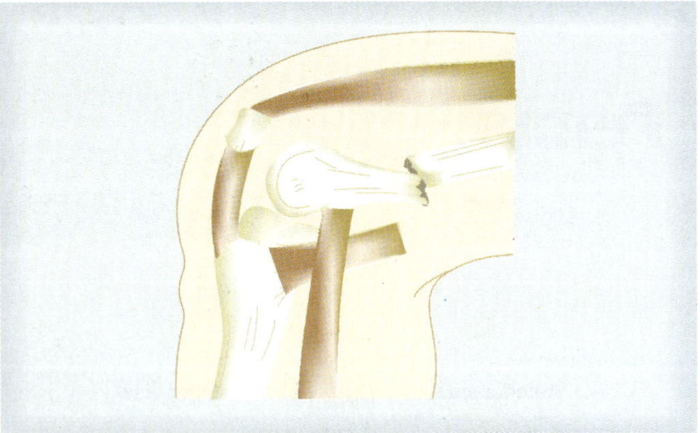

Fig. 18.3: In the distal third the gastrocnemius flexes the distal end of femur

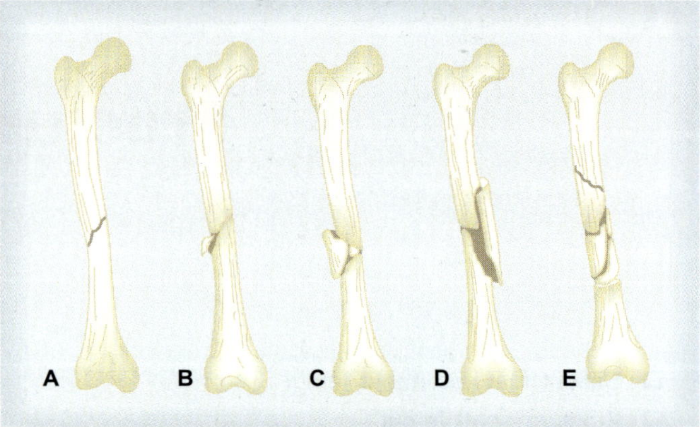

Figs 18.5A to E: Showing varieties of femoral shaft fractures (A and B—Simple fracture, C—Wedge fracture, D—Butterfly fracture, E—Comminution)

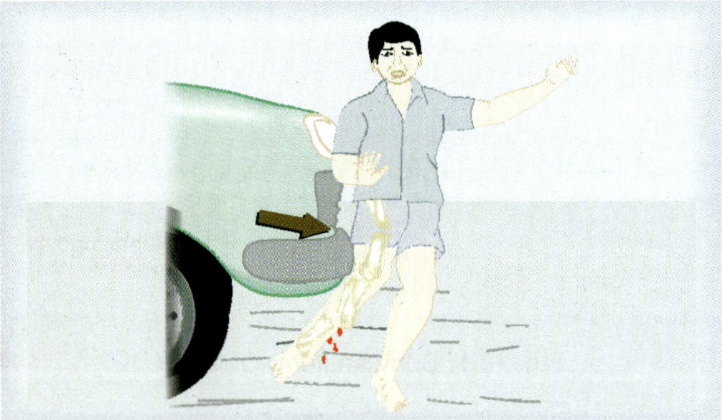

Fig. 18.4: Bumper injuries in RTA commonly cause fracture femur and tibia

and hence the shaft fracture is rare, but fracture of metaphyseal region is common (see box).

Quick facts: Mechanism of Injury

In Adults
- RTA commonest cause
- Industrial accidents
- Fall from height
- Gun shot injuries

In Children
- Fall
- Birth injuries

Male-female ratio = 3 : 1
Average age of occurrence = 25–35 years

Classification of Femoral Fractures (Figs 18.5A to E)

- Femoral fractures could be in the proximal, midshaft or distal fragments.
- Each of the above fractures could be tranverse, oblique, spiral, segmental or comminuted.
- Based on the degree of comminution, Winquist and Hansen have described four types:
  Type I: None or significant comminution
  Type II: <50 per cent comminution
  Type III: 50-100 per cent comminution of the cortex
  Type IV: No contact between major fragments.
- AO/ASIF classification
  Type A: Simple fracture (tranverse/oblique/spiral/minimal comminution)
  Type B: Wedge fractures and greater than one fracture line
  Type C: Extensive comminution

Clinical Features

Apart from all the features of fractures, there could be shortening of the lower limb and complete external rotation deformity such that the lateral border of the foot touches the bed. Since the fracture femur is usually due to major violence, the patient may also present with features of shock, like unconsciousness, pallor, cold nose, tachycardia, cold and clammy skin, hypotension, etc.

Radiography

Routine anteroposterior and lateral views (Fig. 18.6) of the femur suffice, but care should be taken to include the neighbouring joints (hip and knee) to rule out the possibilities of injuries to these joints.

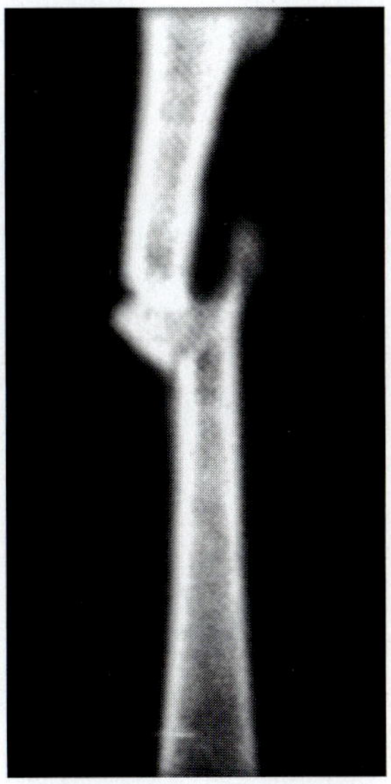

Fig. 18.6: Radiograph showing comminuted fracture shaft femur

Management

General principles

1. Almost 100 per cent union occurs whether fracture is treated by closed or open reduction methods.
2. By internal fixation, hospital stay is reduced.
3. Simpler the fracture, more likely to be treated by open reduction and internal fixation (ORIF).
4. More comminuted the fracture, less likely is the internal fixation attempted. For severely comminuted fracture and extensive soft tissue damage, traction is the safest. Interlocking nailing is the other popular alternative.

Treatment Methods

Children It is mainly conservative in children.

0 to 2 years	—	Plaster spica in human position[1] or modified Bryant's or Gallow's traction (Fig. 18.7).
2 to 10 years	—	Most femoral fractures are seen in this age group. Here split Russel traction (Fig. 18.8) is more useful.
10 to 15 years	—	90 to 90° Femoral skeletal traction or hip spica or both (Fig. 18.9).
More than 15 years	—	Treatment is as in adults.

Note: [1]Human position is 90° of flexion and 45° of external rotation at the hip.

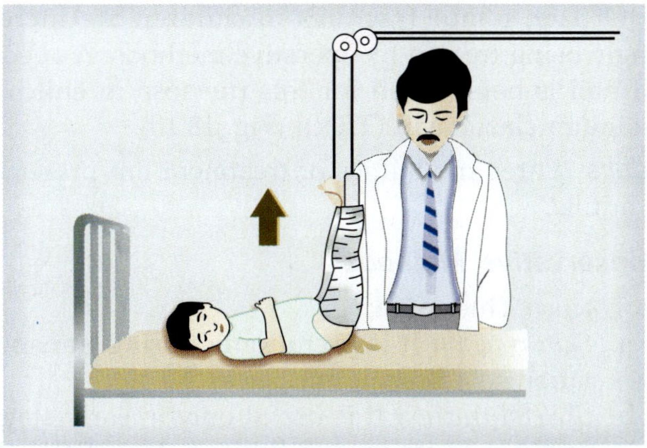

Fig. 18.7: Showing Gallow's traction in children (< 2 years of age)

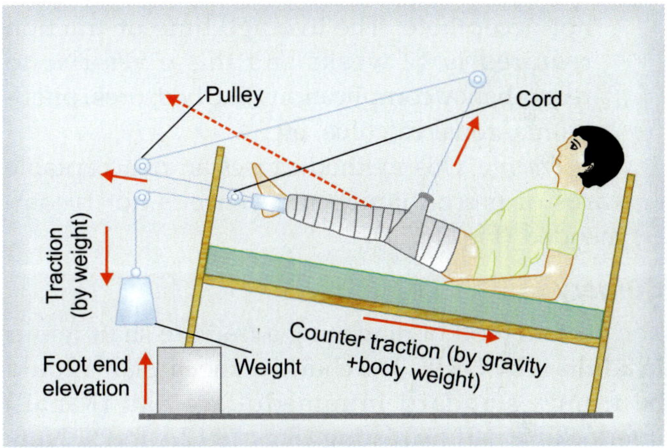

Fig. 18.8: Russel traction

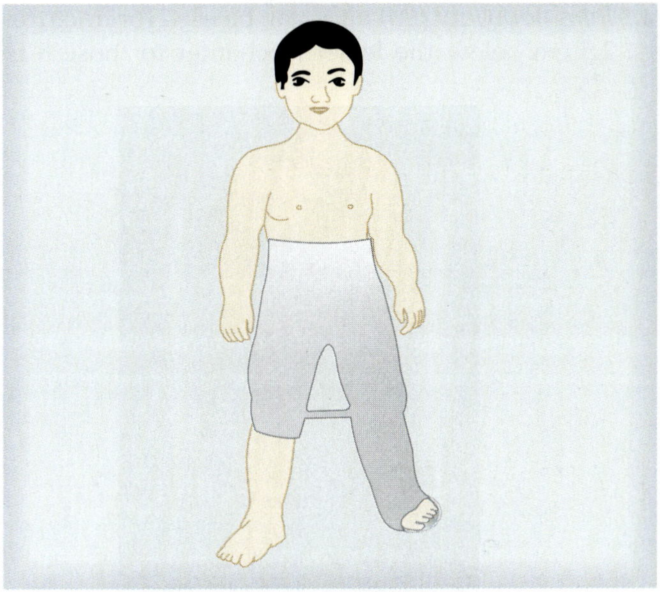

Fig. 18.9: Treatment of fracture shaft femur in children by hip spica

Of late, femur fractures in children are increasingly being treated by operative methods. A special IM nail is being used for this purpose in children [titanium elastic nail (TEN)] (Fig. 18.10).

Adults Three modalities of treatment are preferred in adults.

Conservative Methods

1. *Traction* This could be:
   a. *Skin traction* It is useful only during transportation as a first aid measure.
   b. *Skeletal traction* It is useful only in early stages and hence its role is limited. However, the patient treated in traction shows 100 per cent union, but it causes shortening, and hence is not acceptable. The average time of traction required is 12 weeks and this gives rise to recumbency complications like bedsores, pneumonia, renal calculus, etc.
2. *Cast bracing* This method causes an unacceptable varus of more than 8° and hence is not recommended (Fig. 18.11).

Surgery

The best method of managing a fracture shaft femur in adults is by ORIF. The choice of the implants could be from a standard intramedullary nail (K-nail) interlocking nail or plating (Figs 18.12A to C). Now let us try to know about these in greater detail:

a. *Intramedullary (IM) nails* can be used for fractures 2.5 cm below the lesser trochanter to those 8 to 10 cm above the knee joint. It can be used in simple or comminuted fractures. It can be done immediately or delayed. Infection and nonunion is rare (0.8%).

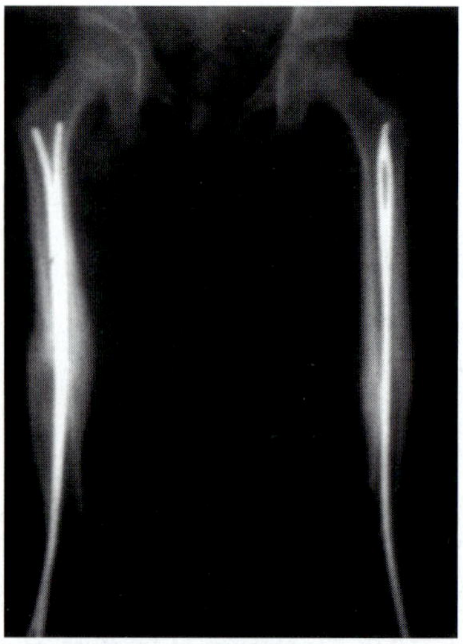

Fig. 18.10: Radiograph showing femur fracture in children treated with titanium elastic nails (TENS)

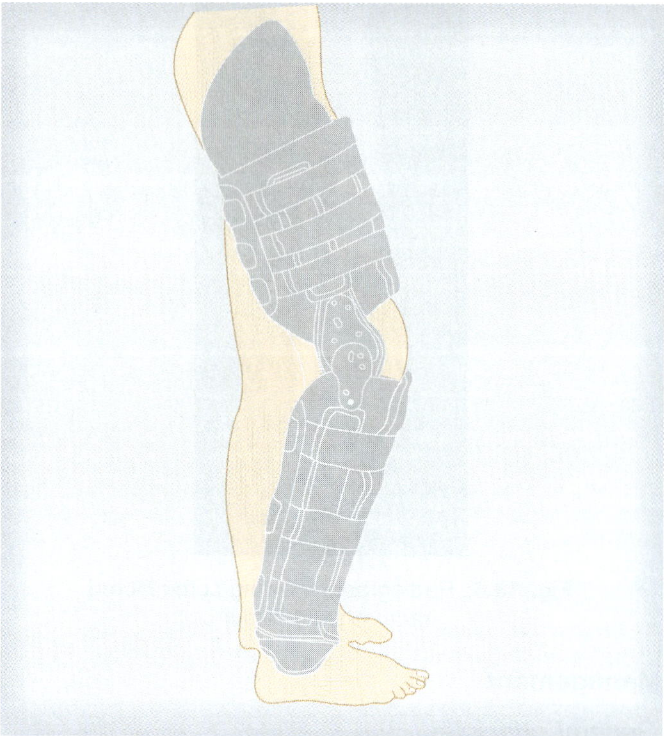

Fig. 18.11: Showing functional cast brace

Types of nails in common usage for fixing fracture shaft femur:

1. *Standard IM nails (Küntscher's nail)*—the ideal indication for this nail is the fracture shaft femur in adults at the level of isthmus.
   Isthmus is the portion of the femoral shaft. It is the junction between the upper and middle one-third and is the narrowest portion of the shaft.
2. *Interlocking nails (Gross-Kempf nail)* These extend the indications of standard IM nail and can be used in the following situations where IM nail is less successful:
   a. Comminuted fractures
   b. Segmental fractures
   c. Proximal and distal fractures
   d. Nonunion, etc.
3. *Flexible medullary nails* like Ender's nail, which is usually passed from below upwards through the distal femur.

What is new in femoral nails?

- UFN: Unreamed femoral nail
- CFN: Cannulated femoral nail
- PFN: Proximal femoral nail
- DEN: Distal femoral nail
- TEN: Titanium elastic nail used in children

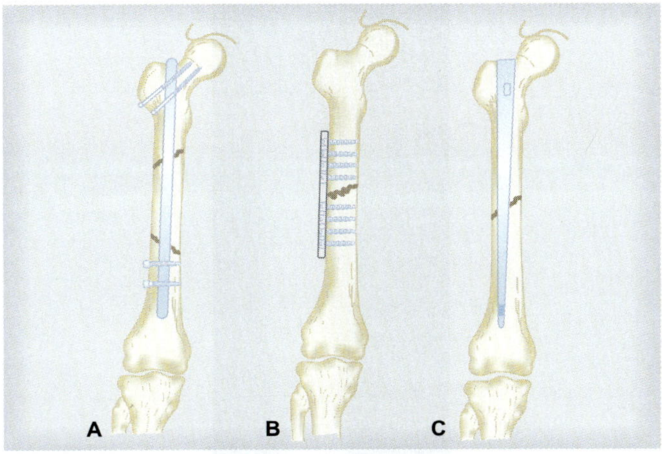

Figs 18.12A to C: Methods of internal fixation for fracture shaft femur: (A) Interlocking nail, (B) DCP plate and screws, and (C) Küntscher's intermedullary nails

Methods of Intramedullary Nailing

Closed method This is the best method, but technically difficult as it requires sophisticated equipment like C-arm, instrumentation, etc.

Open method It allows direct visualisation of fracture site and hence fracture can be anatomically fixed. But the chances of infection are quite high with this technique.

Cardinal Points in IM Nailing Technique

- Full set of nail size and length should be available before surgery.
- K-nails are available in 8 diameters from 8 to 15 mm. Average diameter is 11 to 12 mm.
- Ream the canal by reamers with progressively increasing size.
- Select the nail diameter equal or 1 size more of the reamer to provide a snug fit.
- The open slot of the K-nail is placed anterolaterally on the convex (tension) side of the femur. This helps convert the tensile force into compressive force at the fracture site.
- The eye of the nail should face posteromedially so that extraction can easily be made at a later date.
- The upper end of the nail should be less than 2.5 cm above the trochanter and the distal end should extend to the level of the proximal pole of the patella.
- The clover shape of the K-nail helps prevent rotation in the canal.

Intramedullary nail can be inserted either through the open or closed techniques. A comparative study is presented in Table 18.1.

Technique of Intramedullary Nailing (Open Method) (Küntscher's Nail)

Technique After anaesthesia (preferably spinal), strong traction is exerted on the affected limb to reduce the fracture and the patient is firmly fastened to the operating table. The limb is painted and draped. Through a lateral or posterolateral approach, the fracture is exposed. By using a suitable sized medullary reamers, the proximal and distal fragments are reamed. Appropriate sized snugly fitting Küntscher's nail is chosen and driven in a retrograde fashion through the proximal fragment till it emerges into the subcutaneous tissue through the greater trochanter. The fracture is now reduced under direct vision and the nail is driven down into the distal fragment. The wound is closed in layers over a drain.

Closed IM Nail Technique

In this, the patient is securely fixed to a fracture table (Fig. 18.13). Under C-arm control, a suitable sized IM nail is passed through the trochanter into the proximal fragment and driven down into the distal fragment after reducing the fracture and reaming it.

Table 18.1: Open and closed techniques compared

S.N	*Features*	*Open technique*	*Closed technique*
1.	Equipment required	Less expensive	More expensive
2.	Fracture table	Not a must	Always required
3.	C-arm	Not required	Required
4.	Anatomic reduction	Easier to obtain	Difficult to obtain
5.	Method of nailing	Retrograde	Antegrade
6.	Blood loss	More	Less
7.	Direct visualisation of fracture site	Possible	Not possible
8.	Fracture haematoma	Lost	Preserved
9.	Exposure time	More	Nil
10.	Skin scar	More	Less
11.	Infection rate	High	Less
12.	Tissue trauma	More	Less
13.	Technique	Simple	Demanding
14.	Morbidity	More	Less

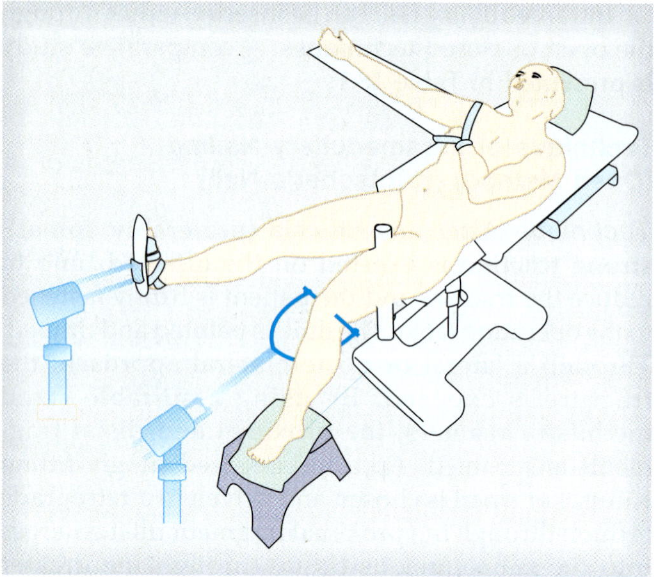

Fig. 18.13: Positioning for ILN femur

Complications of Intramedullary Nails (K-Nail)

The following are some of the well-known complications of K-nail:

1. If the nail size is small—it may bend, break or migrate either in the proximal or distal direction.
2. If the nail size is large—it may splinter the bone or the nail gets jammed in the medullary canal.
3. If the nail is projecting more than 2 to 5 cm in the upper end, it may lead to the development of an adventitious bursa in the gluteal region which if inflamed causes pain and limp.
4. If the nail is extending more into the distal fragment, it may cause a reactionary effusion in the knee joint.
5. Faulty asepsis during insertion leads to infection.

Interlocking Nailing Technique (Gold Standard)

Here, the technique is almost similar to the closed technique except that the interlocking nail has 2 holes in the upper and lower ends unlike the standard IM nails. Transverse screws are passed through the upper and lower holes and the nail is locked into position (Fig. 18.14).

Plates

Dynamic compression plating is used for proximal and distal one-third fractures. However, it is less commonly used nowadays.

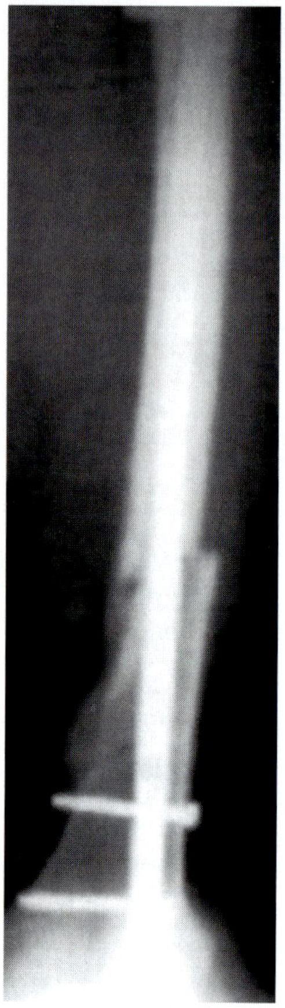

Fig. 18.14: Radiograph showing ILN femur

Vital facts:

Standard IM nailing and plating have fallen into disrepute. Interlocking nail has emerged as the gold standard in treating most of the shaft femur fractures in adults.

Future trends: What does the future hold for fracture femur treatment?

- Titanium metal
- Bio-absorbable polysters (Polyglycolide or polylactide). This eliminates need for extraction.

Complications of Fracture Shaft Femur

- *Immediate complications* These are life threatening and the common ones are shock, fat embolism neurovascular injury to the femoral artery, sciatic nerve, etc.
- *Delayed complications* These are more common and include:
  1. *Refracture* This is the most embarrassing complication and is commonly seen in simpler

fractures due to poor welding of the fracture site by the callus and after plate removal due to the holes left over by the removal of screws which takes time to fill up leaving a potential weak spot for refracture. The incidence of this complication is around 9 to 15 per cent.

2. *Complications of fixation devices* The problems usually encountered with intramedullary nails are breaking, loosening, proximal or distal migration, jamming, bending, infection, etc. These may be due to faulty implants, techniques or choice.
3. *Nerve injury* Injury to the common peroneal nerve is more often seen in these fractures. However, it is not a very common occurrence.
4. *Malunion* This is one of the most common complications seen in fracture shaft femur and is due to the strong and variable muscular forces already described. Malunion is more often seen following conservative treatment and traction than in operative treatment.
5. *Nonunion* It is not that common as, fracture shaft femur is known to unite well.
6. *Joint stiffness* In fracture shaft femur knee joint may become stiff due to quadriceps atrophy following prolonged immobilisation and due to intra-articular or extra-articular adhesions.

FRACTURE DISTAL FEMUR

The distal part of the femur encompasses the lower one-third. It varies between 7.6 cm and 15 cm of distal femur. The supracondylar area is a transition zone between the distal diaphysis and the femoral articular surface. The distal femur is subjected to the quadriceps force anteriorly and the flexion force of the gastrocnemius posteriorly (see Fig. 18.3). The fractures of the distal femur could be classified into supracondylar, intercondylar, unicondylar and comminuted fractures (Figs 18.15A to C). The distal femur fracture accounts for 7 per cent of all femoral fractures.

SUPRACONDYLAR FRACTURE OF FEMUR

Supracondylar region extends from the femoral condyles to the junction of metaphysis with femoral shaft. The distal fragment is displaced and angulated posteriorly due to the pull of gastrocnemius muscle.

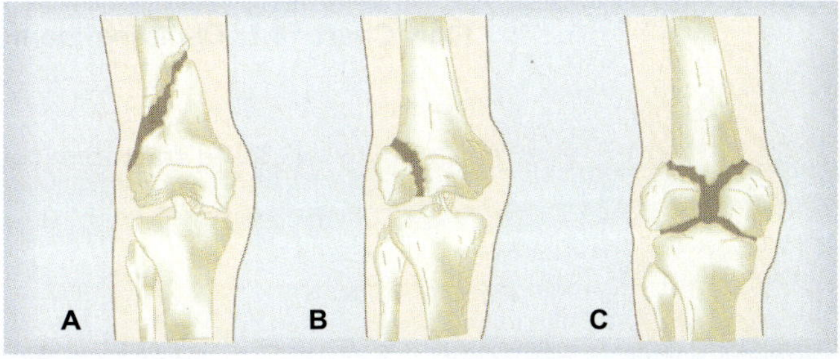

Figs 18.15A to C: Fractures of distal femur: (A) Supracondylar fracture, (B) Unicondylar fracture, (C) Comminuted fractures (Bicondylar)

Mechanism of Injury

It is due to severe valgus or varus forces with axial loading and rotation due to RTA, fall, etc.

Classification

Neer's Classification *(Figs 18.16A to D)*

1. Undisplaced fracture.
2. Displaced fracture:
   a. Medial displacement.
   b. Lateral displacement.
3. Comminuted fractures.

Muller's AO Classification

- Type A: Extra-articular fractures
- Type B: Unicondylar fractures
- Type C: Bicondylar fractures

  Each is further subdivided into 1 to 3 depending on the severity of comminution.

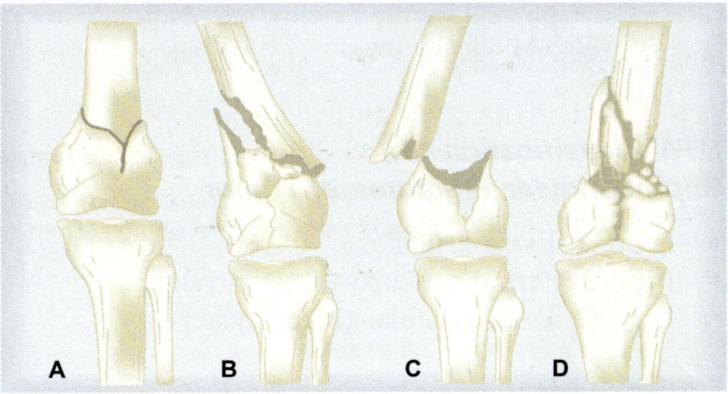

Figs 18.16A to D: Neer's classification for supracondylar fractures: (A) Undisplaced, (B) Displaced and medial, (C) Displaced and lateral, (D) Comminuted

Flow Chart 18.1: Depicting the treatment plan in fracture shaft of femur

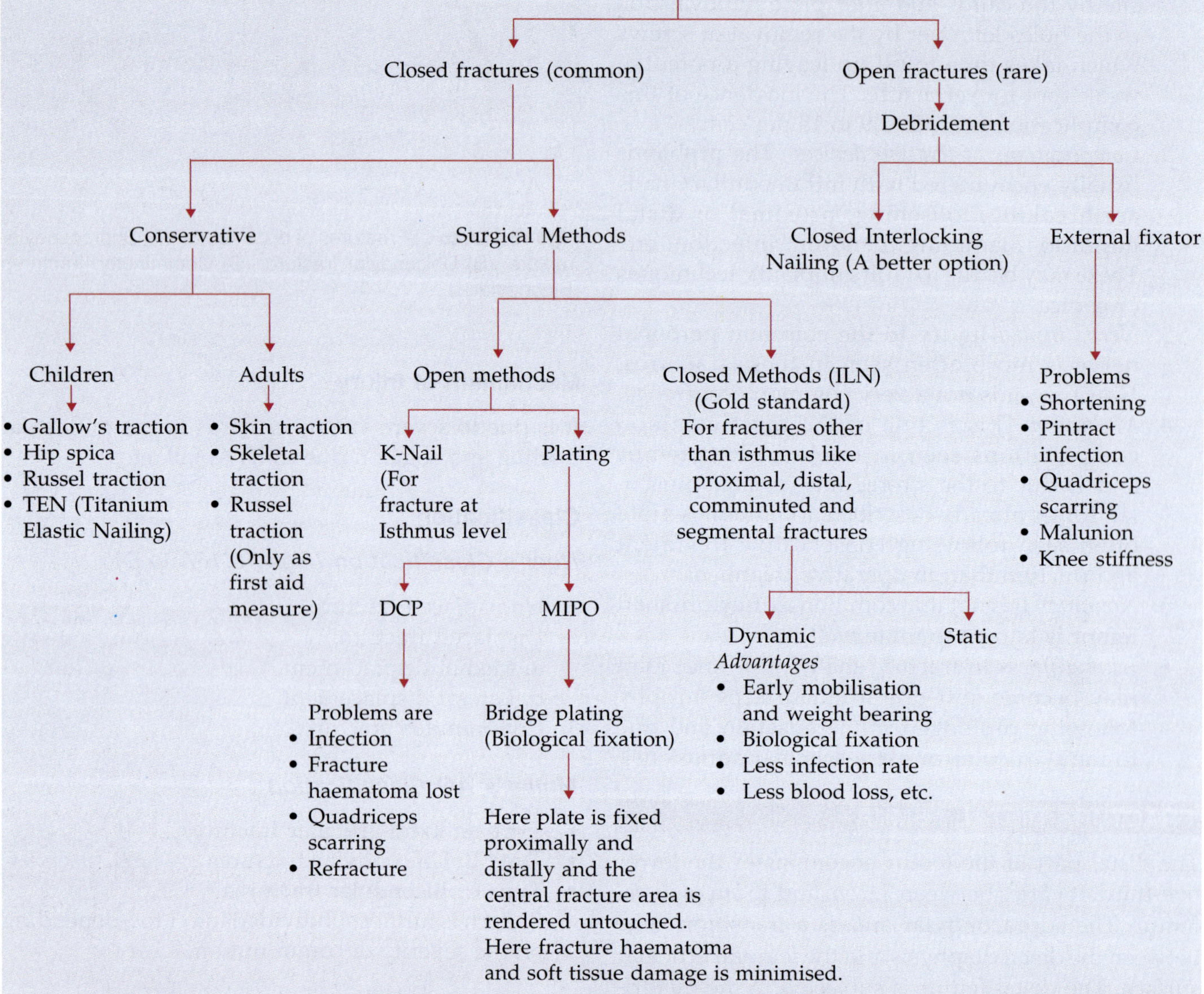

Note: • Metaphyseal fractures are the only indication for primary plating.
• MIPO-Minimally Invasive Plate Osteosynthesis.

OTA Classification of Supracondylar Fractures of Femur

- Type A: Extra-articular
- Type B: Partial articular (Unicondylar)
- Type C: Total articular (Bicondylar)

Further Subdivisions

Type A
- Simple
- Metaphyseal wedge
- Metaphyseal comminution

Type B
- Fracture lateral condyle
- Fracture medial condyle
- Frontal fracture

Type C
- Articular and metaphyseal simple
- Articular simple and metaphyseal comminution
- Total comminution.

Clinical Features

It consists of the usual features of fractures, but what is specific to this fracture is the flexion deformity caused by the pull of gastrocnemius. Haemarthrosis is commonly seen, especially with fractures extending into the joint.

Radiography

Radiograph helps to study the fracture pattern more accurately. Routine AP, lateral and oblique (45°) views are required.

Arteriography: This should be performed in suspected vascular damage or in associated dislocation of the knee joint.

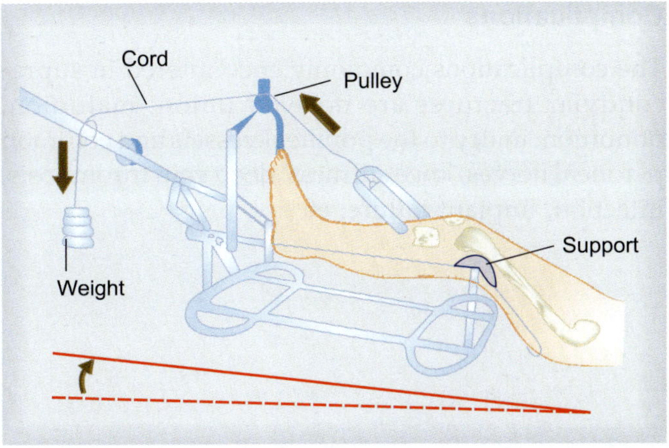

Fig. 18.17: Skeletal traction through Böhler-Braun frame for supracondylar fracture. Note the support is given at the fracture site and not the knee to prevent angulation

Treatment

The treatment usually consists of conservative methods, traction and operative methods.

Conservative methods This has a limited role and is usually useful in impacted and undisplaced fractures. In the former, a long leg or spica cast is sufficient and in the latter a long above knee cast after an initial period of skin or skeletal traction is all that is required.

Traction methods The choice is mainly skeletal traction and two methods are described:

a. *Upper tibial traction* (Fig. 18.17) Here the skeletal traction is applied through the upper end of tibia. Initial weight used is around 15 to 20 lbs and is subsequently reduced. The traction is given for a period of 8 to 12 weeks and the patient is put on cast braces. To prevent the knee stiffness from developing, the patient is encouraged to carry out the knee movements during the traction itself.
b. *Two-pin traction method* In this method, traction is added through the distal femur apart from the traction given through the upper end of tibia. This helps in accurate reduction of the fracture and also maintains the reduction so obtained. The disadvantage of this technique is that it is cumbersome and may cause neurovascular compressions in and around the knee.

Operative methods This consists of ORIF and is preferred as the closed reduction is associated with troublesome complications like limited knee motion, residual varus and internal rotation deformities. The advantages of open reduction are early mobilisation of the knee joint and a fairly accurate reduction and rigid fixation.

Fixation methods The choice is between medullary fixation and blade plate fixation. Rush pins, Ender's nail, medullary nails, split nails, etc. are some of the commonly used medullary fixation methods. While AO plates, Elliott or Jewett plates comprise the blade fixation methods. Dynamic condylar screw (DCS) also gives good fixation. Buttress plate in highly comminuted fractures (Fig. 18.18).

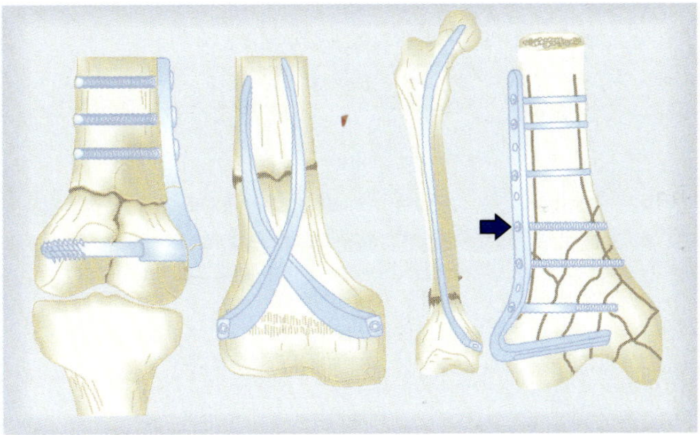

Figs 18.18: Showing different methods of internal fixation of supracondylar fracture of femur

Complications

The complications commonly encountered in supracondylar fractures are delayed union, malunion, nonunion, injury to the popliteal vessels and common peroneal nerves, knee stiffness, deep vein thrombosis, infection, implant failure, etc.

Do you know why fractures of the distal femur are difficult to manage?

- They are frequently comminuted
- Due to distractive muscle forces
- Due to its proximity to the knee
- Due to associated trauma in the young and due to medical problems in the old.

19

Injuries of the Knee

- Brief anatomy
- Knee ligament injuries
- Medial collateral ligament injury
- Cruciate ligament injuries
- Semilunar cartilage injuries
- Fracture of patella
- Injury to the extensor apparatus of knee

BRIEF ANATOMY

THE KNEE JOINT SPEAKS

You will have to agree with me that I am the most remarkable joint in the body by any engineering standards. Being the most heavily stressed joint in the body, I have amalgamated two apparently incompatible properties of stability and mobility. During complete extension I am very stable, and during flexion I am very mobile. I have a *hinge joint* between the lower end of femur and upper end of tibia and a *saddle joint* between the patella and the femur. Hence I am rightly called a *compound synovial joint*.

I am heavily dependent for stability on the following ligaments (Fig. 19.1):

Medial side Here in the anterior third I am supported by the anterior capsule and extensor retinaculum, in the middle third by the superficial and deep layers of tibial collateral ligament, in the posterior third the capsule is reinforced by posterior oblique ligament, expansions from semitendinosus, etc.

Lateral side In the anterior third, capsule and the lateral extensor retinaculum; in the middle third, the iliotibial band; in the posterior third by the arcuate complex formed by fibular collateral ligament, and a slip from the popliteus, biceps femoris, etc.

Anteroposterior stability For this, I have two cruciate ligaments: one anterior and the other posterior who are the primary stabilisers in the anteroposterior plane.

Anterior cruciate ligament (ACL) restrains me during anterior glide. It has two main functional components, the smaller anteromedial bundle supports me best in flexion and the larger posterolateral bundle supports me best in extension. Both are taut at full extension. *Posterior cruciate ligament* (PCL) is thicker and is approximately twice as strong as either anterior cruciate or medial collateral ligaments. It restrains me mainly during the posterior glide and is under tension throughout the whole range of movements.

I have two wonderful structures in the form of *menisci* whose structure and function are discussed in the section on meniscal injury.

Knee stability depends upon

1. Mechanical axes of the joint.
2. The bony contours.
3. Extra-articular stabilisers (synovium, capsules, collaterals, muscles and tendons).
4. Intra-articular stabilisers (menisci and cruciates).

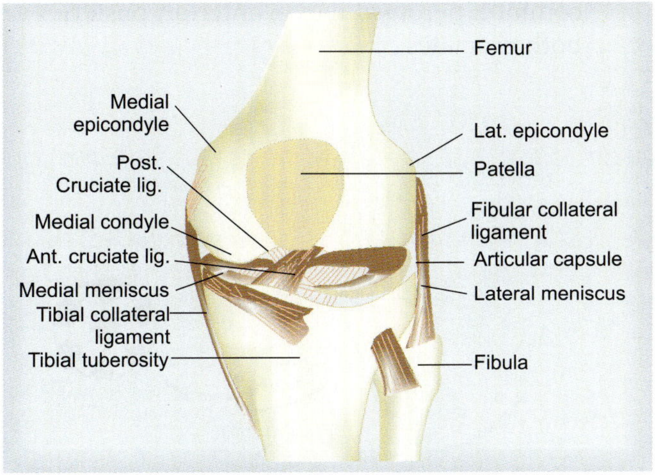

Fig. 19.1: Anatomy of knee joint

KNEE LIGAMENT INJURIES

GENERAL PRINCIPLES

Aetiology

1. *Athletes* Knee ligament injuries are very common in athletes who are involved both in contact and non-contact sports. The injury could be either direct due to the collision with another athlete or indirect due to rotation and twisting injuries.
2. *Road traffic accident (RTA)* Here the mechanism is usually direct and could be due to a dashboard injury.
3. *Fall* from a height with twisting force.

Mechanism of Injury (Palmar)

The following are the common mechanism of knee ligament injuries (Fig. 19.2):

1. Direct valgus force.
2. Rotational or twisting forces.
   - **Abduction, flexion and internal rotation of femur on tibia (Ab FIR)** This causes damage to medial structures, like tibial collateral, medial capsule and if more force is applied ACL and medial meniscus may also tear.
     "O' donoghue's unhappy triad" (Fig. 19.3) Indicate injuries to medial structures + ACL tear + medial meniscus injury.
   - **Adduction, flexion and external rotation of femur on tibia (Ad FER)** Causes damage to fibular collateral, lateral capsule, arcuate complex, popliteus, iliotibial band, biceps, common peroneal nerve, anterior, posterior or both cruciates.

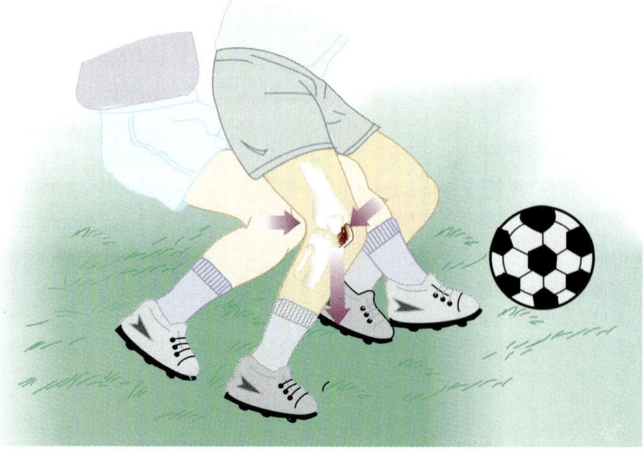

Fig. 19.2: Showing common mechanism of knee ligament injuries

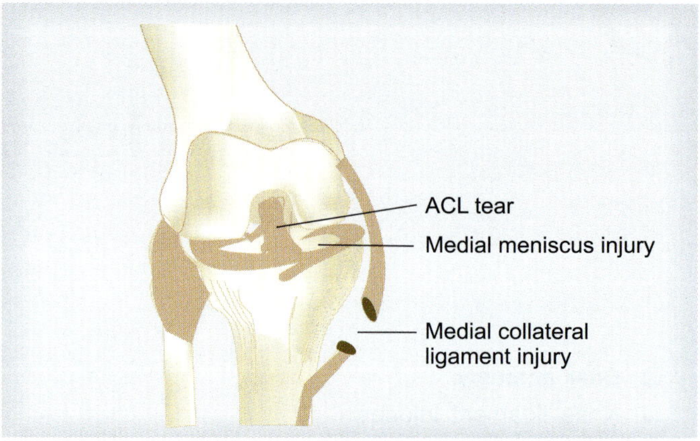

Fig. 19.3: Showing unhappy triad of O'donoghue

3. **Hyperextension force** may cause either anterior or posterior cruciate ligament injury.
4. **Anteroposterior displacement** Either anterior (dashboard injury) or posterior cruciates may be injured due to a direct force in RTA.

Goals of Treatment

The goals of treatment in knee ligament injuries are restoration of anatomy and stability to normal or near to normal.

MEDIAL COLLATERAL LIGAMENT INJURY

Collateral ligament injury is due to direct or indirect violence as described earlier. Medial collateral ligament injury is more common due to the valgus stress caused by striking the lateral aspect of the knee joint during collision in sports. The varus force on the medial side required to cause the lateral collateral ligament injury is less common because of the protection offered by the other leg.

- However, a severe varus force may cause avulsion of the lateral collateral ligament from the head of the fibula (Fig. 19.4A).

Do you know?

- About Pellagrini-Stieda disease: It is a calcification seen at the adductor tubercle visualised on AP X-ray of the knee in MCL injury of greater than 6 weeks.

Mechanism of injury: This has already been described.

Classification

(American Medical Association)

- **Sprain (Fig. 19.4B)** (Ligament injury)
  - *I Degree*
    - Minimal tear (< 1/3)
    - Local tenderness
    - No instability
    - → + If joint separation is < 5 mm
  - *II Degree (1/3–2/3)*
    - More disruption
    - No instability
    - → ++ If joint separation is > 5-10 mm
  - *III Degree*
    - Complete disruption instability
    - → +++ If joint separation is > 10 mm
- **Strain** (Muscle and tendon injuries)

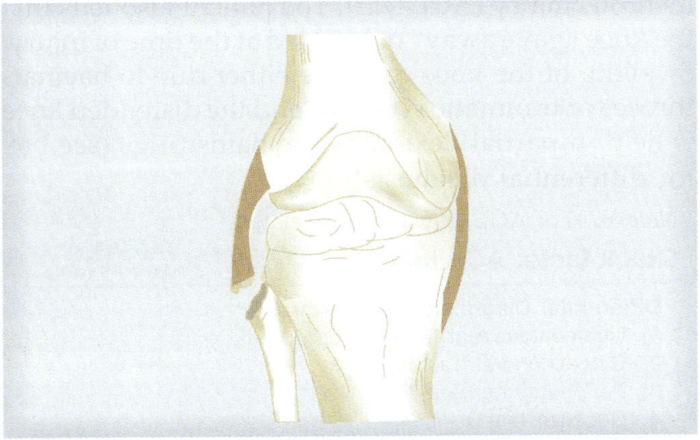

Fig. 19.4A: Avulsion of lateral collateral ligament from the head of the fibula

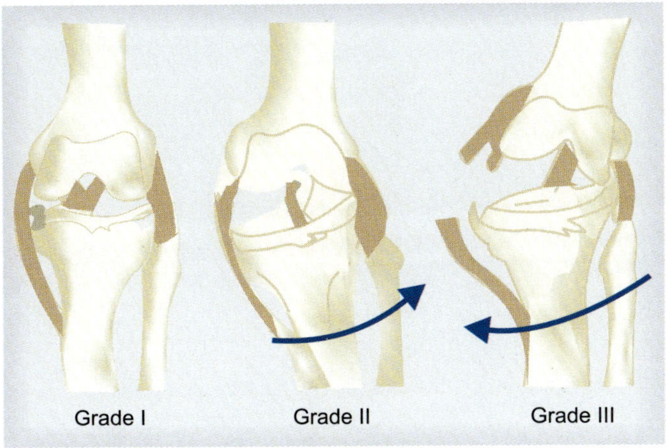

Fig. 19.4B: Showing sprain of medial collateral ligament of the knee

Clinical Features

The patient gives history of valgus and external rotation force in mild sprains. In severe sprains, the patient gives history of valgus stress force due to the direct blow on the lower thigh or upper leg seen commonly in contact sports like football, rugby, etc. It may be associated with ACL tear or meniscal injury and then the patient may present with pain, swelling, haemarthrosis, etc.

On examination, the point of local tenderness could be at adductor tubercle, joint line or at the insertion of tibial collateral ligament (Fig. 19.5). About 10 to 20 per cent of patients have damage to the extensor mechanism of the knee.

Clinical Tests (Figs 19.6A and B)

These are abduction stress in 30° knee flexion and extension. The amount of opening on the medial side should be assessed. To rule out the associated injuries, do the anterior drawer test and Lachman's test (p. 223).

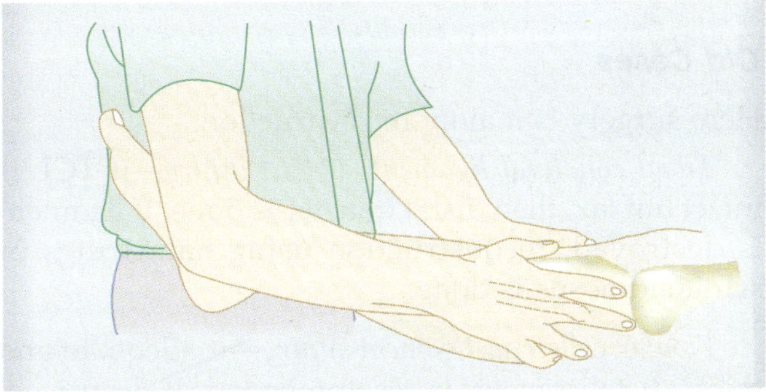

Fig. 19.5: Showing method of eliciting joint line tenderness

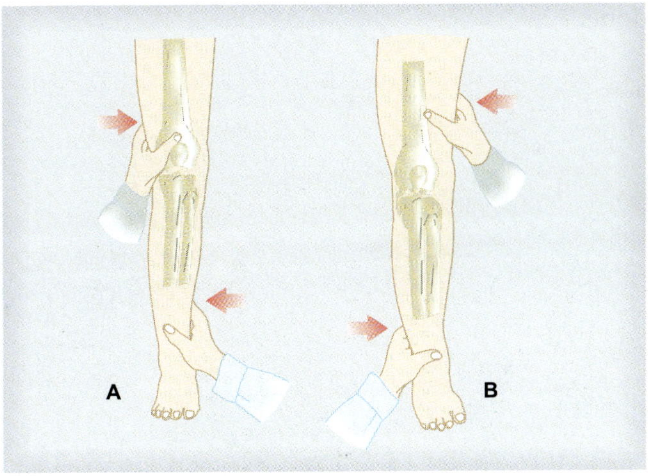

Figs 19.6A and B: Stress tests: (A) Abduction or valgus stress test, and (B) Adduction or varus stress test

Investigations

1. Stress radiographs at 15 to 20° of valgus.
2. MRI helps to localise the MCL tears, ACL, meniscal injuries, etc.
3. Arthrograms and arthroscopy to evaluate and rule out meniscal and cruciate pathology.

Treatment

Nonoperative treatment is the mainstay of treatment.

Fresh Injury

I° Sprain → Symptomatic treatment, nonsteroidal anti-inflammatory drugs (NSAIDs), etc.

II° Sprain → Long leg cast for 4 to 6 weeks with knee in 30 to 40° of flexion.

III° Sprain → Surgical repair in isolated tears. Repair and reconstruction in old tears or in associated injuries (Fig. 19.7). Brace is required for 4 to 7 months.

Old Cases

Here surgery is mainly reconstruction.

Tibial collateral ligament (TCL) injury—if TCL is intact but lax, then distal transfer is done. If ligament is destroyed, reconstruction using hamstrings or semitendinosus is done.

Fibular collateral ligament injury—if adequate and thick, distal transfer is recommended. If destroyed, reconstruction using fascia lata, biceps tendon, etc. is done.

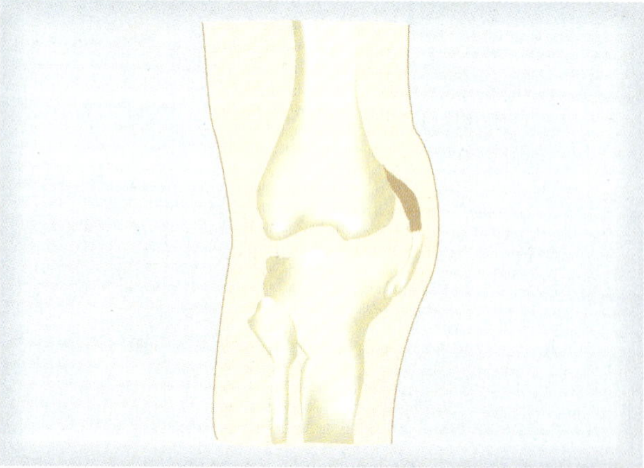

Fig. 19.7: Showing direct ligament repair in fresh tears

CRUCIATE LIGAMENT INJURIES

ANTERIOR CRUCIATE LIGAMENT (ACL) TEAR

Of all the knee ligament injuries, ACL tear is the most common (Fig. 19.8).

Know the role of ACL in your knees

- AP stability
- Proprioception
- Mechanical function

Clinical Features

Mechanism of anterior cruciate ligament (ACL) tear has already been discusssed. The most common mode of injury is external rotation with abduction of the flexed knee or hyperextension of knee in internal rotation. This is a disabling injury and the knee may immediately collapse and is painful. Popping sensation felt or heard at the time of injury signifies ligamentous injury (ACL tear). The patient also tells that the knee "gave away" or buckled at the time of injury. Swelling of the knee could be either due to haemarthroses or traumatic synovitis and the distended knee is held in partial flexion by the hamstrings (see box for differential diagnosis).

Note: 67% of ACL tear is sports related.

Quick facts: ACL tear

Differential Diagnosis: Haemarthrosis

1. Ligamentous tear (ACL, PCL, etc.)
2. Osteochondral fracture
3. Peripheral meniscal tear
4. Capsular tear
5. Patellar dislocation
6. Intra-articular fractures

Note: Commonest cause is ACL tear

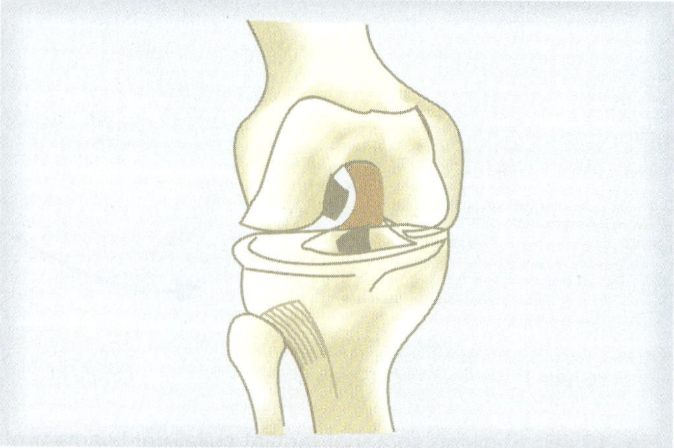

Fig. 19.8: Showing ACL tear

Combined instabilities of knee

• If anterior, medial and lateral structures are torn.	*Anteromedial and anterolateral instabilities.*
• If anterior, posterior cruciates lateral structures are torn.	*Anterolateral and posterolateral instabilities.*
• If anterior, posterior cruciates and medial structures are torn.	*Anteromedial and posteromedial instabilities.*

Did you know?

ACL tear was first described by Galen in AD 170.

Clinical Examination (Figs 19.9A to F)

Always examine the normal knee first and form a basis for "comparison." Clinical findings depend on associated ligamentous injury or meniscal injury or bone damage. Depending on the combination there will be specific instabilities, that will allow anterior displacement of tibia on the uninvolved side. Anterior subluxation of more than 5° suggests lax or disrupted ACL. Isolated injury is rare. Various other clinical tests to detect ACL tear are depicted in Table 19.1 and Figures 19.9B and C.

Table 19.1: Clinical tests to diagnose various knee ligament injuries

Tests	*How to perform*	*Inference*
I. Adduction or varus: **Abduction or valgus stress test** (Fig. 19.9A) 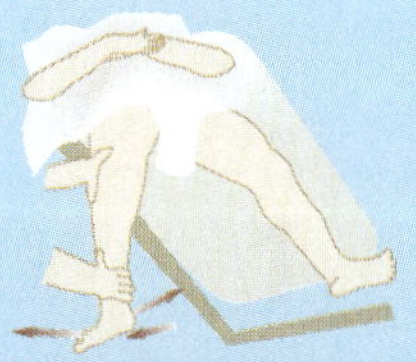	Patient is supine, knee is flexed to 30° **For abduction test** One hand is on the lateral aspect of the knee and the other at the ankle, force is applied outwards. **For adduction test** Change hand to the medial side of the knee and give an adduction force.	Positive in injury to the medial structures of the knee like tibial collateral ligament. Positive in injuries to lateral structures of knee like fibular collateral ligament.
II. Lachman's* test (Fig. 19.9B) 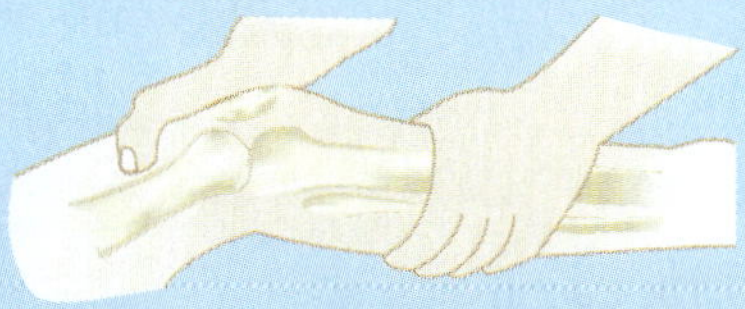	This is an anterior drawer's test done at 20 to 30° of knee flexion with patient in supine position.	Indicates ACL tear. This test is used in acute injuries of knee to test ACL tear where knee cannot be flexed to 90°.
III. Anterior Drawer's test (Fig. 19.9C) 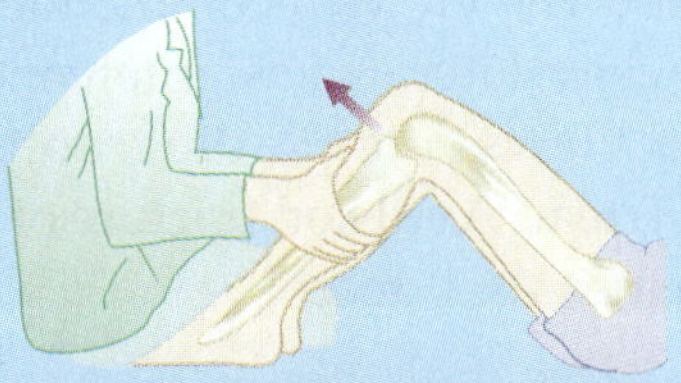	Patient is in supine position. Hip is flexed to 45° and knee to 90°. Examiner sits on the dorsum of the foot and pulls the tibia forwards. The anterior drawer's test is done in 3 positions: a. Foot in neutral position—if positive, it indicates ACL tear, etc. b. Foot in 15° internal rotation—if positive, indicates damage to anterolateral structures. c. Foot in 15° external rotation—if positive, indicates damage to anteromedial structures.	If the tibia shifts anteriorly more than 6 to 8 mm, then it indicates torn ACL and the test is considered as positive. This should always be compared with the normal knee.
IV. Posterior Drawer's test (Fig. 19.9D) 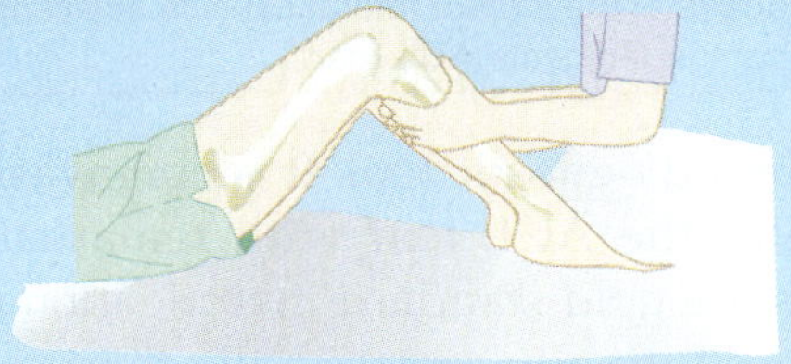	Same as above but tibia is pushed backwards. Positive test is indicated by the movement of the tibia backwards.	Indicates posterior cruciate ligament tear.

Contd...

Section 2

Contd...

Tests	*How to perform*	*Inference*
V. Jerk test of Hughston (Fig. 19.9E) 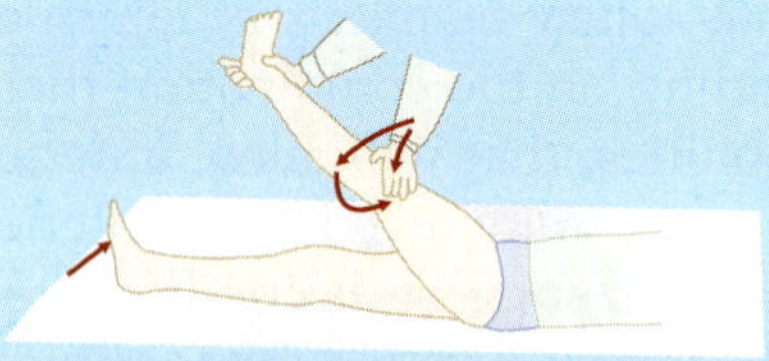	Patient is supine, knee is flexed to 90°. Tibia is internally rotated with a valgus force applied at the knee, it is slowly extended. *Lateral tibial condyle subluxates at 30° and spontaneous relocation occurs as knee extends.*	*Inference* indicates anterior cruciate ligament tear and is more specific than Drawer's test in detecting ACL tear.
VI. Pivot shift test (Fig. 19.9F) 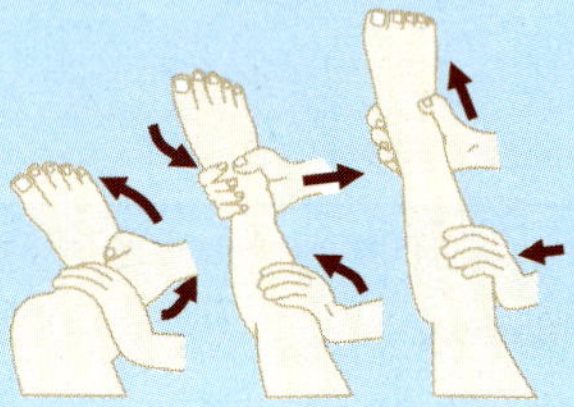	Patient is supine. The knee is extended, with a valgus stress applied on the knee and the tibia is internally rotated. The knee is slowly flexed. Subluxation occurs at 30–40°.	A positive test indicates anterior cruciate ligament tear.

Disturbing facts: About ACL tear

- ACL tear → Knee instability → Repeated episodes of instability leads to damage to menisci, cartilage and other ligaments → This ultimately leads to secondary OA knee

Clinical tests

- **Slocum test** It is an anterior drawer's test (rotary test) performed with 15° of internal rotation and 30° of external rotation. The former is positive in anterolateral instability and the latter in anteromedial instability.
- **External rotation recurvatum test (posterior sag sign)** When the leg is passively lifted by holding the toes, the knee sags posteriorly indicating injury to PCL and posterolateral structures.
- **Lachman's test** (Fig. 19.10) As already described, this is an anterior drawer's test done at 20 to 30° of flexion. It has several advantages over 90° flexion anterior drawer's test. The following are some of them:
  1. It can be done in the presence of effusion and hence is useful in acute cases when knee cannot be flexed up to 90°.
  2. Evokes less pain as full flexion is not required.
  3. Hamstrings and torn menisci will not block forward glide easily.
  4. More specific for posterolateral fibres of ACL tear.

Grading of Lachman's test

- Grade I—end feel appreciation (0–5 mm displacement).
- Grade II—visible anterior movement of tibia (5–10 mm displacement).
- Grade III—gross anterior tibial translation (more than 10 mm displacement).

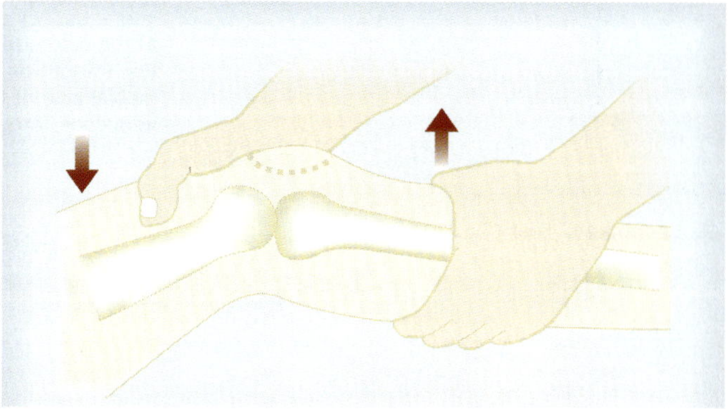

Fig. 19.10: Lachman's test

Investigations in ACL Tear

Radiograph of the knee The views recommended are anteroposterior (AP) view, lateral view, intercondylar notch view, sunrise views, etc. Radiographs are usually normal in ACL tear. Avulsion fracture of tibial spine if present indicates ACL tear.

Did you know what is a Segund fracture?

It is an avulsion fracture of the inferior lateral capsule adjacent to the tibia. If present, it suggests ACL tear.

MRI This is the best diagnostic tool. It is noninvasive and demonstrates the ACL tear with remarkable accuracy. This is the gold standard investigation for ACL tears and has virtually replaced all others.

KT-1000 This is a measuring system that documents anteroposterior tibial displacement by tracking the tibial tubercle in rotation to the patella. More than 3 mm anterior displacement at 20 lbs predicts an ACL tear with 94 per cent accuracy.

POSTERIOR CRUCIATE LIGAMENT (PCL) TEAR

It is less common than ACL tear. It is ruptured due to severe rotational injury, dashboard injury or complete dislocation of the knee.

Note: PCL tear accounts for 3–4% of all knee ligament injuries.

Vital points: ACL tear

- Common in young active people usually athletes, may interfere with activity or it may make activity impossible.
- Usually it does not tear in isolation.
- Associated with other ligament injuries.
- May predispose to meniscal lesions.
- May predispose to OA changes.

Isolated PCL tear is rare and is accompanied with other ligament injuries.

Clinical Features

The patient complains of pain, swelling and tenderness over the popliteal fossa. Clinically, posterior drawer test and sag sign will be positive (Fig. 19.11).

Pearl

90° posterior drawer test is the most important test to diagnose PCL tear.

Rupture of the cruciate and collateral ligaments either singly (rare) or in combination (common) makes the knee unstable. Depending upon the combination of injuries, the knee instability could be either one plane, two plane or both (Tables 19.2 and 19.5).

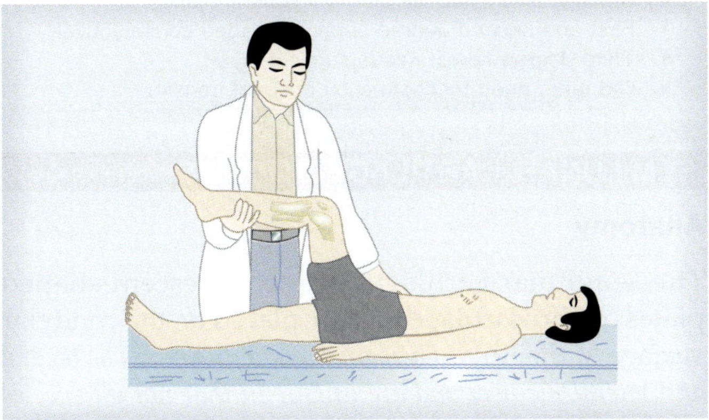

Fig. 19.11: Showing posterior 'sag sign' for PCL tear

Table 19.2: Showing knee instability in different planes

If only medial structures torn	*One plane medial instability*
If only lateral structures torn	*One plane lateral instability*
If ACL and medial structures torn	*Two plane anterior and medial instability*
If ACL and lateral structures torn	*Two plane anterior and lateral instability*
If PCL and medial structures torn	*Two plane posterior and medial instability*
If PCL and lateral structures torn	*Two plane posterior and lateral instability*

Combined instabilities of knee

• If anterior, medial and lateral structures are torn.	*Anteromedial and anterolateral instabilities.*
• If anterior, posterior cruciates lateral structures are torn.	*Anterolateral and posterolateral instabilities.*
• If anterior, posterior cruciates and medial structures are torn.	*Anteromedial and postero-medial instabilities.*

Treatment of ACL Tear

Conservative

This is reserved for Grade I and II tears and consists of rest, long leg casts for 4 to 6 weeks, NSAIDs, physiotherapy, etc.

Surgical

Arthroscopically assisted ACL reconstruction has been universally advocated due to its superior results.

1. *Fresh* Primary repair is indicated in young adults and athletes. Repair is successful if ACL is torn at its femoral or tibial attachments. It is not successful in midposition tears. Failure rate is as high as 50 per cent.
2. *Old cases*
   - Reinforcement of ACL tear should be augmented except when avulsion is with a fragment of bone. Reinforcement could be either intra-articular, or extra-articular or both by using iliotibial band, semitendinosus tendon, etc.
   - Reconstruction in chronic ACL insufficiency, could be either intra-articular or extra-articular replacement by using quadriceps, tendon,

Section 2

patellar tendon (central 1/3) bone patella tendon bone graft (BPTB) (Fig. 19.12), semitendinosus tendon, gracilis, etc.

These autografts are preferred over allografts which are reserved for:
1. Revision ACL reconstruction.
2. Rupture of both ACL and PCL.

Surgical Technique of ACL Reconstruction in a Nutshell

- Graft harness and preparation
- Notchplasty
- Tibial tunnel placement
- Femoral tunnel placement
- Graft passage

Posterior cruciate ligament injuries Most of the Grade I and II PCL tears can be treated nonoperatively.

Surgery This is indicated in Grade III injuries with posterior translation > 10 mm. Reconstruction is done by using medial head of gastrocnemius, etc.

Avulsion of the PCL from the femoral or tibial ends is more common unlike in ACL tears. Here reattachment of the avulsed ligament usually gives good results.

Reconstruction is reserved for:
1. Midsubstance tears.
2. Old tears.

Graft Options for PCL Reconstruction

- Central one-third of patellar tendon.
- Patella tendon allograft.
- Achilles tendon allograft.
- Semitendinosus or gracilis graft.
- Two-tailed femoral graft is the graft of choice.
- Some prefer anterolateral femoral reconstruction with a tibial inlay grafting.

Anterolateral instability This is due to injury of anterolateral structures. Reconstruction is done by using iliotibial band or biceps femoris transfer.

Posterolateral instability This is due to injury to the posterolateral structures. Posterolateral structures repair or reconstruction is recommended.

Remember

Autografts widely used in reconstruction of ACL tear
- Central 1/3 of patellar tendon (BPTB Graft)
- Semitendinous and gracilis tendons

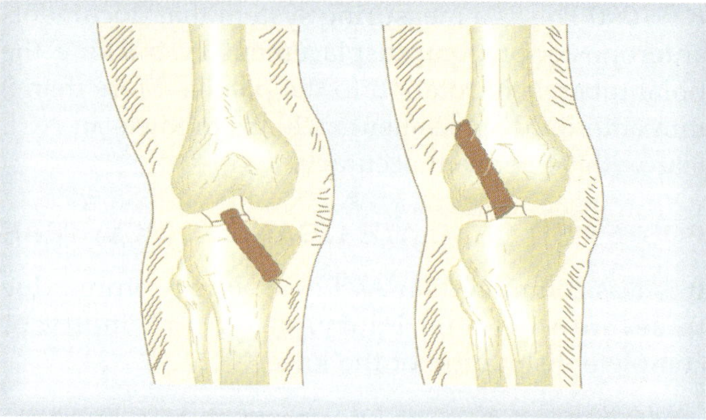

Fig. 19.12: Showing methods of ACL repair

Posteromedial instability This is due to injury to the posteromedial structures. Repair or reconstruction of posteromedial structures is done.

At a glance

Cruciate injuries
- ACL commonly tears than PCL (9:1).
- Commonest mechanism for ACL tear is external rotation with abduction of a flexed knee and for PCL tear dashboard injury.
- Rarely tears in isolation.
- Commonly tears in combinations.
- May tear at midsubstance or femoral and tibial attachments.
- ACL tear is a common cause of haemarthroses (70%).
- Lachman's test is useful in acute ACL tear.
- Drawer's test, rotary test, etc. helps in the diagnosis of combination tears.
- Treatment is by three **R's**
  - **R**epair in fresh cases
  - **R**einforce in old lax ligaments
  - **R**econstruct in old torn ligaments
- Predisposes to instability and osteoarthritis changes.

Collateral injuries
- Medial collateral injury is more commoner than lateral.
- Medial collateral injury is due to valgus force.
- Ligament sprain is graded into three degrees.
- Stress tests help in the diagnosis.
- Usually associated with other ligament injuries.
- First and second degree sprain managed conservatively.
- Third degree sprain needs surgical repair.
- Old tears need reconstruction or distal transfer.

SEMILUNAR CARTILAGE INJURIES

Anatomy

The semilunar cartilages are two crescent-shaped plates of fibrocartilage that are placed on the condylar surface of the tibia. *They are commonly known as medial and lateral menisci and are unique in that not all species have menisci in their knees and not all joints have menisci*

Section 2

(Table 19.3). They are vital for the function of the knee joint (Fig. 19.13). The vascular supply to both the menisci is from the lateral, medial and middle geniculate vessels. The depth of vascular penetration at the periphery is 10 to 30 per cent width of medial meniscus and 10 to 25 per cent width of lateral meniscus. In cross section they appear triangular, the thicker peripheral portion is vascular and heals well and the thin central edge is avascular, receiving nutrition by diffusion and hence heals poorly.

Functions of the Menisci

1. Contributes towards the stability of the knee joint.
2. Weight transmission of 40 to 70 per cent of the load across the knee joint.
3. Acts as a shock absorber.
4. Deepens the tibial condyles on which the femoral condyles roll by increasing the contact area by 40 per cent.
5. Assists in nutrition of the articular cartilage by distribution of the synovial fluid.
6. Helps the knee in locking mechanism.
7. Prevents impingement of synovial membrane, capsule, etc.
8. Assists and controls gliding and rolling motion of the knee.

MEDIAL MENISCUS INJURY

Medial meniscus is more commonly injured than the lateral and is usually associated with other ligament injuries of the knee.

[1]Smillie's Classification

Medial meniscus injury (Figs 19.14A to F) is seen in over 71 per cent of the cases. In 5 per cent of cases injury of medial meniscus is bilateral. Lateral meniscus is less commonly injured than the medial meniscus because it is smaller in diameter, thicker in periphery, wide, more mobile, attached to both cruciate ligaments and stabilised posteriorly to the femoral condyle by popliteus.

1. *Longitudinal tears* (35%)—in these peripheral attachments tear 10 per cent, complete tear 23 per cent (bucket handle tear), and segmental tear 2 per cent (ant/post).
2. *Horizontal tears* (48%)—could be posterior, middle, or anterior.
3. *Cystic degeneration* (12%).
4. *Congenital abnormalities* 5 per cent.
5. *Regenerative lesions.*

Mechanism of Injury

Mechanism of injury is a rotational force when a flexed knee extends.

Table 19.3: Comparative study between medial and lateral meniscus

	Features	*Medial meniscus*	*Lateral meniscus*
1	Shape	Semicircular	Circular
2	Anterior horn	Attached to tibial intercondylar eminence in front of ACL	To intercondylar eminence of tibia lateral to ACL
3	Posterior horn	Intercondylar area in front of PCL and behind posterior horn of lateral meniscus	To the intercondylar eminence
4	Outer aspect	Attached to posterior fibres of TCL	Separated from FCL by capsule and popliteus
5	Mobility	Less mobile	More mobile

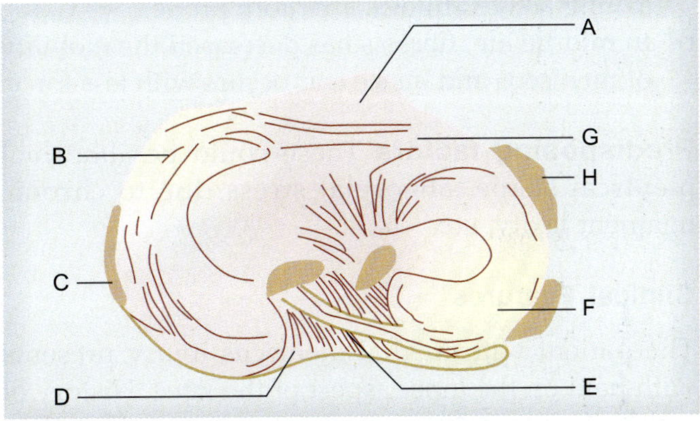

Fig. 19.13: Showing anatomy of two menisci: (A) tibial tubercle, (B) lateral meniscus, (C) fibular collateral ligament, (D) posterior cruciate ligament, (E) ligament of Wrisburg, (F) medial meniscus, and (G) intertransverse ligament, and (H) medial collateral ligament

Section 2

[1]**Smillie IS (1974)** Scotland. His other works: (a) Monograph of knee joint (b) Osteochondritis diseases.

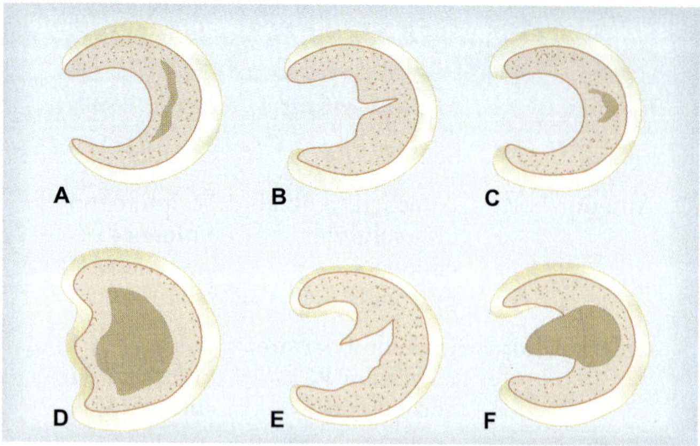

Figs 19.14A to F: Different types of meniscal injuries: (A) Longitudinal tear, (B) Radial tear, (C) Horizontal tear, (D) Bucket handle tear, (E) Parrot beak tear and, (F) Segmental tear

a. In young, it can occur only when weight is being taken, knee is flexed and there is a twisting strain. Young active athletes are more prone.
b. In middle life, fibrosis has decreased the mobility of meniscus and hence tear occurs with less force.

Predisposing factors These could be abnormal meniscal shape, abnormal stress due to chronic ligament laxity, etc.

Clinical Features

The patient with medial meniscus injury presents with pain on the inner aspect of the knee. History of locking is seen in 40 per cent of the cases and swelling if present is minimal. There is remarkable recovery after the initial acute attack and there could be periodic complaints pertaining to the knee. One or more clinical signs mentioned in the flow chart can be elicited with careful examination of the knee.

Investigations

- Radiograph is usually normal. The views recommended are anteroposterior, lateral, intercondylar notch and sunrise views of the patella.
- Arthroscopy helps to identify the torn meniscus (Figs 19.16A).
- Arthrography may reveal the tear. Double contrast arthrography is 95 per cent accurate.
- MRI is expensive but useful.

Clinical features

Symptoms

Signs (Table 19.4)
- *Locking + ve
- McMurray's test +ve (Figs 19.15A to D)
- Apley's grinding test +ve
- Payr's squat test +ve
- Duck waddle test +ve
- Steinmann's sign +ve
- Helfet's sign +ve
- Quadriceps atrophy +ve
- Medial joint line tenderness positive

Initial injury
- Patient complains of pain on the inner side of the knee
- History of locking (+ in 40%)
- Swelling of the knee
- Recovery after the initial episode

Further incidents
- Knee periodically gives trouble
- Locking history ± (unreliable)
- Unlocking (If present is pathognomonic)
- Feeling of something moving within the joint
- Click
- Pain inner side of the knee

Between incidents
- Knee is normal

*Locking is defined as restriction of the last few terminal degrees of extension of the knee.

Differential Diagnosis (Tables 19.5 and 19.6)

Fracture of tibial spine if present may give clue to the possible ACL tear. It also helps to exclude osteochondritis dissecans, osteocartilaginous loose bodies, etc.

Quick diagnostic points

Medial meniscal injuries

Medial joint line tenderness	+ve in 74% of cases
Apley's grinding test	+ve in 46% of cases
Painful hyperextension	+ve in 43% of cases
Steinmann I sign	+ve in 42% of cases
McMurray's	+ve in 35% of cases

Hence, no one test is diagnostic. That is why multiple tests are required for diagnosis. See for tests (Table 19.4 and Figs 19.17A to G)

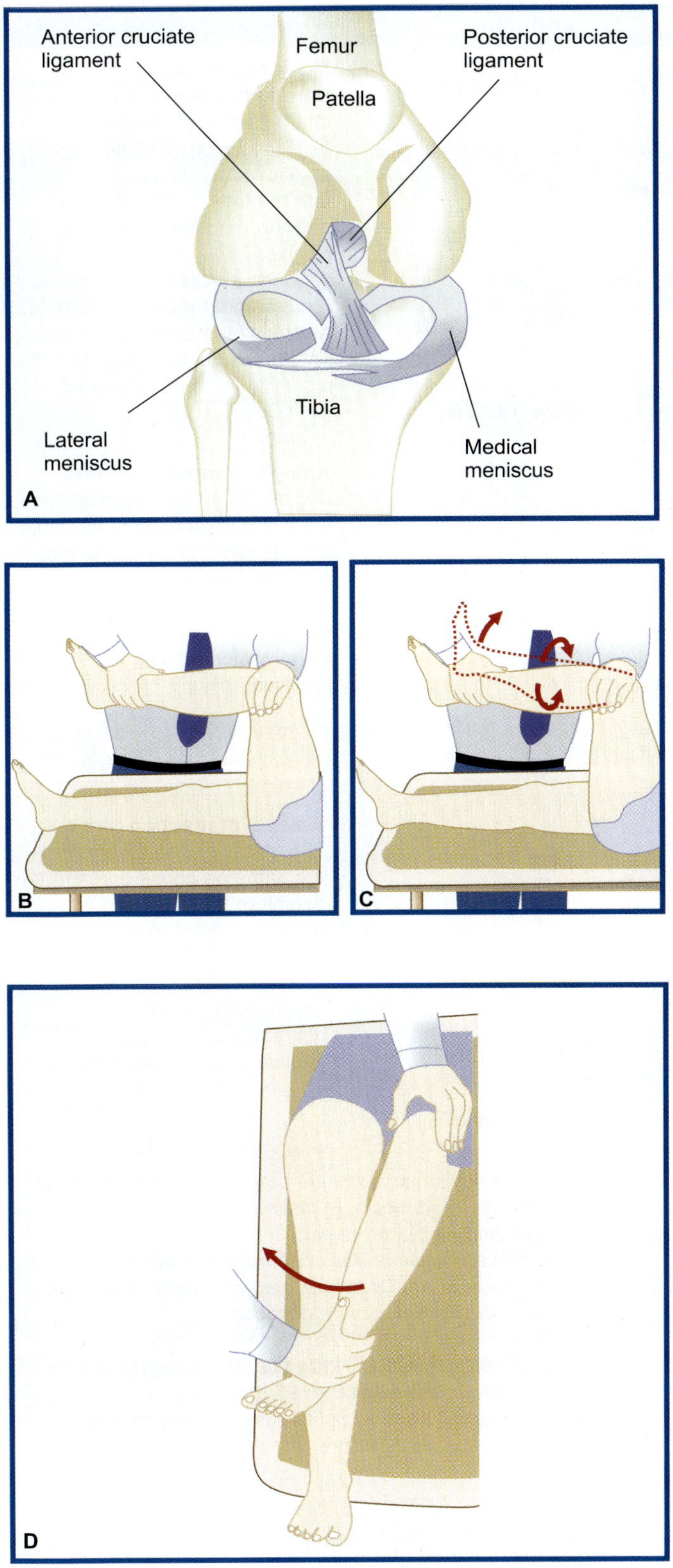

Figs 19.15A to D: (A) Anatomy (B to D) Steps of performing the McMurray's test (see page 230)

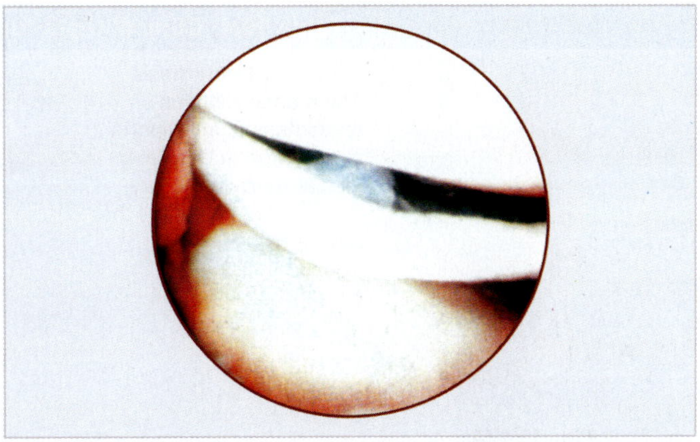

Fig. 19.16: Arthroscopic view of a bucket handle tear of medial meniscus injury

Table 19.5: Differential diagnosis of locking

True locking	*Pseudolocking*
1. Loose bodies	1. Ligament injuries
2. Recurrent dislocation of patella	2. Chondromalaciae patella
3. Fracture of tibial spine	
4. Meniscal injuries	

Treatment

Conservative This is indicated in patients soon after injury with no locking and with infrequent attacks of pain and in tears less than 10 mm, partial thickness tears.

Measures

- Abstinence from weight bearing.
- Rest, ice packs, compressive bandage.
- Buck's skin traction.
- Joint aspiration.
- Quadriceps exercises.
- If symptom persists, a cylindrical cast may be considered.

Manipulation under anaesthesia If joint is locked due to the torn menisci, manipulation under anaesthesia is recommended.

Surgery

Indications Surgery is indicated, if joint cannot be unlocked and if symptoms are recurrent.

Table 19.4: Clinical tests for diagnosis of meniscal injuries

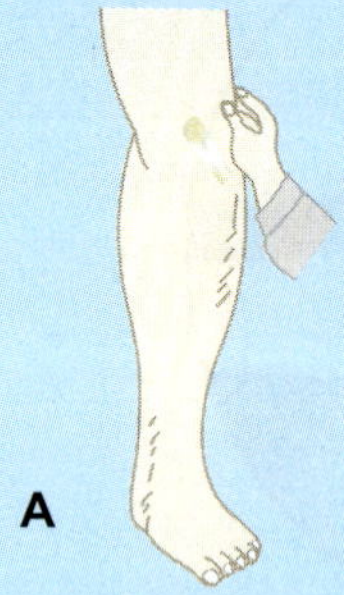

Fig. 19.17A

Joint line tenderness
The medial joint line tenderness is an important clinical sign in detecting medial meniscus injury.
It is positive in 74% of the cases (Fig. 19.17A)

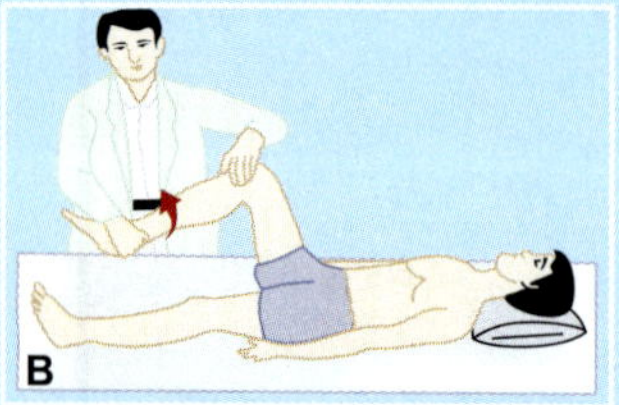

Fig. 19.17B

McMurray's test
Here forced flexion and internal rotation as shown in 1 and external rotation as shown in 2 is done to test the lateral meniscus and the medial meniscus respectively.
A positive McMurray's test requires both pain and clunk to be felt by the examiner's finger on the medial side (Fig. 19.17B).

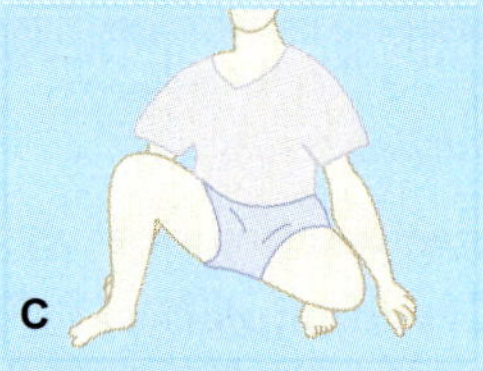

Fig. 19.17C

Duck waddle test (Fig. 19.17C)
The patient assumes a squatting position with heels touching the buttock and is asked to perform a duck walk. The patient will be unable to assume full squatting position in medial meniscus injury This is called as *childress sign* and is a diagnostic test for posterior horn tear of medial meniscus.

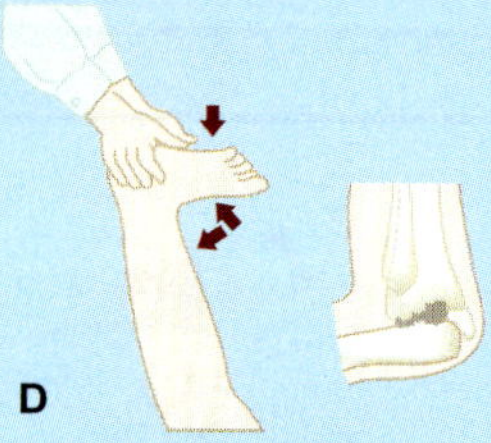

Fig. 19.17D

Apley's compression test
(Fig 19.17D) The patient is prone, fixing the thigh against the table the examiner presses the foot and leg downward while rotating the tibia (grinding test) Pain noted during axial compression implies a meniscal lesion.

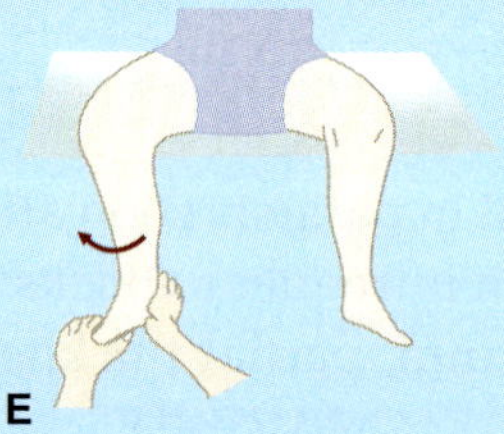

Fig. 19.17E

Steinmann's sign (Fig. 19.17E)
Meniscal pathology may be suspected if medial pain is elicited on lateral rotation (medial meniscus injury) and lateral pain on medial tibial rotation (lateral meniscal injury).

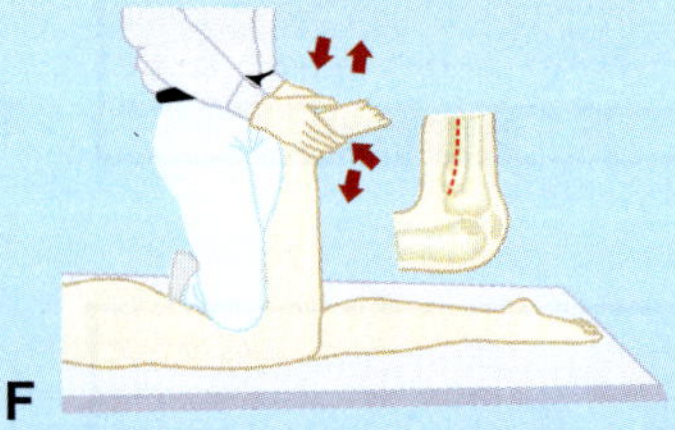

Fig. 19.17F

Apley's distraction test
(Fig. 19.17F) The technique is the same as above but here the examiner pulls the foot and leg upward to distract the joint while again rotating the tibia. Pain noted during axial distraction of joint implies a ligamentous lesion.

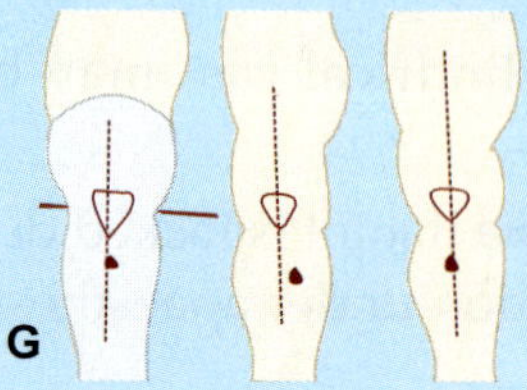

Fig. 19.17G

Helfet's sign (Fig. 19.17G)
In normal knee in sitting position tibial tubercle lies in line with midline of the patella. When extended, lateral tibial rotation puts it in line with lateral border of patella. *Positive sign occurs when the rotation is blocked by a torn meniscus and the tubercle remains centred over the patella in extension.*

Note

1. *The Apley's test is unique among the meniscus tests because of its ability to distinguish between ligamentous and meniscal lesions.*
2. *Positive meniscus test confirms the suspicion of meniscal lesion. However, negative tests do not rule out a tear with absolute confidence.*
3. *No one test is diagnostic, hence a combination of tests are carried out. With this, the accuracy rate* for *diagnosis raises by 60 to 95 per cent.*
4. *The routine work-up could best include joint line tenderness. McMurray's test and Steinmann's sign.*

Table 19.6: Classification of knee instability after performing the various tests mentioned earlier

	Tests	Structures injured
I. One plane instability		
One plane medial →	Abduction stress positive	Tibial collateral ligament + Medial capsule
One plane lateral →	Adduction stress positive →	Lateral capsule + Fibular collateral ligament
One plane posterior →	Posterior Drawer's test positive →	PCL + Arcuate complex
One plane anterior →	Anterior Drawer's test →	ACL + Medial and lateral positive capsular ligament
II. Two plane instability (rotary)		
Anteromedial →	Slocum's test +ve Rotary test +ve →	ACL + TCL + Posterior oblique ligament + Medial capsular tear.
Anterolateral →	Slocum's test +ve Rotary test +ve →	LCL + ACL + Arcuate complex + Lateral capsule.
Posteromedial →	Posterior drawer's, reverse pivot shift test, recurvatum test positive. →	TCL + Medial capsule + Posterior oblique ligament + ACL + Posteromedial capsule
Posterolateral →	Same as above →	FCL + PCL Arcuate complex + Lateral capsule
III. Combined		
a. Anterolateral posteromedial instability: (most common) →	Anterior drawer's test positive in neutral Ext and Int rotation position of the knee →	Anterior posterior lateral and medial structures injured
b. Anterolateral posterolateral instability: →	External rotation recurvatum test positive →	Anterolateral and posterolateral structures
c. Anteromedial and posteromedial instability: →	Knee opens medially Tibia rotates anteriorly at first and then moves posteriorly →	Anteromedial and posteromedial structures

Note: TCL—tibial collateral ligament, ACL—anterior cruciate ligament, PCL—posterior cruciate ligament, FCL—fibular collateral ligament

Methods

- *Arthroscopic meniscal repair:* This is the treatment of choice of late. Repair is indicated if the tear is > 10 mm or is unstable on probing. Repair is successful in the outer third (Red-red zone) edge of the vascular rim (Red-White zone) and even in a few avascular zone (White-White zone) (Fig. 19.18).
- *Closed partial meniscectomy* via an arthroscope is better than total removal of the menisci by open surgery (Fig. 19.19).
- *Meniscal transplant:* In cases with total menisectomies, cadaveric meniscal transplant may be considered. However, this is still in the evolving stage.

Complete removal of the menisci incapacitates the knee, hence, the emphasis is on conservative surgery than the radical removal.

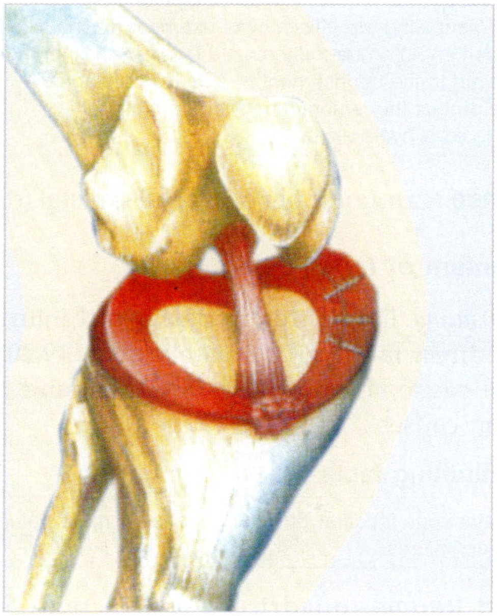

Fig. 19.18: Showing arthroscopic meniscal repair

Fig. 19.19: Smillie's meniscus knife used for meniscectomy

Treatment facts: Meniscal injuries

- Nothing like normal meniscus.
- If minor lesion and asymptomatic better leave it alone.
- Partial meniscectomy better than total.
- Resuturing in appropriate locations.
- *Earlier it was said, when in doubt remove, now the concept is when in doubt, observe do not treat.*

Note: How important are menisci to the knee?
Consider the following facts:
Partial meniscectomy increases stress by 50 to 60 per cent.
Total meniscectomy increases stress by 200 to 235 per cent.
Meniscal repair may normalise the stress.

FRACTURE OF PATELLA

Patella is the largest sesamoid bone in the body. The clinical picture of a patellar fracture is determined by a combination of definite and equivocal signs.

Functions of Patella

1. Increases the mechanical advantage of quadriceps tendon by increasing the efficiency of extensor mechansim by as much as 50% due to increased lever arm.
2. To aid in the nourishment of articular cartilage.
3. To protect the femoral condyles from injury.
4. Acts as a hydraulic brake.

Incidence is around 1 per cent of all skeletal fractures.

Mechanism of Injury

Direct trauma This is due to dashboard injuries and due to direct fall over the patella (Fig. 19.20). They usually cause comminuted fractures, and are the common causes.

Incriminating facts

Subcutaneous location of patella makes it more vulnerable for direct injures.

Indirect trauma (quadriceps contraction) Sudden forceful contraction of the quadriceps as in sports

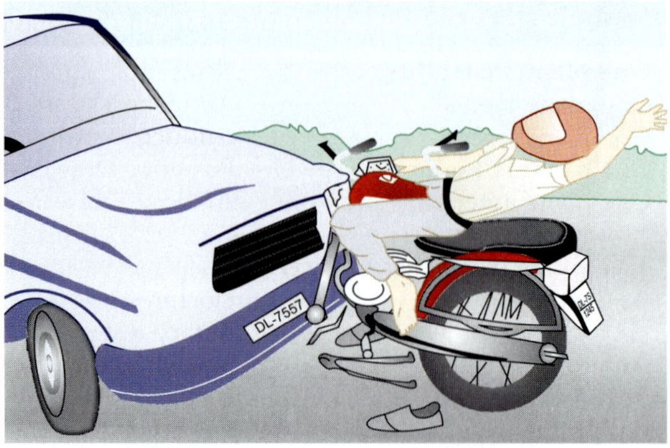

Fig. 19.20: Direct injuries due to road traffic accidents (RTAs) are a common cause of patellar fractures

person and athletes can cause patellar fractures. Here the fracture is usually transverse and sometimes avulsion fractures of the proximal or distal poles may also be seen.

Age Common in 20 to 50 years age group.

Male : Female = 2 : 1.

Classification (Fig. 19.21)

1. Undisplaced:
   a. Transverse fracture—These account for nearly 50 to 80 per cent of cases. About 80 per cent occur in the middle-third.
   b. Stellate fracture
   c. Vertical fracture

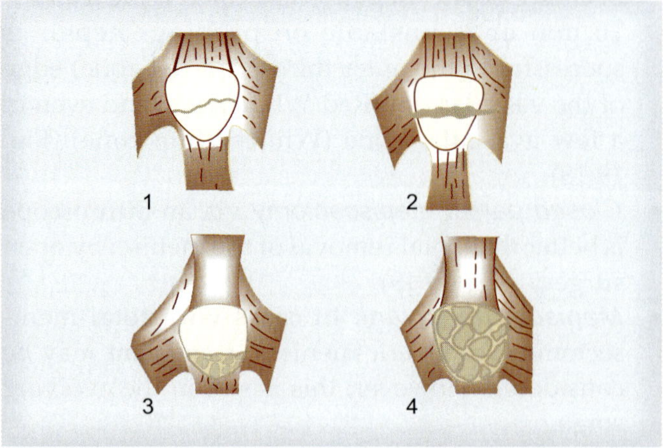

Fig. 19.21: Showing types of patellar fractures: (1) undisplaced fracture, (2) transverse fracture, (3) distal pole fracture, and (4) comminuted fracture

2. Displaced: If displacement is > 3 mm and if articular incongruity > 2 mm:
   a. Transverse—involving upper or lower poles (50 to 85%).
   b. Oblique fracture.
   c. Vertical fracture (12 to 27%).
   d. Comminuted fracture (30 to 35%).
   e. Polar—Could be proximal or distal.
   f. Osteochondral fractures.

Clinical Features

The patient gives history of trauma following which there is pain and swelling at the knee joint. The patient is unable to extend the knee and both the active and passive movements are restricted. On examination, there could be a palpable gap, tenderness, signs of effusion and a positive patellar tap (Figs 19.22A and B).

Investigations

- Radiograph of the knee joint consists of AP view, lateral view, intelcondylar notch view (Fig. 19.23) and skyline or axial view (Fig. 19.24) to rule out undisplaced vertical fracture.
- CT scan, bone scan and tomography are other useful investigations.

Note Bipartite patella and osteochondral fractures cause confusion in the diagnosis (Fig. 19.25).

Mystifying facts

- Do you know which patellar fractures are difficult to diagnose clinically? Well, it is the thin vertical fracture of the patella which has a very few clinical signs and symptoms.

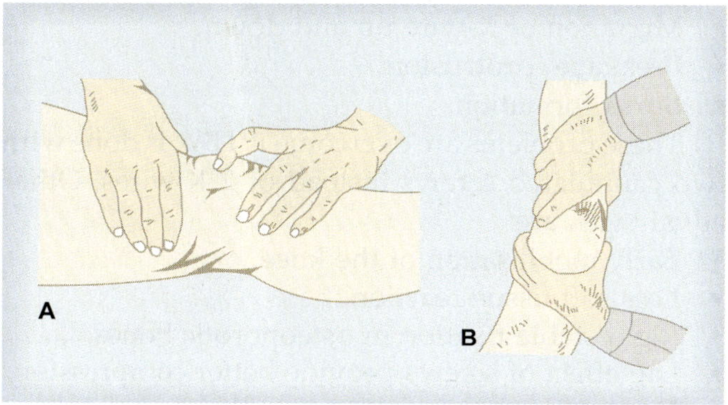

Figs 19.22A and B: Showing method to elicit: (A) Patellar tap, (B) Fluctuation test

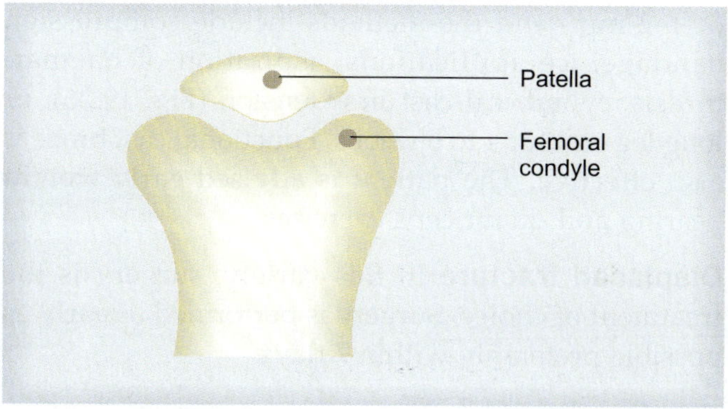

Fig. 19.23: Showing intercondylar notch view of patella

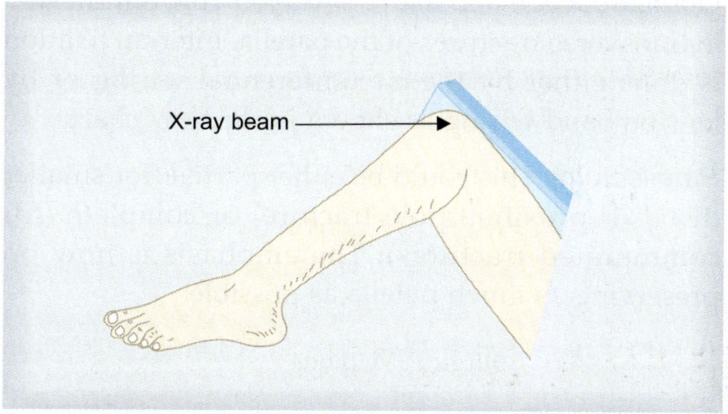

Fig. 19.24: Showing the axial view of the knee

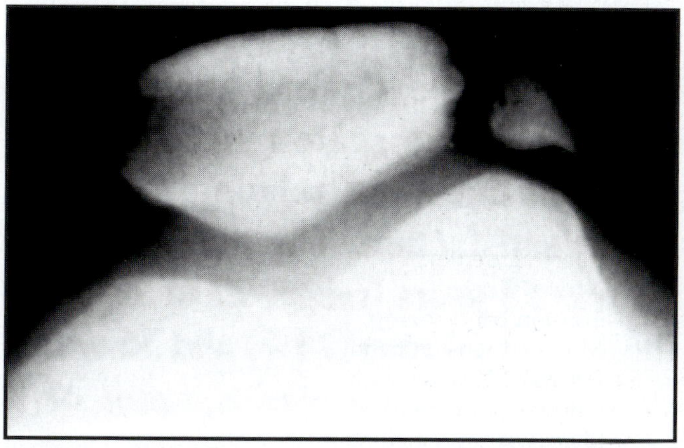

Fig. 19.25: Radiograph showing bipartitie patella (a diagnostic pitfall)

Management

Undisplaced fracture Nonoperative treatment will produce good results in undisplaced fracture and if displacement is less than 1 to 2 mm and in intact extensor mechanism and minimal articular step-off

(< 1–2 mm) and the methods include compression bandage, ice applications, aspiration of haemarthrosis, cylindrical cast in extension (Fig. 19.26), or long leg cast for 4 to 6 weeks. Functional cast brace is also effective. The patient is advised early weight bearing and quadriceps exercises.

Displaced fracture In this variety, surgery is the treatment of choice. Surgery is performed as early as possible preferably within 7 days.

Surgical Methods

Open reduction and internal fixation This is indicated in transverse fractures of the patella. Internal fixation is done either by the circumferential wiring or by tension band wiring as shown in the flow chart.

Patellectomy This could be either partial (for smaller distal or proximal pole fracture) or complete (for communited fractures). The emphasis is now on preserving as much patella as possible.

Surgical Methods

↓

- **Open reduction and internal fixation**
  - **For transverse fracture**
    - Martin's circumferential wiring around the patella through the surrounding soft tissues
    - Magnuson's interfragmentary wiring.
    - Tension band wiring
    - Modified tension band wiring (2-K wires with anterior placement)
    - Shaeuwacker's method: Interfragmentary screws + Fig of 8 tension band wiring
- **Patellectomy**
  - **Partial** For smaller proximal or distal pole
  - **Total** For comminuted fractures

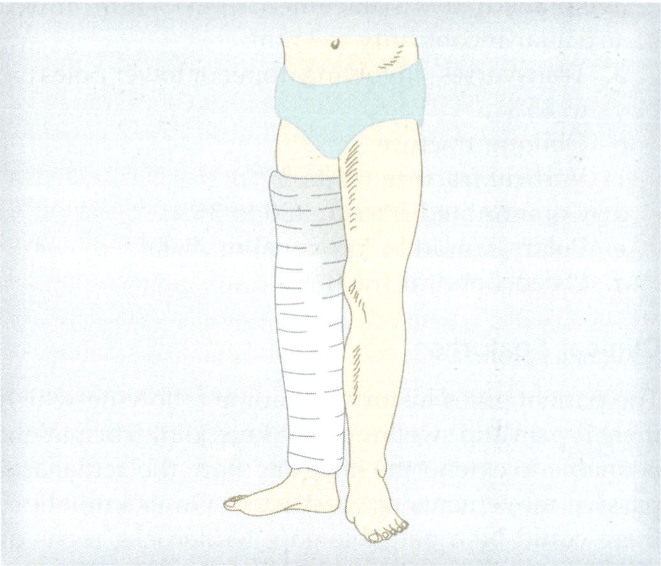

Fig. 19.26: Showing cylindrical cast

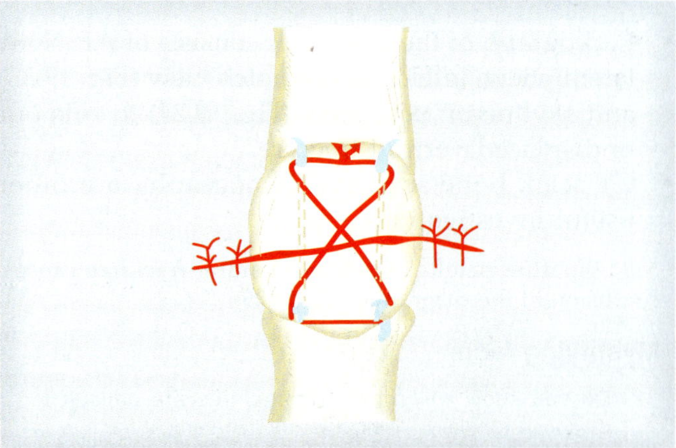

Fig. 19.27: Showing tension band wiring

Anterior Tension Band Wiring (ATBW) (Fig. 19.27)

ATBW though a popular method of stabilisation of patellar fractures, K-wires, offer the following problems:

- Migration of K-wire up and down.
- Breakage/protrusion.
- Bursa formation.

These problems are overcome if TBW is done with two cannulated screws instead of 2 K-wires. Other advantages are:

- Early mobilisation of the knee.
- Less soft tissue reaction.
- Rigid stable fixation in osteoporotic bones.
- Lag effect of screws provide better compression.
- Destructive forces shared equally by screws, and circlage wire, thereby reducing chances of breakage.

Complications

Postoperative complications Early fracture dehiscence, postoperative infection, refracture (1–5%), avascular necrosis (25% incidence in proximal pole) are some of the common postoperative complications.

Delayed complications This is like knee stiffness, osteoarthritis of the patellofemoral and knee joint extensor lag, etc. can also occur. Delayed union, nonunion, loss of knee motion, etc.

Disadvantages of Patellectomy

1. Strength of quadriceps returns slowly although knee motion is regained quite fast.
2. Obvious atrophy of the quadriceps muscle persists for months and often permanently.
3. Protection of the knee by the patella is lost.
4. Pathological ossification may develop where the patella is excised.

Extensor lag (Fig. 19.28) This is inability of the patient to perform the last 10° of extension. About 80 per cent of quadriceps strength is required to bring about the last 20° of extension. After patellectomy, due to the decreased lever arm the efficiency of quadriceps is reduced and the patient will be unable to bring about the terminal extension of the knee. *Thus, an attempt is made to save as much of patella as possible, all of the patella or at least the proximal or distal half, if practical to preserve the quadriceps efficiency.*

Disturbing facts

Do you know the common sequelae of patellar fractures?

- Patellofemoral arthritis
- Instability of the knee
- Decreased ROM of the knee
- Difficulty with stairs, downhill walking and kneeling

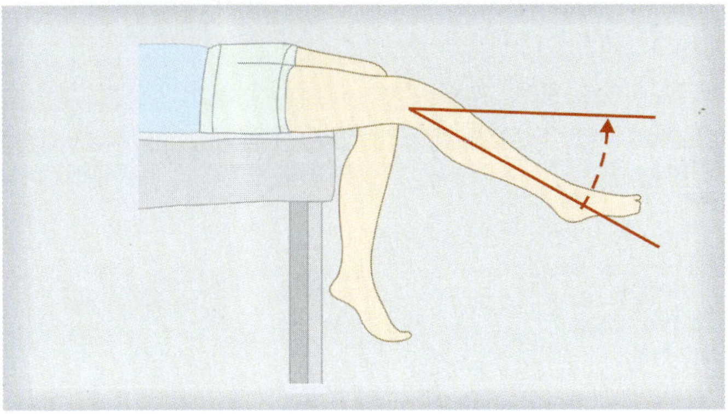

Fig. 19.28: Showing extensor lag

INJURY TO THE EXTENSOR APPARATUS OF KNEE

The extensor apparatus of the knee is comprised of the following six structures:

1. The quadriceps muscle with a group of six extensor muscles and the quadriceps femoris tendon.
2. Patella.
3. Ligamentum patellae (patellofemoral and patellotibial ligaments).
4. Patellar bursae and the fat pads.
5. Capsule and synovial membrane.

Note: The quadriceps muscle consists of rectus femoris, vastus medialis, lateralis intemedius, articularis genu and ligamentum patellae.

QUADRICEPS STRAIN

Causes

- Direct blow to the muscle.
- Indirect forces due to violent sudden contractions.

Sites

- Rectus femoris is the most commonly injured muscle.
- This is followed by vastus medialis, lateralis and intermedius.
- Avulsion may occur at the upper pole of patella or tibial tubercle and rarely through the patella.

Symptoms

- In rectus femoris injury, the patient complains of pain during hip flexion and knee extension as this muscle is known to act on both these joints. Tenderness is present at the site of injury.
- In grade III sprain a gap may be felt at the site of rupture and ambulation is difficult.
- In injuries to the vastus medialis, intermedius and lateralis the patient may complain of pain and limp, terminal stage of flexion and resisted knee flexion is extremely painful.

Treatment

In general, grade I and grade II injuries can be managed conservatively, while grade III injury may require surgical suturing in the event of complete rupture and loss of function (Fig. 19.29).

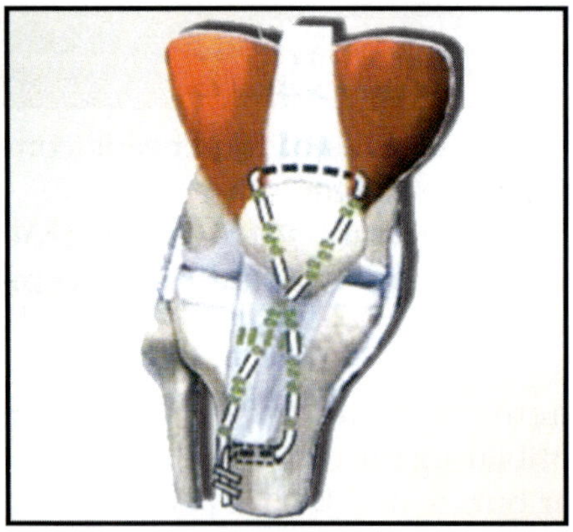

Fig. 19.29: Reconstruction of extensor mechanism

Treatment Methods

Grade I and II Strain

- Ice therapy and ice packs.
- Compression bandaging (Jones).
- Limb elevation.
- Mild isometric exercises.
- Relaxed passive knee movements.
- To improve the strength and mobility of the knee joint, active and active-assisted knee exercises are begun.
- Progressive resistive exercises to increase the endurance of the knee muscles.
- Gradual weight-bearing with assistive devices. The patient should be functionally independent by 6 weeks.

Grade III Strain

- Quadriceps exercises are begun by 5 to 6 days.
- Self-assisted SLR.
- By 2nd or 3rd days nonweight-bearing and partial weight-bearing by 3 weeks, full weight-bearing by 6 weeks
- For extensor lag, electrical stimulation helps.
- Rest of the measures are the same as mentioned above.

20

Fracture of Tibia and Fibula

- ❑ Proximal tibial fracture
- ❑ Fractures of tibia and fibula
- ❑ Open tibial fractures
- ❑ Distal tibial fractures

PROXIMAL TIBIAL FRACTURE

Proximal tibia consists of the medial and lateral condyles along with the upper tibial articular surface and includes the proximal 10 to 12 cm of the tibia (Fig. 20.1). These fractures are frequently intra-articular and usually unite well considering the cancellous nature of the bone.

Incidence 1 per cent of all fractures and 8% of fractures in elderly people.

Mechanism of injury It is due to valgus or varus force with axial loading.

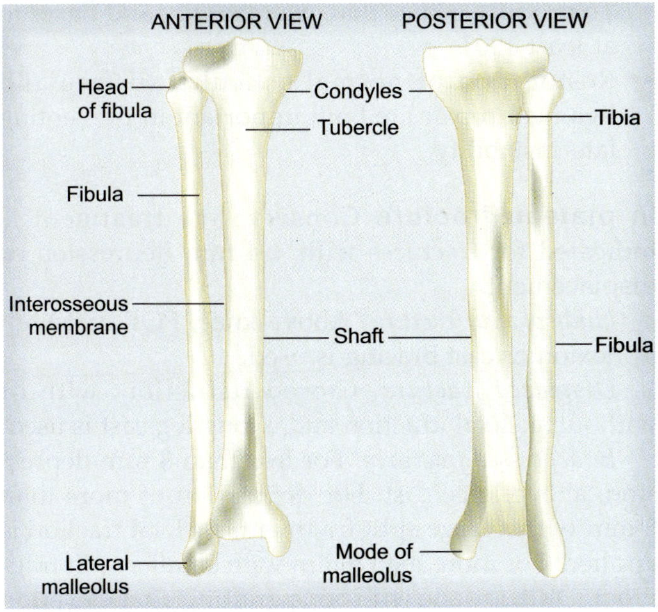

Fig. 20.1: Bony anatomy of tibia and fibula

Causes

- 52 per cent—due to auto-pedestrian injuries (Bumper injuries) (Fig. 20.2).
- 17 per cent—due to fall from heights.
- 31 per cent—miscellaneous causes (football or soccer injuries).

Interesting facts: Associated injuries with condylar fractures:

- Meniscal injury—50%
- Ligament injury—30%
- Peroneal nerve neuropraxia
- Popliteal artery injury.

Types

1. Articular variety
2. Nonarticular variety

Classification

Articular	Non-articular
Hohl and Moore's classification (Figs 20.3A to F)	e.g. fracture of tibial tuberosity

Articular ↓

Plateau Fracture	**Fracture Dislocation**
1. Minimally displaced fracture	1. Split fracture
2. Local compression fracture	2. Entire plateau fracture
3. Split compression fracture	3. Rim avulsion fracture
4. Total condylar depression fracture	4. Four part fracture
5. Bicondylar fracture	*Here soft tissue injuries produce* instability *and require surgery.*

Other Classifications

1. Schatazker's classification: This is widely followed in North America and has six types:
   - Type I — Split fracture of lateral condyle.
   - Type II — Displaced lateral condyle fracture.

Section 2

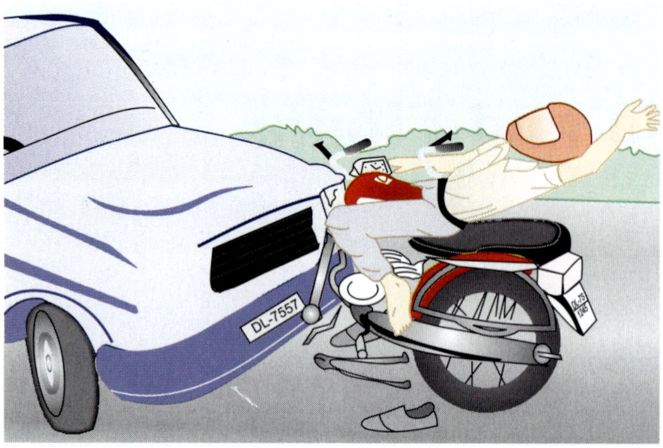

Fig. 20.2: Bumper injuries are a common cause of tibial fractures

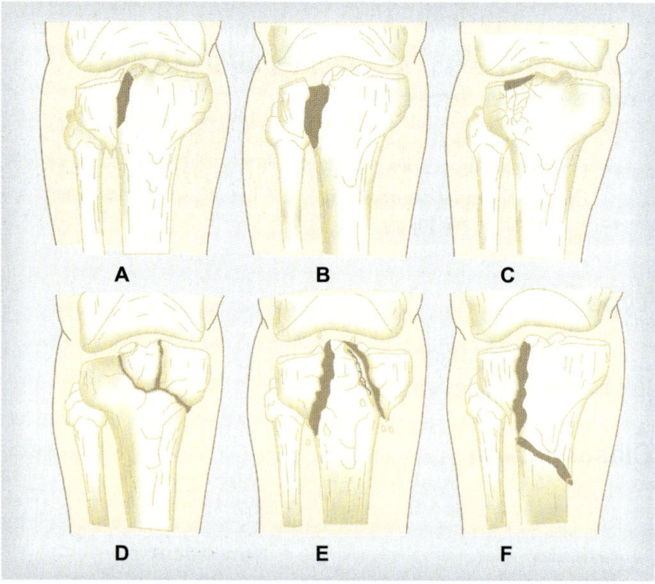

Figs 20.3A to F: Hohl and Moore's classification of proximal tibial fractures: (A) minimally displaced fracture, (B) local compression fracture, (C) split compression fracture, (D) total condylar depression, (E) bicondylar fractures, (F) bicondylar fracture with diaphyseal metaphyseal extension

- Type III — Isolated lateral condyle depression.
- Type IV — Medial condylar fracture.
- Type V — Bicondylar fractures.
- Type VI — Bicondylar fracture with diaphyseal metaphyseal extension.

2. Modified Hohl and Moore's classification.

Did you know?

Lateral condyle is fractured 70–80% more often than the medial condyle.

Interesting facts:

- Isolated lateral tibial condyle # — 55–70%
- Isolated medial tibial condylal # — 10–23%
- Both plateau fractures — 10–30%.

Clinical Features

The patient with proximal tibial fractures presents with pain, swelling, deformity, haemarthrosis, decreased movements of the knee and instability in valgus or varus. There could be features of compartment syndrome of the leg, disturbed peripheral vascular and nerve functions of the leg.

Investigations

The routine AP and lateral radiographs of the knee help to demonstrate majority of tibial condyle fractures. Oblique view may be required to localise the fractures. To study the depth of depression, CT scan is excellent, but 10° caudal plateau view also helps. To know the knee ligament injuries, valgus or varus stress films are required. Aspiration may reveal blood or fat. If fat is present, it indicates an intra-articular fracture. Angiography if pulses are feeble or absent.

Management

Aim

- To produce a knee that extends fully and flexes to at least 120°.
- Restoration of normal articular surface and ligament repair are both important in preventing late instability.

In plateau fracture Conservative treatment is indicated for fractures with < 4 mm depression or displacement.

Undisplaced fracture Above knee, POP cast with 5° flexion or cast bracing is used.

Displaced fracture Closed reduction, with or without skeletal traction and a long leg cast is used.

In depressed fractures For less than 8 mm depression, above knee cast. For depression of more than 8 mm with a large split fragment, skeletal traction is applied. For more than 8 mm with smaller split fragment, ORIF is done with bone grafting after elevation of the depression.

What is new in the treatment of tibial condylar fractures?
Of late lightweight UMEX external fixator frame is being tried with a reasonable success in treating the difficult and comminuted tibial condylar fractures.

Some surgeons advocate dual plating in difficult bicondylar fractures notwithstanding the many complications it opens up as a consequence of extensive exposure.

In split fracture Here closed reduction is not useful. Open reduction and internal fixation with cancellous screws, buttress plate, etc. are used (Fig. 20.4). Skeletal traction is useful in grossly comminuted fractures.

Complications

These include compartment syndrome, peroneal nerve palsy, popliteal artery laceration, nonunion (rare), malunion and degenerative arthritis.

Do you know what is a floating knee?
Well, it is an ipsilateral fracture of lower end of femur and upper end of tibia.

- It is usually compound.
- It is usually associated with vascular injuries.
- Surgery is the treatment of choice.

FRACTURES OF TIBIA AND FIBULA

Tibial shaft fractures are the most common long bone fractures and they are famous for high incidence of open fractures.

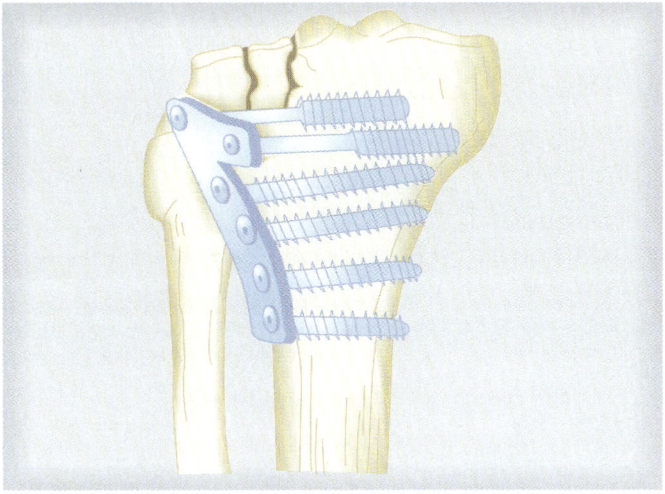

Fig. 20.4: Showing internal fixation of proximal tibial fracture with buttress plate and screws

Features of tibial fractures

- Most common of all long bone fractures. Next common to intracapsular fracture neck femur.
- More controversial, exceeded only by fracture neck femur.
- Subcutaneous and hence incidence of open fracture is high.
- Distal one-third has a deficient blood supply and a fracture in this area is known for delayed union and nonunion.
- Bounded above and below by hinge joints and hence no malunion is acceptable.
- Responds well to conservative treatment.
- Only 5 per cent need operative treatment.

Did you know?

- Isolated tibial fracture—23%
- Both tibia and fibular fractures—77%
- 77% of tibial fractures are closed
- 23% are open fractures
- The common site of tibial fractures due to indirect force is the region of the isthmus.

Mechanism of Injury

- RTA—37.5%
- Sports—24.7%
- Assaults—4.5%
- Falls—rest.

Direct violence due to road traffic accidents (most common mode of injury), fall, assault, etc. (Fig. 20.5). Open fractures are common in this mode of injury.

Indirect violence due to falls, twisting force due to sports injuries, usually cause spiral fractures.

Classification

1. Ellis

	Grades of severity	Features
I	Minor	• Undisplaced • Not angulated • Minor comminution • Minor open fracture
II	Moderate	• Total displacement • Small degreee of comminution Minor open wound
III	Major	• Complete displacement • Major comminution • Major open fracture

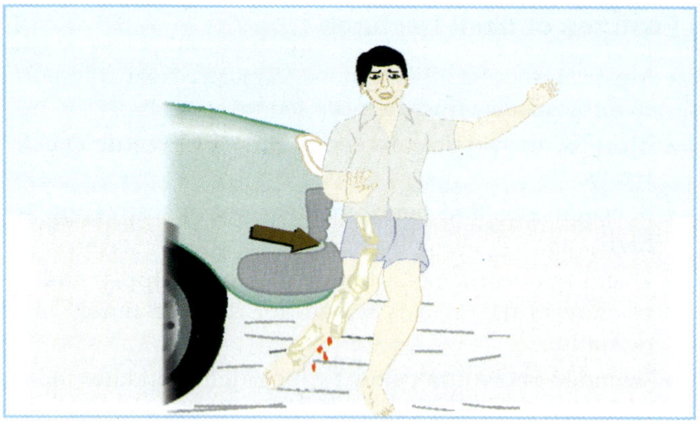

Fig. 20.5: Bumper injuries in RTA commonly cause fracture femur and tibia

2. Tscherne classification (takes into account soft tissue injuries too)
   C_0 — Simple fracture with no soft tissue injury.
   C_1 — Mild to moderate, fracture with superficial abrasions.
   C_2 — Moderately severe fractures with deep contusions.
   C_3 — Severe fracture with severe destruction of the soft tissues.

Interesting facts: What holds the tibial fractures together?

- Intact fibula
- Interosseous membrane intact
- Surrounding calf muscles.

Note: Many classifications like the OTA, Tscherne, Gustilo Anderson classification for open fractures are in vogue.

Clinical Features

In these fractures, the common symptom is pain and the obvious sign is the deformity, apart from other features of fractures. Damage to the blood vessels and nerves is not that common, but fibular neck fracture may injure the lateral popliteal nerve; and if the posterior tibial vessels are injured, compartmental syndrome may develop.

Radiography

Radiograph for acute cases require AP and lateral views. For delayed cases, AP, lateral and oblique views (Fig. 20.6) may be required. Knee joint above and ankle below should always be included.

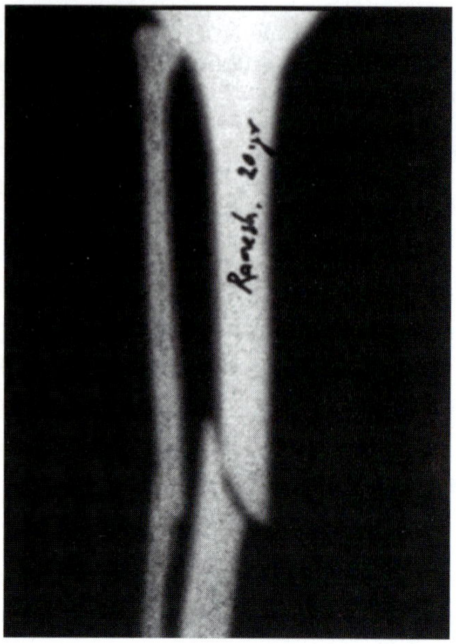

Fig. 20.6: Radiograph showing fracture of tibia and fibula

Interesting facts:

Do you know fibula bears approximately 12% of the body weight?

Methods of Treatment

Conservative management This consists of closed reduction under general anaesthesia and a long leg cast application (Fig. 20.7).

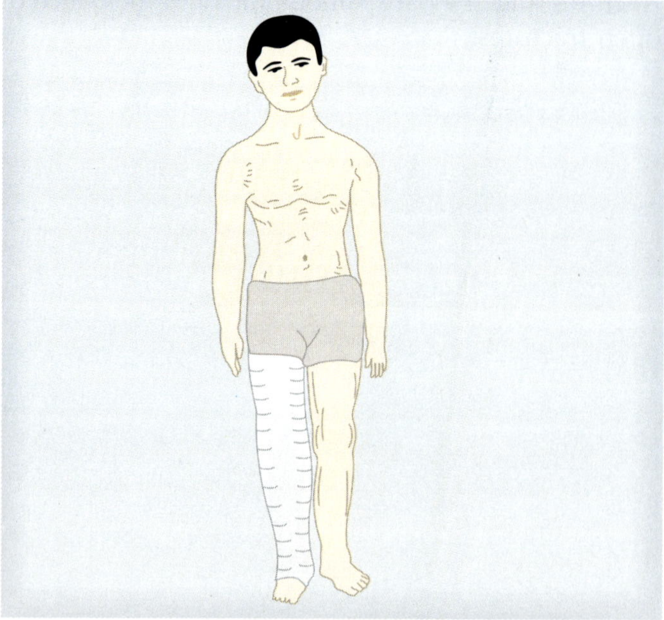

Fig. 20.7: Fracture tibia treated with long leg cast

Long Leg Plaster Casts

Indications

- Most closed fractures.
- Undisplaced fracture.
- Fractures with minor or moderate displacements.
- Young adults.
- Low energy trauma.

Methods of reduction There are two methods of closed reduction. In the first, the patient is supine and is under general anaesthesia. With the limb held parallel to the table, the fracture is reduced by traction and countertraction method (by an assistant) and a long leg cast is applied. The disadvantage with this technique is due to the gravitational forces, posterior angulation develops at the fracture site.

In the second and more commonly followed method (Fig. 20.8), the patient is supine under anaesthesia or sitting. The patient is brought to the edge of the table and both the legs are kept dangling. Through a halter, the clinician holds the leg of the patient and manipulates the fracture. A long leg cast is then put with the knee in slight flexion and the ankle at 90°.

Criteria of acceptable reduction

- Rotation should be nearly perfect.
- Ankle and knee joint surfaces should be parallel.
- Acceptable varus or valgus angulation is 5° in AP view.
- Anterior or posterior angulation of 10° in lateral view.
- Even 50 per cent apposition is acceptable provided there is no rotation.
- Shortening of 5–7 mm is acceptable.

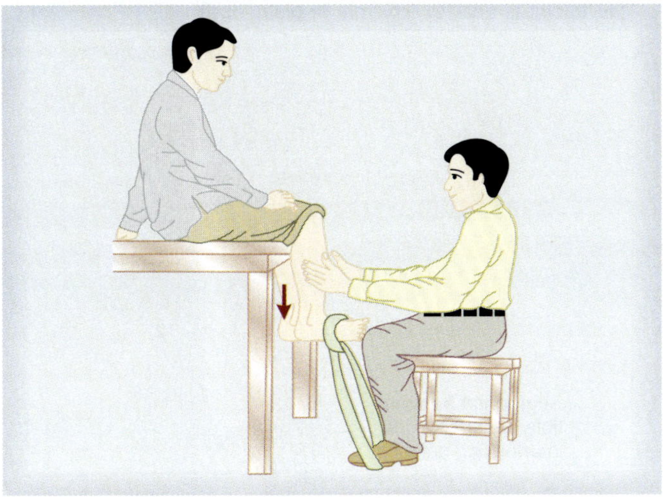

Fig. 20.8: Reduction technique of fracture tibia

The advantages of this method are:

1. Traction and countertraction do not require the services of an assistant.
2. The patient's own weight of the leg provides traction through the gravity.
3. Easy to compare with the normal leg regarding the accuracy of closed reduction by looking at the control of rotation and angle.

Did you know?

Böhler of Vienna was the first person to use and popularise the long leg casts for tibial fractures.

Concept of wedge plaster correction

For postreduction angulation of the fracture tibia which is in a plaster cast, the technique of wedge correction of the plaster will enable the surgeon to correct the residual angulation without removing the original plaster cast.

In a postreduction radiograph, the direction of the angulation whether medial or lateral, anterior or posterior is noted. Then an attempt is made to correct the angulation by either opening a wedge or closing a wedge in the cast. In the open wedge plaster correction, the plaster is cut at the opposite end of the angulation and opened thereby correcting the angulation. In the closed wedge technique, a wedge of plaster cast is removed at the apex of the angulation and the plaster cast is closed correcting the angulation (Fig. 20.9).

The open wedge technique is preferred over closed wedge because of the chances of the skin being caught within the plaster edges in the closed technique. After either procedure, the plaster cast is completed and a check radiograph is taken to confirm the correction.

Sarmiento's Total Contact Below Knee Cast

After reduction of the fracture and application of a long leg cast for 2 to 3 weeks, a total below knee cast which is moulded around the tibial condyles and patella in the fashion of patellar tendon bearing prosthesis is applied (PTB casts or brace) (Fig. 20.10).

Advantages

- Allows early knee movements.
- Sitting can be permitted early.
- Ease of ambulation for patients with bilateral fracture.
- Decreases the incidence of delayed union and nonunion.

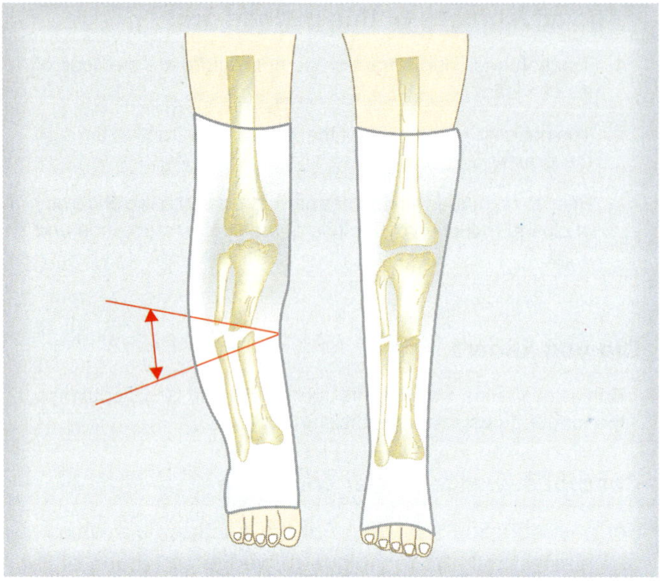

Fig. 20.9: Residual postreduction angulation corrected by closed wedge plaster technique

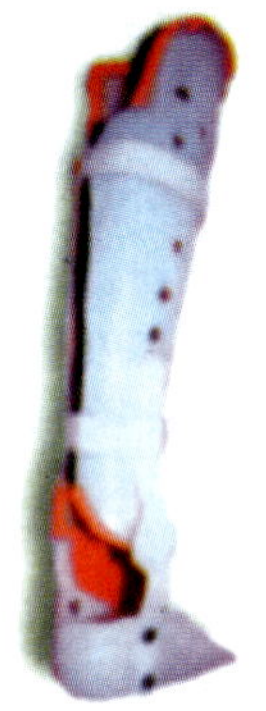

Fig. 20.10: Showing Sarmiento's total contact below knee cast

Functional Braces

This allows movements of both ankle and knee joints, while the PTB cast includes the ankle joint also.

Pins Above and Below the Fracture

Here two Steinmann's pins are passed above and below the fracture site and incorporated within the plaster cast. This method is, however, no longer used except in some remote centres.

Indications

1. For moderate and severe fracture.
2. Unstable fracture.
3. Open fracture.

Surgical Treatment

Open reduction and internal fixation As mentioned earlier, only 5 per cent of the cases require operative treatment in tibial fractures.

Advantages

1. Definitive form of treatment.
2. No loss of position or shortening.
3. No postfracture deformity.
4. Joint movements obtained early.

Absolute indications

1. Tibial fracture with vascular or neural injuries.
2. Segmental fractures.
3. Inadequate reduction.
4. Associated knee problems.
5. Associated tibial plafond fracture.

Internal fixation methods (See flow chart) (Fig. 20.11A).

Not so long ago, plating as the internal fixation methods ruled the roost so much so that tibial fractures were plated right, left and centre.

But slowly interlocking nailing emerged as the *Gold Standard* and pushed the technique of plating into oblivion. It appears that with its obvious advantages interlocking nailing is here to stay (Fig. 20.11B).

The conventional nails are the GK nail and the RT nails with the proximal and distal holes. However, new generation nails are fast emerging as an effective alternative.

Know About Newer Generation Nails:

There are nails with multiple holes in different planes, in order to maximize the options for interlocking and to allow nailing of the fractures near to proximal or distal ends.

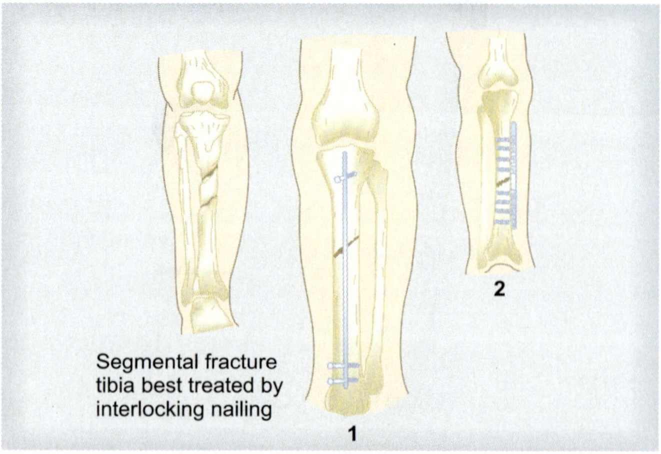

Fig. 20.11A: Methods of internal fixation in tibial fracture (1) interlocking nailing, (2) DCP plate and screws

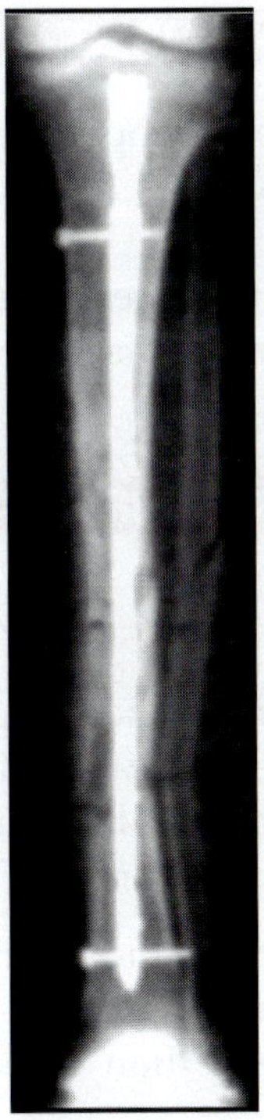

Fig. 20.11B: Radiograph showing ILN tibia

Note: The other most important advantage of ILN nailing is that the fracture need not be opened it can be managed closed.

Internal fixation methods

Compression Plating for ↓ (1970's)	IM nails ↓ (Rare)	Interlocking nails (Recent) ↓
1. Intra-articular fractures	Not as successful as for femur	Done in ↓
2. Arterial injuries with fracture	↓ Done in	1. Proximal ¼ fractures
3. Segmental fractures 4. Some open fractures 5. Short, oblique, lower 1/3 tibial fractures	↓ Noncomminuted transverse or short oblique fracture of the middle 1/3	2. Distal ¼ fractures (up to 5 cm above ankle) 3. Comminuted fractures 4. Segmental fractures

Note: ILN could be reamed or unreamed.

Vital points:

Unlocked IM nail is useful only in transverse or short oblique fracture that too only at the isthmus level. These fractures are few and hence it has limited usage.

Role of external fixators This is useful in compound fractures of the tibia as it enables to stabilise the fracture and also helps to take care of the wound (Fig. 20.12).

Types of External Fixators: Three types

1. Uniplanar: Most popular. Easy to apply. Applied on anteromedial surface with 4 to 6 pins.
2. Multiplanar: Quadrilateral or triangular frame. These increase the usage.
3. Circular frame (Ilizarov).

Complications of Tibial Fractures

1. *Delayed union* This is a common complication and has an incidence of 1 to 17 per cent. If there is no evidence of union of the fracture even after 20 weeks, delayed union is suspected and is treated with cancellous bone graft.
2. *Nonunion* This is a notorious problem usually encountered in fractures at the junction of middle one-third and lower one-third. It can be treated by electric stimulation or rigid internal fixation with compression plating and cancellous bone grafting.
3. *Infected nonunion* It poses a tough challenge to the orthopaedic surgeons and is best managed by Ilizarov's method of external fixation.

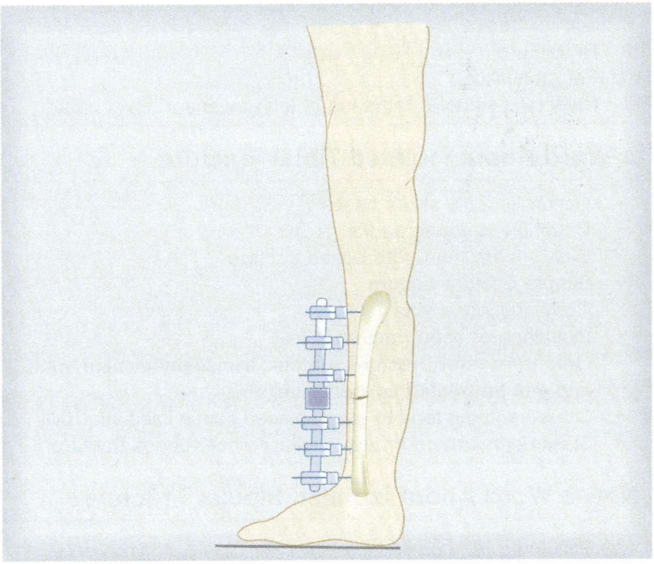

Fig. 20.12: External fixator treatment of choice for open tibia fractures

4. *Malunion* Because of the parallel hinge knee and ankle joints above and below, malunion of tibia is an unacceptable problem as it may cause early degenerative arthritis. Corrective osteotomy is the treatment of choice.
5. *Shortening* This may be due to malunion or overlap of the fracture fragments, less than 2 cm shortening is acceptable and may be corrected by footwear adjustments, while more than 2 cm shortening may require bone lengthening procedures.
6. *Infection* Due to the subcutaneous location of the bone, infection is a fairly common complication in these fractures due to a higher frequency of compound fractures following RTAs.
7. *Other complications* Compartmental syndromes, joint stiffness, refractures, fat embolism and claw toes due to tethering of the long extensors over the callus are the other common complications.
8. Reflex Sympathetic Dystrophy (RSD).

Quick facts

Complications of tibial fracture

1. Delayed union
2. Nonunion
3. Infected nonunion
4. Malunion
5. Shortening
6. Infection
7. Compartmental syndromes
8. Joint stiffness
9. Refracture
10. Fat embolism
11. Claw toes—due to tethering of long extensors over callus

A Word About Isolated Tibial Fracture

- Occurs in 22% of the cases
- Common in young adults
- Less severe than both bones fracture
- Simple fracture pattern
- Comminution is less
- Incidence of open fracture is less
- Only transverse fracture without displacement heal well and can be treated conservatively
- Other fractures tend to get displaced hence fixed internally
- Treatment is more or less similar to both bones fracture.

Now a Word About Isolated Fibular Fractures

- Seen in three situations
  a. Avulsion fracture of proximal fibula.
  b. Syndesmotic fibular fracture on ankle injuries.
  c. True isolated fibular fractures.
- Nonoperative treatment is enough
- Operative treatment if nonunion develops.

OPEN TIBIAL FRACTURES

As mentioned previously, open fractures are frequently seen in tibial fractures due to its subcutaneous location.

The principles of treatment, methods of treatment and complications are as discussed in Chapter 3 *(ref. p. 23)*.

DISTAL TIBIAL FRACTURES

PILON FRACTURES (SYN: TIBIAL PLAFOND FRACTURES)

These are severe injuries and are predominantly due to axial loading forces following the RTA or fall from height unlike the malleolar fractures which are mainly due to rotational forces (Figs 20.13A to C).

Incidence Here are some of the vital statistics concerning the pilon fractures:

- It accounts for less than 10% of all lower limb fractures
- Males are more commonly affected than females
- Mean age is 35 to 40 years.

Classifications The important classifications have been described namely.

1. *Ruedi and Allgower classifications* Till recently, this was the classification that was widely used. Three varieties are described.
   - Type I — Undisplaced cleavage fracture of the joint.
   - Type II—Displaced but minimally comminuted fractures.
   - Type III—Highly comminuted and displaced fractures.
2. *AO/OTA Classification* This is the most recent classification and it consists of the following varieties (Figs 20.14A to C).
   - Type A—Extra-articular fractures.
   - Type B—Partial intra-articular fractures.
   - Type C—Total intra-articular fractures.

Depending upon the amount of comminution, each variety is divided into three groups. Any of these groups are again divided into three subgroups depending on the fracture characteristics.

The associated soft tissue injuries are classified into four categories from 0 to 3 from negligible damage to extensive soft tissue damage. This classification was proposed by Tscherne and Goetzen.

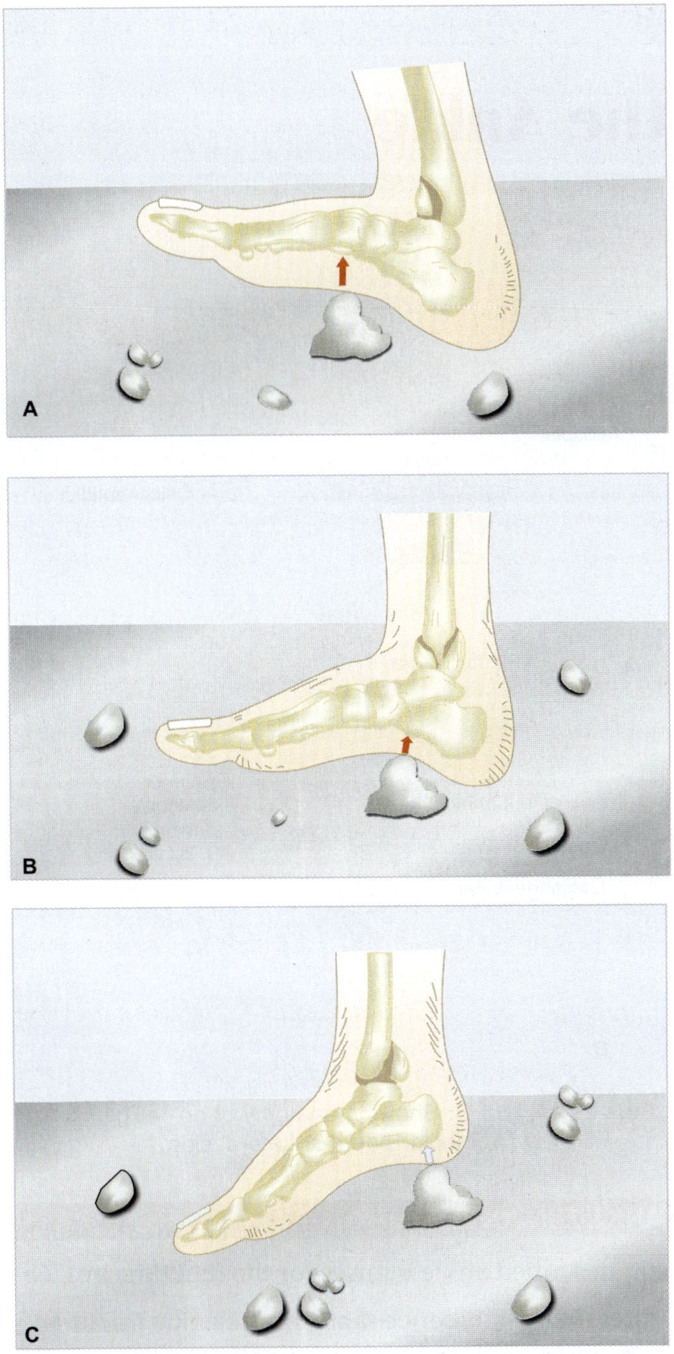

Figs 20.13A to C: Showing mechanism of injury of pilon fractures

Clinical Features

The patient complains of pain, swelling, deformity and inability to bear weight. Open wounds are a

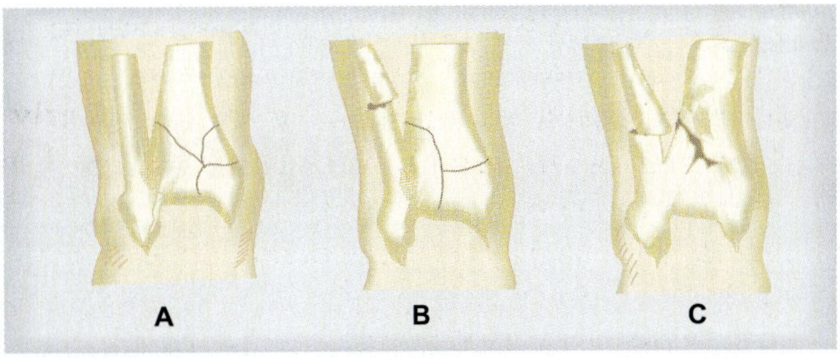

Figs 20.14A to C: Showing varieties of pilon fractures (OTA varieties)

disaster and the patient may complain of cold, clammy feet and loss of sensation.

Findings

Look for the peripheral pulses and the sensations in the foot. There may be gross deformity and swelling of the foot. The open injuries may vary from a small wound to major gush injuries.

Look for local bruising, fracture blisters and if there is a tense calf muscle, it indicates the development of the dreaded compartmental syndrome.

Investigations

Routine X-rays of the ankle consists of the AP, lateral and ankle mortise views.

CT scan is more useful and gives more information about the nature and extent of the injury than mere X-rays.

Treatment

Minimally displaced fractures (Type A variety) can be treated conservatively with a plaster cast on external fixation.

Grossly displaced fractures require surgical treatment consisting of open reduction and internal fixation with plate and screws. Other forms of external fixation methods are:

a. Hybrid fixation
b. Ilizarov's fixation
c. Monolateral fixator.

These external fixators can be used cross ankle or on the same side of the joint.

What is new?

Hybrid external fixator is fast emerging as an effective treatment option for pilon fractures.

21

Injuries of the Ankle

- ❑ Brief anatomy
- ❑ Ankle injuries
- ❑ Ankle sprains
- ❑ Tendo-Achilles injury

BRIEF ANATOMY

THE ANKLE JOINT SPEAKS

I am a complex joint made up of distal ends of tibia, fibula and the talus. The tibiofibular joint functions as a uniplanar hinge joint and in which about 25° of dorsiflexion and 35° of plantar flexion takes place. I am fully congruous in all positions. The stability is provided by the configuration of the ankle mortise and the ligaments which are arranged in the following three groups:

Medial collateral ligament consists of deltoid ligament with a superficial or deep part (Fig. 21.1A).

Lateral collateral ligament is formed by anterior and posterior talofibular ligaments and calcaneofibular ligament (Fig. 21.1B).

Syndesmotic ligaments are formed by anterior tibiofibular ligament, the posterior tibiofibular ligament, the inferior transverse ligament and the interosseous ligament

It is interesting to note that I am surrounded on all sides by the following structures:

1. *Anteriorly* Tendons of tibialis anterior, extensor hallucis longus, tibial vessels and nerves, tendons of extensor digitorum longus, and posterior tibialis in that order. These structures are held in position by the superior and inferior retinaculae.
2. *Posteromedial* Tendons of tibialis posterior, flexor digitorum longus, posterior tibial vessels and nerves and tendon of flexor hallucis longus pass in that order behind and below the medial malleolus. Flexor retinaculae hold them in position.
3. *Posterolateral* Peroneus longus and brevis held in position by superior and inferior peroneal retinaculae.
4. *Posteriorly* It is the tendo-Achilles and plantaris. These tendons are all covered by synovial sheaths. I am the fulcrum at which the leg transmits the body weight to the foot. My peculiarity lies in the fact that I have no muscular covering on any of my sides.

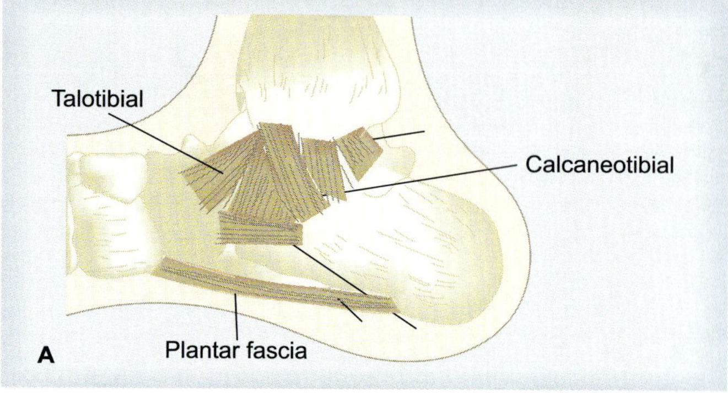

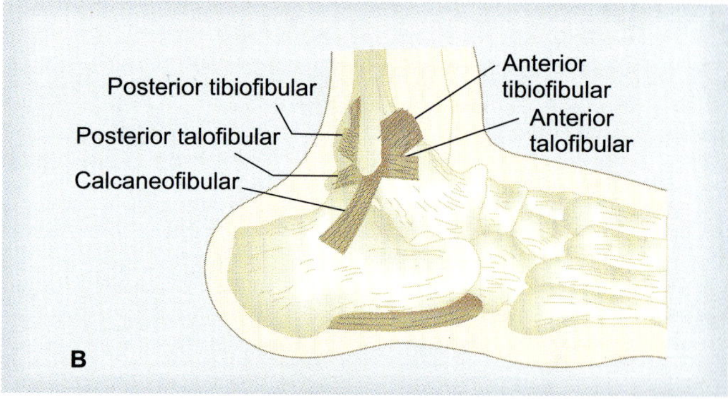

Figs 21.1A and B: Showing anatomy of ankle ligaments: (A) Medial side, (B) Lateral side

ANKLE INJURIES

Pott described ankle injuries for the first time in 1768.

Interesting 'Incidence facts' about ankle fractures

- More commonly in elderly women
- About 2/3—are isolated malleolar fracture
- About 1/4—are bimalleolar fracture
- Trimalleolar fracture—seen only in 7%
- Open fracture—2%

Mechanism of Injury Ankles are usually injured due to low injury rotational forces due to:

- Twisting injury while walking, running, sports, athletes, etc. are the most common mode of ankle injuries (Figs 21.2 and 21.3)

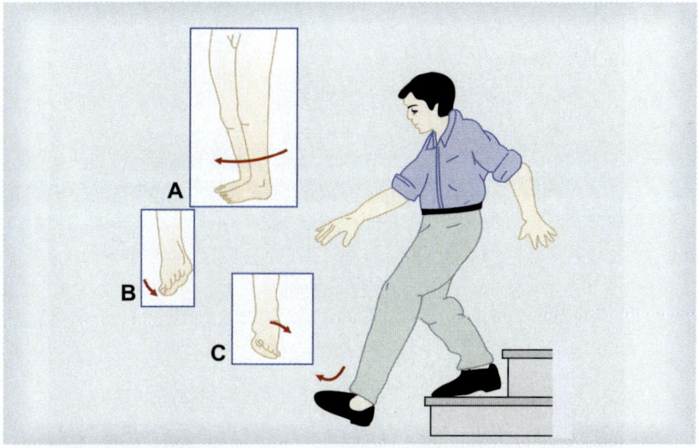

Figs 21.2A to C: Showing common mechanism of ankle injuries: (A) external rotation force, (B) abduction force, (C) adduction force. Inversion injury while getting down the stairs is a common mode of ankle injury

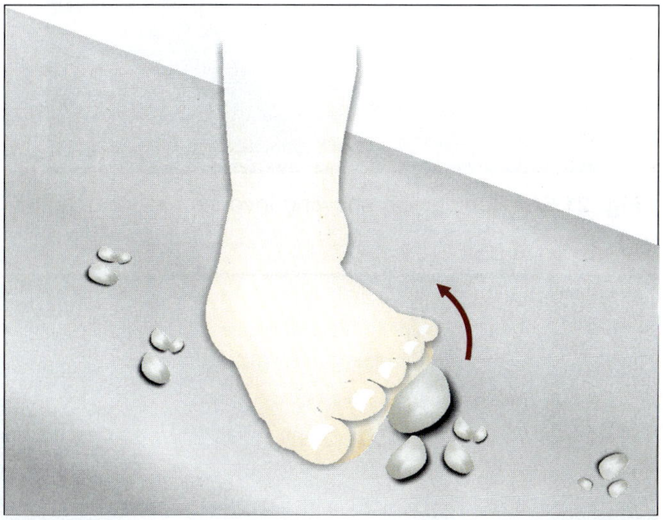

Fig. 21.3: Showing eversion mechanism of ankle injury

- *Fall from a height:* Ankle injuries are indirect injuries here brought about by the displacing talus.

Classification

Ankle injuries are classified after the mechanism causing them. Hence, it is of paramount importance to understand the movement of the ankle to comprehend the classification. What complicates the issue is the practice of using more than one term to describe the same motion.

There are six movements of the ankle and the hindfoot. *Plantar flexion* and *dorsiflexion* are the up and down movements of the foot. Movement causing the toes to point inwards is called *internal rotation* and movement causing the toes to point outwards is called *external rotation. Supination* is the movement which raises the medial aspect of the foot and the heel off the ground. In *pronation,* the motion is to bring the lateral aspect of the foot and the heel from the ground. In *adduction,* the hindfoot is moved towards the midline and in *abduction* is moved laterally. Pure vertical loading position as in landing, jumping, falling, etc. will cause Pylon fracture by the driving of the talus into the tibia (see page).

Lauge Hansen's Classification

Four major types are described. The mechanism of injury could be adduction force, abduction force or external rotation force. The foot could be in supination or pronation (Figs 21.4A to E). The first word refers to the position of the foot at the time of injury and the second to the direction of injuring force.

Supination adduction

Stage I	Transverse fracture of lateral malleolus or tear of lateral collateral ligament
Stage II	Stage I + fracture of medial malleolus

Supination eversion

Stage I	Rupture of anterior inferior tibiofibular ligament
Stage II	Stage I + spiral oblique fracture of the lateral malleolus
Stage III	Stage II + posterior lip of fracture of tibia (posterior malleolar fracture)
Stage IV	Stage III + fracture medial malleolus or tear of deltoid ligament

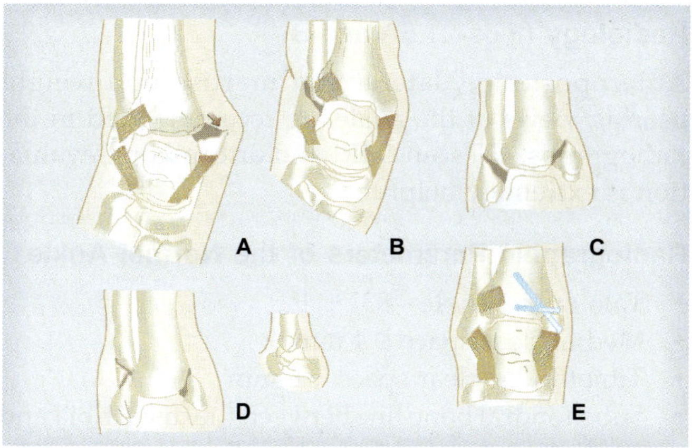

Figs 21.4A to E: Lauge Hansen's classification: (A) Supination adduction, (B) Supination eversion, (C) Pronation abduction, (D) Pronation external rotation, (E) Fracture fixed with malleolar screws

Pronation abduction

Stage I	Fracture medial malleolus or tear of deltoid ligament
Stage II	Stage I + rupture of anteroinferior tibiofibular ligament and posterior inferior tibiofibular ligament with fracture posterior lip of tibia
Stage III	Stage II + oblique supramalleolar fracture of the fibula.

Pronation-external rotation

Stage I	Fracture medial malleolus or tear of deltoid ligament
Stage II	Stage I + tear of anteroinferior tibiofibular and interosseous ligament
Stage III	Stage II + tear of interosseous membrane and spiral fracture of the fibula
Stage IV	Stage III + fracture of posterior lip of tibia due to ligamentous avulsion by posterior inferior and inferior and transverse tibiofibular ligament

Note: About 75 per cent of the cases fall into the first two groups.

Denis Weber Classification

This is the other classification proposed for ankle injuries and it is based on the *level of the fibular fracture,* while the Lauge Hansen's system is based on experimentally verified injury mechansim like adduction, abduction, etc.

Clinical Features

The patient usually gives history of inversion injury, following which there is pain, swelling, deformity of the ankle. Movements are decreased, Drawer's test, inversion and eversion stress tests may be positive. Note the color and condition of the skin. Examine the entire leg.

Radiology (Figs 21.5A and B)

Anteroposterior, lateral and mortise non-weight bearing views of the ankle are recommended in the radiographs. CT scan, MRI and arthroscopy evaluation is extremely helpful.

Radiographic Parameters of the Normal Ankle

- Talo crural angle—83° ± 4°
- Medial clear space ≤ 4 mm
- Tibiofibular clear space < 6 mm
- Subchondral bone line between the distal tibia and medial surface of lateral malleolus should be continuous.

Note: All these parameters are best studied in Mortise views.

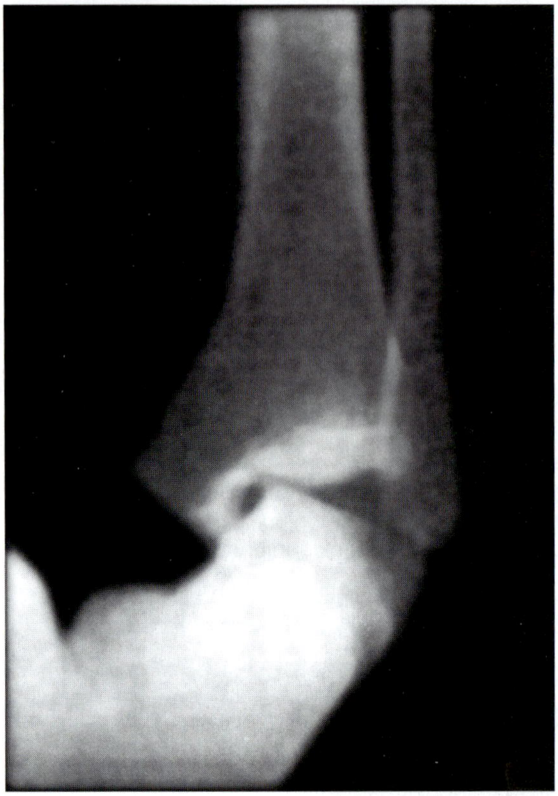

Fig. 21.5A: Radiograph showing inversion injury of ankle

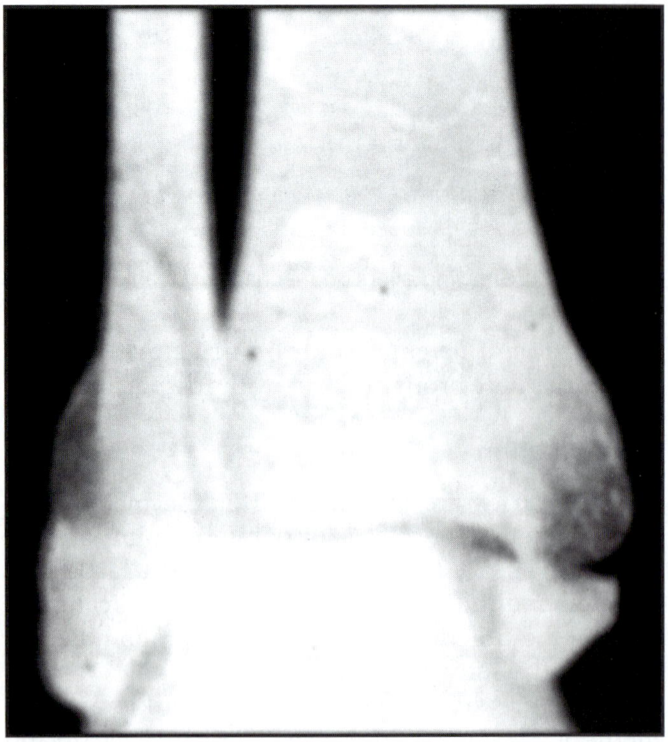

Fig. 21.5B: Radiograph showing bimalleolar ankle fracture

Treatment

Goals

1. Anatomical positioning of the talus beneath the tibia.
2. To obtain a joint line that is parallel to the ground.
3. Smooth articular surface.

If these three things are not achieved, post-traumatic osteoarthritis results.

For stable injuries no reduction is required, immobilisation with only plaster splints till the swelling decreases and then a below-knee plaster cast is applied with foot in neutral position.

Unstable injuries require reduction and immobilisation in plaster casts. The commonly encountered unstable injuries are:

a. *Fracture due to external rotation* This is more common and can be managed both by conservative and operative methods.
   Conservative method This consists of reversal of the injuring forces by closed reduction and a below-knee plaster cast application (Fig. 21.6). A walking cast is applied after a period of one month.
   Surgical method In this, both the malleoli are fixed, first the lateral malleolus is fixed with pin or screws and later the medial malleolar fracture is fixed with a single screw perpendicular to the fracture line. Below knee splint is given initially and later a cast is applied.

b. *Fracture primarily due to abduction* These are less common than the fractures due to external rotation. But, however, the principles of the treatment remains the same. Adduction force is required to bring about reduction and if closed reduction fails, open reduction is preferred. During the open reduction, both the malleoli are fixed.

c. *Fracture primarily due to adduction* Unlike external rotation and abduction, adduction violence is more frequently an isolated event. Wedging of small comminuted fragments into the fracture line often prevents closed reduction, so that open reduction and internal fixation (ORIF) is required more frequently.
   Medial malleolus is approached first, since it is more unstable, and the fracture is fixed with two screws, one at right angle to the tibial cortex and another at right angle to the fracture line (Fig. 21.7). Lateral fibular fracture is stabilised with plate and screws.

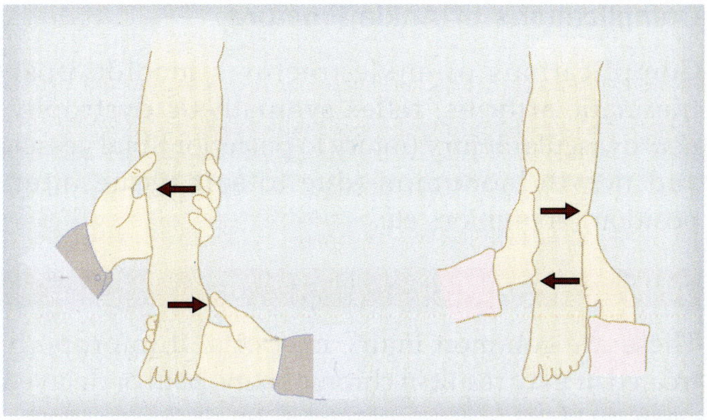

Fig. 21.6: Showing methods of closed reduction of ankle fractures

d. *Fracture resulting from primarily vertical compression* This may be isolated or associated with other forces described above. The anterior and posterior tibial plafond margins are fractured. Two types are described:
   1. *Posterior marginal fracture* For undisplaced fracture, below knee cast is sufficient. For more than 25 per cent of articular surface involvement, ORIF with 2 screws is preferred.
   2. *Anterior marginal fracture (tibial plafond injury)* It may include a crush of the anterior lip or it may include a major fragment. If crushed, calcaneal traction is given and if there is a large fragment, ORIF is required.

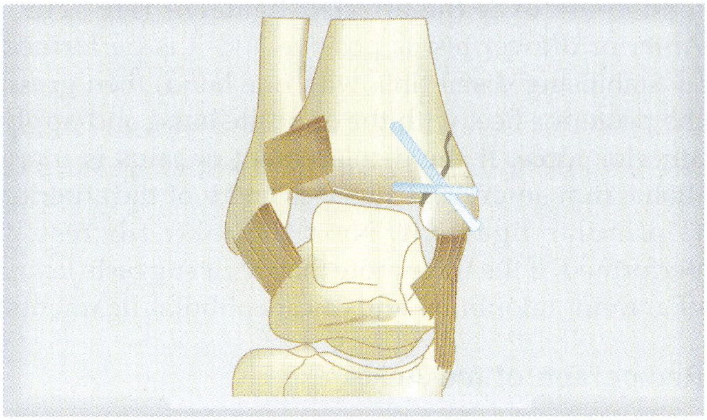

Fig. 21.7: Showing method of internal fixation of medial malleolar fracture

Complications of Ankle Fracture

Complications of ankle fractures include post-traumatic arthritis, reflex sympathetic dystrophy, neurovascular injury (injury to posterior tibial vessels and nerve), nonunion (due to soft tissue interposition), malunion, etc.

ANKLE SPRAINS

These are common injury in sports. If improperly treated, it may result in chronic laxity, pain or delayed recovery.

Quicks facts: Involvement of Various Structures in Ankle Sprain

- Complete rupture of the anterior tibiotibular ligament (ATFL)—65%
- Both ATFL and calcaneofibular ligament—20%
- Anterior inferior tibiofibular ligament (high ankle sprain)—10%
- Deltoid ligament—3%.

Lateral Ligament Sprain (Fig. 21.8)

This is the most common musculoskeletal injury with an incidence of 1/10,000/day. In 85 per cent of cases, it is due to inversion of supinated plantar flexed foot. The lateral ligament commonly injured is anterior talofibular ligament followed by calcaneofibular ligament. The posterior talofibular ligament is rarely sprained (Fig. 21.8).

Note: Lateral ankle sprain is the most common soft tissue limb injury and < 15% actually show a significant fracture.

Clinical Features

The patient complains of pain, swelling and tenderness over the affected ligament (Fig. 21.9). Anterior drawer test is positive and it is performed by stabilising distal tibia with one hand, then grasp the posterior heel with the opposite hand and apply anterior force. If the displacement of talus is more than 8 mm anterior, it suggests laxity of the anterior talofibular ligament. Next the talar tilt test is performed, if the tilt is more than 5°, it suggests laxity of anterior talofibular and calcaneofibular ligaments.

Radiograph of the Ankle

If the talar tilt of the injured ankle is 10° greater than the uninjured ankle, it is considered as significant.

Vital facts: Ottawa Rules (Fig. 21.10)

X-rays are required in ankle sprains if:
- There is bony tenderness in the posterior half of lower end of tibia and fibula
- Tenderness over the V metatarsal and navicular bones
- Inability to bear weight immediately or after 10 days after injury.

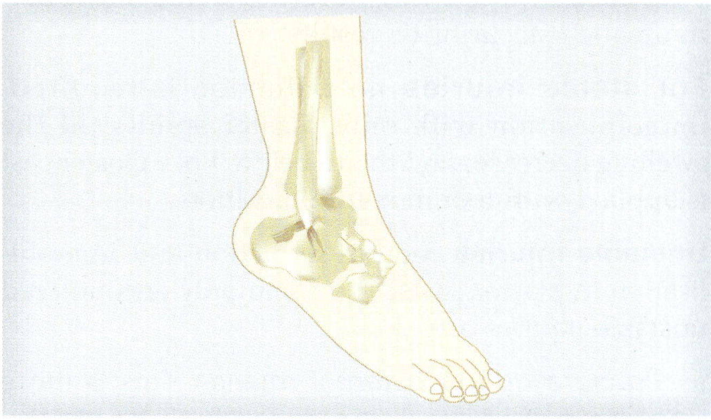

Fig. 21.8: Showing lateral ligament sprain (due to adduction injury)

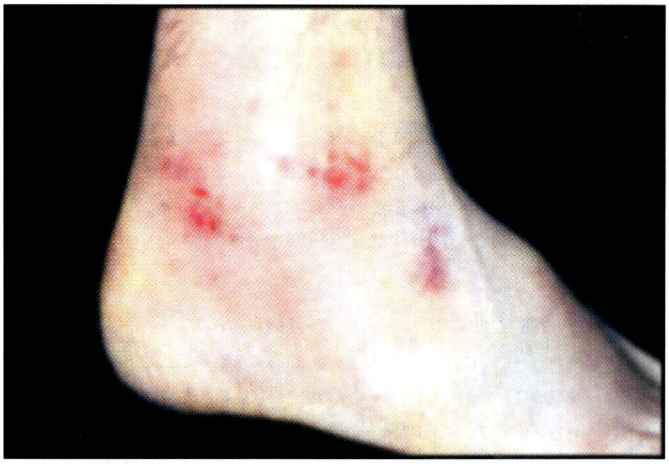

Fig. 21.9: Clinical photograph of ankle sprain

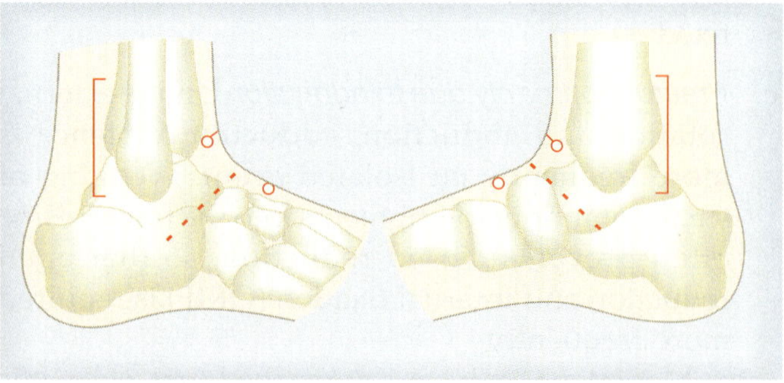

Fig. 21.10: Ankle injuries Ottawa rules

Grading of Ankle Sprains

Grade I No laxity, minimal pain and mild swelling.

Grade II Mild to moderate laxity, soft tissue swelling, anterior drawer and talar tilt is slightly positive.

Grade III Severe swelling and pain, the anterior drawer and talar tilt tests are highly positive.

Treatment

Grade I sprain Ice therapy, compression bandage, foot and elevation, ankle strap nonsteroidal anti-inflammatory drugs (NSAIDs), crutch walking, etc. are the recommended treatment (Figs 21.11 and 21.12).

Grade II sprain Long leg cast, range of motion exercises, strengthening exercises, etc. are helpful (Figs 21.13A and B).

Grade III sprain Same lines as mentioned above and sometimes may rarely require surgical repair.

Quick facts

Treatment of acute ankle sprain in a nutshell (First 48 hours) (PRICE Regime) (see Fig. 21.12)

P – painkillers
R – rest
I – ice therapy
C – compression bandage (Jones bandage)
E – elevation at hip level

Medial Ligament Sprain

This is due to pronation eversion injury. In mild sprains, only the superficial part of the deltoid ligament is torn, but in severe forms, the deep part of the deltoid ligament is also torn resulting in a lateral talar tilt. If this exceeds more than 2 mm, significant alteration in the weight bearing mechanism takes place resulting in post-traumatic arthritis. For mild sprains, conservative treatment is sufficient; and for severe sprains, surgical reduction and repair are considered.

Do you know the sources of pain after acute ankle sprain?

- Superficial peroneal nerve tension neuropathy
- Anterior and lateral ankle impingement syndrome
- Cuboid subluxation.

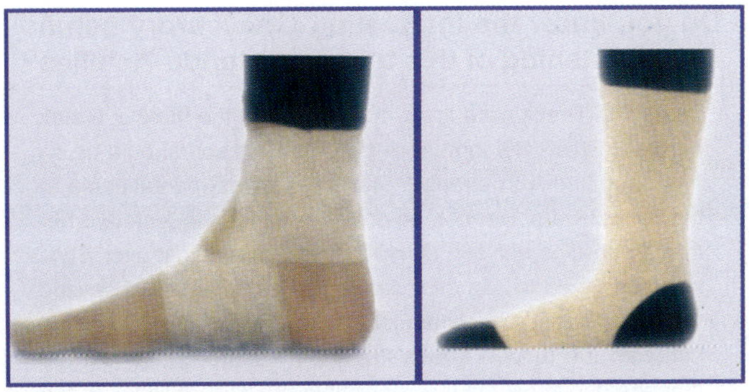

Fig. 21.11: Showing ankle strap

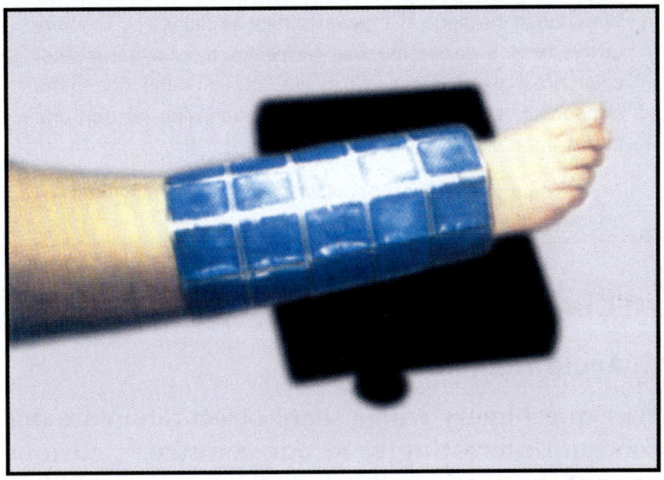

Fig. 21.12: The RICE regimen—rest, ice, compression and elevation

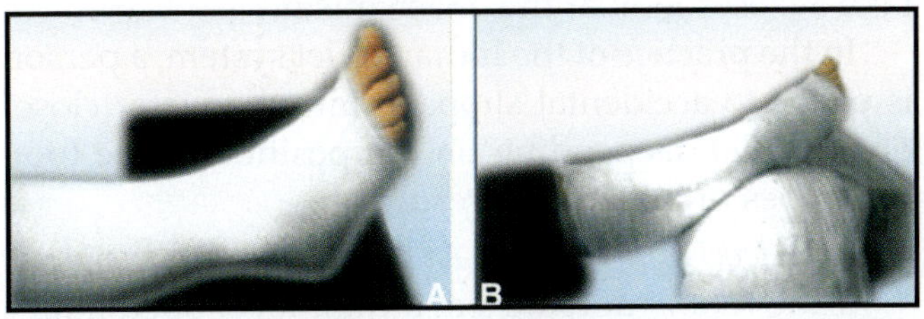

Figs 21.13A and B: (A) Compression bandaging, (B) Elevation for ankle sprain

TENDO-ACHILLES INJURY

There is no other stronger tendon in the body than the tendo-Achilles. It is formed by two powerful muscles, the gastrocnemius and the soleus. It is the powerful plantar flexor of the foot. The origin of the name of this tendon is of tremendous historical significance (See box).

Do you know the interesting Greek story behind the Christening of this tendon as tendo-Achilles?

Pleus and Thetis were the proud parents of the famous Greek hero, Achilles. His mother desired that his son should be so much fortified with strength that he remains indefatigable in the field of wars. Her coterie of well-wishers suggested to her that if she dips her son completely in the magical river Styx, no force on earth can ever defeat him. Completely obsessed with this thought, she immersed her son in that river by holding him with the tendon above the heel. Apparently, it seemed that she had achieved the impossible but was oblivious of the stark reality that the tendon area in the heel held by her remained undipped in the river and hence was deprived of the magical protection. A seemingly omnipotent Achilles met his Waterloo at the siege of Troy when he was slained by an injury to this tendon during the war. Ironically, though her mother could not make him immortal in war, she gave the idea to the orthopaedic surgeons to name this tendon after his son and thus immortalised him.

Note: The moral of this story is whoever tries to play God will be vanquished!

MECHANISM OF INJURY

I. Acute Rupture

Any direct injury with a sharp object can injure this tendon. Interestingly, in our country, a curious mechanism of injury, thanks to the practice of Indian toilet system, is being described to the utter bewilderment and astonishment of the West. Let us take a closer look at this mechanism.

In the practice of the Indian toilet system, a person is prone to accidental slippage into the water closet of the toilet. Depending on the position of the foot, two types of injury may result:

1. *High level injury (68%):* At the moment of slippage, if the foot is dorsiflexed, a high level open injury is an inevitable outcome (about 3–4 cm above the insertion). However, the silverlining is that these injuries will heal well after repair (Fig. 21.14A).
2. *Low level injury (32%):* Here a panic stricken patient tries to extricate his foot trapped in the closet in a plantarflexed position. This indiscretion leads to slicing of the tendon at a low level by the overhanging sharp edge of the closet. However, the problems are compounded due to poor healing after repair and also due to sloughing of the skin (Fig. 21.14B).

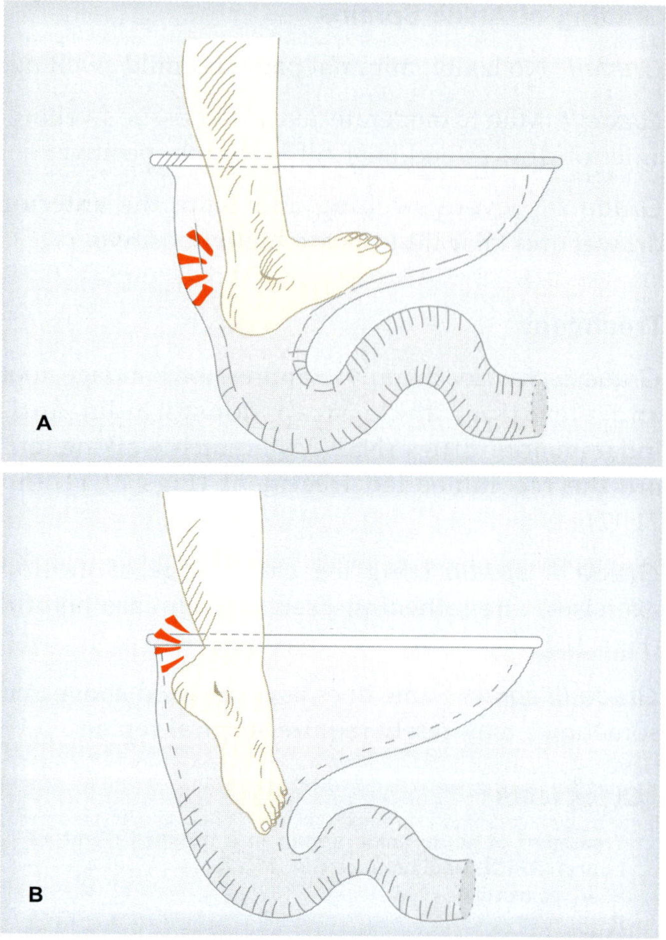

Figs 21.14A and B: Showing mechanism of injury of tendo-Achilles rupture: (A) High level injury (B) Low level injury

II. Chronic Rupture

This is due to gradual weakening of the tendon over the years. Spontaneous rupture may occur in such situations (See box).

Vital facts

Predisposing factors leading to chronic TA rupture:
- Age more than 40 years, people involved in active athletics and sports
- Weakened athletes
- Previous history of tendinitis
- Loss of flexibility of tendo-Achilles

Clinical Features

In acute tears, the patient complains of pain and swelling in the region of the tendon. The patient is unable to walk. However, in incomplete tears, when the patient is instructed to stand over the tip toes, there will be a definite heel lag.

Signs

Tenderness can be elicited and a gap is felt during a complete tear. Dorsiflexon is exaggerated, but plantar flexion is diminished; but never totally absent due to the residual action of tibialis posterior, toe flexors and the peroneals.

Clinical Tests

1. Thompson's test is still the gold standard.
2. O'brium's needle test is also reliable.
3. Tip toe test.

X-Ray of the Heel

- Lateral view of the heel will show soft tissue swelling around the heel.
- MRI scan helps to identify the tears more clearly (Fig. 21.15).

Interesting facts

Do you know the common sites of rupture in chronic tears?
- It is 2–10 cm proximal to the insertion of the tendon in the OS Calcis: This area is weaker than other areas due to relative avascularity

Treatment

I. Conservative

Immobilising the ankle in slight plantar flexion for 6 to 8 weeks. Though the incidence of infection is less, recurrent ruptures are quite common. Hence, it is second best to surgery.

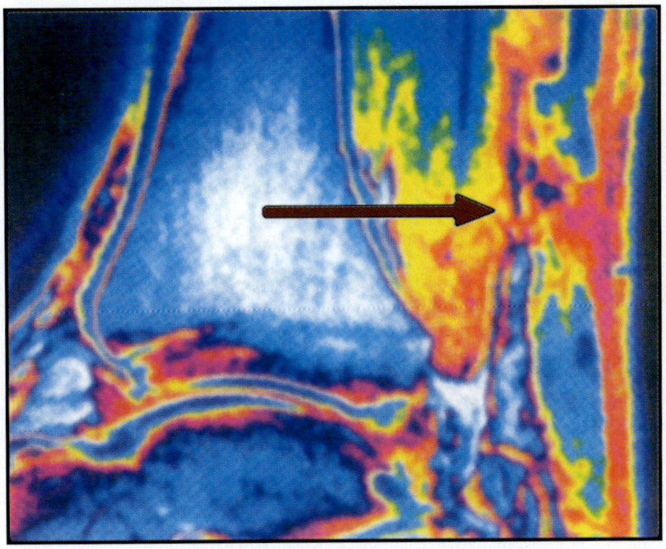

Fig. 21.15: MRI of tendo-Achilles rupture

II. Surgery

Direct surgical repair and immobilisation in a below-knee plaster cast with slight plantar flexion is a better alternative. Though recurrent ruptures are less, the chances of infections are high. Hence, extreme caution needs to be exercised to prevent the dreadful infection.

BIBLIOGRAPHY

1. Harish Gillies. The Management of Fresh Rupture of Tendo-Achilles. JBJS Vol 52-A, 337-343, March 1970.
2. Hooker CH. Rupture of TendoAchilles. JBJS Vol. 45-B, No. 2, 360-363, May 1963.

22

Injuries to the Foot

FOREFOOT INJURIES

The forefoot complex consists of five metatarsals, sesamoid bones and the bones of the five toes (Fig. 22.1). The joints include metatarsophalangeal and interphalangeal joints. Forefoot plays a very important role both in gait and weight transmission. It is frequently injured in sports persons.

CLASSIFICATION

Fracture of the forefoot is classified as shown in Flow chart 22.1.

Now let us analyse the individual forefoot injuries in greater detail.

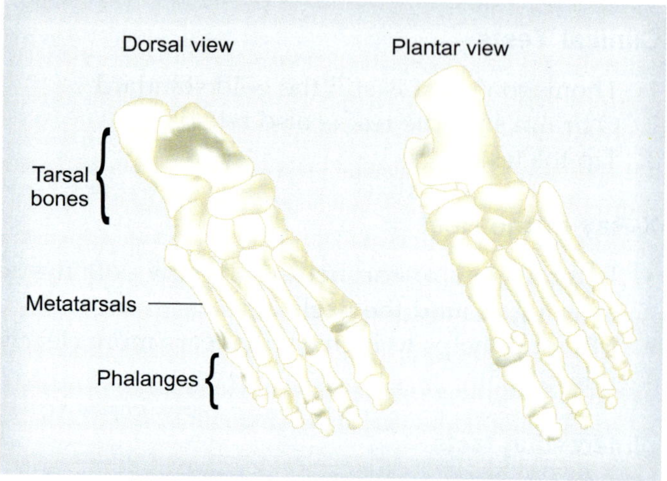

Fig. 22.1: Bony anatomy of the foot

TREATMENT GOALS IN FOREFOOT FRACTURES

Orthopaedic Goals

a. To restore the normal anatomy of the great toe, phalanx, metatarsal and sesamoid bones.
b. In phalanges 2 through 5 toes, perfect alignment is not very crucial
c. Metatarsals two through five, need to be restored as anatomically as possible.

PHALANGEAL FRACTURES

Features

- This is the most common injury of the foot.
- Proximal phalanx is more commonly injured than all other phalanx.
- Proximal phalanx of the fifth toe is most commonly injured.

Flow chart 22.1: Fracture of the foot

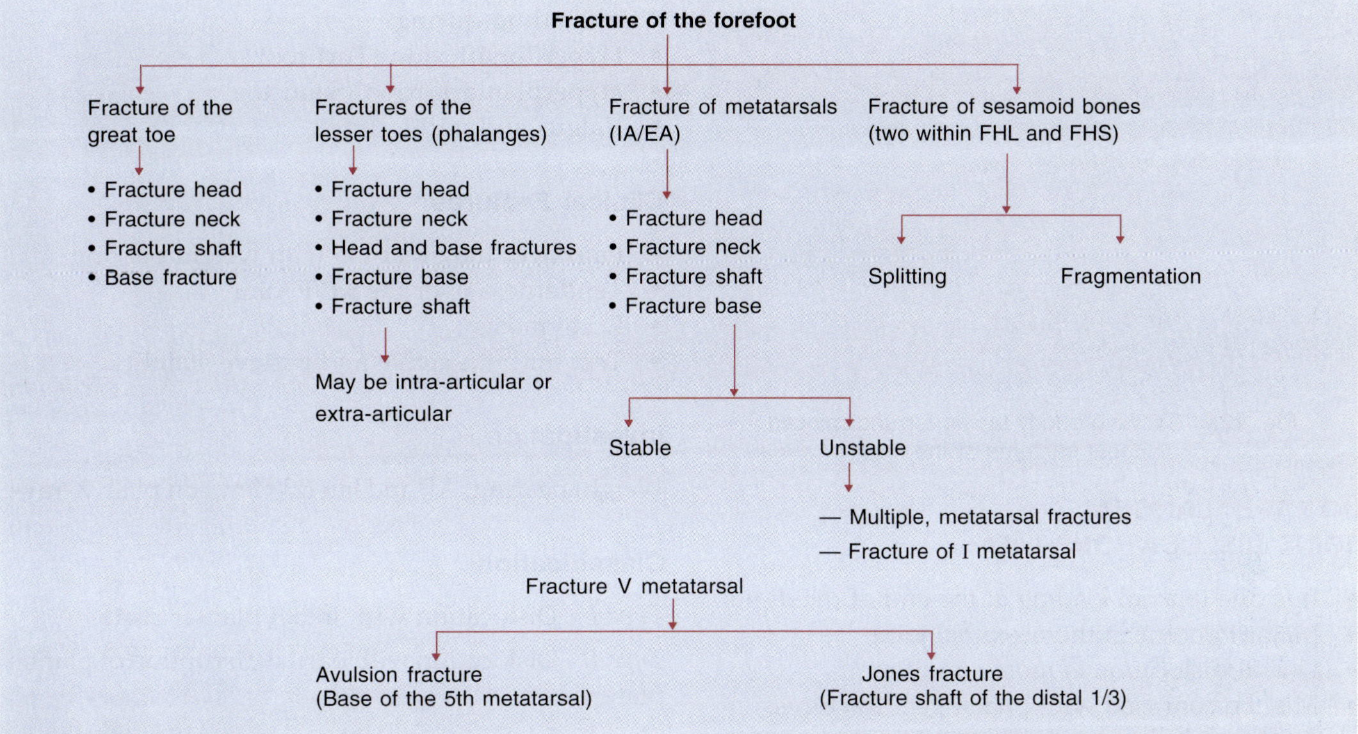

Note: IA—Intra-articular, EA—Extra-articular, FHL—Flexor hallucis longus, FHL—Flexor hallucis superficialis

Mechanism of Injury

- Direct blow due to fall of a heavy object on the toes. This causes transverse or comminuted fractures.
- Indirect forces due to axial loading with secondary varus or valgus forces (stubbing injury). This leads to spiral or oblique fractures.

Clinical Features

The patient presents with pain, swelling, limp and difficulty to wear the footwears.

Investigation

Standard AP and lateral films of the forefoot help to make the diagnosis.

Classification (OTA)

Group A Extra-articular and simple diaphyseal fractures.

Group B Partial articular and diaphyseal wedge fractures.

Group C Complex articular and diaphyseal shaft fractures. Each group is further subdivided into the position and pattern of fractures.

Treatment

Nonoperative Treatment

- *Immobilisation only:* This is indicated for stable closed injuries with no intra-articular extension. The treatment consists of buddy taping and weight bearing with stiff shoes (Fig. 22.2).
- *Closed reduction:* This is indicated for displaced extra-articular or intra-articular fractures. The treatment consists of closed reduction and buddy taping to the medial toe.

Operative Treatment

This is indicated for grossly unstable intra-articular fractures. The treatment method of choice is closed reduction and percutaneous K-wire fixation or open reduction, K-wire or screw fixation.

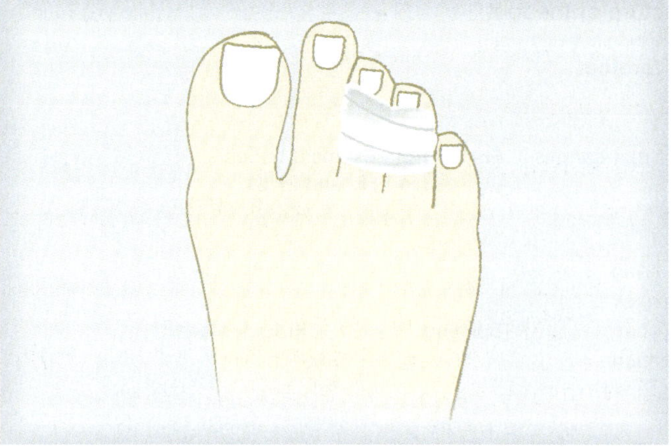

Fig. 22.2: Showing buddy taping for undisplaced phalangeal fractures of the toes

INTERPHALANGEAL JOINT DISLOCATIONS (IJD)

- It is due to axial loading at the end of the digits
- Majority occur in the proximal joint
- Dorsal dislocation is more common
- May be confused with phalangeal fractures.

Clinical Features

- Pain and swelling
- Stiffness of the toes
- Dorsoplantar thickening of the toe on palpation.

Investigation

Plain X-rays AP and lateral views help to make the diagnosis.

Treatment

Closed reduction with longitudinal traction along the toes with plantar flexion of the toes under digital block is the treatment method of choice. This is followed by buddy taping to the adjacent toe.

METATARSOPHALANGEAL JOINT INJURIES

First MTP Joint

- Most commonly injured
- Most commonly affected during sports injury
- Injuries vary from minor sprain to frank dislocations.

Mechanism of Injury

Axial loading during:

- Hyperdorsiflexion (Turf toe)
- Hyperplantarflexion (Sand toe)
- Valgus and varus stress.

Clinical Features

- Pain over the great toe with weight bearing
- Tenderness over the MTP joint
- Ecchymosis
- Test for both active and passive stability.

Investigation

Weight bearing, AP and lateral views on plain X-rays.

Classification

Type I Dislocation with intact plantar plate

Type II Dislocation with partial disruption of plantar plate

Type III Dislocation with complete disruption of plantar plate.

Sprains are classified into Grades I, II and III, depending on the degree of tear.

Treatment

i. *Nonoperative treatment*: For stable injuries, RICE regime.
ii. *Operative treatment*: This is indicated for intra-articular fractures and significant avulsion fractures causing instability. These injuries need open reduction, internal fixation with ligament repair.

INJURIES TO THE OTHER MTP JOINTS

These are hyperdorsiflexion and hyperplantarflexion injuries with axial loading and are rare. The treatment is essentially conservative for minor sprains. Dislocations are treated by closed reduction by finger traps to the affected toe for overcoming the gravitational force. This is successful in 50 per cent of the cases. If this fails, open reduction and pinning may be required.

SESAMOID BONE INJURIES

Two sesamoid bones are present within the flexor hallucis longus and flexor hallucis superficialis tendons of the great toe.

Functions of Seasamoid Bones

- Shock absorber
- Supports weight bearing function of the great toe
- Protects the FHL tendon.

Note: Bipartite sesamoid bones are seen in 9 to 30%
Medial sesamoid is more commonly injured.

Mechanism of Injury

- Due to the impact of the foot on a hard surface while the toes are dorsiflexed.
- Stress fracture due to repeated trauma (as in dancers; runners, etc.)

Clinical Features

Pain, tenderness beneath the plantar surface of the sesamoid bone (Fig. 22.3), limp is present.

Investigations

- Plain X-ray—AP, lateral and tangential (sesamoid) views.
- CT scan or MRI is more accurate but expensive.

Treatment

a. *Acute fractures*—Soft padding, strapping the MTP joint in neutral or in slightly plantar flexed position.

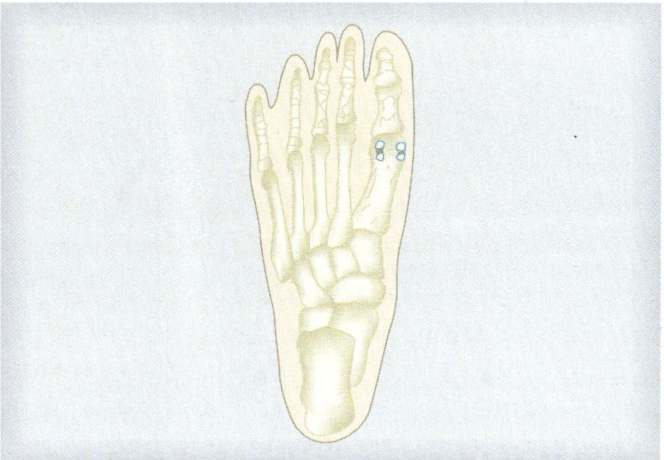

Fig. 22.3: Showing sesamoid bone fractures

b. *Sesamoidectomy*—This is done if casting fails or if there is persisting pain.

METATARSAL FRACTURES

Mechanism of injury

- Direct force—common, due to fall of a heavy object.
- Indirect force—Due to twisting forces, avulsion and spiral fractures are caused.
- Avulsion fractures are common at the base of the 5th metatarsal.
- Stress fractures are common at the II and III metatarsals (march fracture).

Clincial Features

- The patient complains of pain, swelling and tenderness over the dorsum of the foot. There could be considerable soft tissue swelling.
- Limp is present.
- Pain in the foot increases with weight bearing.

Investigations

Plain X-ray with AP, lateral and oblique views helps to make the diagnosis.

Classification (OTA)

Group A Extra-articular and simple diaphyseal fractures.
Group B Partial articular and diaphyseal wedge fractures.
Group C Complex articular and diaphyseal shaft fractures.

Treatment

I. *First metatarsal:*
   a. *Nonoperative methods:* NWB below-knee plaster cast for 6 to 8 weeks for stable fractures with no loss of bone length.
   b. *Operative methods:* Displaced and unstable fractures should be treated by closed reduction and percutaneous fixation with K-wires, screws only or with plate and screws.

II. *Central metatarsals (2–4):* These injuries are more common than the first metatarsal.
   a. *Nonoperative methods* Fractures with < 10 mm long axis angulation and < 4 mm transition

of shaft with hard or stiff-soled shoes for fractures with > 10 degree angulation and > 4 mm translation can be treated with closed reduction and gravity, traction or immobilisation with hand or stiff-soled shoes.

b. *Operative methods* Closed reduction and percutaneous K-wire fixation is done for unstable injuries and for multiple fractures.

FIFTH METATARSAL INJURIES

Mechanism of Injury

a. *Direct force*—Rare and is seen in RTAs, sports, etc.
b. *Indirect force*—Twisting force injury is more common.

Classification

Fifth metatarsal fractures are divided into:

I. Distal spiral or dancer's fracture.
II. Proximal base fractures. These are further subdivided into:
   a. Pseudo-Jones fracture—Tip of the styloid process (avulsion fracture)
   b. Jones fracture—Metaphyseal fracture due to sudden adduction of the forefoot.
III. Stress fracture of the proximal fifth metatarsal.

Treatment

Nonoperative treatment is indicated for undisplaced and stable injuries and it consists of:

a. Tip of the styloid process or Zone Injury—wearing a hard sole or stiff shoes.
b. Metaphyseal fractures (Jones)—Below knee weightbearing plaster cast for 6 to 8 weeks.
c. Diaphyseal fractures—NWB cast for 3 months.

JONES FRACTURE

Definition

It is a fracture of the diaphysis of the 5th metatarsal bone approximately 1.5 cm above the tip of the tuberosity (Fig. 22.4A) at the metaphyseal junction.

Mechanism of Injury

It is an avulsion fracture due to the pull of the peroneus brevis muscle. It is frequently encountered in athletes.

Clinical Features

The patient complains of pain, swelling and limp. On examination, tenderness can be elicited over the base of the 5th metatarsal bone.

Disturbing facts about Jones fracture

- It is often confused with pseudo-Jones fracture
- Delayed union and nonunion is a frequent occurrence due to the poor blood supply
- Surgery may be required if there is nonunion.

Do you know about pseudo-Jones fracture?

- This is an avulsion fracture of the styloid process of the fifth metatarsal bone due to the pull of the peroneus brevis muscle (Fig. 22.4B)
- It heals readily and surgery is rarely required.

Radiology

Radiograph of the foot helps to confirm the diagnosis. It shows a fuzzy periosteal reaction in the metadiaphyseal region after 7 to 10 days.

Treatment

Treatment is essentially conservative and consists of application of a below-knee plaster cast for a period of 3 to 4 weeks.

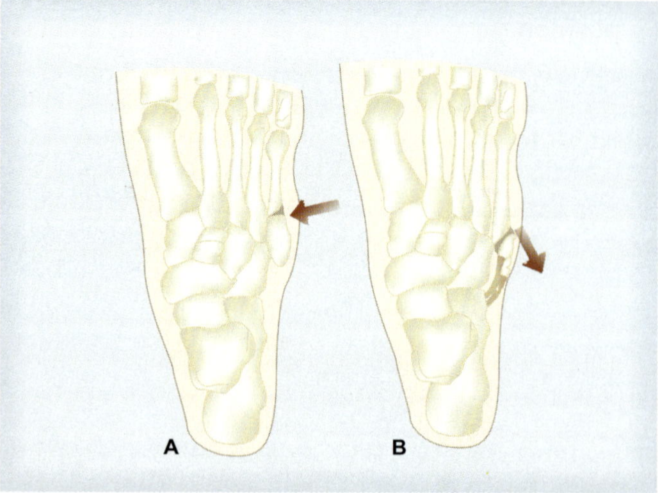

Figs 22.4A and B: Showing (A) Jones fracture, (B) Avulsion fracture of the styloid process of 5th metatarsal bone

MARCH FRACTURE (INSUFFICIENCY FRACTURE)

This is a stress or fatigue fracture of the metatarsals particularly the II metatarsal bone (Fig. 22.5). It is more often encountered in military personnel who indulge in frequent and prolonged marching and hence its name. It is also seen in policemen, dancers, nurses, and surgeons who require to stand or dance for a long duration. Radiograph helps in the diagnosis and the treatment is rest, NSAIDs, splints, elasto crepe bandage application, etc.

This is an important cause of chronic midfoot pain and it requires prompt identification and treatment.

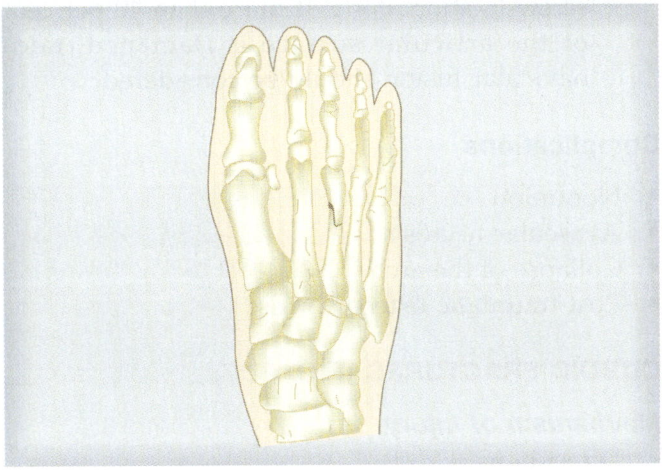

Fig. 22.5: Showing march fracture

MIDFOOT INJURIES

Midfoot consists of the navicular, three cuneiform and cuboid bones with their intervening joints. This region of the foot is fairly susceptible to injuries. Midfoot fractures are depicted in Flow chart 22.2.

Mechanism of Injury

There are three common causes of midfoot fractures:

1. *Twisting of the forefoot*: This usually occurs in an RTA due to forced foot abduction (twisting injury).
2. *Axial loading of a fixed foot*: This can happen in two ways:
   a. Fall on an extremely dorsiflexed foot (here an axial compression is applied to the heel).
   b. Fall on an extremely ankle equinus (here axial compression is from the body weight).
3. *Direct crushing injuries* as in industrial accidents.

Treatment Goals

Orthopaedic goal

a. To restore the keystone of the midfoot (i.e. the first and second metatarsal articulation with the medial cuneiform) as it provides stability between the midfoot and forefoot during gait.

b. To maintain the medial longitudinal arch of the foot by restoring the length and alignment of the

Flow chart 22.2: Midfoot fractures

MIDFOOT FRACTURES

- Tarsometatarsal joint (Lisfranc joint)
  - This may include fractures of metatarsal bases
    - Isolated
      - • 1–2 metatarsal
      - • Fracture displaced
    - Homolateral
      - All the metatarsals are fractured and displaced in the same direction
    - Divergent
      - Displaced in both coronal and sagittal planes
- The cuneiforms
- The navicular bone (Scaphoid)
  1. Cortical avulsion fracture
  2. Tuberosity fracture
  3. Fracture of body
  4. Stress fracture
- The cuboid bone (Nutcracker fracture)
  - Cracked like a nut between the base of 5th metatarsal and calcaneus during forced foot abduction

cuneiforms, cuboid and navicular bones. The longitudinal and transverse arches should be maintained as they control the direct distribution of weight of the body or the foot during gait.

c. To restore the Lisfranc joint complex.

Note: Midfoot extends between the Chopart's joint proximally to Lisfranc joint distally.

NAVICULAR BONE FRACTURES

This is the keystone of the medial longitudinal arch of the foot (Fig. 22.6).

Mechanism of Injury

- *Direct blow* Rare, can cause avulsion or crush injuries.
- *Indirect forces* Due to fall from height, sports-related injuries or due to RTA.

OTA Classification

Group A—Extra-articular fracture
Group B—Involvement of the talonavicular joint
Group C—Involvement of both talonavicular and talocuneiform joints.

Each group is further subclassified depending upon fracture types and position.

Clinical Features

The patient complains of pain, swelling, and limp. Tenderness can be elicited over the navicular bone.

Investigations

AP and lateral X-rays of the joint and CT scan give more reliable information about the fracture pattern.

Treatment

I. *Nonoperative Treatment:* This is indicated in undisplaced fractures and in fracture with less than 2 mm displacement of the talonavicular joint. The treatment consists of short leg NWB cast for 6 to 8 weeks.

II. *Operative Treatment:* This is reserved for displaced fractures with > 2 mm separation. Fixation can be achieved most of the times by screw fixation alone. If more than 40 per cent of the articular surface is damaged, talonavicular fusion should be considered.

Complications

- Nonunion
- Avascular necrosis
- Collapse of the arch
- Post-traumatic osteoarthritis

CUBOID FRACTURES (FIG. 22.7)

Mechanism of Injury

- Direct blow
- Indirect force: Forced plantar flexion and abduction (nutcracker effect).

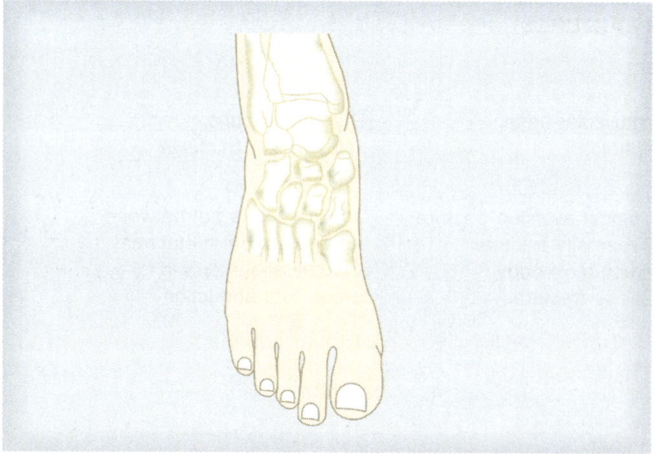

Fig. 22.6: Showing navicular bone fracture

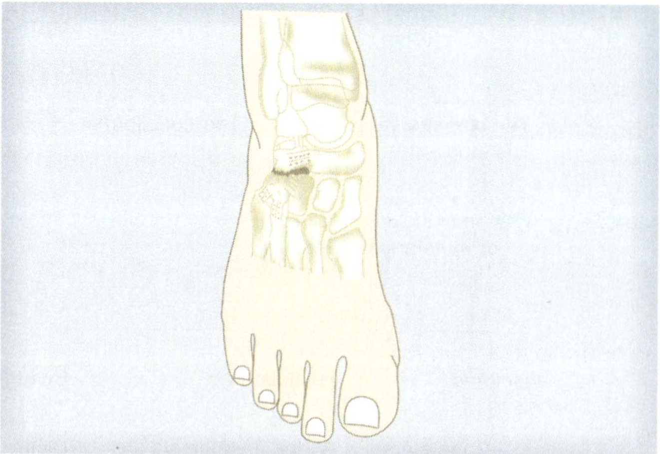

Fig. 22.7: Showing cuboid bone fracture

Clinical Features

The patient complains of dorsolateral pain, swelling and skin discolouration.

Investigations

Plain X-ray with a medial oblique view and CT scan are the recommended investigations.

Classification (OTA)

Group A Extra-articular.

Group B Partly intra-articular involving either the calcaneocuboid or metatarsocuboid joints.

Group C Completely intra-articular involves both the joints.

Each group is further classified depending upon the fracture pattern and position.

Treatment

Nonoperative Method This is indicated in undisplaced and in fractures < 2 mm separation. The treatment of choice is a below-knee cast for 6 to 8 weeks.

Operative Method For displaced fractures, open reduction and K-wire fixation is indicated. External fixation is recommended for the nutcracker fracture.

Note: Cuboid syndrome is a painful subluxation of the calcaneocuboid joint.

CUNEIFORM INJURIES

These are rare injuries and are usually due to indirect forces. More commonly, they are associated with injuries to the tarsometatarsal joints (Fig. 22.8).

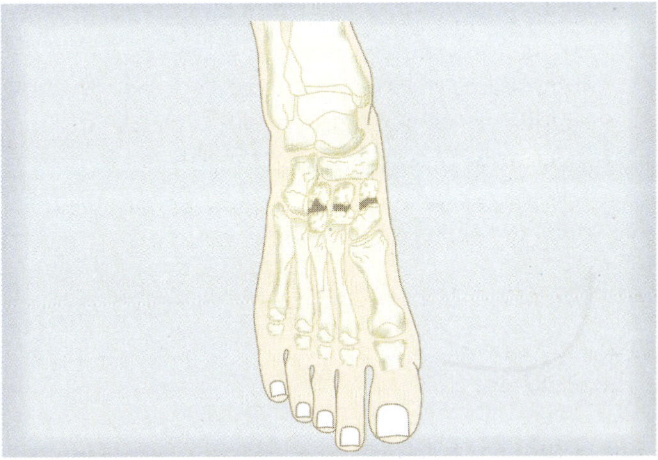

Fig. 22.8: Showing cuneiform bone fractures

Clinical Features

Pain, swelling, tenderness, limp and pain on weight bearing.

Investigations

Plain X-ray (AP, lateral, oblique views) with CT scan of the foot.

Classification (OTA)

Group A Extra-articular

Group B Partly intra-articular (involves other navicular cuneiform or metatarsal cuneiform joints)

Group C Involves both articular surfaces.

Treatment

a. *Nonoperative:* Short leg cast for 6 to 8 weeks for undisplaced fractures
b. *Operative:* For displaced fractures, open reduction and internal fixation with pins or screws.

TARSOMETATATARSAL INJURIES (LISFRANC INJURIES)

Lisfranc joint consists of three cuneiform metacarpal articulations and two cuboid metatarsal articulations of the fourth and fifth metatarsals. It represents the transition bone between the midfoot and the forefoot.

Mechanism of Injury

- *Direct injury:* This is rare and is due to crush injury or direct blow on the dorsum of the foot.
- *Indirect injury:* This is more common and three varieties are described (Figs 22.9A and B):
  a. Axial loading to the foot in fixed equinus (e.g. football injuries).
  b. Axial loading in descending stairs.
  c. Axial loading following fall from height.

The associated injuries could be fracture of second metatarsal (most common), fractures of cuneiforms, cuboids, metatarsals and lateral ligament injuries.

Clinical Features

- Pain in the tarsometatarsal area
- Passive dorsiflexion or plantarflexion produces pain
- Single limb heel lift produces pain in the midfoot
- Plantar ecchymosis.

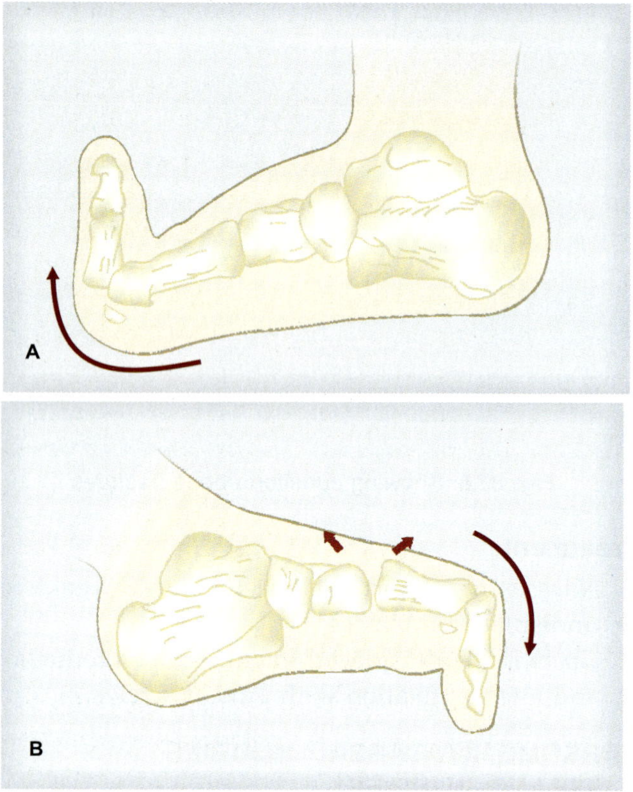

Figs 22.9A and B: Showing mechanisms of Lisfranc injury

Investigations

- Plain X-ray in weightbearing position (AP, lateral and 30° medial oblique position).
- CT scan provides better visualisation and is more accurate in analysing the injuries.

CLASSIFICATION (OTA) (Figs 22.10A to C)

- Type I–Anterior dislocation 1st ray, dorsal and plantar dislocations of the lesser rays.
- Type II–Divergent dislocation.
- Type III–Homolateral dislocation (medial or lateral).

Treatment

a. *Nonoperative Methods:* This is indicated for sprains and for < 2 mm displacement of tarsometatarsal joint in any plane. The treatment of choice is a below-knee POP cast for 6 to 8 weeks. For sprains—RICE regime.

b. *Operative Methods:* For displaced injuries, closed reduction and internal fixation. With K-wires or

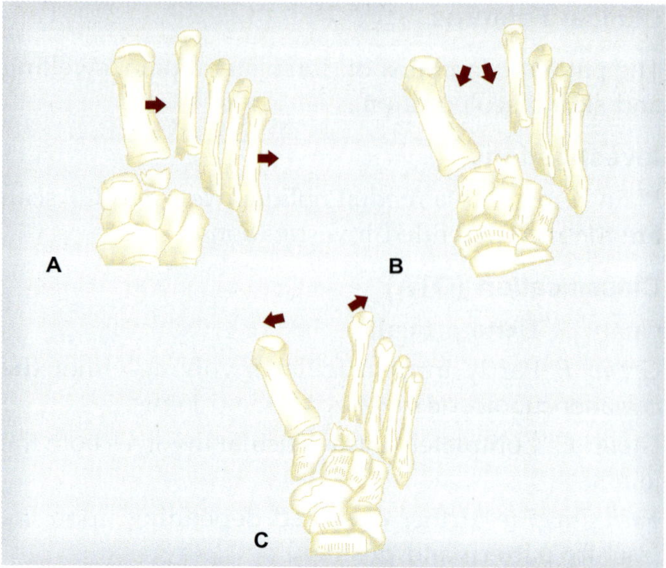

Figs 22.10A to C: Showing different types of Lisfranc: injury: (A) Type I, (B) Type II, (C) Type III

screws is indicated for displacement < 50 per cent. For more than 50 per cent displacement, primary fusion is indicated. Open reduction or internal fixation is indicated for widely displaced fractures (Fig. 22.11).

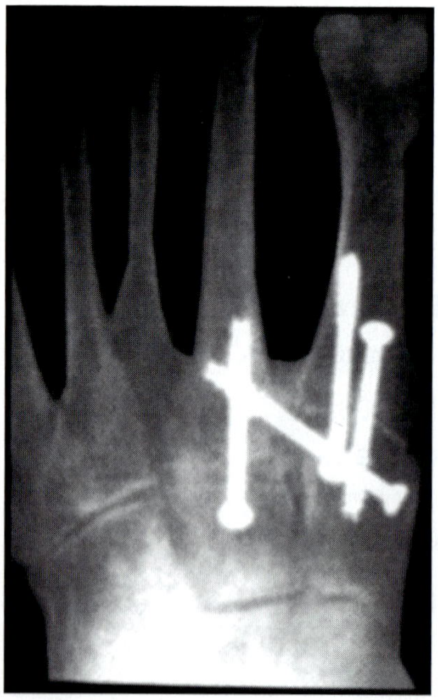

Fig. 22.11: Radiograph showing Lisfranc injury fixed with screws

HINDFOOT INJURIES

FRACTURE CALCANEUM

Calcaneus is the most often fractured tarsal bone. No ideal method of treatment has been described yet.

Functions

1. Supports weight of the body.
2. Acts as a spring board for locomotion.

Structure

It has a thin cortical shell except at the posterior tuberosity. Two types of trabecular pattern are described

1. *Traction trabeculae* This radiates from the inferior cortex.
2. *Compression trabeculae* converge to support anterior and posterior facets.

Vital angles

In the lateral view of the radiograph two angles are important:

1. **Böhler's angle** This is the angle between lines drawn from anterior articular process to the posterior tuberosity. The tuber angle is 25 to 40° (Fig. 22.12).
2. **Crucial angle of "Gissane"** The lateral process of talus is wedged in this angle (Fig. 22.13).

Axial compressive forces with talus acting as a bursting wedge will disrupt the subtalar joint.

Restoration of the above two angles is the aim of the treatment.

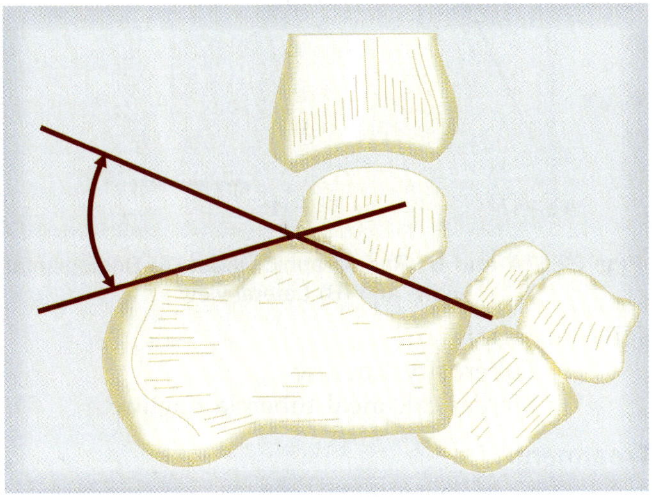

Fig. 22.12: Tuber joint angle (Böhler's angle)

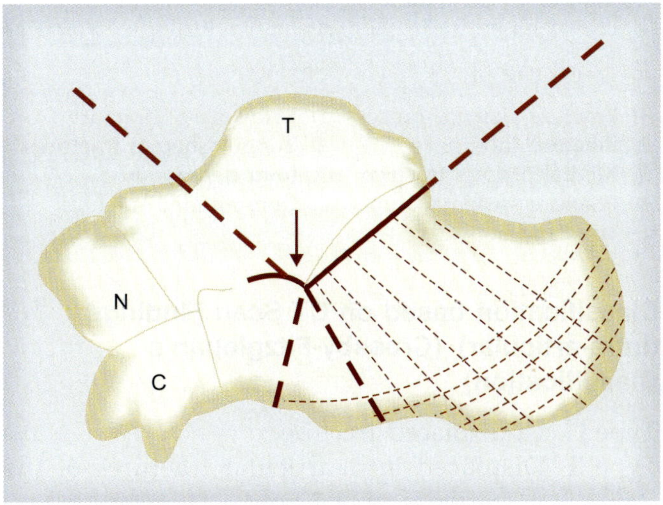

Fig. 22.13: Gissane angle

CLASSIFICATION

Essex-Lopresti's Classification

This is the most accepted classification for fracture calcaneum. It consists of *extra-articular fractures* (Figs 22.14A to D) (less common accounting for only 25% of the cases) and *intra-articular fractures* which is more common (Figs 22.15A to C and Table 22.1).

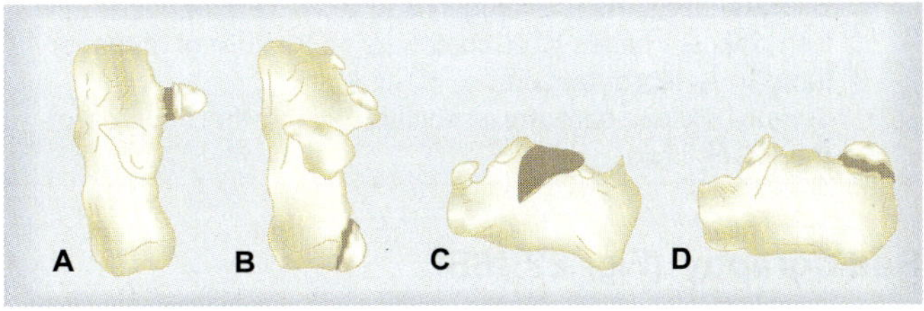

Figs 22.14A to D: Types of extra-articular fractures: (A) S. tali fracture, (B) Medial process fracture, (C) Anterior process fracture, and (D) Tuberosity fracture

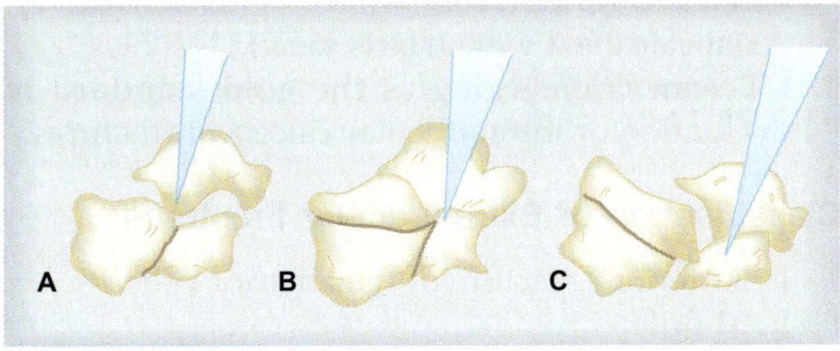

Figs 22.15A to C: Varieties of intra-articular fractures: (A) Undisplaced fracture, (B) Tongue-shaped fracture, (C) Comminuted fracture

Table 22.1: Types of calcaneal fractures	
Extra-articular (25–30%)	*Intra-articular (70–75%)*
1. Fracture anterior process	1. Undisplaced fracture
2. Fracture tuberosity	2. Tongue-shaped fractures
3. Medial process fracture	3. Joint depression
4. Fracture sustentaculum talus and body	4. Comminuted fracture

Classification based on CT Scan Findings (Intra-articular) (Crossby-Fitzgibban's Classification)

Type I Undisplaced fracture
Type II Displaced intra-articular fractures of the posterior facet (< 2 mm)
Type III Comminuted fractures

Note: Type I Nonoperative treatment
Type II Operative treatment

Mechanism of Injury

Twisting forces cause many of the extra-articular fractures.

Fall from height with landing on the heels causes vast majority of intra-articular fractures (Fig. 22.16A).

Vital facts

- Bilateral fractures are seen in 5 to 9 per cent of cases.
- Ten per cent cases have compression fracture of dorsal or lumbar vertebral bodies.
- Twenty-six per cent are associated with other injuries of the lower limbs.

Radiography (Fig. 22.16B)

Three views are recommended:
1. Dorsoplantar or anteroposterior view (Fig. 22.17A).
2. Lateral view helps to study the crucial angle of Gissane (Fig. 22.17B).
3. Axial calcaneal view (Haris view).
4. CT scan is emerging as the gold standard in evaluation of intra-articular calceneal fractures.

Classification of Extra-articular Fractures

I. Anterior—fracture of the anterior process.
II. Middle:
- Body fracture
- Fracture of sustentaculum tali
- Lateral calcaneal process fracture
- Peroneal tubercle fracture

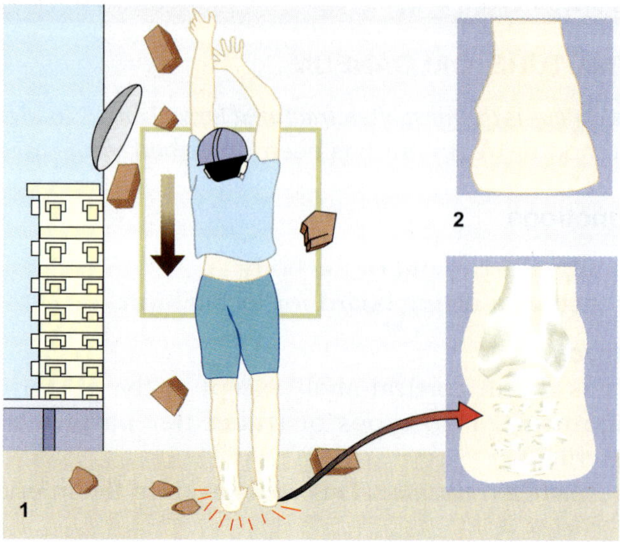

Fig. 22.16A: (1) Fall from height causes intra-articular fracture of calcaneum, (2) Broadening of the heel

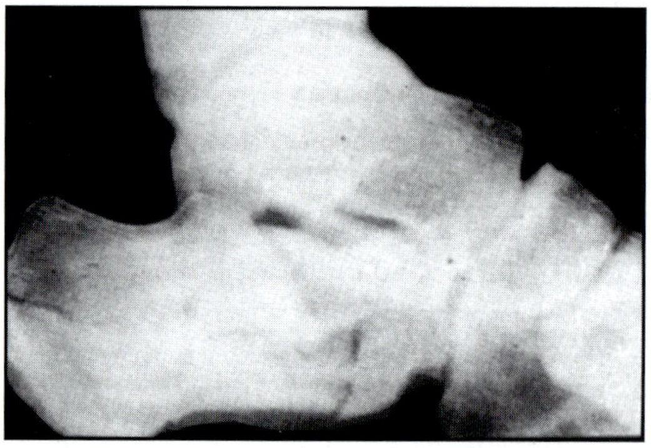

Fig. 22.16B: Radiograph showing calcaneum fracture

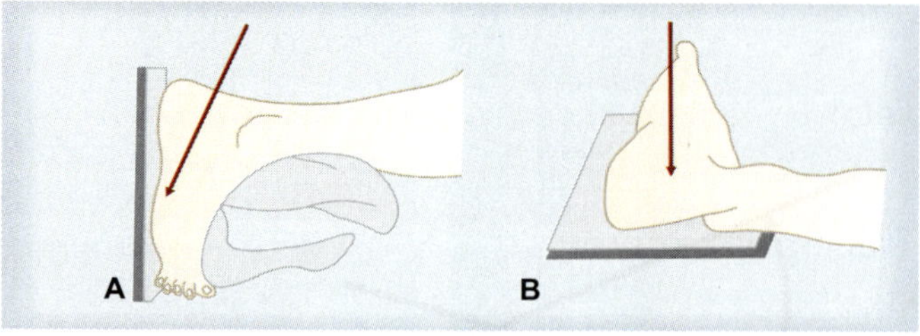

Figs 22.17A and B: Radiographic views: (A) Dorsoplantar view, and (B) Lateral view

III. Posterior:
- Tuberosity fracture
- Medial calcaneal tubercle fracture.

Treatment

Extra-articular fractures

1. Fracture of anterior process:
   a. Avulsion fracture—short leg cast (Fig. 22.18).

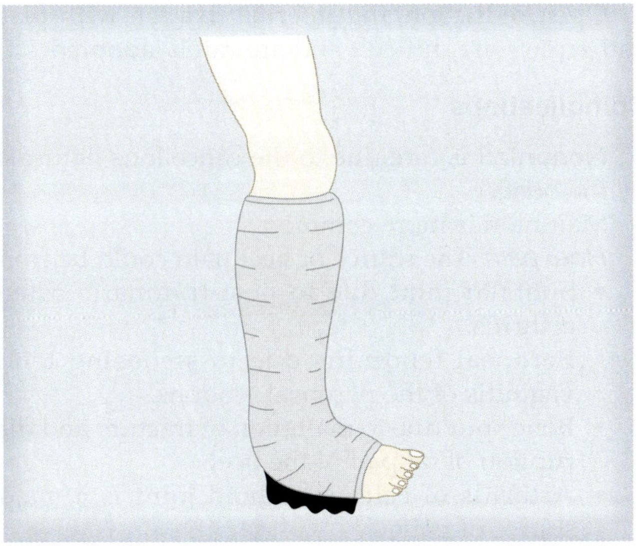

Fig. 22.18: Showing short leg POP cast with walking heel for calcaneal fracture

b. Compression fracture—should be reduced and fixed with K-wire or screw.

2. Fracture tuberosity:
   - Undisplaced fracture—short leg cast.
   - Displaced fracture—open reduction and internal fixation.
3. Fracture medial calcaneal process:
   - Undisplaced fracture—plaster cast.
   - Displaced—open reduction with medial lateral compression and internal fixation.
4. Fracture sustentaculum tali:
   - Undisplaced—plaster cast.
   - Displaced—open reduction and casting.
5. Fracture of the body not involving the subtalar joint: Responds well to conservative treatment.

Intra-articular fractures Account for 60 per cent of all tarsal injuries and 75 per cent of all calcaneal fractures.

Mechanism of Injury

Fall from height Lateral process of talus acts as a wedge and is forced through the Gissane's angle resulting in four fracture patterns:

1. Undisplaced
2. Tongue shaped
3. Joint depression
4. Comminuted.

Clinical Features

- Pain and swelling of the heel.
- The patient is unable to bear weight, stand or walk.
- Pain and difficulty during inversion and eversion of the heel.

Clinical Signs

- Swelling over the heel
- Tenderness over the heel
- Lateral heel compression test elicits pain (Fig. 22.19A).
- Broadening of the heel (see Fig. 22.16B).
- Horse shoe swelling on either side the tendo-Achilles.
- Distance between the heel and malleoli is reduced.

Treatment

Conservative

The following are the basic methods of treatment:

1. No reduction and early motion consists of:
   - Elasto crepe bandage application
   - Foot elevation
   - Weight bearing at the end of 12 weeks.
2. Closed reduction and fixation

Goals

- *Restore congruity of the subtalar joint*
- *Restore Böhler's angle*
- *Restore normal width of the calcaneum.*

Omoto Technique of Calcaneal Fracture Reduction (Fig. 22.19B)

Common Steps of Reduction

- Under anaesthesia (general or spinal), the patient is prone and knee is flexed to 90°.

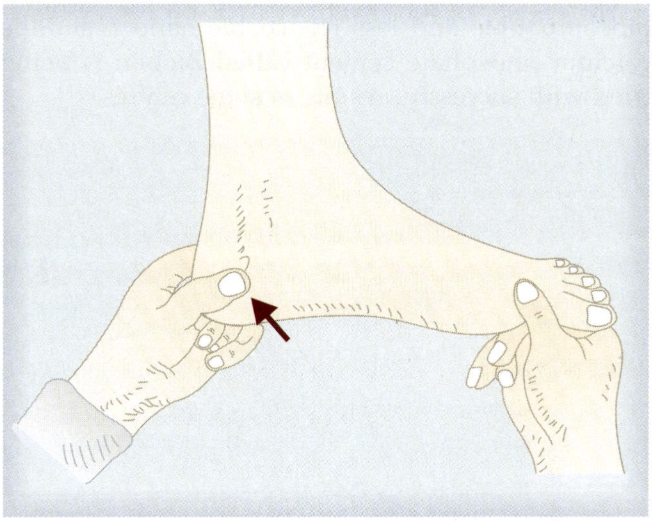

Fig. 22.19A: Showing heel compression test for diagnosing undisplaced or stress fracture of calcaneum

Section 2

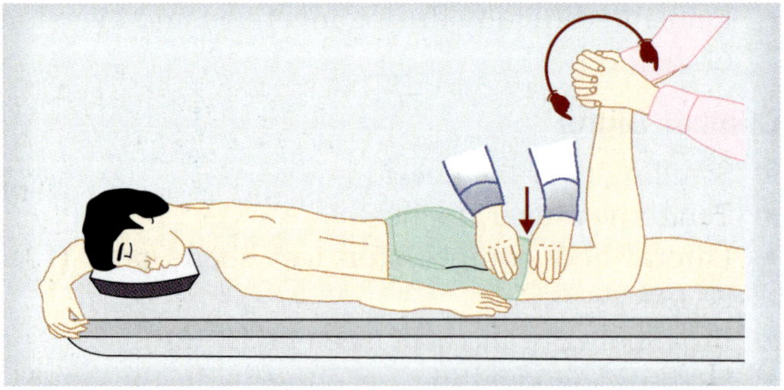

Fig. 22.19B: Showing the method of closed reduction of calcaneal fractures (Omoto technique)

- With the assistant supporting the thigh, the surgeon compresses the medial and lateral sides of the heel.
- Strong longitudinal traction is now applied along the direction of the leg.
- Varus or valgus force is now applied depending on the displacement.
- Lastly the calceneal tuberosity is manipulated in position.
- Compression bandage is finally applied.

Essex-Lopresti method of lifting the fragment with an axial percutaneous pin and retention with K-wires is done (Figs 22.20A and B).

Surgery

Severly comminuted and depressed fracture with subchondral defects require open reduction and internal fixation with cancellous bone graft to fill the gap. Recently, for this purpose, alternatively, a biocompatible and less resorbable nanocrystalline calcium phosphate cement called Bioban is being tried with successful results in some centres.

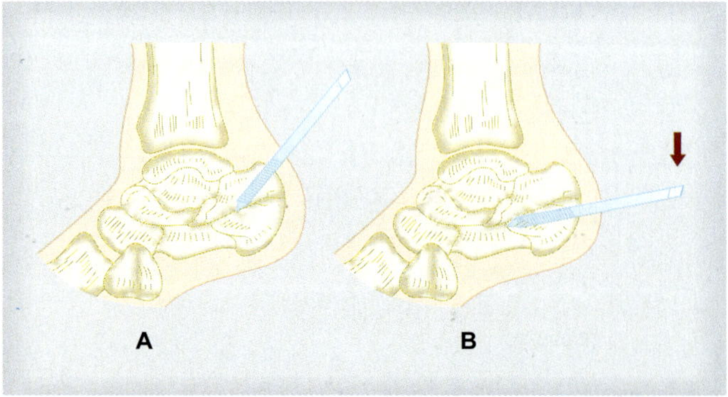

Figs 22.20A and B: Showing Essex-Lopresti method of reduction of calcaneal fractures: (A) Disimpaction, (B) Elevation

Open reduction and internal fixation with plate and screws are difficult and are rarely adopted.

Complications

1. Nonunion is rare due to the cancellous nature of the bone.
2. Malunion is more common.
3. *Heel pain:* The source of heel pain could be from
   - Subtalar joint due to post-traumatic osteoarthritis.
   - Peroneal tendinitis due to stenosing tenovaginitis of the peroneal tendons.
   - Bone spur due to malunion of fracture and disruption of fat pad of the heel.
   - Arthritis of calcaneocuboid joint is a major source of pain.
   - Nerve entrapment is rare. Medial or lateral plantar branches of posterior tibial nerve or sural nerve may be entrapped due to soft tissue scarring.

FRACTURE TALUS

Importance of talus:

- Takes part in weight transmission.
- Has a precarious blood supply.
- 3/5th of the bone is covered by articular cartilage.
- Sudden hyperextension of the forefoot causes fracture neck called "Aviators Astralagus".

Blood Supply of Talus (Fig. 22.21)

- Sixty per cent is covered by articular surface, only limited surface is available for vascular perforation.
- No muscle originates or inserts into talus.
- All the three major arteries of the foot posterior tibial artery, anterior tibial artery and peroneal artery supply talus.
- There is important contribution from capsular and ligamentous vessels.
- The branches of these arteries form an anterosuperior and inferior groups. The posterior inferior surface of the body has no blood supply.

FRACTURE NECK TALUS

This is the second most common of all tarsal bone fractures and is second in frequency to the chip and avulsion fracture of the talus.

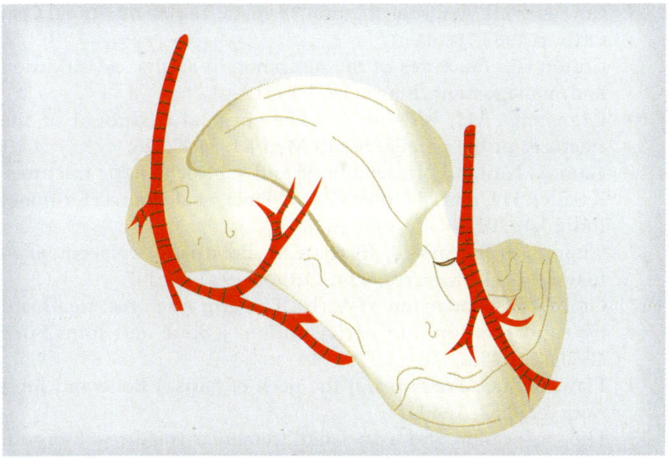

Fig. 22.21: Blood supply of talus

Incidence is 30 per cent of all talus fractures.

Mechanism of Injury

The common mode of injury is hyperdorsiflexion of the foot on one leg (Fig. 22.22). It may be associated with fracture of tarsal bones and fracture of the metatarsal bones.

Earlier, it was more commonly seen in flying accidents, but now it is more commonly seen in RTA due to head-on collision.

Note: Anderson coined the term Aviator Astralgus.

Classification (Hawkin's) (Fig. 22.23)

Type I Undisplaced vertical fracture neck of talus.

Type II Displaced fracture with subluxation or dislocation of subtalar joint.

Type III Displaced fracture neck with dislocation of the body of the talus from both ankle and subtalar joints.

Type IV Displaced fracture neck with dislocation of the head and body of the talus from subtalar/ankle/talonavicular joints.

Clinical Features

The patient usually gives a history of high velocity rudder bar type of accident. The patient complains of pain, swelling and deformity in displaced fractures. The skin may be kinked or stretched.

Radiography

In radiograph of the fracture talus the following views are recommended. Anteroposterior view with foot in maximum equinus and 15° pronation, lateral and oblique views of the ankle.

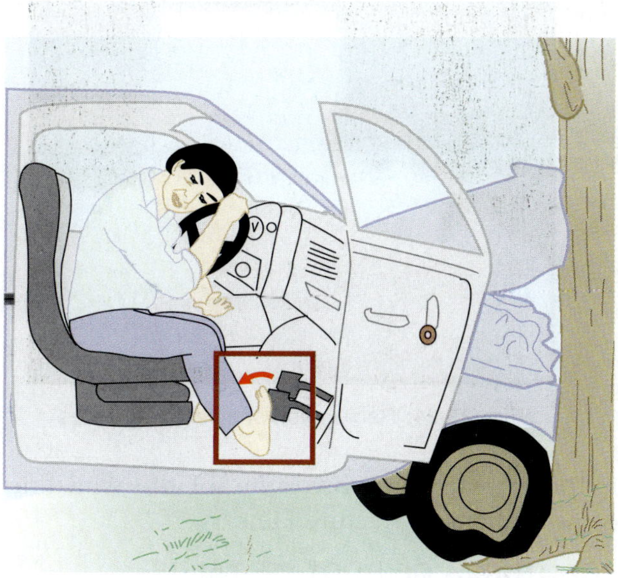

Fig. 22.22: Mechanism of injury of talus neck fractures

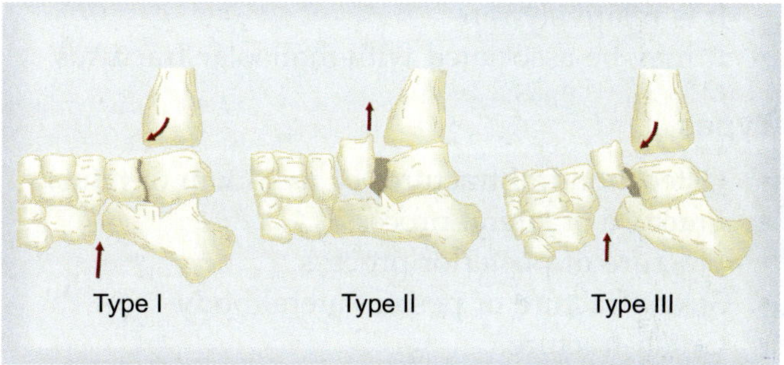

Fig. 22.23: Fracture neck of talus (Hawkin's Types)

Treatment

Type I This is best treated by below-knee plaster cast for 6 to 8 weeks with 6 weeks NWB.

Type II In this, closed reduction is done by traction in plantar flexion and a plaster cast is put in equinus. Alternatively, closed reduction is followed by percutaneous cannulated screw, fixation to prevent redisplacement of the fragments which could be possible with earlier treatment. If this fails, ORIF with lag screws is done.

Type III In these, approximately 25 per cent are open fractures. Debridement is done first and closed reduction is attempted later. If unsuccessful, ORIF with K-wires or open reduction with lag screws is attempted.

Complications

Skin necrosis, infection, delayed union, nonunion, malunion, avascular necrosis (Fig. 22.24), post-trau-

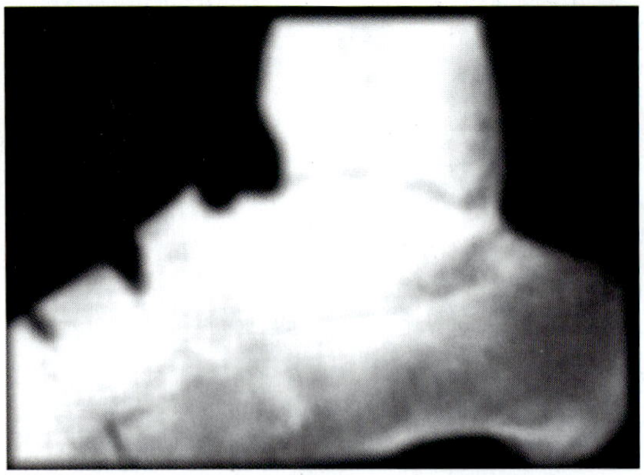

Fig. 22.24: Radiograph showing AVN talus

matic arthritis, etc. are some of the well-known complications of fracture talus.

FRACTURES OF BODY OF TALUS

- Usually due to fall from height
- It is relatively rare
- It may be associated with malleolar fractures.

Types

- Osteochondral fractures of the doom of talus.
- Fracture of lateral process
- Fracture of posterior process
- Stress fracture of posterolateral body
- Crush fracture.

BIBLIOGRAPHY

1. Adams JC. Outline of Fractures, Including Joint Injuries (8th edn). Churchill Livingstone, Ednigburgh, 1983.
2. Amihood S. Posterior dislocation of hip: Clinical observations and review of literature. S Afr Med J 1974;48:1029.
3. Apley AG, Solermm L. Apley's System of Orthopaedics and Fractures (6th edn), Butterworths: London, 1982.
4. Arnold CC, Linderholm H. Fracture of the femoral neck. Clin Orthop 1972;84:116.
5. Bioban in the treatment of talus fracture. Michael RS et al, University of Uhn, Germany, European Journal of Trauma, Dec. 2002.
6. Boyd HB, George LL. Classification and treatment of trochanteric fractures. Arch Surg 1949;58:853.
7. Campbell's operative orthopaedics, 5th volume. Edited by AS Crens Law (8th edn).
8. Cooney WP. External fixation of distal radial fractures. Clin Orthop 1983;180:44.
9. Cotton CL. Fractures of the olecranon in adults: classification and management. Injury 1973;5:121.
10. Crenshaw AH, Wilson FD. The surgical treatment of the fractures of the patella. South Med J 1954;47:716.
11. Gamma Nail in Portrochanteric and subtrochanteric fractures. K Sailer, H Umer, R Hourbesch, C Finta, et al. Source: Orthonet India Jan 2001.
12. Gingras MB, Clarke J, Evarts CM. Prosthetic replacement in femoral neck fractures. Clin Orthop 1980;152:147.
13. Grace TG, Eversmann WW (Jr). Forearm fractures: treatment by rigid fixation and early motion. J Bone and Joint Surg 1980;62-A:433.
14. Hawkins LG. Fractures of the neck of talus. J Bone and Joint Surg 1970;52-A:991.
15. Hip dislocation and associated acetabular fractures. J Orge E Alonso et al. Clinical Orthopaedics and Related Research. August 2000.
16. Hughes JL, Weber H, Wellenegger H, Kuner EH. Evaluation of ankle fractures, non-operative and operative treatment. Clin Orthop 1979;138:111.
17. Karlstrom G, Olereud S. Fractures of the tibial shaft: a critical evaluation of treatment alternatives. Clin Orthop 1974;105:82.
18. Kaufer H. Mechanical function of the patella. J Bone and Joint Surg 1971;53-54:1557.
19. Lisfranc joint injuries—RS Kuo, Tejwani et al. JBJS, Nov. 2000.
20. Mann RJ, Neal EG. Fractures of the shaft of the humerus in adults. South Med J 1965;58:264.
21. Neer CS II. Displaced proximal humeral fracture. J Bone Joint Surg 1970;52-A:1077.
22. Newer Generation Nails for Tibial fractures. Source. Orthnet 2003;56:5.
23. Reckling FW, Cordell LD. Unstable fracture dislocations of the forearm, the Monteggia and Galezzi lesions. Arch Surg 1968;96-999.
24. Reamed Nailing of Gustilo Grade IIIB. Tibial fractures: JF Keating et al. JBJS, British Nov. 2000.
25. Rockwood CA, Green DP, 1975.
26. Sarmiento A. Functional bracing of tibial fractures. Clin Orthop 1974;105:202.
27. Seinshemer F. Subtrochanteric fractures of the femur. J Bone and Joint Surg 1978;60-64:300.
28. Smith L. Deformity following supracondylar fractures of the humerus. J Bone Joint Surg 1960;42-A:235.
29. Stoddard A. Manipulation of the Elbow Joint. Physiotherapy 1971;57:259.
30. Traumatic hip distortions in adults. Edward C Yong, Roger Cornwell. Clinical Orthopaedics and Related Research. August 2000.
31. Watson Jones. Fractures and Joint Injuries (6th edn), 2 volumes. Edinburgh: Churchill Livingstone.

23

Pelvic Injuries, Rib and Coccyx Injuries

BRIEF ANATOMY

THE PELVIS SPEAKS

I am made up of two innominate bones, a portion of spine and sacrum (Fig. 23.1). The innominate bone is formed by fusion of three separate bones, the ilium, ischium and pubis. Ilium forms the superior part, the ischium the posteroinferior part, the pubis the anteroinferior part. These three bones of mine meet to form the acetabulum. Anteriorly, I am connected by a strong minimally mobile fibrocartilaginous joint called the pubic symphysis. Posteriorly, I articulate with the sacrum through the almost immobile sacroiliac joint. I derive my stability in the posterior aspect from the sacroiliac (SI) and the sacrospinous ligament complex, anteriorly by the pubic symphysis and inferiorly by the muscles and ligaments forming the pelvic floor and perineum.

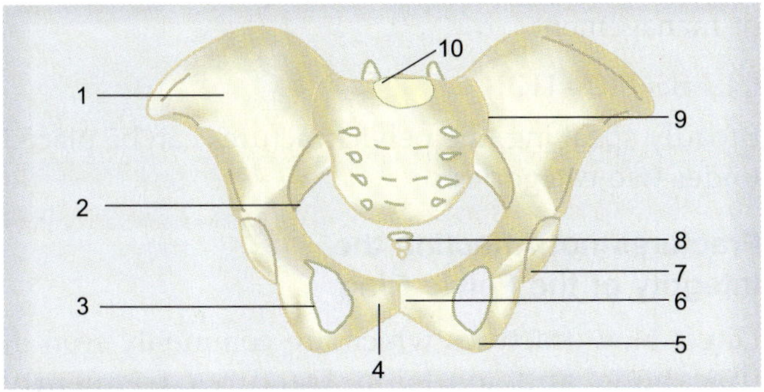

Fig. 23.1: Showing anatomy of pelvis; (1) Ilium, (2) Arcuate line, (3) Obturator foramen, (4) Pubis, (5) Ischium, (6) Pubic symphysis, (7) Acetabulum, (8) Coccyx, (9) Sacroiliac, (10) Sacrum

My main functions are:

1. To transmit the forces from the spine to the lower limbs and vice versa.
2. In the standing position, I transmit the weight through the ilium and in the sitting position through the ischium.
3. I give attachment to the muscles helping in posture and locomotion.
4. I protect the vital genitourinary system and lower abdominal viscera.

FRACTURE PELVIS

STABILITY OF THE PELVIS

Stability of the pelvis depends on both bony and ligamentous structures. Anterior portion of the pelvic ring neither participates in normal weight bearing nor it is essential for maintenance of pelvic stability. The posterior arch is formed by the sacrum, SI joints and ilia and is the weight bearing portion of the pelvis. The posterosuperior SI ligaments provide most of the ligamentous stability of the SI joints.

Stable Pelvic Fracture

These fractures do not involve the pelvic ring and they are minimally displaced.

Unstable Pelvic Fracture

They involve the pelvic ring and are widely displaced. Pelvic fractures pose a problem different from others. Here the emphasis is on recognition of potential complications associated with these fractures, the notable ones being injuries to the major vessels and nerves of the pelvis and major viscera like intestines, bladder and the urethra, severe intrapelvic haemorrhage from fracture of pelvic ring. Mortality from pelvic fracture varies from 10 to 50 per cent. Proper fracture management decreases the blood loss and controls the haemorrhage. A to F management as proposed by Mac Murthy in multiple trauma patients is important in management of the pelvic fractures.

Vital practice points

A to F management of Mac Murthy

A. Airway management
B. Blood and fluid replacement
C. Central nervous system management
D. Digestive system management
E. Excretory system management
F. Fracture management

HISTORY Pelvic fractures usually occur due to high-velocity trauma following a road traffic accident (RTA) or due to fall from a height.

The relative incidences are as follows:

- RTA—80.7 per cent.
- Fall—16.1 per cent.
- Compresssion fracture—rest.

MECHANISM OF INJURY

There are four mechanisms by which pelvic ring fractures are produced:

1. Lateral compression (Fig. 23.2A).
2. Anteroposterior compression (Fig. 23.2B).
3. Vertical shear forces.
4. Inferior forces (e.g. fall on buttocks).

The first two mechanisms are common in RTA and may cause stable or unstable fractures. Vertical shear forces are due to fall from a height and will cause grossly unstable fractures.

Fortunately, most pelvic fractures are stable and respond to nonoperative treatment. Unstable fractures need manipulative reduction and stabilisation by external fixators and sometimes by internal fixation. A proper evaluation of the fracture by radiograph and CT scan helps to determine the best course of management.

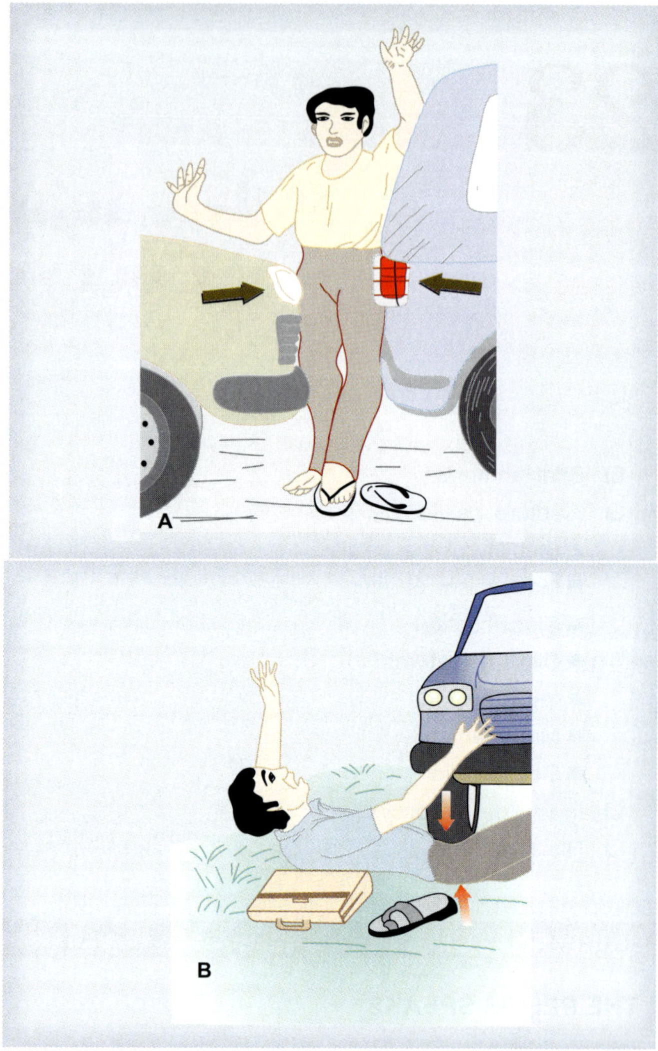

Figs 23.2A and B: Showing mechanism of pelvic fractures in RTA: (A) Lateral compression, (B) Anteroposterior compression

CLASSIFICATION

Broadly speaking, the pelvic fractures can be placed under two categories.

Fractures not Affecting the Integrity of the Pelvic Ring

Direct blow fractures which are commonly seen in iliac bone and avulsion fractures frequently encountered in the young come under this group. Avulsion fractures are commonly seen in antero-superior and inferior iliac spines and ischial tuberosity (Fig. 23.3).

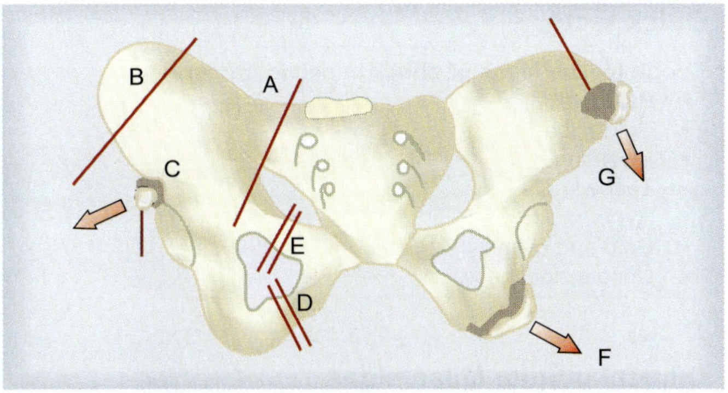

Fig. 23.3: Showing avulsion fractures and fractures of individual bones not affecting the pelvic ring: (A) fracture of the sacrum, (B) fracture of the iliac wing, (C) avulsion fracture of anteroinferior iliac spine, (D) inferior rami fracture, (E) superior ramus fracture, (F) avulsion fracture of ischial tuberosity, and (G) avulsion fracture of anterosuperior iliac spine

Fractures Affecting the Integrity of the Pelvic Ring

These are single or double break fractures in the pelvic ring and could be stable or unstable. A stable fracture is one which resists displacing forces (Fig. 23.4). Obviously, fractures which cannot resist usual forces are called unstable fractures and these pose a major therapeutic challenge (Fig 23.5).

Many classifications have been proposed for pelvic fractures. Key and Conwell's classification is by far the simplest and commonly used classification. It has prognostic importance too.

Key and Conwell's Classification

Fracture of Individual Bones without a Break in the Pelvic Ring

1. Avulsion fracture of the:
   a. Anterosuperior iliac spine
   b. Anteroinferior iliac spine
   c. Ischial tuberosity.
2. Fracture of pubis or ischium.
3. Fracture wing of ilium (Duverney).
4. Fracture sacrum.
5. Fracture or dislocation of coccyx.

Single Break in the Pelvic Ring

1. Fracture of both ipsilateral rami.
2. Fracture near or subluxation of symphysis pubis.
3. Fracture near or subluxation of sacroiliac joints.

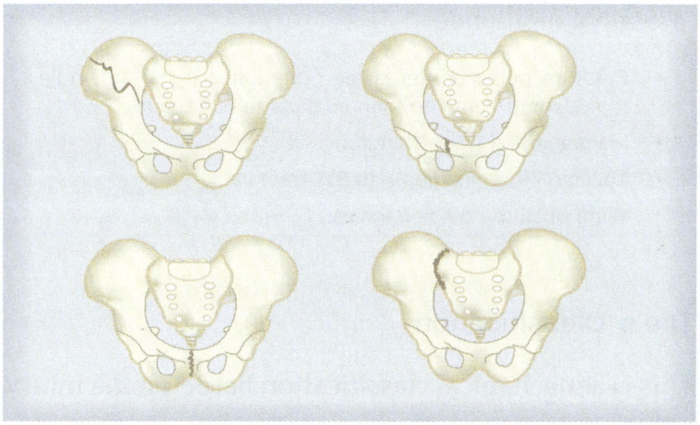

Fig. 23.4: Showing stable pelvic fractures

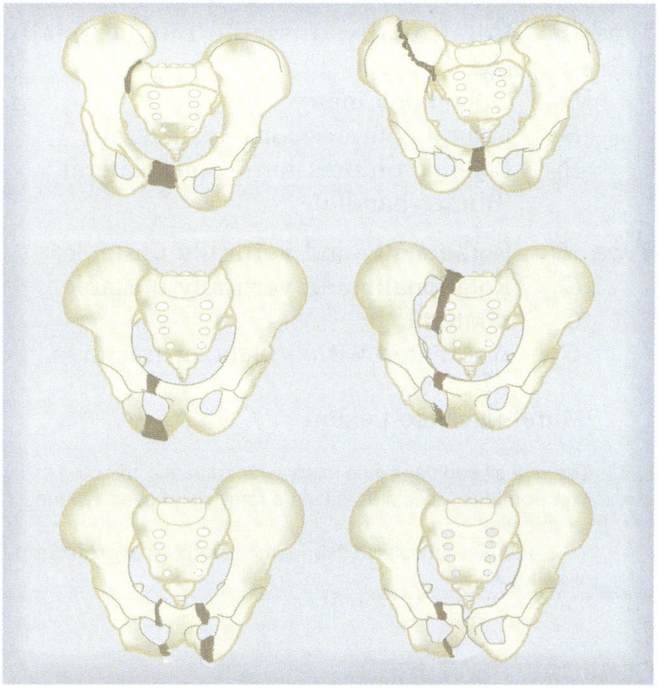

Fig. 23.5: Showing unstable pelvic fractures

Double Breaks in the Pelvic Ring

1. Double vertical fracture or dislocation of pubis *(straddle fracture).*
2. Double vertical fracture or dislocation of pelvis *(Malgaigne's fracture).*

Acetabulum Fractures

1. Undisplaced
2. Displaced.

Relative incidence

- Fracture pubic bones is the commonest > 69%. Single ramus more common than multiple rami fracture.
- Malgaigne—11.8% fracture.
- Multiple crush injuries—10.8% fracture.
- Wing of ilium—5.4% fracture.

Tile's Classification

This is a mechanical classification based on the injury forces.

Type A Stable.
A_1 Fracture pelvis not involving ring.
A_2 Stable, but minimally displaced.

Type B Rotationally unstable but vertically stable.
B_1 Open book injury.
B_2 Lateral compression—Ipsilateral.
B_3 Lateral compression—Contralateral. (Bucket handle).

Type C Rotationally and vertically unstable.
C_1 Rotationally and vertically unstable.
C_2 Bilateral.
C_3 Associated with acetabular fractures.

Murel-Lavallee Lesion

This is a closed degloving injury with traumatic shearing of skin from deep fascia. It leaves a large dead space prone for infection.

Treatment consists of debridement and primary closure of soft tissues.

CLINICAL FEATURES

Symptoms

The patient most often gives a history of high-velocity trauma and usually presents in a state of hypovolaemic shock. Features of intra-abdominal injuries and genitourinary injuries are frequently present.

Clinical Signs

The patient may present with all signs of shock. Tenderness over the fracture site and one has to look for three important signs described by Milch.

Quick facts

Look for the signs of shock in pelvic fracture

- Pale look
- Cold nose
- Sweating
- Tachycardia
- Hypotension
- Cold and clammy skin
- Unconsciousness

Clinical points: Milch signs

1. **Destot's sign**—Large haematoma above inguinal ligament or scrotum.
2. **Roux's sign**—Distance from greater trochanter to pubic spine is ↑ on affected side.
3. **Earle's sign**—On per rectal examination, the bony prominence or a large haematoma can be palpated.

Clinical Tests

Compression test When a compressive force is applied through the two iliac bones, the patient complains of pain in pelvic fracture (Fig. 23.6A).

Distraction test When distraction force is applied to the two iliac bones at the anterosuperior iliac spine, the patient complains of pain (Fig. 23.6B).

Direct pressure test Direct pressure over the symphysis pubis elicits pain (Fig. 23.6C).

Following this, an examination for abdomen and pelvis injuries is carried out and next urethral catheterisation or urethrogram is done.

INVESTIGATIONS

Radiography

Different radiographic views are recommended to study the fracture configuration, displacements, etc. in pelvic fractures:

1. Plain AP view.
2. Oblique view—45° oblique projections.
3. Internal and external rotation view.
4. Inlet view—40° caudad view.
5. Outlet view—40° cephalad view.

Futher radiographic studies include CT scans and 3-dimensional imaging.

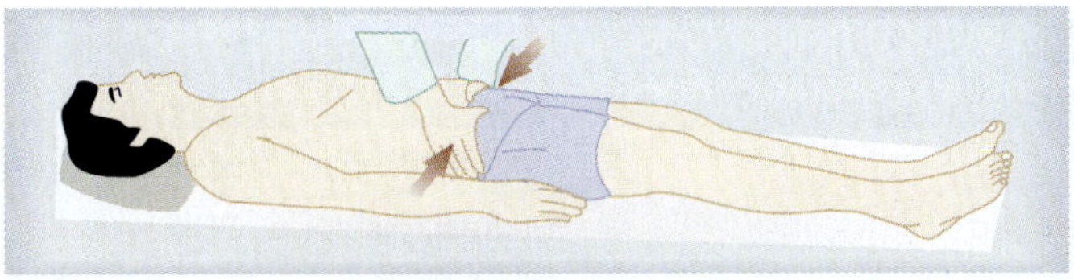

Fig. 23.6A: Showing compression test in pelvic fractures

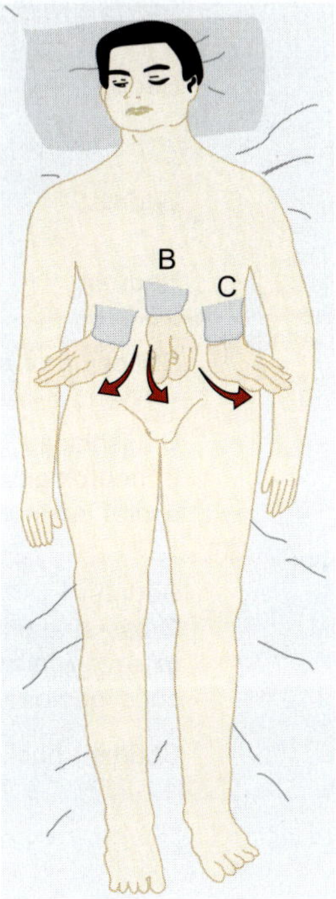

Figs 23.6B and C: Showing (B) direct pressure test, (C) distraction test

MANAGEMENT

One should remember that pelvic fractures are usually due to high-velocity trauma and is associated with multiple fractures and multiple system injuries. Resuscitation and correction of hypovolaemic shock takes precedence over the management of fracture per se. But once the general condition is stabilised attention should be given to treat the fracture which will prevent further blood loss and damage to visceral organs.

Different types of pelvic fractures, their clinical features and treatment are listed in the Table 23.1.

Treatment points

Three main pitfalls in the treatment of pelvic fracture
1. Treating only fracture overlooking visceral injuries.
2. Overtreating a stable fracture.
3. Treating an unstable fracture.

Treatment Methods

Initial treatment is carried out as follows:
- Resuscitation and other general measures, to improve the general condition of the patient.
- Blood transfusion and other medical and surgical emergency measures are carried out.
  1. *Avulsion fractures* Conservative treatment like bedrest, traction, physiotherapy, etc. gives good results. They rarely need surgery.
  2. *Undisplaced fractures* Respond to bedrest, traction, pelvic slings (Fig. 23.7), nonsteroidal anti-inflammatory drugs (NSAIDs), etc.
  3. *Displaced fractures* Reduction by lateral compression methods as described by Watson Jones is very helpful. Retention is either by spica cast, canvas sling or external fixators.
  4. *Role of external and internal fixators* The above methods usually suffice, but the fractures associated with multiple system injuries need to be stabilised either by external fixators or by open reduction and internal fixation (ORIF) (Fig. 23.8). These two methods have the following advantages:
     - Gives firm stability.
     - Helps early mobilisation.
     - Reduces period of bedrest.
     - Helps early control of osseous bleeding.

COMPLICATIONS

Pelvic fracture is a dreaded injury as it is associated with a plethora of complications. The following are some of them.

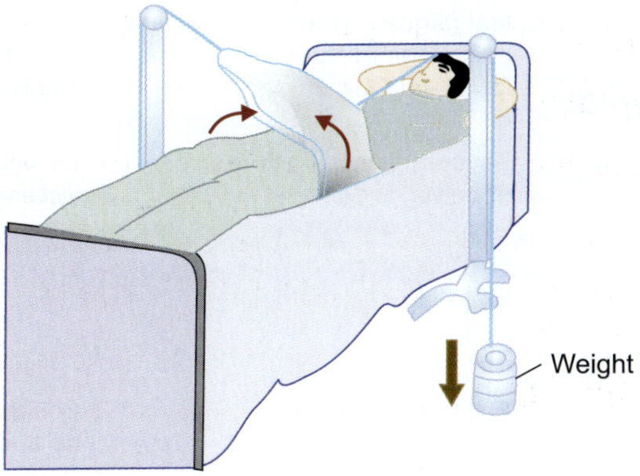

Fig. 23.7: Pelvic sling as a mainstay of conservative treatment in fracture pelvis

Table 23.1: Key and Conwell's types: A comparative study of different types of pelvic fractures, their clinical features and treatment is presented here

Sl No	*Type of pelvic fracture*	*Clinical features*	*Treatment*
Type I	1. Avulsion of anterosuperior iliac spine	Pain on trying to flex and abduct the thigh	Bedrest, hip spica, ORIF rarely done
	2. Avulsion of anteroinferior iliac spine	Rare	Rest with hip flexed for 2 to 3 weeks
	3. Avulsion of ischial tuberosity	Flexion of thigh with knee in flexion ↑ pain	Conservative treatment
	4. Single ramus fracture of pubis or ischium	Commonest fracture seen in elderly, confused with fracture neck of femur	Bedrest
	5. Fracture body of ischium	Pain when hamstrings are put in tension	Bedrest
	6. Stress fracture pubis or ischium fracture	Can occur in last trimester of pregnancy	Bedrest
	7. Fracture iliac wing (6%)	Lateral compression force ↑ pain Walking is painful	Strapping of pelvis
	8. Fracture sacrum	Neurological deficits due to involvement of higher sacral roots	Undisplaced fracture; bedrest In neurological lesions posterior sacral laminectomy is done
	9. Fracture coccyx	Fall in sitting position	Bedrest Cross-strapping of buttocks In severe disability, coccygectomy
Type II	1. Fracture of two rami ipsilateral	Flexion, abduction and external rotation (FABER) test is positive. This fracture is common **FABER—Flexion abduction and external rotation**	Bedrest; bucks traction
	2. Fracture or subluxation near symphysis pubis	Tenderness over symphysis pubis + palpable gap + injury to genitourinary tract common.	Circumferential strapping
	3. Fracture or subluxation near SI joint	FABER test is positive Straight leg raising test is painful	Symptomatic treatment and bedrest, pelvic sling, belt
Type III	1. Double vertical fracture **(Straddle fracture)**	Urethral injury—20% Abdominal injury—38%	Symptomatic treatment, bed-rest, etc.
	2. **Malgaigne's fracture** (ipsilateral pubic rami fracture with ipsilateral SI joint dislocation)	Shortening, external rotation deformity, limb shortening, umbilicus displaced	Postural reduction + traction + pelvic slings
	3. Severe multiple fracture of pelvis	Associated with severe visceral damage	• In compound fracture external fixators preferred • Open reduction and internal fixation if associated with multiple system injuries • Rest in bed with sand bags, pelvic slings and traction
Type IV	Fracture acetabulum	Could be displaced or undisplaced, could be a rim fracture or central floor fracture	Skeletal traction through the greater trochanter

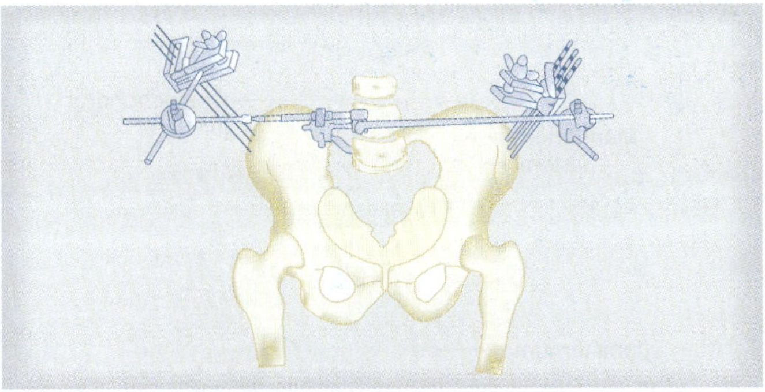

Fig. 23.8: Showing treatment by external fixation methods in pelvic fractures

Haemorrhage It is usually intra-abdominal and the incidence is around 20 per cent. The patient usually presents with features of shock. If the pulse is greater than 100/min, it suggests 20 per cent blood volume deficit; if the blood pressure is less than 100 mm systolic, it suggests 30 per cent volume deficit. Diagnostic peritoneal lavage and open paracentesis has an accuracy rate of 98 per cent in intra-abdominal injuries. CT scan is also sensitive and specific.

Treatment is by laparotomy and is indicated if there is continuing blood loss, visceral perforation, expanding palpable suprapubic haematoma.

Injuries of lower urinary tract Rupture of urethra and rupture of urinary bladder are the common lower urinary tract injuries frequently seen in separation of pubic symphysis and fracture pubic rami. It has an average incidence of 13 per cent. The dictum is *"All pelvic fractures must be assumed to have urinary tract injuries until proved otherwise."*

Presence of haematuria is not pathognomonic, but its presence calls for three radiographic studies like retrograde urethrogram, cystogram and IVP. Rupture of anterior urethra is seen in straddle fractures and is not very common. Rupture of posterior urethra is relatively more common and is limited to male. Suprapubic cystostomy, direct repair, rail road repair, urethroplasties are some of the treatment methods.

Bladder injuries are seen in 4 per cent of the cases and are associated with symphysis pubis injuries and rami fracture. Eighty per cent injuries are extraperitoneal and calls for direct surgical intervention as quickly as possible.

Other injuries Testicular injuries and vaginal lacerations, bowel and rectal injuries and urethral injuries are all common and require immediate surgical intervention.

Other Complications

Loss of reduction, sepsis, thrombophlebitis, delayed union, nonunion, post-traumatic arthritis, fat embolism, major arterial injuries, abdominal wall injury, neurological injuries usually L_5, S_1 roots due to sacral fracture are the other common complications.

Recap

Pelvic fractures

- A fracture feared for its complications.
- RTA accounts for 80% of cases.
- Fracture broadly classified into not affecting and affecting integrity of the pelvic ring.
- Fracture pubic rami, usually single, is the commonest pelvic fracture (69%).
- Usual presentation is hypovolaemic shock.
- Correction of hypovolaemia and other general measures takes precedence over fracture management.
- Conservative treatment usually gives good results.
- External and internal fixation is done for specific indications
- Intra-abdominal and genitourinary injuries are common possibilities and need early recognition and prompt treatment.
- Mortality is 20%.

Note: Mortality in closed pelvic fractures is 10 to 30 per cent and open fractures is 40 to 50 per cent.

INJURY TO THE COCCYX

These are relatively rare injuries, but could be quite troublesome to the patients.

Mechanism

Due to a direct fall on the buttocks (Fig. 23.9). The patient usually complains of chronic pain in the

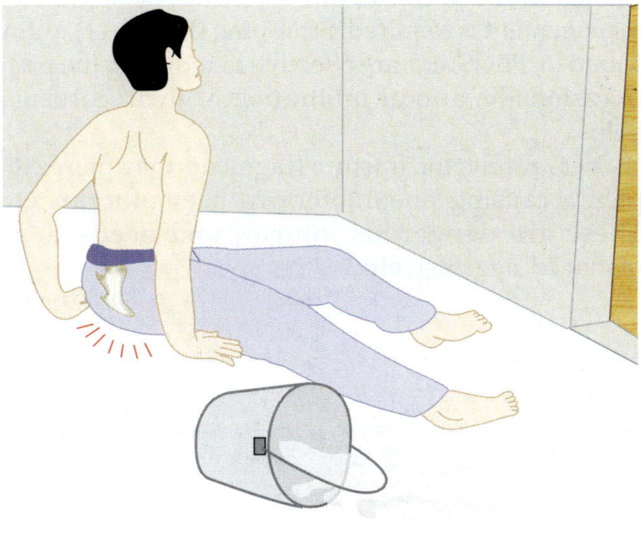

Fig. 23.9: Showing mechanism of injury in coccyx fractures

buttocks. The treatment is essentially conservative in nature with periods of bedrest and symptomatic treatment for pain and inflammation.

Physiotherapy Management

Consists of the following steps:

1. To relieve pain, thermotherapy like ultrasound and TENS.
2. To relieve prolonged pressure on the buttocks, sitting on a ring cushion and sitting on alternate buttocks is advised.
3. Isometric exercises to the glutei maximus muscle in sitting, lying and prone positions is advisable.
4. *Sitz bath helps to relieve pain.

> *Note* These injuries are difficult to tackle.
> *Reasons*
> 1. Due to the position of coccyx which is deep and covered by thick muscles on either side.
> 2. Due to the pressure from sitting. Hence long sitting posture needs to be controlled.

Note: *Sitz bath—This consists of sitting in a shallow tub of warm water. Commonly advocated in Piles patients after surgery.

RIB FRACTURES

These are relatively rare injuries and are usually due to direct trauma. The rib usually breaks at the angle which is a point of maximum convexity (Fig. 23.10).

Intercostal muscles provide natural immobilisation to the fractured ribs and hence no aggressive management is required. Strapping (Fig. 23.11), ultrasound or TENS, etc. are effective in reducing the pain. Occasionally, a local infiltration of hydrocortisone helps.

Very rarely, the fracture fragments may pierce the pleura causing pneumothorax, haemothorax, etc. These are dangerous injuries and needs to be managed aggressively.

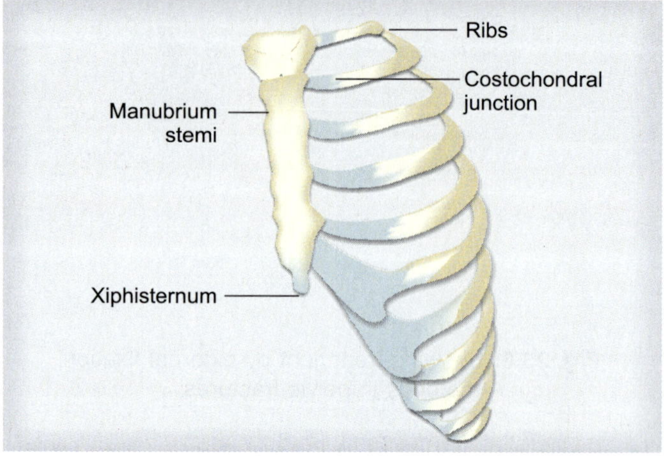

Fig. 23.10: Showing anatomical features of the ribs

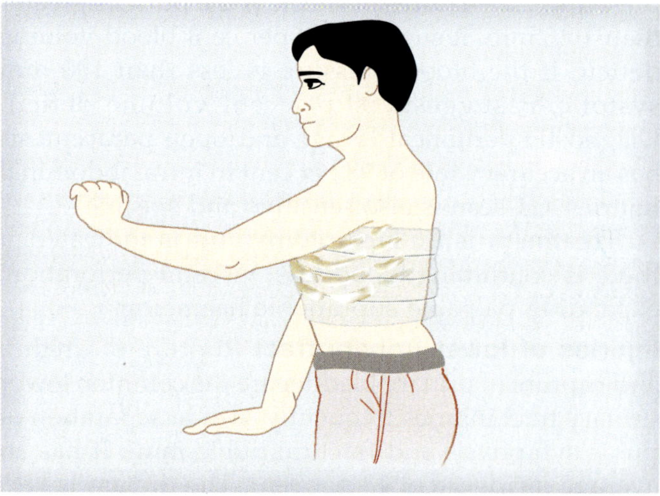

Fig. 23.11: Showing strapping method for treatment of fracture ribs

Physiotherapy Management

This essentially consists of deep breathing exercises which are progressively made more vigorous to improve the mobility of the thorax.

BIBLIOGRAPHY

1. Murel-Lavallee Lesion. Source: Orthonet, 2003;5-58.

24

Injuries of the Spine

- Brief anatomy
- Injuries of the cervical spine
- Thoracic and lumbosacral spine injuries
- Spinal cord injury
- Cauda equina syndrome

BRIEF ANATOMY

THE SPINE SPEAKS

I am a family of 33 bones running from the skull to the pelvis (Fig. 24.1). I have been assigned the twin responsibility of carrying the load of the body and head, thanks to the two-legged posture human beings enjoy and the still more important responsibility of protecting the vital spinal cord.

My neck bones (Fig. 24.2) are called *cervical vertebrae*, bones of upper back and in line with the chest are called *thoracic vertebrae* and the bones of the lower back are called *lumbar vertebrae*. Each vertebra of mine rest on the vertebra above and below. At these points, they articulate with each other through the *facet* joint which keeps all my vertebrae in their correct position and in alignment with each other. I have a spinal shock absorber called the *disc* which separates each vertebra from the next (see page 279).

Each vertebra of mine has an *anterior body* and a *posterior neural arch* (Figs 24.3 and 24.4). The body has a tough outer cortex and a cancellous middle portion. It is supported in front and back by anterior longitudinal ligament and posterior longitudinal ligament respectively. The posterior neural arch consists of two pedicles, two transverse processes, a posterior spinous process and a pair of lamina which together form the spinal canal along with the posterior surface of the body. In this canal of mine lies the all-important spinal cord.

While ligamentum flavum binds the laminae together, the interspinous ligament binds the spinous processes, and the supraspinous ligament binds the tip of the spinous process. All the structures of mine mentioned so far help me in providing the much needed stability.

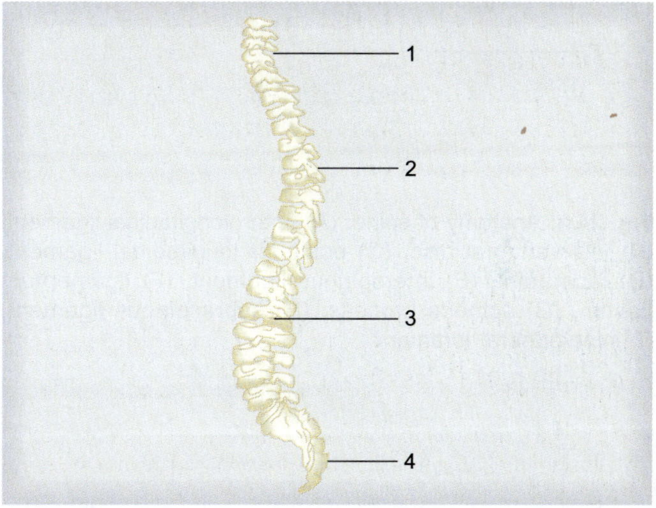

Fig. 24.1: Normal spinal curves: (1) cervical lordosis, (2) thoracic kyphosis, (3) lumbar lordosis, and (4) sacral kyphosis

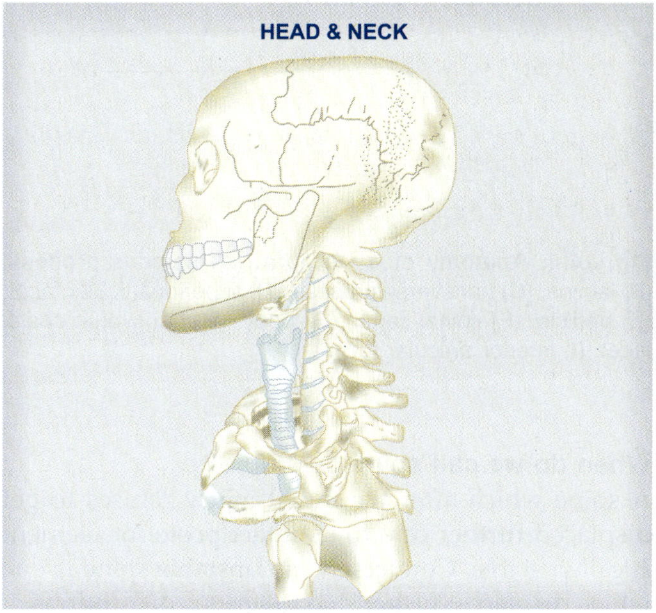

Fig. 24.2: Arrangement of the neck bones

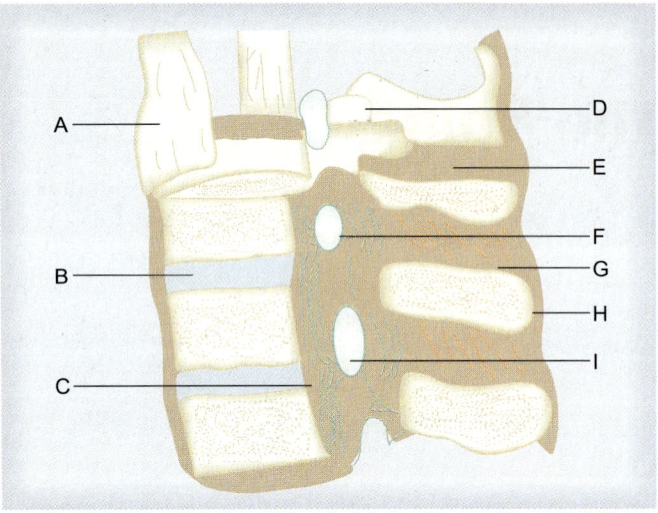

Fig. 24.3: Anatomy of spine: (A) anterolongitudinal ligament, (B) intervertebral disc, (C) posterior longitudinal ligament, (D) facet joint, (E) interspinous ligament, (F) ligamentum flavum, (G) spinous process, (H) supraspinous ligament, (I) intervertebral foramen

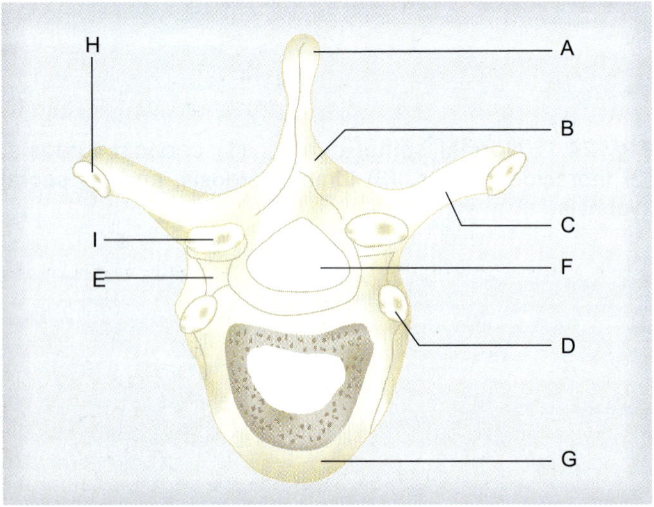

Fig. 24.4: Anatomy of a vertebra: (A) spinous process, (B) lamina, (C) transverse process, (D) superior articular facet, (E) pedicle, (F) spinal canal, (G) body, (H) transverse costal facet, (I) inferior articular facet

When do we call spine as stable?

A spine which after the initial injury refuses to get displaced further due to its intact posterior element is called stable. Conversely, an unstable spine is one which displaces further due to serious disruptions of the structures jeopardising the spinal cord.

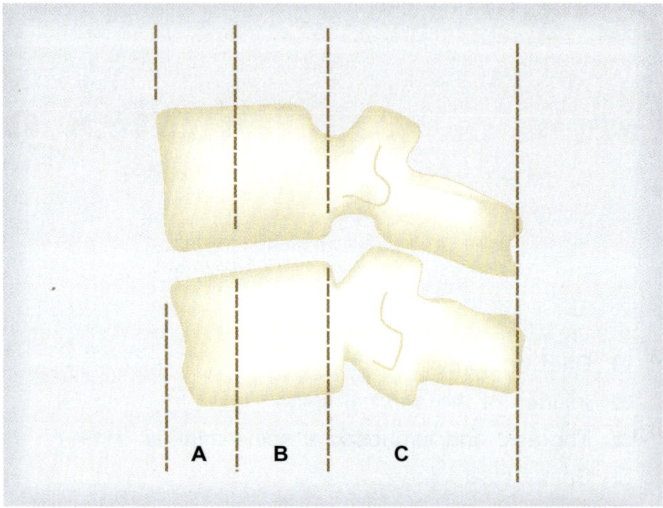

Fig. 24.5: Three-column concept of spine: (A) anterior column, (B) middle column, and (C) posterior column

The *three-column concept* (Fig. 24.5) is the latest description of the spine stability. The *anterior column* consists of anterior half of the vertebral body, anterior part of the disc and anterior longitudinal ligament. The *middle column* consists of posterior half of the body and the disc, the posterior longitudinal ligament. The *posterior column* consists of the posterior vertebral arch consisting of transverse process, spinous process and the accompanying ligaments. One-column injury is stable, two-column injury is unstable and three column is invariably unstable. Unstable spine is a dangerous spine for it may injure the spinal cord.

About spine

- It is the principal load bearing structure of the head and torso.
- Each portion of the spine has specific functions:
  - **Cervical spine** provides head with limited mobility and protects proximal part of the spinal cord.
  - **Thoracic spine** provides mobility to the upper torso and rib cage and protects the cord.
  - **Lumbar spine** provides the lower torso, its mobility and protects the cord.
- Like the skull which protects the brain, spinal column protects the cord.
- Spine should be flexible yet strong.
- Spinal cord injury could result in death, quadriplegia or paraplegia.

Disc facts

Functions of disc

- A disc has in the centre nucleus pulposus and annulus fibrosus at the periphery.
- Binds vertebra together.
- Allows motion.
- Absorbs shock.
- Distributes load between the segments.
- Contributes to lordosis.
- Comprises approximately 25 per cent of the total length of the spinal column.

Incidence of Spine Injuries

- About 1 million/year in the USA alone.
- Male : Female = 4 : 1
- Injury is common at the cervicothoracic and thoracolumbar regions
- Modes of injury:
  a. RTA — 45 per cent
  b. Falls — 20 per cent
  c. Sports injuries (diving) — 15 per cent
  d. Acts of violence — 15 per cent.

INJURIES OF THE CERVICAL SPINE

Injuries of the cervical spine are dangerous; and if associated with neurological damage, the results can be devastating. Though diagnostic and treatment methods have vastly improved over years, still injuries of the cervical spine pose the greatest challenge to the skill and acumen of orthopaedic and neurosurgeons.

Jefferson pointed out two areas commonly involved in cervical spine injuries, C_{1-2} and C_{5-7}. According to Meyer, C_2 and C_5 are commonly involved. Neurological damage is seen in 40 per cent of cases. In 10 per cent of cases, radiographs are normal.

Causes

1. Fall from height—it is the most common cause in developing countries.
2. Diving injuries—diving into water with insufficient depth or in an inebriated condition.
3. Road traffic accidents (RTAs)—common cause in developed countries, e.g. whiplash injury (Fig. 24.6).
4. Gunshot injuries, etc. These injure the cervical spine and the cord directly.

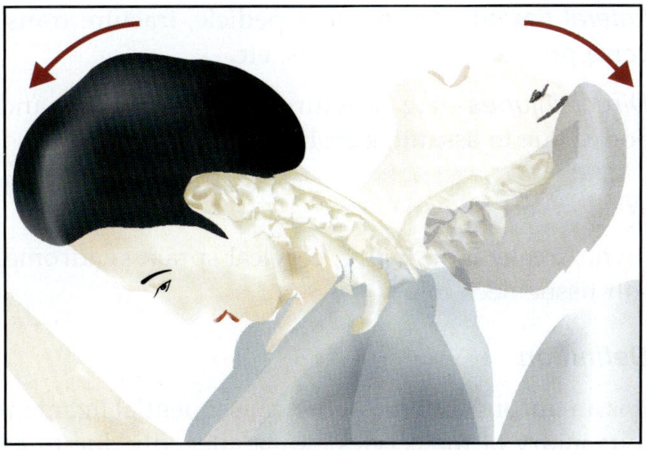

Fig. 24.6: Whiplash injury: due to sudden deceleration, forceful hyperextension is followed by flexion of the neck

Mechanism of Injury (Figs 24.7A to D)

Pure flexion force—e.g. compression fracture of vertebral body, e.g. fall from height.

Flexion rotation force—e.g. fall on one side of the shoulder, disruption of facet capsule is seen.

Axial compression—e.g. fall of an object on the head results in load compression, e.g. explosive comminuted fracture of C_5 body.

Extension force—e.g. avulsion fracture of superior margin of vertebral body, e.g. whiplash injury.

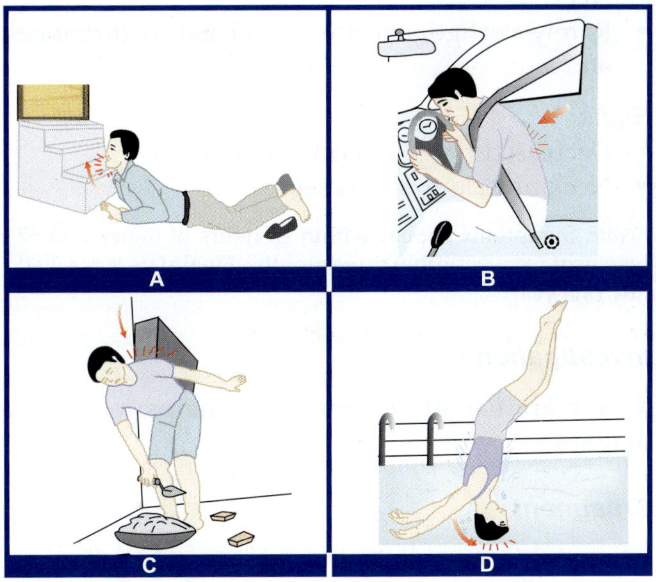

Figs 24.7A to D: Common mechanism of cervical spine injuries: (A) Hyperextension injury, (B) Flexion extension injury, (C) Flexion rotation injury, (D) Hyperflexion injury

Section 2

Lateral flexion—e.g. fracture pedicle, fracture transverse process and facet joints, etc.

Direct injuries—e.g. fracture spinous process and body. Due to assault, gunshot injury, etc.

WHIPLASH INJURY

(Syn: Acceleration injury, cervical sprain syndrome, soft tissue neck injury)

Definition

It is an unconventional and inconsequential ligamentous injury of the cervical spine allegedly due to an extension injury following a rear-end collision in an RTA (Fig. 24.6).

Incidence

- It is seen in about 25 per cent of rear-end collision of RTAs
- Seventy per cent of those affected are women.
- It is common in the 3rd or 4th decades.

Clinical Features

Symptoms
- Upper neck pain that becomes worse with movement
- Occipital headache
- Neck stiffness
- Rarely vertigo, auditory or visual disturbances, etc.

Signs
- Decreased range of neck movements
- Neck muscle spasm is seen.

Note: Symptoms appear within 48 hours of injury and 57 per cent recover within three months. Final state is reached by one year.

Investigations

X-rays are usually normal. MRI helps to make a diagnosis.

Treatment

It is mainly conservative and consists of the following:
- *Drugs:* NSAIDs, muscle relaxants, etc. are given
- *Collars:* These are recommended for the first three days.
- Short arc active movements are slowly begun
- Active ROM exercises are slowly commenced
- After the pain subsides, isometric strengthening exercises are slowly commenced
- Other modalities take ultrasound, traction, manipulation, massage, etc. also helps.

Allen's Classification of Cervical Spine Fractures (Figs 24.8A to D)

Compressive flexion (5 stages) Ranges from blunting of anterosuperior vertebral margin to posterior displacement into the spinal canal. It is usually a stable fracture but may become unstable if compression is more than 50 per cent.

Vertical compression (3 stages) Ranges from fracture of superior or inferior endplate with centrum fracture of the vertebral body. Stable fracture if compression is less than 50 per cent of the vertebral body.

Distractive flexion (4 stages) Ranges from failure of posterior ligamentous complex to full-width vertebral body displacement. This is an unstable fracture.

Compression extension (5 stages) Ranges from unilateral vertebral arch fracture to bilateral vertebral arch fracture with full-vertebral body displacement anteriorly. It is unstable.

Distractive extension Ranges from failure of anterior ligament complex to posterior ligament complex. This is also an unstable fracture.

Lateral flexion Ranges from asymmetric compression and ipsilateral vertebral arch to fracture without displacement and with displacement. May become unstable.

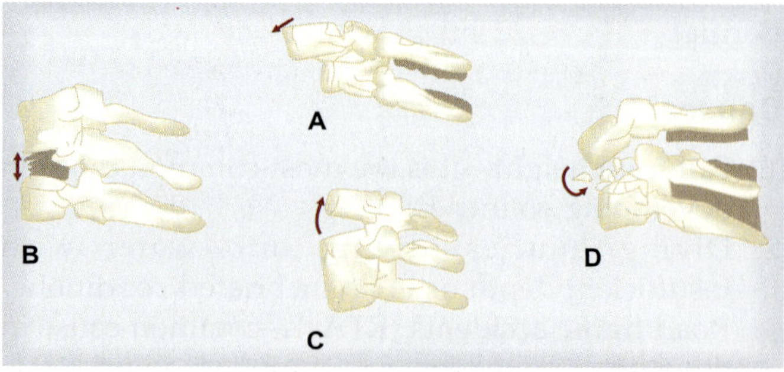

Figs 24.8A to D: Cervical spine injuries: (A) distraction injury, (B) compression injury, (C) hyperextension injury, (D) compression and distraction injury

1. The lowermost functioning muscle is documented and a functional level is established.
2. Next the sacrally innervated skin is examined. Perianal, anal, scrotal, labia, and plantar surface of the toes are examined.
3. *Perianal sensation may be the only sign to indicate an incomplete lesion.*

Table 24.2: Cervical spinal cord injury

↓ **Root injury**
- At the neural foramen
- Essentially a peripheral nerve injury (flaccid paralysis) (see Table 24.1)

↓ **Cord injury**

↓ **Incomplete** (sparing distal to the injury)
1. *Brown-Sequard syndrome* Injury to lateral half of the spinal cord.
2. *Central cord syndrome*—most common. Results in gross quadriplegia, with sacral sparing.
3. *Anterior cord syndrome*—complete motor paralysis and sensory anaesthesia except deep pressure and proprioception.
4. *Posterior cord syndrome*—motor power, deep pressure, pain and proprioception lost.

↓ **Complete**

Complete loss of sensation and motor power below the level of injury.

Other Examinations

1. *Rectal sensation*—loss of sensation around the anus.
2. *Rectal motor*—sphincter contracts, over a gloved finger.
3. *Bulbocavernosus reflex* involves S_1, S_2 and S_3 nerve roots. Squeeze the glans penis, anal sphincter contracts around the gloved finger.

Initially, following the injury, the above reflexes are absent, indicating spinal shock. Usually, it returns within 24 hours. If not a presumptive diagnosis and determination of a root or cord lesion is made.

A diagnosis of a complete or incomplete syndrome is documented.

Cord concussion

A state of "spinal shock", i.e. temporary electrical dysfunction

Features
1. Sensory loss.
2. Flaccid paralysis.
3. Visceral paralysis.
4. Reflexes are in abeyance.
5. Anal reflex lost (anal wink lost).

Usually
- 8 hours later concussion regresses.
- 7–10 days later complete recovery. If the reflexes, do not return within 24 hours to 10 days a diagnosis of complete cord transection is made.

Investigations

Radiography (Fig. 24.17) Lateral view is important. If an adequate lateral radiography reveals no fracture or dislocation, then a complete radiographic examination including anteroposterior, open mouth and oblique projections are performed.

Myelography is of value in incomplete lesion who fail to show progressive improvement.

CT scan makes an accurate diagnosis of hidden fracture. It is not helpful in assessing the soft tissue injury.

MRI evaluates cord injuries better. MRI is found to be very reliable and helpful in assessing the bony, soft tissue damages and injury to the cord very accurately.

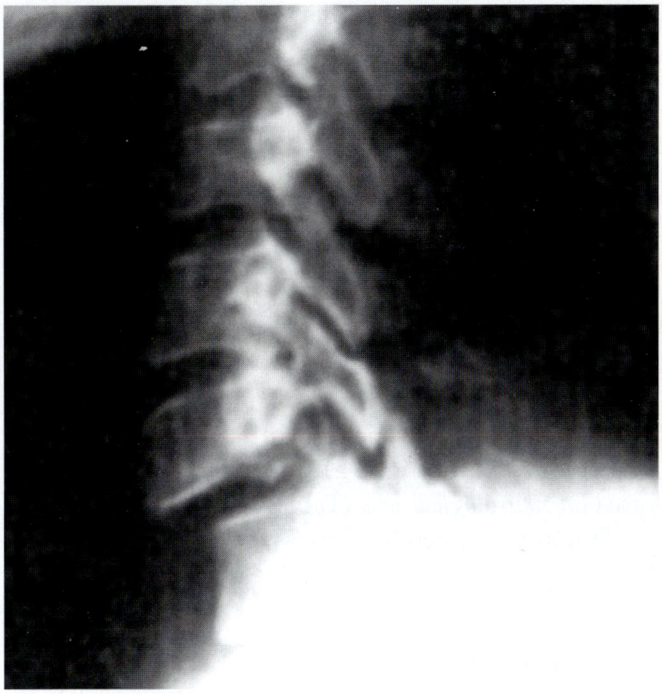

Fig. 24.17: Radiograph showing fracture dislocation of C6 over C7

General laboratory investigations—like Hb percentage, blood group, bleeding time, clotting time, electrolyte status, etc. are done.

Treatment facts

Goals of treatment of cervical spine injury
1. Realign the spine.
2. Prevent further neurological damage.
3. Aid neurological recovery.
4. Obtain and maintain spinal stability.
5. Aim at early functional recovery.

Treatment Methods

At the accident site Resuscitation and transport is important. *In a person lying still without using his neck after an RTA, a cervical spine injury is always suspected until proved otherwise.*

The patient is transported with utmost care over a stretcher to the hospital. All unnecessary neck movements should be totally avoided. If the patient needs resuscitation, it has to be carried out with a lot of care.

At the hospital

Nonoperative treatment Most cases can be treated nonoperatively by halovest, four postcervical collars, minerva jacket, cervical collars, etc. (Figs 24.18A to C).

Indications

1. Stable cervical spine with no neurological injury. A rigid cervical brace or halo for 8 to 12 week is usually sufficient.
2. Stable compression fracture of vertebral bodies and undisplaced fracture of laminae, lateral masses or spinous process.
3. Unilateral facet dislocations reduced in traction may be immobilised in a halovest for 8 to 12 weeks.

Skeletal traction Reduction with traction is done for unstable fracture (Fig. 24.19). *Urgency of reduction is based on neurological loss* (Table 24.3).

Traction is given for 3 to 6 weeks; and once satisfactory reduction is achieved, the patient is mobilised with a collar, corset or jacket.

Surgical treatment

Indications Unstable injuries with or without neurologic damage require surgery.

Table 24.3: Skeletal traction

Neurologic loss	No neurologic loss
↓	↓
Urgent skeletal traction through Crutchfield tongs (Fig. 24.20) or Gardner-Wells tongs	No urgency Only maintenance of reduction of skeletal traction.
↓	
10 lbs weight for head, 5 lbs weight for each vertebra to a maximum of 40 lbs.	

If reduction is obtained, weight is ↓ by 50 per cent. If reduction is not obtained, open reduction is attempted.

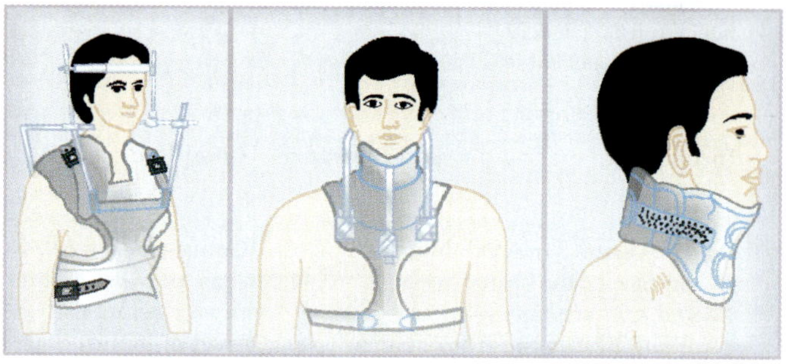

Figs 24.18A to C: Methods of cervical immobilisation: (A) Halo-vest traction, (B) Four postcervical collar (C) Cervical collar

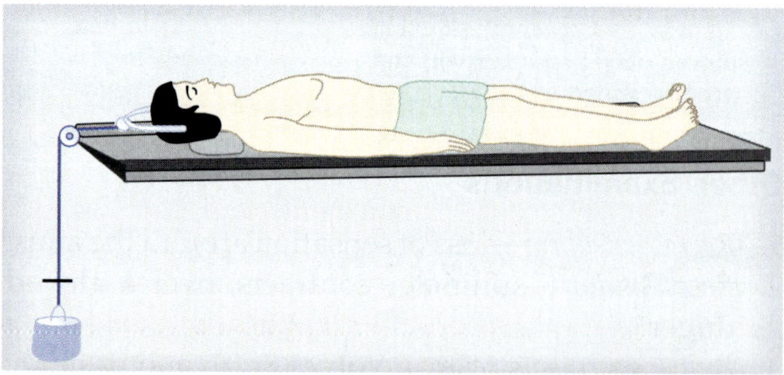

Fig. 24.19: Showing skeletal traction applied through Crutchfield tongs

Methods

- In most patients early open reduction and internal fixation (ORIF) is indicated to obtain stability. Cervical spine is stabilised through an anterior or posterior approach. Usually, a posterior approach is used with triple wire stabilisation and fusion with iliac bone grafting. This allows rapid mobilisation of the patient in a cervical orthosis.
- Anterior decompression consists of removal of the disc and is recommended when disc prolapse is present.

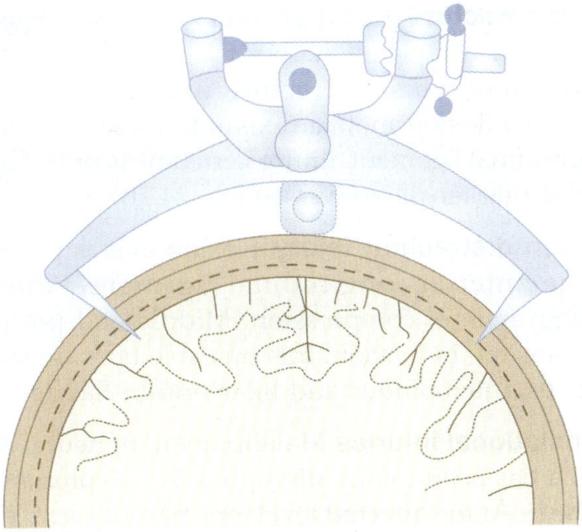

Fig. 24.20: Crutchfield tongs

- Posterior approach preferred for ligamentous instability.
- Anterior approach and corpectomy (removal of the crushed body) for burst fracture with cord compression. After corpectomy, the gap is filled up by a bone graft or a cage.
- Combined anterior and posterior decompression for posterior instability and anterior compression of the neural elements.

Laminectomy has limited role in the treatment of cervical fracture.

INDIVIDUAL CERVICAL FRACTURE OF INTEREST

Fracture of C_1 This is popularly known as Jefferson's fracture (Fig. 24.21). Here the patient usually presents with neck pain without neurologic deficit. This can be radiologically diagnosed by open mouth odontoid view.

Treatment

For stable fracture Rigid cervicothoracic brace for three months with a Philadelphia cast.

For unstable fractures Skeletal traction or halo cast for three months.

Rotary subluxation of C_1 or C_2 Here the patient presents with torticollis and neck pain and is diagnosed radiologically. Treatment is usually by reduction and skull traction.

Odontoid process fracture (Also called Dens) (Figs 24.22A to C) Anderson and D'olonzo's classification.

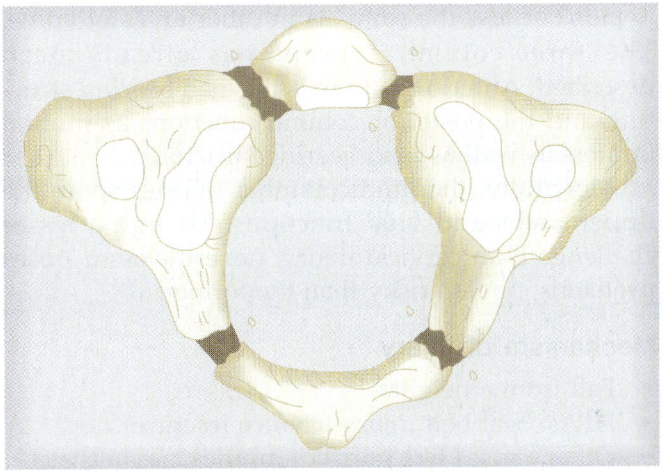

Fig. 24.21: Jefferson's fracture

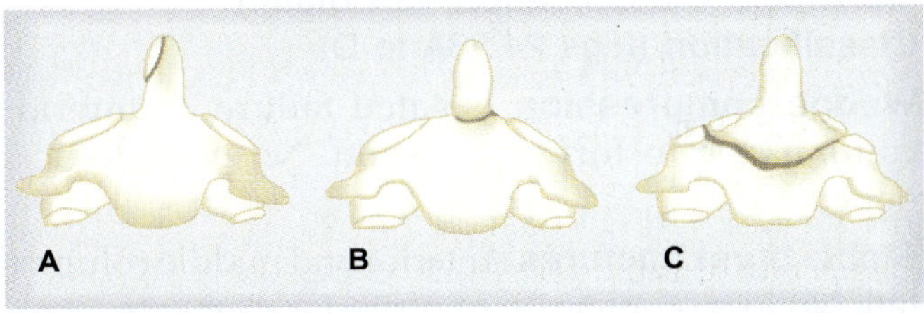

Figs 24.22A to C: Odontoid process fracture: (A) Type I, (B) Type II, and (C) Type III

Type I Oblique fracture of the upper part of the odontoid process. It is uncommon and is treated by cervical cast.

Type II Junction of odontoid process and body. Common with a nonunion rate of 36 per cent. Requires surgical wiring and fusion.

Type III fracture is through the upper part body of the body of vertebra. Cancellous area hence fracture unites well with a halo cast.

Hangman's fracture It is a fracture through pedicle at parsinterarticularis of C_2 and is due to distraction extension force. There is no neurological deficit and the patient needs rigid cervical support usually through a Philadelphia collar immobilisation.

THORACIC AND LUMBOSACRAL SPINE INJURIES

Thoracolumbar spine is generally regarded as extending from 10th thoracic vertebrae to 2nd lumbar vertebrae and is the transitional area between the kyphotic upper thoracic spine to the lordotic lumbar spine. The general anatomy of the vertebral column is more or less the same as in other areas of spine. The three-column concept has already been described. Anterior column is the load bearing structure and the posterior column functions as motion limiters as well as load bearing structures.

Mercifully, the thoracolumbar injuries spare the upper limbs and vital functions. Though a lesser challenge than cervical injury, nevertheless it poses problems, no less risky than the former.

Mechanism of Injury

- Fall from a height.
- RTAs: Seat belt injury (chance fracture).
- Other causes like gunshot injuries, assault, etc.

Mc Afee's Classification—3-Column Classification (Figs 24.23A to D)

Wedge compression Isolated failure of anterior column due to forward flexion. No neurological deficit.

Stable burst fractures Anterior and middle columns fail. No loss of integrity of posterior elements.

Unstable burst fractures Anterior and middle column fail in compression. Posterior column fail in compression, lateral flexion or rotation. Post-traumatic kyphosis and neural symptoms are present.

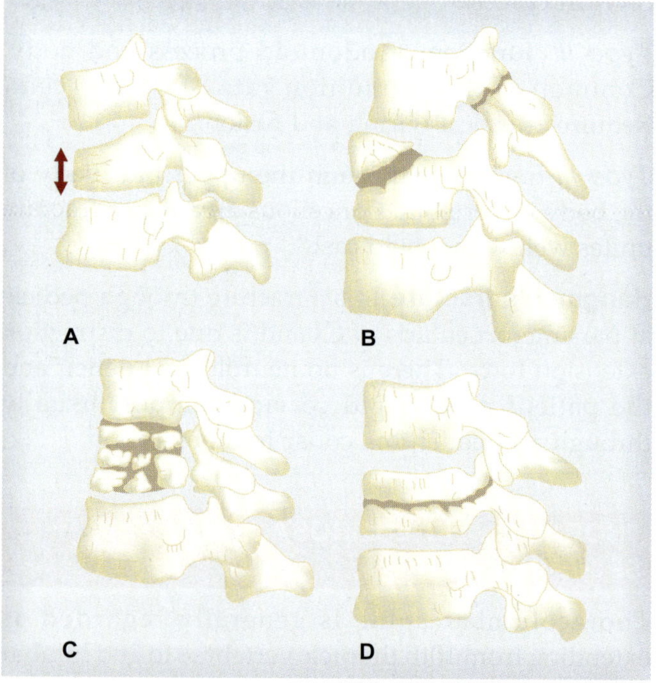

Figs 24.23A to D: Thoracolumbar fractures: (A) Wedge compression, (B) Stable burst fracture, (C) Unstable burst fracture, (D) Chance fracture

Chance fracture (Seat belt injury) It is seen in people who wear a lap belt without a shoulder harness. Horizontal avulsion fracture of vertebral bodies caused by flexion about an axis anterior to the anterior longitudinal ligament. Entire vertebrae is pulled apart by a strong tensile force (see Fig. 24.7B).

Flexion distraction injury Flexion axis is posterior to the anterior longitudinal ligament. Anterior column fails in compression. Middle and posterior columns fail in tension. It is unstable because supraspinous, interspinous and ligamentum flavum fail.

Translational injuries Malalignment of neural canal which has been totally disrupted. All 3 columns fail in shear. At the affected level, one part of sacral canal has been displaced in the transverse plane.

Modified Magerl Classification (AO/ASIF)

Type A—Compression varieties:
1. Wedge.
2. Split.
3. Burst.

Type B—Distraction:
1. Through posterior soft tissues (subluxation).
2. Through the posterior arch (chance fracture).
3. Through the anterior disk.

Type C—Multidirectional with translation:
1. Anteroposterior dislocation.
2. Lateral (lateral shear fracture).
3. Rotational (rotational burst).

Clinical Features

The patient gives history of trauma due to RTA or fall from a height and complains of pain, posterior swelling, tenderness, palpable interspinous gap or a step may be felt. Neurological involvement may vary from paraplegia to individual nerve root involvement. Spinal shock is present for 24 hours during which all the reflexes are lost. Cauda equina paralysis is present if the lesion is below L_1. Exaggerated lumbar lordosis may be seen in old cases.

Investigations

Radiography of the affected spine (Figs 24.24A and 24.25) This is the preliminary investigation and all 3 views (AP, lateral and oblique) are taken. Fracture of the vertebral body, pedicles lumbar transverse

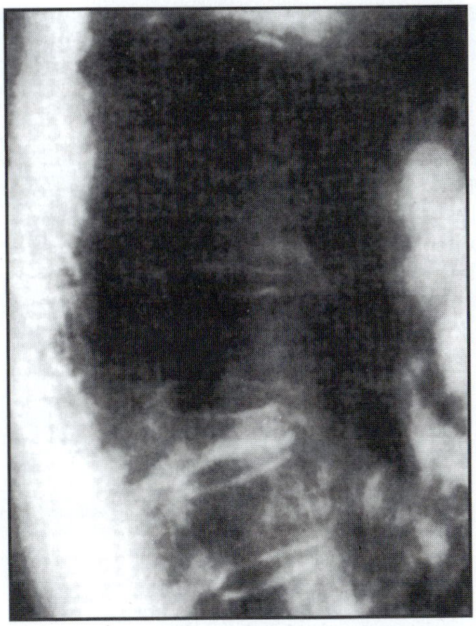

Fig. 24.24: Radiograph showing flexion compression fracture of T_{12} vertebra

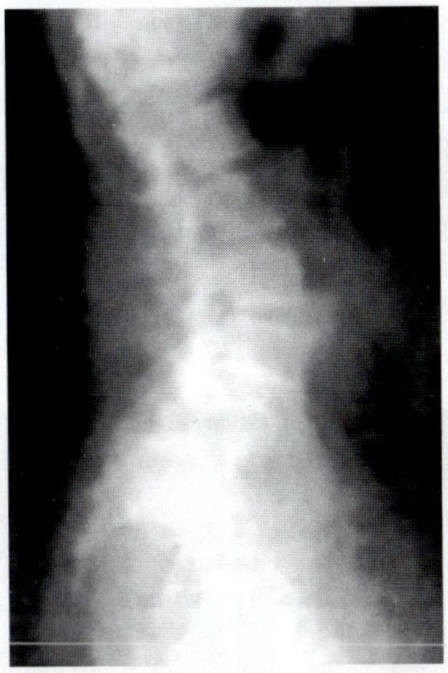

Fig. 24.25: Radiograph showing exaggerated lumbar lordosis due to L_1 fracture

process, pedicles spinous process, etc. are looked for. Disc space and neural canal narrowing is also looked for. With the advent of MRI and CT scan, the role of radiography appears to be diminishing in importance.

CT scan and MRI Both CT scan and MRI are found to be more useful than radiographs in evaluation of spinal trauma. While CT scan helps in studying the bony elements, MRI helps in the study of both bone and soft tissue elements. The damage to the cord is detected fairly accurately and is now being considered as the "gold standard" in the investigation of spine injury.

Mystifying Facts: Radiological clues about an unstable spine:

- Loss of vertebral height > 50 per cent
- Kyphosis > 30 per cent
- Spondylolisthesis > 3 mm

Management

This is discussed under two heads.

Management at the site of accident This consists of careful handling of the patient suspected to have spine injury. Consider all patients with spine injury to have neurological damage and shift them to the hospital with utmost care and caution avoiding all unnecessary movements.

Definitive treatment at the hospital This varies depending upon the nature of injury and the presence or absence of neurological damage (Table 24.4).

a. *For stable fracture without neurological deficit* Less than 30 per cent anterior wedge, lateral, central compression fracture of the vertebral body is considered as stable fracture. In these injuries, there is no fracture of the posterior cortex of the vertebral body, and there is no disruption of the neural arch.

   Treatment This is essentially conservative and consists of bedrest, NSAIDs and external spine supports like brace, corsets, etc. If the vertebral body compression is less than 30 per cent, only corset is used; and if the compression is more than 30 per cent but less than 50 per cent, a plaster jacket along with a corset is preferred (Fig. 24.26).

b. *For stable fracture with neural deficit* It has to be first determined whether the neurological deficit is complete (loss of motor power, sensory loss and absent reflexes) or incomplete (only cord or only spinal nerve roots).

   If neurological damage is incomplete, IV steroids are given for 4 days. Anterior decompression and anterior interbody fusion is done in the first stage, followed by posterior segmental spinal stabilisation by either pedicle screws, Hartshill rectangle frame, Luque instrumentation, etc. can be done one week later. Laminectomy has less role as it makes the spine less stable.

Table 24.4: Treatment plan for thoracolumbar injuries

Thoracolumbar fractures

- *Stable* (Anterior wedge, lateral and central compression fracture)
  - *Without* neurological deficit →
    - Bedrest for 3–6 wk
    - External spine supports (e.g. collar brace, etc.)
  - *With* neurological deficit →
    - *Incomplete*
      - IV Decadron
      - Anterior decompression
      - Anterior and posterior fusion

      → Early rehabilitation regime
    - *Complete*
      - IV Decadron
      - Early operative decompression and fusion to mobilise the patient early and help nursing care

      → Rehabilitation
- *Unstable* (Flexion rotation, flexion distraction, translational injuries, etc.
  - *Without* neurological deficit → Early OR + IF and bony fusion
  - *With* neurological deficit →
    - Systemic steroids
    - Early OR + IF and spinal fusion both in incomplete or complete paralysis to permit early uninhibited rehabilitation

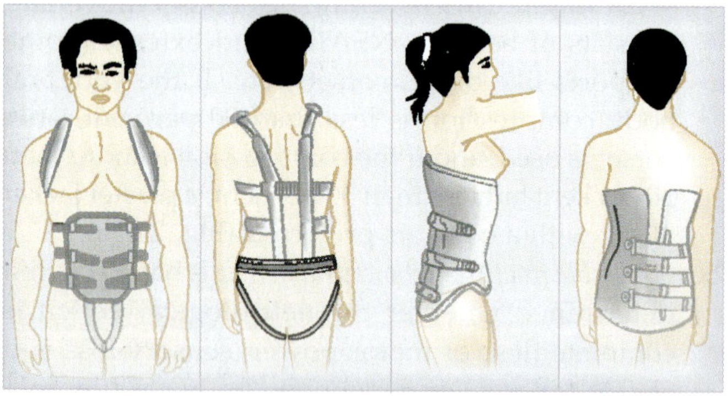

Fig. 24.26: Showing spinal braces for the treatment of stable thoracolumbar injuries

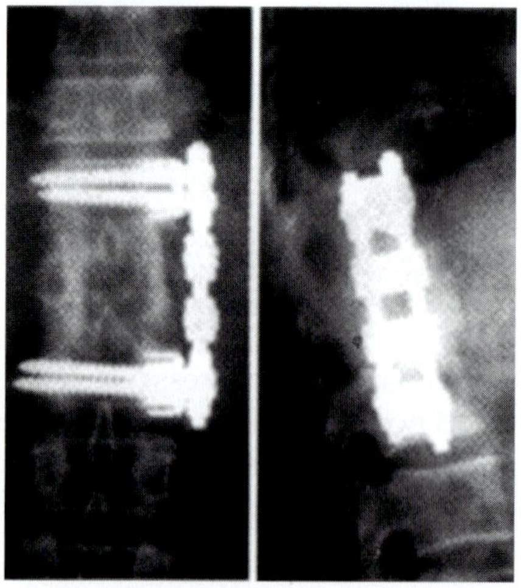

Fig. 24.27: Radiographs showing fixation of thoracolumbar fractures

c. *Unstable fracture without neurological deficit* This is best treated by early open reduction, internal fixation and fusion is done preferably within 12 to 24 hours. It is done with spinal cord monitoring. Internal fixation is either by VSP plates, Hartshill frame, Harrington instrumentation, etc. (Fig. 24.27).

d. *Unstable fracture with neurological deficit* Systemic Decadron 4 to 6 mg/every 6 hours IV for 3 days is given. Early open reduction and internal fixation and fusion is done in incomplete neurologic deficit cases. This is also desirable in complete neurologic deficit to permit early uninhibited rehabilitation.

Segmental spinal stabilisation with Luque or Hartshill frame is recommended.

What is new in the treatment of spine injuries?

Vertebroplasty: Injection of liquid cement into the vertebra through a key hole technique. This can be used along with the usual fixation methods to improve the stability.

SPINAL CORD INJURY

Spinal cord could be damaged due to injuries of spine extending from cervical vertebrae to the thoracolumbar junction. Below this, the cord ends and the cauda equina begins.

Incidence

- Spinal cord injuries are seen in 10 to 25 per cent of cases of spinal column injuries.
- They are more common at the cervical level (40%) than the lumbar level (20%).

Pathology

The pathology may vary from extradural haemorrhage to cord concussion, laceration to cord crushing. Lesion has longitudinal, sagittal and coronal dimensions. Amount of neural damage has no relationship to radiographic appearance (Fig. 24.28).

Clinical Classification of Neurological Damage

1. Complete paralysis.
2. Sensory paralysis.
3. Motor paralysis useless.
4. Motor paralysis useful.
5. Recovery.

Injury at the cervical level This has already been discussed and may vary from concussion, root injuries, incomplete and complete cord transection.

Injuries at the thoracic level This could result in paraplegia.

Injuries at the thoracolumbar region Due to injuries at the thoracolumbar junction, three things can occur:

1. Complete cord division and nerves intact.
2. Complete cord division and partial nerve division.
3. Complete cord division and complete nerve division.

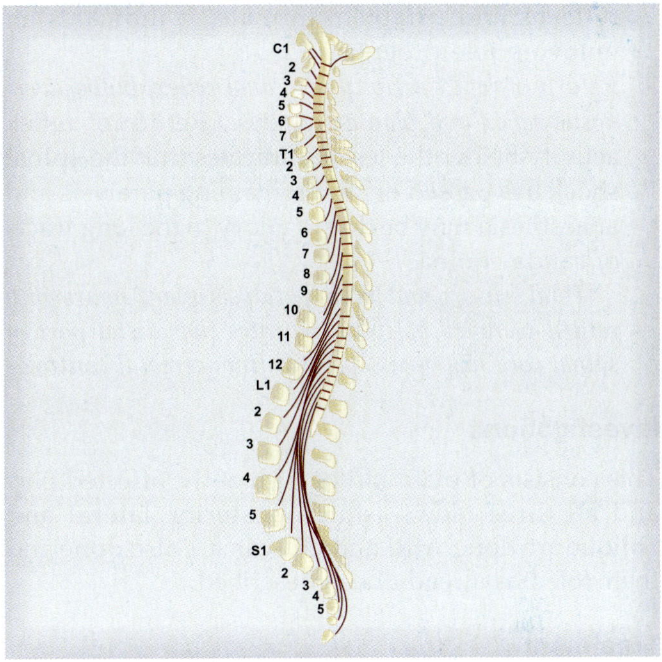

Fig. 24.28: Showing spinal cord ending at L_1 cauda equina starting at this point

Injuries below L_1 causes cauda equina paralysis.

Clinical Assessment

1. *General examination* This consists of examination of the head, chest, pelvis and other systems for incidence of injuries and also recording the vital statistics.
2. *Neurologic examination* Each muscle group and dermatome has to be checked. In cases of cervical cord injury, survival is impossible if the cord is injured above C_4 level due to paralysis of the diaphragm and respiratory muscles. In injuries below C_4 and above C_7, the level of lesion can easily be detected by examining the respective myotome, dermatome and reflexes *(ref p. 281 and 282)*. In cases of injury at the thoracolumbar junction, a mixed picture of both cord and root lesion may emerge and there could be an UMN and LMN feature in the lower limbs. Below the L_1, it is the nerve roots which are damaged and it is easy to identify the injured nerve root by a careful examination of myotome, dermatome and reflexes of the lower limb *(ref p. 422)*. Slightest voluntary movement and sensation below the level of cord lesion indicate cord continuity with better prognosis. If paralysis is complete even after 8 hours and if there is symmetrical returning of

reflexes and priapism in male, it indicates an unfavourable prognosis.

3. *Return of reflex activity (e.g. anal reflex, bulbocavernosus reflex and plantar response)* Return of reflex activity below the lesion indicates that the spinal shock has passed off and remaining paralysis and anaesthesia may be due to injury to the long tracts of cauda equina.

   Total sensory and motor paralysis after 8 hours with return of reflex activity indicates that distal part of spinal cord has been separated from cerebral control.

Investigations

This consists of plain radiograph of the affected part and all three views—anteroposterior, lateral and oblique are done. MRI and CT scan are also done and their role has already been described.

Treatment

- First aid as already discussed.
- Management of vertebral fracture and dislocations as discussed in individual injuries.
- Rehabilitation programmes in neurological injury following spinal fracture are as shown in Table 24.5.

Paralysed bladder Bladder injuries could be either UMN type or LMN type (Table 24.6).

Table 24.5: Rehabilitative measures for neurological injury

Level	*Disabilities*	*Measures*
$S_{2,4}$	Only bowel and bladder injured	Bladder and bowel programme
L_4-S_1	Bladder, bowel and prolonged sitting impaired	Short leg braces
$L_{1,2,3}$	Bladder, bowel and walking impaired	Walking with long leg brace
$T_{7\text{-}12}$	UMN bladder	Long leg brace and wheel chair
T_2-T_6	Bowel, bladder, walking, sitting impaired	Wheel chair is a must
C_7-T_1	Up to the level patient can become independent in all activities of daily living	Wheel chair is a must
C_5	Assistance to all activities of daily living required	Electrical chair is required
Above C_5	Total dependence + impaired breathing	

Table 24.5 shows the level of spinal injuries, their corresponding disabilities and the measures to be followed

Table 24.6: Characteristic features of UMN and LMN bladder injuries

	Bladder	*Automatic*	*Autonomous*
1.	*Type*	UMN	LMN
2.	*Level*	Above S_2	S_2 and below
3.	*Reflex centre of bladder*	Takes over	Lost
4.	*Controlled by*	Reflex centre	Intrinsic plexus of bladder
5.	*Emptying by*	Involuntary	Voluntary
6.	*Residual urine*	Minimal	Large > 200–300 cc

Goal in either case is to attain an automatic reflex emptying of the bladder

UMN type (automatic bladder) This is seen in injury above S_2 due to complete transection of the cord. Here the bladder is distended and there is no real sensation of vesical filling and the bladder is controlled by the reflex centres. There is automatic involuntary emptying and no residual urine is left.

LMN type (autonomous bladder) This occurs in injuries at or below S_2. The bladder reflex centre is destroyed. It now depends on the intrinsic plexus in the musculature of the bladder wall (detrusor ganglion). Here, emptying is to be done by manual pressure or by trained contraction of abdominal musculature. There is a large amount of residual urine in this condition.

Treatment In either conditions mentioned above, the treatment method aims at obtaining automatic reflex emptying. This is done as follows:

- Urinary retention catheter is placed in the bladder for 24 to 48 hours.
- After 48 hours, intermittent catheterisation is started, to develop the automatic reflex emptying of the bladder.
- Persons with traumatic quadriplegia have an UMN bladder controlled by reflexes through conus medullaris.
- If intermittent catheterisation is not available, bladder range of motion exercises are performed by clamping the catheter tube for 50 minutes and opening for 10 minutes every hour to allow the bladder to develop a reflex pattern of emptying.
- If reflex emptying with residual bladder urine volume of less than 100 cc does not occur within 6 to 9 months, urological procedures like external sphincterotomy or bladder neck resection is done to achieve a balanced bladder.

- Urinary diversion through ileal loops, etc. is not superior to reflex emptying of the bladder and hence is not recommended.

All possible attempts should be made to remove the catheter and have a catheter-free reflex emptying of the bladder.

Bedsore Management

Nursing goals Education of the patients and relatives.

- Only sure method of preventing pressure ulcers is strict nursing care and gradual shifting of responsibility of the skin to the patient's family.
- Spinal beds, mattresses and pads are not reliable to prevent pressure sores.
- Sleeping in prone position with a pillow bridging the bony prominences is the most reliable method of preventing bedsores. Sidelying postures are also equally effective (Fig. 24.29).
- Using water bed also helps prevent bedsores (Fig. 24.30).

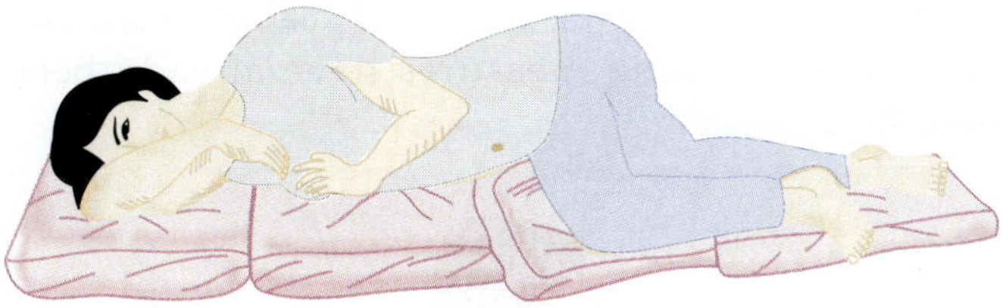

Fig. 24.29: Bed posture (sidelying) to prevent formation of bedsores

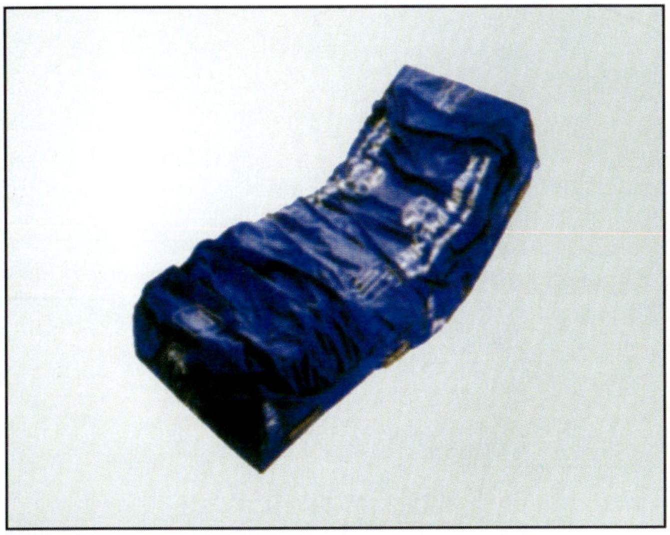

Fig. 24.30: Water bed, a boon for prevention of bedsores

Bowel Programme

Reflex emptying of the bowel with suppository stimulation is the goal of bowel training Every 2nd or 3rd day bowel reflex is stimulated by insertion of glycerine or Dulcolax suppository with digital stimulation. Enemas should not be given as this destroys the bowel reflex. Stool softeners and mild laxatives may be necessary.

Beds A conventional hospital bed and pillow is preferred. Side-to-side rotating bed is used during the first week. Proper positioning of the patient with supportive pillows, frequent turning in the bed and care towards personal hygiene is very much needed.

Concept of Rotating Beds

- All spine injuries are placed on rotating beds in the casuality
- The bed rotates 40° on either side
- Rotation stopped only for 2 hours in 8 hours
- Safety straps and pads are applied firmly
- Extremity exercises are permitted
- Compression stockings to prevent thromboembolism
- Spirometry is done every 2 hours
- All investigations, MRI, X-ray, etc. can be carried out
- The patient can be mobilized once the condition and the spine are stable

Vital facts:

Who require rotating bed treatment?

- 2-3 column injury patients
- Bony injuries without posterior ligamentous disruption
- For individuals who are neurologically normal and improving.

Advantages

- The patient is comfortable.
- Nursing care becomes easy.
- Investigations, exercises, etc. can safely be done.

Family education The family members of the victim are trained to take care of the victim's bowel, back, bladder and bed. They are also encouraged to give all the necessary moral support which is so essentially required to rehabilitate the patient back to normalcy.

Physical therapy This consists of putting joints through all the range of movements by passive

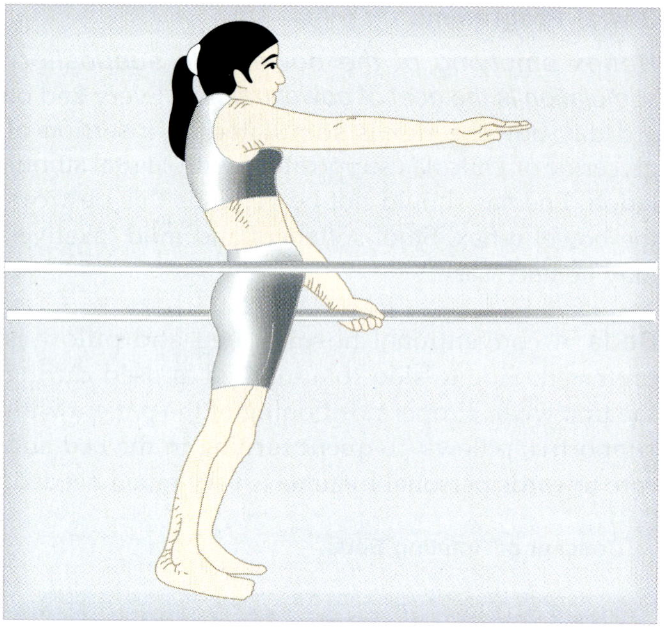

Fig. 24.31: A paraplegic patient learning to balance and walk within a parallel bar

stretching and exercises. Parallel bar walking, walking with the help of walkers or crutches is encouraged (Fig. 24.31). Wheel chair transfer activities are encouraged for injuries from C_6 level onwards.

Occupational therapy If possible, the patient is allowed to return to his original work with minor adjustments if necessary. But, if the patient, however, is unable to return to his original work, an alternative employment depending upon his present status of health is suggested.

Social therapy The attitude of the people towards these patients should not be of sympathy, but of support and encouragement. The right attitude of the society towards these unfortunate victims will go a long way in rehabilitating them back to normal.

CAUDA EQUINA SYNDROME

Cauda equina syndrome is seen in injuries below the level of first lumbar vertebra. It is essentially injury to the nerve roots below L_1.

Causes

1. Tumours of the spine.
2. Pott's disease.
3. Protrusion of disc—large midline disc prolapse at 4–5.
4. Fracture dislocation of the thoracolumbar spine.

Clinical Features

Signs

The patient complains of back pain, perineal pain, difficulty in micturition, impotence in male, etc.

Sensory signs The most salient feature of a cauda equina lesion is an area of *saddle-shaped hyperaesthesia and later anaesthesia* (involving both buttocks, anus and perineum) (Fig. 24.32).

Motor signs Flaccid paralysis below the knee.

Reflexes Ankle jerk is lost and the knee jerk is increased due to the weakness of the opposing hamstrings.

Bladder symptoms Common problems are retention of urine with overflow. Even after a severe cauda equina lesion reflex micturition is established later, reflex being mediated through the vesical plexus.

Anal Sphincter Relaxation

Treatment Prompt surgical intervention is the treatment of choice. This consists of operative stabilisation of the fractures, bowel, back and bladder care and other rehabilitating measures have already been described above.

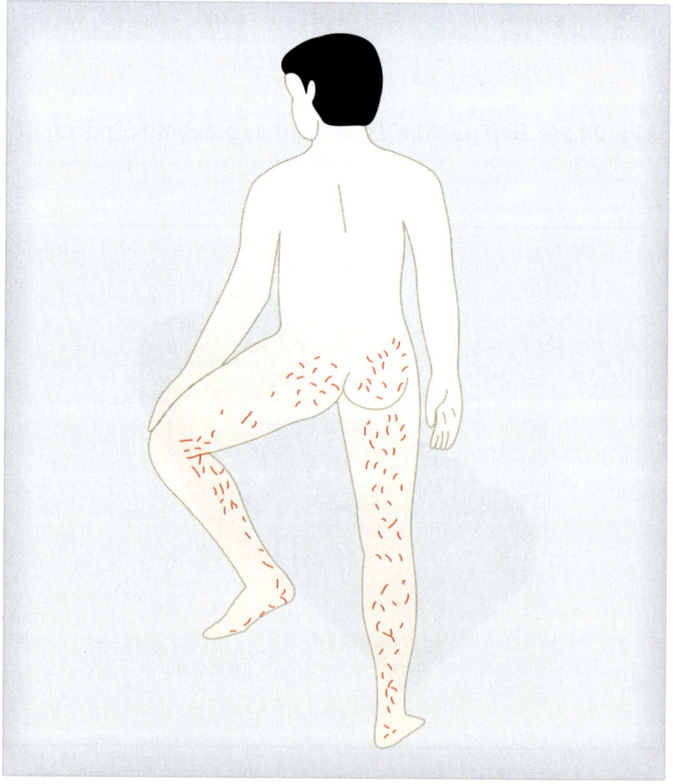

Fig. 24.32: Showing cauda equina lesion

Prognosis in Spinal Cord Injuries

Ten-year survival rate in spinal cord injury is 86 per cent.

Vital facts

Do you know the chief causes of death in spinal cord injuries? Well it is:

- Pneumonia
- Suicides

Interesting facts

Do you know what is 'SCIWORA'?
Well it is Spinal Cord Injury Without Radiological Abormality.
It is more common in children < 10 years.

BIBLIOGRAPHY

1. Crutchfield WG. Fracture dislocations of cervical spine. Am J Surg 1937;38:592.
2. Crutchfield WG. Skeletal traction in the treatment of injuries to the cervical spine. JAMA 1954;155:29.
3. Davis L. Treatment of spinal cord injuries. Arch Surg 1954;69:488.
4. Diskson JH, Harrington PR, Erwin WD. Harrington instrumentation in the fractured, unstable thoracic and lumbar spine. Texas Med 1973;69-91.
5. Holdsworth FW. Traumatic paraplegia. In Platt H (Ed), Modern Trends in Orthopaedics (2nd series), New York: Paul B, Hoeber, Inc 1956.
6. Holdsworth FW. Fractures, dislocations, and fracture-dislocations of the spine. J Bone Joint Surg 1970;52-A:1534.
7. Jefferson G. Fracture of the atlas vertebra: report of four cases and a review of those previously recorded. Br J Surg 1920;7:407.
8. Kelly RP, Whitesides TE (Jr). Treatment of lumbodorsal fracture dislocations. Am Surg 1968;167:705.
9. Maffee PC, Youn HA, Lasada NA. The unstable burst fracture. Spine 1982;7:365.
10. Watson-Jones R. Fractures and joint injuries (4th edn), Baltimore: Williams and Wilkins Co 1952;1,1955,2.

25 Peripheral Nerve Injuries

BRIEF ANATOMY

ABOUT SPINAL NERVE

The dorsal and ventral nerve roots arising from the spinal cord join at the intervertebral foramen to form a spinal nerve. In the thoracic segments, these mixed spinal nerves retain their autonomy and supply one intercostal segment both dermatomal and myotomal. In virtually all other segments spinal nerves join with others to form a plexus. There are 31 pairs of spinal nerves consisting of 8 cervical, 12 thoracic, 5 lumbar, 5 sacral and 1 coccygeal.

A spinal nerve has got three components: motor, sensory and sympathetic. The sympathetic components of all 31 mixed spinal nerves leave along the 14 motor roots (12 thoracic and 2 lumbar roots). Each spinal nerve now divides into an *anterior and posterior* rami. The anterior rami of the upper four cervical nerves form the *cervical plexus* and the lower four cervical together with upper thoracic nerves form the *brachial plexus*. The anterior rami of the first three lumbar nerves and part of the fourth lumbar nerve form the *lumbar plexus*. The sacral anterior rami along with the anterior rami of the fifth lumbar and part of fourth lumbar form the *lumbosacral plexus*.

The posterior rami supply the paraspinal muscles and the skin of the back. They are smaller than anterior rami except for upper three cervical posterior rami. The spinal nerves are then distributed to the limb buds through several peripheral nerves. *So basically a peripheral nerve is also a mixed nerve like the spinal nerve* (Fig. 25.1).

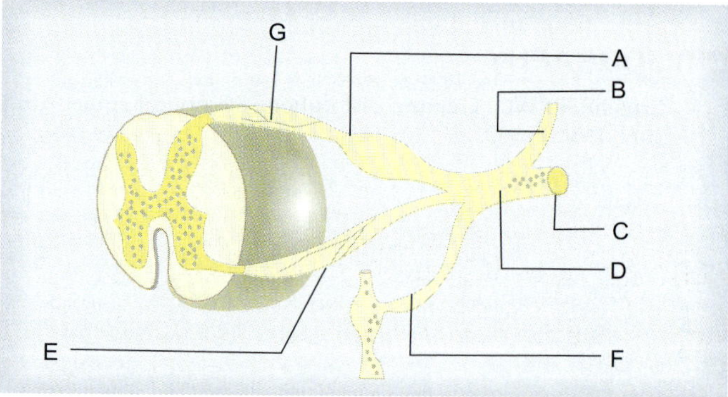

Fig. 25.1: Components of a mixed spinal nerve: (A) dorsal root ganglion on the sensory root, (B) posterior rami, (C) anterior rami, (D) mixed spinal nerve, (E) motor root, (F) grey ramus communicans from the sympathetic ganglion, (G) sensory root, (G) scurvy root

Dermatome is an area of skin supplied by a single spinal root.

Myotome represents a muscle unit supplied by a single spinal root.

MICROSCOPIC ANATOMY (Fig. 25.2)

Each nerve fibre or axon with a diameter greater than 1 μ has a myelin sheath. The axon is a direct continuation of dorsal root ganglion cell, an anterior horn cell, or postganglionic sympathetic cell. It is encircled by its Schwann cell sheath. In the unmyelinated fibres the Schwann cell alone acts as a sheath and in myelinated fibres it forms a multilaminated structure that encloses the myelin sheath. The axon with its Schwann cell and myelin sheath is surrounded by a delicate fibrous tissue called the *endoneurium*. A bundle of these fibres (called funiculi) are enclosed by a denser layer of fibrous tissue called the *perineurium*. The entire group of funiculi with their

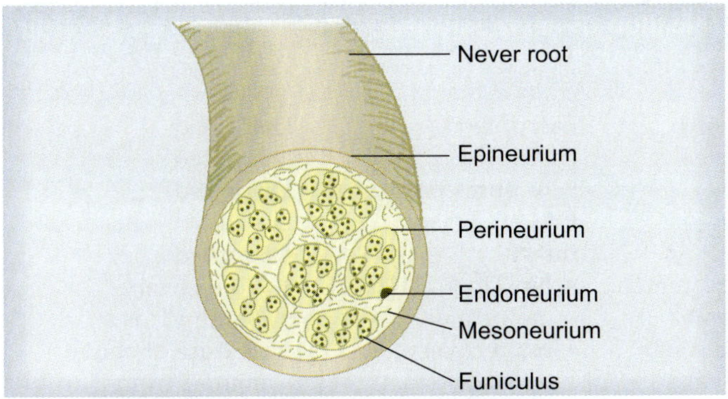

Fig. 25.2: Cross-section of a spinal or peripheral nerve root

surrounding perineurium is encased as a mixed spinal or peripheral nerve in a denser *epineurium*.

Blood supply to the nerve fibres enters through the *mesoneurium*.

GENERAL PRINCIPLES OF NERVE INJURY

NERVE DEGENERATION

Any part of the neuron detached from its nucleus degenerates and is destroyed by phagocytosis. This process of degeneration distal to a point of injury is called *secondary* or *wallerian degeneration*. Reaction in proximal end is called *primary* or *retrograde degeneration*. Time required for degeneration varies between sensory and motor and is related to the size and myelination. In secondary degeneration response is obtained to faradic stimulation up to 18 to 72 hours. After 2 to 3 days, distal segment is fragmented and the myelin sheath starts degenerating. By seven days, macrophages clear the axon or debris and is completed within 15 to 30 days. Schwann cells undergo mitosis from seventh day onwards and start filling the areas previously occupied by axon and its myelin sheath. Primary retrograde degeneration proceeds for at least one internode or more. Histologically, it is identical to wallerian degeneration. More proximal the site of injury, more pronounced will be the changes.

NERVE REGENERATION

Axonal sprouting starts from 24 hours after the injury. Unmyelinated initially but later on it gets myelinated. Now if the endoneurium is intact, sprouts will readily pass along their former courses and after regeneration may innervate their previous end organs. If the endoneurium is interrupted, then the sprouting axons may migrate aimlessly throughout the damaged area into the epineurial, perineurial regions forming a *stump neuroma* or *neuroma in continuity* or they may enter into the other empty endoneural tubes or newly formed endoneural tubes only to terminate in myotomal or dermatomal areas of their own. Hence, recovery is difficult if entire axon is transected and filled with scar tissue.

CLASSIFICATION OF NERVE INJURIES

Seddon's (1943) Classification (Table 25.1)

Seddon identified three types of nerve injuries: the first one is a mere contusion, the second is the transection of axons only, and the third complete transection of the nerve. This classification is less accepted clinically.

Table 25.1: Seddon's classification

Neuropraxia	*Axonotemesis*	*Neurotemesis*
• Minor contusion of the peripheral nerve	• Axon breakdown • Endoneurium is intact	• Complete anatomic section • No recovery
• Axis cylinder is preserved	• Spontaneous recovery is expected	
• Temporary		
• Recovery is complete		

Sunderland's Classification

Accepted clinically Arranged in ascending order of severity from 1 to 5. Various degrees represent injury to myelin, axon, endoneurium, perineurium and the entire trunk (Table 25.2).

Aetiology

General causes Metabolic diseases, collagen diseases, malignancies, endogenous or exogenous toxins, thermal, chemical or mechanical trauma, etc. can cause injury to the peripheral nerves.

Local causes Forty per cent of bone and joint injuries are associated with peripheral nerve lesions.

Table 25.2: Sunderland's classification of nerve injuries

Degrees	*I°*	*II°*	*III°*	*IV°*	*V°*
Axon	Contusion	Disrupted	Disrupted	Disrupted	Disrupted
Endoneurium	Intact	Intact	Disrupted	Disrupted	Disrupted
Perineurium	Intact	Intact	Intact	Few fibres preserved	Disrupted
Entire nerve	Intact	Intact	Intact	Intact	Disrupted
Myelin	Intact	Intact	Intact	Intact	Disrupted
*Motor march: Recovery of the motor innervation in a progressive manner from proximal to distal	• No motor march* • No Tinel's sign • Complete restoration of function	• Motor march present • Tinel's sign present • Good recovery	• Motor march present • Tinel's sign present • Incomplete recovery	• No Tinel's sign or motor march • No recovery	• No recovery • Grade VI° is a mixture of above injuries from I° to V°

Types

Primary This is due to injury of a peripheral nerve resulting from the same trauma that has injured a bone or joint.

Secondary This is due to involvement of the nerve in infection, scar, callus, etc.

Incidence of peripheral nerve injuries

1. Radial nerve is commonly injured.
2. Ulnar nerve 30 per cent.
3. Median nerve 15 per cent.
4. Peroneal nerve.
5. Lumbosacral plexus 3 per cent.
6. Tibial nerve.

Clinical Diagnosis

It is difficult to evaluate a nerve injury immediately after a severe trauma. However, typical attitudes and simple screening tests help clinch the diagnosis with reasonable accuracy (see box).

Vital facts:

Typical deformities

- Wrist drop → Radial nerve injury.
- Claw hand → Ulnar nerve injury.
- Foot drop → Lateral popliteal nerve injury.
- Ape thumb → Median nerve injury.
- Winging of scapula → Thoracodorsal nerve injury.
- Pointing index → Median nerve injury.
- Policeman tip → Brachial plexus injury.

Simple screening tests

1. In ulnar nerve injury, loss of pain at tip of the little finger.
2. In median nerve injury, loss of pain on the tip of index finger.
3. In radial nerve injury, inability to extend the thumb (hitch-hiker's sign).

Diagnostic Tests

Electromyography

Electromyography (EMG) helps to record the electrical activity of a muscle at rest and during activity.

Intact muscle There is no electrical activity in an intact muscle at rest. During a weak contraction, the electrodes record a single action potential. In powerful muscle contractions these motor action potentials superimpose to give an interference pattern.

Injured or denervated muscle These muscles show denervation potentials which are spontaneous electrical activity at rest. These are primitive responses which is normally suppressed by the stronger nerve action potentials. These denervation potentials normally appear by 1 to 2 weeks after injury. If they have not appeared by 15 to 20 days after muscle denervation, it indicates a good prognostic sign.

Quick facts: EMG (Figs 25.3A to C)

- Normal insertional activity immediately after section.
- Positive waves seen after 5 to 14 days.
- Denervation fibrillation after 14 days.
- Spontaneous fibrillation after 15 to 30 days of interruption.

Uses and limitations of EMG Electromyography helps to detect the presence or absence of nerve injury if present whether it is complete or incomplete and whether any regeneration is taking place or not. EMG does not give the level of injury or the degree of injury accurately.

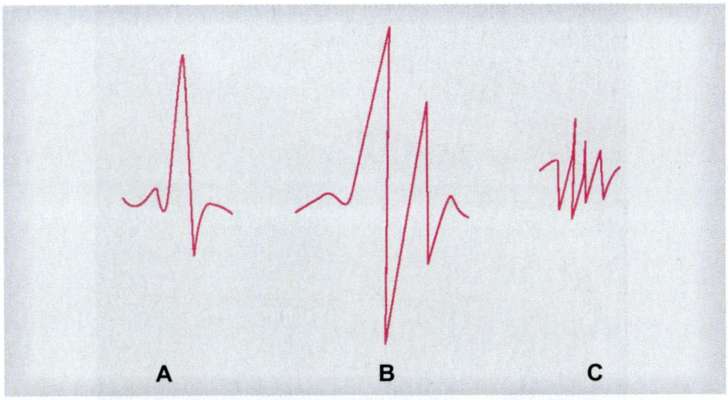

Figs 25.3A to C: Pattern of electromyography curves: (A) Normal insertional activity, (B) Positive waves (5–14 days), and (C) Denervation fibrillation after (15–30 days)

Strength duration curve A muscle usually responds to an electric stimulus. However, greater strength of current is required to excite a denervated muscle than normal muscle. Minimum current required to elicit a muscle contraction is called the "rheobase" and is expressed in milliamperes. The "chronaxie" is the duration of current required to excite a muscle with a current strength of double the rheobase. This is expressed in milliseconds.

To know the excitability of a muscle in relation to the current strength and its duration, the muscle is stimulated by decreasing the duration of the current from 300 milliseconds to 1 millisecond and a consequent increase in the strength of the current required is detected and plotted on a graph as the strength duration curve.

Utility of strength duration curve (SDC)

Normal muscle A normal muscle responds to stimuli from duration of 300 millisecond to 1 second without any increase in the strength of the current. However, if it is less than 1 millisecond, increase in the strength of the current is required. This curve is called the *nerve curve*.

Completely denervated muscle records a muscle curve and here either more strength or longer duration stimulation is required to produce a contraction.

Partially denervated muscle The curve here lies in between the two curves mentioned above. However, there is an upward kink which denotes the superimposition of the two basic types of curves.

Limitations of EMG EMG merely indicates whether the muscle is innervated or not. It gives no specific indications as to the level of injury or degree of injury.

Nerve Conduction Studies

Stimulation of a peripheral nerve by an electrode placed on the skin overlying the nerve will readily evoke a response from the muscle innervated by that nerve. Immediately after section, stimulation distal to the point of injury will elicit an essentially normal response for 18 to 72 hours after injury till wallerian degeneration sets in. This failure of response after about 3 days excludes "neuropraxia". Slowed conduction at a specific point indicates "compression neuropathy".

Tinel's Sign

This is an important sign which helps in recording the rate of regeneration of the nerve clinically.

Procedure Gentle percussion is done along the course of injured nerve. Tingling sensation is experienced by the patient in the distribution of injured nerve rather than the area percussed, and the sensation should *persist* for several seconds following the stimulation. Positive Tinel's sign indicates regenerating axonal sprouts have not obtained complete myelinisation. Response fades as myelinisation takes place. Distal progression of the response and the rate of the progression have been used by some to establish prognosis (rate of recovery should be 3 cm per month). Presence of this sign is encouraging. Even a few regenerating sensory fibres can result in positive Tinel's sign. *Thus, its presence cannot be taken as an absolute evidence of recovery.*

Sweat Test (Starch Test)

Presence of sweating within *autonomous zone suggests that complete interruption of the nerve has not occurred.

Skin Resistance Test

It is another method of evaluating autonomic interruption by using Richter's thermometer.

*Note *Small area of complete anaesthesia after section of a peripheral nerve or root*

Electrical Stimulation

Faradic stimulation is of little value (because even normally innervated muscles may fail to respond).

Galvanic stimulation Recording of chronaxie and strength duration curve by galvanic stimulation are more helpful in evaluating nerve injuries.

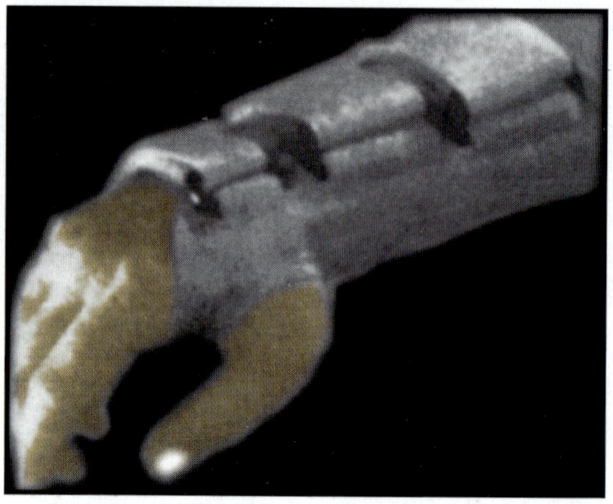

Fig. 25.4: Wrist cock-up splint (static type)

Management

General principles Resuscitation is carried out first, if the patient is in shock. General condition is improved by the emergency management measures. A thorough debridement of the wound is carried out; and if the wound is clean, primary repair of the nerve is carried out by direct suturing of the perineurium or epineurium or epiperineurium of both the cut ends. If the wound is contaminated, nerve is repaired after 3 to 6 weeks. In closed fractures with peripheral nerve injuries, conservative management is the treatment of choice. Careful assessment of the recovery is made and early surgical exploration is done if the recovery is not satisfactory.

Conservative management This consists of the following essential steps:

1. *Splinting of the limbs.* Different splints are required to immobilise the limbs in various nerve injuries.
   a. *Upper limb*
      - Brachial plexus injury—aeroplane splint.
      - Axillary nerve injury—shoulder abduction splint.
      - Radial nerve injury—cock-up splint (Fig. 25.4).
   b. *Lower limb: common peroneal nerve injury*—foot drop splint (see Fig. 25.26).
2. *Passive movements* of all joints are done to prevent contractures.
3. *Physiotherapy* Massage, exercises, stimulation, etc.
4. *Care of the skin,* etc.

Operative management This consists of various types of nerve repair (Figs 25.5A to D), tendon transfers, arthrodesis, etc.

Types of nerve repair

1. Primary repair is done within 6 to 8 hours after injury and if the wound is clean cut.
2. Delayed primary repair is done between 7 and 18 days after injury and if the wound is contaminated.

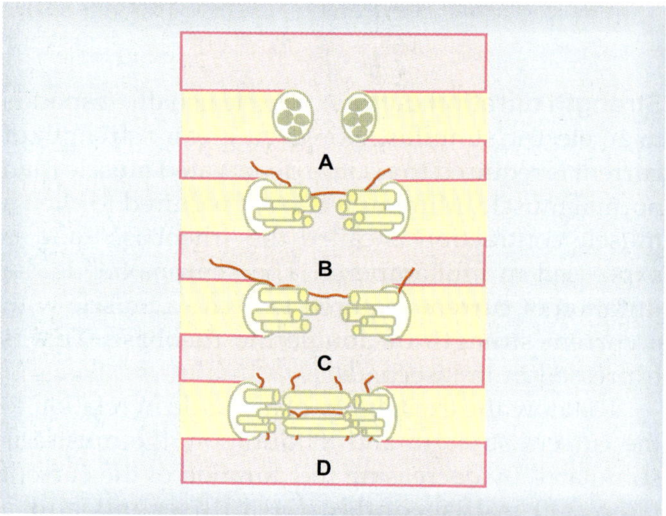

Figs 25.5A to D: Types of nerve repair: (A) epineural neurorrhaphy, (B) perineural neurorrhaphy, (C) epiperineural neurorrhaphy, and (D) interfascicular nerve grafting

3. Secondary repair is carried out 18 days after injury, if the injury is seen late, failure of conservative treatment, incomplete injury, etc.

Techniques

1. *Endoneurolysis:* It is freeing of the nerve entrapped within the scar tissue either external scar (external neurolysis) or within nerve (internal neurolysis).
2. *Partial neurorrhaphy:* This is advisable if one-half of a large nerve is disrupted, e.g. sciatic nerve injury.
3. *Neurorrhaphy and nerve grafting* if there is a gap after injury.
4. Methods of closing the gaps between the nerve ends if the nerves cannot be approximated end to end

- Mobilisation of the nerves by sectioning its cutaneous branches and freeing it from the fibrous tissue around.
- Positioning of the extremities in functional position.
- Transposition of the nerves, e.g. ulnar nerve transposition.
- Bone resection.
- Nerve grafting by using sural nerve.
- Nerve crossing.

By these above methods the cut ends of the nerves can be brought together and sutured by any one of the techniques mentioned above.

5. Tendon transfers are contemplated after 18 months of injury when there is no recovery after various nerve repair techniques or if the patient presents late.
6. Arthrodesis is considered if no tendons are available for transfers and if there is no hope of recovery.

Quick Recap:

Methods of nerve suture (Figs 25.5A to D)

- Epineural repair
- Epiperineural repair
- Perineural repair
- Fascicular repair

Quick summary

- Peripheral nerve is a mixed nerve.
- Sunderland's classification is clinically accepted
- Forty per cent of bone and joint injuries are associated with peripheral nerve lesions
- Radial nerve is the most common peripheral nerve to be injured
- Screening test helps in quick diagnosis
- In closed injuries conservative management is the treatment of choice
- In open injuries, primary nerve repair if the wound is clean and if the wound is contaminated delayed primary nerve repair or secondary repair is done

ULNAR NERVE INJURY

THE ULNAR NERVE SPEAKS

I am the largest branch of the medial cord of the brachial plexus with a root value of C_8-T_1. I arise at the level of pectoralis minor muscle, run through the axilla and lie in the medial compartment of the arm. I pierce the medial intermuscular septum at the level of coracobrachialis and lie in the posterior compartment of the arm. I pass over the posterior aspect of the medial epicondyle and enter the forearm through the two heads of flexor carpi ulnaris via the elbow. I lie beneath the flexor carpi ulnaris muscle within the forearm. At the junction of middle and lower one-third of forearm, I give a dorsal sensory branch which winds round the forearm and passes dorsally to supply the dorsum of the ulnar border of the hand, the little finger and medial half of ring finger. Later, I pass through the Guyon's canal at the wrist formed by the pisohamate ligament and the hook of the hamate. On the exit from the canal, I split into a superficial and deep branch. I supply the following muscles during my course:

- In the arm—Nil.
- In the forearm—Flexor carpi ulnaris and medial half of flexor digitorum profundus (Fig. 25.6) I supply both these muscles at the proximal third. As already mentioned, I give off a dorsal sensory branch at the distal third.
- In the hand—Superficial branch supply palmaris brevis and digital branches to volar aspect of little finger and medial half of ring finger. Through the deep branch, I supply the hypothenar, the dorsal and the palmar interossei, two medial lumbricals and the adductor pollicis muscles.

  In short, I supply ulnar flexors of the wrist, deep finger flexors of the little and ring fingers and mainly I supply the intrinsic muscles of the hand comprising hypothenar, lumbricals and interossei muscles.

Role of lumbricals Mainly flexes the metacarpophalangeal joints and extends the proximal interphalangeal joint.

Role of interossei Palmar interossei adducts the fingers and dorsal abducts the fingers. Through the dorsal digital expansion, they aid the action of lumbricals.

Role of hypothenar Abducts and helps in the movement of apposition of little finger.

Causes of Ulnar Nerve Injury

General causes are as described in the general principles of peripheral nerve injury.

Local causes are more important and could be in the following areas:

Causes in the axilla

- Crutch pressure.
- Aneurysm of the axillary vessels.

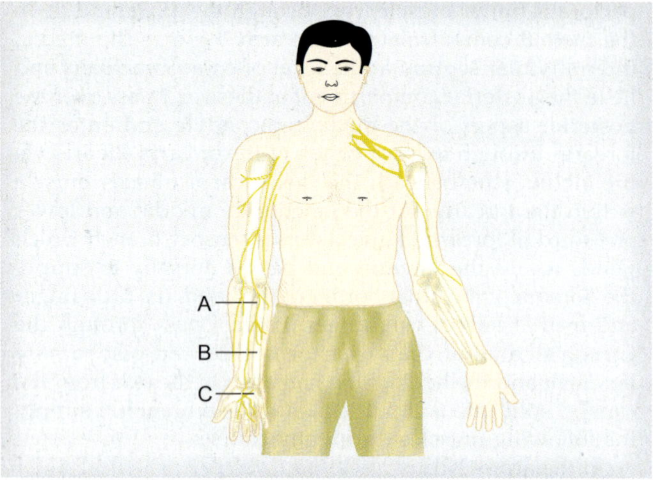

Fig. 25.6: Showing the course of the median and ulnar nerves and their supply, (A) Flexor carpi ulnaris, (B) Flexor digitorum profundus, (C) Intrinsic muscles of the hand

Causes in the arm

- Fracture shaft of humerus.
- Gunshot and penetrating injuries.

Causes at the elbow

- Compression by the accessory muscle (anserina epitrochlearis).
- Fracture lateral epicondyle of humerus.
- Repeated occupational strains.
- Recurrent subluxation of the nerve.
- Compression by the osteophytes as in rheumatoid and osteoarthritis.
- Cubitus valgus deformity due to various causes results in repeated friction of the nerve giving rise to tardy (late) ulnar nerve palsy.

Causes in the forearm

- Fracture both bones forearm.
- Incised wounds, gunshot wounds and penetrating injuries of the forearm.

Causes at the wrist

- Compression by osteophytes.
- Fracture hook of the hamate.
- Compression by ganglion.
- Wrist injuries.

Causes in the hand

- Blunt trauma
- Penetrating injuries
- Occupational—people operating high-speed drills in rock mining, etc.
- Associated ulnar artery aneurysm.

Ulnar nerve injuries give rise to *claw hand* deformity either true type or ulnar claw hand.

CLAW HAND DEFORMITY

Definition It is a deformity with hyperextension of the metacarpophalangeal joints and flexion of the interphalangeal joints of the fingers.

Types and Causes

Two varieties are described: one is a true claw hand involving both median and ulnar nerves and the second an ulnar claw hand or claw-like hand due to ulnar nerve injury (Table 25.3).

Table 25.3: Types and causes of true claw hand and ulnar claw hand

Types and causes of claw hand	
True claw hand (both median and ulnar nerve involved)	**Ulnar claw hand** OR A claw-like hand
↓	↓
Syringomyelia, amyotropic lateral sclerosis, progressive muscular atrophy, VIC, leprosy, peripheral neuritis, anterior poliomyelitis, etc.	Here only ulnar nerve is involved (causes already mentioned)

Pathomechanics

Loss of intrinsic muscle function due to ulnar nerve injury results in loss of flexion at MP joints and extension of IP joints of the fingers.

In a bid to bring about the flexion of the MP joints, the long finger flexors overact pulling the IP joints and wrist into more flexion. This causes a tenodesing (pulling) effect on the long finger extensors. The extensors cannot extend the IP joints without the stabilisation of the MP joint in neutral or slightly flexed position which is normally brought about by the intrinsics. This along with the compensatory overaction of the long finger extensors to bring about the lost extension of the MP joints results in hyperextension of the MP joints and the classical deformity.

This is called the intrinsic minus hand. The thumb is also adducted by its long extensors because the intrinsics and the abductors are paralysed.

Problems of claw hand

1. Hyperextension of MP joints (not the only primary or most disabling deformity).
2. Grasp decreased by 50 per cent due to loss of power of flexion at MP joints.
3. Pinch decreased due to loss of stabilising effect from the intrinsics.
4. Roll up manoeuvre lost.

Many surgical procedures are devised to block hyperextension of MP joints as it is still considered as the primary deformity.

Note: MP—Metacarpophalangeal, IP—Interphalangeal.

Clinical Features

These include the classical deformity, loss of sensation along the ulnar nerve distribution and wasting of the hypothenar muscles, intrinsic muscles of the hand leading to hollow intermetacarpal spaces on the dorsum of the hand (Figs 25.7A to C).

A test for loss of sensation along the distribution (Figs 25.8 and 25.9) of the ulnar nerve in the hand and fingers is carried out. However, the clinical features vary depending upon the level of lesion (Table 25.4).

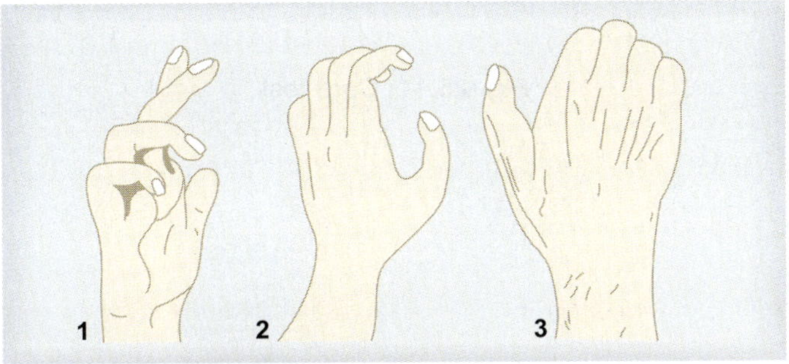

Fig. 25.7A: (1) Ulnar clawing, (2) total clawing, and (3) wasting of intermetacarpal spaces

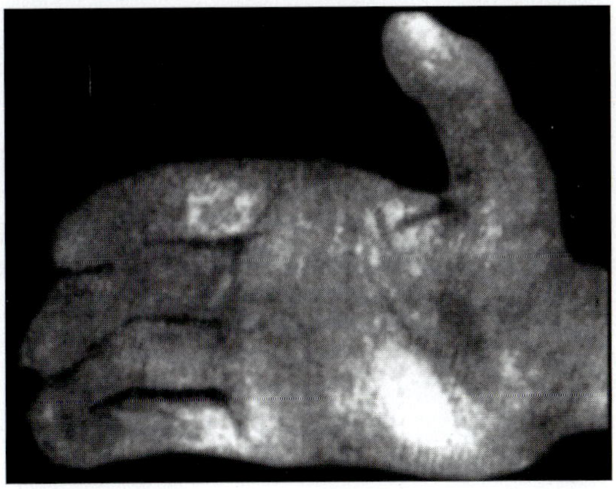

Fig. 25.7B: Claw hand deformity with thenar muscle wasting

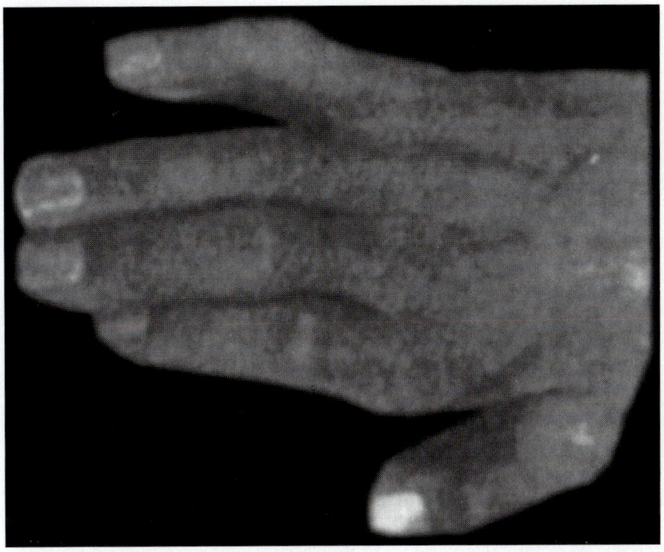

Fig. 25.7C: Wasting of intermetacarpal spaces

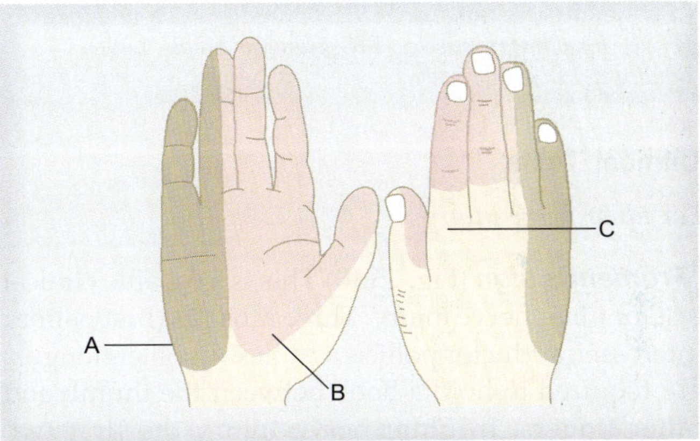

Fig. 25.8: Sensory distribution of the hand: (A) ulnar nerve distribution, (B) median nerve distribution, and (C) radial nerve distribution

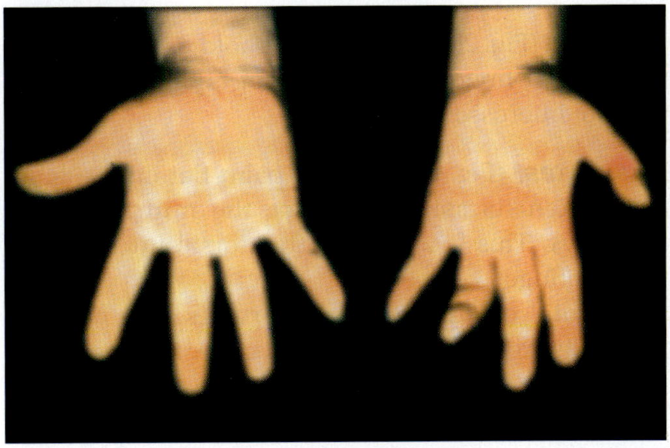

Fig. 25.9: Ulnar nerve palsy

Table 25.4: Levels of lesion

Level	
High Above the level of elbow, entire nerve function is lost	
Low	
1. *Below the elbow* at the junction of middle and lower third of forearm	*Spared*: Function of FDP and FCU *Lost*: Motor-HTM, Its, Lum, PB. • Sensory—dorsal aspect of hand (medial border) and one and half fingers.
2. *Proximal to Guyon's canal*	*Spared*: FDP, FCU and dorsal sensation. *Lost*: Same as above + loss of volar sensation.
3. *Distal to Guyon's canal*	*Spared* FDP, FCU, HTM, PB, dorsal and volar sensations *Lost*: Interossei and lumbricals.

FCU—flexor carpi ulnaris, FDP—flexor digitorum profundus, HTM—hypothenar muscles, PB—palmaris brevis, Lum—lumbricals, Its—interossei.

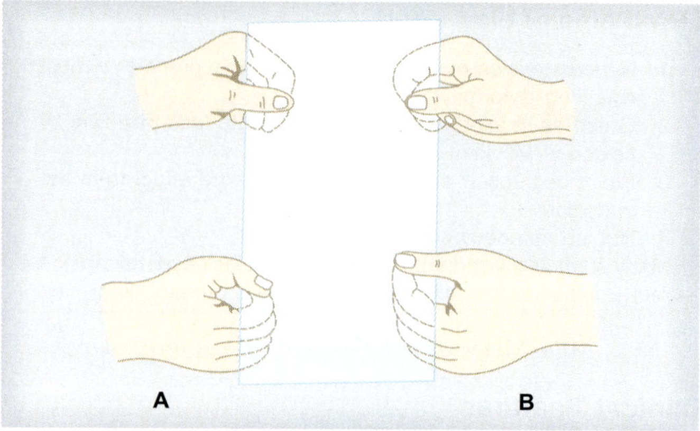

Fig. 25.10: Froment's sign: (A) normal, and (B) ulnar nerve injury

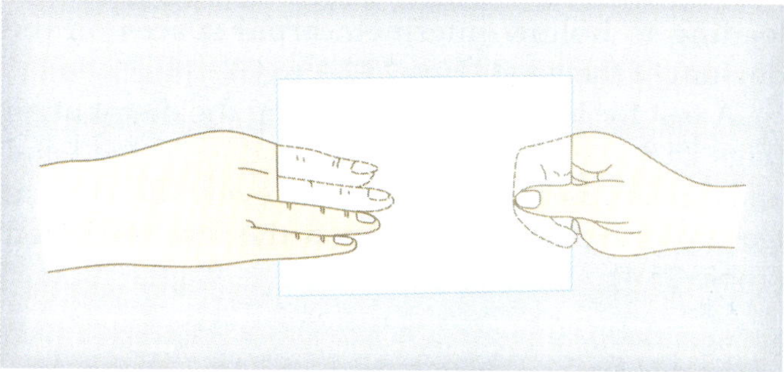

Fig. 25.11: Card test

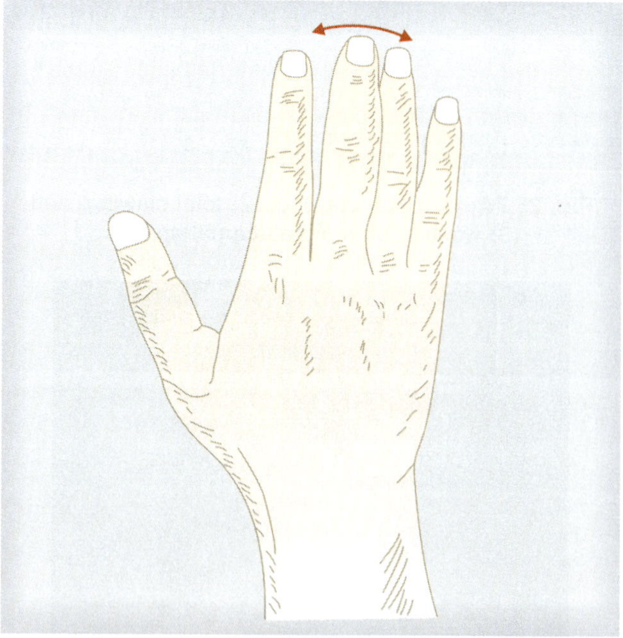

Fig. 25.12: Egawa test

Clinical Tests

For ulnar nerve injury

[1]***Froment's sign*** (Fig. 25.10) This is a reliable clinical test for ulnar nerve injury. Three muscles (first palmar interossei, adductor pollicis and flexor pollicis longus) are required to hold a book between the thumb and other fingers. In ulnar nerve injury the first two muscles are paralysed and now to hold the book, the patient has to depend only on flexor pollicis longus which flexes the thumb prominently. This is the positive Froment's sign.

Card test (Fig. 25.11) Inability to hold a card or paper in between fingers due to loss of adduction by the palmar interossei.

Egawa test (Fig. 25.12) With palm flat on the table the patient is asked to move the middle finger sideways. This is a test for the dorsal interossei of middle finger.

In total clawing median nerve is also injured. Following tests will help to detect the median nerve injury.

[1]**Jules Froment** (1878-1946) France. He was a Professor of Clinical Medicine.

Pen test (Fig. 25.13) The patient is unable to touch the pen due to the loss of action of abductor pollicis brevis.

Pointing index or Oschner's clasp test (Fig. 25.14) When both the hands are clasped together, index and middle fingers, fail to flex due to the loss of action of long finger flexors of the index and middle fingers which are supplied by the median nerve.

Benediction test (Fig. 25.15) For the same reason mentioned above, the patient is unable to flex the index and middle finger on lifting the hand (this is the position a clergyman uses to bless the couple during marraige. Hence called the benediction test).

Note Median nerve supplies the following muscles:
- *In the forearm* Pronator teres, flexor carpi radialis, palmaris longus, flexor digitorum superficialis, flexor digitorum profundus, flexor pollicis longus and pronator quadratus.
- *In the hand* Abductor and flexor pollicis brevis, opponens pollicis middle and index lumbricals.

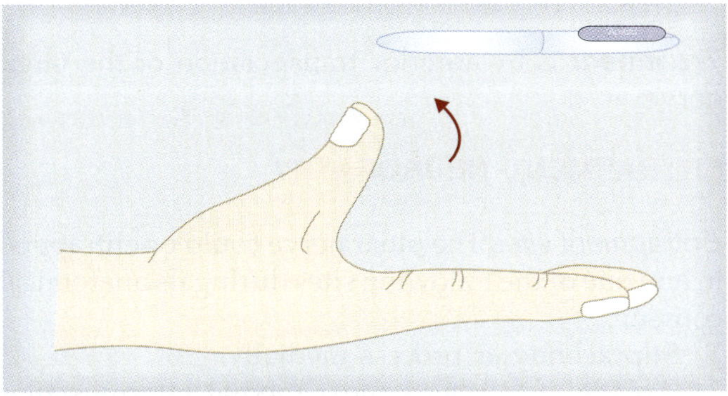

Fig. 25.13: Pen test

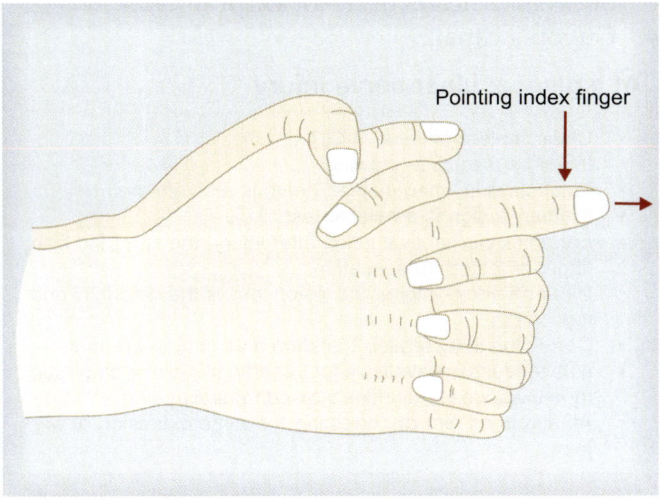

Fig. 25.14: Oschner's clasp test

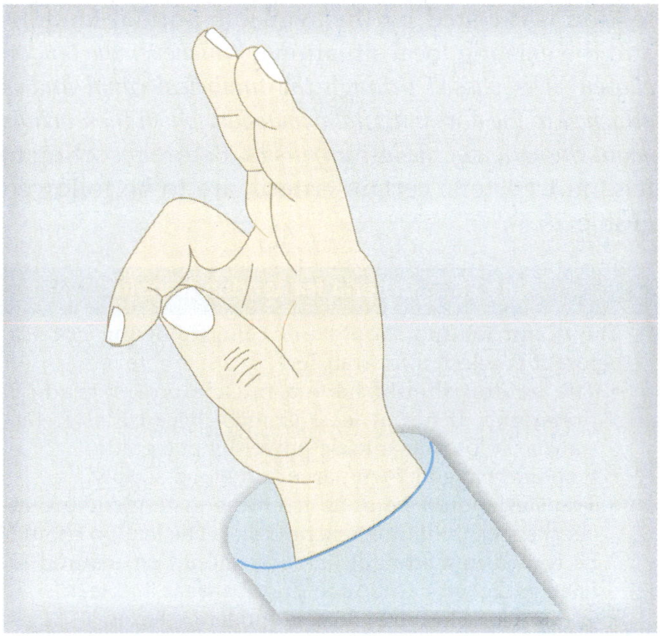

Fig. 25.15: Benediction test

What is ulnar paradox?

The higher the lesion of the median and ulnar nerve injury, the less prominent is the deformity and vice versa. This is because in higher lesions the long finger flexors are paralysed. The loss of finger flexion makes the deformity look less obvious.

Treatment of Ulnar Nerve Injury

In acute injuries the treatment is as discussed in the general principles.

For Claw Hand Deformity

Principles of treatment All the treatment measures aim at blocking the hyperextension at the metacarpophalangeal joint. Once this joint is stabilised, the long extensors will bring about the extension of IP joints. The long finger flexors will help in flexion of the MP joints along with their action of finger and wrist flexion.

Methods of Stabilisation of MP Joints

This can be done by the *active method* which involves tendon transfer or by *passive method* which involves arthrodesis, capsulodesis or tenodesis.

Active method This is by tendon transfers. A neighbouring healthy tendon is brought to replace the action of the lost intrinsics. The choice of the tendon is dictated by the available normal tendons and the existing local situations. *Whichever the tendon chosen, it is passed through the lumbrical canal and is attached to the dorsal digital expansion which then brings about the action of the lost intrinsics*. Before resorting to tendon transfers, certain criteria are to be followed (Table 25.5).

Table 25.5: Criteria for tendon transfer

The donor tendon should fulfil the following criteria before it is selected for transfer:
- The tendon should have a muscle power grade 5 preferably. If not at least grade 4 because after the transfer it loses its muscle power by one grade.
- It should have its own nerve and blood supply.
- Transfer should be done from the synergistic group because rehabilitation will be easier. The tendon should be routed in a straight line and should be ensured to have sufficient padding to prevent wear and tear.
- Tendon should be sutured in moderate tension.
- Prior to tendon transfer, joint stiffness, contractures and malunion of bones should be corrected.
- Age of the patient should be minimum of 5 years.
- The disease should not progress.
- Any infection of bone and joints should be controlled.
- There should be good range of passive movements available at the joints.

Choice of Surgery

Modified [2]S. Bunnel's operation When finger flexors are strong, wrist flexors and extensors are strong, and if there is no habitual flexion of the wrist, modified S. Bunnel's operation is preferrred in which *flexor digitorum superficialis of the ring finger* is transferred through the lumbrical canal into the dorsal digital expansion.

Riordan's operation When flexion of the wrist has become habitual or if there is a flexion contracture of the wrist, a wrist flexor can be spared to overcome the above-mentioned problems. In Riordan's operation the *flexor carpi radialis muscle* is removed and transferred with a free tendon graft leaving behind the flexor carpi ulnaris to bring about the wrist flexion.

Brand's operation When the finger flexors are weak, the wrist flexors are also weak and when the wrist extensors are strong *extensor carpi radialis longus* or *brevis* is transferred by a free tendon graft.

Fowler's operation When finger flexors, wrist extensors and wrist flexors are not available for transfer, extensor digitorum longus tendon of the index and little fingers are transferred by the Fowler's technique.

When no muscle is available for transfer and if the joints are supple, capsulodesis of MP joint or tenodesis is done. If the joints are not supple, arthrodesis in functional position is done.

Tardy ulnar nerve palsy It is a late onset ulnar nerve palsy and could be due to the following causes:
1. Malunion or nonunion of lateral condyle fracture of humerus.
2. Fracture medial epicondyle of humerus.
3. Dislocation of elbow.
4. Nerve contusions.
5. Cubitus valgus.
6. Shallow ulnar groove.
7. Hypoplasia of humeral trochlea.
8. Recurrent subluxation due to inadequate fibrous arch.

Treatment is by anterior transposition of the ulnar nerve.

ENTRAPMENT NEUROPATHY

Entrapment sites The ulnar nerve could be entrapped in any one of the following sites during its anatomical course:
1. Supracondylar process medially.
2. Arcade of Stuther's (near medial intermuscular septum).
3. Between 2 heads of flexor carpi ulnaris.
4. Guyon's canal.

At a glance: ulnar nerve injury

- Ulnar nerve root value is C_8T_1.
- Injury causes ulnar clawing.
- Total clawing when median nerve is also affected.
- Froment's sign is a reliable test.
- For quick clinical evaluation after injury, the tip of the little finger is tested for sensation.
- Ulnar paradox—higher the lesion less is the deformity and vice versa.
- Correction is by tendon transfers if all criteria are met.
- If no tendons are available for transfer, MP joint is stabilised by capsulodesis, tenodesis or arthrodesis.
- All surgeries aim at correcting the hyperextension at MP joint.

[2]**Sterling Bunnel** (1949) UK.

RADIAL NERVE INJURY

THE RADIAL NERVE SPEAKS

I am the continuation of the posterior cord of the brachial plexus and I am its largest branch. My root value is C_{5-8} T_1. In the axilla I lie behind the axillary artery and pass posterior to the humerus beneath the teres major and enter in the interval between the long and medial head of triceps. I wind round the spiral groove and pierce the lateral intermuscular septum at the junction of the distal third and the middle third and come to lie in the anterior compartment of the arm. Here I lie between the brachoradialis and extensor carpi radialis longus and at the level of the lateral epicondyle I split into superficial branch and posterior interosseous nerve. Superficial branch is my direct continuation which runs distally in the forearm under cover of brachoradialis and about two inches above the wrist it pierces the deep fascia, turns dorsally and laterally and reaches the dorsum of the hand supplying three and half fingers till the level of middle phalanges. My posterior interosseous branch penetrates the supinator muscle through the arcade of Frohse and runs distally in the forearm and lies on the interosseous membrane. It ends as a pseudoganglion over the wrist joint. I supply the following muscles in my course (Fig. 25.16):

- **Above the spiral groove** All the three heads of triceps and anconeus.
- **In the spiral groove** I give off three cutaneous branches, posterior cutaneous nerve of the arm, posterior cutaneous nerve of the forearm and lower lateral cutaneous nerve of the arm.
- **Between the spiral groove and lateral epicondyle** I supply brachialis, brachoradialis and extensor carpi radialis longus.
- **Before piercing the supinator** I supply extensor carpi radialis brevis and part of supinator.
- In the supinator I supply the rest of it. After emerging out of the supinator, I supply all the remaining extensor muscles of the forearm and abductor pollicis longus.

Thus, you can say that I supply all the muscles on the lateral and dorsal aspects of the forearm, except the brachoradialis and extensor carpi radialis longus, through the posterior interosseous branch of mine.

Radial nerve can be entrapped at the following sites:

In the arm—fibrous arch of lateral head of triceps.

In the forearm—arcade of Frohse.

At the elbow—radial tunnel syndrome at origin of extensor carpi radialis brevis.

At the wrist—scar tissue compressing the superficial radial nerve.

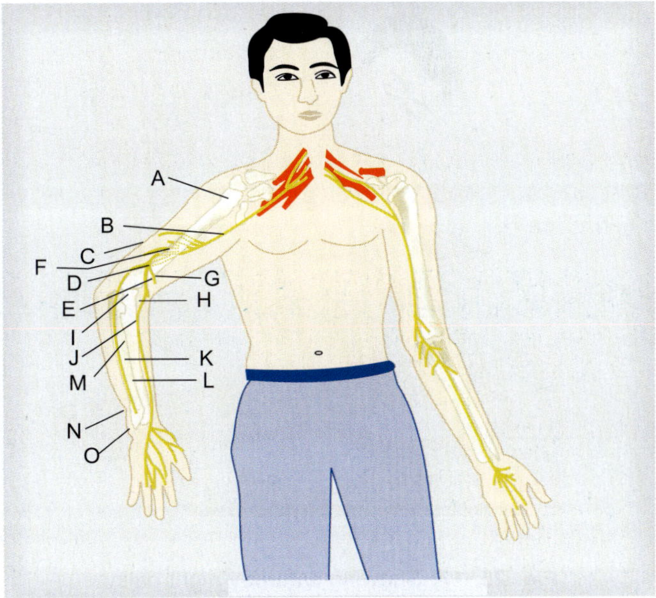

Fig. 25.16: (A) medial head of triceps, (B) long head of triceps, (C) lateral head of triceps, (D) brachioradialis, (E) extensor carpi radialis longus, (F) extensor carpiradialis brevis, (G) anconeus, (H) supinator, (I) extensor digitorum longus, (J) extensor digitorum minimi, (K) extensor carpi ulnaris, (L) abductor pollicis longus, (M) extensor pollicis longus, (N) extensor pollicis brevis, and (O) extensor indices

Causes for Radial Nerve Injury

General already discussed *(ref. p.295)*

Local

In the axilla

- Aneurysm of the axillary vessels
- Crutch palsy

In the shoulder

- Proximal humeral fractures
- Shoulder dislocation

In the spiral groove 5'S

- Shaft fracture
- Saturday night palsy (Fig. 25.17)
- Syringe palsy (Fig. 25.18)
- Surgical positions (Trendelenburg)
- 'S'march's (Esmarch) tourniquet palsy

Saturday night palsy (also called weekend palsy)

In this condition there is compression of the radial nerve between the radiospiral groove and the lateral intermuscular septum.

It is known after an event which typically happens on a saturday night weekend when in an inebriated

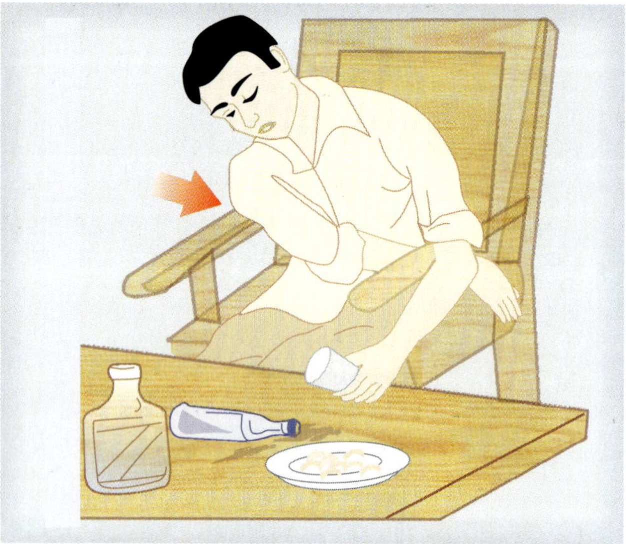

Fig. 25. 17: Showing saturday night palsy *(patient's mistake)*

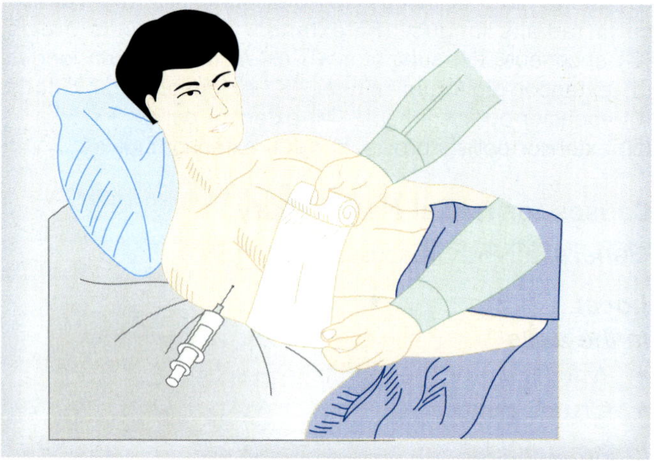

Fig. 25,18: Showing injection and tourniquet palsy *(doctor's mistake)*

condition, a person slumps with his midarm compressed between the arm of the chair and his body (See Fig. 25.17).

Did you know about Honeymoon Palsy

You have heard about saturday night palsy, but have you heard about honeymoon palsy?
Well, it is another sleep palsy and is seen in young couples where a bed partner's head compresses the radial nerve, while resting in the crook of the partner's arms!

Between spiral groove and lateral epicondyle

- Fracture shaft humerus (Fig. 25.19).
- Supracondylar fracture humerus.

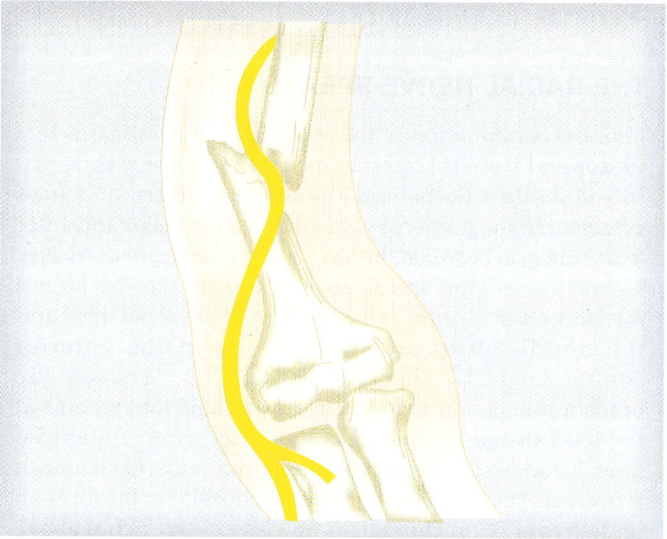

Fig. 25.19: Showing entrapment of radial nerve in between the fracture fragments of the humerus *(nobody's mistake)*

- Lateral epicondyle fracture of the humerus.
- Penetrating and gunshot injuries.
- Cubitus valgus deformity .

At the elbow

- Posterior dislocation of the elbow.
- Fracture head of radius.
- Monteggia fractures.

Causes in the forearm

- Fracture both bones forearm.
- Penetrating and gunshot injuries.

Levels of lesion

	Features
High Above spiral groove	Total palsy
Low: Type I Between the spiral groove and the lateral epicondyle	*Spared:* Elbow extensor *Lost:* Motor • Wrist extensor • Thumb extensor • Finger extensors *Sensory:* Dorsum of first web space.
Low: Type II Below the elbow	*Spared* • Elbow extensor • Wrist extensor *Lost* : Motor • Thumb extensor • Finger extensor *Sensation* first web space

Clinical Features

If the lesion is high, the patient will present with wrist drop (Fig. 25.20), thumb drop and finger drop. He will be unable to extend the elbow. If the lesion is low the elbow extension is spared; but the wrist, thumb and the finger extensions are lost, but *the patient, however, can extend the IP joints of the fingers because of the action of the intrinsic muscles of the hand.* Sensation along the posterior surface of the arm and forearm is lost in high lesions and in low lesions the above sensations are spared, but there is loss of sensation over the first dorsal web space.

In acute injuries it is difficult to evaluate the injury to the radial nerve. In such situations, the hitch-hiker's sign (inability to extend the thumb) is used as the screening test.

Investigations

Radiograph of the injured part and all other investigations mentioned in the general principles are carried out.

Treatment

Early cases As mentioned in the general principles for closed fractures, conservative treatment is adopted. The patient is put on a cock-up splint or dynamic splints (see Figs 25.4 and 25.21). This is followed by active and passive physiotherapy. In failed conservative treatment operative treatment is considered after a period of 12 to 18 months.

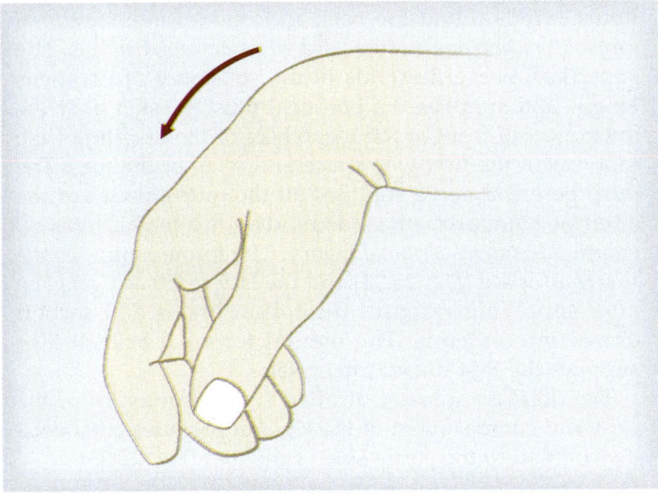

Fig. 25.20: Showing wrist drop

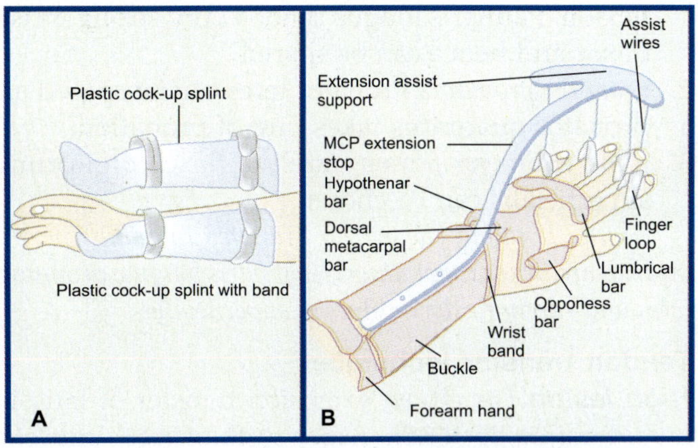

Figs 25.21A and B: Wrist drop splints: (A) Static or cock-up splint, (B) Dynamic splint

In open fractures, surgery is the treatment of choice. If the wound is clean, primary nerve repair is done, and if the wound is contaminated, delayed primary or secondary nerve repair is resorted to.

Treatment

↓ ↓

General management ↓

Closed fracture
1. Conservative
2. Splints dynamic preferred over static
3. Physiotherapy: Active/passive
4. Surgery: If there is failure of conservative treatment by 12 to 18 months

Local management ↓

Open fracture
Surgery is the treatment of choice
↓ ↓
Clean wound → Primary repair, splint, physiotherapy
Contaminated wound → Delayed primary repair, Secondary repair, Delayed secondary repair

Late cases
Tendon transfers
Arthrodesis

Treatment of Late Cases: (> 1 year)

Broad principles

Active treatment If neighbouring tendons are intact and if all the criteria for tendon transfers mentioned earlier are met, then tendon transfer is the treatment of choice.

Passive method If no tendons are available for transfer, then tenodesis or wrist arthrodesis in functional position is preferred.

Choice of tendons in active treatment

1. *From the wrist flexors* Flexor carpi ulnaris can be spared. Flexor carpi radialis takes care of the wrist

flexion. Palmaris longus is not a very strong wrist flexor and hence can be spared.

2. *From the pronators* Pronator teres can be spared as pronator quadratus takes care of pronation.
3. *From the finger flexors*, rarely a flexor digitorum superficialis can be chosen.

So the tendons chosen for transfer in radial nerve injuries are flexor carpi ulnaris, palmaris longus, pronator teres and rarely flexor digitorum superficialis.

Tendon transfer techniques

High lesion For elbow extension transfer of latissimus dorsi or pectoralis major to the triceps muscle can be done, if the patient needs active extension to use the crutches. Otherwise, gravity alone helps in passive extension of the elbow and is sufficient if the patient does not prefer to use the crutches.

Low lesions

Type I

- For wrist extension→pronator teres transfer.
- For finger extension→flexor carpi ulnaris split into four slips and transferred dorsally into four fingers.
- For thumb extension and abduction→palmaris longus transfer.

Type II Here wrist extension is spared and hence the plan is

- For finger extension→flexor carpi ulnaris transfer (split into 4 slips).
- For thumb extension→palmaris longus transfer
- For thumb abduction→pronator teres transfer.

Omer's technique consists of splitting flexor carpi ulnaris into five slips and transferring into all the five fingers instead of four.

Boye's technique uses flexor digitorum superficialis instead of flexor carpi ulnaris to bring about extension of four fingers.

Problems in radial nerve injury

- Wrist drop.
- Thumb drop.
- Finger drop only at MCP joint but extension at IP joint is possible due to action of interossei.
- Sensation over dorsal first web space is lost.
- In high lesions inability to extend the elbow and loss of sensations over posterior surface of arm and forearm are additional problems.

Radial nerve injury at a glance

- Continuation of posterior cord of the brachial plexus.
- Most common peripheral nerve to be injured.
- Most common site of injury is the distal end of humerus.
- Thumb extension test (hitch-hiker's sign) is the screening test.
- In radial nerve injury extension at finger IP joint is still possible.
- For early cases in closed fractures conservative treatment.
- For open fractures operative treatment and repair.
- For late cases, tendon transfers if neighbouring tendons are available and if all the criteria are met.
- If no tendons are available, wrist arthrodesis is done in functional position.

Interesting nerve palsies concerning radial nerve

Did you know about hand cuff palsy, dog handler's palsy or Cheralgia paraesthetica?
Well, all these are due to compression of the sensory branch of the superficial radial nerve at the level of the distal one third of the forearm where it pierces the deep fascia and becomes dorsal.

INJURY TO SCIATIC NERVE

THE SCIATIC NERVE SPEAKS

I am the **thickest** nerve in the body with a root value of $\mathbf{L_{4,5}\ S_{1,2,3}}$. I enter the gluteal region through the greater sciatic notch and pass between the greater trochanter of femur and ischial tuberosity. From here I enter the thigh and in the middle I divide into *common peroneal* and *the tibial part*. Before doing so, I supply biceps, semitendinosus, semimebranosus and adductor magnus. The *common peroneal part is the smaller of* my two terminal divisions. This runs along the medial border of biceps, leaves the popliteal fossa at the lateral angle, passes behind the head of the fibula, winds round the neck and divides into *superficial (musculocutaneous nerve)* and *deep peroneal nerve*. The superficial nerve descends in the substance of peroneus longus and supplies the peroneal muscles, skin over the lower part of front of the leg, whole of the dorsum of the foot except the first web space and most of the toes. The deep peroneal nerve supplies all the four muscles of the anterior compartment and divides into *medial terminal branch* and *lateral terminal branch*. The former supplies the first web space (Fig. 25.22) and the latter *ends as a ganglion* after supplying extensor digitorum brevis and second dorsal interosseous. The medial terminal branch also supplies the first dorsal interossei.

The tibial component of mine supplies muscles of the posterior compartment of the leg and provides cutaneous distribution to the entire sole of the foot (Fig. 25.23).

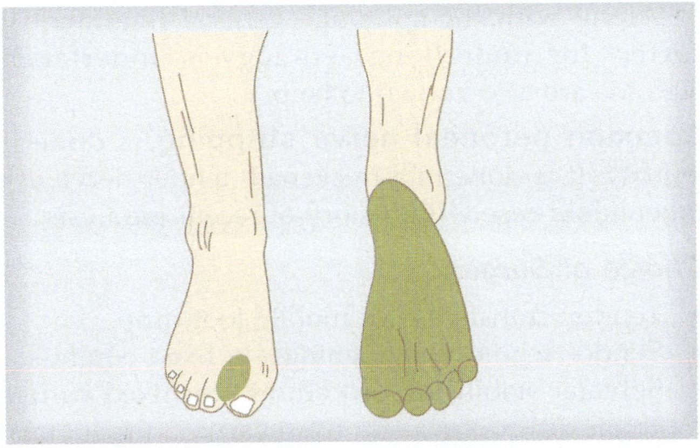

Fig. 25.22: Dorsal web space is supplied by anterior tibial nerve. Sole of the foot is by posterior tibial nerve

FOOT-DROP

Causes of Foot-Drop

General causes have been already mentioned, *the important one being leprosy as a cause of foot-drop.*

Local causes are seen along the course of the nerve

At the spine
- Spina bifida
- Tumours
- Disc prolapse, etc.

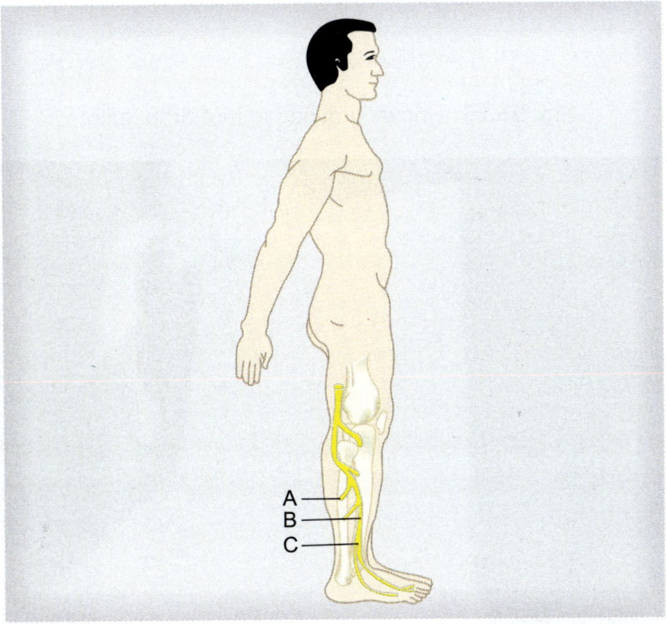

Fig. 25.23: Showing course of common peroneal (lateral popliteal) nerve; (A) tibialis anterior, (B) extensor hallucis longus, (C) extensor digitorum longus

At the hip
- Posterior dislocation of the hip (Fig. 25.24).
- Fractures around the hip.
- Fracture acetabulum.

At the gluteal region
- Deep intramuscular injections.

At the thigh
- Fracture shaft femur.
- Penetrating injury and gunshot injury.

At the knee (common causes)
- Forcible inversion of the knee.
- Dislocation of knee.
- Fracture lateral condyle of tibia.
- Lateral meniscal cysts and tumours.
- Dislocation of superior tibiofibular joint.
- Tight plaster casts around the knee.
- Poor padding during traction.
- Surgical damage during application of skeletal traction.
- *Direct injuries*—gunshot injuries, incised and penetrating injuries, etc.

Levels of lesion

• **High lesion** (above knee)	Both tibial nerve and common peroneal nerve are paralysed.
• **Low lesion** (below knee)	*Spared:* Peroneus longus and brevis.
Type I Anterior tibial nerve injury	*Lost:* Tibialis anterior, extensor hallucis longus, extensor digitorum longus and peroneus tertius. *Sensation:* Over first web space is lost.
Type II Musculocutaneous nerve injury	*Spared:* All the above muscles innervated by anterior tibial nerve. *Lost:* Peroneus longus and brevis. *Sensation:* over outer leg and foot.

Clinical Features

The resulting deformity following injury to the above nerves is *foot-drop* (Fig. 25.25). This could either be *complete* (in sciatic nerve or lateral popliteal nerve injury) or *incomplete* (injury to either superficial or deep peroneal nerve).

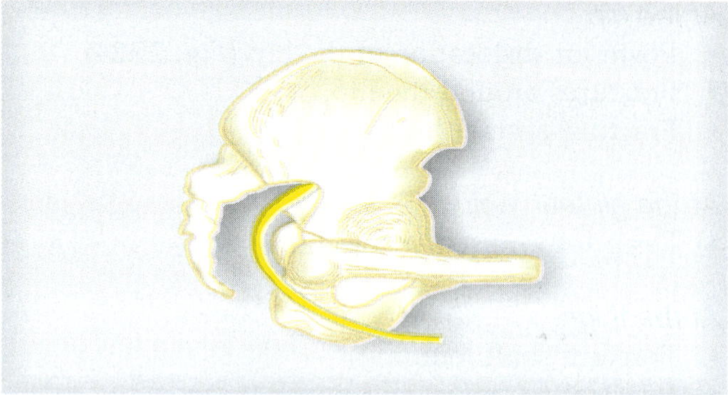

Fig. 25.24: Showing injury to sciatic nerve due to posterior dislocation of hip joint

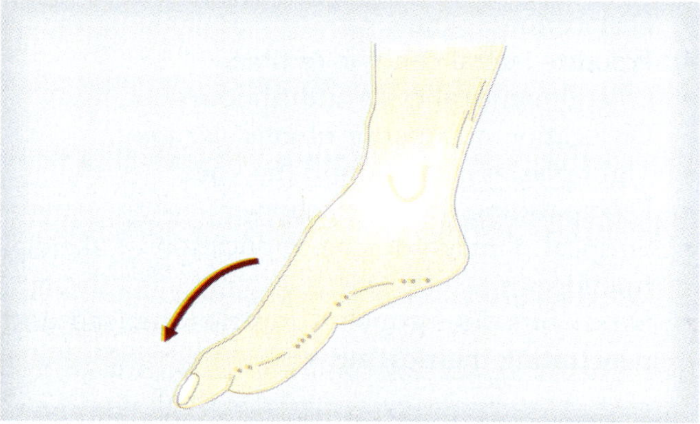

Fig. 25.25: Showing foot-drop

In high lesions it is a total foot-drop and in low lesions the foot-drop is usually incomplete. In low type I, the patient cannot dorsiflex and invert the foot but eversion is possible, front of the leg is wasted. In low type II, the patient cannot evert but can dorsiflex and invert the foot. There is wasting of the outer half of the leg. In type I injury sensation over the dorsal web space is lost and in type II injury it is lost over outer leg and foot.

The gait typical of foot-drop is a *high stepping gait.*

Treatment of Early Foot-drop

The lesions show a high incidence of recovery. Hence, conservative treatment with a view to encourage recovery (at least for 1 year) should be carried out.

Splintage of knee in 20° of flexion and ankle in 90° for night time. In the daytime, walking is allowed by using a "Foot-drop appliance".

Foot-drop appliances are of two varieties:

- Dynamic—spring shoe (Fig. 25.26).
- Static—back stop shoe (Fig. 25.27).

Along with the splintage general treatment to correct the underlying aetiology is undertaken. Steroids are also known to help.

Common peroneal nerve stripping is done in leprosy. It is done in a thickened, tender nerve in a tuberculoid case with history of recent paralysis.

Choice of Surgery

- Tendon transfers—for mobile foot-drop.
- Tendo-Achilles lengthening—in fixed equinus.
- Subtalar stabilising procedure—for fixed varus.
- Triple arthrodesis—for fixed varus at the subtalar joint.

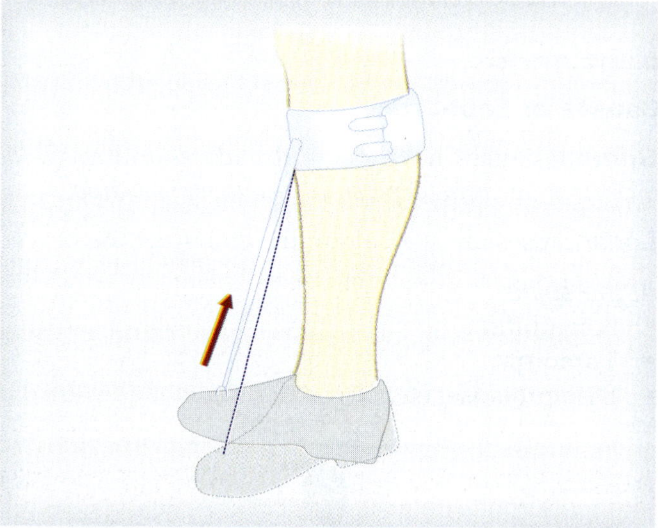

Fig. 25.26: Showing dynamic foot-drop splint

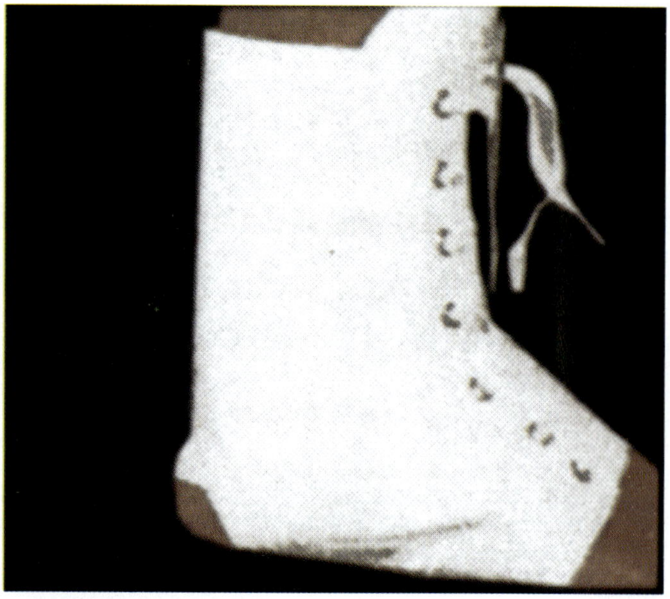

Fig. 25.27: Showing foot-drop splint (static variety)

Treatment of established foot-drop (more than one year)

Complete foot-drop (common peroneal nerve palsy)	Incomplete foot-drop
• Operation of choice is tibialis posterior transplant	• Commonest variety is anterior tibial nerve injury (loss of dorsiflexors and presence of evertors)
• Two methods employed: a. Circumtibial route (preferred method) b. Interosseous route	• Method of correction Anterior transposition of tibialis posterior (fixed to extensor hallucis longus) combined with peroneus brevis transfer to prevent excessive valgus due to strong evertors

At a glance

- Sciatic nerve is the thickest nerve in the body.
- Common peroneal nerve also called as lateral popliteal nerve is commonly injured at the fibular neck.
- Leprosy is the commonest general cause.
- Foot-drop could be complete or incomplete.
- High stepping gait is characteristic.
- Dynamic foot-drop splint is the mainstay of conservative treatment.
- Conservative treatment is indicated up to one year.
- Tendon transfer for mobile foot-drop contemplated after 1 year.

MERALGIA PARAESTHETICA

This is characterised by pain, numbness and paraesthesia along the anterolateral aspect of the thigh due to compression neuropathy or neuroma of the lateral femoral cutaneous nerve (Fig. 25.28).

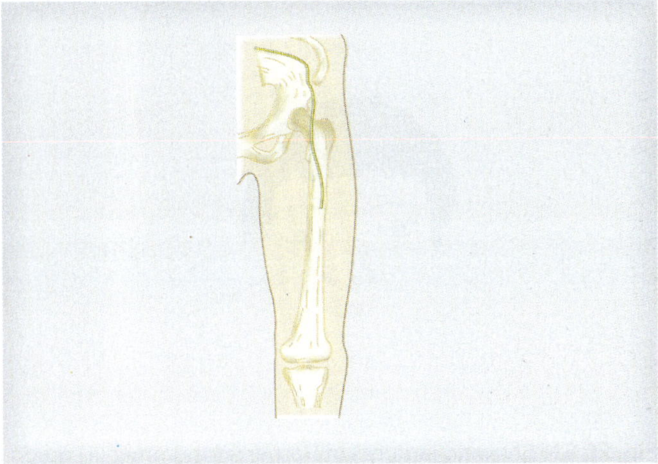

Fig. 25.28: Showing the course of the lateral femoral cutaneous nerve

Types

1. *Idiopathic:* Here, the exact cause is unknown.
2. *Spontaneous:* This is due to mechanical compression anywhere throughout the course of the nerve. The common site of injury is at the exit of the nerve at the pelvis.
3. *Iatrogenic:* This is commonly seen after orthopaedic surgeries like anterior iliac crest bone grafting and anterior pelvic procedures and prone positioning for surgeries.

Diagnostic test: If there is relief of pain and paraesthesia after injecting local anaesthetic, the diagnosis is clinched.

Treatment

1. *Conservative:*
   Idiopathic type: Improves by removal of the compressive agents, nonsteroidal anti-inflammatory drugs and local steroid injection.
   Iatrogenic type: Care should be exercised during pelvic surgery.
2. *Operative*: If pain persists in spite of the above treatment, surgery is indicated. The procedures include neurolysis or transection of the nerves.

BRACHIAL PLEXUS INJURIES

Everything about brachial plexus is complex, its anatomy (Fig. 25.29), mode of injury, the diagnosis, management and prognosis. It is a harrowing experience both for the patient and the surgeon. Among the more famous causes of brachial plexus injury is the birth injury in children and bike injury in adults.

Causes

Brachial Plexus injuries (Figs 25.30A and B) could be

Closed Here the injury could be due to birth trauma or bike trauma as mentioned above.

Open It is a rare injury and could be due to penetrating or gunshot injuries.

Note: Other less important causes of brachial plexus injuries:
- Traction injuries
- Tumour removal
- Abnormal pressures due to faculty postures
- Postirradiation scenario
- Surgical excision of cervical ribs
- Shoulder dislocations.

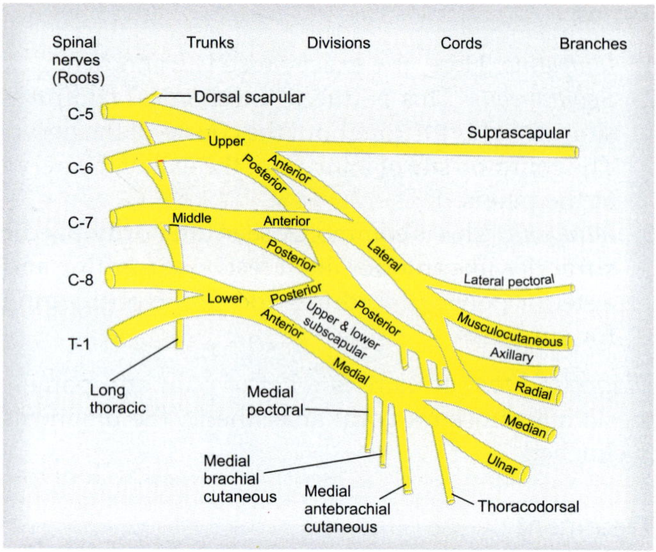

Fig. 25.29: Showing the normal anatomy of brachial plexus

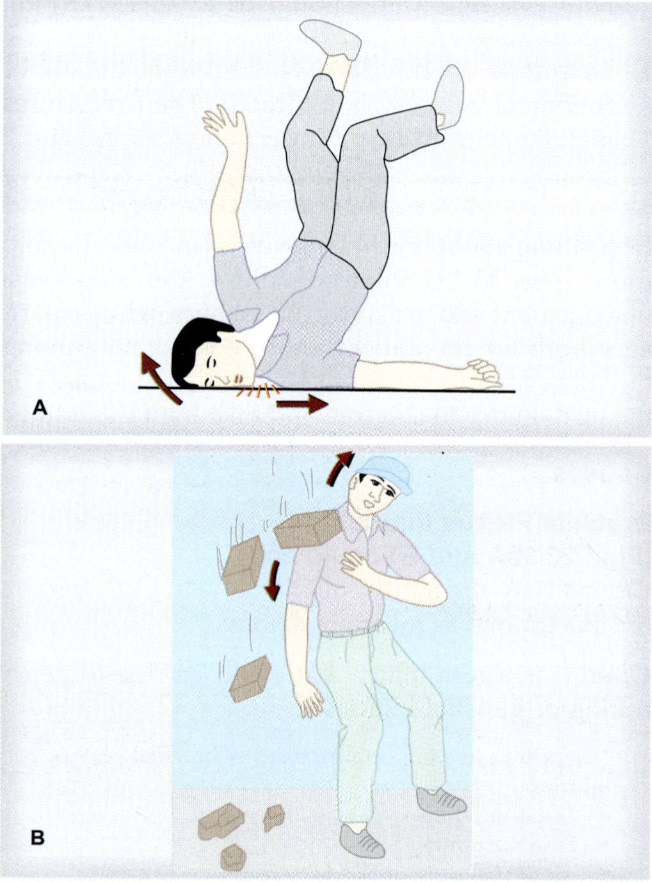

Figs 25.30A and B: Showing mechanism of brachial plexus injury

> **Interesting facts: Causes of brachial plexus injuries**
>
> Remember **"B"** in
> Brachial plexus injuries:
> **B**—*Birth* injury due to faulty forceps application.
> **B**—*Bike* injury-fall on the shoulder in young adults, usually from a speeding bike.
> (A combination of depression of the shoulder and forced lateral flexion of the neck).
> **B**—*Bad* prognosis most of the times.

TYPES OF LESIONS

Supraclavicular Lesion

1. **Preganglionic lesion** This is an unfortunate situation wherein the nerve roots are avulsed from the spinal cord. The cause could be either birth or bike trauma as mentioned earlier. The characteristic feature of this lesion is the presence of Horner's syndrome (Fig. 25.31).

> **Interesting facts**
>
> *About Horner's syndrome*
> What constitutes a Horner's syndrome? (All P's)
> - Ptosis of the eyelid.
> - Pupils which are small and constricted.
> - Protrusion of the eyeball which is slight.
> - Pain even at rest.
> - Positive sensory action potentials.
> - Poor prognosis.

2. **Postganglionic lesions** Here there is no Horner's syndrome. The prognosis is slightly better than the preganglionic lesion. A positive Tinel's sign may be elicited in this lesion.

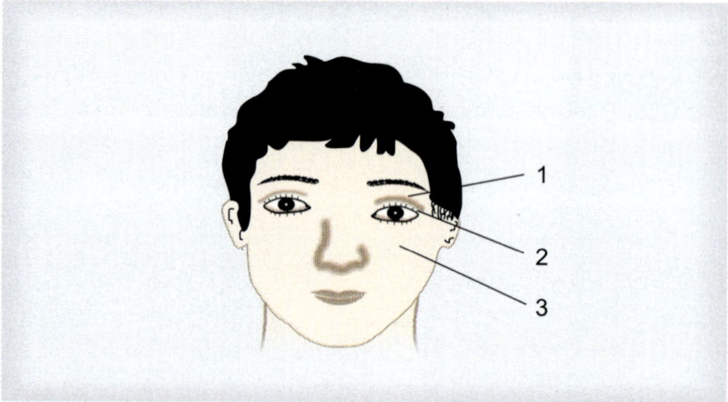

Fig. 25.31: Showing features of Horner's syndrome: (1) drooping of the eyelid, (2) constricted pupil, (3) absence of sweating in the surrounding skin

Assessment of Brachial Plexus Injury

It is important to assess whether the brachial plexus injury is preganglionic or postganglionic.

1. *In preganglionic lesions*
   - Horner's syndrome is present (Fig. 25.31).
   - The patient is unable to elevate the scapula (due to the disruption in the nerve supply to the Rhomboids and L. scapulae).
2. *In postganglionic lesions*
   - No Horner's syndrome.
   - The patient is able to elevate the scapula.
   - Tinel's sign is present in the later stages.

(Tapping above the clavicle, produces tingling sensation in the anaesthetic limb).

Investigations

These are less reliable than the clinical tests. However, X-ray to rule out neck fractures, CT scan to study the cross-section anatomy, MRI to study the soft tissue damages, myelogram (shows meningocoele in avulsion, but hazardous) and electrical studies are some of the investigations which give useful information during a brachial plexus injury.

The electrodiagnostic tests include EMG, nerve conduction study, SEP (somatosensory-evoked potential), percutaneous electrical stimulation, etc. EMG is by far the most reliable and effective test which successfully identifies the roots involved.

Treatment

During the initial stages

1. *Splinting*
   a. *For complete paralysis* A flail arm splint (FAS) designed by Framton is advised.

Quick facts

About FAS
- It immobilises the shoulder in abduction.
- It prevents glenohumeral joint subluxation.
- It permits five different positions of the elbow.
- It provides a platform for the forearm on which split hook, etc. can be applied.
- It can be operated through a cable to the shoulder strap attached to the opposite normal limb.
- It is cosmetically acceptable.

   b. *For incomplete lesions* Here splints with necessary modifications as per the situations can be used.
2. For pain control, TENS is best suited.
3. To prevent contractures and deformities, a careful passive ROM exercises under suitable guidance is recommended.

During the later stages

a. *Measures to strengthen the muscles* If there are movements, efforts are made to strengthen the muscles by repeated self-resistive exercises, PNF techniques, etc.
b. *Re-education of the muscles* This is done by encouraging movements of the shoulder, percutaneous electrical stimulation, stimulating techniques like icing, brushing, etc.
c. Modifying the splints and dynamising it helps
d. TENS to control pain
e. After 2 years, reconstructive surgeries are planned for the residual paralysis and deformities.

Surgical Measures

Acute phases In preganglionic lesions wherein the roots have avulsed from the cord, surgical exploration serves no purpose. However, suture or nerve grafting can be considered in postganglionic lesions.

Late stages (> 2 years) Reconstructive surgeries are planned after 2 years when the recovery can no longer take place. Surgeries are planned according to the residual paralysis.

a. *For shoulder function* Trapezius transfer to the neck of the humerus to improve abduction is advised.
   Arthrodesis of the shoulder is done in functional position.
b. *For elbow function* Steindler's flexorplasty (transfer of latissmus dorsi or pectoralis major to biceps).
c. *For wrist and finger extension* After the surgery, the patient is put on a detailed regime for re-educating the transplanted muscle.

ERB'S PALSY

This is due to injury to the C_5 nerve root and rarely the C_6 nerve root is also injured. It occurs either very early in life due to birth trauma (obstetric palsy, due to faulty application of forceps) or in young adults due to bike trauma (Fig. 25.32).

The Effects of the Injury

At the shoulder Here there is paralysis of the deltoid, rhomboids, supra and infraspinatus and teres minor

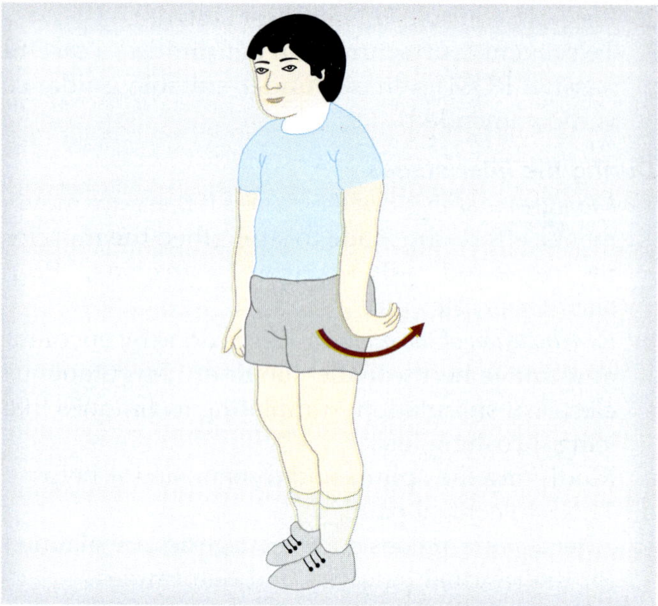

Fig. 25.32: Showing Waiter's or Porter's tip position in Erb's palsy

muscles. This results in the loss of shoulder abduction and external rotation.

At the elbow Biceps and brachialis muscles are paralysed. This results in loss of flexion of the elbow joint.

At the forearm Supinator muscles are paralysed resulting in loss of supination of the forearm.

The combined effect of the injury is an arm hanging loosely by the side of the trunk. The shoulder is internally rotated, the elbow is in extension, the forearm is pronated and the wrist is in flexion. This characteristic posture is popularly known as *"Policeman or Waiter's tip."*

Apart from this, there may be sensory loss on the outer aspects of the arm and forearm both in the front and back.

Management

Splinting This is done by using an abduction or aeroplane splint. The shoulder is maintained in abduction and external rotation, elbow in 90° of flexion, forearm in supination and wrist in extension.

Measures to prevent contractures A full range of passive movements to the affected joints helps prevent the contractures. This is a home treatment programme and should be taught to the mother.

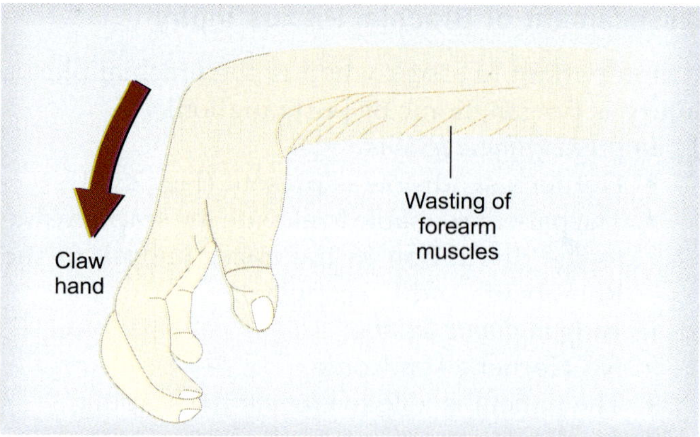

Fig. 25.33: Klumpke's paralysis

Electrical Stimulation of the affected muscles by using bilaterally symmetrical PNF stimulus helps to activate them.

Surgery This is rarely indicated as most of the cases recover spontaneously with the above treatment. Some of the recommended surgical measures are:

a. Exploration and repair of the nerve roots.
b. Tendon transfers to improve abduction and external rotation of the shoulder.
c. Release of soft tissue contractures.
d. De-rotation osteotomy for the rotational deformity.

KLUMPKE'S PARALYSIS (Fig. 25.33)

This is also due to either a birth trauma or a bike trauma.

The C_8T_1 nerve roots are involved and there will be paralysis of the wrist flexors, finger flexors and intrinsic muscles of the hand. This results in a claw hand deformity. The clinical features and management are discussed in the section on ulnar and median nerve injuries (see page 301).

BIBLIOGRAPHY

1. Bunnel S. Surgery of the Hand (3rd edn), Philadelphia: JB Lippincott Co, 1956.
2. Kahn EA. Direct Observation of Sweating in peripheral nerve injuries. Surg Gynecol Obstet 1951;92:22.
3. Leffert RD. Brachial plexus traction injuries. Clin Orthop 1988;237:24.
4. Lewi SD, Miller EM. Peripheral nerve injuries associated with fractures. Ann Surg 1922;76:528.
5. Mark D Grossman MD, Stephen A Ducey MD et al. Meralgia Paraesthetica.

6. Moldarcer J. Tind's sign: Its characteristics and significancies: J Bone JA Surg 1978;60-A:412.
7. Mukherjee SR. Tensile strength of nerves during healing. Br J Surg 1953;41:192.
8. Ober FR. Tendon transplantation in the lower extremity. N Engl J Med 1933;209:52.
9. Omer GE, Spinner M. Peripheral nerve testing and suture techniques. In American Academy of Orthopaedic Surgeons, Instructional Course Lectures. St Louis: CV Mosby Co, 1975;24.
10. Perry WB. Rehabilitation of the Hand (4th edn). Butterworths: London 1981;126-44.
11. Seddon HJ. Three types of nerve injury. Brain 66: 237, 1943.
12. Seddon HJ. The practical value of peripheral nerve repair. Proc R Soc Med 1949;42:427.
13. Seddon HJ. Nerve grafting. J Bone Joint Surg 1963;45-B:447.
14. Sunderland S. A classification of peripheral nerve injuries producing loss of function. Brain 1951;74:491.
15. Suderland S. Nerve and nerve injuries, Baltimore. The Williams and WIlkins Co, 1968.
16. Watson-Jones R. Primary nerve lesion injuries of the elbow and wrist. J Bone Joint Surg 1930;12:121.

SECTION THREE

NON-TRAUMATIC ORTHOPAEDIC DISORDERS

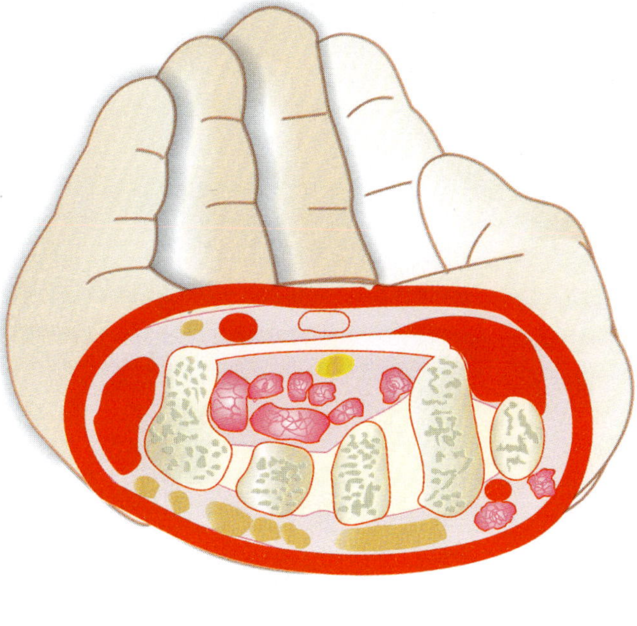

26 Approach to Orthopaedic Disorders

- History
- Examination
- Investigations

As in other branches of medicine, the diagnosis of orthopaedic disorders revolves around the following fundamentals (Fig. 26.1).

So we will try to discuss in brief the three steps of diagnosis in orthopaedics.

HISTORY

History is "His- Story", as told by the patient. History taking is an art. Caution has to be exercised in the story "told" and the story "untold." Everything told should be taken with a pinch of salt lest the examiner is misled.

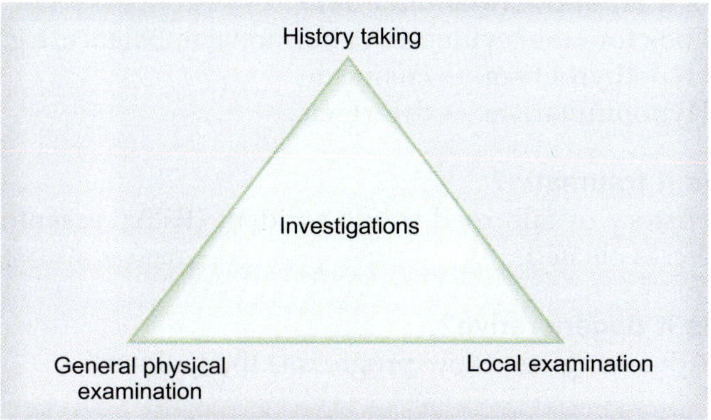

Fig. 26.1: Fundamentals of diagnosing orthopaedic disorders

Certain Points of Importance in the History

Age Certain diseases have predilection for certain age groups, e.g. Perthes' disease and acute osteomyelitis are common in children. Avascular necrosis and degenerative disorders are common in the elderly. Some diseases may be seen in all the age groups, e.g. tuberculosis of bone and joints.

Quick facts: age *vs* orthopaedic disease

< 1 year	Congenital dislocation of hip and cerebral palsy
1–2 years	Nutritional rickets Poliomyelitis Ewing's tumour
5–10 years	Tuberculosis of hip Perthes' disease
15–20 years	Slipped capital epiphysis
<15 years	Osteomyelitis
10–20 years	Bone malignancies
30–40 years	Rheumatoid arthritis
> 40 yeas	Degenerative disorders Prolapsed intervertebral disc (PIVD) Multiple myeloma, etc.

Sex Congenital dislocation of hip (CDH) is common in females. Congenital talipes equinovarus (CTEV) is more common in males.

Quick facts—sex vs orthopaedic disease

- Males: Perthes, slipped epiphysis, traumatic disorders, multiple myeloma, etc.
- Females: Rheumatoid arthritis, CDH, osteoporosis, etc.

Onset It may be sudden or gradual.

Trauma It could be a predisposing factor or the causative factor.

Traumatic points

Role of trauma vs orthopaedic disorders—trauma as a causative factor
- Fracture
- Dislocation
- Sprain
- Strain
- Subluxation

Trauma as a predisposing factor
- TB hip
- Perthes' disease
- Slipped capital epiphysis
- Osteogenic sarcoma
- Acute osteomyelitis, etc.

Fever It may be high as in acute osteomyelitis or low grade as in tuberculosis.

Pain This could be continuous or intermittent, low or high grade. One should be on guard about the radiating pains as these often mislead the examiner (Fig. 26.2).

Facts—about radiating pains

Region	Radiation sites
1. Cervical spine	Shoulder, arm, forearm, and fingertips.
2. Upper limbs	
a. Shoulder	Arm and elbow.
b. Elbow	Forearm.
3. Thoracic spine	Girdle pains.
4. Lumbar spine	Groin, buttocks, posterior thigh, legs and foot.
5. Hip	Knee.

Any constitutional problems like weight loss, anorexia, etc. if present is a pointer towards neoplasm, tuberculosis, etc.

Seasonal variation If present, it is suggestive of rheumatoid disorders. Apart from these points, relevant past history, socioeconomic status and personal history should be taken into account.

An attempt should be now made to place the problem into one of the following categories at the end of history taking.

Is the problem congenital?
If so, it will be present since birth or seen within a few years from birth. A strong family history is elicitable.

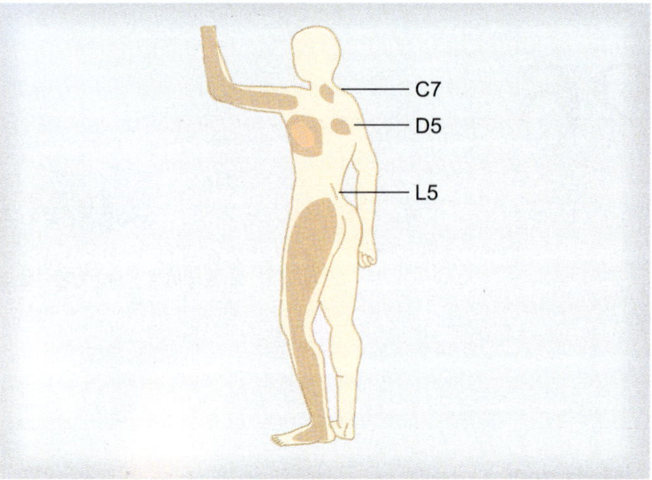

Fig. 26.2: Showing radiating pain at the upper limbs, chest and lower limbs

Is it developmental?
Here the disease gets manifested during the process of development.

Is it an infective disorder?
History of fever, chills, rigors, sweating, etc. are present.

Is it inflammatory disorder?
Seasonal variation, remissions and exacerbation, multiple joint involvement, etc. are present.

Is it a metabolic disorder?
Nutrition, socioeconomic status, generalised skeletal disorder, etc. assume importance in this group.

Is it an endocrinal disorder?
Look for other evidences of hormonal imbalance, e.g.
Hypothyroidism → cretinism
Hypopituitarism → dwarf, etc.

Is it traumatic?
History of fall, road traffic accident (RTA), assault, etc. is elicited.

Is it degenerative?
Advancing age, slow progress is the hallmark.

Is it neoplastic?
Look for the features of either benign or malignant bone tumours.

If it cannot be categorised into any of the above, then it could be *idiopathic*.

Having made a tentative diagnosis at the end of history, next important step is resorted to.

Diagnostic facts

• Present since birth	**Congenital**
• During the development process	**Developmental**
• History of fever, chills, rigors	**Infective**
• Nutrition, socioeconomic status	**Metabolic**
• Other evidences of hormonal imbalance	**Endocrinal**
• Seasonal variation, multiple joint involvement, etc.	**Inflammatory**
• H/o RTA, fall, assault	**Traumatic**
• Features of either benign or malignant	**Neoplastic**
• Advancing age, etc.	**Degenerative**
• If no obvious complaints	**Idiopathic**

EXAMINATION

A good systematic clinical examination will help to clinch the diagnosis with certainty. *No sophisticated technology can replace the value of a good clinical examination*. A good clinician will make the diagnosis clinically and will make use of the investigation armamentarium judiciously. *A clinician should command the investigation and not vice versa.*

Examination of the locomotor system involves four steps.

STEP I

Examination of Gait

An examination of the gait is extremely important as it gives vital clues regarding the diagnosis.

Definition *It is a term used to describe the style of walking.* This is dependent not only on normal muscles and joints but also upon an intact central nervous system (CNS), peripheral nervous system and normal labyrinthine function.

Walking is divided into two phases.

The stance phase (Figs 26.3A to C) This forms 60 per cent of the gait and here the foot is on the ground. It is further subdivided into:

1. *Heel strike*—i.e., heel striking the ground.
2. *Mid-stance*—here the foot is flat on the ground.
3. *Push off*—here the foot is off the ground.

The swing phase (Figs 26.4A to C) This forms 40 per cent of the gait cycle and here the foot is not in contact with the ground. It is further subdivided into:

1. *Acceleration*—here leg is in front of the body.
2. *Swing through*—here leg continues to swing forward.

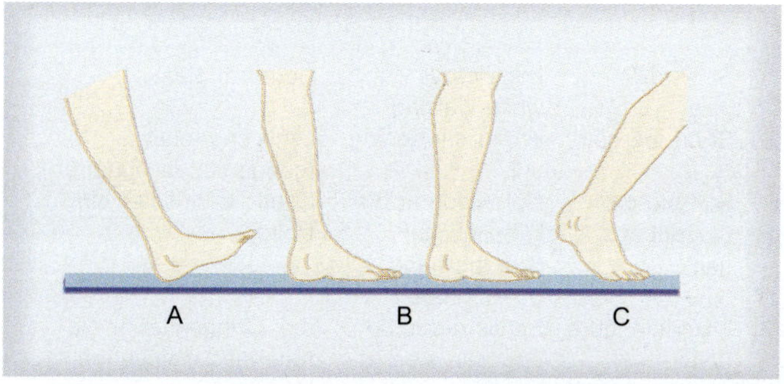

Figs 26.3A to C: Stance phase of gait: (A) heel strike, (B) midstance, and (C) push-off

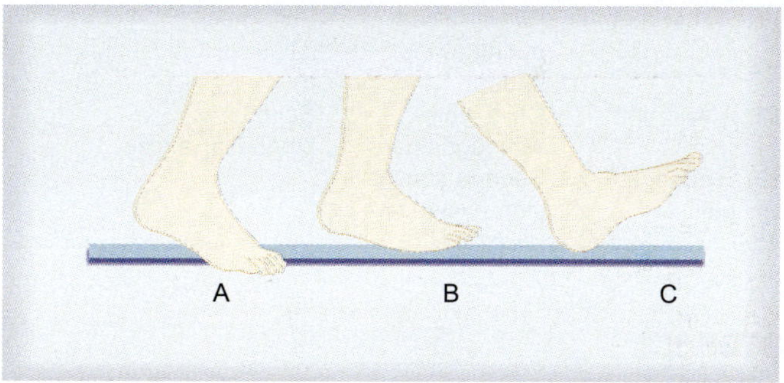

Figs 26.4A to C: Swing phase of gait: (A) acceleration, (B) swing through, and (C) deceleration

3. *Deceleration*—swing slows down and the heel is ready for the strike.

In normal gait, each leg alternatively goes through a stance phase and a swing phase. Thus, the body is carried forward in normal walking by these rhythmic cycles.

Running gait Here the sequences are the same as in walking but are faster.

Types of gait and probable diagnosis

Types	What happens	Probable diagnosis
1. Antalgic gait	Duration of stance phase decreased	Any painful lesion of foot, knee, hip, etc.
2. Gluteus medius gait	Lurch of body towards the affected side during every stance phase.	Paralysis of gluteus medius.
3. Gluteus maximus gait	Backward lurch	Anterior polio.
4. High stepping gait	To clear the dropped foot from the ground	Foot drop.

Contd...

Section 3

Contd...

5. Scissors gait	Legs cross while walking	Cerebral palsy.
6. Short leg gait	When shortening > 2"	Limb shortening (congenital or acquired).
7. Stiff hip gait	No flexion at hip	Septic arthritis at hip.
8. Quadriceps gait	Limping gait with the hand on the knee	Polio.
9. Trendelenburg gait	Pelvis drops on opposite side of the hip	e.g. Congenital or old traumatic dislocation of hip joint, nonunion fracture neck of femur
10. Calcaneus gait	No push off	Calf weakness.
11. Stiff knee gait	Pelvis raised during swing phase	Stiff knee.
12. Ataxic gail	Child walks with legs apart	Spinal cerebellar ataxia.
13. Hysterical gait	Seen in conversion hysteria	

STEP II

General Physical Examination

A good general physical examination (GPE) from head to toe gives vital clues in the diagnosis of most of the orthopaedic disorders, particulary generalised disorders of the skeleton, e.g.

- Metabolic disorders, e.g. rickets, etc.
- Developmental disorders, e.g. osteogenesis imperfecta, etc.

STEP III

Clinical Examination

Symptoms

The following are the usual presenting symptoms in a patient with orthopaedic disorder.

1. *Pain* This is the first and the most common complaint. It is a highly subjective complaint and can be classified as mild, moderate or severe.

   The must-ask questions regarding the pain are: How did it start? Is it related to trauma? Site of pain? Does it radiate? What are the aggravating and relieving factors? Does it interfere with sleep? etc.
2. *Swelling* It may precede or follow pain. Relevant questions to be asked are: Site of the swelling, painful or painless? Is it rapidly growing (e.g. malignancy) or slow growing (benign growth)? Is it associated with fever, chills, etc. (e.g. infective origin), single or multiple (e.g. neurofibromas, etc.)?
3. *Deformity* Sudden onset of deformity is usually seen in fresh fractures and dislocations. Longstanding deformities are usually seen in old fractures and other nontraumatic disorders like congenital, developmental, and metabolic conditions. The patient may complain of cosmetic and functional impairment due to the deformity.
4. *Limitations of joint movements* In the initial stages, it may be due to muscle spasm; and in the later stages, it may be due to intra-articular adhesions (e.g. TB, septic arthritis, rheumatoid arthritis, etc.) or extra-articular contractures (like postburn contractures, Volkman's ischaemic contracture, etc.).
5. *Limp* This could be painful (e.g. arthritis of hip, trauma, etc.) or painless (e.g. CDH, coxa vara, etc.).The patient may complain of difficulty or alteration in various day-to-day activities like walking, squatting, running, working, etc.
6. *Limb weakness* This may be due to disuse atrophy, motor problems like polio, motor neuron disease, etc., muscle problems like muscular dystrophies, etc., or due to peripheral or diabetic neuropathies.

Signs

General Look for the signs of anaemia, fever, weight loss, etc.

Local

1. **Deformity** Deformity may be due to an abnormality of bone or joint. If a joint is out of its anatomical position, a deformity is said to exist. And in case of bone, deviation from its normal anatomy is deformity. In cases of old fractures and dislocations, the deformity may be fixed.

Remember

- A fixed deformity is the angle between the neutral position of the normal joint and the position the deformed joint will reach.

2. **Temperature** This is always compared with the normal side. Check with dorsum of the hand as this is the most sensitive part.

3. **Tenderness** This is elicited by examining from the normal to the affected area and is graded I to IV (Fig. 26.5). Also see page no. 20.
4. **Swelling** The following things are noted in the examination of a swelling.
   - Decide the anatomical plane. The plane of the swelling could be either bone (swelling decreases in size when muscle is put into contraction) or could be in the muscle (swelling slightly decreases in size and gets fixed on muscle contraction) or could be between the muscle and the skin (no change in the size at the swelling when muscle is put into contraction). Also, examine the level of the swelling and identify whether it is epiphyseal, metaphyseal or diaphyseal (Figs 26.6A to D).
   - Describe the shape as globular, oval or round, etc.
   - Grade the consistency (*see* below).
   - Decide whether it is congenital, neoplastic, etc. (*see* diagnostic fact p. 321).
   - Look for slipping sign, sign of emptying, indentation sign and expansile impulse.

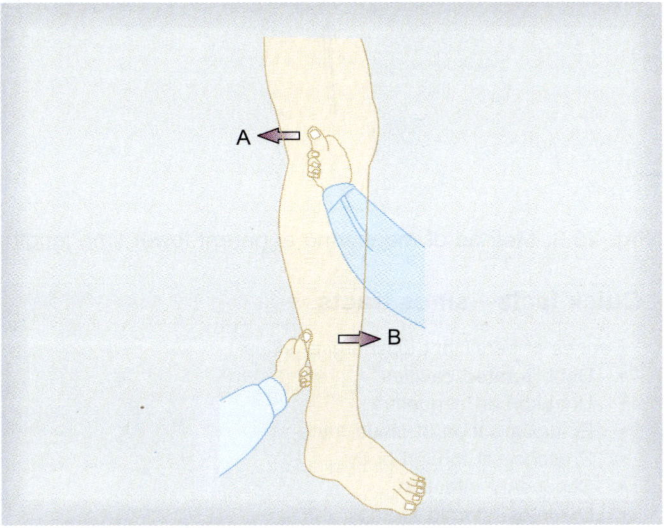

Fig. 26.5: Showing method of eliciting joint line tenderness (A) and bony tenderness (B)

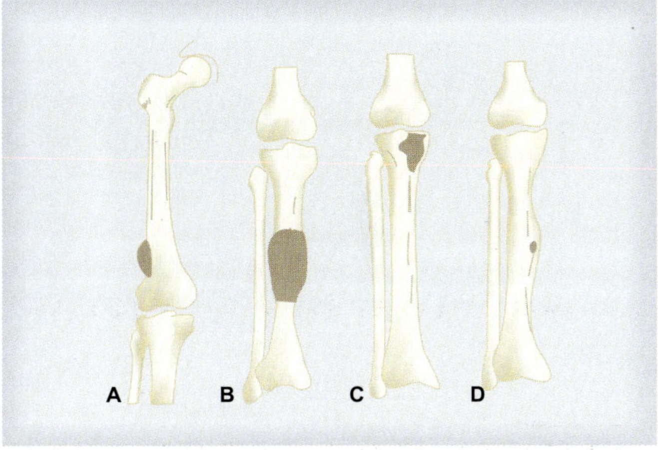

Figs 26.6A to D: Showing different levels of bony swelling (A) Metaphyseal, (B and D) Diaphyseal, (C) Epiphyseal

Remember

Grading of consistency
- Grade I — Very soft (like jelly).
- Grade II — Soft (as relaxed muscle).
- Grade III — Firm (like a contracted muscle).
- Grade IV — Hard (as a contracted biceps).
- Grade V — Stony and bone hard.

5. **Movements of joint**
   Active movement The patient himself moves the joint in one direction and later in the other. The extent of active movement is noted. Both the joints should be tested.
   Passive movement of the joint is tested by the examiner without causing pain. The extent of passive movement is noted (Fig. 26.7).

Remember
- Limitation of all movements of a joint indicates arthritis.
- Limitation of certain movements of a joint indicates an extra-articular lesion or mechanical block.
- If passive movements exceed active movements, paralysis of muscle is likely.

6. **Measurements** Accurate limb length measurements give vital clues regarding the diagnosis. Measurement should be taken for two purposes.

To know the limb length For this, measurement is taken between two fixed bony points and is always compared with the normal.

Upper limbs
- *Arm length* From the angle of acromion to the lateral epicondyle of humerus (Fig. 26.8).
- *Forearm length* From the lateral epicondyle of humerus to the radial styloid process.

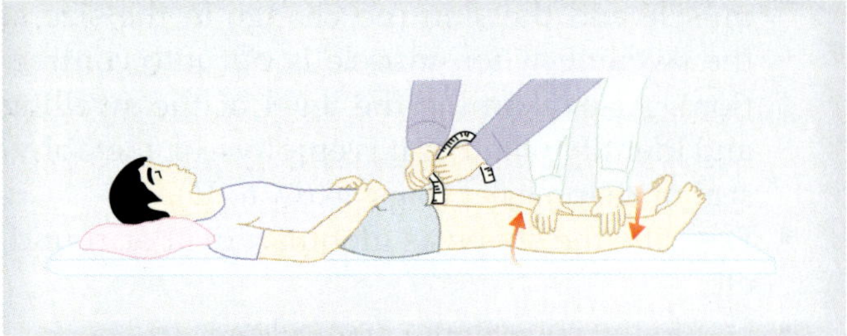

Fig. 26.7: Method of measuring the girth of a limb and checking the movements

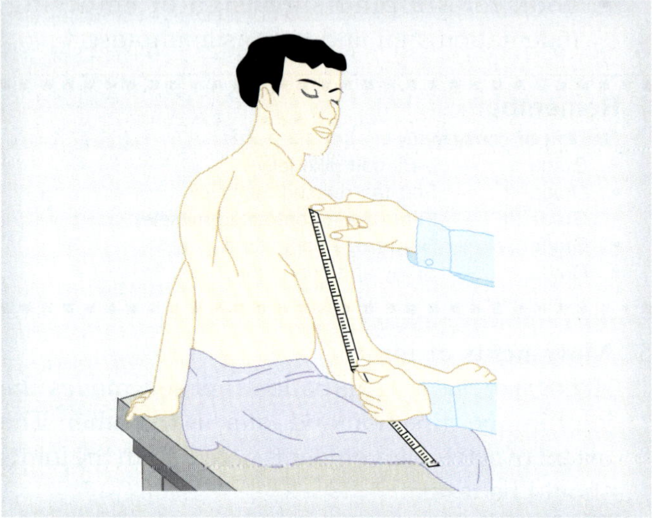

Fig. 26.8: Showing the method of upper arm length measurement

Lower limbs

- *Thigh length* From anterior superior iliac spine to the medial knee joint line.
- *Leg length* From the medial knee joint line to the medial malleolus.

To know the apparent length of the lower limbs measurement is taken from the xiphisternum to the medial malleolus (Fig. 26.9).

To know the girth of the limb To detect wasting of muscles, the circumference of the limb is measured at fixed points on both sides, e.g. 18 cm above joint line in the thigh (see Fig. 26.7).

7. **Irregular thickening of bone and persistent discharging sinus** If this is present along with scars fixed to bone, it indicates chronic osteomyelitis (see box for causes of persistent sinus) (Fig. 26.10). *Peripheral, vascular and nervous system examination* should be done next. This is discussed in appropriate sections.

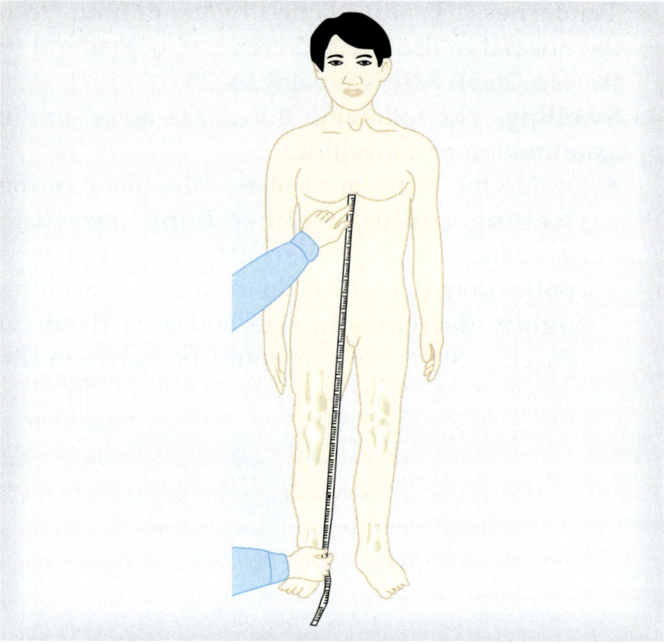

Fig. 26.9: Method of measuring apparent lower limb length

Quick facts—sinus tracts

Causes of persistent discharging sinus:

- Unobliterated cavities.
- Unabsorbed sequestra.
- Epithelialisation of sinus tract.
- Presence of foreign body.
- Secondary infection.
- Diabetes, steroid therapy, etc.
- Malignant change in the sinus.

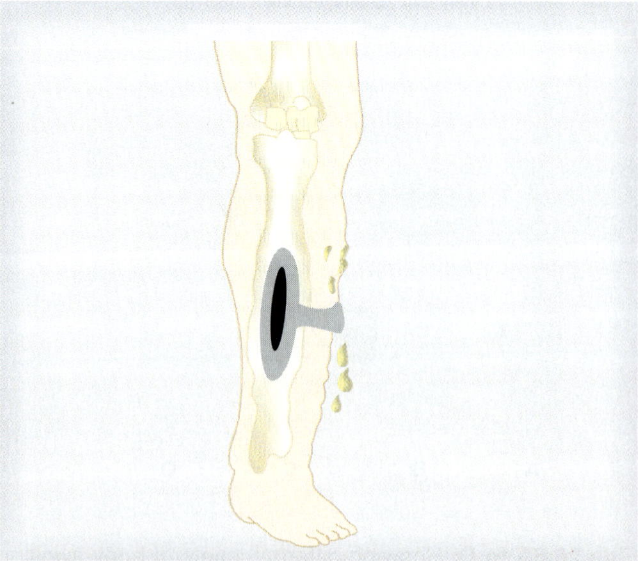

Fig. 26.10: Showing irregular thickening of bone and discharging sinus due to chronic osteomyelitis

INVESTIGATIONS

These help to confirm the diagnosis and in some cases help to make the diagnosis (e.g. crack fracture, etc. can be diagnosed only by X-ray). One has to choose carefully from the following vast armamentarium:

- *Laboratory investigation* This consists of blood investigations like routine haemogram, urine examination, ECG, chest X-ray, etc.
- *Special investigations:*
  1. *Radiography* At least two views of the affected part should be taken, oblique views and some special views are required in some cases.
  2. *CT scan* to study the cross section of the limb anatomy and bones.
  3. *MRI* This is the recent gold standard in the investigative armamentarium of bone disorders. It helps to study the bone, soft tissues, medullary spread, etc. with greater accuracy. The only problem is its prohibitive cost.
  4. Angiography and biopsy help in tumour diagnosis.

Thus, a reasonably accurate diagnosis can be made by following the guidelines discussed above.

Steps in the process of diagnosis

At the end of investigation	**Final**
At the end of examination	**Provisional**
At the end of history	**Guess**

27

Deformities and their Management

- ❑ Definition
- ❑ Classification
- ❑ Deformities since birth (congenital)
- ❑ Acquired deformities
  - ■ Bone causes
  - ■ Joint causes
  - ■ Soft tissue causes
  - ■ Treatment options

DEFINITION

Any deviation from the normal anatomy of a bone and joint is called a deformity.

CLASSIFICATION

The deformities can be classified as shown in the flow chart:

Deformity
- Congenital
- Acquired
  - **Bone**
    1. Fractures
    2. Variations in bone growth
    3. Diseases of the bone
  - **Joint**
    1. Dislocations
    2. Subluxations
    3. Muscle imbalance
    4. Muscle and tendon contractures or tethering
    5. Arthritis
    6. Poor posture
    7. Idiopathic
  - **Soft tissue**
    - Contractures of skin, deep fascia and muscles

Acquired deformities are more commonly encountered than the congenital variety.

DEFORMITIES SINCE BIRTH (CONGENITAL)

These are due to some genetic abnormalities or environmental variations or both. They may be obvious at birth or may be seen a few years later. Incidence is around 2 to 3 per cent. They may be so severe that the child is still born or may be so minor that it is not noticeable.

(See section on Congenital deformities for details).

ACQUIRED DEFORMITIES

These could be due to problems in the bone, joint or soft tissues (Figs 27.1A to G).

Clinical facts: Famous orthopaedic deformities due to fractures

1. S-shaped deformity	Supracondylar fracture humerus.
2. Gunstock deformity	Malunited supracondylar fracture humerus.
3. Cubitus valgus	Malunited lateral condyle fracture of humerus.
4. Dinner fork deformity	Malunited Colles.
5. Mallet finger	Avulsion tip of base of distal phalanx.
6. Genu varum/valgus	Tibial condylar fractures.
7. Varus-valgus at ankle	Ankle injuries.
8. External rotation lower limb	Fracture neck femur, trochanteric fracture, fracture shaft femur, fracture tibia.

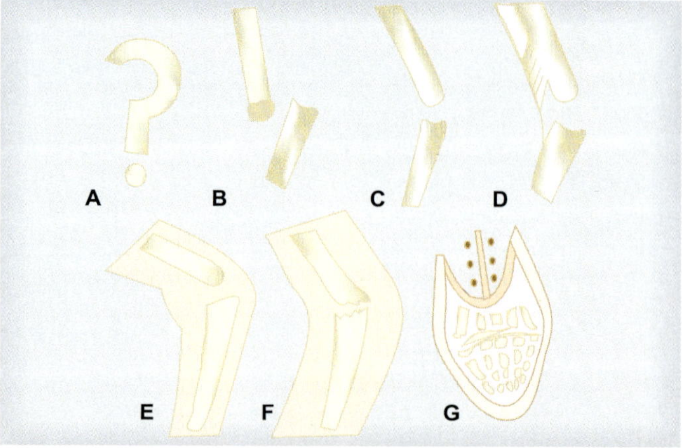

Figs 27.1A to G: Causes for deformity: (A) Idiopathic, (B) Dislocation, (c) Muscle imbalance, (D) Muscle tethering, (E) Soft tissue contractures, (E) Fractures, and (G) Postural

BONE CAUSES

The following causes are responsible for deformities in the bone.

a. *Growth disturbances* Tumour, infections or trauma near the growth epiphysis can cause either unequal stimulus, suppression or stimulation of growth. This results in bending, shortening or lengthening of a bone respectively, e.g. osteomyelitis, epiphyseal injuries, tumour, etc.
b. *Bone disorders* Endocrine disorders, metabolic disorders, developmental disorders are some of the examples with bone deformities.
c. *Fractures* This is by far the most important cause for a bone deformity. All displaced and fresh fractures cause temporary deformity while malunion or nonunion of fractures lead to deformities at a later date.

JOINT CAUSES

The causes for the deformities due to joint are varied.

a. *Dislocation or subluxation* This is usually due to trauma. It may also be seen due to pathological conditions of the hip, e.g. TB hip.
b. *Muscle imbalance* Muscles balancing the joint on either side, if they are either overactive (e.g. cerebral palsy) or underactive, e.g. polio, deformity of the joint results.
c. *Tethering of muscles and tendons* This can take place due to the growth of fibrous tissue following infections or due to callus following fractures. Tethering restricts the joint movements and if held for some time deformity results, e.g. VIC, tenosynovitis of finger flexors etc.
d. *Arthritis* of any joint may give rise to muscle spasm in the initial stages and fibrous or bony ankylosis in later stages giving rise to deformities, e.g. TB knee, rheumatoid hand, TB hip, etc.
e. *Postural* This is due to improper postural habits like hallux valgus in women due to tight and rigid shoes.
f. *Idiopathic* Here, there is no apparent cause for the joint deformities, e.g. idiopathic scoliosis.

SOFT TISSUE CAUSES

Soft tissue contractures (skin and deep fascia) other than the muscle contractures can also cause joint deformities, e.g. Dupuytren's contractures, postburn contracture, etc.

TREATMENT OPTIONS

Conservative Measures

These include manipulative correction under anaesthesia and retention by splints or casts, gradual correction by traction or splints, etc. (e.g. turn buckle splints). Correction by plaster wedging is hazardous.

Surgical Measures

There are various surgical options available:

1. *Ilizarov* This is the gold standard for deformity correction in recent times.
2. Soft tissue release by surgical methods.
3. Tenolysis, tendon lengthening or tendon transfers are successfully employed in polio, cerebral palsy, etc.
4. *Arthroplasty* can be crude as a salvage procedure (e.g. girdle stone excision in TB hip) or sophisticated as in total hip replacement or total knee replacement in osteoarthritis, rheumatoid and other disorders.
5. *Corrective osteotomy* This is a simple but effective procedure to correct joint deformities, e.g. French osteotomy in cubitus varus deformity, etc.
6. *Arthrodesis* fusion of the joints in functional positions in badly damaged joints, e.g. TB knee, rheumatoid arthritis, etc.
7. *Epiphyseal growth arrests* When potential for growth is still left, stapling of the epiphysis can be attempted on one side to correct the bending deformity, e.g. in genu varum or valgum.

Section 3

28 Treatment of Orthopaedic Disorders

- Masterly inactivity
- Conservative methods
- Operative treatment methods

There are three time-tested and time-honoured treatment methods (i) masterly inactivity, (ii) conservative methods, and (iii) operative treatment methods of treating an orthopaedic disorder.

MASTERLY INACTIVITY

It is interesting to observe that nearly 50 per cent of the orthopaedic disorders can be managed best by '*not doing anything*'. To allay the doubts, fears, myths, and misconceptions, a patient has regarding his ailment and assuring him that nothing is seriously wrong with him is all that is required.

This is more of a 'mind' management than 'orthopaedic' management and is more a 'human' care than 'health care'!

CONSERVATIVE METHODS

This is the next commonly advocated and recommended method of treatment.

Rest This implies not total rest but selective rest with avoidance of unnecessary activities and strain. This was first advocated by HO Thomas and of late due to improved methods of treatment and technology, emphasis is now on early restoration of activities and not passive rest.

Support This enables the diseased part to heal, provides rest, prevents deformities, relieves pain and also supports the patients psychologically, e.g. plaster splints for fractured limbs, lumbosacral belts and corsets for low backache, callipers in polio, cervical collars for neck pains, knee cap, ankle binders, etc. (Figs 28.1 and 28.2).

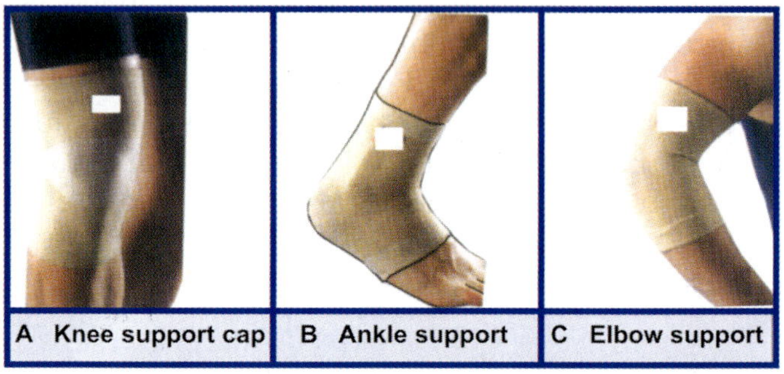

Figs 28.1A to C: Showing supportive braces

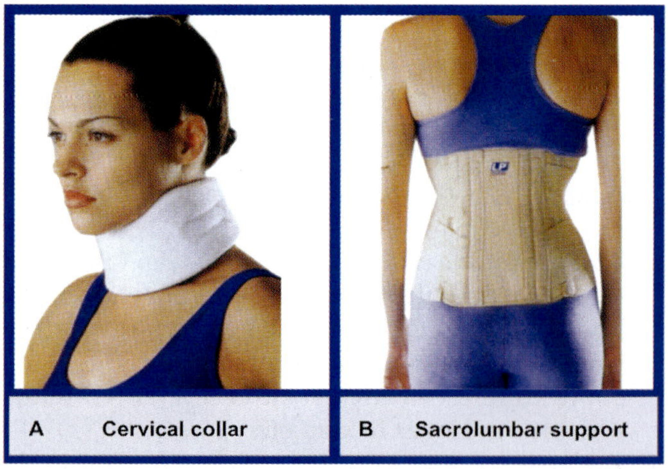

Figs 28.2A and B: Showing neck and back supports

Traction This is a popular method of treating certain chronic orthopaedic conditions like low backache, cervical spondylosis, etc. In these conditions, it is known to reduce pain, muscle stiffness, spasm, etc. (Figs 28.3 and 28.4).

Physiotherapy

Physiotherapy, if properly understood and skilfully executed by trained persons, gives excellent results in treating orthopaedic disorders and in postoperative rehabilitation. For optimum results, physiotherapy should be pursued systematically till

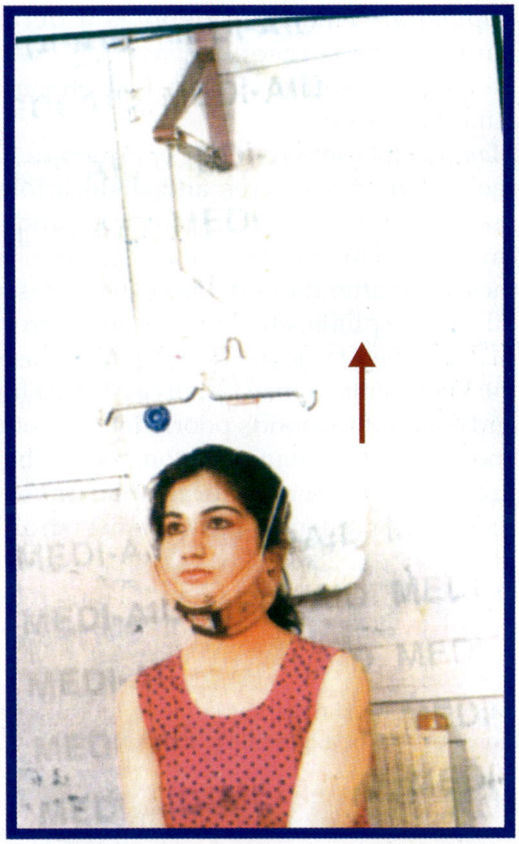

Fig. 28.3: Showing cervical traction

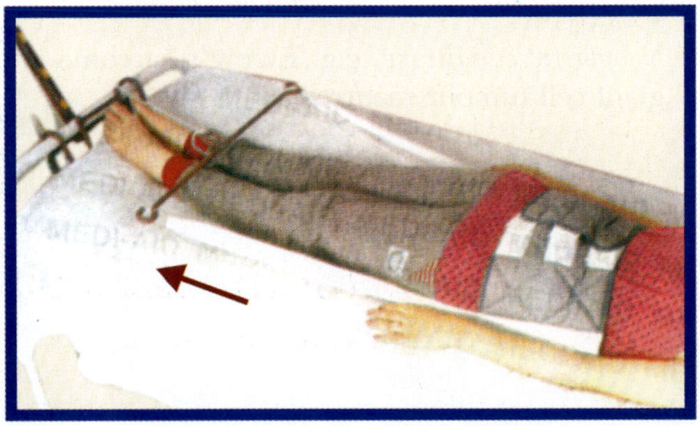

Fig. 28.4: Showing lumbar traction

its final logical conclusion and should not be abandoned in between. Physiotherapy has a great role to play and sometimes is the only treatment option in diseases like polio, cerebral palsy, hemiplegia, paraplegia, etc.

The following are the various physiotherapy options:

1. *Active exercises* Here the patient is made to actively contract his or her muscles and joints against resistance and weight. This helps to mobilise the joints, strengthen the muscles and to improve coordination or balance (Fig. 28.5).
2. *Passive exercises* This can be given by the physiotherapist normally or by machines which can provide continuous passive movements of the joints. This is of immense help to maintain the mobility of all the joints when active movements are not possible due to paralysis or injury to the muscles. Thus, the joints are kept supple and deformities are prevented (Fig. 28.6).

Note: Active muscle strengthening exercise could be either isometric (here muscle does not move and hence no change in length, e.g. pushing against a static object) or isotonic (here muscle actually moves, e.g. quadriceps exercises).

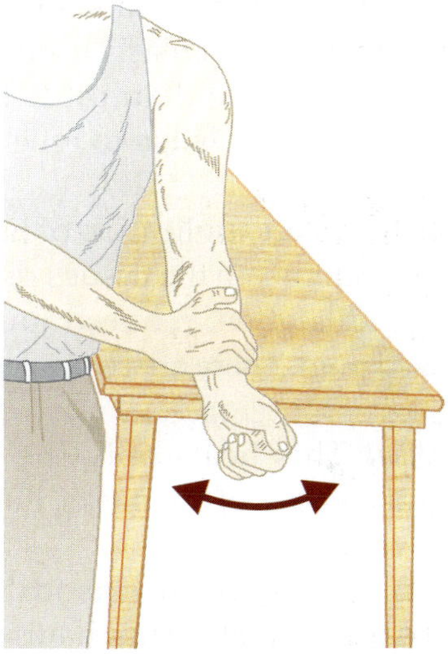

Fig. 28.5: Showing method of active wrist dorsal and palmar flexion of the wrist joint

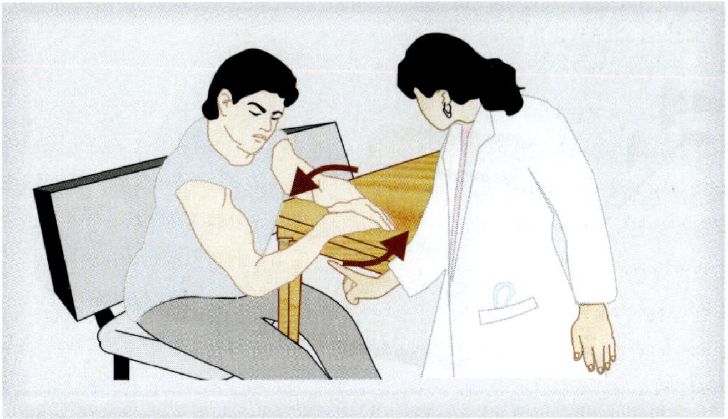

Fig. 28.6: Self-assisted passive wrist flexion and extension with the hand at the edge of a table

3. *Electrical muscle stimulation* Depending upon whether the nerve supply of a muscle is intact or not, two types of electrical stimulation is chosen:
   a. *Faradism* In this, the nerve supply of the muscle should be intact. In faradism, an electronic stimulator delivers shocks at shorter duration at a frequency of 1 mm at 50 Hg to the muscle through its intact motor nerve root, e.g. for regaining the strength of intrinsic muscles of the hand and foot, quadriceps muscle and to retain the tendons after tendon transfers.
   b. *Galvanism* Here the muscle is stimulated directly with shocks of longer durations (100–1000 mm at frequency of 5–15 Hg). When the muscle is denervated after a peripheral nerve injury, etc. this treatment modality helps.
4. *Hydrotherapy* This is particularly useful in patients suffering from rheumatoid arthritis. The warmth and buoyancy of water helps to relieve pain and muscle spasm.
5. *Heat therapy* By direct application of heat the local temperature underneath the tissues rises up to 10° inducing vasodilatation, reduced muscle spasm and decreased pain. There are two varieties of heat therapies.
   a. *Surface heat* This heats only the superficial tissues and consists of hot packs, infra-red heat, paraffin wax bath, etc.
   b. *Deep heat* Apart from vasodilatation, it stimulates the circulatory mechanism and helps in heating the deeper structures. It is also helpful in treating joint disorders, e.g. shortwave diathermy, ultrasound, interferential heat therapy, etc. (Fig. 28.7).

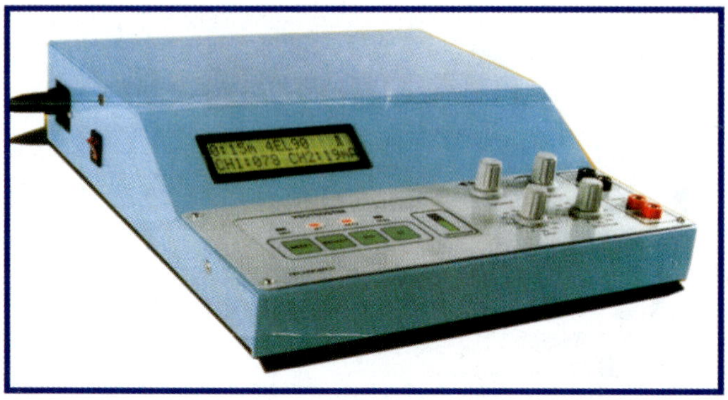

Fig. 28.7: Equipment for interferential therapy (IFT)

6. *Manipulation* This term denotes a deliberate attempt by the surgeon to passively move the joints bone or soft tissues. It is useful in three specific purposes:
   a. *Manipulation for correction of deformity* Closed reduction of fractures and dislocations and manipulation of a club-foot falls under this category. This is done under general anaesthesia and after the correction, the part is immobilised in splints, etc. to retain the correction.
   b. *Manipulation for joint stiffness* This is useful in the knee joints, it may be successful in shoulder and foot but responds poorly in cases of elbow and hand. The manipulation should be done gradually under general anaesthesia and forcible or abrupt movements should be avoided (Fig. 28.8).
   c. *For relief of chronic pain* Manipulation may help in chronic pain of shoulder tarsal, spine or sacroiliac joints.

Note: Manipulation should not be done in acute painful conditions for fear of aggravating the problem.

Radiotherapy

It has a role in:

a. *Inflammatory conditions* like recalcitrant ankylosing spondylitis.
b. *Neoplastic conditions,* e.g. Ewing's sarcoma and giant cell tumour recurrence.

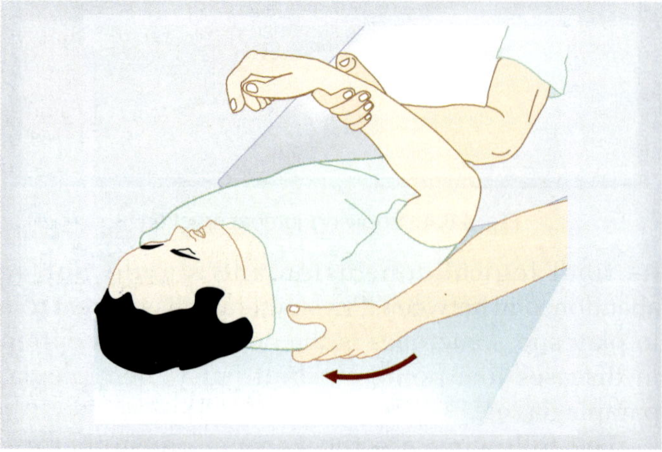

Fig. 28.8: Active assisted shoulder abduction with gravity eliminated

Massage Delicate, continuous and systematic massage if done regularly has a lot of beneficial effects like relief of pain, soothening, etc. (Fig. 28.9).

Drugs

Drugs though limited have an important role to play in orthopaedic practice. The commonly used ones are:

a. *Analgesics and anti-inflammatory agents* These help relieve pain and inflammation. Long-acting drugs are preferred in chronic disorders like rheumatoid arthritis, etc. while short-acting drugs are preferred in acute infections, trauma, etc.
b. *Muscle relaxants* These are useful to relieve painful muscle spasms.
c. *Sedatives and anxiolytics* These are used to induce sleep, alleviate anxiety and also to relieve muscle spasm.
d. *Antibiotics* These are extremely useful in acute and chronic infections of bones and joints. Broad-spectrum, bactericidal agents are usually preferred.
e. *Hormones* Growth hormones, stilboesterol for metastatic carcinomas, anabolic steroids and oestrogens for osteoporosis are some of the examples.
f. *Specific drugs* Vitamin C for scurvy, vitamin D for rickets are some of the examples.
g. *Cytotoxic drugs* These are used as chemotherapeutic agents for malignant tumours.

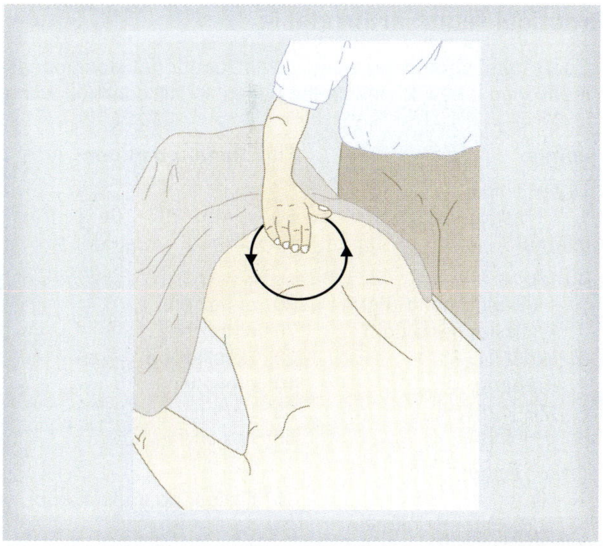

Fig. 28.9: Showing technique of back massage

OPERATIVE TREATMENT METHODS

Operative treatment should be resorted after great deliberations and when all other treatment options have been tried or thought of. Once undertaken, it should not worsen the condition of the patient.

A brief account of various orthopaedic surgical techniques are presented here.

OSTEOTOMY (Figs 28.10A and B)

This is a procedure of creating a surgical fracture to achieve the following objectives:

a. To correct excessive angulation, bowing or rotation of a long bone.
b. To compensate and correct the malalignment of a joint.
c. To correct leg length inequality either by shortening or by lengthening.
d. To alter the line of weight bearing and increase the stability at the hip joint, e.g. abduction osteotomy.
e. To relieve the pain in an arthritic hip, e.g. displacement osteotomy, high tibial osteotomy, etc. (Fig. 28.11).

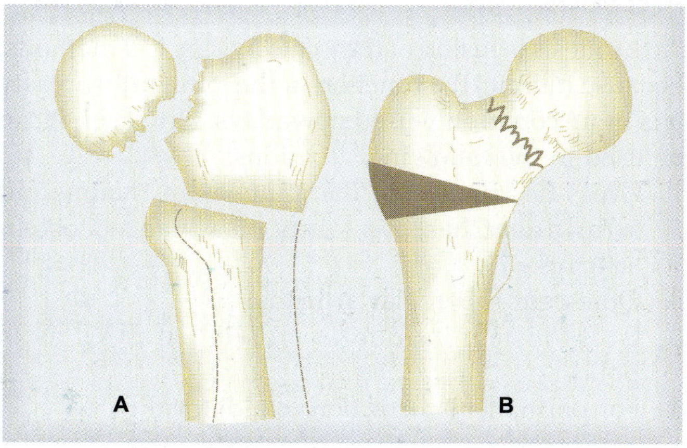

Figs 28.10A and B: Different types of osteotomies: (A) McMurray's displacement osteotomy, (B) Angulation osteotomy

For greater detail on physiotherapy and rehabilitation methods for various orthopaedic disorders, students are requested to read Essentials *of Rehabilitation for Orthopaedic Surgeons* by Dr John Ebnezar.

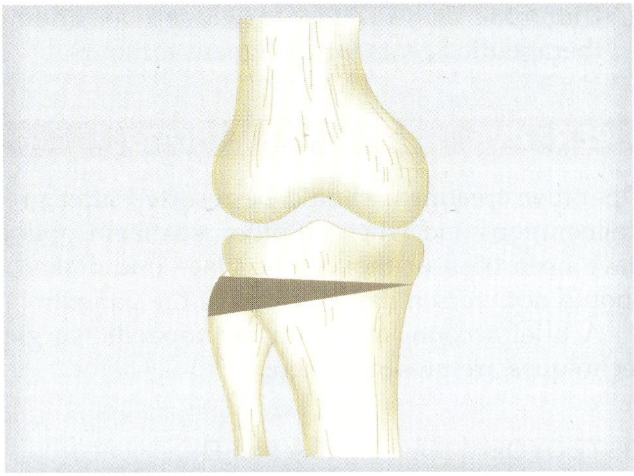

Fig. 28.11: Showing high tibial osteotomy done in OA knee

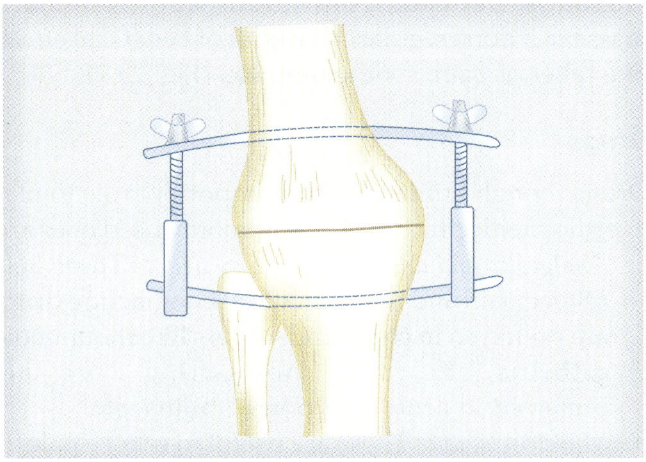

Fig. 28.12: Showing Charnley's compression arthrodesis

A quick glance at famous osteotomies

Upper limbs	*Done for*
• French osteotomy	Malunited supracondylar fracture humerus
• Fernandez and Campbell osteotomy	Malunited Colles' fracture
Lower limbs	
• Salter, Chiari, Pemberton	CDH
• McMurray's, Shanz	Fracture neck femur
• Pauwel's	OA Hip
• High tibial osteotomy	OA Knee
• Dwyer's osteotomy	Club foot
Spinal osteotomy	Ankylosing spondylitis

ARTHRODESIS

Arthrodesis is fusion of the joints by surgical methods. Because it limits the function of the joint, arthroplasty it is more commonly used nowadays. However, it can be used in the following situations:

1. Gross destruction of the joints as in rheumatoid arthritits, Charcot's joints or advanced osteoarthritis.
2. Quiescent tubercular arthritis.
3. Gross instability due to muscle paralysis as in polio.
4. For permanent correction of a deformity.

Methods

There are three methods:

Intra-articular arthrodesis Here joint is opened, articular cartilage is denuded, cancellous bone grafts are packed, joint is kept in a functional position and either fixed internally or externally by plaster, etc. (Fig. 28.12).

Extra-articular arthrodesis This is indicated in infective condition of the hip, shoulder or spine. In this, there is no risk of reactivating or spreading the infection as the joint itself is not opened, but bone-to-bone fusion is obtained above or below the joint.

Combined arthrodesis This is a combination of the above two procedures.

Note: Arthrodesis of a joint gives it stability but takes away its mobility. It is like robbing Peter to pay Paul.

Practical facts: arthrodesis

Each joint should be fixed in its functional position as mentioned below to enable the patient to still continue using it:

Joints	**Functional positions**
Upper limbs	
1. Shoulder internal	30° Abd/30° flexion/40° rotation
2. *Elbow*	
• Eating hand (right)	90° of flexion
• Toilet hand (left)	70° of flexion
3. Wrist	20° dorsiflexion
4. Forearm	10° pronation
5. MP joint	35° flexion
6. IP joints	45° flexion
Lower limbs	
1. Hip abduction or rotation	15° flexion, no adduction or
2. Knee	20° flexion
3. Ankle (men)	90° or neutral position
• Ankle (women)	15–20° of plantar flexion
4. Metatarsophalangeal joints of big toe	Slight extension

ARTHROPLASTY

Arthroplasty is an operation to construct a new mobile joint. The following are the indications:

1. Advanced osteoarthritis or rheumatoid arthritis of hip, knee, shoulder, elbow, hand and foot.
2. Quiescent destructive tuberculous arthritis of hip and elbow.
3. Fracture neck nonunion in patients of more than 60 years.
4. Rarely to correct deformity, e.g. hallux valgus.

Types

There are three varieties of arthroplasties (Figs 28.13 to 28.16) namely:

1. *Excision arthroplasty* (Fig. 28.13A) Here one or both the articular surfaces are excised, fibrous tissue fills up in the gap thus created and provides mobility. It is usually done in hip, elbow and metatarsophalangeal joint of the great toe.
2. *Hemireplacement arthroplasty* (Fig. 28.13B) Either of the articulating surface is removed and replaced by a prosthesis of similar shape and size, e.g. Austin Moore's prosthesis in fracture neck nonunion.
3. *Total replacement arthroplasty* (Fig. 28.13C) Here both the articular surfaces are excised and replaced by prosthetic components, the larger joint is replaced by a metallic prosthesis, and the smaller joint by high-density polyethylene. Both the components are fixed by acrylic cement, e.g. total hip replacement for osteoarthritis or rheumatoid hip and partial or total knee replacement for advanced intractable osteoarthritis or rheumatoid arthritis (Figs 28.14 to 28.16).

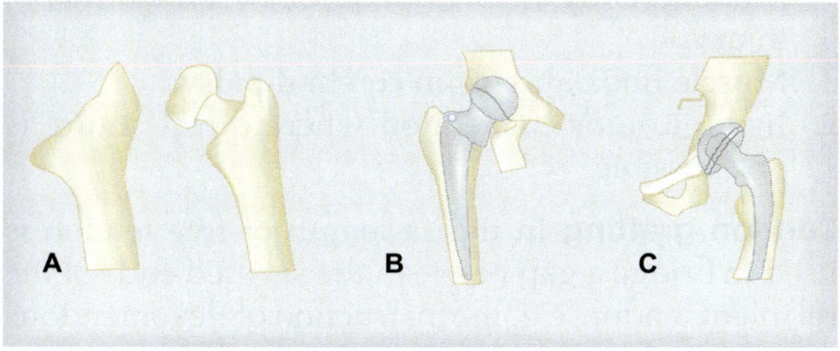

Figs 28.13A to C: Different types of arthroplasties: (A) Excision arthroplasty, (B) Hemireplacement arthroplasty, and (C) Total hip replacement

BONE GRAFTING OPERATIONS

Bone grafting is used in the following situations in orthopaedic practice:

1. To promote union in cases of nonunion or ununited fractures.
2. In arthrodesis of joints for intra-articular or extra-articular fusion.
3. To fill a defect or cavity in a bone.

Types

There are three types of bone grafts.

1. *Autogenous grafts or autografts* These are bone grafts either cancellous or cortical obtained from different parts of the patient's own body. Cancellous bone grafts are obtained from the iliac

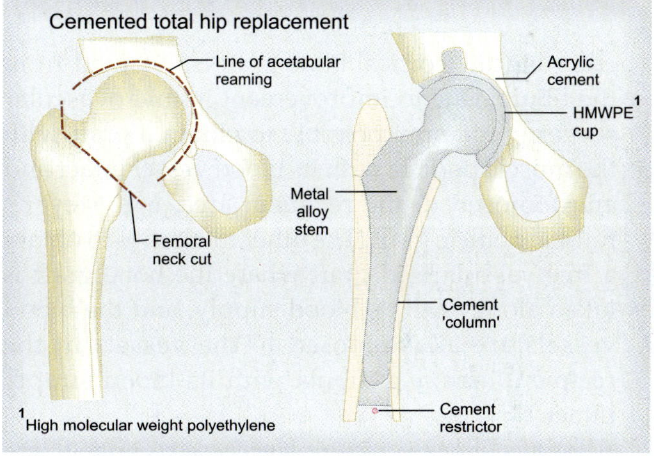

Figs 28.14A and B: Total hip replacement

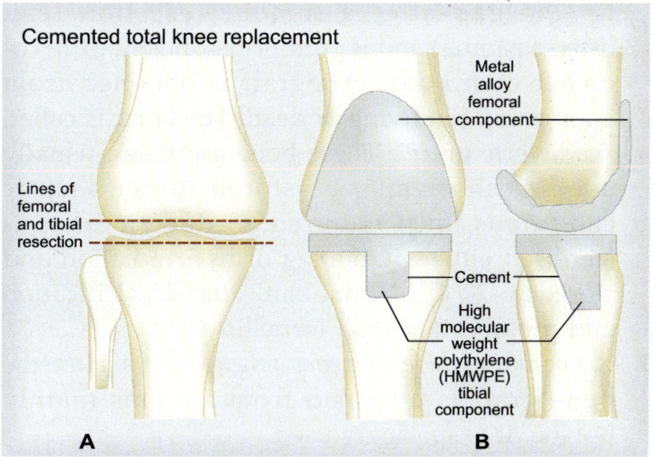

Figs 28.15A and B: Total knee replacement

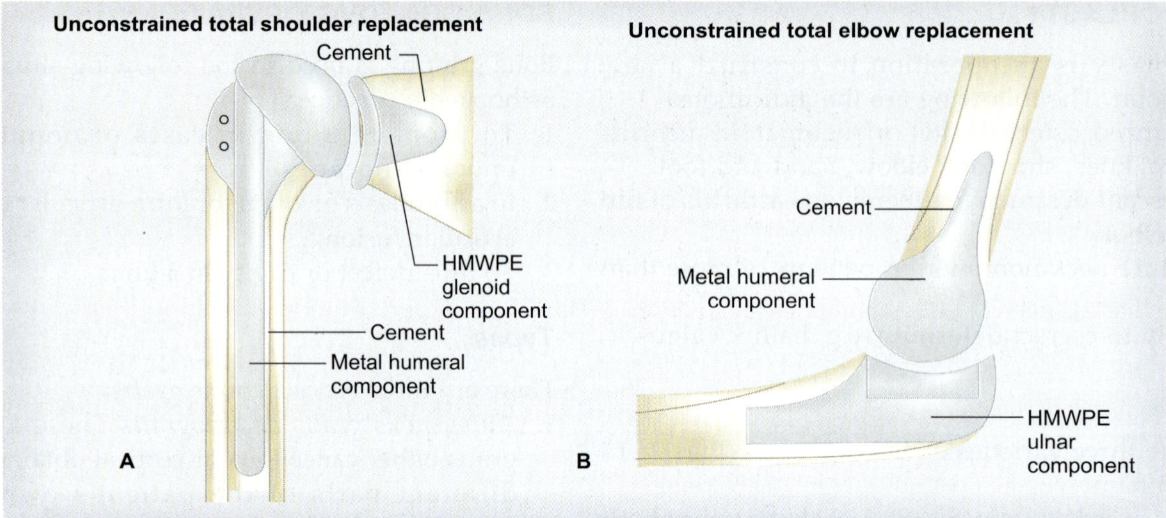

Figs 28.16A and B: Total shoulder replacement and total elbow replacement

crest and the cortical bone graft is obtained from the fibula. Due to improvement in microvascular surgery, it is now possible to obtain a graft with the muscle pedicle with its blood vessel intact and anastomosed to the recipient area, e.g. Meyer's muscle pedicle graft. The other method is to obtain a free vascularised graft where the bone graft is taken along with its blood supply, and the blood vessels are anastomosed to the vessels in the recipient area, e.g. fibula with its blood supply intact.

2. *Allografts or homografts or homogeneous grafts* Here the bone graft is obtained from another person's body usually if the requirement is large as in filling up the gap after a tumour resection (e.g. osteoclastoma) and if graft is insufficient from his or her own body. Allograft is obtained from another person living or dead. The latter is called "cadaveric graft". These bone grafts are usually used fresh or may be stored under aseptic conditions until required. Cadaveric bone is sterilised either by boiling or by irradiation and stored at –70°C in a bone bank after decalcification and preservation with formalin.
3. *Xenografting (heterogeneous or heterografts)* Here the bone graft is obtained from animals mainly bovine. It is sparingly used.

Artificial bone This is made up of hydroxyapatite and is now being used in some centres.

Role of a Bone Graft

It provides a scaffold or a temporary bridge upon which a new bone is laid down. Thus, the bone cells of the graft die and are eventually replaced by a new living bone. Vascularised grafts get incorporated very rapidly.

Tendon Surgeries

This includes:

Tendon transfers In this operation the insertion of a healthy functioning muscle is moved to a new site, so that it has a different action. Other intact tendons will take care of the original function of the transferred tendon.

Indications

1. Muscle paralysis as in polio or peripheral nerve injury.
2. Muscle imbalance as in cerebral palsy.
3. In rupture or cut tendon where direct suture is not possible.

Tendon grafting In this, a length of free tendon is used to bridge a gap between the severed ends of the recipient tendon, e.g. reconstruction of flexor tendons severed in the fibrous digital sheaths of the hand.

Free tendon graft is usually obtained from the palmaris longus or from one of the toe extensors at the dorsum of the foot (Fig. 28.17).

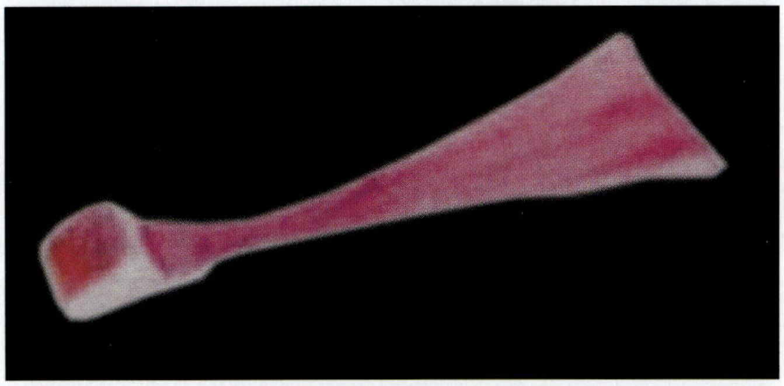

Fig. 28.17: Tendon graft

Equalisation of leg length In patients with unequal leg length as in polio, equalisation of leg length can be obtained by:

1. Leg lengthening by Ilizarov's technique.
2. Leg shortening, especially in femur or tibia. Not advocated as a routine procedure.
3. Arrest of epiphyseal growth by stapling in children.

Excision of tumours This has been discussed in chapter on bone neoplasias.

Amputations See discussions on amputations.

A Quick Recap

Treatment method in orthopaedics

1. *Masterly inactivity*
2. *Conservative methods*:
   - Rest
   - Support
   - Traction
   - Physiotherapy
   - Radiotherapy
   - Massage
   - Drugs
3. *Operative methods:*
   - Osteotomy
   - Arthrodosis
   - Arthroplasty
   - Bone graft procedures
   - Tendon surgeries
   - Equalisation of leg length
   - Excision of tumours
   - Amputations

29 Regional Conditions of the Neck

- Torticollis (Wryneck)
- Thoracic outlet syndrome
- Cervical rib
- Cervical disc syndromes

Regional orthopaedics deals with a vast array of interesting orthopaedic problems. Each region has its own peculiar problems depending on various factors like anatomical, physiological, occupational and others operating in that region. An effort is made in this section to highlight the various regional orthopaedic problems. However, a detailed description of the regional disorders is avoided as it is outside the scope of this book. The student is requested to refer bigger books in orthopaedics in case he or she desires a detailed study of the regional problems.

TORTICOLLIS (WRYNECK)

Torticollis is defined as the rotational deformity of cervical spine that causes turning and tilting deformity of the head and neck (Fig. 29.1).

Causes

- *Congenital* (see the chapter on Congenital Disorder for description).
- *Infective* Tuberculosis of cervical spine, acute respiratory tract infection, etc.
- *Traumatic* Sprain, dislocation and fracture of the cervical spine.
- *Myositis or fibromyositis* of sternocleidomastoid, exposure to cold causes myositis.
- *Spasmodic* painful, persistent or intermittent sternomastoid muscle contraction.

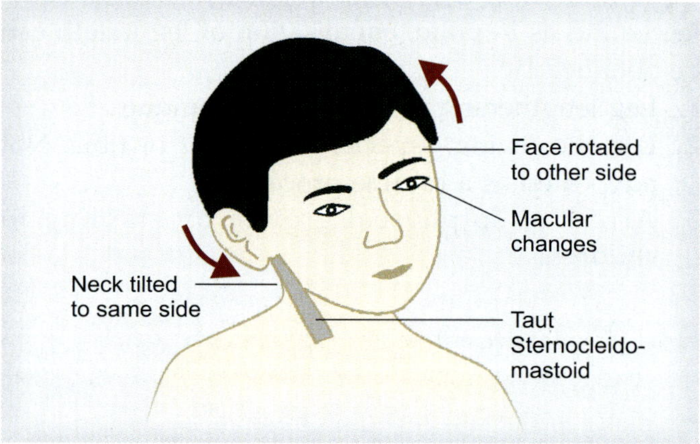

Fig. 29.1: Features of wryneck

- *Unilateral muscle paralysis,* e.g. polio.
- *Neuritis* of spinal accessory nerve.
- *Ocular disturbances* child turns head to one side to compensate for defective vision.

Clinical Features

Head of the patient is tilted towards the affected side while the chin points to the other side. Sternocleidomastoid muscle is prominently seen. In the later stages, the patient may develop facial asymmetry and macular disturbances in the eye.

Among the acquired causes of torticollis, spasmodic muscle contraction of the sternocleidomastoid is the most common cause.

Management

Conservative Initially conservative line of treatment is observed. This consists of nonsteroidal anti-inflammatory drugs (NSAIDs), muscle relaxants drugs, etc.

Physiotherapy like ultrasound, heat, massage is advocated. In acute pain, the patient is encouraged to wear a collar. Gradual neck stretching exercises are advised once the acute symptoms subside.

Surgical management is advised after the failure of conservative treatment. It consists of release of sternomastoid muscle from its clavicular attachment as in congenital torticollis and intradural section of both spinal accessory and three cervical roots in cases of torticollis due to spasmodic or neural causes.

THORACIC OUTLET SYNDROME

The space at the thoracic outlet or inlet when it is less than adequate, subjects the neurovascular structures seeking to gain entry into the upper limbs via this space, to undue pressure (Fig. 29.2). The blame for the neurovascular complaints should be placed at the doorstep of the decreased space and not at the structures producing the problems.

This syndrome results from the compression of neurovascular bundle comprising of subclavian artery and vein, axillary artery and vein and brachial plexus at the thoracic outlet. Thoracic outlet is a space between the first rib, clavicle and the scalene muscles. The above structures are liable to be compressed (Fig. 29.3) when this space gets narrowed either due to hypertrophy of the existing muscles or due to any other cause like congenital, trauma, etc.

Sites of Compression

The sites of compression could be either supra-clavicular, subclavicular or infraclavicular.

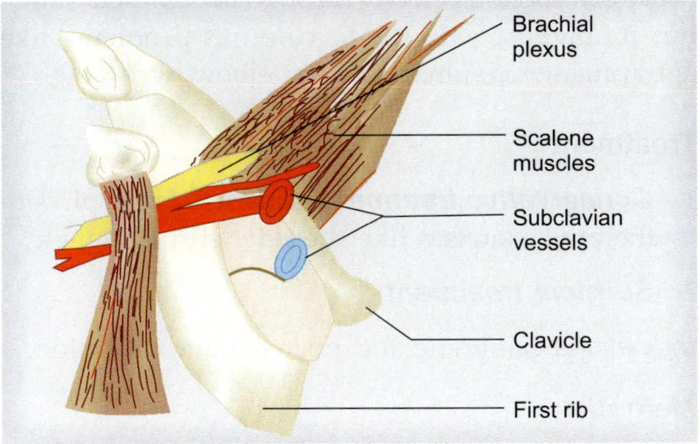

Fig. 29.2: Anatomy of the thoracic outlet

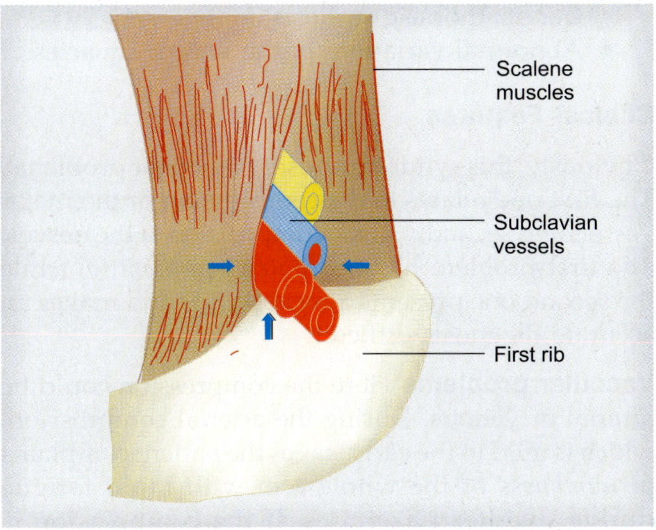

Fig. 29.3: Abnormal scalene muscle insertion causing compression of neurovascular structures

Supraclavicular Interscalene triangle between the anterior scalene muscles.

Subclavicular Interval between the second thoracic rib, clavicle and subclavius.

Infraclavicular Beneath an enclosure formed by the coracoid process, pectoralis minor, and costocoracoid membrane.

Rare cause Scissor-like encirclement of axillary artery by the median nerve.

Contributing Factors

Dynamic factors Arm when in full abduction pulls up the artery by 180° causing compression in the short retroclavicular space.

Static factors

1. *Vigorous occupation*—increases the muscle bulk and thereby decreases the space.
   Inactive occupation—decreases the muscle bulk and thereby increases the space.
2. *Congenital* Cervical rib decreases the interscalene space and thereby decreases the retroclavicular space.
3. *Traumatic* Malunion or nonunion of fracture clavicle.
4. *Arteriosclerosis.*
5. *Anomalies of the first thoracic rib.*
6. *Miscellaneous*
   - Tumour arising from the upper lobe of the lung.

- Cervicothoracic scoliosis.
- Abnormal variations of the scalene muscles.

Clinical Features

Obviously, this syndrome poses two major problems. The first one relates to the compression of the major vessels and secondly to the compression of the nerves. The first problem has a *definite clinical entity*, while the second one presents a *vague picture* and makes an accurate diagnosis difficult.

Vascular problems Here the compression could be arterial or venous. During the arterial compression, which is mild in the early stages the patient complains of *numbness* of the whole arm with rapid fatigue during overhead exercises. If the compression is significant, the patient will complain of *cold, cyanosis, pallor* and *Raynaud's phenomenon.*

Venous compression leaves the limb *swollen* and *discoloured* after exercises which disappears slowly with rest.

Neurogenic problems This involves C_8 T_1 segment (Klumpke's paralysis). Patients complain of *paraesthesia* along the medial aspect of the arm, hand, little and ring fingers. There is *weakness* of the hand also.

Tests

Intermittent claudication test The arm is abducted and elevated and fingers are exercised. The inference:

- If pain develops after 1 minute; it is negative (normal)
- If pain develops before 1 minute; the test is positive.

Compression of subclavian artery in the neck Radial pulse decreases.

Allen's test To determine the adequacy of radial and ulnar arteries, by compressing each one at a time and checking for adequacy.

Costoclavicular manoeuvres The patient's shoulder is braced down and back. The reproduction of the symptoms, change in the radial pulse, bruit heard in infraclavicular area are the positive findings.

Provocative tests

Adson's test The radial pulse is felt and the patient is asked to take a deep breath and turn the head to the same side (Fig. 29.4B). Decrease in the radial pulse indicates positive test.

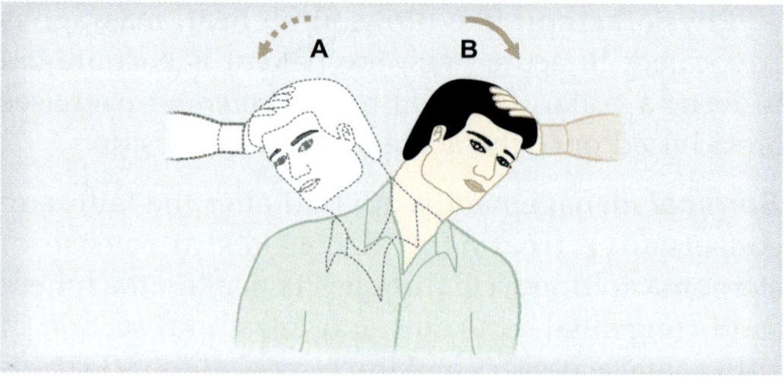

Fig. 29.4: Showing methods of performing: (A) Wright's test, (B) Adson's test

Wright's test The same manoeuvre as above but the head is tilted towards the opposite side (Fig. 29.4A). It should be noted that thoracic outlet syndrome is a diagnosis of exclusion. First the cervical pathology should be excluded and later the above tests should be performed as the initial screening procedures.

Complications

Subclavian artery compression → results in post-stenotic dilatation → stasis favours thrombosis → the thrombi break and migrate distally causing embolisation → this results in the distal artery blockade causing ischaemia and gangrene of the upper limbs.

Investigations

X-ray neck to rule out intrinsic causes like cervical spondylosis, cervical rib, etc.

Nerve conduction studies Difficult to determine the nerve conduction velocity through the thoracic outlet, but its biggest value is to rule out problems like entrapment, e.g. ulnar nerve at elbow, wrist, etc.

Treatment

1. ***Conservative treatment*** consists of rest, physiotherapy, exercises like shoulder shrugging, etc.
2. ***Surgical treatment***

Indications Gangrene and post-stenotic dilatation.

Methods

- *Removal of the first thoracic rib* this is the most efffective treatment as it deals with both supraclavicular

and infraclavicular aetiological factors in this syndrome.
- *Removal of cervical rib* If this is the cause of compression.
- *Scalenotomy* is indicated in scalenus anticus syndrome.

Quick facts

- Sites of compression—could be supra, sub, or infraclavicular.
- Clinical manifestation—could be neural, vascular or both.
- Diagnosis is usually by exclusion and the screening test helps.
- Excision of the first thoracic rib is the most effective surgical procedure.

CERVICAL RIB

Cervical rib problem is akin to the story of the "Return of the Prodigal Son". But unlike the chastened prodigal son, cervical rib returns to torment the unfortunate victim!

It is a rib arising from the 7th cervical vertebra, rarely 6th and 5th cervical vertebra.

Incidence is 0.46 per cent. Nearly 50 per cent of those are unilateral.

Side It is more frequent on the right side.

Developmental Factors

In the embryo nerves larger than the ribs interfere with the development of the costal process. When brachial plexus is prefixed, well developed 4th cervical root and small 2nd thoracic root offer little resistance to the costal process at the 7th cervical root.

In postfixed brachial plexus, well-developed 1st thoracic root offers resistance to costal process of 7th cervical root. Obviously, cervical rib is more common in prefixed variety.

Types

Four varieties are described:
- *Complete* The cervical rib reaches up to the first thoracic rib.
- *Bulbous end* In this, the cervical rib has a bulbous end.
- *Tapering end* In this, the cervical rib tapers.
- *Fibrous band* In this, the rib is represented by a thick fibrous band.

Pathological Anatomy

The neurovascular structures, the brachial plexus and subclavial vessels are hung up by the cervical rib that is inserted into the scalene tubercle of the 1st rib space.

Pronounced drooping of the shoulder in women after middle age, trauma, unusual lifting operations, acute illness make the muscles weak, pulling the plexus and artery distally giving rise to symptoms.

Clinical Features

1. *Cervical rib with local symptoms* Show presence of a lump and tenderness in the supraclavicular fossa.
2. *Cervical rib with vascular symptoms* This gives rise to pain in the upper limbs, temperature and colour changes, radial pulse is feeble or absent and a feeling of numbness is present.
3. *Cervical rib with nerve pressure symptoms* The nerve pressure symptoms are due to the angulation of the first thoracic nerve root. The patient complains of paraesthesia along the medial aspect of the arm, hand and little fingers. There is weakness of the hand muscles also.

Investigations

X-ray of the neck (AP and lateral views) helps to detect the presence of cervical rib (Fig. 29.5). However, the absence of the rib on the X-ray does not rule out the possibility of the presence of cervical rib.

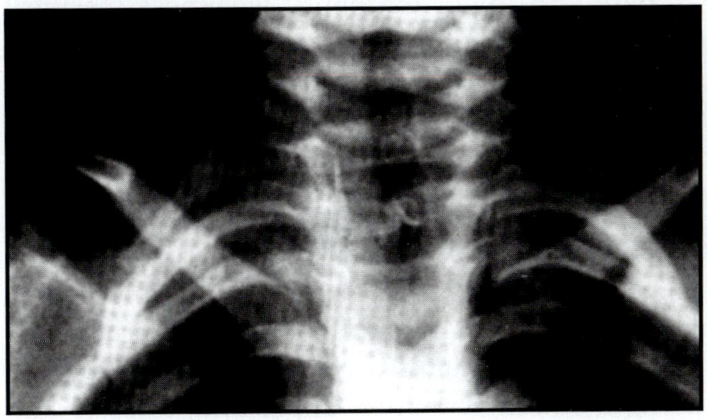

Fig. 29.5: Radiograph showing unilateral cervical rib

Section 3

Treatment

In mild cases, sling exercises often help. In more severe cases, scalenotomy (resection of scalenus anterior muscle) may be required and is successful in 70 per cent of the cases. In troublesome cases removal of the cervical rib or the first rib surgically with its periosteum to prevent its regeneration is advocated.

CERVICAL DISC SYNDROMES

The cervical region consists of seven cervical vertebrae with their intervening discs. The disc is made up of central nucleus pulposus and annulus fibrosus at the periphery. The disc functions as an effective shock absorber and also gives the cervical spine more mobility. If the disc material herniates (Fig. 29.6) because of trauma or old age, it gives rise to the cervical disc syndrome.

More than 90 per cent of the disc lesions in the cervical spine occur at the C_5 and C_6 levels as these are the most mobile segments. About 70 percent of the people are affected with these changes by the age of 70 years.

Types

1. *Soft disc lesions* It is common in young adults and is usually following trauma. In this, there is only a nuclear herniation through the wide annulus fibrosus of the disc.
2. *Hard disc lesions* This is more common than the first, seen in older age group, gradual in onset and is usually due to cervical spondylosis. Rarely large posterior osteophytes may cause pressure on the anterior portion of the spinal cord and produce mixed symptoms of the upper limb nerve root pain and lower extremity weakness (cervical spondylosis with myelopathy).

Clinical Features

Symptoms The patient complains of *pain* in the neck which is gradual or acute in onset. There is history of morning stiffness. Extension of the neck increases the pain. *Tingling* and *numbness* develop if the nerve root is compressed, but it does not follow the dermatomal pattern. Patients may also complain of radiating pain along the neck, shoulder, upper arm, forearm and hand (Fig. 29.7).

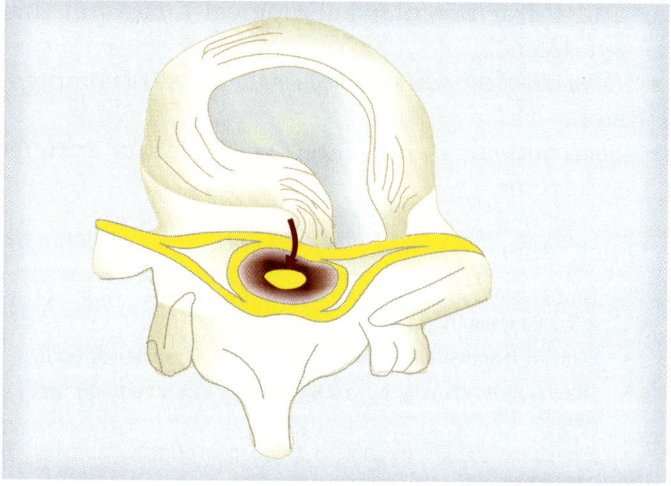

Fig. 29.6: Cervical disc herniation compressing the nerve root

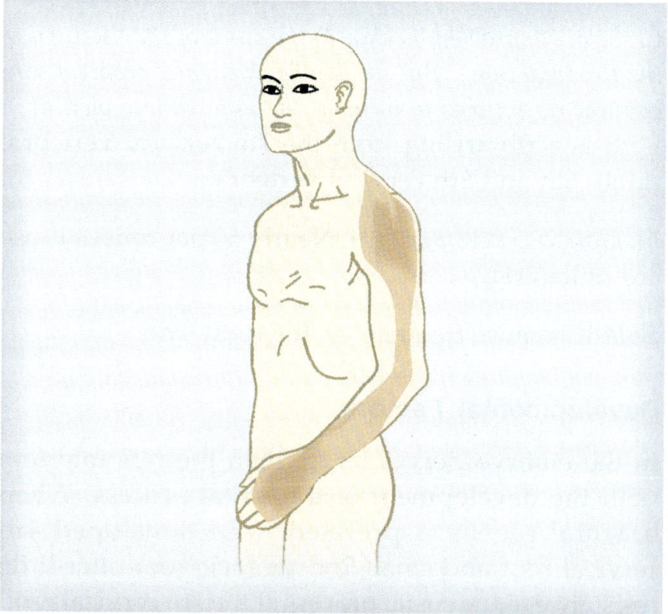

Fig. 29.7: Showing distribution of radiating pain in cervical sypondylosis

Signs Movements of the neck are decreased due to pain. Pain increases on hyperextension. There is localised tenderness over the spinous process. Trigger point tenderness at the scapular region is present. Pressure against the top of the head increases pain. If the nerve root is compressed by the disc herniation (see Fig. 29.6) sensory, motor and reflex changes occur and follow the dermatomal pattern (Table 29.1 and Fig. 29.8). *Rarely symptoms referrable to the lower limbs*

Table 29.1: Showing dermatomal and myotomal pattern

Root	*Motor*	*Reflex*	*Sensation*
C_5 ($C_{4\text{-}5}$ lesion)	Deltoid↓	Biceps reflex↓	Numbness in the deltoid region
C_6 ($C_{5\text{-}6}$ lesion)	Wrist extension↓	Brachioradialis reflex↓	Dorsolateral aspect of the thumb and index finger
C_7 ($C_{5\text{-}6}$ lesion)	Wrist flexion↓	Triceps reflex↓	Index, middle and dorsum of the hand
C_8	Finger flexion↓	None	Ring, little finger, medial border of forearm

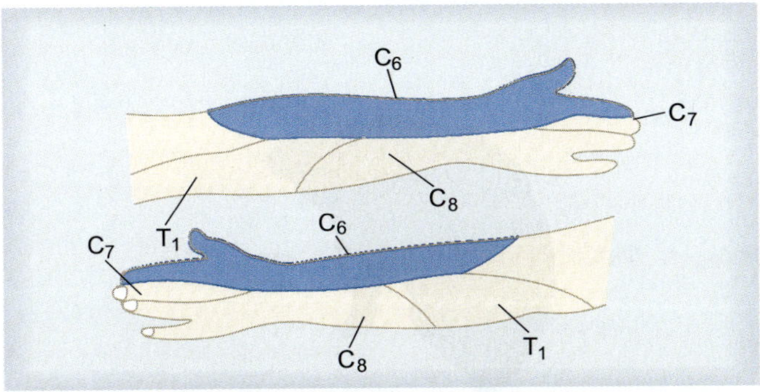

Fig. 29.8: Dermatomal pattern of upper limb

develop due to pressure of posterior osteophytes on the anterior portion of the cervical cord. This symptom complex appears as a combination of cervical roots and cord symptoms [LMN upper limbs + UMN lower limbs].

Do you know?

At what levels does cervical spondylosis most typically occur? Well it is:

$C_{5\text{-}6}$ > $C_{6\text{-}7}$ > $C_{3\text{-}5}$ > C_7T_1

Investigations

X-ray Normal in soft lesions but in hard lesions it shows, narrowing of disc space, anterior and posterior osteophyte formation, and narrowing of IV foramen (Figs 29.9A and B).

Myelography It helps in localising the lesion but is invasive.

MRI This is useful, as it is non-invasive, and helps localise the lesion, but its high cost is prohibitive.

CT scan It is more useful in evaluating traumatic conditions of the neck than degenerative conditions.

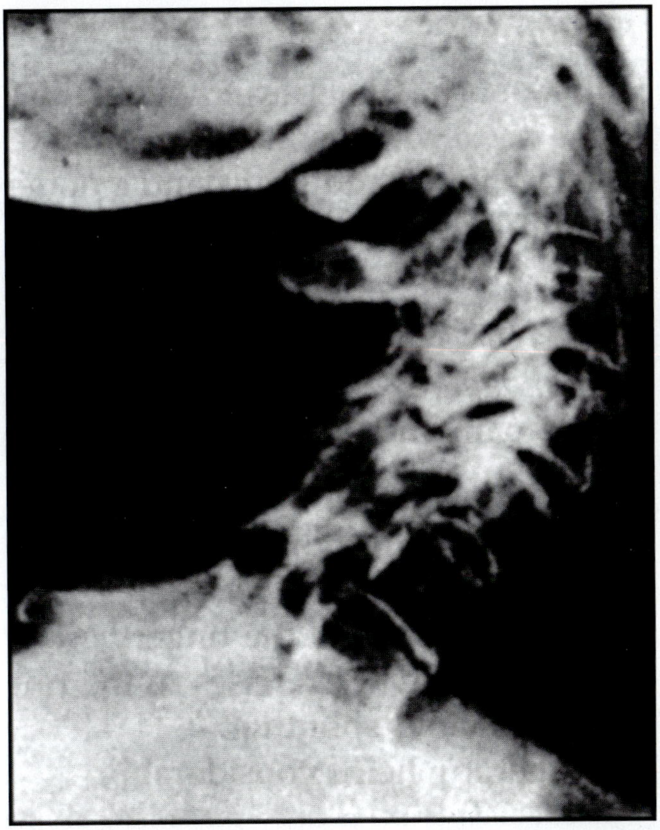

Fig. 29.9A: Radiograph showing cervical spine: Loss of intervertebral disc space and osteophyte formation seen in cervical spondylosis

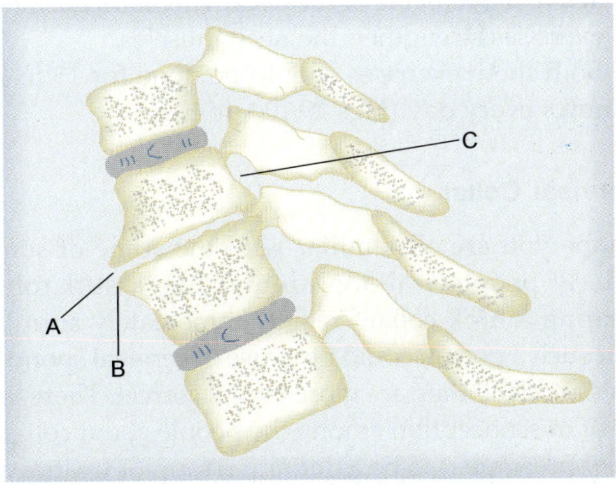

Fig. 29.9B: Pictorial display of a radiograph in cervical disc syndrome: (A) disc space narrowing, (B) osteophyte formation, and (C) narrowing of intervertebral foramina

EMG, discography, thermography are occasionally used.

Treatment

Conservative treatment is the more accepted form of treatment in cervical disc syndrome. It consists of rest which is the cornerstone of the treatment as it allows soft parts to heal by reducing the inflammation. Cervical traction could be continuous or intermittent depending on the severity of the symptoms. Traction helps by reducing the muscle spasm, increasing the disc space and reducing the tension on the nerve roots. Physiotherapy like short wave diathermy, ultrasound, infrared rays are useful. NSAIDs once a day are usually preferred. After the pain decreases, patients are encouraged to perform gradual graded isometric neck exercises.

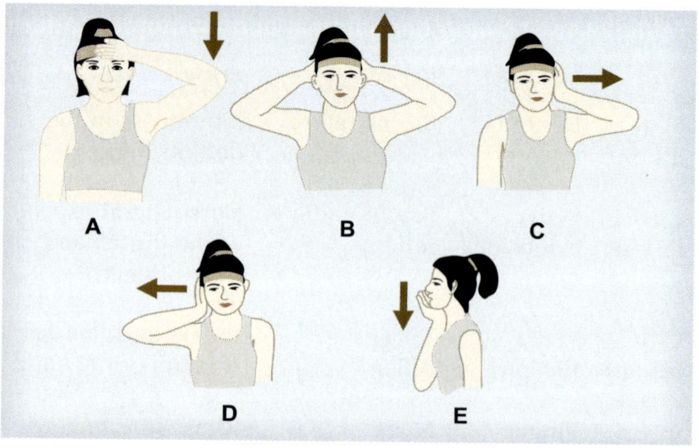

Figs 29.10A to E: Different self-resistive isometric neck exercises (A) Neck flexion, (B) Neck extension, (C) Lateral flexion (D) Neck rotation, (E) For neck flexion

Neck Exercises

Neck exercies aim to improve the mobility of the stiff neck and strengthen the weakened neck muscles. Hence, the following two sets of exercises are recommended:

1. *Mobilisation exercises* This consists of gradual active mobilisation of the neck by performing all the movements of the neck.
2. *Strengthening exercises* Here the patient is instructed to offer resistance by the other hand to all the active movements of the neck. This self-resistance exercises strengthen the neck muscles.

   Both these exercises should be done for 15 to 20 minutes every day (Figs 29.10A to E).

Cervical Collar

I hope you are all familiar with the scene of some elderly people walking around like a stiff robot wearing a neck collar. People immediately surmise that such a person could be a case of cervical spondylosis and well they are more or less correct. There is a lot of misconception among the people about collars. They presume it to be a definitive form of treatment, while it is only supportive (Fig. 29.11).

It is indicated during acute exacerbation of chronic spondylosis and should be worn only for a short duration. If used for long, it weakens the neck muscles, thereby nullfying the beneficial effects of neck exercises.

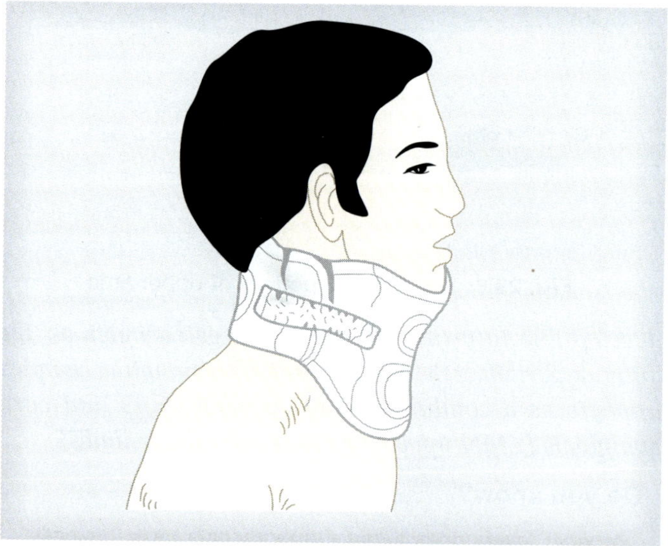

Fig. 29.11: Wearing a cervical collar is a popular method of treatment of cervical spondylosis

Did you know?
Cervical collar was discovered by HO Thomas.

Surgical treatment Less than 5 per cent of the cases of cervical spondylosis require surgery and is usually indicated in cases of chronic pain, failed conservative treatment and neurological deficits due to root or cord compressions.

The surgical procedure usually consists of removal of the cervical disc through an anterior approach and

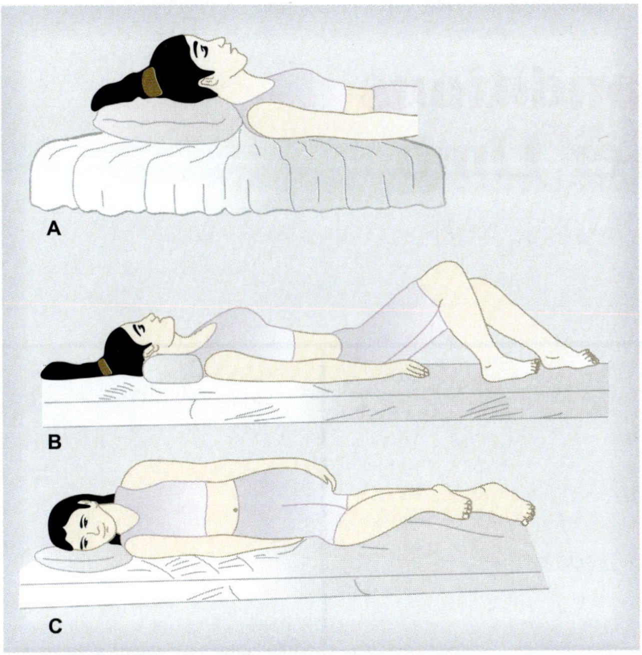

Figs 29.12A to C: (A) Improper neck posture during lying down. Correct neck posture: (B) During supine position, (C) During side-lying

cervical interbody fusion by placing an autologous iliac bone graft. Excision of large osteophytes can also be done through this route. Excision of one or two cervical bodies (corpectomy) may be justified in multiple level disc pathology. Laminectomy usually does not produce the desired results.

Quick facts

Surgical Treatment of Cervical Spondylosis

- Anterior cervical discectomy with interbody fusion for single or 2 level disc involvement.
- Corpectomy and strut graft or cages for multiple level disc involvement.
- Laminectomy has a doubtful role.
- Surgery is required in less than 5 per cent of cases.

Preventive Measures

This can be done by good postural habits and using proper sized pillows of 7.5 to 10 cm thickness and should be placed under the neck rather than the head (Figs 29.12A to C).

30 Regional Conditions of the Upper Limb

- Regional conditions of the shoulder
  - Frozen shoulder
  - Rotator cuff lesions
  - Rotator cuff tears
  - Deltoid contracture
- Regional conditions of the elbow
  - Tennis elbow
  - Golfer's elbow
  - Olecranon bursitis (Student's elbow)
- Regional conditions of the wrist and hand
  - de Quervain's disease
  - Trigger fingers and thumb
  - Ganglia
  - Dupuytren's contracture
  - Carpal tunnel syndrome
  - Compound palmar ganglion

REGIONAL CONDITIONS OF THE SHOULDER

FROZEN SHOULDER (SYN: PERIARTHRITIS, ADHESIVE CAPSULITIS)

Paradoxically shoulder joint privileged as the most mobile joint in the body has its nemesis because of this very advantage. Its mobility makes it very vulnerable to problems which ultimately "freezes" its movements. Unable to come to terms with the paucity of liberal movements hitherto enjoyed, the hapless patient resigns himself or herself to suffer the agony in silence!

It is defined as a clinical syndrome characterised by *painful restriction* (Figs 30.1A and B) *of both active and passive shoulder movements* due to causes within the shoulder joint or remote (other parts of the body).

History **Dupley** first described it in 1872 and called it as *humeroscapular periarthritis*. In 1934, **Codman** coined the term *Frozen shoulder*, and in 1945, **Neviaser** gave the name *adhesive capsulitis*.

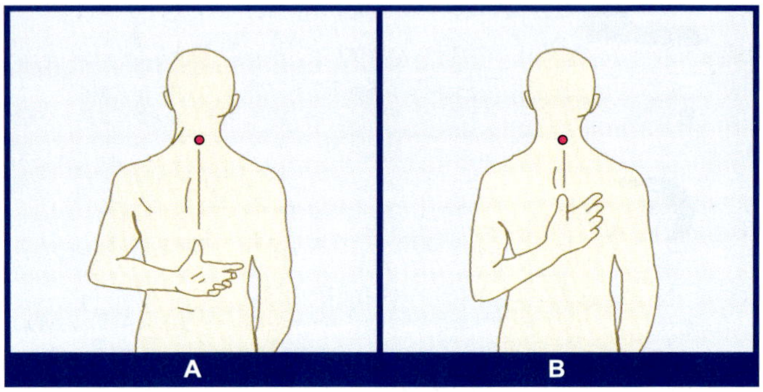

Figs 30.1A and B: Test to detect frozen shoulder (note the distance between the thumb): (A) Frozen shoulder, (B) Normal

Epidemiology of Frozen Shoulder

- Incidence in general population is 2%
- Incidence in diabetics is 10 to 35%
- More common in females than males
- Mean age is 40 to 60 years
- Bilateral 12%.

Causes

The causes for frozen shoulder could be:

I. ***Primary*** Here the exact cause is not known and it could be idiopathic.

II. ***Secondary*** According to **Lumberg,** the secondary causes could be:
   a. *Shoulder causes* Problems directly related to shoulder joint which can give rise to frozen shoulder are tendinitis of rotator cuff, bicipital tendinitis, fractures and dislocations around the shoulder, etc. (Figs 30.2A and B).
   b. *Nonshoulder causes* Problems not related to shoulder joint like diabetes, cardiovascular diseases with referred pain to the shoulder which keeps the joint immobile, reflex sympathetic dystrophy, frozen hand shoulder

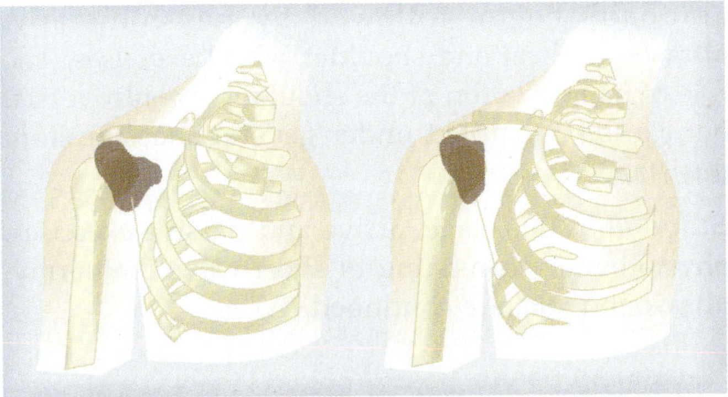

Figs 30.2A and B: Showing: (A) Normal capsular pattern, (B) Shrinkage of the capsule in frozen shoulder

syndrome, a complication of Colles' fracture can all lead to frozen shoulder. The reason could be prolonged immobilisation of the shoulder joint due to referred pain, etc.

Pathology

1. During abduction, and repeated overhead activities of the shoulder, long head of biceps, and rotator cuff undergo repeated strain. This results in inflammation, fibrosis and consequent thickening of the shoulder capsule which results in loss of movements. *If the movements are continued, then the fibrosis gradually breaks, movements return but never come back to normal.*
2. Prolonged activity causes small scapular and biceps muscles to waste faster, load on joint increases and degenerative changes sets in. Capsule is fibrosed and shoulder movements are decreased.

Clinical Features

A patient with frozen shoulder clinically presents as follows:

- Decreased range of both active and passive shoulder movements.
- The patient demonstrates a capsular pattern of movement restrictions (i.e. external rotation > abduction > internal rotation).
- Pain is noted at the end stage of stretch.
- Accessory joint play is reduced.
- Resistive tests are generally pain free in the available range of motion.

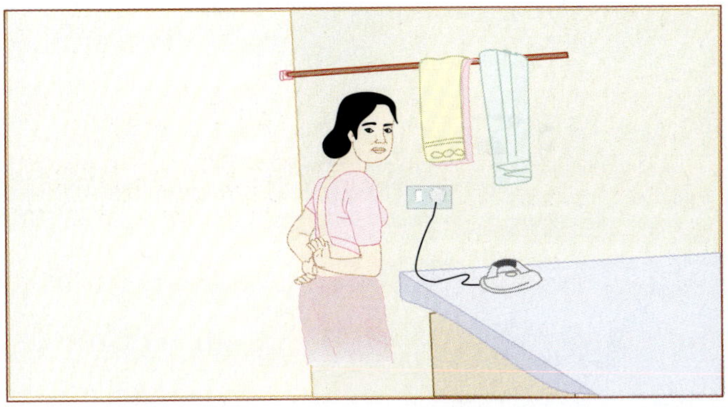

Fig. 30.3: A patient of frozen shoulder is unable to do the daily routine activities like these

- Patient is unable to do routine daily activities like combing the hair, in case of women wearing the buttons of their blouse, (Fig. 30.3), doing overhead activities, etc.

Facts you must know

Diagnosis of frozen shoulder is primarily by clinical examination which records capsular type of rectriction of both the active and passive range of motion of the shoulder.

Clinical Stages

There are three classical stages in frozen shoulder, according to **Reeves:**

Stage I *(stage of pain)* Patient complains of acute pain, decreased movements, external rotation greatest followed by loss of abduction and then forward flexion. *Internal rotation is least affected*. This stage lasts for 10 to 36 weeks.

Note: Pain in frozen shoulder does not radiate below the elbow (Fig. 30.4).

Stage II *(stage of stiffness)* In this stage, pain gradually decreases and the patient complains of stiff shoulder. Slight movements are present. This lasts for 4 to 12 months.

Stage III *(stage of recovery)* Patient will have no pain and movements would have recovered but will never be regained to normal. It lasts for 6 months to 2 years.

Radiology

X-ray of the shoulder is usually normal; but in a few cases, 'sclerosis' may be seen on the outer edge of greater tuberosity (***Golding's sign***) (Fig. 30.5).

Section 3

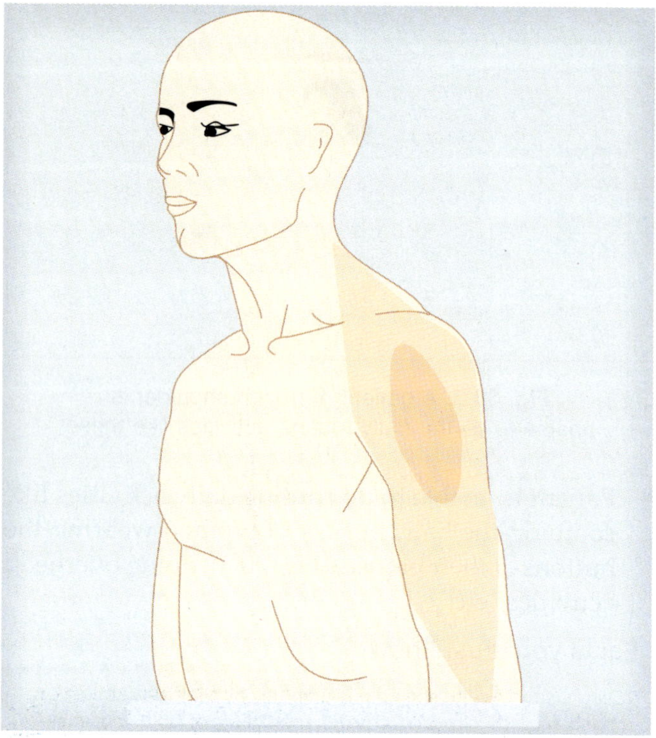

Fig. 30.4: Showing region of distribution of pain in frozen shoulder

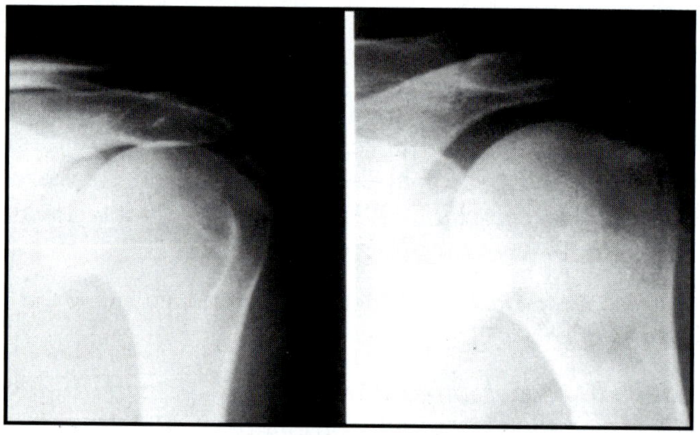

Fig. 30.5: Radiographs showing features of frozen shoulder

Treatment

Stage I In this stage, long-acting once a day NSAIDs are usually preferred as this condition usually runs a long course (10–36 weeks). Intra-articular steroids may help to provide transient relief of pain only.

Stage II In this stage, since the pain will have reduced considerably, exercises both active and passive are gradually begun followed by physiotherapy, ultrasound, heat and shoulder wheel exercises. The role of manipulation of the shoulder is controversial but can be attempted under general anaesthesia in this stage.

Stage III In this stage, active and passive exercises, physiotherapy consisting of short wave diathermy, ultrasound, etc. are continued.

Treatment pearls

- Exercises are most effective than modalities, drugs and steroid injection.
- Mobilisation techniques are the other effective method.
- Traditional manipulation under GA is a previous successful method.
- Traditional manipulation under GA is more successful than traction manipulation.
- Arthroscopic distension (Bruisement technique): This helps to increase ROM after several weeks or months.
- *Arthroscopic releases:* This is indicated in recalcitrant cases where the above measures have all failed.

ROTATOR CUFF LESIONS

This includes both rotator cuff tears and impingement syndrome.

Fine adjustments of the humeral head within the glenoid is achieved by coordinated activity of four interrelated muscles (Fig. 30.6) arising from the scapula and is called *rotator cuff.*

Note: Rotator cuff comprises supraspinatus, infraspinatus, subscapularis and teres minor (Mnemonic SITS).

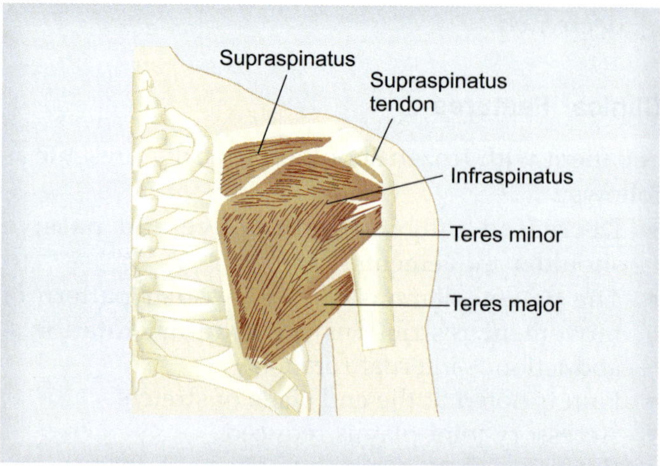

Fig. 30.6: Showing muscles of the rotator cuff

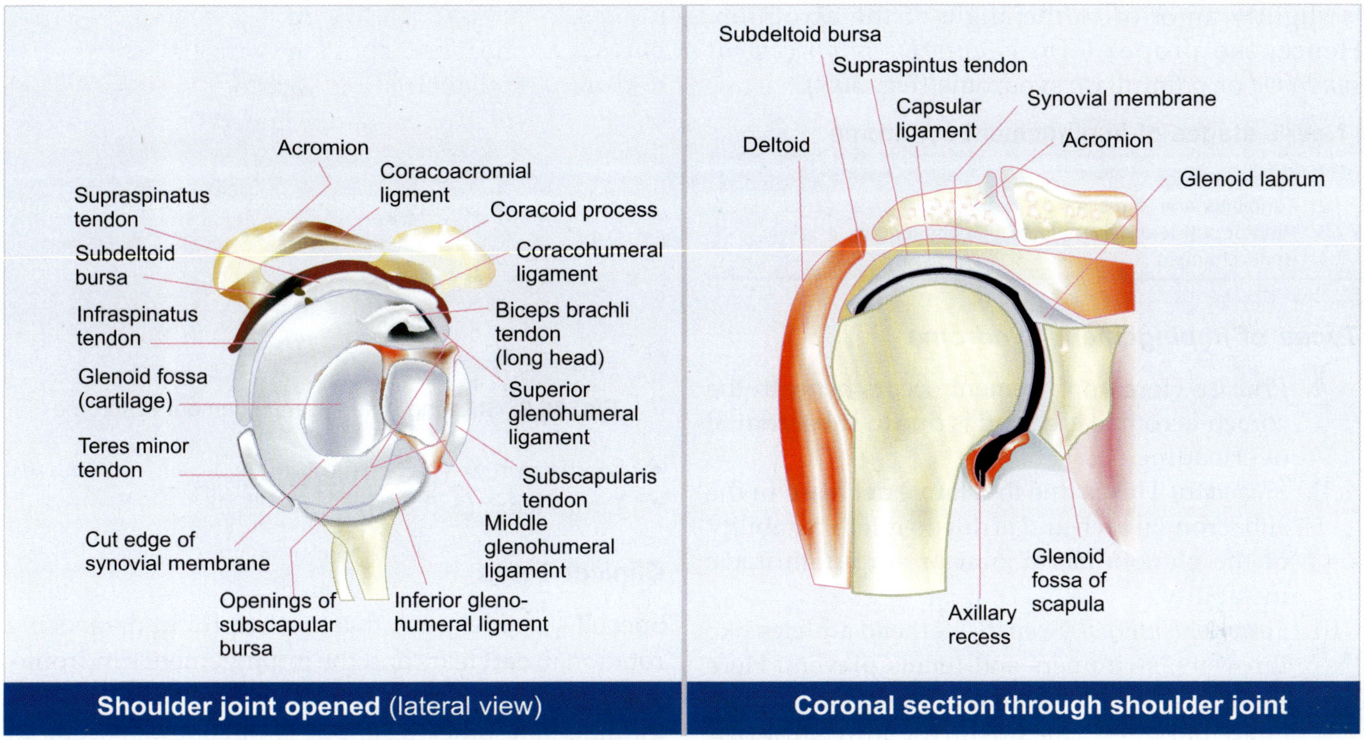

Figs 30.7A and B: Anatomy of the shoulder joint (internal structures)

Role of Rotator Cuffs

In the movement of abduction, supraspinatus steadies the head from above, infraspinatus depresses the head, subscapularis steadies the head in front paralleling the action of the infraspinatus. *This combined action allows the deltoid muscle to swing up the arm from a steady fulcrum irrespective of the position of the scapula* (Figs 30.7A and B).

Impingement Syndrome

It is a problem which is commonly associated with supraspinatus tendon. Other causes like bicipital tendinitis, and intraspinatus tendinitis, subacromial bursitis, etc. may give rise to rotator cuff problems, but they are not that common (see box).

Causes of impingement syndrome

- Complete or partial rupture of rotator cuff (Fig. 30.8)
- Supraspinatus tendinitis
- Calcific deposits
- Subacromial bursitis
- Subdeltoid bursitis
- Periarthritis
- Bicipital tenosynovitis
- Fracture greater trochanter

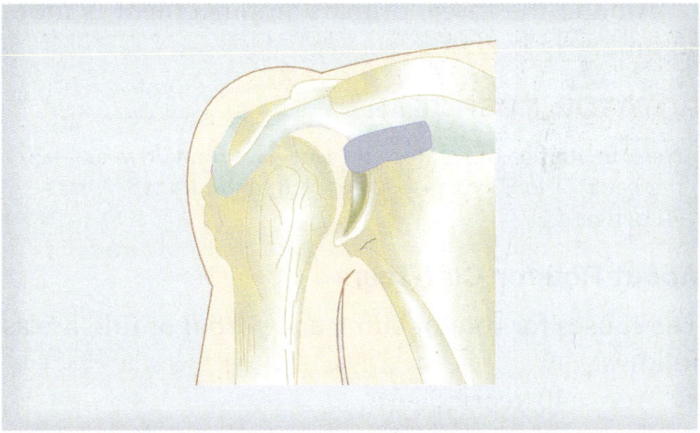

Fig. 30.8: Showing supraspinatus tear

Among the various causes mentioned above, supraspinatus tendinitis is the one that is commonly encountered and this gives rise to the *impingement syndrome.* Impingement occurs beneath the coraco-acromial arch. The most vulnerable structures for impingement between the undersurface of the acromion and the head of the humerus are the greater tuberosity, the overlying supraspinatus tendon and the long head of biceps. The major site of compression is slightly anterior to the angle of the acromion. Hence, the proper term is *anterior impingement syndrome* or painful arc syndrome (Fig. 30.9).

Neer's stages of impingement syndrome

1. Oedema stage
2. Tendinitis and fibrositis
3. Rotator cuff tear and rupture of biceps tendon
4. Bone changes

Types of Impingement Syndrome

I. *Primary* Here impingement occurs beneath the coraco-acromial arch and is due to subacromial overloading.

II. *Secondary* This is due to relative decrease in the subacromial arch and is due to microinstability of the glenohumeral joint or scapulothoracic instability.

III. *Posterior (Internal)* Seen in overhead athletes like throwers, swimmers and tennis players. Here the supra- and infraspinatus tendons are pinched between the posterior and superior aspects of the glenoid when the arm is in elevated and externally rotated position.

Among the three, primary impingement is more common.

ROTATOR CUFF TEARS

Note: Incidence of rotator cuff tear, less than 70 years—30 per cent; 71 to 80 years—60 per cent; more than 89 years—70 per cent.

About Rotator Cuff Tears

The causes for rotator cuff tears, partial or full, are as follows:

- Age > 40 years
- Occupations requiring repetitive and excessive overhead movements
- Overhead sports and athletes like throwers, swimmers, tennis players, etc.
- Degenerative etiology is the major cause
- Dislocation of shoulder joint in 40 to 60 years of age
- About 2/3rd cases are seen in male population.

Classification of Rotator Cuff Tears

(According to American Arthroscopic Orthopaedics)

- Small tear (< 1 cm)

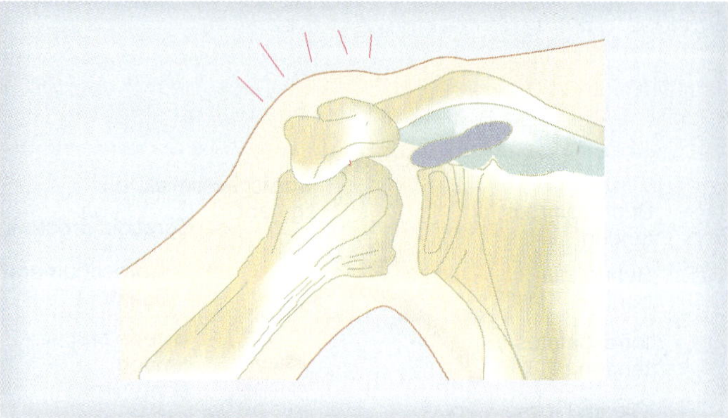

Fig. 30.9: Showing anterior impingement syndrome

- Medium tear (1–3 cm)
- Large tears (3–5 cm).

Clinical Tests

Special shoulder tests that are helpful in diagnosing rotational, cuff tears and the impingement syndrome, is the ***painful arc sign*** (It is 81% specific). There are innumerable other tests but is outside the scope of this book.

Interesting facts

Do you know the clinical facts leading to the diagnosis of RCL tear?

- Age > 40 years
- Previous history of minor trauma
- Degenerative changes on the X-rays (Figs 30.10A and B)
- Various clinical tests

How accurate are these tests?

There are 91% sensitive and 75% specific.

Pearl: Clinical tests are ***more*** accurate and cost effective than a battery of investigations in diagnosing an RCL.

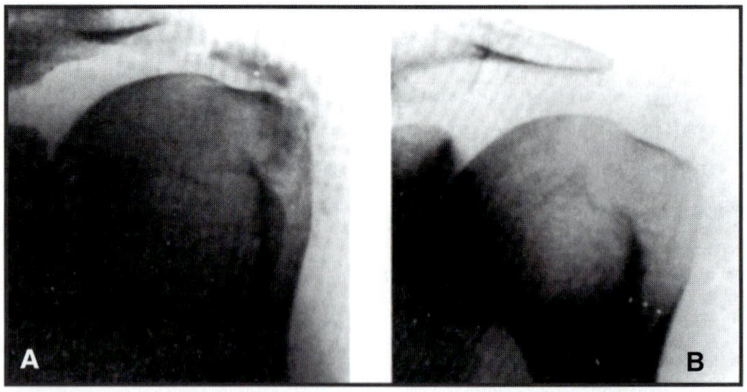

Figs 30.10A and B: Radiographs showing changes in the rotator cuff tears: (A) Calcific depositis, (B) Degenerative changes

Clinical Features

All patients with impingement syndrome have similar clinical features like pain, swelling, limitation of shoulder movements, muscle atrophy (supraspinatus and infraspinatus), tenderness over the greater tuberosity, etc. The following grades are described in anterior impingement syndrome.

Grade I This is common in young adults and athletes in the age group of 18 to 30 years. Due to overstress and repeated overhead activity, impingement occurs and supraspinatus is inflamed. The painful arc appears here (Fig. 30.11).

Grade II This is seen in age group of 40 to 45 years and may be due to supraspinatus tendinitis or subacromial bursitis. The cause could be either overuse or degeneration and osteophyte formation.

Grade III It is seen in patients over 45 years of age and may be due to occupational overuse, fall, sudden increase in activity, atrophic degenerative changes in the cuff and rarely due to acute tear of the rotator cuff.

Investigations to Diagnose Rotator Cuff Lesions

1. *X-rays of the shoulder* This helps to detect bony avulsions, spurs, calcific deposits, sclerotic areas, etc. (see box).

Mystifying facts about X-ray changes in Rotator Cuff Lesions

- ↓ Subarachnoid space ↓ 6 mm.
- Anterior spurring of ACM joint.
- Humeral head degeneration.
- Sclerotic inferior acromion (eyebrow sign).
- Hooking of the acromion.

2. *Arthrogram* Single contrast arthrogram is considered as the gold standard in diagnosing rotator cuff tears.
3. *Ultrasonography* This is highly reliable in diagnosing rotator cuff pathology with a sensitivity of 98 per cent.
4. *MRI* This is also very accurate (81%) but expensive.

Management

Conservative Treatment It consists of heat, massage, NSAIDs, local infiltration of hydrocortisone, subacromial steroid injections, exercises both active and passive, temporary immobilisation, etc. *Ninety per cent will recover with these measures.*

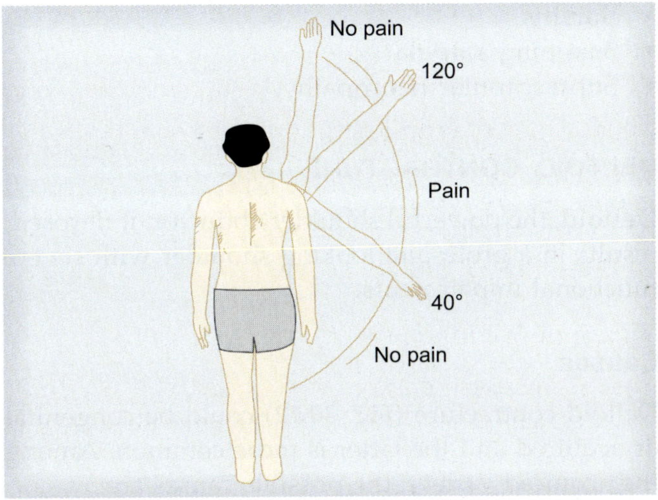

Fig. 30.11: Pain occurs in the impingement syndrome between 40 to 120° of shoulder abduction as it is in this position that the supraspinatus tendon is impinged against the undersurface of the acromion and head of the humerus. Rest of the movements are painless (painful are syndrome)

Surgical treatment

Indications Failure of conservative treatment for three months, if the patients are young and active, and if there is increasing loss of shoulder function, surgery is indicated.

Methods

a. Arthroscopic repair in small and partial tears.
b. Open methods in major tears.

Depending upon the aetiological factors, the following surgical techniques are described: excision of adhesions and manipulation of shoulder, excision of calcium deposits, repair of incomplete tear, acromioplasty, acromionectomy for more disabling pain with normal range of movements, direct suture for complete rupture of rotator cuff, rotation and transposition of flap, free graft, etc. Results are good in 85 to 90 per cent.

Differential Diagnosis of Impingement Syndrome

- Frozen shoulder
- Cervical spondylosis
- ACM and shoulder joint arthritis

- Bursitis
- Snapping scapula
- Suprascapular neuropathy.

DELTOID CONTRACTURE

Deltoid, the powerful shoulder abductor, if fibrosed, results in a grotesque looking shoulder with severe functional impairments.

Causes

Deltoid contracture (Fig. 30.12) could be congenital or acquired and the latter is more common. Among the acquired variety, the possible causes are:

1. Due to anatomical aberration of multiple intramuscular septae in the intermediate portions of the deltoid, repeated intramuscular injection into the deltoid results in fibrosis.
2. Chronic infection due to the injected drugs.
3. Pressure ischaemia.

Disturbing injection facts: The muscles commonly used for IM injections

- Deltoid muscle
- Triceps muscle
- Anterior abdominal muscles
- Gluteal muscles
- Quadriceps muscle

Among these, deltoid, gluteal and quadriceps are the commonly injected muscles. However, postinjection contractures are more common in quadriceps followed by deltoid.

Do you know?

The most common cause of muscle contracture in our country is PPRP (Post polio residual paralysis).

Interesting facts about postinjection muscular contractures (Indian contribution)

- Postinjection muscle contractures are not very common.
- Though reported all over the world, India is perhaps the leader.
- The credit of 'first reporting' in India belongs to Bhattacharya.
- The largest number reported is by TK Shanmugasundaram.
- No specific injectable has been incriminated but tetracycline was found to be the culprit in most number of cases by Shanmugasundaram.

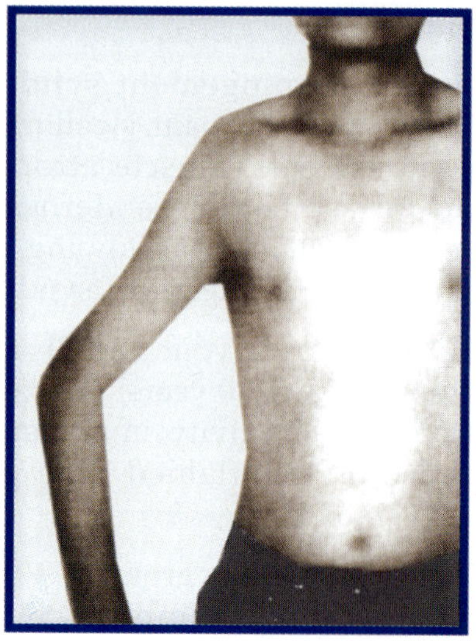

Fig. 30.12: Showing features suggestive of deltoid contracture

Clinical Presentations

A patient with deltoid contracture typically presents as follows:

- Inability to keep the arm in contact with the chest in the anatomical plane of the scapula.
- When the arm is forcibly brought into contact with the chest, winging of the scapula happens.
- Dimple or puckering of the skin over the deltoid may or may not be seen.
- On palpation, a thick intermediate fibrotic deltoid muscle can be felt.
- Shoulder function is not severely affected.

If the above clinical findings are supported by a strong history of repeated IM injections into the deltoid muscle, the diagnosis is more or less certain.

Mystifying facts

Beware of the diagnostic pitfalls:

- Neglected ADS (Anterior dislocation of shoulder)
- Serratus anterior palsy
- Old injury to the proximal humeral epiphysis
- Poliomyelitis

Treatment

Prevention

This is better than the best of curative measures and consists of avoiding unnecessary and indiscriminate deltoid IM injections.

Curative

Surgical release of the fibrotic bands by closed fasciotomy technique of Shanmugasundaram gives excellent results.

Rehabilitation

To facilitate faster recovery of shoulder function and to correct winging of the scapula, repeated stretching and straightening exercises are recommended.

REGIONAL CONDITIONS OF THE ELBOW

TENNIS ELBOW

I am sure every one is fascinated by tennis. We may not get a place under the sun with Steffi Graff, Monica Seles, Boris Becker, Sania Mirza and others, but certainly we may get an appointment with an orthopaedic surgeon for a problem common in them, that too without playing tennis! Yes, the obvious reference is towards *tennis elbow*.

Note: Sachin Tendulkar should be credited for popularising and creating lots of awareness and controversies about tennis elbow at least in our country!

History

It was first described from the *Writer's cramps* by Range in 1873. It was Madris who called it as "tennis elbow" shortly thereafter.

Definition

Tennis elbow syndrome encompasses lateral, medial and posterior elbow symptoms. The one commonly encountered is the lateral tennis elbow which is known as the ***classical tennis elbow*** and is the *pain and tenderness on the lateral side of the elbow*, some well defined and some vague, that results from repetitive stress.

Tennis Elbow

Classical tennis elbow
- It is the lateral tennis elbow

Other varieties
- Medial tennis elbow *(golfer's elbow)*
- Posterior tennis elbow around the margins of the olecranon process

Vital points

Location of pain in tennis elbow
- Lateral epicondyle (75%)
- Lateral muscle mass (17%)
- Medial epicondyle (10%)
- Posterior (8%)

Lateral Tennis Elbow

It is a lesion affecting the tendinous origin of common wrist extensors (Fig. 30.13). It is more common in men than women and is believed to be a degenerative disorder.

Causes

1. *Epicondylitis* This is due to single or multiple tears in the common extensor origin, periostitis, angiofibroblastic proliferation of extensor carpi radialis brevis (ECRB), etc.
2. *Inflammation of adventitious bursa* between the common extensor origin and radiohumeral joint.
3. *Calcified deposits* within the common extensor tendon.
4. *Painful annular ligament* is due to hypertrophy of synovial fringe between the radial head and the capitulum.
5. *Pain of neurological origin,* e.g. cervical spine affection, radial nerve entrapment, etc.

Mystifying fact

- ECRB is the most commonly involved structure in lateral epicondylitis

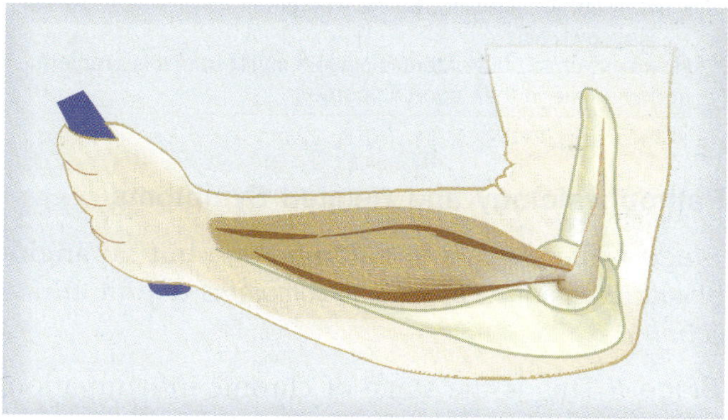

Fig. 30.13: Repetitive stress at common extensor origin in tennis players

Seen in

- All levels of tennis players.
- In world class players "SERVE" appears to be the cause.
- In less than world class players "backhand stroke".
- Seen in other sports also.
- May be occupational, etc.
- More common in the dominated arm.

Causes in tennis players More than one-third tennis players all over the world are affected with this problem over 35 years of age.

- Novice
- Playing several games per week
- > 35 years of age
- Equal sex incidence
- Backhand stroke (38%)
- Serve (25%)
- Forehand stroke (23%)
- Backhand volley (7%)
- Overhead smash (4%)
- Forehand volley (3%)

Contributing factors

- Little playing experience.
- Consistent missing of "*sweet spot*" while hitting.
- Poor stroke techniques: use of arm instead of body.
- Poor power or flexibility.
- Heavy stiff racket, large handle size, too tight racket stringing.
- Heavy duty wet balls.
- Playing surface—balls bounce quicker off the cement court.

Did you know?

Though called tennis elbow, it is more common in non-tennis players (95%). Causes can be:

- Throwing sports
- Swimming
- Carpentry, plumbing, textile workers
- Housewives

However, up to 50% of tennis players suffer from this problem at some time in their sporting career.

Pathophysiology and Related Symptoms

Stage I There is acute inflammation but no angioblastic invasion. *The patient complains of pain during activity.*

Stage II This is the stage of chronic inflammation. There is some angioblastic invasion. *The patient complains of pain both during activity and at rest.*

Stage III Chronic inflammation with extensive angioblastic invasion. *The patient complains pain at rest, night pains, and pain during daily activities.*

Clinical Tests

1. Local tenderness on the outside of the elbow at the common extensor origin with aching pain in the back of the forearm (Fig. 30.14).
2. *Cozen's test:* Painful resisted extension of the wrist with elbow in full extension elicits pain at the lateral elbow (Fig. 30.15).
3. Elbow held in extension, passive wrist flexion and pronation produces pain.
4. *Maudsley's test:* Resisted extension of the middle finger (Remember the letter 'M') elicits pain at the lateral epicondyle due to disease in the extensor digitorum communis.

Radiograph for Tennis Elbow

The AP, lateral and radiocapitellar views are the recommended views. In most cases it is normal. However, in 16 per cent of the cases, a faint

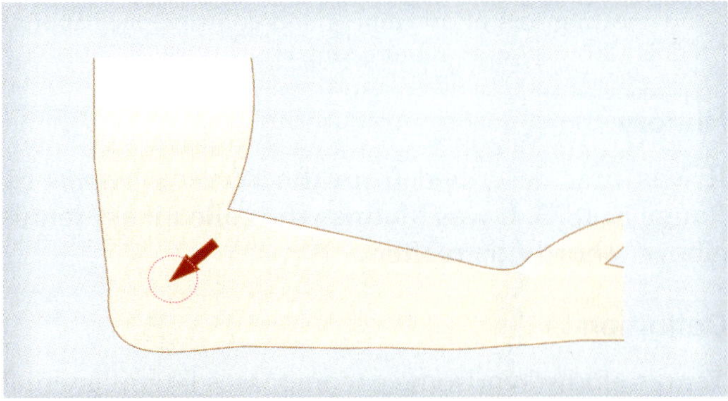

Fig. 30.14: Arrow showing site of tenderness in tennis elbow

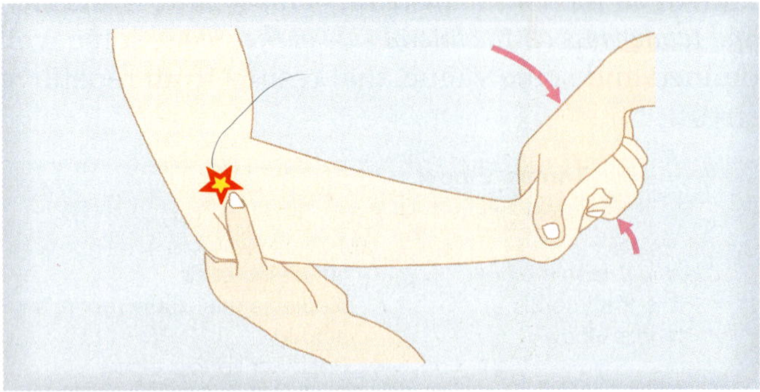

Fig. 30.15: Method of performing the Cozen's test

calcification along the lateral epicondyle can be detected.

Treatment

Conservative Management

It consists of rest and physiotherapy. In tennis players exercises, light racket, smaller grip, elbow strap, etc. are helpful (Fig. 30.16). Injection of local anaesthetic and steroid are useful in 40 per cent of cases.

Mill's Manoeuvre

This is the final option before surgery. About 10 per cent of the cases do not respond to conservative treatment. In them, a forceful extension of a fully flexed and pronated forearm after injection may be attempted.

Surgical Management

Indications

- Severe pain for 6 weeks at least.
- Marked and localised tenderness over lateral epicondyle.
- Failure to respond to restricted activity or immobilisation for at least 2 weeks.

Surgical Methods

1. Percutaneous release of epicondylar muscles.
2. Bosworth technique of excision of the proximal portion of the annular ligament, release of the origin of the extensor muscles, excision of the bursa and excision of synovial fringes.

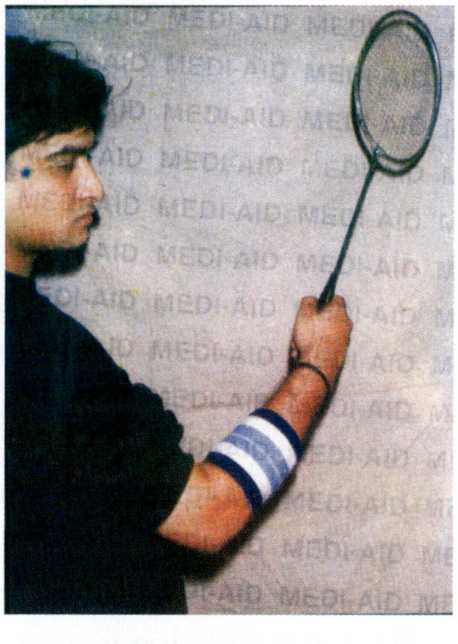

Fig. 30.16: Showing the elbow supports to be used in tennis elbow

What is new in the treatment of Tennis and Golfer's Elbow?

- *The use of extracorporeal shock wave therapy (ESWT):* About 2,000 shock waves of 0.04 to 0.12 nj/mm^2, three times at monthly intervals for 6 months is found to be effective in cases with failed conservative treatment for at least 6 months.
- *Arthroscopic release:* Of ECRB with failed conservative treatment for nearly 6 months. It is minimally invasive and helps in early rehabilitation.
- *Autologous blood injections:* In refractory cases, injections of 2 ml of autologous blood and 0.5% bupivicaine has been tried with good success in some centres.
- *Counterforce bracing (called the tennis elbow or forearm band):* These forces release the forces in the ECRB region.
- *Rehabilitative exercises:* These are wrist flexion, extension, forearm supination and pronation, wrist radial and ulnar deviations at 3 sets of ten repetitions everyday for 2 to 6 months is known to give good results.
- *Ultrasound-guided percutaneous needle therapy:* This consists of ultrasound-guided corticosteroid injection and needle debridement of the structures around lateral epicondyle.

Indications: In small tears, not responding to conservative therapy and if too small for surgery.

Advantages

- Minimally invasive procedure
- Restoration of function is rapid
- The option of surgery is still open.

In experts hands, it has a success rate of 65%.

Quick facts

Significant relief of symptoms in tennis elbow

• Changing tennis strokes	92 per cent
• Stretching exercises	84 per cent
• Use of splints	83 per cent
• NSAIDs/steroid	85 per cent
• Physiotherapy	50-75 per cent
• Rest more than 1 month	72 per cent

GOLFER'S ELBOW (SYN: EPITROCHLEITIS, MEDIAL TENNIS ELBOW)

Did you know?

Golfer's elbow is also called Swimmer's elbow.

Definition

It is a tendinopathy of the insertion of the epitrochlear muscles [flexors of the fingers of the hand flexor carpi radialis (FCR) and pronators].

Epitrochleitis is very similar to lateral epicondylitis (tennis elbow) but occurs on the medial side of the elbow, where the pronator teres and the flexors of the wrist and fingers originate. Tensing of these muscles by resisted wrist and finger flexion in pronation will provoke the pain (Fig. 30.17).

Tenderness is often less well localised than in tennis elbow.

Do you know?

Tennis elbow is nine times more comon than golfer's elbow.

Treatment

It is the same as for tennis elbow, but the treatment is even less satisfactory.

Lesser known but interesting elbow conditions:

You know about tennis and golfer's elbow, but do you know about:

1. *Boxer's Elbow:* This is also called as hyperextension overload syndrome or olecranon impingement syndrome and is due to the repetitive valgus hyperextension by a boxer during jabbing.
2. *Little Leagues Elbow:* This is a medial epicondyle avulsion fracture. It is seen commonly in children and adolescents involved in throwing sports.

OLECRANON BURSITIS (STUDENT'S ELBOW)

(Sign: Miner's elbow or Draughtsman elbow)

This is a chronic inflammation of the olecranon bursa. It may be the result of repetitive minor injuries or irritation, microcrystalline deposition. Infection occurs due to chronic friction as in students who tend to keep their elbows repeatedly over the table, bench, etc. over long periods during writing, reading, etc. (Fig. 30.18).

Clinical Features

It usually manifests as a swelling over the tip of the olecranon (Fig. 30.19). There may be pain, if there is inflammation. Inspection or palpation usually easily detects it (Fig. 30.20).

Investigations

Aspiration and culture of the bursal fluid is necessary in order to exclude the possibility of an infectious aetiology.

Treatment

Treatment is essentially conservative and consists of NSAIDs, local steroids, etc. Surgical excision is done in chronic cases. Microcrystalline-induced bursitis has a good prognosis and the symptoms usually resolve after a few days, whether treated or not. But bursitis due to repeated minor irritation is more difficult to treat.

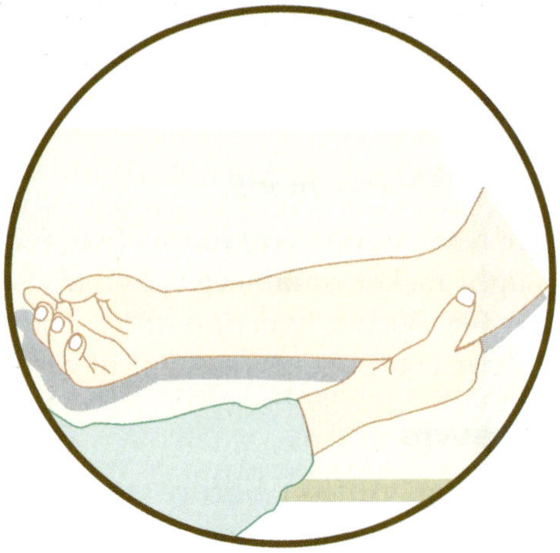

Fig. 30.17: Method of eliciting tenderness in Golfer's elbow

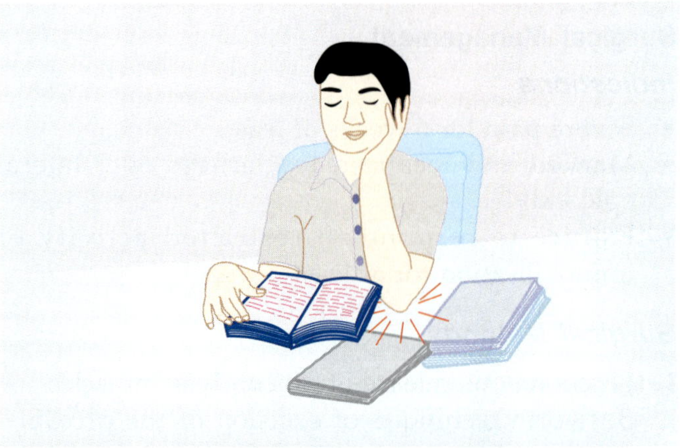

Fig. 30.18: Are you guilty of reading like this? Well you could develop student's elbow!

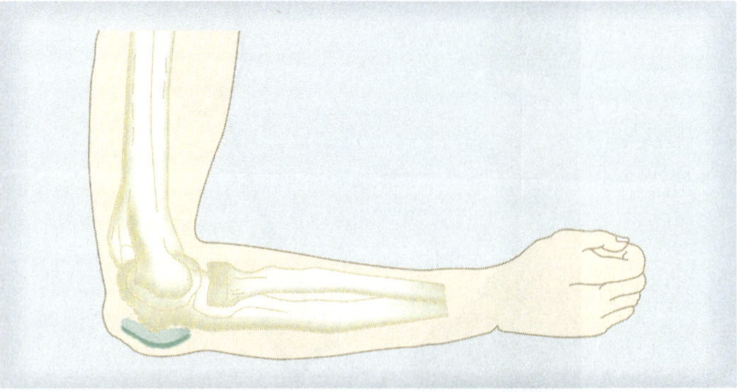

Fig. 30.19: Showing the olecranon bursa

Section 3

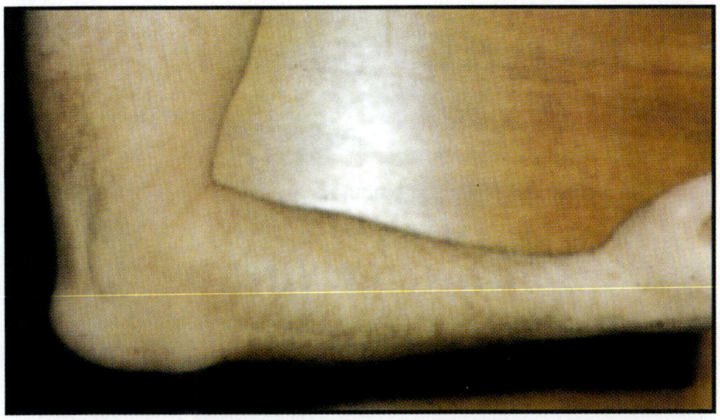

Fig. 30.20: Clinical picture of olecranon bursitis

REGIONAL CONDITIONS OF THE WRIST AND HAND

DE QUERVAIN'S DISEASE

It is also called as stenosing tenosynovitis of the first dorsal compartment of the wrist involving the abductor pollicis longus and extensor pollicis brevis tendons.

Aetiology

Exact cause is not known. [1]de Quervain's disease is commonly seen in women between 30 and 50 years of age, and may be due to repeated overuse of the wrist (Fig. 30.21). Trigger finger is common in conditions like rheumatoid arthritis.

Clinical Features

Pain and limitation of the movements of the involved tendons are the presenting features. In this, the common sheath of abductor pollicis longus and extensor pollicis brevis tendons at the wrist are involved. Tenderness can be elicited by sudden ulnar deviation of the flexed hand [Finkelstein's test—with the thumb tucked inside the palm (Fig. 30.22)].

Pitfalls

Do you know that Finkelstein's test is not pathognomonic of de Quervain's disease. It is also positive in:

- First carpomatacarpal arthritis.
- Warrenberg's syndrome
- Arthritis of radiocarpal and intercarpal joints

Interesting facts

Do you know about Intersection syndrome? Well, it is tenosynovitis of the II dorsal compartment.

Treatment

Conservative methods This treatment consists of rest, NSAIDs, local infiltration of hydrocortisone, wrist immobilisation, etc.

Surgery Division of the appropriate retinaculum if the above measures fail.

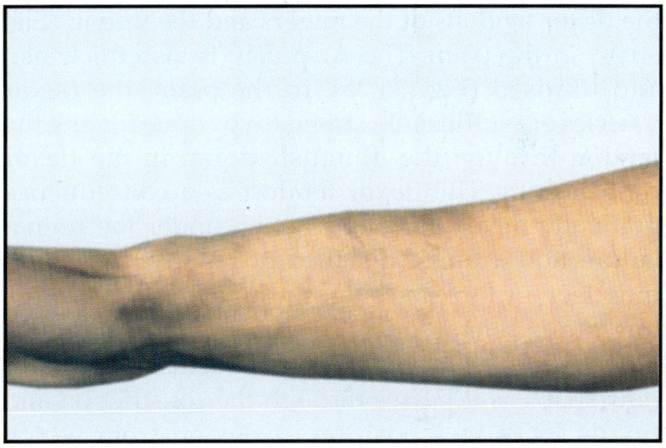

Fig. 30.21: Clinical photograph of de Quervain's disease

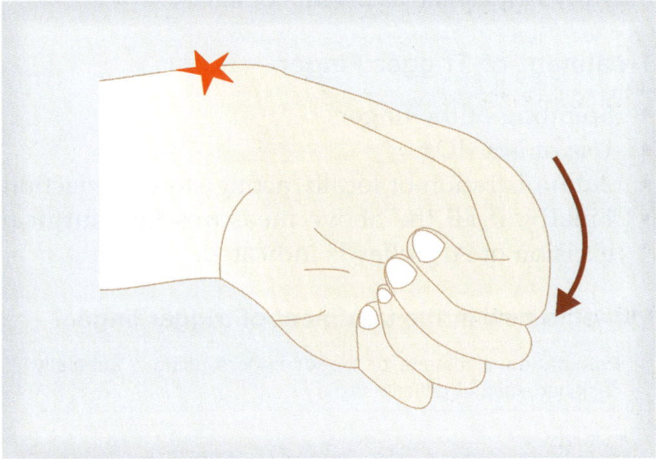

Fig. 30.22: Showing Finkelstein's test

[1]**Fritz de Quervain** (1968-1940) Switzerland. Described the condition in 1940.

Mystifying facts

Do you know the reasons for failure of conservative treatment in de Quervain's disease?

- Anomalous tendons
- Multiple slips of abductor pollicis longus tendon
- Multiple subcompartments within the first wrist compartment. This is seen in 75% of the cases.

TRIGGER FINGERS AND THUMB

It is a stenosing tenovaginitis, in which the sheath of a flexor tendon thickens, apparently spontaneously, so as to entrap the tendon.

It is locking of the finger in a position of flexion, (Figs 30.23A and B) that occurs at the retinaculae of the flexor tendons of the fingers and the thumb (Fig. 30.24) in the palm. The A_1 pulley is also thickened and fibrosed (Fig. 30.25). In the palm, the flexor muscles are sufficiently strong to continue forcing the tendon through the diminished gap in the flexor retinaculum. The flexor tendon as a consequence gradually develops a constriction under the retinaculum and a bulge distal to it. Finally, the flexor muscles may force the bulge through the retinaculum, but the extensor muscles may be insufficiently powerful to extend the finger hereafter. The finger now snaps as it passes through the constriction and finally locks in a position of flexion from which attempts to passively extend the fingers are painful (Fig. 30.26). These are common in women. Congenital trigger fingers are seen in 25 per cent of cases and may present as late as 2 years of age.

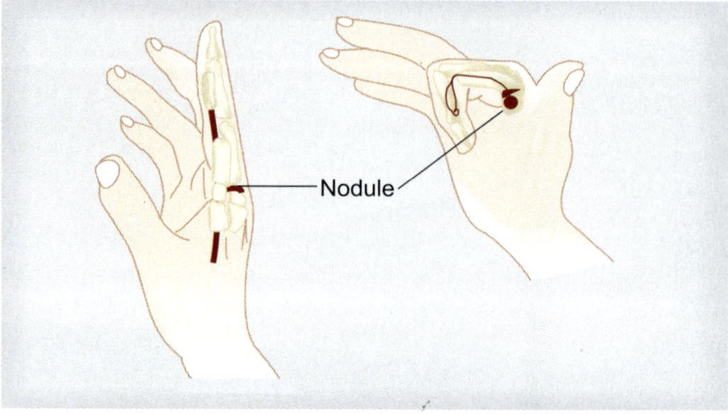

Figs 30.23A and B: Showing trigger finger

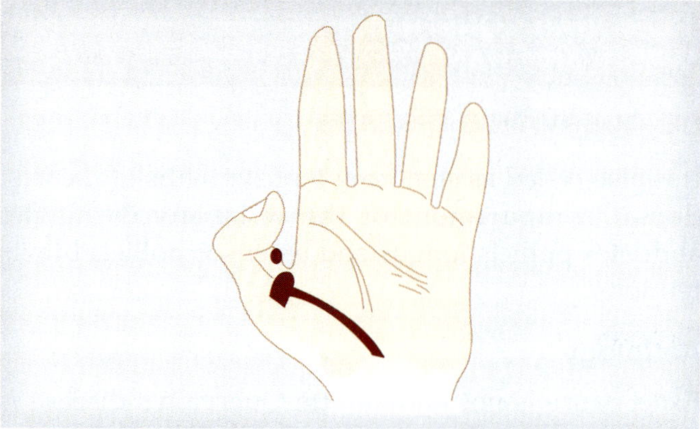

Fig. 30.24: Showing trigger thumb

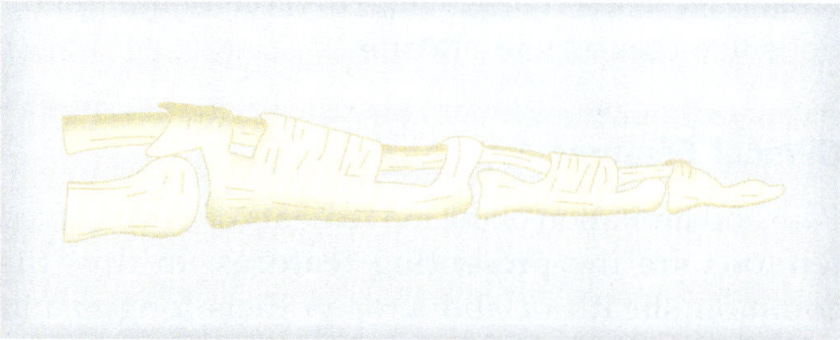

Fig. 30.25: Showing the flexor retinaculae (pulleys) of the finger which may be responsible for trigger fingers

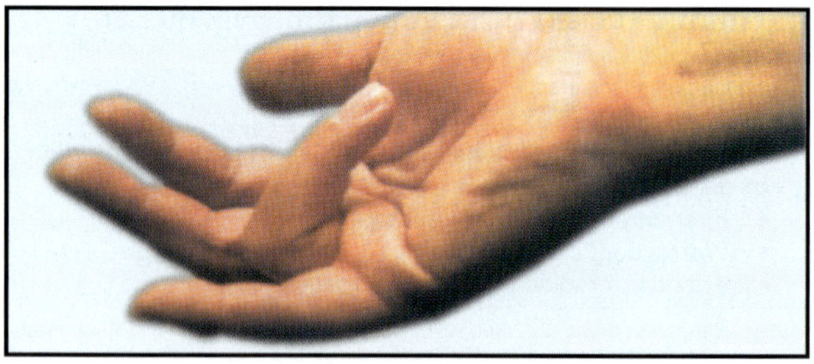

Fig. 30.26: Clinical photograph of a trigger finger

Treatment of Trigger Finger

- Splinting of the fingers
- Use of NSAIDs
- Administration of locally acting steroid injection
- Finally, if all the above measures fail, surgical excision of A_1 pulley is indicated.

What is new in the treatment of trigger finger?

Percutaneous release of trigger fingers using a specially designed knife in difficult cases.

GANGLIA (ALSO CALLED GANGLION CYST)

The term *'Ganglia'* is derived from a Greek term meaning *'Cystic tumour'*.

Definition

It is defined as a localised, tense, painless, cystic, swelling, containing clear gelatinous fluid (Fig. 30.27A). It accounts for 50 to 70 per cent of all soft tissue tumours of the hand and wrist.

Origin The clear gelatinous fluid may be due to leakage or subsequent fibrous encapsulation of synovial fluid through the capsule of a joint or a tendon sheath (Fig. 30.27B).

Sites It is commonly seen over dorsum of the wrist, flexor aspects of the fingers and dorsum of the foot.

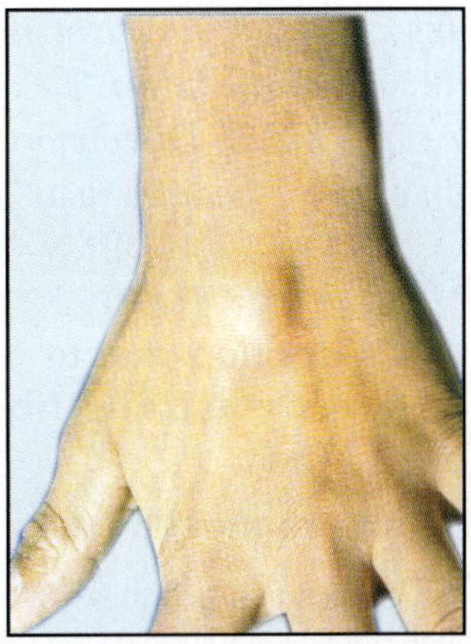

Fig. 30.27A: Clinical photograph showing a ganglion

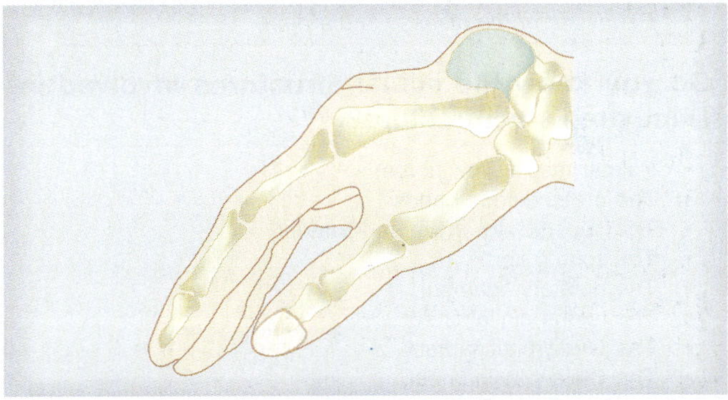

Fig. 30.27B: Showing origin of a ganglion

Quick facts: ganglion

- Dorsal wrist ganglia accounts for 60 to 70 per cent of all hand ganglia. It arises from scapholunate ligament.
- Volar ganglion—18 to 20 per cent.
- Ganglion at the flexor tendon.
- Sheath at A_1 pulley—10 to 12 per cent.

Predisposing factors Chronic repetitive stress and sometimes injury. It is more prevalent in women (M: F = 1:3).

Treatment

It may resolve spontaneously over a period of time. Excision is indicated if it is causing symptoms.

Biblical facts

What role the Holy Bible has in orthopaedics? Well in ancient days it was used to bang the ganglion into submission!

What is new?

Treatment of Ganglia: Arthroscopic release of the dorsal wrist ganglia is a sensible option than open excision for the following advantages:

- Minimal scarring
- Safe
- Faster rehabilitation
- Early mobility

Did you know?

In some dorsal wrist ganglia is usually due to capsular abnormality in the region of interosseous scapholunate ligament

DUPUYTREN'S CONTRACTURE

[2]Dupuytren's contracture is defined as a proliferative fibroplasia of the subcutaneous palmar tissue, forming nodules of cords along its ulnar border. *This fibroplasia results in finger contractures, thinning of subcutaneous fat, adhesions of skin to the lesion, pitting of skin, and knuckle pads on the dorsum of proximal interphalangeal (PIP) joints.*

The following lesions may be associated with Dupuytren's, lesions in medial plantar fascia in 5 per cent and plastic induration of penis (3%).

Causes

Exact cause is not known but may be due to:

- Heredity
- Trauma of chronic repetitive in nature.
- Occupational, seen in people employed in rock drilling due to the vibrations of the machine.
- Males—10 times more common in males.
- Whites are affected more than Blacks.
- Frequent and severe in epileptics and alcoholics (42%).
- Onset is usually less than 40 years of age.

[2]**Baron Guillaume Dupuytren** of France (1817). His other contributions: (1) Described neurological manifestation of spina bifida occulta. (2) Subungual exostosis. (3) Callus and its formation. (4) Upward and outward dislocation of foot.

Usually begins with ring finger at the distal palmar crease and later involves little finger. Flexion of MCP and PIP joints occur (Fig. 30.28). Discomfort is rare, itching or occasional pain over the nodules may be present.

Pathogenesis

Nodules and cords develop due to fibroplasia and hypertrophy of already existing fibres of palmar fascia on its ulnar border.

Prognosis: Poor prognostic facts

- *Hereditary* In patients with family history the lesion progresses fast. Hence heredity is a poor prognostic factor.
- *Sex* In women it begins late and progresses slow.
- *Alcoholics or epileptics* Severe, rapid and recurs.
- *Bilateral.*
- *Behaviour of the disease in the past.*

Do you know the actual structures involved in Dupuytren's contracture?

- Palmar fascial (few fibres).
- The pretendinous bands.
- The superficial transverse ligament.
- The spiral band.
- The natatory ligament.
- The lateral digital sheet.
- The Grasym's ligament.
- The Cleland's ligament.

Treatment

Observation consists of no treatment with observation being done at every three months interval.

Radiotherapy is given only during early fibroblastic phase.

Surgery It is the best known treatment and is delayed until actual contractures develop.

Procedures chosen It depends upon the degree of contractures, age, occupation, status of the palmar skin, presence or absence of arthritis of the finger joints, etc. More severe the involvement, more extensive is the surgery.

Surgical Methods

Subcutaneous fasciotomy This is preferred in elderly, arthritis patients and if the general condition is poor. Results are good when lesion is mature than diffuse. It may be used as a preliminary step to fasciectomy. This procedure has a 72 per cent recurrence rate.

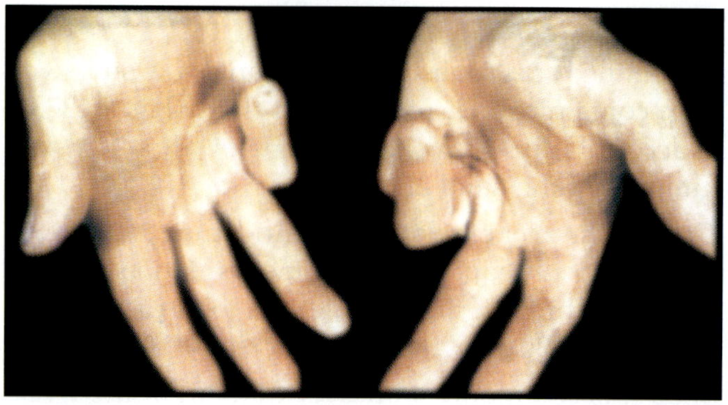

Fig. 30.28: Showing contractures of MCP and PIP joints of ring and little fingers in Dupuytren's disease

Partial selective fasciectomy This is indicated only when the ulnar two fingers are involved. This is a commonly done procedure, morbidity is less and is associated with less complications. Recurrence rate is 50 per cent, needs another surgery in 15 per cent of the cases.

Complete fasciectomy This is rarely done and is associated with haematoma, joint stiffness, delayed healing and recurrence.

Fasciectomy with skin grafting This is done in young people with epilepsy, alcoholism, and in cases of recurrence after excision.

Amputation may be considered if flexion contractures of PIP joint are very severe.

Resection and arthrodesis is indicated for severe contractures of the PIP joint. This is better than amputation as it prevents amputation neuroma.

CARPAL TUNNEL SYNDROME

Carpal tunnel syndrome was first described by [3]Sir James Paget in 1854, but the term was coined by Moerisch.

Anatomy

The carpal tunnel is bounded by bones on three sides and a ligament on one side (Fig. 30.29). The floor is

[3]**Sir James Paget**, London (1814-1899). His other contributions: (a) Paget's disease, (b) Apophysitis of tibial tubercle.

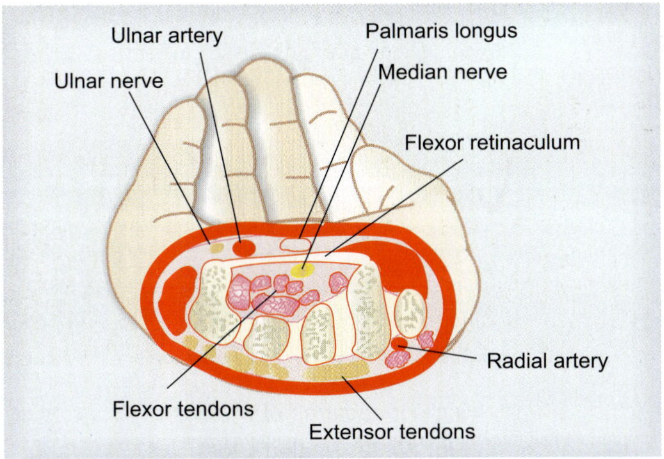

Fig. 30.29: Anatomy of the carpal tunnel

an osseous arch formed by the carpal bones and the roof is formed by the transverse carpal ligament.

Contents

Tendons of flexor digitorum superficialis and profundus in a common sheath, tendon of flexor pollicis longus in an independent sheath and the median nerve (Fig. 30.30).

Synovitis of the above tendons can generate pressure on the nerve.

> Know that 9 tendons and 1 nerve pass through the carpal tunnel.

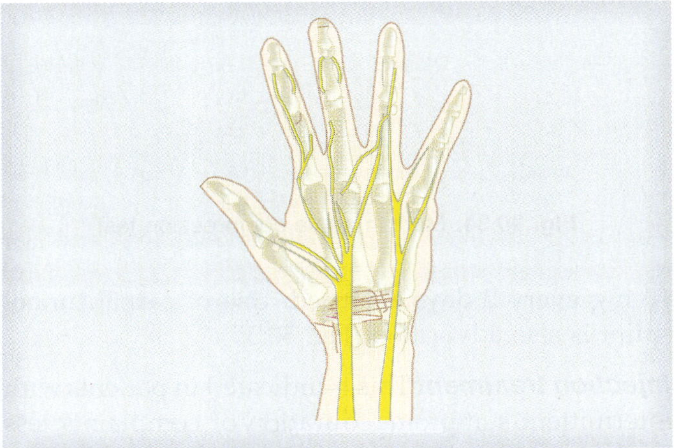

Fig. 30.30: Median nerve coursing through the carpal tunnel

Causes

General

1. Inflammatory—e.g. rheumatoid arthritis.
2. Endocrine—hypothyroidism, diabetes mellitus, menopause, pregnancy, etc. are some of the important endocrine causes.
3. Metabolic cause—gout.

Local These cause crowding of the space. Malunited Colles' fracture, ganglion in the carpal region, osteoarthritis of the carpal bones, and wrist contusion, haematoma, etc. are some of the important local causes.

> **Remember**
> Mnemonic PRAGMATIC for causes of carpal tunnel syndrome [(*P*—Pregnancy, *R*—Rheumatoid arthritis, *A*—Arthritis degenerative, *G*—Growth hormone abnormalities (acromegaly), *M*—Metabolic (gout, diabetes myxoedema, etc.), *A—Alcoholism, T*—Tumours, *I*—Idiopathic, *C*—Connective tissue disorders (e.g. amyloidosis)].

Clinical Stages or Features (Fig. 30.31)

Stage I In this stage, pain is usually the presenting complaint and the patient complains of characteristic discomfort in the hand, but there is no precise localisation to the median nerve. There may be history of morning stiffness in the hand.

Stage II In this stage, symptoms of tingling and numbness, pain, paraesthesia, etc. are localised to areas supplied by the median nerve.

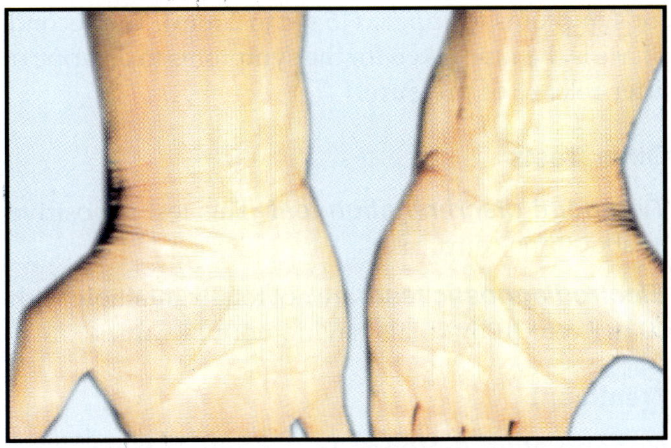

Fig. 30.31: Clinical photograph of bilateral carpal tunnel syndrome

Stage III Here, the patient complains of clumsiness in the hand and impairment of digital functions, etc.

Stage IV In this stage, sensory loss in the median nerve distribution area can be elicited and there is obvious wasting of the thenar eminence.

Clinical Tests

These are provocative tests and act as important screening methods and as an adjunct to the electrophysiologic testing.

Wrist flexion (Phalen's test) The patient is asked to actively place the wrist in complete but unforced flexion. If tingling and numbness are produced in the median nerve distribution of the hand within 60 seconds, the test is positive. It is the most sensitive provocative test (Fig. 30.32). It has a specificity of 80 per cent.

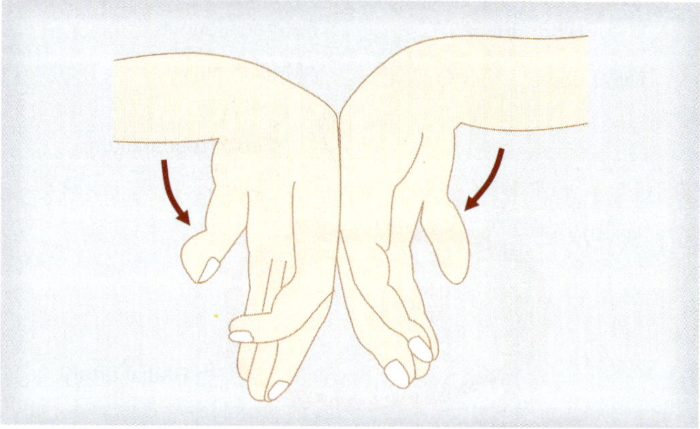

Fig. 30.32: Phalen's test

Tourniquet test A pneumatic blood pressure cuff is applied proximal to the elbow and inflated higher than the patient's systolic blood pressure. The test is positive if there is paraesthesia or numbness in the region of median nerve distribution of the hand. It is less reliable and is specific in 65 per cent of cases only.

Median nerve percussion test (Fig. 30.33) The examiner gently taps the median nerve at the wrist. The test is positive if there is tingling sensation. Seen only in 45 per cent of cases.

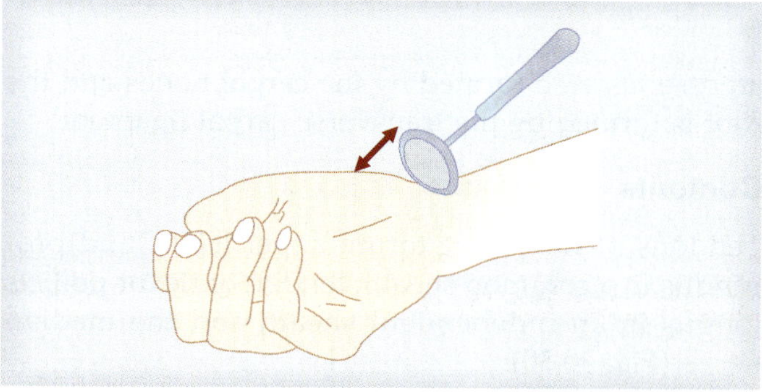

Fig. 30.33: Median nerve percussion test

Median nerve compression test (Fig. 30.34) Direct pressure is exerted equally over both wrists by the examiner. The first phase of the test is the time taken for symptoms to appear (15 sec to 2 min). The second phase is the time taken for the symptoms to disappear after release of pressure.

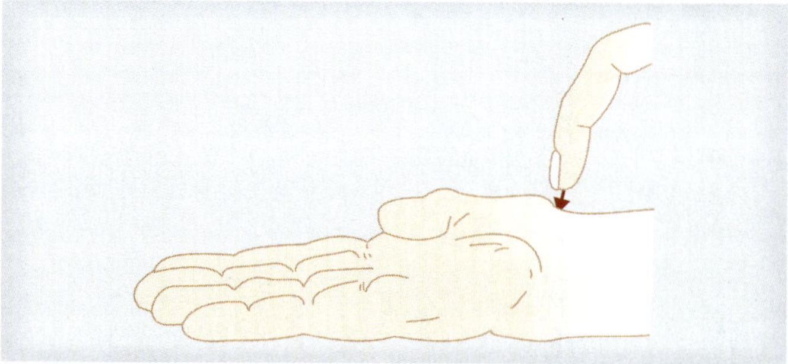

Fig. 30.34: Median nerve compression test

Other Tests

Two-point discrimination test This test is positive in about one-third cases.

Electrodiagnostic tests are not totally infallible with 10 per cent individuals having normal values.

Treatment

Nonoperative methods In the initial stages, nonsteroidal anti-inflammatory drugs NSAIDs are given. If it is unsuccessful, steroids like prednisolone for 8 days starting with 40 mg for 2 days and tapering by 10 mg every 2 days are tried. Use of carpal tunnel splint is also advocated (Fig. 30.35).

Injection treatment This is indicated in patients with intermittent symptoms, duration of complaints less than one year and if there is no sensory deficits, no marked thenar wasting, etc.

In the injection therapy a single infusion of cortisone with splinting for 3 weeks is tried.

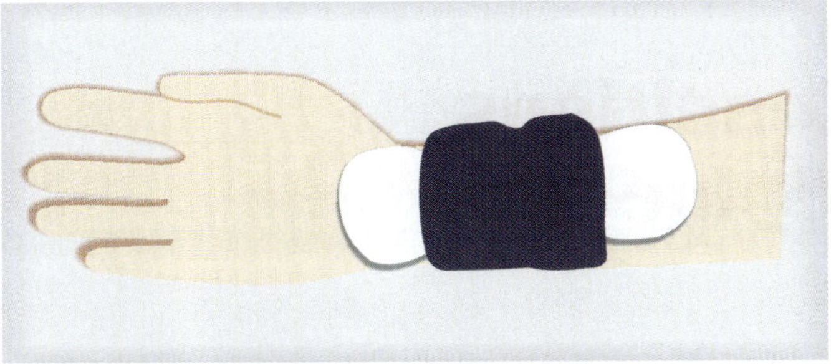

Fig. 30.35: Carpal tunnel splint

Surgery This consists of division of flexor retinaculum and transverse carpal ligament and is indicated in failed nonoperative treatment, thenar atrophy, sensory loss, etc. (Fig. 30.36).

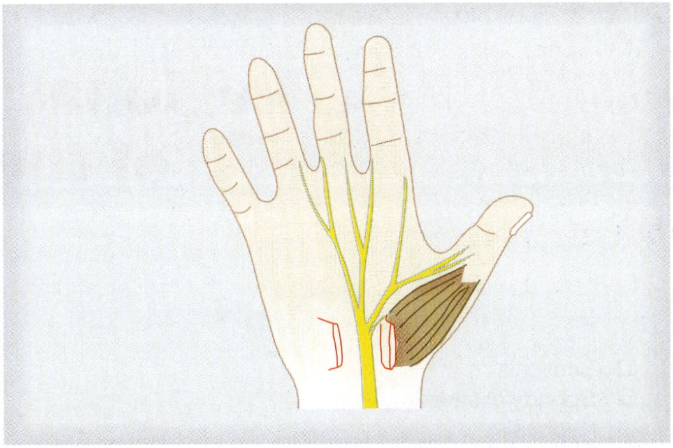

Fig. 30.36: Showing surgical division of the transverse carpal ligament

What is new in the treatment of Carpal Tunnel?

Chow's Technique
This is an endoscopic release of the carpal ligament. It is a reliable alternative for the open procedure and has a success rate of 93.3 per cent.

COMPOUND PALMAR GANGLION

This is a condition which affects the flexor tendons of the fingers mainly the ulnar bursa. It is usually due to tuberculosis though rheumatoid arthritis may also be a cause. The term *compound* is derived from a swelling one above and below the flexor retinaculum (Fig. 30.37).

Here, the endothelial lining of the sheath is substituted by granulation tissue containing miliary tubercles. The presence of *melon seed* bodies is a hallmark of this condition. Effusion may be seen and in the late stages the tendons may rupture.

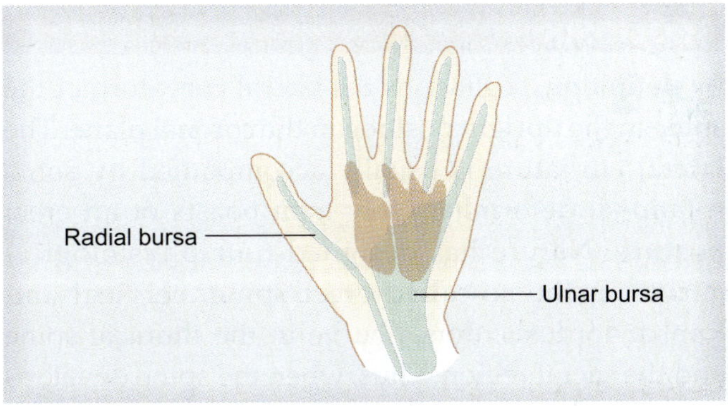

Fig. 30.37: Showing ulnar bursa site of compound palmar ganglion

Quick facts: About melon seed bodies

- Hallmark of compound palmar ganglion.
- Resemble grains of boiled sago.
- Gives rise to a soft, coarse crepitations.
- Made up of fibrin, cellular debris and occasional TB bacilli.

Clinical Features

Those affected with this condition are usually less than 40 years and pain is not a feature. An hourglass swelling with cross-fluctuation may be noticed. There may be features of median nerve compression, but there is definite evidence of wasting of the hand and forearm muscles.

Treatment

Antitubercular treatment, splinting of the forearm and exercises in the late stages, if it is due to tuberculosis. Complete excision forms the treatment in rheumatoid.

BIBLIOGRAPHY

1. Bhattacharya S. Abduction of contracture of shoulder from contracture of intermediate part of deltoid. Report of 3 cases. J Bone Joint Surg (BE) 1966;48B:127-31.
2. Shanmugasundaram TK. Post injection, fibrosis of skeletal muscle: a clinical problem. A personal series of 169 cases. Int Orthop 1980;4:31-37.

Section 3

31

Regional Conditions of the Spine

SCOLIOSIS

By definition, scoliosis is the lateral curvature of the spine in the upright position in the coronal plane. The lateral curvature is usually accompanied by some rotational deformity. Only man boasts of an erect posture. Nature has designed four physiological curves in the so-called erect spine, cervical and lumbar lordosis, dorsal curve in the thoracic spine and the sacral region. Thus, when the spine develops a lateral curve, it is abnormal. It throws the well-adjusted spinal mechanism out of gear and poses the following problems:

1. A cosmetically unacceptable deformity.
2. Deranges the load and force transmission mechanism through the spine.
3. Jeopardises the functions of vital organs like lungs, heart by overcrowding the ribs.
4. Managing it is cumbersome and unrewarding experience most of the times.

Thus, a scoliotic curve makes the spine 'crooked' and a 'crooked spine is a wicked spine', if one considers the above problems it poses.

Mystifying facts

Do you know the difference between scoliosis and spinal asymmetry:

- Lateral curve < 10° - Is spinal asymmetry
- Lateral curve > 10° - Is scoliosis

Varieties

Structural scoliosis *In structural scoliosis, the curves are fixed and nonflexible and fail to correct with side bending.* Lateral bending of spine is asymmetric or involved vertebrae are fixed in a rotated position or both.

Nonstructural scoliosis In nonstructural scoliosis, the curves are flexible and readily correctible with side bending. It is frequently seen as a compensatory mechanism to a leg length discrepancy, fixed flexion deformity of the hip (compensatory scoliosis), local inflammation or irritation due to acute lumbar disc disease and prolapsed disc (sciatic scoliosis) or due to poor postural habits (postural scoliosis).

Note:

1. Postural scoliosis is the most common variety of nonstructural scoliosis.
2. Idiopathic scoliosis is the most common variety of structural scoliosis.

Structural scoliosis may occur from a variety of causes. Idiopathic scoliosis accounts for 90 per cent of all scoliosis and appears to represent a hereditary disorder, but the exact mechanism of its production is unknown. Broadly speaking, there are two types of scoliosis:

1. Idiopathic (unknown cause)
2. Known cause. The important among these are:
   a. *Congenital scoliosis* This is due to defect in segmentation which is usually due to a lateral bar or due to a defect in the formation, including hemivertebrae or double hemivertebrae. These curves usually progress very fast and require surgical fusion on both the convex and concave sides of the curve.
   b. *Paralytic scoliosis* This is due to muscle imbalance on either side of the trunk, the most common cause being anterior poliomyelitis. Cerebral palsies, muscular dystrophies, etc. are the other common causes.

Some of the other causes are mentioned at the end of the chapter.

Idiopathic scoliosis (unknown cause) This is the most common (75–90%) and three varieties are recognised—infantile, juvenile and adolescent (Table 31.1). Though the exact cause is not known, role of genetics is hotly debated. Overall incidence is 1 to 4 people/ thousand.

Table 31.1: Types of idiopathic scoliosis

Infantile	Juvenile	Adolescent
• > 70–90% • < 3 years • Curve is progressive or resolving	• 15% • 4–10 years • Thoracic curve usually to the right	• 2–3% • 10–16 years F:M = 3.6:1
Treatment	**Treatment**	**Treatment**
• Curves < 20° observation • > 20° Bracing • If severe surgical fusion	• < 20° observation • > 20% Milwaukee brace • If > 60° surgical correction and fusion	• Surgical correction

Clinical Features

Though idiopathic scoliosis can occur at any age, it usually appears clinically between 10 and 13 years. It is more common in females (10%). The disease is usually asymptomatic and is usually accidentally discovered. The diagnosis is usually made on routine physical examination (Fig. 31.1).

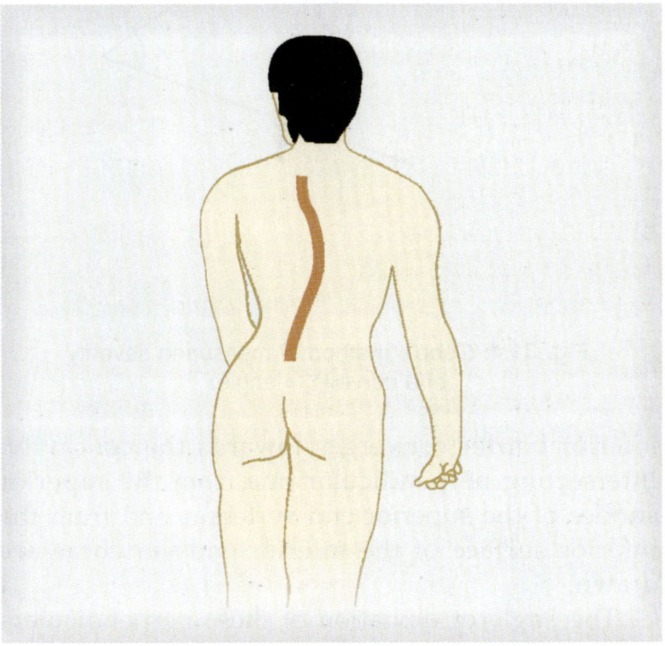

Fig. 31.1: A scoliosis patient should be examined from the back

For the examination, the patient should be undressed to the waist or wear a bathing suit and a routine should be followed. The shoulders and iliac crest are inspected to determine whether they are at the same level. The scapulae, rib cage and flanks are then observed for symmetry. The spinous processes are palpated to determine their alignment. Rib hump or abnormal paraspinal muscular prominence indicates spinal rotation. Rib hump leads to asymmetry of the trunk and is also called angle trunk rotation (ATR). It is measured by using a scoliometer. The patient is then made to bend forward to see for the disappearance of the curve (Adam's test).

Radiographic evaluation of the spine is the only available method to determine the severity of the curve. It is repeated at intervals to determine the progression of the curve.

Scoliotic Facts

Structural curve is a laterally curved spine that lacks normal flexibility.

Primary care This is the earliest curve to appear.

Compensatory curve or secondary curve This is the curve which develops above or below the primary curve in an effort to balance the spine.

Major curve This is the largest structural curve.

Minor curve This is the smallest curve.

Apical vertebra This is the most deviated vertebra from the vertical axis of the patient.

End vertebrae

a. The uppermost vertebra whose superior surface tilts maximally towards the concavity of the curve.
b. The lowermost vertebra whose inferior surface tilts maximally towards the concavity of the curve.

Quick facts

Curve Patterns in Idiopathic Scoliosis (Figs 31.2A to D)

Curve	*Apical Vertebra*
1. Cervical	C_1-C_6
2. Cervicodorsal	C_7-T_1
3. Thoracic	T_2-T_{11}
4. Thoracolumbar	T_{12}-L_1
5. Lumbar	L_2-L_4
6. Lumbosacral	L_5-S_1

How to describe a scoliotic curve?

Remember the mnemonic PLEAD
P—Pattern (primary, secondary, etc.)
L—Location (thoracic, thoracolumbar lumbar)
E—Etiology (idiopathic, congenital, paralytic, etc.)
A—Apex (thoracic lumbar)
D—Direction (right, left)

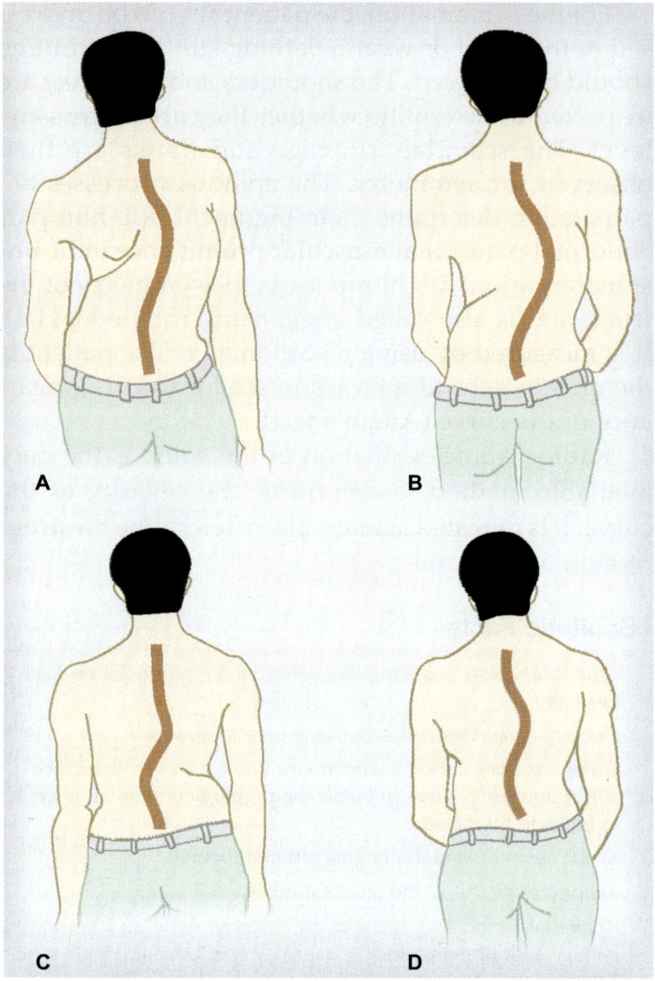

Figs 31.2A to D: Various types of scoliosis: (A) Thoracic, (B) Thoracolumbar, (C) Double curve thoracic and lumbar, (D) Lumbosacral

Radiology

In radiography of the spine, the following views are taken.

PA view of the spine (Fig. 31.3), standard lateral radiography of the spine, right and left bending films of spine and the Stagnara derotation view which is an oblique view of the spine. The radiological parameters of importance are:

Cobb's method to measure severity of the curve (Fig. 31.4) The upper and lower vertebrae are identified. The upper end vertebra is the highest one whose superior border converges towards the concavity of the curve and the lower end vertebra is the one whose inferior border converges towards the concavity. Intersecting perpendicular line from the superior surface of the superior end vertebrae and from the inferior surface of the inferior end vertebrae are drawn.

The angle of deviation of these perpendiculars from a straight line is the 'angle of the curve'.

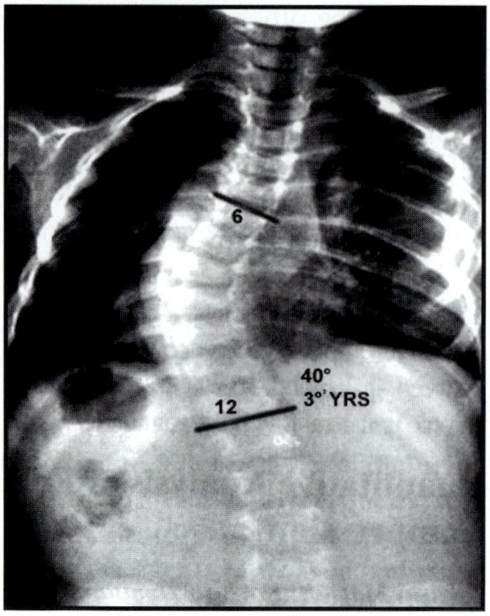

Fig. 31.3: Radiograph showing a paralytic scoliosis

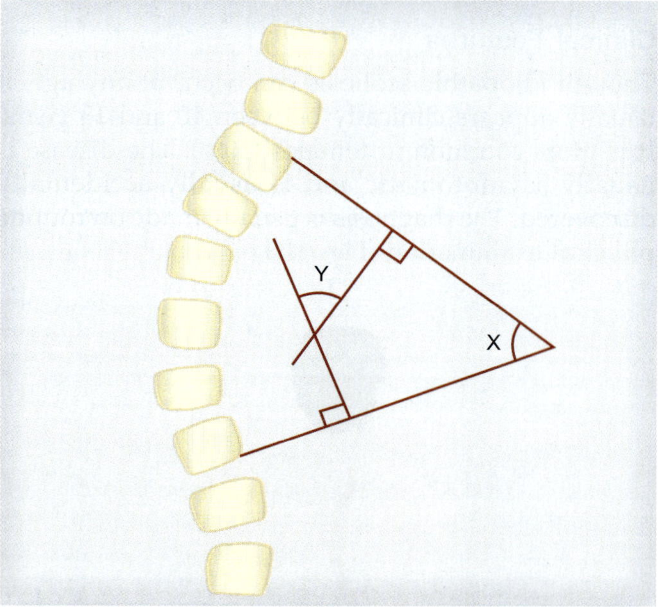

Fig. 31.4: Cobb's method of measuring severity of a curve (Y = angle)

Nash and Moe's method to measure vertebral rotation In the PA view (Figs 31.5A and B) the positions of the spinous process and the pedicles are noted. Normally, the spinous process lies in the centre. The apical vertebrae are graded for rotation on a scale from 0–4, depending upon the pedicle shadows and the position of spinous process. The spinous processes are identified and classified according to the amount of rotation.

Reisser's sign This is a classification of the ossification of the iliac epiphysis which usually starts from the anterior superior iliac spine and progresses posteriorly towards the posterior iliac spine. Reisser's stage 4 corresponds with cessation of spine growth and stage 5 correlates with cessation of height increase. *The importance of this sign is the completion of growth can be radiologically assessed which indicates no possibility of the curve progression.*

Reisser's classification

It uses ossification of iliac apophysis to grade the remaining skeletal growth. The ossification progresses from lateral to medial:

Type I	—	Ossification of lateral 25%
Type II	—	Ossification of lateral 50%
Type III	—	Ossification of lateral 75%
Type IV	—	Ossification of lateral 100%
Type V	—	Fusion of ilium

Rib angle of Mehta The rib vertebral angle is constructed by the intersection of a line perpendicular to the apical vertebral end plate with a line drawn from the midneck to the midhead of the corresponding rib. The rib vertebral angle difference (RVAD) is the difference between rib vertebral angle of the convex and concave side of the apical vertebra. If the initial RVAD is less than 20°, progression is unlikely; and if initial RVAD is more than 20°, the curves tend to progress (Fig. 31.6).

Original structural curves are distinguished from secondary curves by the following criteria:

- Vertebrae in structural scoliosis are displaced to the convexity of the curve; but in secondary curve, they are displaced to the concavity of the secodary curve.
- When there are three curves, *middle* one is structural.
- When there are four curves, *two middle* ones are structural.
- The greater curve or the one towards which the *trunk is shifted is the structural curve.*
- The curve that is flexible and corrective is the non-structural curve.

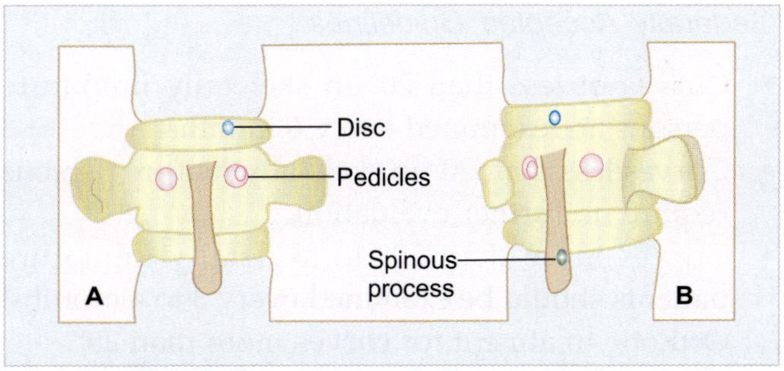

Figs 31.5A and B: (A) Normal PA view of the spine showing the normal positions of the pedicles and spinous processes, and (B) The pedicles and spinous processes shadows are altered and indicate vertebral rotation in scoliosis

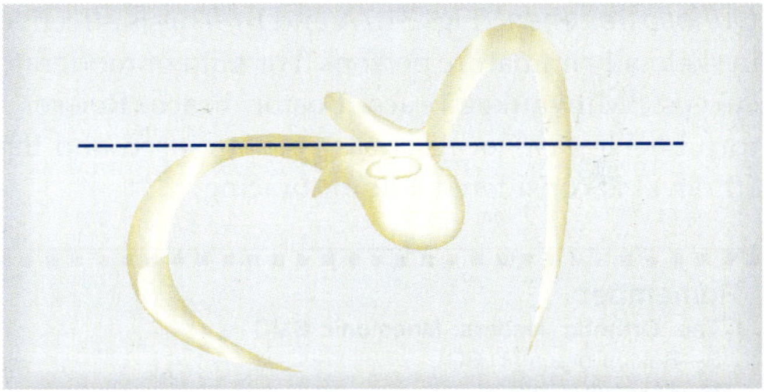

Fig. 31.6: Showing rib distortion due to vertebral rotation

Compensation

If head is to be balanced above the pelvis when the patient is erect, it is done so by any curve or curves that develop in the opposite direction. *The formation of curves in the opposite direction is called compensation.* The angle of the secondary curves should be equal to that of the primary curve. If it exceeds, it is called overcompensation.

Treatment

The most important aspect in the treatment of scoliosis is early detection of the curve. A curve that is obvious in standing position has already approached 30 to 40°. *Detecting a curve before it reaches 20° is of utmost importance because curves over 20° tend to progress.* Frequent re-examinations are essential. The treatment depends on the age of the patient and the severity of the curve.

Non-surgical treatment Observation is the primary treatment of all curves. *At present, radiography is the only definite documentation of curve size and progression.*

Generally Accepted Guidelines

- Curves of less than 20° in skeletally immature persons are examined every 6 months.
- Curves less than 20° in skeletally mature persons require no further evaluation.
- Curves more than 20° in skeletally immature patients should be examined every 3 to 4 months. Orthotic treatment for curves more than 25°.
- Curves more than 30 to 40° in skeletally mature persons do not require treatment. But they are examined radiographically for progression every 2 to 3 years.

Orthotic treatment (Figs 31.7A and B) This is effective in skeletally immature persons. For mild or moderate curves, [1]Milwaukee brace, Boston brace, Reisser's turn buckle cast, localiser cast, etc. are used and the 20° level is considered still for bracing.

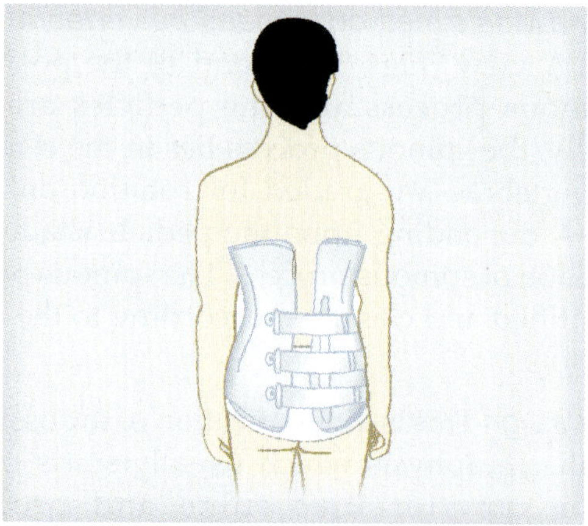

Fig. 31.7A: Showing orthotic treatment of structural scoliosis with Boston brace

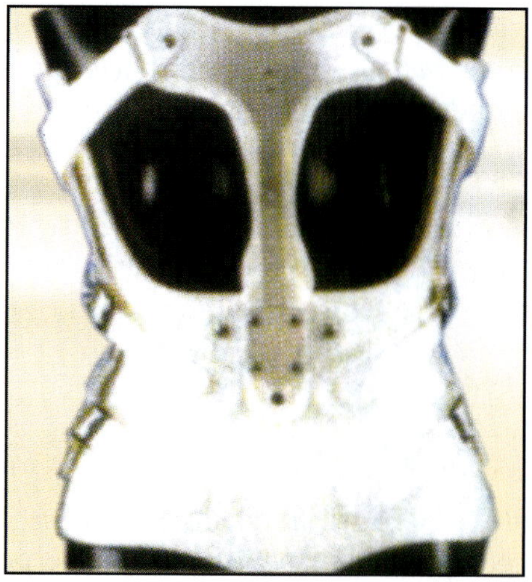

Fig. 31.7B: Brace for scoliosis

Remember

The 'Orthotic' leaders: Mnemonic BMC

B—Boston brace (TLSO)
M—Milwaukee brace
C—Carleston brace
Most effective among these is the Boston brace

Do you know
Complications of bracing?

- Most Common: Discomfort and rejection due to poor appearance.
- Skin breakdown
- Excessive sweating
- Allergic skin reaction
- Increased gastric pressure and gastroesophageal reflex
- Spontaneous sternum fracture

Other non-operative measures Exercises and electrical stimulation have been unsuccessfully tried in adolescent variety.

Traction

Traction helps to stretch the contracted structures prior to surgery. Methods of traction could be either non-skeletal or skeletal. Skeletal traction is provided by halopelvic or halofemoral traction (Fig. 31.7C).

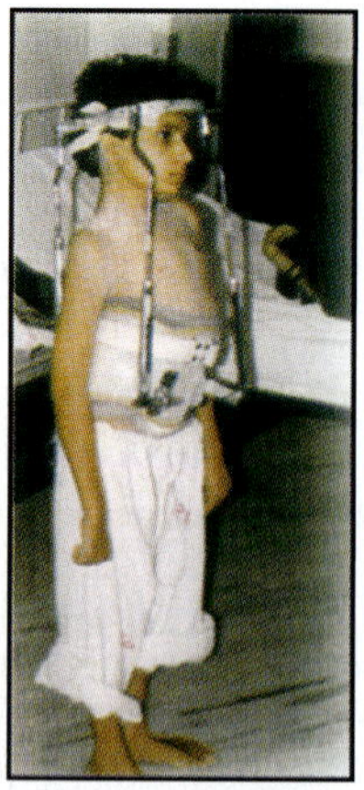

Fig. 31.7C: Showing halopelvic distraction apparatus used for skeletal traction in correction of structural scoliotic curves

Section 3

[1]**Milwaukee brace** was developed in 1945 for more efficient and comfortable passive correction of the scoliosis.

Mystifying facts: About braces

1. Do you know what curves respond best to bracing?
   - Curves < 40°
   - Less severe lumbar hyperlordosis
   - Curves with thoracic lordosis
   - Hyperkyphosis
   - Risser's curve is 0
2. How much is the efficacy of bracing?
   It is about 74 to 81% when worn for 23 hours/day till skeletal maturity.
3. How do braces act?
   By derotating the spine using the rib or transverse process as the lever
4. What are the corrective forces?
   The primary corrective forces are the 'lateral forces' in the braces.

Surgical treatment is indicated for high degree thoracic curve which is inflexible and is associated with secondary changes in the ribs. Casts are not effective in thoracic spine. Spinal surgery is also indicated when the curve is over 60° and aims at obtaining fusion at the spine (see box) (Fig. 31.8).

Do you know in scoliosis?

1. **The proper indications for surgery?**
   - Curves > 50° in the mature patients
   - Curves > 10° with marked rotations
   - Double major curves > 30°
2. **The most common form of surgical intervention in idiopathic scoliosis?**
   Well, it is the segmental instrumentation with multiback system (CD)

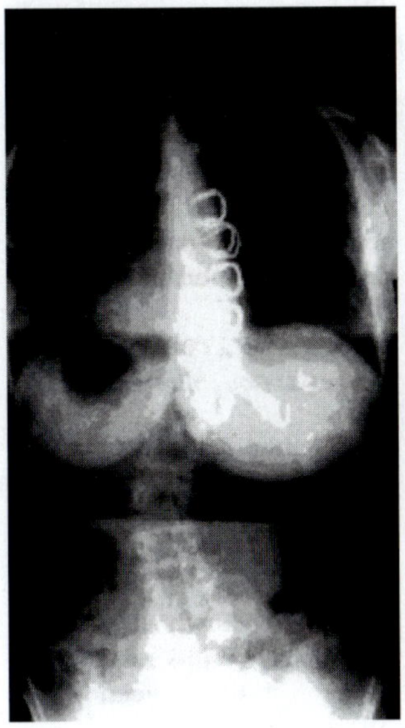

Fig. 31.8: Radiograph showing scoliosis surgical correction by segmental instrumentation

Flowchart showing Methods of Scoliosis Treatment

Methods

Distraction Techniques
- Rarely used
- Spinal instrumentation and spinal cord monitoring have been developed

Methods
1. Halopelvic distraction
2. Halofemoral distraction

Indications
- Kyphosis
- Rigid scoliosis > 100°
- Salvage procedure following failed spinal surgery.
- Unstable spine due to laminectomy.

Surgical Fusion (Indications)
- Too late for Milwaukee brace, > 15 years, > 50° curves.
- Failure to respond to Milwaukee brace.
- Curves > 60°
- Pain in adults
- Paralytic and congenital scoliosis (Fig. 31.6)

Methods

Anterior Fusion

Posterior Fusion
- Harrington's instrumentation
- Dwyer's instrumentation
- Zielke's instrumentation.
- Hartshill rings, etc.
- Segmental (Cotrel-Duboucet System)

Quick facts

- Scoliosis is lateral curvature of the spine.
- Idiopathic variety accounts for 90% of the cases.
- Female preponderance.
- X-ray is the only definite documentation of curve size and progression.
- The most important aspect of treatment is early detection.
- Curves < 20° need observation.
- Curves > 20° require treatment.
- Curves between 20 and 40° can be treated by Milwaukee brace which has to be worn 23 hours per day for a period of at least two years.
- Curves > 40° need surgical correction and fusion.

Facts about curve progression

- Curves < 20° will improve spontaneously in over 50 per cent of cases.
- No accurate method to predict the outcome of curve.
- 20 per cent curves <30° will progress.
- Progression is more common in young children.
- Bigger the curve at detection, higher is the chance of curve progression.
- Curve in females and double curves are more likely to progress.

Scoliosis of known cause Congenital/paralytic

Neuromuscular scoliosis

- *Neuropathic causes* Spinal cord injury, poliomyelitis, progressive neurological disorders, syringomyelia, myelomeningocele and cerebral palsy are some of the neuropathic causes.
- *Muscular* AMC and muscular dystrophy are some of the important muscular causes.
- *Neurofibromatosis*
- *Miscellaneous* Multiple epiphyseal dysplasias, osteogenesis imperfecta, etc.

Interesting facts

Remember 3 'O's in the treatment of idiopathic scoliosis:
- Observation for curves < 20°
- Orthosis for curves for > 20°–50°
- Operations for curves > 50°

In a nutshell

Treatment options in scoliosis

1. Congenital — Surgery/Bracing
2. Paralytic — Wheel chair seating systems
   — Bracing, Surgery
3. Idiopathic — 3Os mentioned earlier
4. Marked rotation — Bracing
5. Degenerative
   < 60 years — Postural correction, exercises, corset, etc.
   > 60 years — Surgery

Alternative therapies: Exercises, electric stimulation, biofeedback, tractions, manipulations, etc.

Unfavourable prognostic facts in scoliosis

- Congenital/juvenile/paralytic
- > 20-40° curve
- Thoracic curve
- 2-4 degree of rotation
- Risser's sign 0/immature
- Female
- Premenarchial
- Presence of osteoporosis
- Rapid increase in curve size
- Single short curve
- Previous discectomy, laminectomy, etc.

SPONDYLOLISTHESIS
(Spondylos—spine; Olisthein—to slip)

It is the story of a "slipping" spine causing "gripping" problems both to the patient and the clinician. That animals never suffer spondylolisthesis is proof enough to declare that this condition is a curse of erect posture which only man prides to possess!

Definition

It is defined as slow anterior displacement of a vertebra at the lower lumbar spine, generally accepted as the lowermost vertebra L_5 slipping forward on the first sacral segment S_1 (Figs 31.9A).

Essential lesion is the interruption in the concavity of the pars interarticularis.

Spondylolysis In this, the defect in the pars exists but without the forward slipping. This could be due to a fracture, stress fracture or nonunion.

Interesting facts about spondylolysis

- About 50% of the patients who present with isthmic spondylolysis do not progress to spondylolisthesis.
- Spondylolisthesis is the most common cause of low backache in childhood

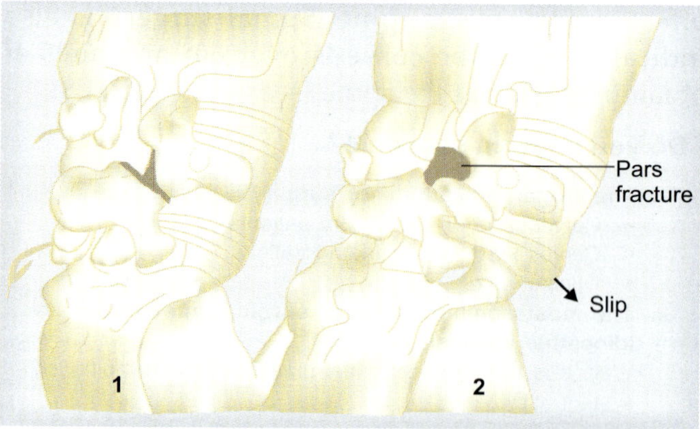

Fig. 31.9A: (1) Fracture or discontinuity in the pars (spondylolysis), (2) spondylolisthesis

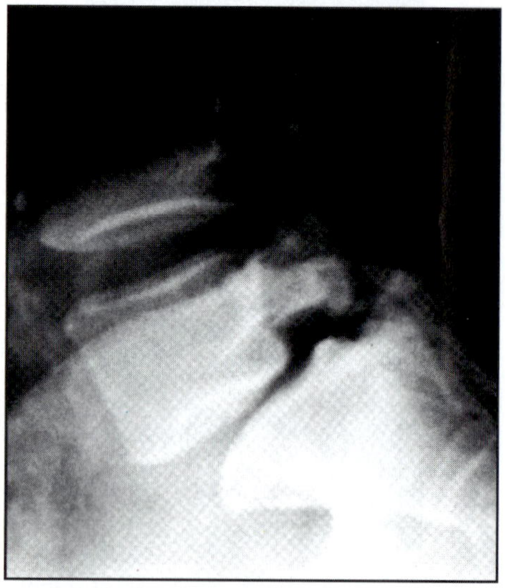

Fig. 31.9B: Radiograph showing spondylolisthesis

Classification (Wiltse, Macnab and Newman)

Five varieties are described (Figs 31.10A to F).

Dysplastic Congenital abnormalities of the upper sacrum or the arch of L_5. These permit the olisthesis to occur.

Isthmic (true) The lesion is in the pars and is the most common variety. Common in children. Rarely seen before 8 years. At adolescent growth spurt, sudden increase in activity, gymnastics, carrying heavy bags, etc. may lead to a fatigue or stress fracture of the pars which may give rise to the slip.

Types

- Lytic fatigue fracture of the pars in children.
- Elongated but intact pars.
- Acute fracture of the pars due to trauma.

Degenerative This is due to long-standing intersegmental instability. Here pars is intact but the facet joints degenerate and allow the forward slip.

Traumatic This is due to fracture in other areas of the bony hook rather than the pars.

Pathological There is a generalised or localised bony disease in this variety.

Clinical Features

The clinical features of different varieties of spondylolisthesis are shown in Table 31.2.

However, increased lumbar lordosis and transverse furrow over the lower back are unmistakable features of spondylolisthesis (Fig. 31.11).

Investigations

Radiograph of the spine is the investigation of choice (see Fig. 31.9B). Anteroposterior and lateral films are helpful. But oblique view of the lumbar spine demonstrates the defect in the pars very accurately as a "Scottie dog" sign. The Scottie dog's neck, which represents the pars defect, is broken in the isthmic variety (Fig. 31.12). The edges of the defect are smooth and rounded and suggest a pseudarthrosis rather than acute fracture.

RADIOLOGICAL GRADING

Meyerding's Grading* (Fig. 31.13)

G1	25 per cent forward displacement
G2	25–50 per cent
G3	50–70 per cent
G4	> 75 per cent

*Percentage of slip calculated by the upper vertebral displacement over the lower vertebral body, on a lateral view plain X-ray of the LS spine.

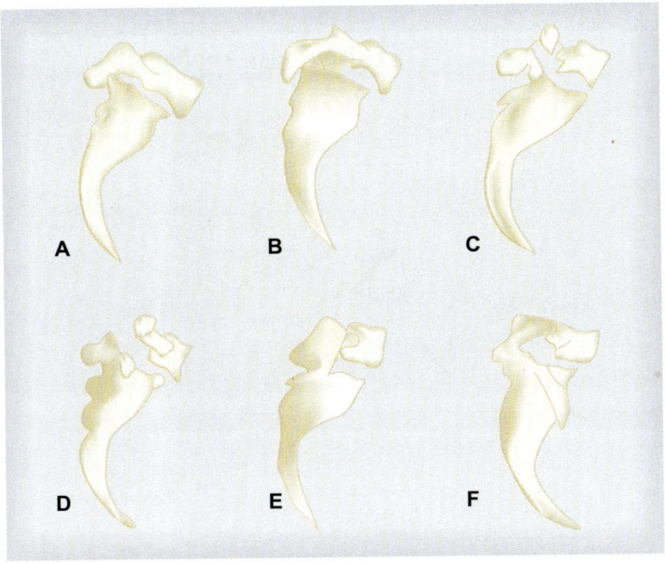

Figs 31.10A to F: Showing varieties of spondylolisthesis: (A) Normal, (B) Congenital, (C) Isthmic, (D) Traumatic, (E) Degenerative, and (F) Pathological

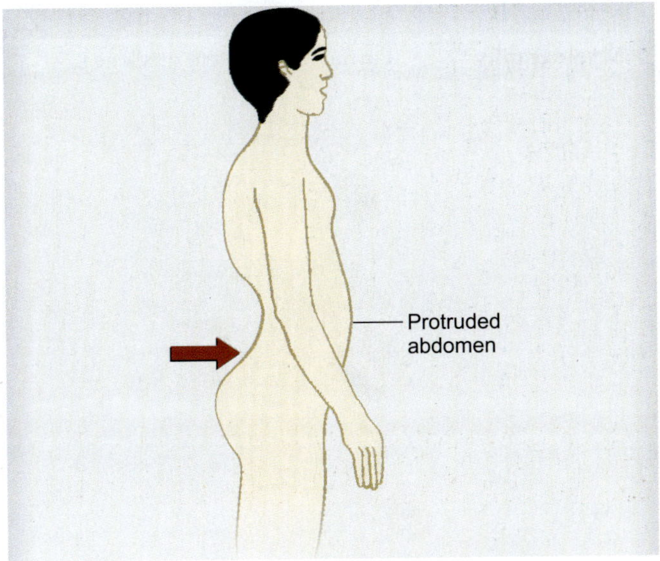

Fig. 31.11: Showing increased lumbar lordosis in spondylolisthesis

Table 31.2: Clinical features of different spondylolisthesis

	True Spondylolisthesis (Isthmic)	*Congenital*	*Degenerative*
1. **Clinical features**	• Asymptomatic or low backpain. H/o Trauma present in 50 per cent • Common history of injury in adults and children	• Pain—low backache, buttocks, feet, toes, thighs and legs	• Known as pseudospondylolisthesis • Intermittent symptoms and is common in the elderly patients Five times more common in women and affects 4 to 10 per cent of the population
2. **Deformity**	• ↑ Lumbar lordosis • Palpable step at L_5–S_1 (Fig. 31.14) • Torso is short • Abdomen protruded forwards • Transvere furrow at L_5 • Sacrum is more vertical • Buttocks flat and hamstring tightness • L_5 spinous process prominently felt. Scoliosis in 13%	• Scoliosis, pelvic waddle present • Buttocks are flat • Stiffness of spine present • Cannot bend beyond the lower thigh	• Pain in the back, buttock or thigh
3. **Neurology**	• L_5 nerve root is involved but rare	• L_5 or S_1 nerve root is involved	• L_5 rare • Neurologic claudication may be present. • L_{3-4} common
4. **Obstetrics**	• Narrowing occurs at the outlet		
5. **X-ray**	• Lateral view is characteristic • Oblique view—shows **"Scottish terrier's sign"**	• Development of sacral neural arch, superior sacral articular process is defective. • Sacral root is not well developed.	• Hyperdactility at L_{4-5} • No motion at L_5-S_1 • Displacement is < 30 per cent
6. **Myelography**	• Partial or complete block at L_5		• Hour glass configuration

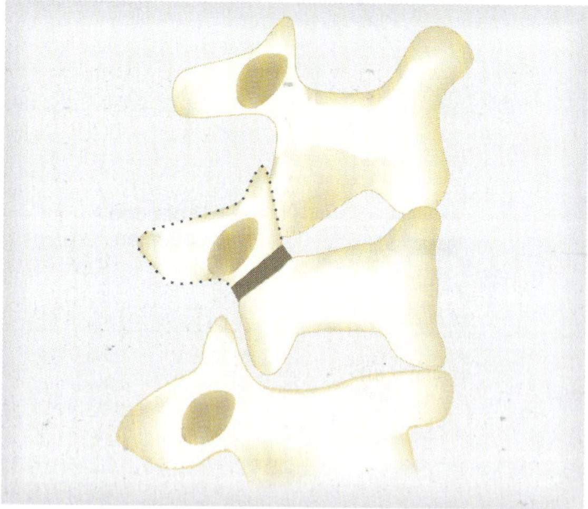

Fig. 31.12: Showing fracture of the pars. In true spondylolysis familiarly known as "Scottish terrier's sign"

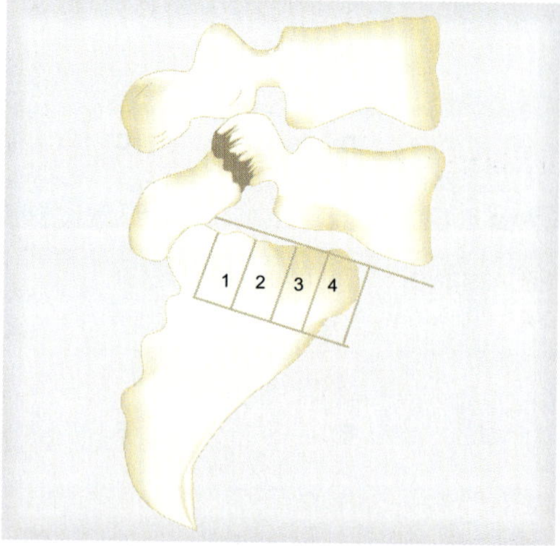

Fig. 31.13: Meyerding's grading (1932) of spondylolisthesis. The amount of slippage is graded 1–4 on a plain lateral X-ray of the spine

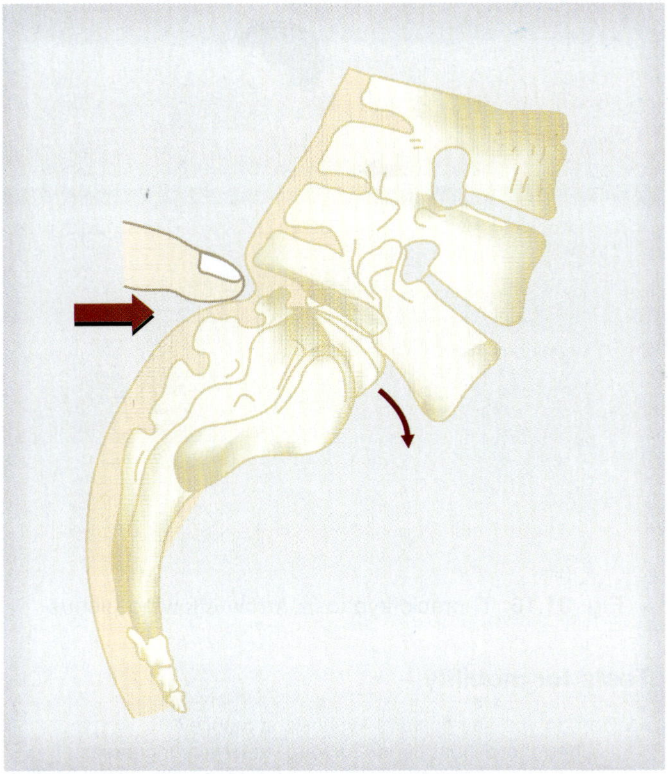

Fig. 31.14: Clinically a step can be palpated at the back in spondylolisthesis and is called a "step sign"

Table 31.3: Different methods of conservative treatment		
Asymptomatic	*Mild to Moderate*	*Severe*
• Correction of poor posture • Elimination of stressful occupation • To avoid certain special sports activities	• Alleviation of anxiety • Analgesics and muscle relaxants • Deep heat • Exercises	• Rest • NSAIDs • Gradual exercises to strengthen the trunk and hamstring muscles

Treatment

Conservative treatment Clinically, spondylolisthesis is divided into three groups, asymptomatic, mild to moderate, and severe varieties, based on the severity of symptoms. Table 31.3 shows the different methods of conservative treatment to be employed in the above three clinical varieties of spondylolisthesis.

Surgical Management

Indications

- Failure of conservative therapy.
- Signs of root compression.
- Progressive slipping.
- Slip of more than 30 per cent even when painless.
- Persistent pain in the back, thigh or persistent sciatica.

Methods of Surgery

1. *Posterolateral fusion* This is the best method of fusing the slipped vertebra because it preserves the supporting soft tissues and has a high rate of fusion.
2. *Posterior fusion* In this method, postoperative and additional slip is frequent till the fusion is solid. This also has a high rate of pseudarthrosis and has to be done with intertransverse fusion.
3. *Laminectomy* This mainly helps to relieve the neurological deficits and has to be followed by posterolateral fusion.
4. Laminectomy and intertransverse fusion.
5. *Anterior interbody fusion.*

This is indicated for subtotal spondylolisthesis and is a risky and difficult procedure with doubtful efficacy.

Fusion is achieved in spondylolisthesis by putting autologous cancellous bone graft and stabilisation is obtained by Hartshill rectangle frame or Steffee plate and screws (Fig. 31.15).

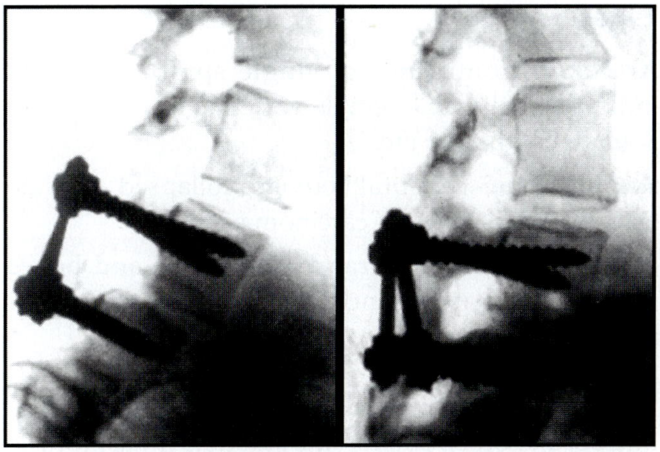

Fig. 31.15: Radiographs showing posterior spinal stabilisation by Steffee plate and screws

KYPHOSIS

Definition

It is defined as increase in normal posterior convexity of the thoracic spine and is referred to as 'hyper-kyphosis' (Fig. 31.16).

Causes

Localised injury or disease like fracture, Potts disease, secondaries in the spine, etc.

Generalised bone diseases ankylosing spondylitis, osteomalacia, Paget's disease, acromegaly, etc. are some of the examples.

Defective Growth or Poor Postural Habits

Children—Stooping posture while reading.

Adolescents—Vertebral epiphysitis (Scheurmann's) seen in boys 14 to 17 years of age.

Adults—Bending occupation, e.g. porter, cobbler, etc.

Old men and women —Senile osteoporosis.

Vital facts: About Scheurmann's disease

- Adolescent kyphosis
- Cobb's angle > 45°, wedging of 5° and at least three adjacent apical vertebrae involved
- Slightly more common in females
- Cause unknown, familial
- Deformity is the main complaint than pain
- Typical X-ray finding—Schmorl's node
- ***Treatment:*** Milwaukee brace in immature spine. In severe deformity and in adults, surgical decompression and stabilisation is advised

Types

Knuckle Prominence of single spinous process indicating collapse of single vertebra, e.g. TB spine/ Kummel's disease, etc.

Angular 2 to 3 vertebral body are collapsed, e.g. late stage of TB, secondary carcinoma, etc.

Round Several vertebrae are involved and hence gives a round appearance, e.g. in children—Scheurmann's disease, in old age—senile kyphosis.

Methods of Examination

Inspection Look from the side and note if the thoracic curvature is regular, now determine if the kyphosis is mobile or fixed.

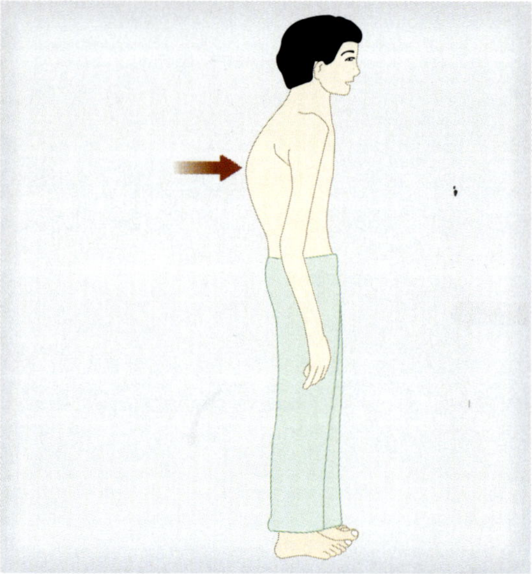

Fig. 31.16: Thoracic kyphosis arrow showing gibbus

Tests for mobility

When do you say postural kyphosis is mobile?

1. When the patient bends forward, deformity increases.
2. When the patient braces the shoulder back, deformity decreases.

   If the above two tests are negative, kyphosis is fixed.

What is Gibbus?

Acute kyphosis is called gibbus and is due to single or two level vertebral involvement.

Investigations

Plain X-ray of the thoracic spine, CT scan, MRI, laboratory tests are some of the important investigation methods to evaluate the severity of kyphosis.

Treatment

In mild deformities, anterior hyperextension bracing is indicated. In severe deformities, surgical decompression and stabilisation is advised.

LUMBAR CANAL STENOSIS

Canal stenosis is common in lumbar vertebrae. One or more roots of the cauda equina may be affected due to the constriction in spinal canal before it exits through the foramen.

This condition was first described by Portal in 1803.

Definition

Lumbar canal stenosis is a cauda equina compression in which the lateral or anteroposterior diameter of the spinal canal is narrow with or without a change in the cross-sectional area (Fig. 31.17). The nerve root canals and the I-V foramen may also be narrowed.

Classification

1. Generalised/localised.
2. Segmental (local area of each vertebral spinal segment is affected):
   a. Central
   b. Lateral recesses
   c. Foraminal
   d. Far out
3. Anatomical area:
   - Cervical (seen)
   - Thoracic (rare)
   - Lumbar (most common)
4. Pathological (Arnold's classification):
   - Congenital—e.g. achondroplasia
   - Acquired—degenerative, iatrogenic, and spondylitic.
5. Other causes:
   - Paget's disease
   - Fluorosis
   - Kyphosis
   - Scoliosis
   - Fracture spine
   - DISH (diffuse idiopathic skeletal hyperostosis) syndrome.

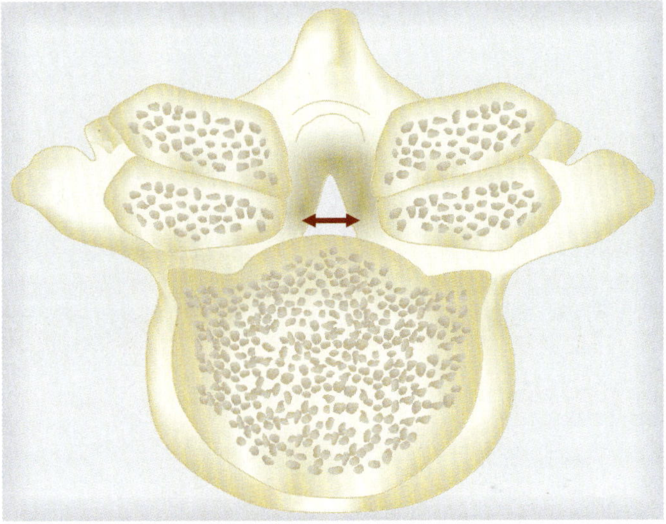

Fig. 31.17: Lumbar canal stenosis

5. Iatrogenic causes, e.g. hypertrophy of posterior bone graft, incomplete treatment of stenotic condition, etc.

Clinical Features

Lumbar canal stenosis is common in males above 50 years. Usually, the symptoms are fewer in number, but the patient may complain of low backache.

Cauda equina claudication is the common symptom. Here, the patient complains of pain in the buttocks and legs after walking, which decreases on sitting, rest and forward bending. Patient may complain of hypoaesthesia and paraesthesia. Usually, the patient finds no problem walking uphill or riding a bicycle. Nerve root entrapment in the lateral recess causes claudication and sciatica. Stoop test is positive.

Difference between ischaemic claudication and cauda equina claudication (neurogenic claudications) is mentioned below (see Table 31.4).

Table 31.4: The features of different types of claudications

Cauda equina claudication	*Ischaemic claudication*
• Pain in the buttocks and lower extremities after walking • Relieved by sitting forward for 20 minutes • Hypoaesthesia, paraesthesia precipitated by walking, walking uphill, cycling, etc. • Pulses are felt • No trophic changes. • Walking downhill worse • Walking uphill better	• Pain in the legs appears on walking • Appears and diappears fast • Decreases in standing • No neurological deficit • Absent pulses • Trophic changes in foot and toes • Walking downhill unchanged or better • Walking uphill unchanged or worse

Stoop test It is positive in lumbar canal stenosis.
Ask the patient to walk briskly → pain develops → continues to walk → patient assumes a stooped posture → symptoms disappear. The pain decreases by forward bending because the canal length increases by 2.2 mm.

Other important tests

- **Bicycle Test:** The patient is made to pedal a stationary bicycle first in an upright position and later in a forward flexed position. If he pedals more during the latter event, the test is positive.
- **Walking Test:** The patient is made to walk on a level surface first in an upright position and then in a flexed position. If he walks more during the latter event, the test is positive.

Investigations

Radiographs of the lumbar spine consisting of AP, lateral and oblique views are recommended.

Radiographs of pelvis are done also. The following points are looked for:

1. Reduced interpedicle distance.
2. AP or midsagittal diameter of the affected vertebra (Normal—15 mm), absolute midsagittal diameter of the canal is decreased.
3. Measurement of the lateral sagittal diameter.
4. Hypertrophy and sclerosis of the facet joints.
5. Reduced interlaminar space and short, stout spinous process.
6. Associated features like presence of listhesis, prolapsed disc, osteophytes, etc.

Myelographic findings consist of waist-like narrowing of the dural sac at the level of facet joint and indentation of the dural tube due to disc prolapse, etc.

MRI and CT scan Help to diagnose lateral recess stenosis, facet hypertrophy, midsagittal distance, etc.

Treatment

Conservative Methods

- Drug therapy like the NSAIDs, etc.
- Epidural steroids may help in some cases
- Physiotherapy with heating modalities helps
- Pelvic traction may help relieve compression.
- ***Exercises:*** General conditioning exercises like walking, swimming and flexion-oriented exercises are useful
- ***Deweighted Treadmill ambulation:*** This consists of applying vertical traction with a harness while doing the treadmill exercises. This offers twin benefits of both exercises and traction.
- ***Belts and corsets*** (soft)—These may offer some relief.

Surgical Methods

Most of the surgical methods described for lumbar canal stenosis aim at decompressing the constricted lumbar canal. Laminectomy is useful in central canal stenosis. Discectomy and osteotomy of inferior articular process to remove the hypertrophic elements.

For lateral canal stenosis laminotomy, disc excision, partial medial facetectomy and foraminotomy helps. Spinal fusion to stabilise the lumbar spine is usually not required as instability is less commonly seen in lumbar canal stenosis.

It should be noted that neurogenic claudication responds poorly to the conservative treatment but responds well to surgical decompression.

Did you know?

That lumbar canal stenosis is the most common reason for undergoing spinal surgery after the age of 65 years.

32

Regional Conditions of the Lower Limb

REGIONAL CONDITIONS OF THE HIP

COXA VARA

Definition It is an abnormality of the proximal end of femur, which is characterised by decreased neck shaft angle (Fig. 32.1).

Normal coxa vara is due to differential growth pattern of capital femoral and greater trochanteric epiphysis. In coxa valga the neck shaft angle is increased (Fig. 32.2).

Classification

Congenital

1. Congenital coxa vara.
2. Congenital short femur with coxa vara.
3. Congenital bowed femur with coxa vara.

Acquired (according to the site of disturbance)

1. *Capital coxa vara* This is seen in Perthes' disease, chondro-osteodystrophy, cretinism, septic arthritis of hip, etc.
2. *Epiphyseal coxa vara* Slipped capital femoral epiphysis.
3. *Cervical coxa vara* This is seen in malunited trochanteric fracture, pathological hip conditions like:
   a. Children—Rickets, bony dystrophies, etc.
   b. Adults—Osteomyelitis, osteoporosis, Paget's disease, fibrous dysplasia, etc.

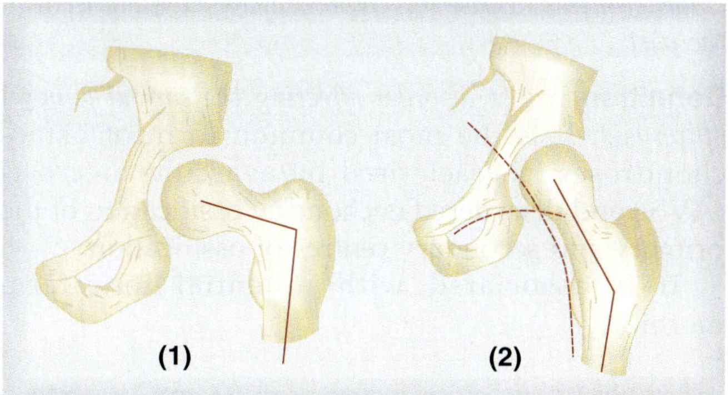

Figs 32.1 and 32.2: Showing (1) Coxa vara, (2) Coxa valga

Part of generalised skeletal dysplasias This is seen in mucopolysaccharidosis, multiple epiphyseal dysplasias, achondroplasia, cleidocranial dysostosis, etc.

Disadvantages of coxa vara

1. Normal apposition between joint surfaces is lost.
2. Trochanter is displaced upwards, impinges on the side of pelvis.
3. Marked shortening of the limb.
4. Waddling gait.

Clinical Features

Small stature, limp, waddling gait, upward shift of greater trochanter, decreased rotation and abduction of hip, pain, stifffness and flexion contractures are some of the important clinical features of coxa vara.

Radiography

Radiographic features are: neck shaft angle is less than 90°, length of the neck is decreased, head is unusually translucent, and triangular fragment of bone is seen occupying lower part of the head close to the neck.

Treatment

It consists of corrective osteotomy at the intertrochanteric level. Usually, a lateral wedge osteotomy is preferred. Macewen and Shands' corrective osteotomy corrects both coxa vara and retroversion of the femoral neck.

LEGG-CALVÉ-PERTHES DISEASE (SYN: OSTEOCHONDRITIS DEFORMANS JUVENILIS AND COXA PLANA)

[1]*Legg-Calvé-Perthes disease is a complex paediatric hip disorder and has some controversial aspects. Although its precise aetiology remains unknown, the pathogenesis and pathology are farely well understood. The prognosis for a child with this disease has improved considerably than in the past.*

Definition It is *a disorder affecting the capital femoral epiphysis*. It is the most common form of osteochondroses, characterised by avascular necrosis (AVN) and disordered enchondral ossification of the primary and secondary centres of ossification.

It is associated with potential long-term morbidity.

Pathogenesis of Legg-Calvé-Perthes disease

Idiopathic capital femoral epiphyseal ischaemia (initial infarction)

↓

Temporary cessation of epiphyseal growth

↓

Epiphyseal revascularisation occurs from periphery

↓

Resumption of growth and ossification

↓

No subchondral **fracture**

Potential form

- No epiphyseal resorption
- No subluxation
- No deformity of femoral head
- Child is asymptomatic
- Good range of hip movements
- X-ray shows **head within head** appearance

Subchondral **fracture**

True form

- Due to trauma and is usually from vigorous activity
- *The painful pathological subchondral fracture heralds the onset of true Perthes' and only the true form produces the characteristic clinical and radiographic features*

Predisposing Factors

1. *Genetic aspects* Increased incidence of 2 to 20 per cent in families of Perthes'.
2. *Abnormal growth and development* Perthes' disease may be a manifestation of an unknown systemic disorder rather than an isolated abnormality of the hip joint. The bone age of children with Perthes' disease is typically lower than their chronological age by 1 to 3 years; as a result, the affected children are shorter than normal.
3. *Environmental factors* Majority of children belong to the poorer class.
4. *Sex* Eighty per cent affected are males (4:1).
5. Trauma to the hip joints.

Aetiology

The aetiology remains unknown, but it is *currently accepted that the disorder is caused by an interruption of the blood supply to the capital femoral epiphysis, causing avascular necrosis.*

[1]**George Clemens Perthes** (1869-1927), a German Orthopaedic Surgeon described it independently. Legg, Arthur Thornton, Massachusetts (1910) and Jacques Calve (1910) of France also described it and called it as coxa plana.

Changes in

1. *Capital femoral epiphysis* The following are the changes seen in the capital femoral epiphysis: Initial ischaemia is followed by revascularisation and pathological subchondral fracture occurs due to trauma or vigorous active movements. This results in a second mechanical ischaemic episode which heralds the onset of true form of Perthes. Again, slow revascularisation called *creeping substitution* takes place and the head is moulded due to the forces acting on it (biologic plasticity).
2. *Epiphyseal growth plate changes* The two ischaemic episodes mentioned above also take place here.
3. *Metaphyseal changes* Four characteristic changes are seen in the metaphyseal area: presence of adipose tissue, osteolytic lesions, disorganised ossification, and extrusion of growth plate.

Ultimate result Following the epiphyseal growth plate and metaphyseal changes, the following end results are seen:

- Altered longitudinal growth of the proximal femur.
- Coxa vara and coxa magna.
- High greater trochanter and short femoral neck results in functional coxa vara.
- Shortening by 1 to 2 cm.
- Trendelenburg gait is due to disturbed hip abductor mechanism.

Clinical Features

It is usually common in boys between 4 and 8 years (mean age 7 years) but can also occur less than 2 years and more than 12 years. *If the child is older than 12 years, it is not true Perthes' disease but rather adolescent avascular necrosis.*

Symptoms

- Painless limp (classical presentation).
- Mild pain in the hip or anterior thigh or knee.
- History of trauma may be present or absent.
- Onset of pain may be acute or insidious.

Signs

- Antalgic gait
- Muscle spasm (detected by roll test).
- Proximal thigh atrophy (by 2–3 cm).
- Limitation of abduction and internal rotation.
- Short stature.

Clinical Tests

- *Internal rotation test* (Fig. 32.3) for hip shows decreased internal rotation.
- *Trendelenburg test* is positive.
- *Abduction test* abduction is limited on the affected side (Fig. 32.4).
- *Roll test* (Fig. 32.5) passive rotation of the lower limb is done to detect the muscle spasm. This is positive.
- *Thomas test* reveals typically 15° fixed flexion deformity (FFD) of hip (Fig. 32.6).

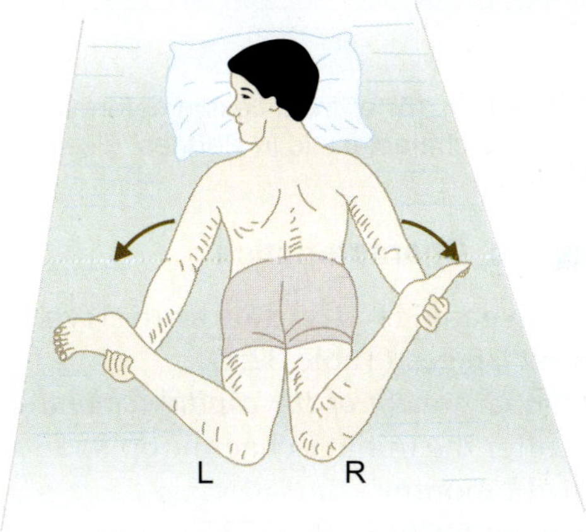

Fig. 32.3: Showing limitation of internal rotation of right hip. Hip rotation is best assessed in prone position because any restriction can be measured easily

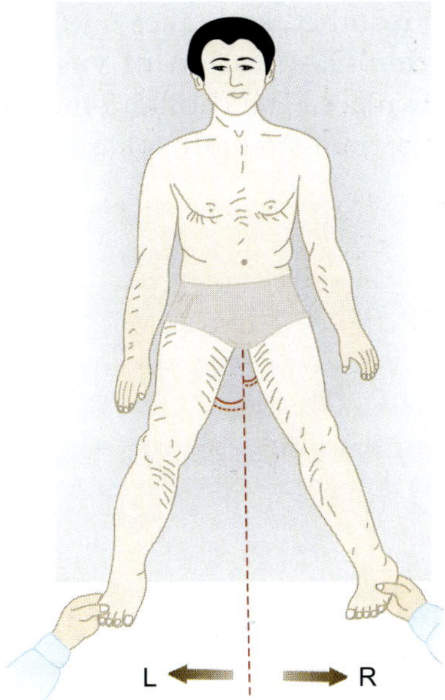

Fig. 32.4: Showing limitation of abduction of the right hip in Perthes' disease

Section 3

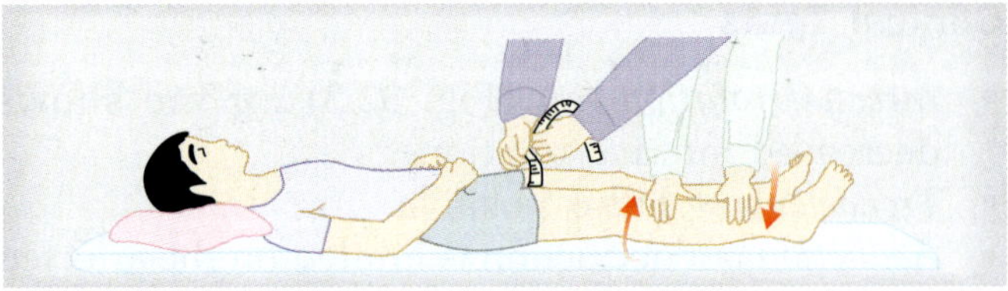

Fig. 32.5: Showing roll test to detect muscle spasm in Perthes' disease (right) and recording of muscle wasting (left)

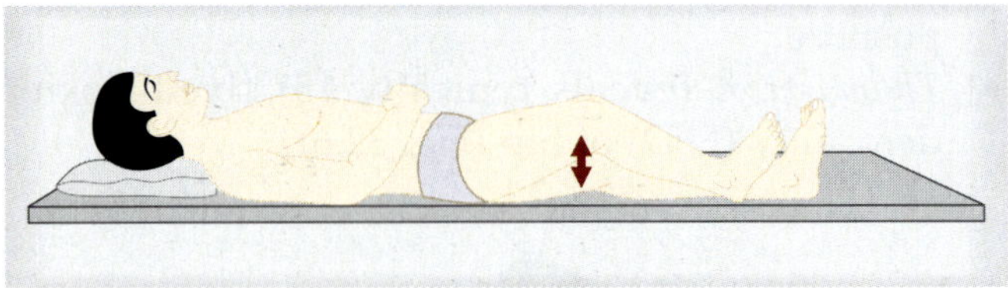

Fig. 32.6: Showing 15° of fixed flexion deformity of the hip which is characteristic in Perthes' disease

Radiographic Characteristics

Perthes' disease is divided into five distinct radiographic stages (Table 32.1).

1. *Cessation of growth of the capital femoral epiphysis* occurs after the initial ischaemic episode and lasts for 6 to 12 months.
2. *Subchondral fractures* (Fig. 32.7) causes collapse of the head and causes ischaemia. Visible on the radiograph for an average of three months.
3. *Resorption* The necrotic epiphyseal bone beneath the subchondral fracture is gradually and irregularly resorbed and takes 6 to 12 months.
4. *Re-ossification* Ossification of vascular fibrous tissue takes place. The capital femoral epiphysis regains its normal strength, takes 6 to 24 months.

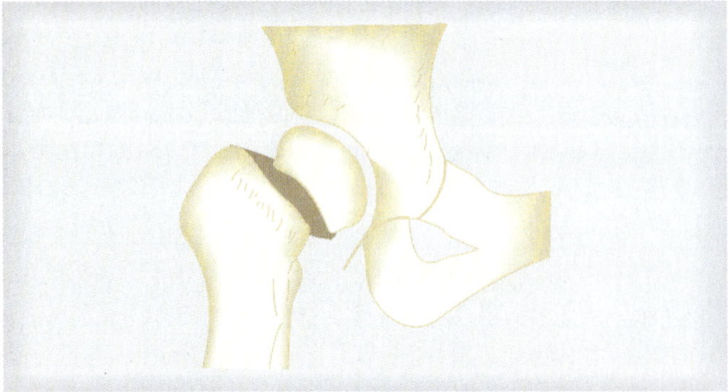

Fig. 32.7: Showing subchondral fracture in Perthes' disease

Table 32.1: Major radiographic characteristics in Perthes'

Group I	Involvement is limited only to the anterior portion of epiphysis.
Group II	Whole epiphysis is involved with the exception of intact lateral margin of epiphysis.
Group III	Involvement of even the lateral margin of epiphysis.
Group IV	Whole head involvement.

5. *Healed or residual stage* The femoral head is healed with or without residual deformity.

Classification

[2]Catterall in 1971 proposed a four group classification system for Perthes' disease based on the radiographic appearance of the femoral head. *This classification has been extremely useful in retrospective analysis of the results of treatment and has a very limited prognostic value (Table 32.2).*

Salter-Thompson's Classification

It simplifies the radiographic criteria and permits early diagnosis of the extent of capital femoral epiphyseal involvement. It is an accurate method to determine the prognosis and decide the form of treatment.

This classification is based on the presence of subchondral fracture:

Group A (Catterall Gr I and II) In this, less than half of the capital femoral epiphysis is involved.

Group B (Catterall Gr III and IV) In this, more than half of the capital femoral epiphysis is involved.

Table 32.2: Catterall's radiological classification of Perthes'

Group	*I*	*II*	*III*	*IV*
Epiphysis				
Anterior	–ve	Part	+ve	+ve
Posterior	–ve	–ve	+ve	+ve
Medial	–ve	–ve	+ve	+ve
Lateral	–ve	–ve	+ve	+ve
	Subchondral fracture			
AP view	–ve	seen	# seen	# seen
Lateral	+ve	# seen	# seen	# seen
Prognosis	Good	Good	Less favourable	Poor

+ve → Affected, –ve → Not affected, # → Fracture

[2]**Anthony Catterall** (1971) described the natural history and monograph of this disease.

The presence of an intact and viable lateral margin of capital femoral epiphysis indicates good prognosis and its absence suggests poor prognosis.

Assessment

Radiographic assessment is necessary to determine the progress of the disease, sphericity of the femoral head, epiphyseal extrusion or collapse, and response to the treatment (Fig. 32.8). Plain radiographs are usually adequate but rarely arthrography, MRI may be required.

Salter's extrusion angle (Fig. 32.9) This angle helps to assess the femoral head extrusion. A horizontal line is drawn from the bottom of acetabular "tear drop" and a perpendicular line is drawn at the lateral ossified margin of the acetabulum. Lines drawn from intersections of these lines through the midpoint of physis give extrusion angles. Normal is 50° or more.

Arthrography It may be useful in the early resorption stage of the disease.

Radionuclide bone scan is used to detect potential form of Perthes' disease.

MRI may be helpful in defining area of epiphyseal infarction and femoral head contour.

Management

Perthes' disease is a local, self-healing disorder of the femoral head. Prevention of the femoral-head deformity and secondary degenerative osteoarthritis is the only justification for treatment.

Treatment Methods

1. *Elimination of hip irritability* can be done by 1 to 2 weeks period of bedrest, sling, suspension, traction, etc.
2. *Restoration and maintenance of hip motion* This can be done by physical therapy active and passive. Abduction exercises may be helpful.
3. *Prevention of the extrusion and collapse* by bedrest, abduction splints, etc.
4. *Attainment of spherical femoral head* to prevent femoral head deformity and can be done by containment methods (see Flow chart) which may be non-surgical or surgical. The following are the four currently accepted forms of management:

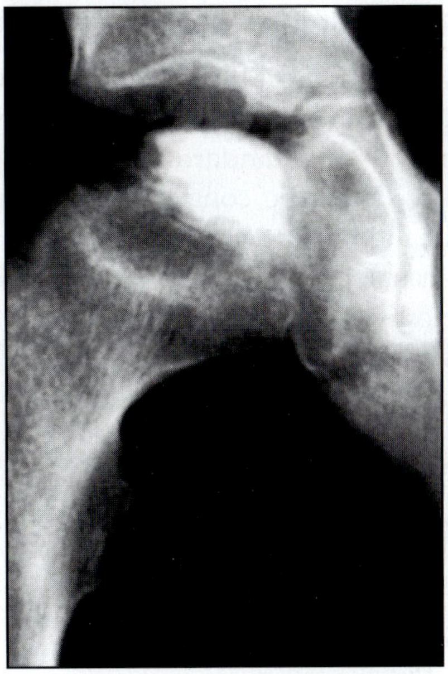

Fig. 32.8: Radiograph showing Perthes' disease

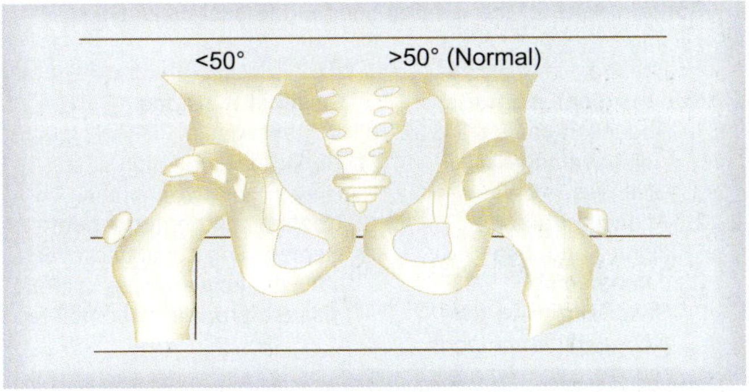

Fig. 32.9: Showing Salter's extrusion angle

a. *Observation* is indicated for children less than 6 years, and for more than 6 years in Caterall I and II.
b. *Intermittent symptomatic treatment* consists of observation, bedrest and abduction exercises.
c. *Definitive early treatment* Non-surgical or surgical containment of the femoral head early in the course of the disease is indicated when the:
   - Age at onset is more than 6 years or older.
   - Catterall III and IV grades.
   - Lateral extrusion of the capital femoral epiphysis.

Prerequisites are good to full range of hip motion, no residual irritability, and the femoral head must also appear round or almost round.

Late Surgical Management for Deformity

For a significant femoral head deformity which prevents reduction into the acetabulum or remodelling after treatment with standard containment methods, an alternative must be considered and may consist of one of the following techniques: muscle release and abduction casts, partial excision of the femoral head or cheillectomy, proximal femoral valgus osteotomy and greater trochanter advancement.

Prognosis

Poor prognostic factors are:

1. Sex—female
2. Age of the clinical onset if more than 6 years
3. Catterall group III and IV
4. Loss of femoral head containment
5. Persistent loss of motion
6. Premature epiphyseal growth plate closure

Flow chart: Treatment plan of Perthes' disease

Containment (of the femoral head in the acetabulum)

↓ ↓

Non-surgical methods

1. Abduction casts (Fig. 32.10) (disadvantage stiffness, etc.)
2. Abduction brace (lighter and less cumbersome)
3. Salter stirrup crutch

Non-surgical methods require approximately 1 year of containment, but eliminates the possible surgical *complications*

Surgical methods

Advantages

1. Period of restoration is less than two months
2. Containment is permanent
3. Remodelling continues even after the active phase of the disease process is completed

↓

Methods

↓ ↓

Femoral varus osteotomy (Fig. 32.11)

↓

- For angulation < 110°
- Osteotomy is fixed with screws and side plates

Problems: ↑ Coxa vara
Shortening

It is technically less demanding procedure than innominate osteotomy. But it has problems like increase in leg length, coxa vara, Trendelenburg gait, etc.

Innominate osteotomy (Fig. 32.12)

↓

- Better coverage
- No further shortening

Disadvantages: It is technically difficult, but it gives a better anterior and lateral coverage of the femoral head and has no disadvantages mentioned in the femoral varus osteotomy.

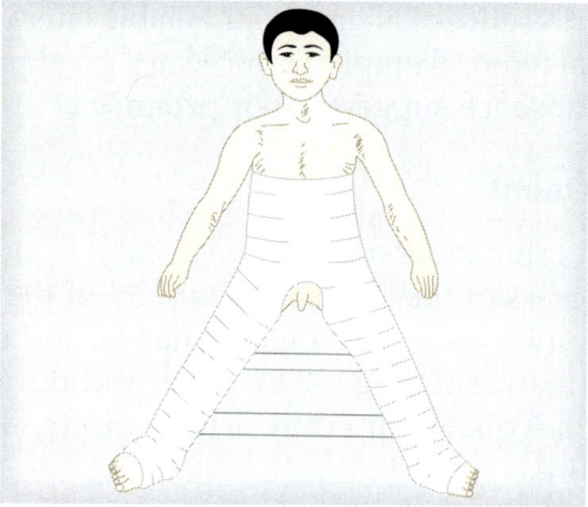

Fig. 32.10: Abduction cast is a non-surgical method of containment in Perthes' disease

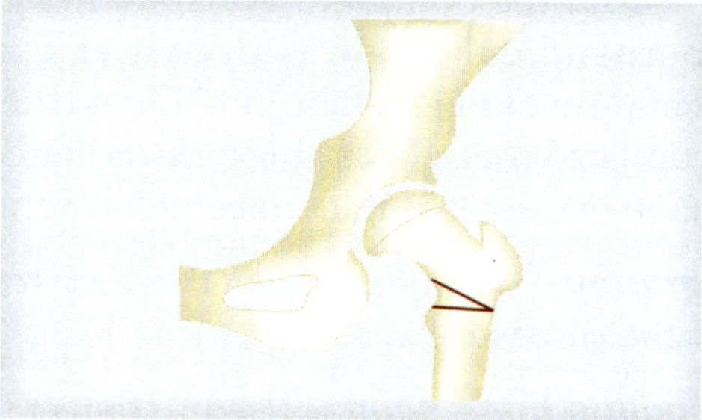

Fig. 32.11: Showing femoral varus osteotomy

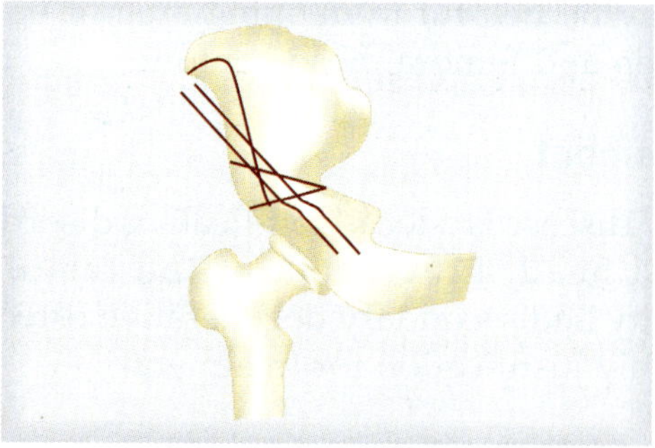

Fig. 32.12: Showing innominate osteotomy

Quick facts: Perthes' disease

- Commonest osteochondroses.
- 80 per cent affected are males between the age group 4 to 8 years.
- Two episodes of infarction.
- First episode cause is not known.
- Second episode is due to subchondral fracture.
- Subchondral fracture heralds onset of true Perthes'.
- Painless limp is the characteristic symptom.
- Decreased abduction, internal rotation is present.
- Catterall's grading helps plan the treatment.
- Salter and Thompson's grading has prognostic value.
- It is a local self-healing disorder.
- The main goal of treatment is to attain a spherical femoral head either by non-surgical or surgical methods.

SLIPPED CAPITAL FEMORAL EPIPHYSIS (SYN: EPIPHYSEAL COXA VARA; ADOLESCENT COXA VARA)

Slipped capital femoral epiphysis (SCFE) occurs during adolescent rapid growth preiod when epiphyseal plate is weak and the capital epiphysis is displaced down and back (Fig. 32.13). It was first described by **Muller** in 1889.

Aetiology

Predisposing factors

1. *Age* It is common in 10 to 17 years of age
2. *Sex* Male:Female is 5:2 ratio
3. *Body type* Female—slender long built, and male—obesity type
4. *Location* Left hip is involved in 58 per cent of the cases.
5. *Trauma* Trivial or none at all.

Theories of causations

1. **Harris hormonal theory** Due to hormonal imbalance between the increased growth hormone and decreased sex and thyroid hormone.
2. **Traumatic theory** Epiphyseal line is the weakest part of the normal adolescent bone.
3. **Theory of periosteal thinning** Periosteum which is thick in children, thins out during adolescence.

Clinical Features and Investigations

a. *Acute (11%)* Sudden onset and the symptoms are less than two weeks duration
b. *Chronic (60%)* Symptoms are present for more than two weeks. X-ray shows callus and remodelling
c. *Acute on chronic (23%)* Symptoms are present for one month and there is a recent sudden increase in pain following trivial injury.
d. *Preslip (6%)* X-ray shows irregular wide epiphysis.

Stages

For clinical stages see Table 32.3.

Radiographic changes

Early changes

- Marginal blurring of the proximal metaphysis.
- Lower margin of metaphysis is included within the acetabulum normally but excluded in the early epiphyseal slip.
- *Trethovan's line* (Figs 32.14A and B) Line drawn along the superior margin of the neck, transects the epiphysis normally, but will be above it in slip.

Table 32.3: Showing stages in SCFE and clinical features

Pre-slipping stage	*Chronic slipping stage*	*Stage of fixed deformity*
• Discomfort in the groin • Stiffness/limp • No objective finding • Medial rotation of the hip is decreased.	• Pain ↑ • Antalgic gait • All movements ↓ particularly. Abduction and internal rotation • Varus + Adduction + External rotation deformity is present • Shortening is present • Extension and external rotation ↑ • Waddling gait is present • Trendelenburg's gait is positive	• No pain • No spasm • Limb shortening + • External rotation + • Adduction deformity

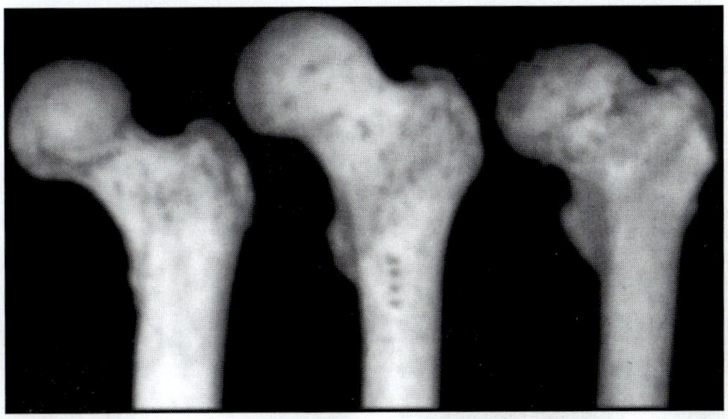

Fig. 32.13: Radiographs showing cadaveric specimen of a slipped capital femoral epiphysis

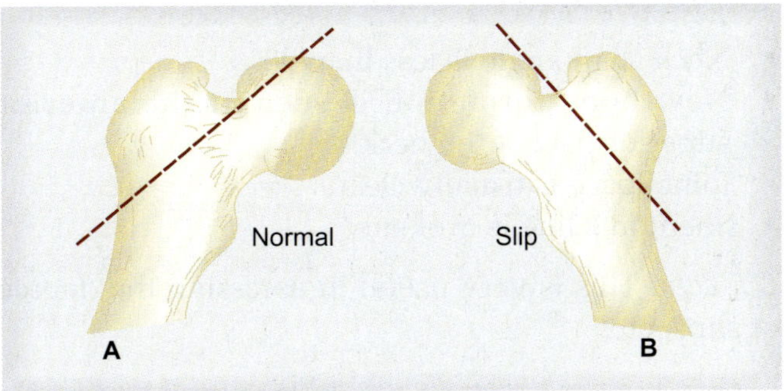

Figs 32.14A and B: Showing Trethovan's sign

- Depth of epiphysis is reduced.
- There is a step between the metaphysis and the epiphysis (Fig. 32.15).

Late changes (Figs 32.16A and B)

- Trethovan's sign is present.
- Head is atrophic.

Section 3

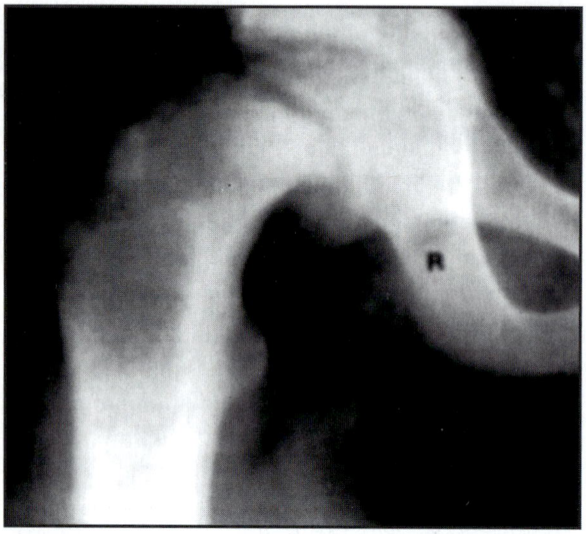

Fig. 32.15: Radiograph showing SCFE (early changes)

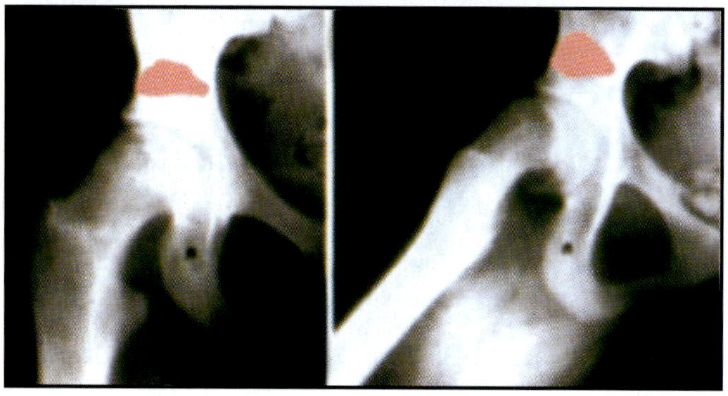

Figs 32.16A and B: Radiographs showing SCFE (late changes)

- Neck shaft angle is less than 90°.
- New bone formation is seen at the anterior superior part of the neck.
- Joint space is usually clear.
- Shenton's line is broken.

CT scan This is very useful in assessing the degree of slips, etc.

Classification of Slipping

1. *Mild slipping: (51%)* Neck is displaced less than one-third of the diameter of the head or head-shaft angle deviates from the normal by less than 30°.
2. *Moderate slipping: (22%)* Neck is displaced more than one-third to one-half of the diameter of the head or the head shaft angle deviates from the normal between 30 and 60°.
3. *Severe slipping: (17%)* Neck is displaced more than one-half diameter of the head or head shaft angle is more than 60° from normal.

Principles of treatment are as follows:

- If epiphysis has begun to displace, there is no safety till the epiphyseal line has fused.
- When there is minor displacement, epiphysis is fused at once by pining in displaced position.
- Acute major slip: Emergency reduction is done under (GA) or reduction is obtained by traction and fixed with pins.
- Irreducible displacement: This is treated by open reduction and cervical osteotomy.
- Old fixed displacement: This is treated by a corrective osteotomy at the intertrochanteric or subtrochanteric level.

Complications

Avascular necrosis (13%) of the femoral head and chondrolysis are the usual complications. Secondary osteoarthritis may be seen at later stages.

Hip Pointer This is a contusion over the iliac crest due to a fall directly on it in sports like football, gymnastics, basketball, etc.

REGIONAL DISORDERS OF THE KNEE

Deformities around the knee joint could be in two planes. In the coronal plane, we may encounter genu valgum and genu varum deformities; and in the sagittal plane, antevertum and recurvatum deformities (Figs 32.17A to E).

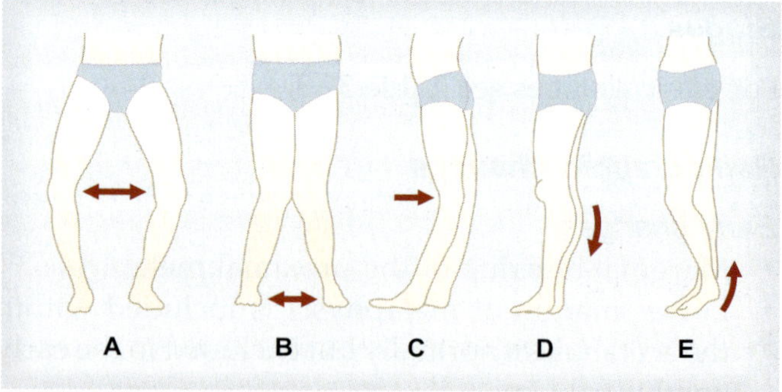

Figs 32.17A to E: Various knee deformities (A) Genu varum, (B) Genu valgum, (C) Genu recurvatum, (D) Triple deformity, (E) Fixed flexion deformity

Strange it may seem but a normal knee is a crooked knee. Nature identifies a 6° physiological outward deviation of the knee (valgum) as normal and not a straight knee! Only when the crookedness of the knee increases (genu valgum) or decreases (genu varum) or when it bends backwards (recurvatum) that it is considered abnormal and is a cause of worry. A person affected by any one of these conditions is brought on his "knees" and is forced to seek remedial measures to be up on his "knees" normally again!

GENU VALGUM (KNOCK KNEE)

Definition It is an outward deviation of the longitudinal axes of both tibia and femur. Apex of the curve or angulation of the knee is medial (Fig. 32.18).

Incidence

Seventy-five per cent children have genu valgum up to 4 years of age. This is called physiological genu valgum which usually disappears by 7 years.

Types

It is broadly classified into physiological and pathological, the latter could be unilateral or bilateral (Table 32.4).

Table 32.4: Causes of genu valgum

Unilateral	*Bilateral*
• Trauma • Osteomyelitis • Tumours	• *Physiological* (disappears by 4 yr) • *Pathological* • Congenital disorders • Idiopathic (most common) • Developmental disorders (e.g., epiphyseal dysplasia) • Endocrine disorders (e.g. thyroid disorders) • Metabolic disorders (e.g. rickets) • Paralytic disorders • Traumatic disorders • Infective disorders • Degenerative disorders • Inflammatory disorders (e.g. rheumatoid arthritis)

Clinical Features

Genu valgum complex The primary deformity in a genu valgum is *a medial angulation of the knee*. In response to this, secondary deformities develop in the femur, tibia and foot. Primary and secondary deformities together form the genu valgum complex.

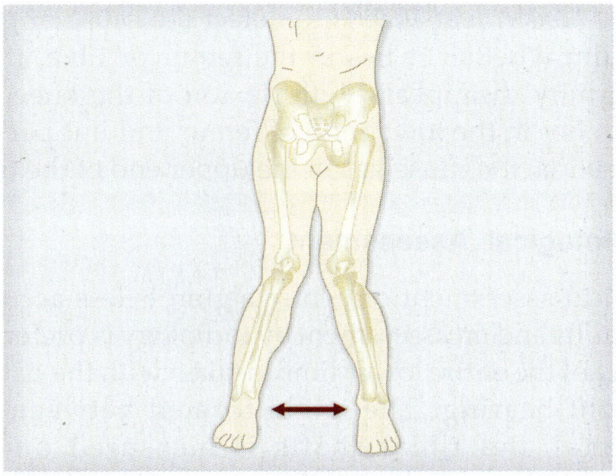

Fig. 32.18: Genu valgum or knock knee deformity

Genu valgum complex

Primary deformity
Medial angulation of the knee

Secondary deformities
1. Distal ends of femur and proximal ends of tibia are rotated externally by pull of biceps and tensor fascia lata.
2. Distal end of tibia develops a compensatory internal torsion.
3. Lateral dislocation of patella.
4. Lateral structures shortened, medial structures elongated (of knee).
5. Pronated flat foot.

Quick facts

Idiopathic genu valgum
The following are its features:
- Commonest variety
- Invariably bilateral
- Deformity is the only complaint
- Occurs at the age of 2 to 3 years and
- Recovers by the age of 6 years

Assessment of Genu Valgum Deformity

Clinical Assessment

Intermalleolar gap The severiy of the deformity is measured by noting the intermalleolar distance.

Method In the spine position the patella is brought to vertical by rotating both the legs and made to touch lightly at the knee. Then holding both the knees in position, the distance between the two malleoli is measured. The acceptable normal limit is 8 to 10 cm. In genu valgum deformity it will be more than 10 cm.

Plumbline test Normally, a line drawn from anterior superior iliac spine (ASIS) to middle of the patella, if extended down strikes the medial malleolus. In genu valgum, the medial malleolus will be outside this line.

Knee flexion test This is to detect the cause of genu valgum whether it lies in the femur or tibia. If the deformity disappears with flexion of the knee, the cause lies in the lower end of femur and if it persists on flexion, the cause lies in the upper end of the tibia.

Radiological Assessment

Clinical assessment of genu valgum is less accurate in adults and an assessment by radiology is preferred. X-ray of the entire lower limb is taken with the patient weight bearing. The angle formed between the femoral and tibial shafts is measured on the radiographs and allowing for a normal angle of 6°, genu valgum is calculated.

Treatment of Genu Valgum (Table 32.5)

1. **Mild cases** Child is seen at intervals of 3 months and the progress is recorded. These cases usually require no treatment, and raising the inner side of the heels by 4 to 5 mm may possibly relieve strain on ankles. The knock knee braces may be useful. If by the age of 4 years, intermalleolar distance is 10 cm or more, operation may become necessary and unless deformity is increasing rapidly, operation is best postponed till the child is 10 years old.
2. **Severe cases**
   a. If lateral portion of epiphyseal plate is intact as seen in the radiographs, it contributes to the longitudinal growth at a reduced rate. This situation is suitable for stapling of the medial epiphysis which arrests the growth on the medial side and allows the growth on the lateral side and thus helps to correct the deformity.
   b. After skeletal maturity, an osteotomy must be performed at the site of maximum deformity of tibia or femur. If limb is long, *medial close wedge osteotomy* is done. If limb is short, *lateral open wedge osteotomy* is done. *Knock knee deformity more than 10 cm at the age of 10 years is an indication for surgery.*

Treatment facts of genu valgum
- < 4 yr—No treatment
- 4–10 yr—Heel raise, knock knee brace
- 10–14 yr—Epiphyseal stapling
- 14–16 yr—Wait till skeletal maturity as it is too late for stapling and too early for osteotomy, as it may recur
- > 16 yr—Osteotomy

Table 32.5: Treatment of genu valgum

Mild (< 8 cm IM distance at 4 yr)	*Severe (> 10 cm IM at 10 yr)*
• **No treatment** • Raise medial heel by 4–5 mm • Knock knee brace (outer iron bar, inner strap) ↓	**Surgery** • Unilateral genu valgum • Intermalleolar distance > 10 cm at 10 yr ↓
Epiphyseal arrest • Done before skeletal maturity • Lateral epiphysis should be intact as seen in X-ray • Staple the medial epiphysis to arrest the growth	**Osteotomy** • Done after skeletal maturity • Medial closed wedge osteotomy if limb is longer or normal • Lateral open wedge osteotomy if limb is short

Note: IM = Intermalleolar

Quick facts: genu valgum
- Medial angulation of the knee
- 75 per cent is physiological up to 4 years of age
- Idiopathic is the most common type
- Deformity is the only complaint

GENU VARUM (BOW LEGS)

Definition It is defined as *a lateral angulation of the knee. The longitudinal axis of femur and tibia deviates medially.*

The deformity involves tibia alone or the femur or tibia and fibula (Fig. 32.19) both.

Types and Causes

Unilateral
1. Due to growth abnormalities of upper tibial epiphysis.
2. Infections like osteomyelitis, etc.
3. Trauma near the growth epiphysis of femur.
4. Tumours affecting the lower end of femur and upper end of tibia.

Bilateral
1. Physiological (gets corrected by four years).
2. Pathological:
   - Congenital causes
   - Postural abnormalities
   - Developmental disorders
   - Metabolic disorders (rickets rare)
   - Endocrine disorders

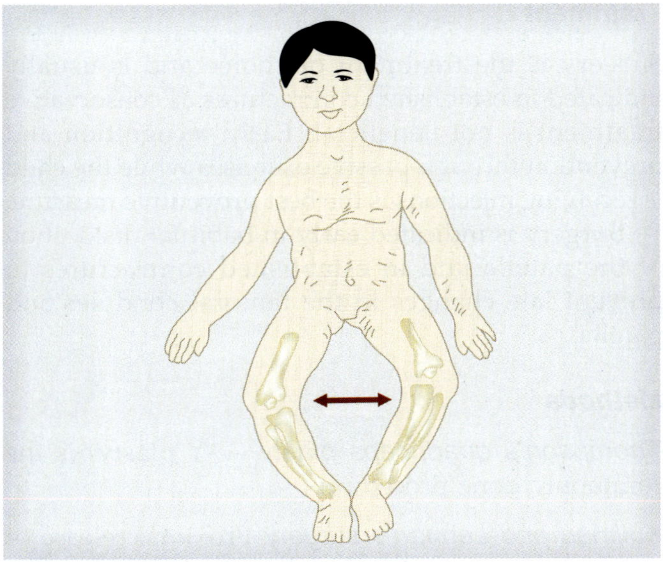

Fig. 32.19: Showing genu varum with increased intercondylar distance. Genu varum is said to exist if there is approximately 3 cm gap between the medial femoral condyles when the malleoli are together

- Degenerative disorders (e.g. osteoarthritis of knee). This is a common cause.
- Occupational disorders (e.g. in jockeys)
- Idiopathic
- Paget's disease
- 'Blounts' disease (tibia vara).

Clinical Measurements of the Deformity

Child

1. The patient is examined supine with knee extended, patella facing the ceiling and the medial malleoli touching each other. If the separation of knee exceeds more than 3 cm or if it is unilateral, it should be investigated.
2. A line is drawn from anterior superior iliac spine through centre of patella to medial malleolus. Normally, all the structures are in the same line but in genu varum medial malleolus is medial to this line.

Adults The angle of genu varum is calculated on a standing radiograph of the whole limb.

Clinical Features

Genu varum complex The primary deformity in genu varum is *lateral angulation of the knee*. In response to this secondary deformities develop in the tibia and the foot. This together is known as genu varum complex (Table 32.6).

Table 32.6: The primary and secondary deformities in genu varum

Primary deformity	*Secondary deformity*
Lateral angulation of the knee	**Associated abnormalities** 1. An internal torsion of distal tibia 2. Intoeing of both the feet 3. Patella face outward while walking 4. Tight medial and lax lateral structures of the knee

Note:
What is apparent genu varum?
Due to anteversion of femoral neck, there is medial rotation of the femur and the child looks bow-legged. But with the patella facing forwards, the "varus deformity" disappears.

Treatment

- Treatment should be conservative till four years of age. Knee-ankle-foot orthoses with the medial bar and the lateral strap is used.
- Correction of early deformity is done by dynamic bracing or splints. After four years, significant deformity should be corrected by surgery. Lateral epiphyseal stapling when the child is within the growth period and supracondylar medial open or lateral closed wedge osteotomy is done after skeletal maturity.

GENU RECURVATUM

Genu recurvatum is defined as *backward bending of the knee*. Up to 5° of genu recurvatum is sometimes seen in women with lax ligaments and is usually generalised. Here, the popliteal fossa is convex instead of concave.

Causes

1. *Congenital* discusssed in congenital disorders.
2. *Quadriceps contracture* is the most common cause in acquired genu recurvatum and is discussed below.
3. *Neurological disorders* Polio, cerebral palsy, etc.
4. *Malunited fractures* around the knee.

Quadriceps contracture There are two varieties:

1. Congenital variety.

2. Postinjection contractures of infancy and childhood.

Quadriceps contracture in early childhood has an age of onset between one and seven years.

Features

1. Limitation of knee flexion from mild to severe.
2. Effusion and other evidence of knee abnormality is absent.
3. Sometimes a dense band that becomes tense during flexion of the knee could be palpated in the proximal part of the patella.
4. Patella is always located more proximally and sometimes laterally.
5. Other features include; it is usually bilateral, common in identical twins, more common in females, and extremely resistant to conservative treatment.

Clinical Tests to Measure Genu Recurvatum

- It is to be measured in the weight bearing position from the lateral side
- The long axis of the thigh (from the tip of the trochanter to the midpoint of the lateral femoral condyle) is drawn
- The long axis of the leg is drawn next (from the middle of the lateral tibial condyle and the lateral malleolus).
- The angle between these two lines is the angle of recurvatum.

Post-injection contractures in infancy First described in 1962 by Miki.

Features

1. Repeated injections and infusions to the thigh soon after birth.
2. Dimples present in the skin at the sites of injections.
3. Common in twins and prematurity (because they often make injections necessary and in infants anterior thigh is commonly the preferred site).
   The muscles usually involved are:
   a. Vastus lateralis
   b. Rectus femoris
   c. Vastus intermedius: *Vastus medialis is not involved because injections are not given to this muscle.*

Treatment

Surgery is the treatment of choice and is usually indicated in established contractures as conservative treatment is not beneficial. Early recognition and prevention through passive exercises while the child is receiving injections is the best preventive measure.

Surgery is indicated early in habitual dislocation of the patella and in established contractures to prevent late changes in the femoral condyles and patella.

Methods

Thompson's quadriceps plasty (V-Y plasty) is the commonly done procedure.

Kullman and Leonart's surgery Proximal release of rectus femoris in an isolated contracture of rectus femoris.

BURSAE AROUND THE KNEE (Figs 32.20A and B)

Knee is a complex joint in the body subserving complex functions. To do so, it requires a host of ligaments, muscles, menisci, etc. To serve the knee efficiently and longer, these structures need to be cushioned properly from the bony surfaces. As long as the knee is being used normally, no problems are encountered. Violation of the physiological actions by way of over and abnormal use frustrates and irritates these cushions which are nothing but bursae around the knee giving rise to various interesting clinical problems.

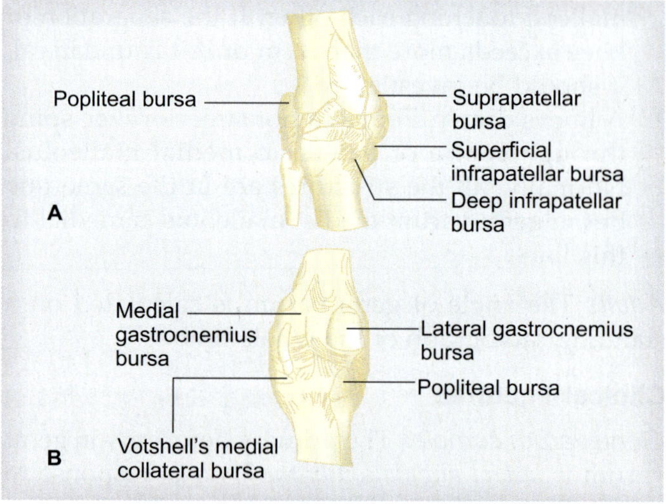

Figs 32.20A and B: Bursae around the knee

Bursae are sacs lined with membrane similar to synovium. They are located over the joints and bony prominences and may or may not communicate with the joint. They reduce the friction and protect the delicate structures from pressures. When subjected to repeated pressure, they give rise to bursitis. There are two types of bursae, one that is normally present and second, an adventitious bursa which develops due to trauma, friction, pressure, etc. Adventitious bursae differ from true bursae by the lack of true endothelial or synovial lining.

Bursae around the knee are as follows.

Anterior

a. *Suprapatellar* Always communicates with the knee joint.
b. *Prepatellar bursitis* (housemaid's knee) (Figs 32.21A and B) is seen in the lower half of patella and upper half of ligamentum patella.
c. *Infrapatellar* seen in the lower half of ligamentum patella (clergyman's, Parson's, or Carpet layer's knee or Vicar's knee) (Fig. 32.22).

Lateral Cyst of lateral meniscus.

Medial

a. Cyst of medial meniscus.
b. Bursa anserina—Between the tibial collateral ligament and tendons of the semimembranosus, gracilis, semitendinosus.

Posteriorly

a. Semimembranosus bursitis
b. Baker's cyst
c. Lymphangiectsia
d. Aneurysm of popliteal artery
e. Neuromyxofibroma.

POPLITEAL CYST (BAKER'S CYST)

This was first described by Adam in the year 1840 and later by [3]Baker in 1877.

What is Baker's cyst?

The exact origin is not known, but it is a distended bursa arising from any one of the structures below:
- Between hamstrings and collateral ligaments.
- Between hamstrings and tibial condyles.
- Each head of gastrocnemius.

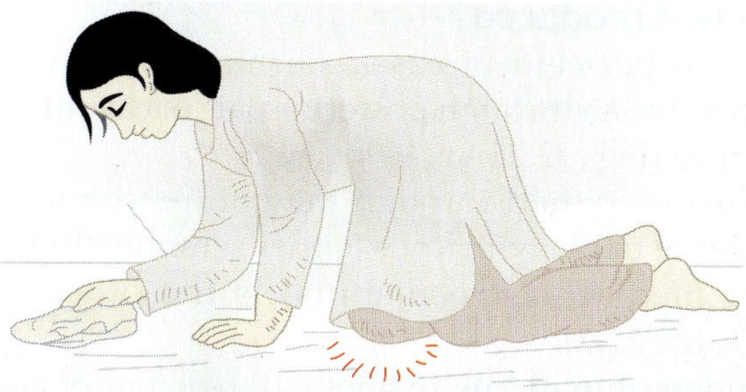

Fig. 32.21A: This is how a housemaid insults her knee

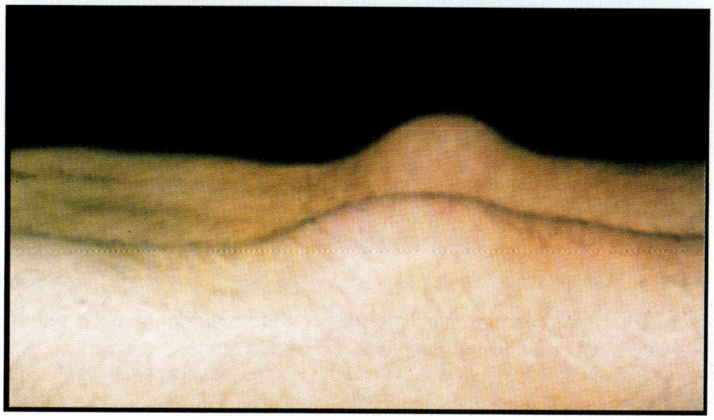

Fig. 32.21B: Clinical photograph of a prepatellar bursitis

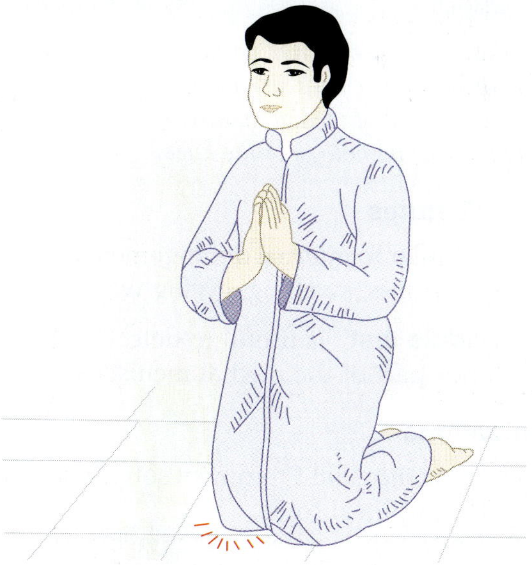

Fig. 32.22: When a clergyman prays for others, his knee weeps in silence

Commonly symptoms are seen in bursa of the medial head of gastrocnemius and semimembranosus bursa.

[3]**William Morrant Baker** (1838-1896) of England. Described Baker's cyst in 1877.

How is it produced?

1. In 30 per cent of cases, herniation of synovial membrane through posterior part of capsule takes place (Fig. 32.23A).
2. Escape of fluid through the normal communication of bursa with knee (either semimembranosus or medial gastrocnemius) is the other mode (Table 32.7).
3. Indeterminate site in about 10 per cent of cases.

What is a giant cyst?

It is a huge popliteal cyst commonly seen in rheumatoid arthritis.

Treatment

- 1 to 2 days of non-surgical treatment.
- Later, arthrography and cyst is excised.
- Synovectomy is done later to prevent recurrence.

Table 32.7: Difference between Baker's cyst in children and adults

Children	*Adults*
• No communication with the joint	• Communication is present
• Intra-articular pathology is rare	• Commonly seen in 50 per cent of cases
• No recurrence even with complete removal of the cyst	• Recurrence is common
• Postoperative immobilisation is not required	• Postoperative immobilisation is required

In adults, intra-articular pathology is seen in 50 per cent, of these 50 per cent are caused by a lesion in the posterior one-third of medial meniscus and the remaining from some other pathology of the knee.

Clinical Features

These are similar to internal derangement of the knee, like pain, stiffness, swelling, giving way, etc.

"Duck waddle test" is useful to detect pathology in the posterior part of the medial meniscus.

Investigations

- *X-ray of the knee joint* Prominent soft tissue swelling over the popliteal fossa.
- *Ultrasound* This is a very effective diagnostic tool with 100% sensitivity.
- *MRI* This is the next best.
- *Arthrography* This is invasive but very effective (Fig. 32.23B).

Treatment

The treatment of choice is excision of the bursa and closure of the capsular orifice by:

1. Scarrification of the edges and suture.

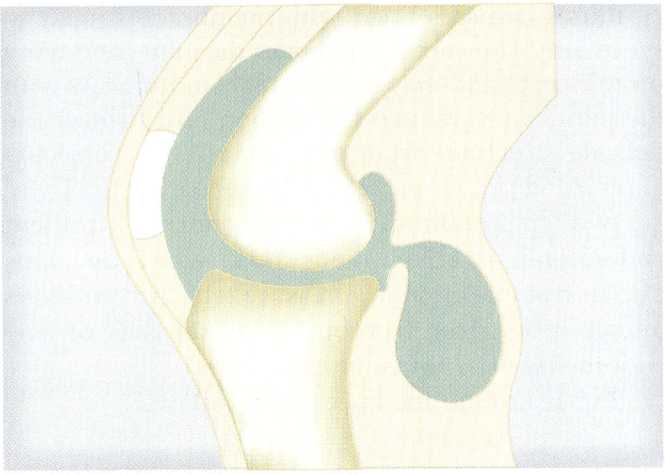

Fig. 32.23A: Baker's cyst arises from the herniation of the synovial membrane through the capsule

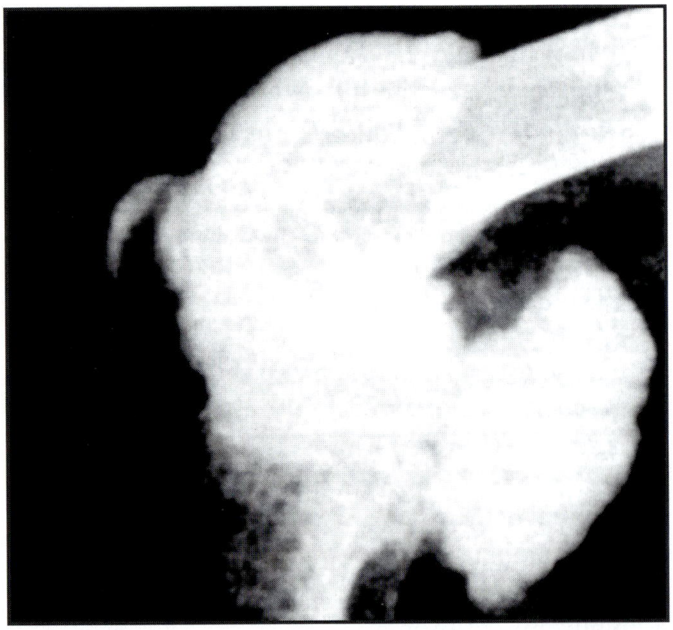

Fig. 32.23B: Arthrography showing ruptured popliteal cyst

2. To close the gap by a graft from tendinous part of the gastrocnemius, etc.
3. Arthroscopic Treatment: This is found to be very effective treatment of popliteal cyst and associated intra-articular pathology with 95% success rate.

It helps in curing the intra-articular pathology and also correcting the valvular mechanism responsible for formation and recurrence of the popliteal cyst.

One-third to one-half of patients with Baker's cyst are children. It is rare after seventh year of life. Hence, delay in excision is followed by gradual disappearance of the cyst.

RECURRENT DISLOCATION OF PATELLA

It is a condition caused by recurrent dislocation of patella usually to the lateral side. This is usually preceded by an episode of acute traumatic dislocation of the patella and probably has not healed properly after the initial trauma.

It has to be diffentiated from another entity called habitual dislocation of patella in which the patella dislocates with each flexion and extension movements of the knee.

The following are the predisposing factors responsible for recurrent dislocation of patella:

1. Patella alta
2. Genu valgum
3. Hypoplastic lateral condyle of femur
4. Tight lateral structures of the knee joint
5. Lax medial patellar retinaculum
6. Femoral anteversion
7. External femoral torsion
8. Genu recurvatum
9. Abnormal insertion of vastus medialis
10. Patellar tendon laterally inserted
11. External tibial rotation
12. Hypoplastic patella
13. Atrophy of vastus medialis
14. Hypertrophy of vastus lateralis
15. Generalised joint relaxation.

Clinical Features

The patient gives history of diffuse pain in the knee joint which gets worsened by going up and down the stairs or hills. He or she complains of a feeling of insecurity in the knee and may feel the joint is about to give way or the patella is about to go out! On examination in addition to the predisposing factors mentioned above, there may be a mild swelling and crepitus in the joint. The apprehension test is positive. In this test the patient's knee is held flexed at 30° and an attempt is made to push the patella laterally. In a positive test the patient complains of pain and resists the attempt. Next the Q-angle (Fig. 32.24) is determined. If the Q-angle is more than 10°, medial transplantation of the patellar tendon is recommended.

Interesting facts: About 'Q'-Angle

Do you know what is Malicious Malalignment Syndrome? Well, when all of the following are present together, it constitutes the MMS:

- Excessive femoral arteversion
- External tibial torsion
- Genu valgum
- Increase in Q-angle.

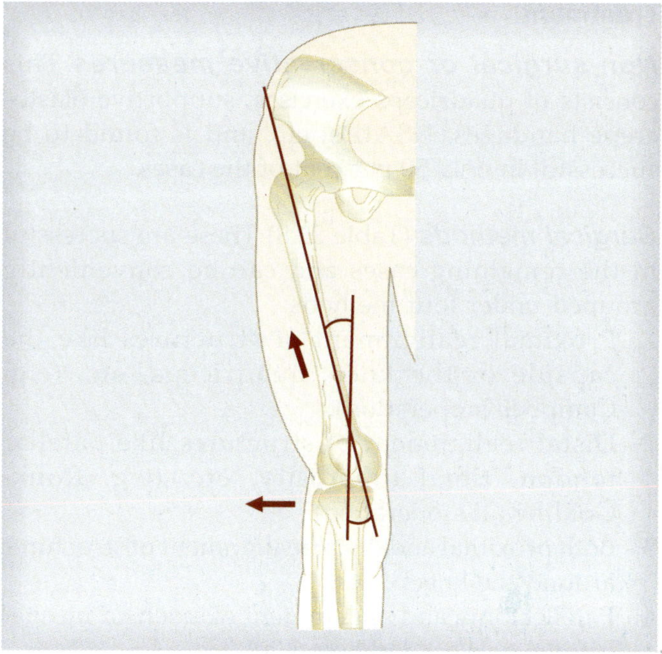

Fig. 32.24: Showing the 'Q'-angle

Radiography

Radiograph of the knee The following radiographic views are necessary: AP view, lateral view, infrapatellar view and the intercondylar notch view or the tunnel view. In the lateral view, the Blumensaat's line (Fig. 32.25) is drawn which represents the bony roof of the intercondylar notch. Normally, the lower pole of the patella just touches that line. If the patella is above this line, a diagnosis of high riding patella is made.

Again, in the lateral view, the ratio between the length of the patella and the length of the patellar tendon is determined. If it is more than 1, it suggests patella alta. This is also known as Insaal's line.

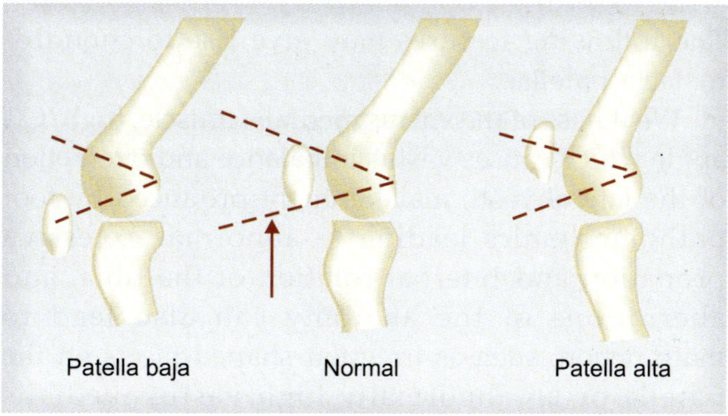

Fig. 32.25: Showing the Bluemensaat's line

Treatment

Non-surgical or conservative measures This consists of quadriceps exercises, supportive elasto-crepe bandages, NSAIDs, etc. and is found to be successful in only 50 per cent of the cases.

Surgical methods (Table 32.8) These are successful in the remaining cases and can be conveniently grouped under four methods:

1. Proximal realignment of structures like the capsule of the knee, quadriceps, etc. (e.g. Campbell's operation).
2. Distal realignment of structures like patellar tendon, tibial tuberosity, etc. (e.g. Roux-Goldthwait's operation).
3. Both proximal and distal realignment of structures around the knee.
4. Patellectomy and realignment of extensor mechanism, e.g. West and Soto Hall.

Table 32.8: A brief account of the surgical procedures

Surgery	What is done?
1. *Campbell's*	Proximal to the knee, the capsule is stripped and carried from medial to the lateral side.
2. *Roux-Goldthwait's procedure*	Here lateral structures of the knee are released and the patellar tendon is split and the lateral half is transferred medially.
3. *Galeazzi's procedure*	Here the semitendinosus tendon is tenodesed to patella.
4. *Houser's procedure (Fig. 32.26)*	Here the tibial tuberosity is shifted down and medial.
5. *Elmsllie-Trillat procedure*	Here release of lateral knee structures, plication of medial structures and medial transfer of tibial tuberosity is done.
6. *Hughston's procedure*	It is a combination of the above procedures.
7. *West and Soto Hall procedure*	This includes patellectomy and is done as a last resort.

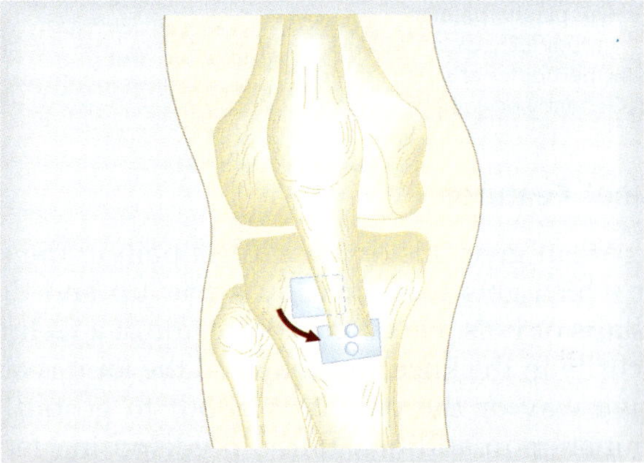

Fig. 32.26: Showing surgical method of treating recurrent dislocation of patella (Houser's method)

CHONDROMALACIA PATELLA

It is defined as a blistering, cystic change of the patellar cartilage and it usually affects the medial facet of the patella. This condition is commonly associated with vastus medialis tendinitis.

It is caused by the combination of several factors which ultimately push the patella out of its groove on the femur. It is attributed to a decrease in sulphated mucopolysaccharide in the ground substance.

> **Did you know?**
> The term 'chondromalacia patella' was coined by Aleman in 1928.

Factors

The following features may give rise to chondromalacia patellae.

Weakness of the vastus medialis muscle, high 'Q'-angle which causes vastus imbalance and overaction of the lateral vasti, malalignment produced by foot pathomechanics leading to abnormal excessive pronation and internal rotation of the tibia, and aberrations of the anatomy can also lead to malfunction, such as irregular-shaped facets on the patella or an abnormally high vastus medialis insertion.

Clinical Features

The patient complains of generalised deep pain in the knee. The knee may be swollen with a chronic effusion of synovial fluid and there will be a positive patellofemoral grinding test when the condition is severe (Fig. 32.27). The patella will appear out of alignment and there may well be a high 'Q'-angle. The vastus medialis will be weak, radiographs will occasionally show spurring and the patient will be unable to do squats. In this condition the typical complaint is that of pain in the knees after prolonged sitting as in watching a movie or while travelling.

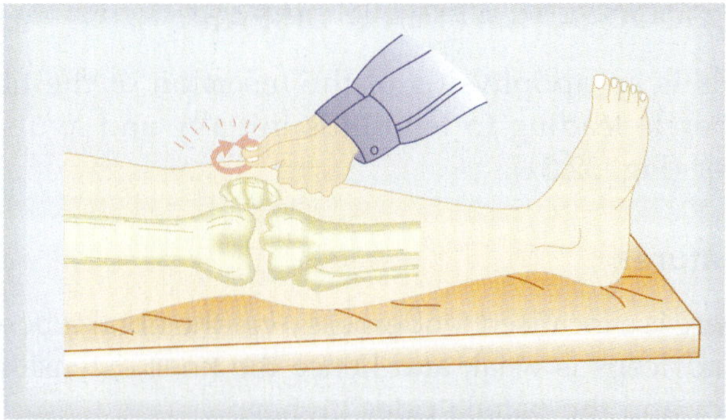

Fig. 32.27: Showing method of performing grinding test in chondromalacia patella

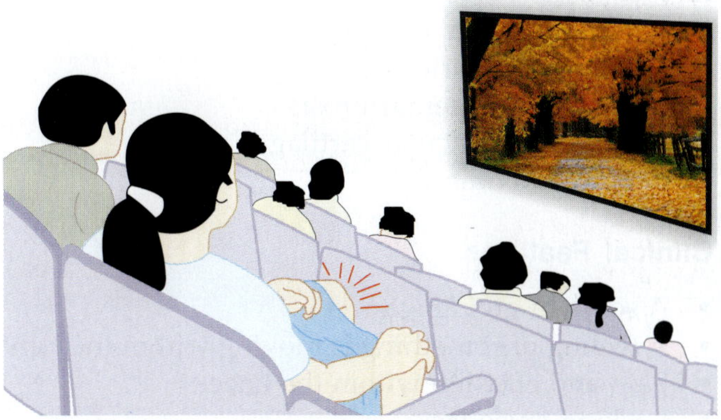

Fig. 32.28: Showing the 'Movie' Sign, a hallmark of chondromalacia

Interesting facts: About Movie sign

If your knees play a spoilsport while you are engrossed watching a movie, watch out, you may be suffering from the irksome chondromalacia patellae! (Fig. 32.28)

Investigations

Radiographs of the knee shows irregular retropatellar surface (Fig. 32.29). Arthroscopy is an extremely useful diagnostic technique. MRI is another very useful investigative option (Figs 32.30A and B).

Differential Diagnosis

Chronic synovitis of the knee, sprain of the retinacula, etc.

Treatment

Treatment consists of ice and ultrasound massage of the painful area, realignment of the maltracking of the patella by orthotic therapy and arthroscopic shaving of the retropatellar surface gives excellent results.

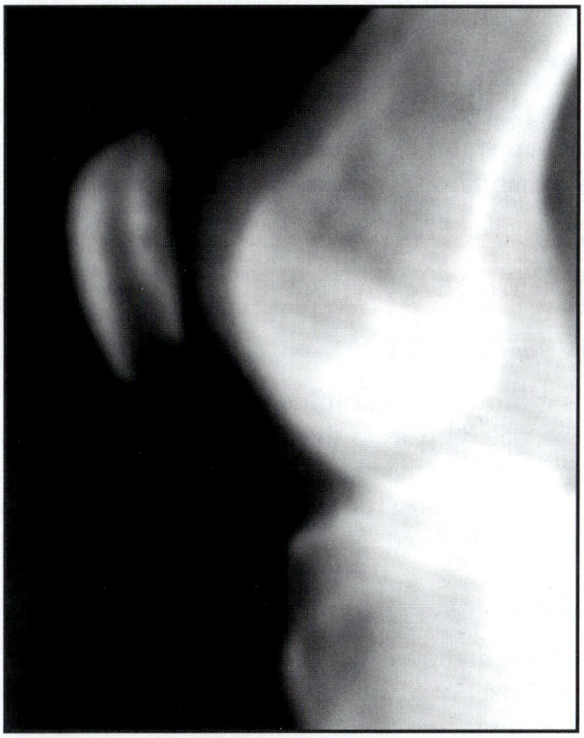

Fig. 32.29: Radiograph showing chondromalacia

LOOSE BODIES IN THE KNEE (JOINT MICE)

Important causes of loose bodies in the knee are:

I. *Non-Traumatic*
- TB arthritis
- Rheumatoid arthritis
- Osteoarthritis
- Osteochondritis dissecans
- Synovial chondromatosis
- Haemarthrosis
- Haemophilia.

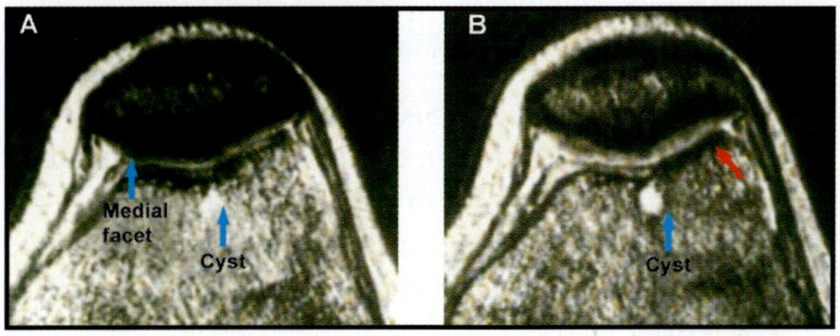

Figs 32.30A and B: MRI showing chondromalacia

II. *Traumatic:*
- Intra-articular fracture
- Meniscal injuries
- Organised haemarthrosis
- Detached articular cartilages
- Foreign bodies.

Clinical Features

- A sense of giving way
- A feeling of something is moving within the joint
- Pain and effusion within the knee
- Locking episodes.

Investigations

This consists of X-ray, diagnostic arthroscopy, MRI etc.

Remedy Arthroscopic removal of the loose bodies is the treatment method of choice and is considered the Gold Standard.

LESSER KNOWN BUT IMPORTANT REGIONAL CONDITIONS OF THE KNEE

JUMPER'S KNEE

This is a patellar tendinitis involving the lower pole of the patella due to overuse of the patellofemoral extensor mechanism. Superior pole of the patella and the site of the insertion at the tibia tubercle can also be rarely involved.

Features

The presentation is very typical and consists of pain at the onset of activity, this reduces during activity and again recurs at the completion of the activity.

Treatment

Some of the recommended measures are:
- Rest to the knee
- RICE regimen and NSAIDs
- *Exercises*: Isometric quadriceps exercises, inferior pateller glides, isotonic quadriceps exercises, hamstring stretching and eccenteric quadriceps stretching are some of the recommended exercise measures.
- Proper orthotic shoes and orthotics to correct hyperpronation.

OSGOOD-SCHLATTER'S DISEASE

This is an apophysitis of the insertion of the tibial tubercle leading to tendinitis initially and avulsion later (Fig. 32.31).

Features

There is a localised tenderness over the tibial tubercle, quadriceps is weak and hence the knee extension is poor and the patella rides higher.

Treatment

It is the same as for jumper's knee. In recalcitrant cases, local steroid injections may help.

SINDING-LARSON-JOHANSSEN SYNDROME

This is an apophysitis of the patellar tendon at the insertion of the patellar tendon into the distal pole of the patella.

ILIO-TIBIAL BAND (ITB) SYNDROME

You already know that ITB is a tendinous and fascial continuation of the tensor fascia latae. It is often inflamed in over-the-hill runner due to repeated friction.

Later, knee pain, tenderness over the ITB band and positive Ober's test all help to clinch the diagnosis.

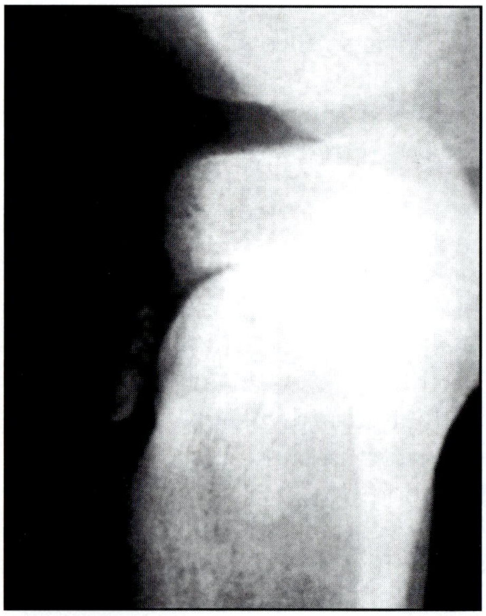

Fig. 32.31: Radiograph showing Osgood's disease

PLICA SYNDROME

This is a fold of synovium present in the suprapatellar, infrapatellar and mediopatellar aspects of the knee. It could be injured during knee trauma, ACL tear and haemarthrosis leading to knee pain. However, it is unclear whether it is the cause or sequelae of other knee pathologies mentioned above.

OSTEOCHONDRITIS DISSECANS (Fig. 32.32)

In this condition, avascular necrosis occurs in an area of subchondral bone followed usually by degenerative changes in the overlying cartilage. Though it can occur in any joint, it is most commonly seen in the knee joint. This avascular bone undergoes necrosis, gets detached and forms a loose body. In fact, this is the most common cause for loose bodies within the knee (see box).

'Loose' facts: Do you know the sources of loose bodies within the knee?

- Osteochondritis dissecans—50%
- Fractured articular surfaces—11%
- Synovial chondromatosis—2%
- Source unknown in 33%
- Osteophytes, damaged menisci, etc. in a few cases.

Causes

Many causes are cited and are controversial:
- Exogenous trauma
- Endogenous trauma
- Ischemia
- Abnormal ossification within the epiphysis
- Genetics
- Combination of these.

Common site Lateral aspect of the medial femoral condyle near the attachment of posterior cruciate ligament.

Age groups
- In young patients before epiphyseal closure. Treatment outcome is good.
- In adults, here treatment outcome is poor.

Note: It is rare in patients < 10 years and older> 50 years of age.

Sex Male to female ratio is 2:1.

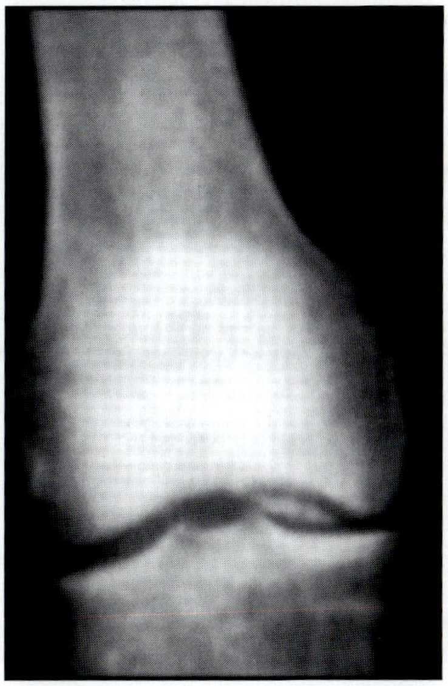

Fig. 32.32: Radiograph showing osteochondritis dissecans

Clinical Features

It is different in the two age groups and consists of vague pain and discomfort in the knee, swelling, catching, popping and locking could occur. After complete separation, loose bodies can be palpated. Tenderness can be elicited over the anteromedial surface of the femoral condyle by deep palpation after flexing the knee.

Investigations

Plain X-rays of the knee (AP, lateral and tunnel view), Arthrogram, arthroscopy, bone scan, MRI, etc. are some of the important investigation tools.

Treatment

This depends on the age of the patient and degree of involvement. Treatment method varies from conservative in children to operative in adults.

The operative methods are arthroscopic excision, curettage, pinning, debridement, grafting, etc. The outcome of the treatment is good in children and is not so good in adults.

HOFFA'S SYNDROME (Syn: Fat Pad Syndrome)

It is affection of the infrapatellar fat pad due to direct trauma to the anterior knee. It could also be due to sudden entrapment following forced knee extension.

Clinical Features

The patient complains of pain and swelling of the infrapatellar fat pad. Tenderness can be elicited on either side of the patellar tendon and at the anteromedial and anterolateral joint lines.

Treatment

This is essentially conservative and consists of the following measures:
- Protection of the anterior knee
- Physiotherapy measures: TENS, Ultrasound, SWD, etc. Heat therapy helps.
- Quadriceps strengthening exercises is helpful.

REGIONAL DISORDERS OF THE FOOT

ARCHES OF THE FOOT

The tarsal and metatarsal bones of the foot are bound by ligaments and arranged in the form of two arches, longitudinal and transverse. Integrity of these arches are maintained by:
1. Shape of the bones.
2. Tension of the ligaments and plantar aponeurosis.
3. Muscular action of both short and long muscles through bracing action of their tendons.

Longitudinal Arch

Longitudinal arch is of greater height and has a wider span along the medial side of the foot than the lateral. It has got two pillars, anterior and posterior. The posterior pillar is short and solid and is formed by calcaneus alone. Rest of the tarsal bones and metatarsal form the anterior pillar. The anterior pillar has got two columns, medial and lateral. Head of the talus forms the keystone of the summit and is situated between the deep socket formed by anterior end of calcaneum and navicular and is supported by the plantar calcaneo-navicular ligament called the spring ligament.

All other ligaments on the plantar surface of the bones of foot play a part in maintaining the arches of the foot and they are assisted by extensive insertion of tibialis posterior and peroneus longus and especially by the plantar aponeurosis which joins the two ends of the arch and acts as a "tie beam" (Fig. 32.33A).

Transverse Arches of the Foot

Transverse arches of the foot lie along the line of tarsometatarsal articulations. Inferior surfaces of the cuneiforms and metatarsal are narrow transversely and are held tightly together by plantar and interosseous ligaments and by tendons of peroneus longus. This arrangement gives the plantar surface in this region a much smaller transverse radius of curvature than the dorsal surface, thus, forming a well-defined transverse arch (Fig. 32.33B).

Two conditions of clinical importance discusssed in this chapter relates one to exaggerated longitudinal arch called the ***pes cavus*** and the other to loss of medial longitudinal arch called the ***pes planus*** (Figs 32.34 and 32.26).

PES CAVUS

Pes cavus is a deformity characterised by an excessively high longitudinal arch that results from an equinus position of the forefoot in relation to the hindfoot (Figs 32.34B).

In this condition finger can be slipped under the navicular bone and it penetrates a distance of greater than 2 cm from the vertical edge of the foot.

Theories of Pathogenesis

1. Weakness of intrinsic muscles of the foot.
2. Overactivity of the intrinsics.
3. Muscle imbalance:
   - Weak anterior tibial muscle and normal peroneus muscle.
   - Weakness of the calf muscles.

Pathologic anatomy This consists of dropping of the foot, contractures of the plantar fascia, varus of the heel and clawing of the toes.

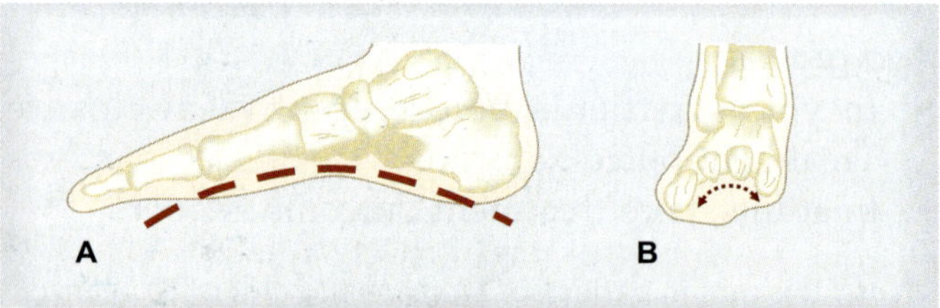

Figs 32.33A and B: Arches of the foot, (A) longitudinal, (B) Transverse

Classification

This is depicted in detail in Table 32.9.

Clinical Features

This consists of high medial longitudinal arch, first metatarsal drop and pronation, tight plantar fascia, cock-up deformities of all the toes at the MTP joints, varus heel, and clawing (Fig. 32.35) of the toes (late feature).

Radiography

AP view Talocalcaneal angle is decreased.

Lateral view Angle betweeen two lines, one through the first metatarsal and another through the talus or calcaneus is decreased.

Treatment

Correction of the primary deformity which is equinus and pronation of the foot is done first. Secondary deformities like contracted plantar fascia, clawed toes and varus of the heels are corrected next.

Early stages require conservative treatment

Late stages Surgery is required, soft tisssue release in children, bony surgeries in adults. *See Table 32.10 for degree of claw toes corresponding deformities and for their respective treatment.*

Table 32.9: Classification of pes cavus

Idiopathic	*Secondary*	*Trauma*	*Others*
• Commonest type (80%) • Develops after 3 years of age • Male : Female 1 : 1 • May be seen in spina bifida	• Spinocerebellar hereditary degeneration • Freidreich's ataxia • Poliomyelitis • Diseases of conus medullaris • Spina bifida • Cerebral palsy • Progressive peroneal palsy	• Direct trauma to the foot or the leg. • Compart-mental syndromes	• Myopathies • CTEV • Plantar fibromato-sis

PES PLANUS

Definition Pes planus (flat foot) (Fig. 32.36B) refers to loss of medial-longitudinal arch of the foot (see Fig. 32.34C).

Associated abnormalities

1. Heel valgus
2. Mild subluxation of the subtalar joint
3. Eversion of the calcaneus at the subtalar joint
4. Lateral angulation at the metatarsal joint
5. Supination of the forefoot
6. Shortened tendocalcaneus.

Table 32.10: Showing degrees of pes cavus, their corresponding deformities and treatment

	Degree	*Deformities*	*Treatment*
1.	**First**	• Foot is normal • Deformity appears when foot is relaxed. • Flexible and corrected by pushing I MT bone manually up	• Daily manipulations • Exercises • Anterior arch bar • Night splint
2.	**Second**	• Equinus and pronation of I MT is fixed • Clawing of large toe • Early contractures of the plantar fascia	• Stiendler's operation • Jones transfer • EHL is transferred to the neck of I MT • Arthrodesis in adults
3.	**Third**	• All five metatarsals are in equinus • Calcaneus begins to invert • No bony deformities	• Extensor shift operation • Dwyer's osteotomy in children
4.	**Fourth**	• All the components of deformities become pronounced and resist passive correction • Some midtarsal movements are preserved	• Japa's 'V'-shaped osteotomy • Anterior tarsal wedge osteotomy
5.	**Fifth**	• Extreme degree of cavus foot • All components are fixed • Toes are dislocated dorsally • Plantar fascia is markedly contracted	• Bone wedge corrections of hindfoot and midfoot and triple arthrodesis

MT—Metatarsal, EHL—extensor hallucis longus

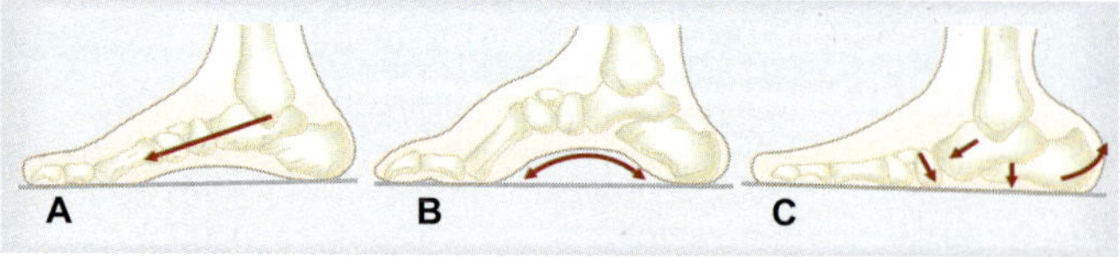

Figs 32.34A to C: Foot arch deformities: (A) normal foot, (B) high-arched foot, (C) flat foot

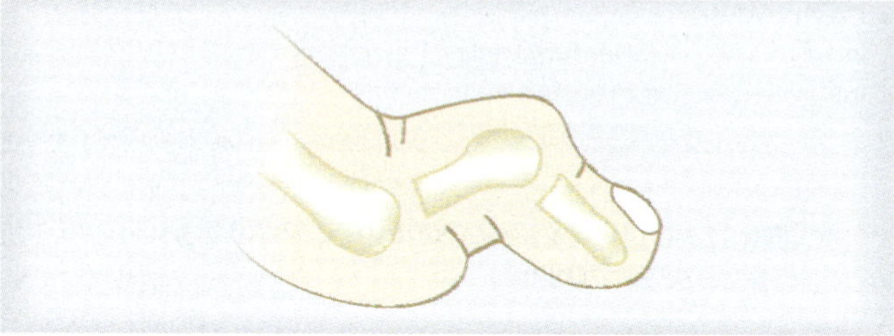

Fig. 32.35: Claw toes (extension of the first phalanx and plantar flexion of second and third)

Types

Flat foot is essentially congenital and acquired and has been depicted in Table 32.11.

Clinical Features

Medial arch is obliterated, navicular bone is prominent, fingers cannot be inserted under the arch, and sole of the foot and area of weight bearing increases and may show increased callosity. Pes planus could be:

Flexible On non-weight bearing, normal appearing arch develops.

Rigid Could be semirigid or fixed. During non-weight bearing, normal acceptable medial arch does not develop.

Static type This is the most common type, the reasons could be faulty postural activity of muscles, equinus deformity of the foot, and varus deformity of the foot.

Predisposing factors

1. General muscle hypotonia
2. Excessive fatigue of the foot muscles due to prolonged standing
3. Unsuitable footwear.

Types

1. Foot strain or incipient flat foot
2. Mobile flat foot
3. Rigid flat foot.

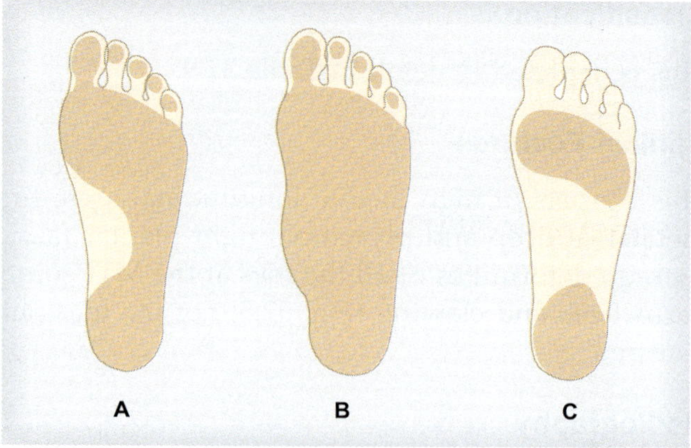

Figs 32.36A to C: Podoscopic appearance of: (A) Normal foot, (B) Flat foot (C) Pes cavus

Table 32.11: Varieties of pes planus

Congenital causes	*Acquired causes and varieties*
• Calcaneovalgus foot	• *Traumatic flat foot* (fracture calcaneus; traumatic Potts' fracture)
• Vertical talus deformity	• *Relaxed or static* flat foot (commonest)
• Talocalcaneal bar	• *Rigid flat-foot,* fibrous or bony ankylosis from any cause
• Congenital ligament laxity	• *Spasmodic flat-foot* due to spasmodic contraction of the peroneal muscles

Peroneal or spasmodic flat foot It is common in young adolescents. Patient complains of acute onset of pain, the tightness, spasm of peroneal muscles, and eversion of foot. It is commonly associated with calcaneonavicular bar. It can also be associated with conditions like tuberculosis, rheumatoid arthritis, which causes spasm due to reflex muscle reaction.

Treatment Plan

Fifteen to twenty per cent adults have flexible pes planus which are asymptomatic.

Up to 3 years Orthopaedic shoes with Thomas heels, medial heel wedges and navicular pads.

Between 3 and 9 years of age

- *Asymptomatic* cases need parent education
- Symptomatic cases require:
  —Orthopaedic shoes for mild cases
  —Custom prosthesis for severe cases.

10–14 years age group

- *Asymptomatic* cases require no treatment
- *Symptomatic* cases require moulded orthroses worn in a sturdy shoe.

Surgical Correction

Principles

1. This is done to relieve the disabling pain after exhausting every means of conservative management and not for cosmesis alone.
2. The patient should accept loss of inversion and eversion.
3. Subtalar joint should be included for arthrodesis of the painful flat-foot.

Techniques

1. Miller's flat foot procedure.
2. Modified Hoke-Miller's flat foot procedure.
3. Durbans flat foot plasty.
4. Triple arthrodesis.
5. In congenital variety displacement osteotomy of calcaneum.

Except for the calcaneal osteotomy, all these procedures require arthrodesis of at least one metatarsal joint.

FOOT PAIN

The following are the causes of foot pain

Pain in the forefoot
- Transverse flat foot
- Morton's metatarsalgia
- March or stress fracture

Pain in the midfoot
- Strain of inferior calcaneonavicular ligament
- Weakness of the short muscles of the sole of the foot
- Fracture base of II Metatarsal

Pain in the heel

Pain within heel
- Calcaneus stress fracture
- Osteomyelitis
- Tumours

Pain behind the heel
- Retrocalcaneal bursitis
- Retroachilles bursitis
- Sever's disease
- Rupture and paratendinitis of the tendo-Achilles

Pain beneath the heel
- Infracalcaneal bursitis (policeman's heel)
- Plantar fascitis
- Fat pad insufficiency
- Calcaneal spur

METATARSALGIA

Definition It is defined as pain beneath the metatarsal heads or shafts. It may be due to trauma, inflammation and static causes.

Types

1. *Static metatarsalgia* Found with developmental anomalies like metatarsus primus varus, hallux valgus, metatarsus hypermobilis, obesity and debilitating illness.
2. *Relaxation metatarsalgia* Interosseous muscle flex the MTP joints → extend the toes → draw the metatarsals together. Failure of these muscles causes splaying of the foot. The extra-weight borne by the metatarsal heads throws a strain on the transverse ligament of the metatarsal heads and pain results.
3. *Compression metatarsalgia* is due to crowded footwear and this causes neuritis.
4. *Fracture of II metatarsal bone* An old fracture of the base of the second metatarsal bone (transverse and undisplaced) is a common cause of chronic midfoot pain. It usually remains undetected. Treatment ranges from immobilisation, electrical stimulation to surgical bone grafting.

Clinical Features

In relaxation metatarsalgia (commonest variety) the patient complains of pain beneath the metatarsal heads, compression of the foot increases the pain (Fig. 32.37). Splay foot, atrophy of the interosseous muscles, and clawing of the toes are the other features.

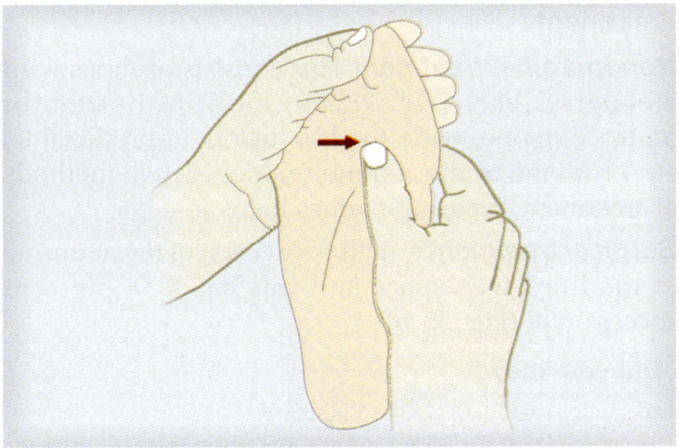

Fig. 32.37: Showing method of eliciting tenderness in metatarsalgia

Treatment

Treatment consists of intrinsic muscle exercises, well-designed shoes, pad and strapping changed at intervals of one week, support of inner sole with pad, and oblique osteotomy of the metatarsal necks for metatarsalgia associated with metatarsal head prolapse.

MORTON'S NEUROMA

In 1876, [4]Morton described a condition of pinching of the lateral plantar nerve in the fourth web space between the mobile fourth to fifth metatarsal heads of the foot (Fig. 32.38). However, it is more common in the III web space and rare in the first. Neuroma is secondarily due to the irritation of the intermetatarsal plantar digital nerve as it travels beneath the metatarsal ligament.

Clinical Features

The patient complains of pain in the region of the third and fourth metatarsal heads, by walking pain increases and decreases by rest. There could be deep burning pain and extension of paraesthesia into the toes.

Tests

1. **Mulder's click** When neuroma is squeezed between the metatarsal heads, a click is felt. This is common in women and is usually unilateral.
2. **Extension test** Passively extend the MTP joints. This tightens the ligament and compresses the nerve eliciting pain.
3. **Provocation tests** Deep palpations in the intermetatarsal space provokes pain.

Treatment

Nonoperative treatment This consists of shoes with metatarsal bars (Fig. 32.39), local infiltration of hydrocortisone, wide toe box use is unpredictable, etc. are some of the common nonoperative methods of treatment. Neurodynamics helps in some cases.

Surgical treatment is mainly excision of the neuroma in the third web space and this has a 83 per cent success rate (Fig. 32.40).

Did you know?

Metatarsal bar was discovered by HO Thomas.

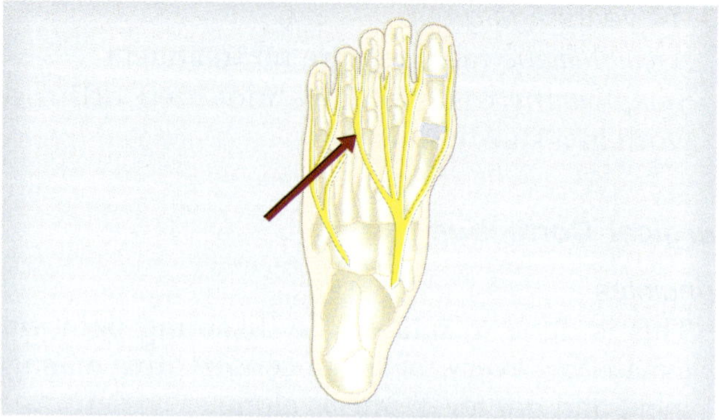

Fig. 32.38: Showing Morton's neuroma

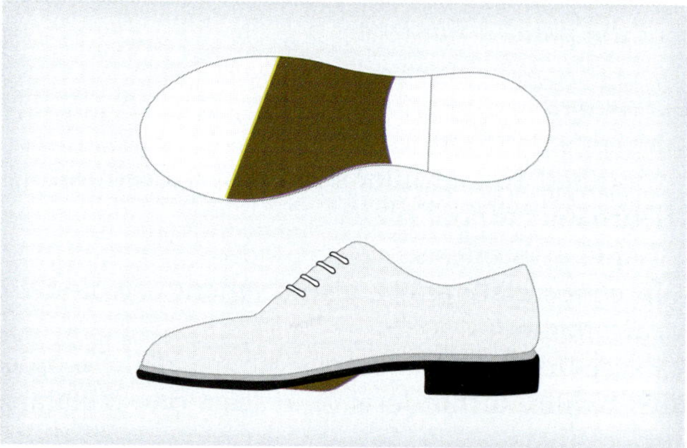

Fig. 32.39: Showing incorporation of metatarsal bars, under the sole of the footwear

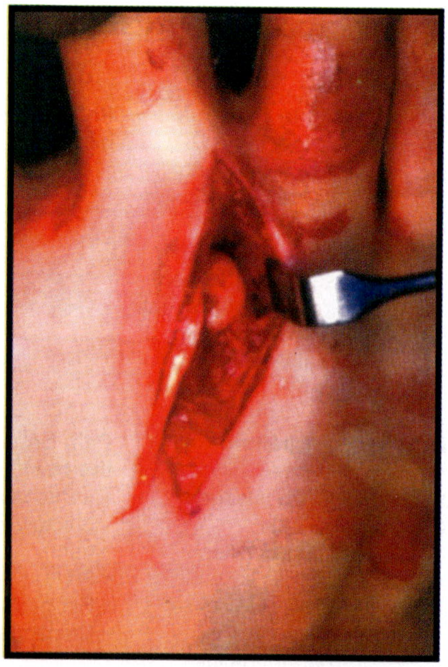

Fig. 32.40: Operative exposure Morton's neuroma

[4]**George Thomas Morton** (1835-1903) of Philadelphia, USA.

PAINFUL HEEL

The following are some of the causes of pain in the heel (see Fig. 32.41):

1. Traumatic disturbances.
2. Developmental and pathological disturbances.
3. Epiphysitis of the calcaneum (Fig. 32.42).

Differential Diagnosis of Heel Pain

Posterior Heel Pain

- Retrocalcaneal bursitis
- Hageland's deformity (Pump-bump)
- Achilles tondinitis or tendinosis
- Calcification within the Achilles tendon
- Referred pain from a soleus muscle trigger point
- Radiculopathy of S_1.

Plantar Heel Pain

- Inflammation or microtrauma of the plantar fascia.
- Entrapoint neuropathy of tibial nerve or its branches and sciatic nerve
- Fat pad atrophy
- Heel spur
- Stress fracture of calcaneum
- Tarsal tunnel syndrome
- Systemic problems like rheumatoid, etc.
- Radiculopathy of S_1
- Irritatum of the first branch of lateral plantar nerve or nerve to abductor digiti minimi (Baxter's nerve)
- Plantar heel bursitis
- Thrombosis of the plantar medial venous plexus
- Post-traumatic fat pad insufficiency (after due to calcaneal fracture)

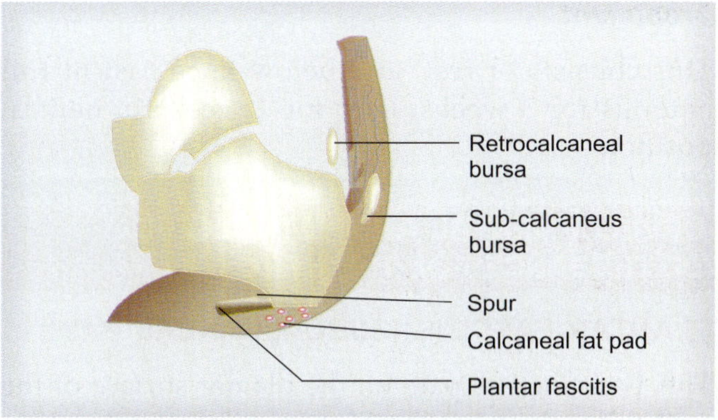

Fig. 32.41: Showing causes of heel pain

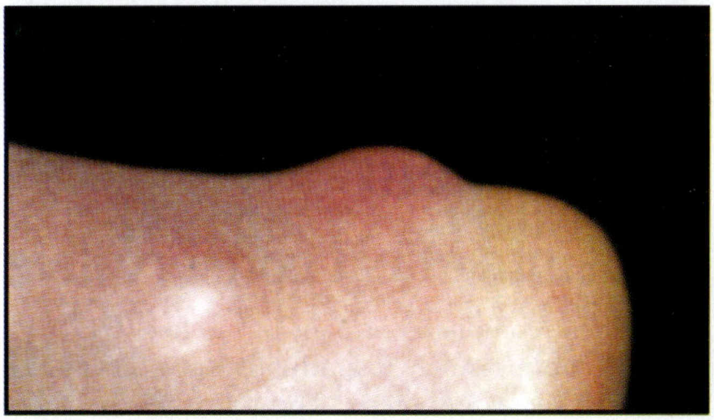

Fig. 32.42: Pump-bump due to friction from the back of the pump shoes

TRAUMATIC DISTURBANCES

Trauma to the back of heel, around insertion of the tendocalcaneus, and plantar aspect of the heel.

Trauma Around the Region of Tendo-Achilles

Tenosynovitis of tendo-Achilles, formation and initiation of enlarged bursae, and partial tendon tears.

In all the above cases, pain increases on movements and decreases by rest.

Hageland's Disease or Winter Heel

In this condition, tenosynovitis leads to fibrous deposits which press on the back of the tendo-Achilles of the heel on wearing a boot and cause pain.

Bursal Enlargements

Normal bursae are present between the tendon and the calcaneus.

Adventitious bursa is subcutaneous and forms over the most prominent part of the posterior surface of the bone. It accounts for early 39 per cent of the cases of pain in the heel. A tender hard lump usually forms over this and is called the "*knobby heels*". It is seen in children and adolescents in whom it is liable to develop due to friction by the ill-fitting boot.

Treatment

Conservative treatment consists of beating out the lateral half of the counter of the shoe at the back of the heel.

Surgery is the treatment of choice and consists of removal of the prominent posterosuperior angle of the calcaneum and any exostoses.

In younger children, excision of a large wedge shape of bone is found to be useful.

Partial Tears of Tendo-Achilles

Here pain is due to fibrous tissue or periostitis.

Treatment

This consists of rest, and below-knee cast in full equinus for 3 weeks, later for 2 weeks in neutral position.

DEVELOPMENTAL AND PATHOLOGICAL DISTURBANCES OF THE HEEL

PLANTAR FASCITIS (SUBCALCANEAL PAIN)

This is defined as pain on the plantar surface of the heel and is the most common cause of posterior heel pain (Fig. 32.43).

Do you know the source of pain in plantar fascitis?

- Plantar fascia
- Subcalcaneal bursa
- Fat pad
- Tendinous insertion of the intrinsic muscles
- Long plantar ligament
- Medial calcaneal branch of tibial nerve
- Nerve to abductor digiti minimi

Clinical Features

The patient complains of pain in the heel which is more in the morning. It gradually subsides as the patient takes a few steps. The pain increases on prolonged standing, walking, etc.

Clinical Tests

Tenderness can be elicited on the medial aspect of the posterior heel. Passive stretching of the toes increases pain in the heel (Figs 32.44A and B).

Mystitying Facts: Why is plantar heel pain more in the morning?

During sleep, foot is in plantarflexed position causing shortening of the plantar structures. Sudden dorsiflexion in waking up from the night's sleep, stretches the structured abruptly causing pain.

Types of Plantar Fascitis

- Insertional plantar fascitis → Called the heel pain syndrome → Pain is felt at the medial calcaneal tubercle (Point tenderness)
- Diffuse plantar fascitis → Pain felt diffusely over the heel and the sole of the foot

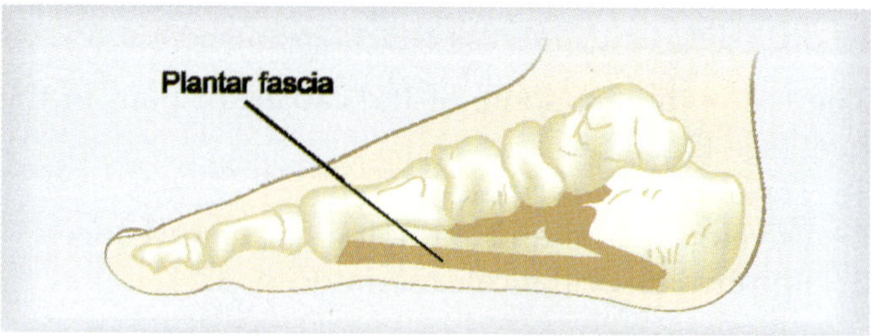

Fig. 32.43: Showing the plantar fascia

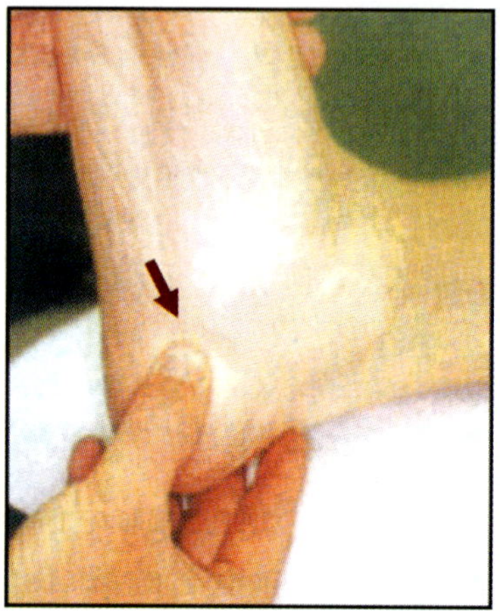

Fig. 32.44A: Method of eliciting tenderness in plantar fascitis

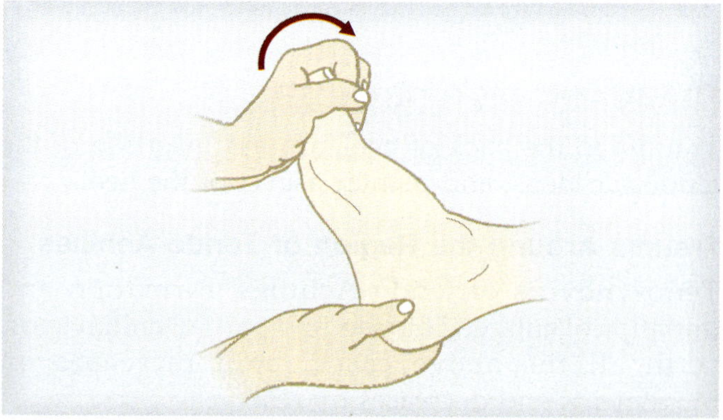

Fig. 32.44B: Passive stretching of toes increases pain

Treatment

1. *Measures to reduce pain and inflammation* Taping, temporary or permanent shoe orthosis, heel cushion, weight management, etc.
2. *Measures to improve the neurodynamics of the tibial nerve* Active calf muscle stretching and calf soft tissue mobilisation.
3. Joint mobilisation with talocalcaneal glides.

4. Strengthening the muscles that support the arch namely the posterior tibial, peroneal and intrinsic muscles.
5. No response to conservative treatment for three months—LIHC (local infiltration of hydrocortisone) is indicated.
6. No response to conservative treatment for 6 months—surgery (partial plantar release) is advised.

Rehabilitation Methods

- Massage the heel by hand.
- Rolling of the foot over a tennis ball.
- Stretching exercises of the tendo-Achilles and hamstrings and intrinsic muscle exercises of the foot.
- Wearing heel cups helps to reduce shock and thus pain (see Fig. 32.49).

What is new?

- Endoscopic plantar fasciotomies have a success rate of 85%.
- For recalcitrant heel pain instead of surgery 1000 impulses of low energy extracorporeal shock wave treatment (3 applications) is found to be effective.

Quick facts: Treatment of plantar fascitis in a nutshell

I line:
- NSAIDs
- Heel pad/Cushion
- Stretching exercises of the ankle and foot.

II line:
- LIHC
- Custom moulded foot orthosis
- Soft supportive shoes
- Foot strapping
- Stretching exercises
- Night brace or AFO or short leg walking cast

III line: Surgery if all the regime mentioned above fail after one year.

CALCANEAL SPURS

It is a spike of bone at the anterior edge of the calcaneal tuberosity (usually medial).

It may be seen on the posterior aspect of the calcaneum also and is called the retrocalcaneal spur (Fig. 32.45).

Causes

1. Due to repeated attacks of plantar fascitis.
2. Due to repeated trauma.

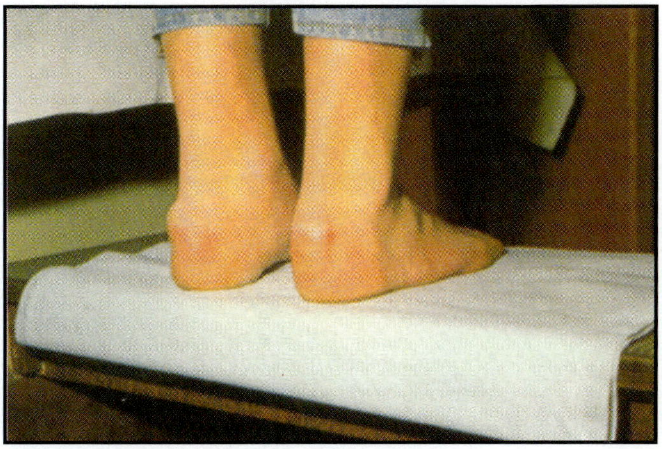

Fig. 32.45: Showing retrocalcaneal spur

3. Constant pull of the shortened plantar fascia.
4. Ill-fitting footwear (Figs 32.46A and B).
5. Fibromatosis of the plantar fascia.

Important spur facts

- Nearly 80% of patients with plantar fascitis have plantar heel spurs
- About 10% of the general population have asymptomatic heel spurs
- Though believed, it is actually not the source of pain
- Many patients with "suspected painful heel spur syndrome" have actually plantar fascitis
- Spur has no therapeutic or prognostic significance.

Clinical Features

The patient complains of pain over ball of the heel, tenderness on plantar aspect of the heel (Fig. 32.47), slight swelling at the attachment of plantar fascia. *It is due to fibrositis or traumatic detachment of plantar fascia and does not give rise to symptoms perse and the pain when present is due to the causative condition and not the spur.*

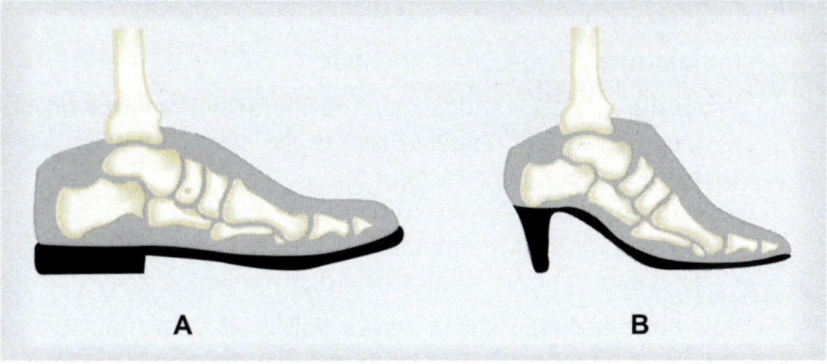

Figs 32.46A and B: Showing (A) Correct footwear, (B) Improper footwear which distorts the normal arches of the foot

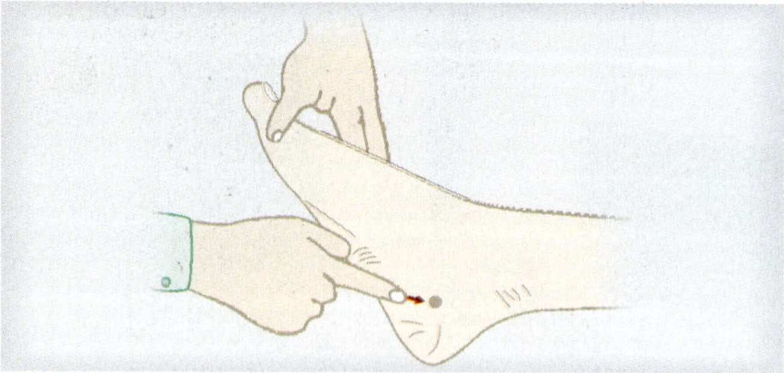

Fig. 32.47: Showing the point of tenderness in plantar fascitis and calcaneal spur

X-ray of the Heel Lateral view of the heel show prominent bone spike arising from the calcaneum (Fig. 32.48).

> **Pitfall:** Only 50 per cent of the patient with heel pain show calcaneal spurs on X-ray.

Treatment

Conservative methods include treating the causative factor, rest, NSAIDs, local infiltration of hydrocortisone and microcellular rubber (MCR) used for the sole of the footwear (Fig. 32.49).

Surgery is indicated when no relief is seen with the conservative treatment.

Methods

1. Osteotomy of the calcaneus.
2. Decompressing operation with multiple drill holes in the calcaneus.
3. Excision of the medial inferior tuberosity.

What is new in the the treatment of calcaneal spur?

1. Endoscopic treatment of calcaneal spur syndrome.

   Indications: Recalcitrant heel pain

   Procedure: Medial endoscopy and lateral instrumentation.
   - Debridement of posterior roof of the calcaneal arch.
   - Removal of calcaneal spur.
   - Lateral to medial release of plantar fascia.
   - Debridement of the periosteum of calcaneal tuberosity.
   - Release of nerve to abductor digiti minimi.
2. Low-dose acoustic shock waves delivered by a machine called an Ossatron. The acoustic waves may work by stimulating increased blood flow to the area, decrease inflammation and help the tissue to heel.

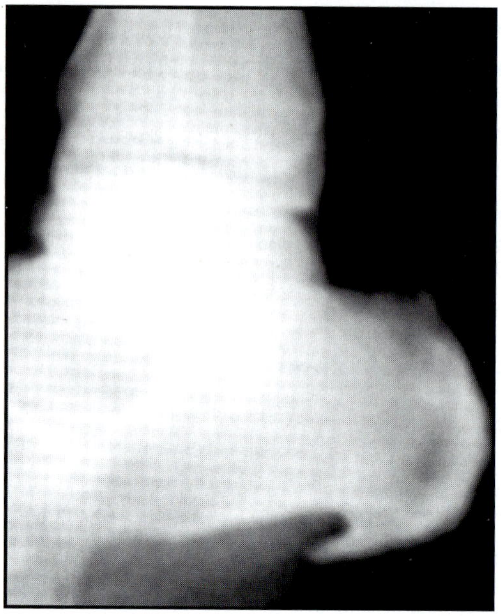

Fig. 32.48: Radiograph showing calcaneal spur (best seen in the lateral view)

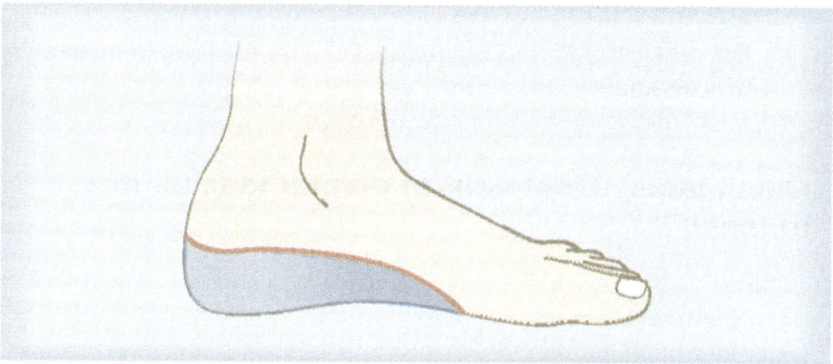

Fig. 32.49: UC-BL shoe inserts to relieve heel stress in plantar fascitis and calcaneal spur

FAT PAD INSUFFICIENCY (ATROPHY OF FAT PAD)

Features

- Seen in older athletes.
- Also seen in younger athletes with multiple cortisone injections.
- Pain and tenderness is diffuse over the heel.
- Flattening of the fat pad on standing.

Clinical Features

Patient complains of pain in the heel, limp, difficulty in standing for a long time, etc. On examination, there is flattening of the heel, broadening and the calcaneum can be easily felt.

Treatment

- NSAIDs
- Ice therapy.
- Polythylene or polypropylene heel cup for increased cushion and support.

CALCANEAL STRESS FRACTURE

This is common in athletes who jump and run repeatedly and faulty training techniques. Patient complains of diffuse heel pain and the heel compression test is positive. Treatment is essentially conservative in nature.

Traumatic subtalar joint arthritis develops due to calcaneal fracture or due to TB, syphilis, gonococcal arthritis, etc.

EPIPHYSITIS OF THE CALCANEUM

[5]**Sever's disease** (Fig. 32.50) This is commonly seen in 9 to 13 years. It is common in boys and is due to inflammation of bursa beneath the tendo-Achilles tendon.

Treatment consists of rest and footwear correction and this usually helps.

Fibromatosis of the plantar fascia In this condition, nodule formation is seen which becomes painful with pressure and weight bearing. It is similar to Dupuytren's contracture, and is seen commonly in patients with antiepileptic drugs.

LESSER KNOWN BUT IMPORTANT FOOT CONDITIONS

PLANTAR FIBROMATOSIS (Lederham Syndrome)

Definition

It is a proliferative fibroplasia of the plantar aponeurosis similar to Dupuytren's contracture.

Presentation

Nodules can be felt on the medial non-weight bearing side of the aponeurosis.

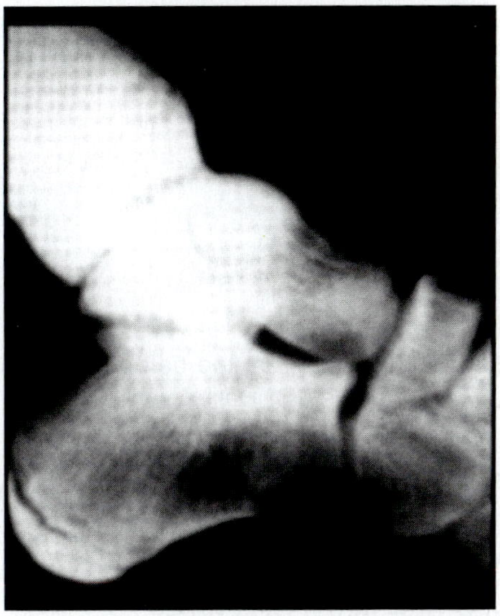

Fig. 32.50: Radiograph showing Sever's disease

Treatment

For small lesions, conservative treatment including shoe modifications are recommended. For large painful lesions, wide surgical excision is recommended.

PUMP-BUMP

Features

- It is not a true tendinitis.
- It is an inflammation of the superficial bursa situated over the insertion of the tendo-Achilles (see Fig. 32.42).
- It is usually due to rubbing of the back part of the pump shoes and is more common in women.

DANCER TENDINITIS

It is tendinitis of the flexor hallucis longus and is seen in ballet dancers.

IMPORTANT BUT LESSER KNOWN CONDITIONS OF THE FOREFOOT

HALLUX VALGUS

Definition It is a deviation of the great toe at the metatarsophalangeal joint away from the midline (Fig. 32.51).

[5]**James Warren Sever, Boston, USA** (1878-1964). Described this condition in 1912.

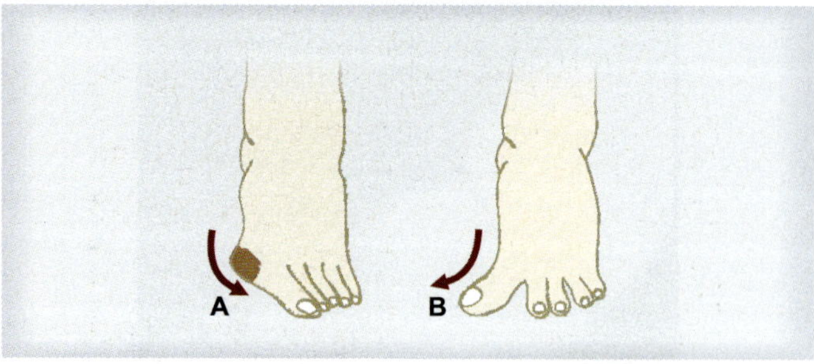

Figs 32.51: Prominent great toe deformities: (A) Hallux valgus, (B) Hallux varus

Secondary Problems

Due to primary problem, some secondary changes develop namely:

1. Varus of first metatarsal bone.
2. Adduction of the phalanges.
3. A protective adventitious bursa may develop over the medial aspect of the joint (called the bunion)
4. Hypertrophy of the medial end of the first metatarsal head.
5. OA changes in the first MTP joint.
6. New bone formation at the end of the I MTP joint.
7. Extensor hallucis tendon may be displaced laterally.
8. The bunion may get ulcerated and infected due to friction from a tight footwear.

Causes

These are some of the important causes of hallux valgus:

- Wearing of tight socks and footwears
- Diseases like gout, rheumatoid arthritis, etc.
- More commonly seen in women (Male: Female = 1:10).
- Congenital.

Clinical Features

Often, deformity is the only complaint. However, in some longstanding cases, there could be pain in the great toe and there could be a significant swelling on the medial side due to bunion. Friction of the bunion due to the ill-fitting footwear could lead to skin ulceration.

Treatment

Mild cases Physiotherapy measures and footwear correction suffices in mild cases.

a. Relaxed passive stretching of the abductors of great toe.
b. Active exercises to the foot intrinsic muscles.
c. Proper weight-bearing methods.
d. Footwears with straight inner border with a wedge between the I and II toe helps.
e. Faradic foot bath is recommended.

Severe cases Surgery is the treatment of choice and includes:

a. *Keller's operation* Excision of the head of the first metatarsal and proximal portion of the proximal phalanx.
b. *Mayo's operation* Here only head of the I metatarsal bone is excised.
c. *Arthroplasty* Excision of the I MTP joint with bunion.
d. *Arthrodesis* of the I MTP joint is also done.

Physiotherapy Measures after Surgery

This is the same as mentioned above except that it is done more vigorously and patients need training in weight bearing, gait and transfers.

HALLUX RIGIDUS

Definition In this condition, there is pain and stiffness in the MTP joint of the great toe.

Causes

- Repeated injuries to the great toe.
- Improper footwear.
- Familial and common in females.

There may be erosion of the articular cartilage and formation of exostosis.

Treatment

Mild cases

- Conservative measures like pain killers, etc.
- Thermotherapy helps to reduce pain and spasm.
- Footwear modifications like metatarsal bars, soft soles, etc.
- POP cast may be required in some cases.

Severe Cases

This may be treated by:

- Arthroplasty of the I MTP joint
- Arthrodesis of the I MTP joint.

Physiotherapy Measures following Surgery

This is the same as mentioned for hallux valgus.

HAMMER TOES

Definition It is a toe deformity with PIP joint flexion. It could be flexible or fixed (Fig. 32.52).

Clinical Features

Most often, deformity is the only complaint. Pain sometimes results from a callus on the dorsum of the PIP joint or under the head of the metatarsal. Hamering of the second toe often is accompanied with hallux valgus deformity (Figs 32.53 and 32.54B).

Treatment

This includes:
- Stretching of the dorsal extrinsics in a position of plantar flexion and MTP extension
- Intrinsic muscle strengthening exercises.
- Extra depth shoes.

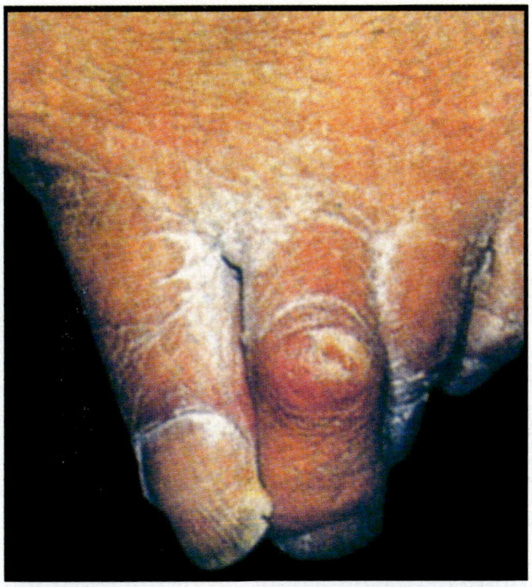

Fig. 32.52: Clinical photograph of hammer toe

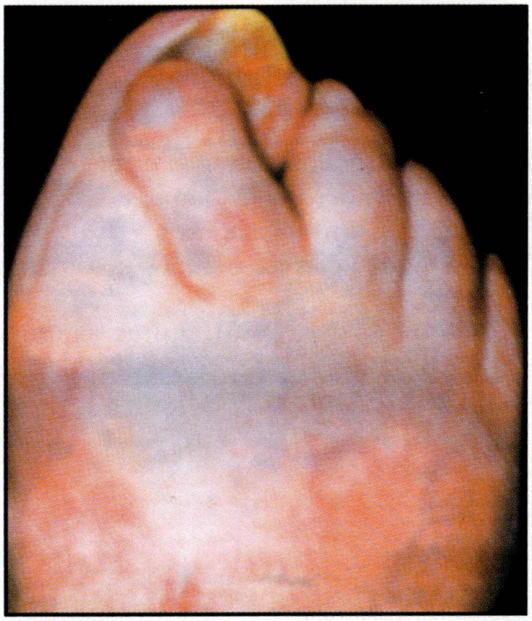

Fig. 32.53: Clincial photograph of hallux valgus

CLAW TOES

Definition It is an extension deformity of the MTP joint with simultaneous flexing or clawing of the toes at both the proximal and distal interphalangeal joints (Fig. 32.54A).

Causes

It is due to muscle imbalance in which the active extrinsics are stronger than the deeper intrinsics (lumbricals and interosseous). This happens usually in a neurologic disorder. It is usually seen in pes cavus.

Treatment

In flexible claw toes, the treatment is similar to hammer toes (Fig 32.55).

SESAMOIDITIS

Definition This is an inflammation in the two small sesamoid bones that are situated in the tendon of the flexor hallucis brevis muscle under the first MTP joint.

Associated problem Since the medial digital plantar nerve runs close to the medial sesamoid bone, it is often irritated.

Clinical Features

- Ambulating is extremely painful
- First MTP joint is tender to palpate

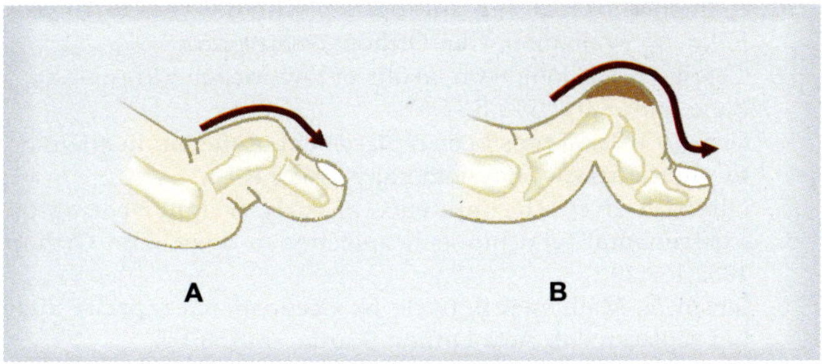

Figs 32.54A and B: Showing (A) Claw toe, (B) Hammer toe

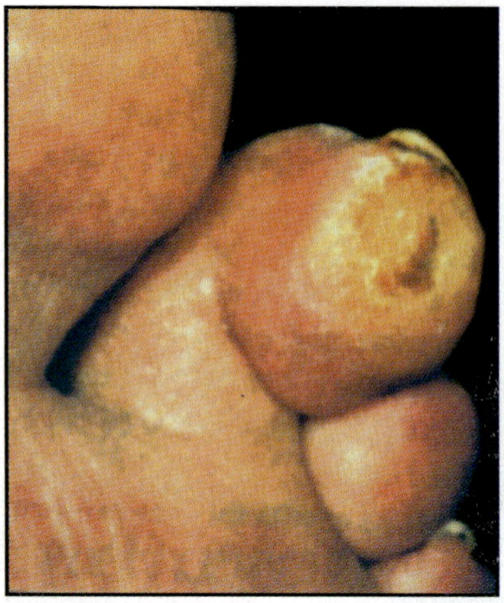

Figs 32.55: Clinical photograph of mallet toe

- Pain increases on extension of the great toe
- There could be swelling at the head of the first metatarsal.

Effective Conservative Treatment for all Forefoot Conditions

- Metatarsal pad or cut-out under orthosis to change the pressure under the tender area
- Changing the ill fitting shoes
- Maintaining the correct arch position by support and exercises
- Intrinsic muscle strengthening exercises to improve flexion and extension of the MTP and IP joints.

BIBLIOGRAPHY

Arthroplasty

Hip

1. Bakenbaugh RD, Ilstruip DM. Total hip arthroplasty: a review of 333 cases with long term follow-up. J Bone Joint Surg 1978;60-A:306.
2. Berrin T, Dorr LD, Perry J, Grontley J, Hull DB. Functional evaluation of total hip arthroplasty with a 5 year to 10 year followup evaluation. Clin Orthop 1985;195:252.
3. Charley J. The long term results of low friction arthroplasty. J Bone Joint Surg 1972;54-B:61.
4. Charley J. Total prosthetic replacement of the hip in attention to physiotherapy. Physiotherapy 1968;54:406.
5. Gitelis S et al. The influence of early weight bearing on experimental total hip arthroplasties in dogs. Clin Orthop 1982;169:29.
6. Jensin JS, Mathiesen B, Jvede N. Occupational capacity after hip replacement. Acta Orthop Scarda 1985;56:135.
7. Johnstan RC, Smidt GL. Hip motion measurements for selected activities of daily living. Clin Orthop 1970;72:205.
8. Mcbeath AA, Bahrke MS, Batra Batze B. Walking efficiency before and after total hip replacement as determined by oxygen consumption; Bone Joint Surg 1980;62A:807.
9. Yoslow W, Simone HD. Hip replacement rehabilitation. Arch Phys Med and Rehab 1976;57:175.

Total Knee Arthroplasty

10. Ewald FC et al. Kinematic total knee replacement. J Bone Joint Surg 1984;66-A:1032.
11. Goodfellow J, O'Connoor J. The mechanism of the knee and prosthetic design. J Bone and Joint Surg 1978;60-B:358.
12. Insall JN, Binnazzi R, Soudry M, Mestriner WA. Total knee arthroplasty. Clin Orthop 1985;192:13.
13. Kapanji LA. The physiology of the joints. New York, Churchill Livingstone 1971;2.
14. Laughman RK, Stauffer RN, Istrup DM, Chao EYS. Functional evaluation of total knee replacement. J Orthop Res 1984;2-307.
15. Morrison JB. Function of the knee joint in various activities. Biomed Eng 1969;4:573.
16. Scott WN, Tria AJ. Principles of surgical technique in knee arthroplasty. Orthop Clin North Am 1982;13:131.

Total Ankle Arthrosplasty

17. Alexakis P, Smith RC, Wellisch M. Irradiations for ankle fusion vs total ankle replacement versus plantar fusion. Orthop Trans 1977;1:87.
18. Morris JM. Biomechanics of the foot and the ankle. Clin Orthop 1977;122:10.
19. Newton SE III. Total ankle arthroplasty: a 4 year study. Orthop Trans 1977;1:86.
20. Sammaroo GJ, Burstein AH, Frankel VH. Biomechanics of the ankle: a kinematic study. Orthop Clin North Am 1975;4:1.
21. Stauffer RN. Total joint arthroplasty of the ankle. Mayo Clin Proc 1979;54:570.

Total Shoulder Arthroplasty and Elbow

22. Cofield RH. Total shoulder arthroplasty. The Neer prosthesis. Orthop Trans 1979;3:262.
23. Neer CS. Reconstructive surgery and rehabilitations of the shoulder. In Kelly et al Textbook of Rheumatology. Philadelphia, 1981.
24. Saunders WB, Bryan RS. Total replacement of the elbow joint. Arch Surg 1977;112:1092.

Painful Heel Syndrome

25. Campher JW, Inman VT. Treatment of plantar fascitis and calcaneal spurs with 4C-BL shoe insert. Clin Orthop 1974;103:57.
26. DuVris HL. Heel spur (Calcaneal spur). Arch Surg 1957;74:536.
27. Furey JG. Plantar fascitis, the painful heel syndrome. J Boneard Joint Surg 1975;57-A:672.
28. Graham CE. Painful heel syndrome: rationale and treatment Foot Ankle 1983;3:261.
29. Hicks JH. The mechanics of the foot. part II. The plantar aponeurosis and the arch. J Anat 1954;88:25.

Arthrodesis

30. Ahank I. Arthrodesis and arthroplasty of hip joint. Acta Orthop Gland 1963;33:253.
31. Barr JS, Record EE. Arthrodesis of the ankle joint. Indications, operative technic and clinical experience. N Engl J Med 1953;248:53.
32. Carnesale PG. Arthrodesis of the hip; a long-term study. Orthop Digest 1976;4:12.
33. Charnley J. Compression arthrodesis. Edinburgh, 1953, E&S, Livingstone Ltd.
34. Charnley J, Lowe HB. A study of the end results of compression arthrosis of the knee. J Bone Joint Surg 1958;40-B:633.
35. Clawson RS, McKay DW. Arthrodesis in the presence of infection. Clin Orthop 1976;114:209.
36. Moure FH, Smith JS. Arthrodesis of the knee joint. Clin Orthop 1959;13:215.
37. Nelson CL, Evarts CM. In Arthroplasty and Arthrodesis of the Knee Joint. Orthop Clin North Am 1971;2:245.
38. Putt V. Arthrodesis for tuberculosis of the knee and of the shoulder. Chir Organ Mov 1933;18:217.

Regional Disorders

Frozen Shoulder

39. Bosworth DM. Supraspiratus syndrome. Symptomatology, pathology and repair. JAMA 1941;117:422.
40. Delta Prota RJ, Evarts M. Rotator cuff tears. Contemp Orthop. 1982;4:327.
41. Duncan BF. The frozen shoulder syndrome rehabilitations approach to treatment. Contemp Orthop 1983;6:69.
42. Grey RG. The natural history of idiopathic frozen shoulder. Journal Bone Joint Surg 1978;60-A:564.
43. Haggart GE, Dignam RJ, Sullivan TS. Management of the frozen shoulder. JAMA 1956;161:1219.
44. Lee M Haq, Wright V, Longron EB. Periarthritis of shoulder controlled trial of physiotherapy. Physiotherapy 1973;59:312.
45. Maitland GD. Treatment of glenohumerab joint by passive movement. Physiotherapy 69:3.
46. Mosley HF. Ruptures of the rotator. GH Br J Surg 1951;38-340.
47. Neer CS II. Impingement lesions. Clin Orthop 1983;173:70.
48. Neviaser RJ. Painful conditions affecting the shoulder. Clin Orthop 1983;173:63.
49. Depalima AF. The painful shoulder. Postgrad Med 1957;21:368.

Tennis Elbow

50. Coonrad RW, Hooper WK. Tennis elbow: its coarse natural history conservative and surgical management. J Bone Joint Surg. 1973;55-A:1177.
51. Cyriax JH. The pathology and treatment of tennis elbow. J Bone Joint Surg 1936;18:921.
52. Dungar BF. Rehabilitation of the tennis elbow syndrome. Contemp Orthop 1983;7:61.
53. Field FW, Field SM. Treatment of tennis elbow. Use of a spenal trace. JAMA 1966;195:67.
54. Gardner RC. Surgery for tenis elbow: a five year followup. Orthop Rev 1974;3:45.
55. Norklood LA, Shock JA, Andrews JK. Acute medial elbow ruptures. Am J Sports Med 1981;9:16.
56. Carpal Junnel. Chow technique. James EY Chow, AMD. Source: Orthonet, May-June 1999.

Olecranon Bursitis

57. Canoso JJ. Idiopathic or traumatic olecranon bursitis; clinical features and bursat fluid analysis. Arth Rheum 1977;20:1213.
58. Jaffe L, Fetto JF. Olecranon bursitis. Contemp Orthop B (5) 51:1984.

Cervical Disc

59. Bloom MH, Ranaji FL. Anterior anterotebral fusion of the cervical spine: A technical note. J Bone and Joint Surg 1981;63-A:842.
60. Bucy PC, Heinburger RF, Oberhill HK. Compression of the cervical spinal cord by herniated intervertebral discs. J Neurosurg 1948;5:471.
61. Bun JWD. Rupture of the intervertebral disc in the cervical region. Proc R Soc Med 1948;41:513.
62. Coventry MB, Ghormley RK, Kernohan JW. The intervertebral disc, its microscopic anatomy and pathology part II: Changes in the intervertebral disc concomitant with age. J Bone and Joint Surg 1945;27:233.
63. Garna A. Cervical traction, an ancient modality. Orthop Rev 1984;13:429.
64. Scoville WB. Types of cervical disc lesions and their surgical approaches. JAMA 1966;196:105.
65. Shertz HH, Watters WC III, Zeiger L. Evaluation and treatment of Natz pain. Orthop Clin North Am 1982;13:439.

Scoliosis

66. Blount WP, Schmidt AC, Bidwell R. Making the Milwaukee brace. J Bone Joint Surg 1958;40-A:526.
67. Cobb JK. Outline for the study of scoliosis. In American Academy of Orthopaedic Surgeons. Instrumental Course Lectures, Vol 5, Ann Arbor, 1948, JW Edwards.
68. Drummond D' et al. Interspinous process segmental spinal instrumentation. J Paediatr Orthop 1984;4:397.
69. Goldstein LA. The surgical management of idiopathic scoliosis. Clin Orthop 1973;93:131.
70. Harrington PR. Treatment of scoliosis. Correction and internal fixation by spine instrumentation. J Bone and Joint Surg 1962;44A:591.
71. Kisser JC. The iliac apophysis; as invaluable sign in the management of scoliosis. Clin Orthop 1958;11:111.
72. Kleinberg S. Scoliosis: pathology, etiology and treatment, Baltimore: Williams and Willkins Co, 1951.
73. Mehta MH. Radiographic estimation of vertebral rotation in scoliosis. J Bone Joint Surg 1973;55-B:513.
74. Moe JH. Methods of correction and surgical techniques in scoliosis. Orthop Clin North Am 1972;3:17.
75. Stagnara P. Scoliosis in adults: surgical treatment of severe forms. Excerpts Med Found International Congress Series No. 1969;192.
76. Thulbourne T, Gillespie R. The rib-hump in idiopathic scoliosis measurement, analysis and response to treatment. J Bone and Joint Surg 1976;58-B:64.
77. Wyer AF. Experience of anterior correction of scoliosis. Clin Orthop 1973;93:191.

Kyphosis

78. Blackborne JS, Velikas EP. Spondylolithesis in children and adolescents. J Bone Joint Surg 1977;59-B:490.
79. Bosworth DM, Fielding JW, Demarest L, Bonaquist M. Spondylolisthesis: a critical review of a consecutive series of cases treated by arthrodesis. J Bone Joint Surg 1955;37-A:767.
80. Bradtord DS et al. Anterior strut-grutting for the treatment of kyphosis. Review of experience with 48 cases. J Bone Joint Surg 1982;64-A:680.
81. Kiriluwto O, Sartavirta S, Salenius P, Morri P, Pytkkanen P. Posterolateral spine fusion, a 1-4 year follow up of 80 consecutive patients. Acta Orthop Siard 1985;56:152.
82. Mezerding HW. Low badghe and sciatic pain associated with spondylolisthesis and protruded intervertebral disc; incidence, significance and treatment (symposium). J Bone and Joint Surg 1941;23:461.
83. Moe JH. Treatment of adolescent kyphosis by non-operative and operative methods. Mantoba Med Rev 1965;75:481.
84. Wiltse LL, Newman PH, Macnab I. Classification of spondylolysis and spondylolisthesis. Clin Orthop 1976;117:23.
85. Witlse LL, Jackson DW. Treatment of spondylolisthesis and spondylolysis in children. Clin Orthop 1976;117:92.
86. Wittse LL, Winter KB. Terminology and measurement of spondylolisthesis. J Bone Joint Surg 1983;65-A:768.

Hallux Valgus

87. Albrechkht E. Pathology and treatment of hallux valgus. Russki Vrach 1911;10:14.
88. Bragman J, Corless J, Gross A, Langer F. A review of surgical procedures for hallux valgus, Foot Ankle 1980;1:39.
89. Clutton HH. The treatment of hallux valgus St Thomas Rep 1994;21:1.
90. Writhton J. A ten-year review of Keiler's operation at the Princes Elizabeth Orthopaedic Hospital-Exeter. Clin Orthop 89:207-1972.

Knee

Arthroscopic treatment of popliteal cyst

91. Valerio Samsone, MD Allesantra DC Ponti, Orthonet, Arothroscopy, May-June 1999.

Pesplanus

92. Harris RT, Beath J. Etiology of peroneal spastic flat foot. J Bone Joint Surg 1948;30-13:624.
93. Jay Kumar S, Cowell HR. Rigid flatfoot. Clin Orthop 1977;122:77.
94. Jones RL. The human foot: an experimental study of its mechanics and the role of its muscles and ligaments in the support of the arch. Am J Anat 1941;68-1.
95. Milkstrom J, Williams RA. Shoe correction and orthopaedic foot supports. Clin Orthop 1983;70:30.
96. Stabeli LT, Griffin L. Corrective shoes for children: A survey of current practice. Pediatrics 1980;65:13.

Morton's Neuroma

97. Cohen HH. Mortan's metatarsalgia (interdigital neuroma). Bull Hosp Joint Dis 1952;13:206.
98. Morris MA. Morton's metatarsalgia. Clin orthop 1977;127:203.
99. Metatarsalgia: Morris G Nix K, Goldmann PP, Dept. of Paediatrics, Philadelphia 2000.

Sesamoid Bones of the Forefoot

100. Jahss MH. The sesamoids of the hallux. Clin Orthop 1981;157:88.
101. Morris JM. The biomechanics of the foot and the ankle. Clin Orthop 1977;122:10.
102. Orr TG. Fracture of great toe sesamoid bones. Ann Surg 1918;48:609.
103. Parra G. Stress fractures of the sesamoids of the foot. Clin Orthop 1960;18:218.

Chronic Heel Pain

104. Open heel surgery Vs Endoscopic plantar fasciotomies. Praveen K. Vohra DPM, Journal of American Pediatric Medical Association Feb 1999.
105. Chronic heel pain - Treatment by Ossatron by Dr. Isadore Rosenfeld. Source: Readers' Digest Feb 2001.

SECTION FOUR

HAND DISORDERS AND LOW BACKACHE

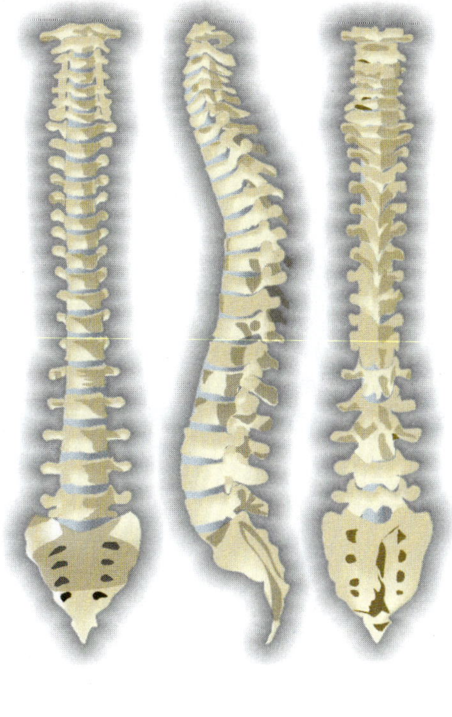

33

Disorders of the Hand

- Congenital anomalies of the hand
- Infections of the hand
- Arthritic hand
- Paralytic hand

Hand is a very important organ of the body. Disorders affecting the hand could lead to loss of hand function in various forms and degrees. Thumb itself accounts for over 40 per cent function of the hand. It is imperative that the problems affecting the hand should be diagnosed and managed correctly. The following are the various disorders affecting the hand.

CONGENITAL ANOMALIES OF THE HAND

Some of the important congenital anomalies of the hand are:

Polydactyly It is a duplication of one or more digits and may require amputation for cosmetic purposes.

Syndactyly This is fusion of digits and usually occurs between the middle and ring fingers and is 3 times more common in males. The fusion may be only in the skin or all the structures. In the latter case surgery is done early at 18 months age and in the less severe former case surgery is done after 5 years.

Macrodactyly This is a rare congenital anomaly and is characterised by enlargement of all structures especially of the nerves of a single or more digits. It is often associated with neurofibroma, lymphangioma, arteriovenous malformation, etc.

Congenital trigger digits Thumb is more commonly involved. It is frequently bilateral and is due to flexion contracture of the distal joint of the thumb. More than 30 per cent of these cases resolve after first year and the remaining may require surgical release after 2 years of age.

Streeter's dysplasia This is a syndrome of congenital constrictions which may affect any part of the body. In the hand, it may range from simple constriction to congenital amputation. To prevent distal circulatory compromise, it frequently requires surgical release by Z-plasty.

Camptodactyly This is a flexion contracture of the proximal interphalangeal joint especially of the little finger. It may rarely be seen in other fingers too. Severe deformity in older patients requires tendon lengthening procedures. Clinicodactyly is angulation of the finger in radioulnar direction. Mild clinicodactyly is seen in normal childrens, while the severe ones are associated with mental retardation.

Cleft hand (also called Lobster claw hand) This is frequently bilateral and is associated with cleft foot, cleft lip, cleft palate, etc. There are two varieties: in the first line, a deep palmar cleft separates the two central metacarpals; and in the second type, the central rays are absent. Both the varieties require surgical excision and Z-plasty.

Mirror hand (reduplication of ulna) Here the ulna and carpus are reduplicated and there may be seven or eight fingers with no thumb. Pollicisation of a finger solves the problem of the absent thumb.

Congenital radioulnar synostosis *(ref. p. 442)*

Madelung's deformity *(ref. p. 443)*

Congenital absence of radius or ulna Congenital absence of radius is more common than that of ulna. The radius may be completely absent or in parts. The forearm is short, wrist is highly unstable and the hand is deviated radially. It requires a complex and difficult surgical corrections.

This deformity of radius absence is also called radial club hand and the absence of ulna is called the ulnar club hand (1:4).

Kirner's deformity This is a spontaneous injuring of the terminal phalanx of the fifth digit. It is a rare disorder and is more often seen in females.

INFECTIONS OF THE HAND

The effects of hand infection can be as devastating as major trauma. Trivial injuries like a scratch, a prick, small punctured wounds, etc. cause hand infections. *Staphylococcus aureus* (80%), *Streptococcus pyogenes* and gram-negative bacilli are the famous trio who inflict the infective unmitigated disaster in the hand. The sequelae of these infections are oedema, abscess, necrosis, fibrosis and lastly contractions leading to a grotesque, debilitating hand. The presence of an abscess seems to send a message to the surgeons, *"Drain me or I'll drain myself!"* Hence, an abscess caused should be drained, the surgeon only has to decide the proper time and incisions. Early use of potent antibiotics has considerably downed the threat of serious hand infections.

As elsewhere before we dwelve into the discussions on individual hand infections, it helps considerably to know the principles of treatment:

1. Hands should be kept elevated to facilitate gravity to drain and thereby prevent oedema and swelling of the hand.
2. Following the treatment, the hand needs to be placed in functional position (*see* Fig. 33.2) for optimum results.
3. Early and appropriate use of IV antibiotics prevents pus formation (within 24–48 hours).
4. If pus is formed, let it out through proper incisions at the appropriate time.
5. Local anaesthetic may help the spread of infection and adds more fluid to the already existing swelling. Hence, general anaesthesia or regional block is preferred.
6. Tourniquet is indicated, but exsanguination is not preferred as it helps spread the infection (alternatively elevation of hand for three minutes is ideal).
7. Do not forget the all important hand aftercare which has a direct bearing on the final outcome of the hand function.

With the principles of treatment as a backdrop, let us now consider the important hand infections in order of importance.

PARONYCHIA

Paronychia (Fig. 33.1) is an infection of the eponychium and could be acute or chronic. Acute paronychia has the distinction of being the most common infection of the hand. *S. aureus* is the culprit and it is usually due to a hangnail, unsterile manicure instruments and reckless nail pairing. The infection normally begins at one corner, tracks down to the opposite end via the eponychium or nail (40%).

Clinical Features

Agonising pain, marked tenderness and a conspicuous red looking swelling are the hallmarks of acute paronychia.

Treatment

Conservative measures and early antibiotic therapy are the mainstay of initial treatment. However, if abscess has formed and if the pus is at one end, incise it, if under one nail corner, remove that corner; and if it has shifted to the opposite end, excise proximal one-third of the nail. If encountered with a floating nail, write its obituary by taking it out totally as it is dead and gone!

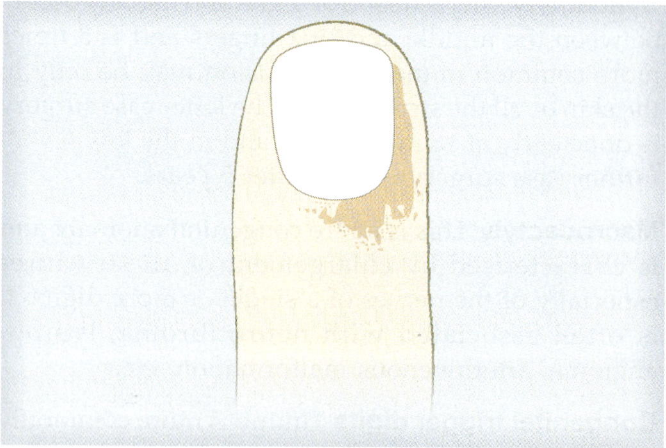

Fig. 33.1: Showing paronychia

Note: Chronic paronychia which is regarded as a complication of acute paronychia is usually not so! It is usually seen in syringomyelia or in people who do not wear rubber gloves during washing!

DISTAL PULP SPACE INFECTION (SYN: FELON)

Next to acute paronychia, this is the most common hand infection. It usually follows a pin prick, with the index finger and thumb being the common unfortunate victim.

Surgical anatomy Multiple fibrous septae travel from skin to bone partitioning the fat-filled distal pulp space into tiny compartments (Fig. 33.2). One such septum also cordons of the space at the distal finger flexor crease. The terminal branches of the digital artery after giving a branch to the basal epiphyseal plate runs through this compartment. The evil effects of this arrangement could lead to the following undesirable consequences:

a. Since it is a tight compartment, any swelling increases the pressure causing excruciating pain.
b. If superficial, penetrates the skin causing skin necrosis and if deep penetrates the periosteum causing osteomyelitis.
c. Thrombosis of the digital arteries leads to osteomyelitis.
d. It may in rare events cause flexor tenosynovitis or infective arthritis of the DIP joint.

Clinical Features

The patient initially complains of dull pain more so in the dependent position and swelling. Loss of sleep due to nocturnal pain is an usual feature after about 2 days. Pressure over the involved part increases pain. Abscess may develop in later stages if left unattended.

Treatment

Treatment consists of antibiotics in the initial stages and if the pain lasts for more than 12 hours, incision helps (Fig. 33.3). If the abscess is pointing volarwards, a longitudinal midline incision is taken; and if the abscess is deep, a longitudinal incision at the side cutting through the partitions is preferred. If osteomyelitis develops in the distal phalanx, sequestrectomy is done if the sequestrum is well formed and separated.

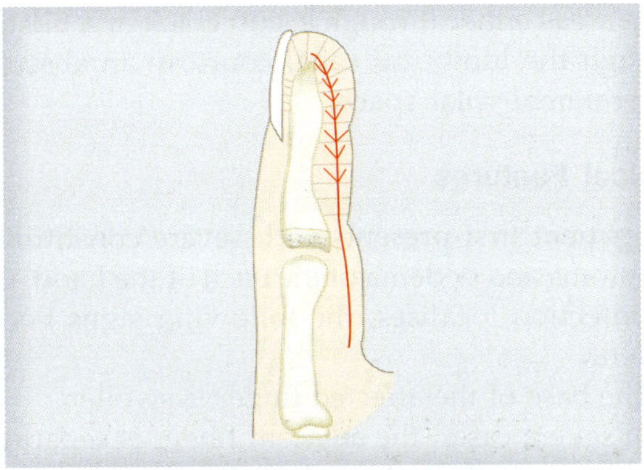

Fig. 33.2: Showing multiple fibrous septa in distal pulp space

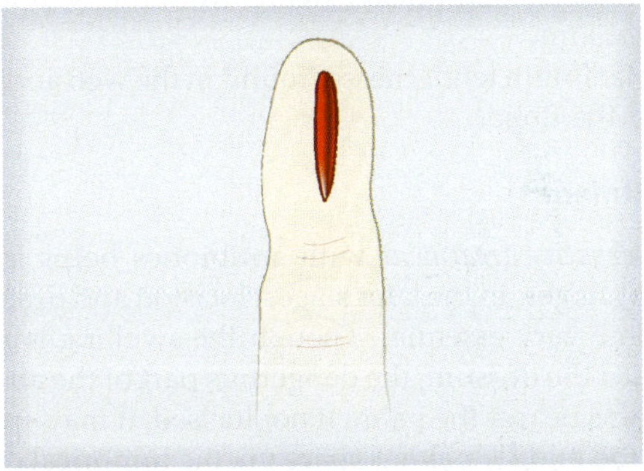

Fig. 33.3: Showing surgical incision for draining felon

MIDDLE AND PROXIMAL VOLAR SPACE INFECTION (Fig. 33.4)

These also follow pin pricks and may be confused with tenosynovitis of the flexor tendons. Spread to the adjacent web space is fairly common. Clinical features and treatment are almost similar.

INFECTION OF THE WEB SPACES

What are these web spaces?

These are three triangular areas filled with loose fat between the ends of the fingers. Infection reaches

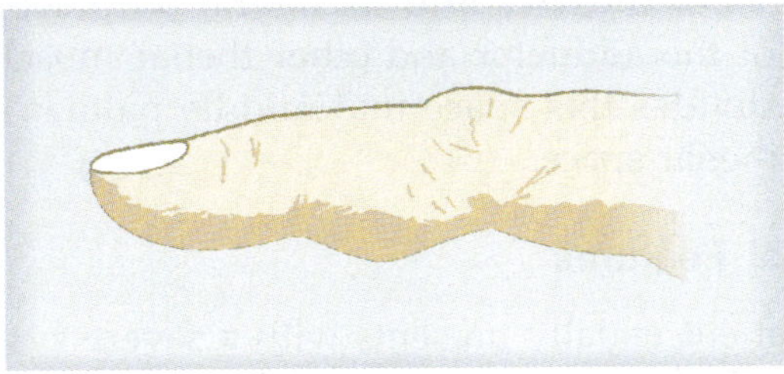

Fig. 33.4: Showing middle volar space infection

these areas either through a skin crack or a blister or through the lumbrical canal courtesy an abscess in the proximal volar space.

Clinical Features

The patient first presents with severe constitutional symptoms and oedema of the back of the hand. Once the infection localises, the following signs become evident:

1. The base of the affected finger is swollen.
2. In severe cases, the adjacent finger is separated.
3. Skin over the affected space shows purplish discolouration.
4. A fan-shaped blush extends from the web to the dorsum.
5. Maximum tenderness is found in the web and base of the finger.

Treatment

Conservative treatment with antibiotics helps in the initial stages. In the later stages, incision and drainage become very essential. Though the swelling is more toward the dorsum, the dangerous part of the abscess remains nearer the palm. If not incised, it may spread into the middle palmar space via the lumbrical canal. Two incisions may be required for drainage, one on the dorsal surface between the metacarpal heads and the other on the palm distal to the distal palmar crease. The web should be left unincised.

DEEP PALMAR ABSCESS

This is rare and accounts for only 1 per cent of all hand infections.

Surgical Anatomy

This is a space lined by fascia and in between the flexor tendons above and metacarpal bones below. Its medial border is formed by the fascia of the hypothenar muscles and its lateral border by the fascia of the adductor and other thenar muscles. A fascia divides this space into middle palmar space and a thenar space.

Clinical Features

The patient usually presents with a severe systemic reaction. There is a local pain, tenderness, loss of active movements of the middle and ring fingers and there is generalised gross swelling of the hand and fingers which resemble an inflated rubber glove (also called Froghand). Similar symptoms are seen in a thenar abscess, but the thumb web is more swollen, index finger is held flexed and active movements of both the index and thumb is lost. With the increasing swelling, the concavity of the palm becomes flat and later convex before it bursts open (Fig. 33.5).

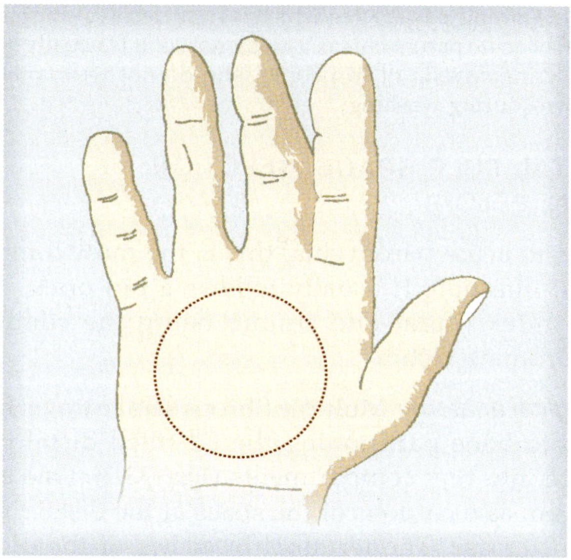

Fig. 33.5: Showing deep palmar abscess

Diagnostic Test

In a deep palmar abscess, passive stretching of the metacarpophalangeal joint is painful while that of interphalangeal joint is painless. In tenosynovitis of the flexor tendons, the passive stretching of both the MP and the IP joints are painful.

Treatment

After the initial conservative treatment, the abscess in the middle palmar space is drained by a central transverse incision at the level of the distal palmar crease in line with the middle finger extending ulnarwards towards the hypothenar eminence. Abscess in the thenar space is drained by a curved incision in the thumb web parallel to the border of the first dorsal interosseous muscle.

TENOSYNOVITIS

These are serious infections and are due to infection of the fibrous sheaths and synovial lining of the flexor tendons of the hand.

Surgical Anatomy

The fibrous and synovial sheaths of the flexor tendons of the hand are arranged in two groups: the radial and ulnar bursae (Figs 33.6A and B). The radial bursa is the smaller of the two and it lines the flexor tendon of the thumb and extends 1 to 2 cm above the wrist up to the distal end of the tendon. The ulnar bursa encloses the synovial sheaths of the index, middle, ring and little fingers. Distally, those for the index, middle and ring fingers, it extends up to the level of transverse palmar cause; and for the little finger, it extends throughout the length of the tendons. The ulnar bursa encloses tendons of flexor digitorum superficialis and profundus of the above fingers. These two bursae may communicate with each other.

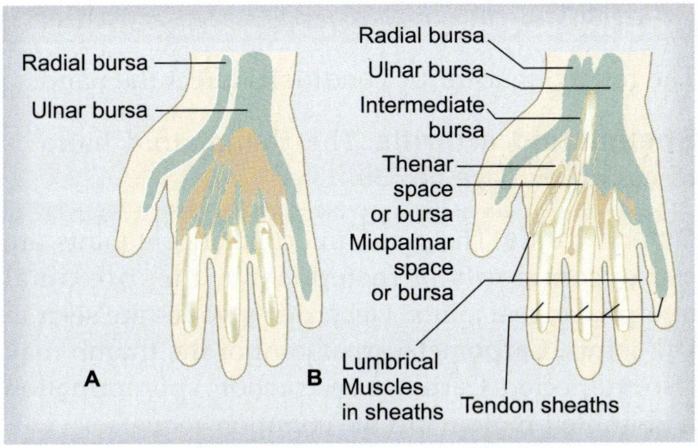

Figs 33.6A and B: Showing (A) Radial (B) Ulnar bursae of the hand

Aetiology

The causative organisms are almost always due to *S. aureus* or *S. pyogenes*. Penetrating injuries of the tendon sheaths, extension of the infection from its terminal pulp space, etc. are some of the common modes of infection. The consequences of teno-synovitis are disastrous, as it may lead to adhesions, rupture if infection is severe and loss of gliding movements.

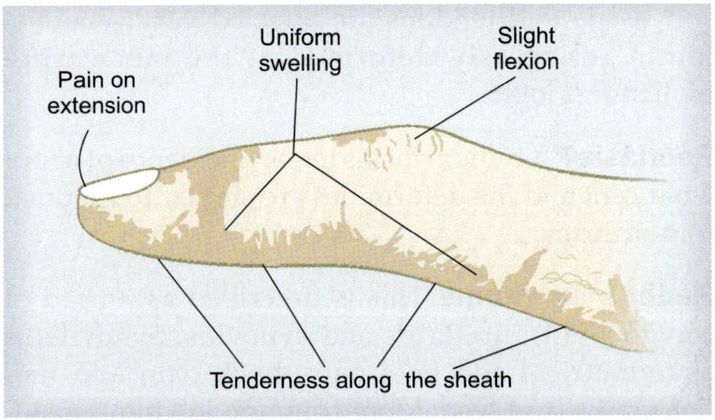

Fig. 33.7: Showing tenosynovitis of a finger showing its four typical features

Clinical Features

The patient complains of pain, swelling, and the affected finger is motionless. Active or passive extensions of the fingers is very painful. The classical local signs include the swelling of the finger through its entire length, flexion of the finger with marked pain on extension, and tenderness over the sheath.

In tenosynovitis of the little finger (Fig. 33.7) tenderness can be elicited at a point in between the two palmar crease. This is called the 'Kanavel's sign' (Fig. 33.8).

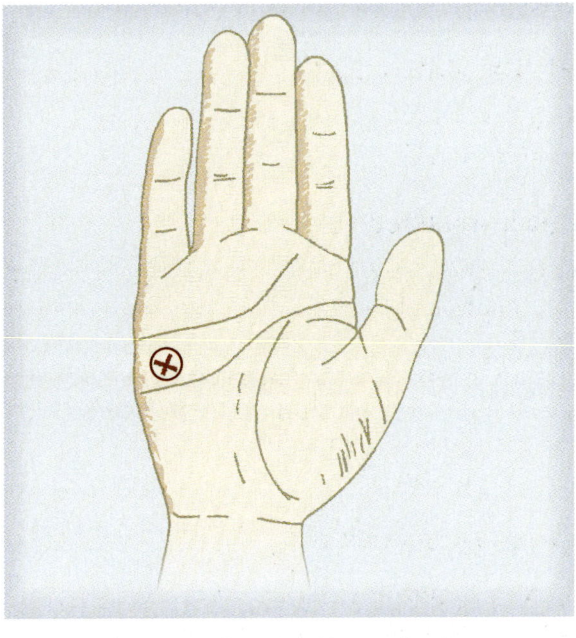

Fig. 33.8: Showing Kanavel's sign

Treatment

Early treatment with antibiotics is started. In the early stages of pus formation abscess is drained by a trans-verse incision at the distal palmar crease and the proximal edge of the sheath is opened. Then the sheath is opened distally through a midcarpal incision over the middle phalanx. If the infection has progressed far, then a full midlateral incision may be required. Sloughed tendons require excision.

ARTHRITIC HAND

The following arthritic conditions affect the hand.

Rheumatoid arthritis The rheumatoid hand is discussed on page no 530.

Osteoarthritis The distal interphalangeal joints are more commonly affected than the proximal interphalangeal joints. Heberden's nodes are seen in DIP joints. Carpometacarpal joint of the thumb may also be affected. Cartilage destruction, spur formation and limited motion are the common sequelae.

Lupus erythematosus This involves the skin over the nose as well as tendons and joints. Periarticular soft tissue and tendons are affected very severely, joints get grossly deformed at the metacarpo-phalangeal joints.

Psoriasis Psoriatic arthritis has an incidence of about 7 per cent and the deformities are similar to rheumatoid arthritis.

Reiter's syndrome This is described as a triad of conjunctivitis, urethritis and synovitis. Synovitis is asymmetrical and heel pain, back pain and nail deformities are seen. More common in young males it attacks the lower limbs more than the upper limbs. More than 90 per cent resolve on its own.

Gout It usually presents as a single, painful, red joint in an adult male. The joint is swollen, hot and tender and is usually confused to a cellulitis or abscess and drained. This is a disease due to massive deposits of monosodium urate crystals around the joints.

PARALYTIC HAND

This is mainly due to peripheral nerve involvement of the upper limbs. Discussed at great length in the chapter on peripheral nerve injuries.

BIBLIOGRAPHY

1. Beasley RW. Principles of tendon transfer. Orthop Clin North Am 1970;2:433.
2. Beasley RW. Surgery of the hand and finger amputations. Orthop Clin North Am 1981;12:763.
3. Carter SJ, Mersheimer WL. Infections of the hand. Orthop Clin North Am 1981;455.
4. Clinkscales GS (Jr). Complications in the management of fractures in hand injuries. South Med J 1970;63:704.
5. Jones JM, Schenck RR, Chesney RB. Digital replantation and amputation: comparison of function. J Hand Surg 1982;7:183.
6. Riordan DC. Tendon transfers in hand surgery. J Hand Surg 1983;8:748.
7. Verdan CE. Practical considerations for primary and secondary repair in flexor tendon injuries. Surg Clin North Am 1964;44:951.
8. Wakefield AR. The management of flexor tendon injuries. Surg Clin North Am 1960;40:267.

34

Low Backache

- Introduction
- Lumbar disc disease and disc prolapse
- Approach to a patient with low backache
- Backache in special situations

INTRODUCTION

Low backache is a very common problem and has an ubiquitous distribution. Among the galaxy of causative factors, both spinal and extraspinal, the most common cause of low backache seems to be the lumbar disc disease. Bad posture plays a very significant role in the genesis of this disease. So much is the contribution of bad posture towards this problem that one can categorically conclude that low backache is all about disc degeneration predisposed by poor posture. A thorough knowhow of the posture, disc disease and back care will enable the student to understand and treat this malady both in his or her patients and household. Other causes of low backache are merely mentioned and the students are suggested to refer suitable chapters for details.

Note: Low backache refers to pain from the low lumbar areas, lumbosacral area and both the SI joints.

EPIDEMIOLOGY OF BACKACHE

Backache which was known as an ancient curse is now known as a modern international epidemic. Eighty per cent of the population are affected by this symptom at some time in life. Impairments of back and spine are ranked as the most frequent cause of limitation of activity in people younger than 45 years. In 2 per cent of the population, backache is the presenting complaint in general practitioner's clinic. In 78 per cent men and 89 per cent women, specific cause was not known. It was believed that bad posture was responsible for most of these cases. The cost to the society and the patient for treatment, compensation, etc. is very high.

POSTURE

Posture is defined as the positional relationship of the different regions of the body to each other. It is divided into:

1. Standing
2. Sitting, and
3. Recumbent positions.

The features of normal posture are as follows:

- Moderate lordosis of cervical and lumbar spines.
- Kyphosis of the thoracic and sacrococcygeal sections.
- Forward pelvic inclination of 30°.
- Neutral rotation of femur.
- Plumb line dropped from the mastoid process passes through the middle of the shoulder and hip, just anterior to the knee and lateral malleolus of the ankle.

PATHOLOGICAL PHYSIOLOGY

In the course of evolution from quadruped to orthograde animal, the relatively straight spine develops forward (neck and low back) and backward curves (thoracic and sacral) as it yields to the forces of gravity. Paraspinal and glutei muscles maintain the erect posture. There is a continuous minimal muscular contractions called the postural tone.

These physiologic curves give the spine its S shape. It is imperative to maintain this S curve in all our erect activities failing which spine becomes unbalanced (Fig. 34.1).

When the spine becomes displaced and unbalanced, a greater number of muscle fibres are called into play at more frequent intervals to keep the spine straight. Thus fatigue develops earlier. This fatigue causes muscle insufficiency as a result of which the spine sags putting the strain on the ligaments and posterior articulating facets. Changes occur at the facet joints and the lumbosacral junction.

Posture of the hip joint is the key to that of the whole body because it determines the pelvic inclination, the pelvis being the foundation for the spine and rotation of the legs. Normal angle is 28 to 31°.

FUNCTIONAL ANATOMY

In the upright position spine has a stabilising function. The body weight is transmitted through the shoulder girdle to the thorax and abdominal cavity, the hydraulic action of which enables the weight to be carried towards the pelvis. Bad posture with lax abdominal muscles impairs the function of the hydraulic system overloading several segments of the spine (Figs 34.2A and B). In all upright position other than that of the physiological vertical axes, the strain on the structures like discs and ligaments is quite high. Furthermore, stabilisation of the muscles is less good during movements, especially if performed abruptly or associated with lifting of a weight. Thus, it can be concluded that postural defects, overloading and abrupt unbalanced movements are frequently responsible for backache.

Remember

- Posture is an entity seen only in human beings, thanks to the two-legged posture.
- Backache is a very common malady next only to headache and affects nearly 80 per cent of the population.
- Most common cause of backache is bad posture which increases the strain on the discs and ligaments causing faster disc degeneration.
- Any abrupt, unbalanced and unwarranted movements upset the stabilising function of the back muscles increasing load on the discs.
- Hence, bad posture, overloading and abrupt unbalanced movements are the causes of disc rupture or prolapse.

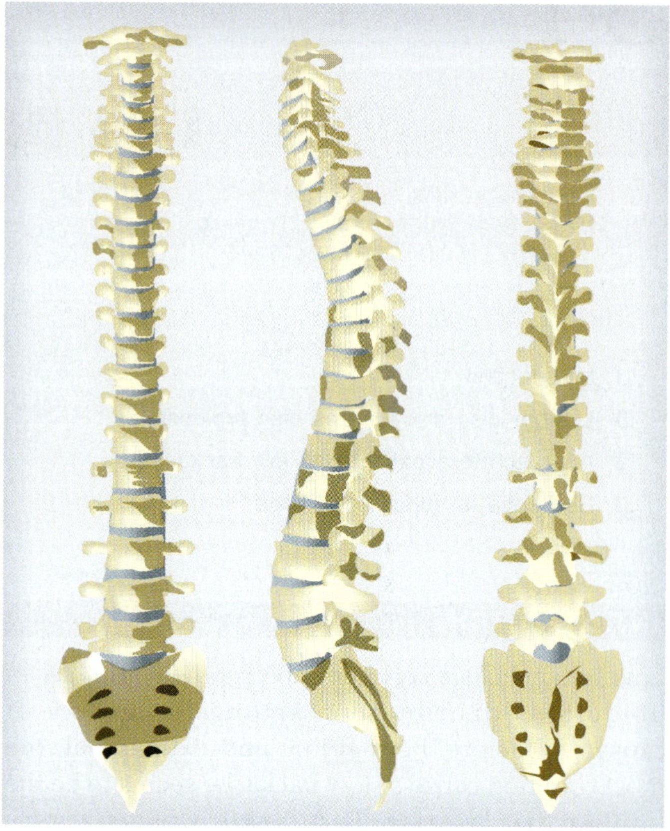

Fig. 34.1: Normal appearance of vertebral column

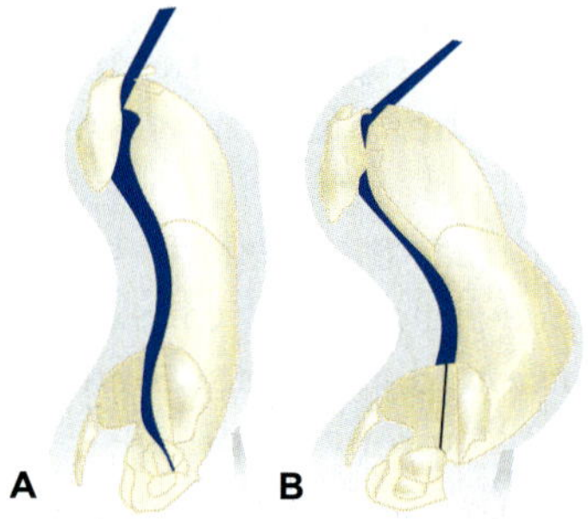

Figs 34.2A and B: Posture: (A) Normal posture, and (B) Bad posture

Structures Involved in Backache (Figs 34.3A to C)

1. *Vertebral bodies*—microcrush fractures, and spondylosis.
2. *Intervertebral discs*—disc degeneration and prolapse.
3. *Posterior intervertebral joints*—degenerative lesions, synovitis, sprain, etc.

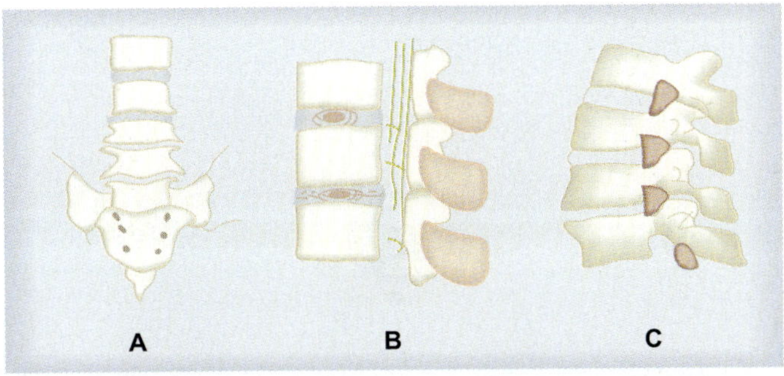

Figs 34.3A to C: Structures involved in low backache: (A) Osteophytes seen in lumbar spondylosis, (B) Compression on PLL and nerves due to disc protrusion, and (C) Disc disease and facet joint arthritis

4. *Ligaments and small intervertebral muscles*—elongation, excessive use, reflex contractures.
5. *Posterior longitudinal ligament*—elongation and irritation by discal protrusion.
6. *Nerves*—irritation or compression of the spinal nerve roots by disc herniation or irritation of the sensory nerves of the various paravertebral structures.

Remember

Factors keeping the spine healthy

- Genetics
- Muscle strength and balance
- Flexibility
- Posture
- Body weight
- Adaptation to stresses

LUMBAR DISC DISEASE AND DISC PROLAPSE

GENERAL DISC AND SPINE ANATOMY

Development of spine starts from the third week of intrauterine life and continues till third decade of life. There are 23 discs throughout the spine, absent only in atlantoaxial articulation. It is thinnest in the thoracic region and thickest in the lumbar. Each disc is interposed between the bodies of a pair of vertebrae (see Fig. 34.2). Body of each vertebrae is covered by a thin end plate of a bone which is perforated by numerous tiny holes. This in turn is covered by a hyaline cartilage which may be considered as the outermost portion of the disc.

Anteriorly and laterally, the bodies and the discs are bounded firmly by the anterior longitudinal ligament and posteriorly by the posterior longitudinal ligament which is weak. The intervertebral discs in adults are avascular, the cells within it are sustained by diffusion of nutrients into the disc through the pores in the bodies. Movements and weight bearing help in diffusion. Degeneration of the disc may be prompted by changes in the permeability of the cartilage end plate.

The disc consists of two parts; centrally, it is *nucleus pulposus* which is made up of collagen fibrils, fibrocytes, chondrocytes, gelatinous matrix, water and salt. Peripherally, it has *annulus fibrosus* which is a fibrocartilaginous tissue. It is thick anteriorly and thin posteriorly more so in the posterolateral aspect. *Hence, posterolateral disc prolapse is more common*. The fibres of annulus are joined by diagonal fibres also known as Sharpe's fibres.

Neural fibres in the outer rings of the annulus contain branches of the sinovertebral nerve dorsally and ventrally branches from the sympathetic chain.

With age, water content of the disc decreases, fibrous tissue and cartilage cells increase, and the nucleus becomes granular and friable.

Mystifying facts about the discs

- There is no disc between C_1 and C_2
- It is avascular and gets its nutrition through local diffusion
- The nutrition of the disc is best in side lying position
- 80% of the nutrition process takes place in the first one hour of night's rest
- The outer annulus fibrosus of the disc is innervated by the sinovertebral nerve and a gray ramus communicans of the sympathetic chain.

DISC PHYSIOLOGY

Disc apart from giving the spine its mobility functions as a shock absorber. Following loss of disc, the vertebral body reacts to abnormal pressure forces by hypertrophic bone formation at the surface revealed as sclerosis and osteophyte formation. Schmorl's node is the disc material which has escaped into the body through the pores and is walled off by the fibrous tissue.

Section 4

Remember

About disc

- It gives spine the mobility.
- It acts as a shock absorber.
- It is fibrocartilaginous.
- It increases the height of the spine by 25 per cent.
- Centrally, it has a nucleus pulposus and peripherally annulus fibrosus.
- It is avascular.
- Annulus fibres are weak posteriorly, hence posterolateral disc prolapse is more common.
- With age, water content of the disc falls.

NATURAL HISTORY OF LUMBAR DISC DISEASE

All spines degenerate with advancing age and so does the intervertebral discs. Degenerative process is divided into three stages:

1. **Stage of dysfunction**
   - Seen between 15 and 45 years of age.
   - Circumferential and radial tears are seen in the disc annulus.
   - Localised synovitis of the facet joints is seen.
2. **Stage of instability**
   - Seen between 35 and 70 years of age.
   - There is an internal disruption of the disc.
   - Progressive disc resorption takes place.
   - Degeneration of facet joints with lax capsules, subluxation and joint erosions are seen.
3. **Stage of stabilisation**
   - Seen over 60 years of age.
   - Progressive development of hypertrophic bone about the disc and facet joints leading to segmental stiffening or frank ankylosis are seen.

Disc herniation (Fig. 34.4) is considered as a complication of disc degeneration in Stages I and II. Spinal stenosis is a complication in late instability and early stabilisation stages. Disc can herniate either into the body as Schmorl's node or posteriorly towards the canal compressing the nerve roots.

CLASSIFICATION OF PROLAPSED INTERVERTEBRAL DISC (Fig. 34.5)

Disc bulging or protrusion This refers to some eccentric accumulation of nucleus with slight deformity of the annulus.

Prolapsed disc is the one in which eccentric nucleus produces a definite deformity as it works through the fibres of the annulus.

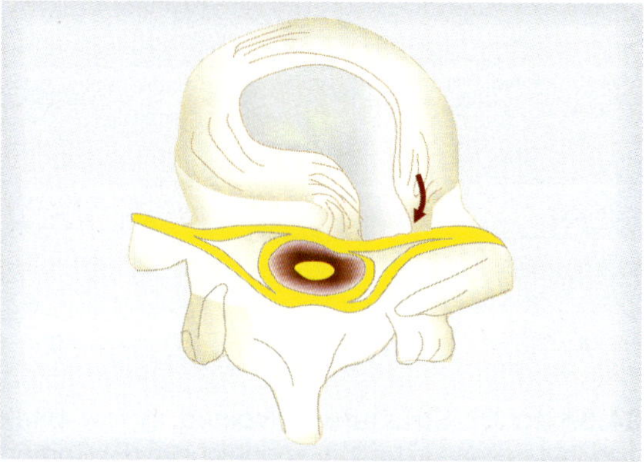

Fig. 34.4: Showing posterolateral disc herniation

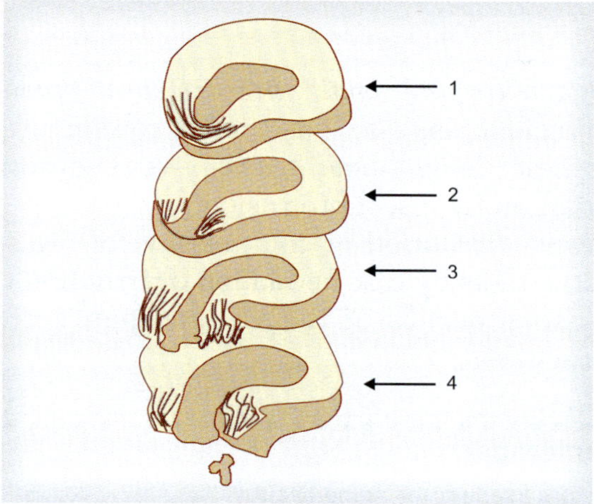

Fig. 34.5: Showing types of prolapse disc: (1) bulge disc, (2) prolapse disc, (3) extruded disc, and (4) sequestrated disc

Extruded disc Here, the disc comes out into the canal and impinges on the adjacent nerve root (Fig. 34.6).

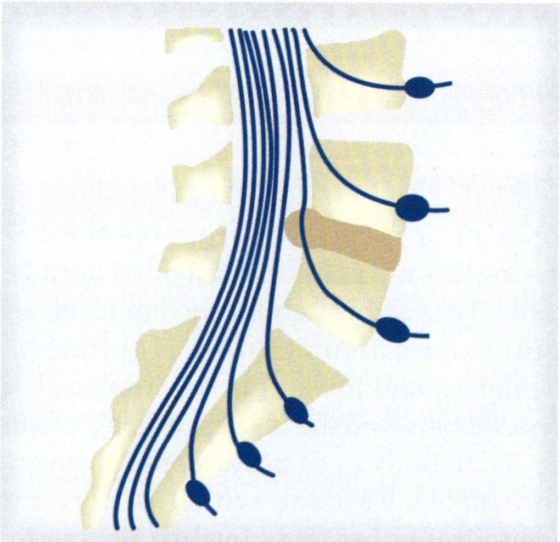

Fig. 34.6: Disc prolapse compressing the nerve root

Sequestrated disc Here the nuclear material has separated from the disc itself and potentially migrates.

Interesting facts

Do you know at what levels does lumbar disc prolapse most commonly occur?

$L_{4-5} > L_5S_1 > L_{3-4} > L_{2-3} > L_{1-2}$

AETIOLOGY OF DISC HERNIATION

The aetiology consists of risk factors and the definitive causes resulting in disc herniation.

Risk factors

- Jobs requiring heavy and repetitive weightlifting (Figs 34.7 and 34.8).
- Use of machine tools.
- Operation of motor vehicles.
- Cigarette smokers and tobacco consumers.
- Anxiety and depression.
- Stressful occupation as in doctors, police, etc.
- Women with greater number of pregnancies.
- Obesity and other cardiovascular risk factors.
- Monotonous work, working overtime, etc.
- Improper postural habits.

Do you know the relative load on your spine measured at L_{3-4}?

- Lying on the sides (25%)
- Standing 100%
- Seated 145%
- Standing with forward bend — 150%
- Sitting with forward bend — 180%

Generally,

- Load is better in supported sitting than unsupported sitting
- Lumbar support decreases the load.

DEFINITIVE CAUSES

- Degenerative changes make the disc susceptible to trauma. Any trauma which suddenly increases the pressure will result in rupture of the posterior fibres of the annulus, e.g. weightlifting, fall on the buttocks, direct trauma to the back, twisting movements and occupation involving flexion and lifting motions.
- Disc may also rupture during pregnancy, labour and after prolonged bedrest due to disc softening.
- Disc rupture without any cause is due to degenerative process.

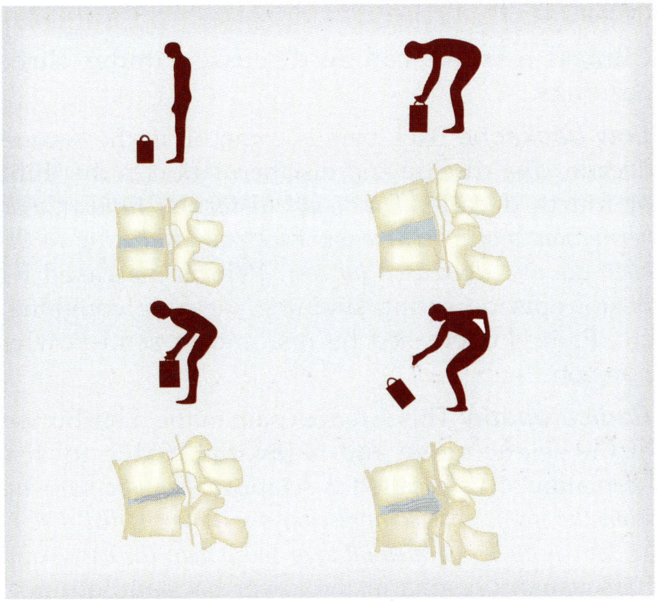

Fig. 34.7: Showing common mode of disc prolapse due to sudden and improper weightlifting

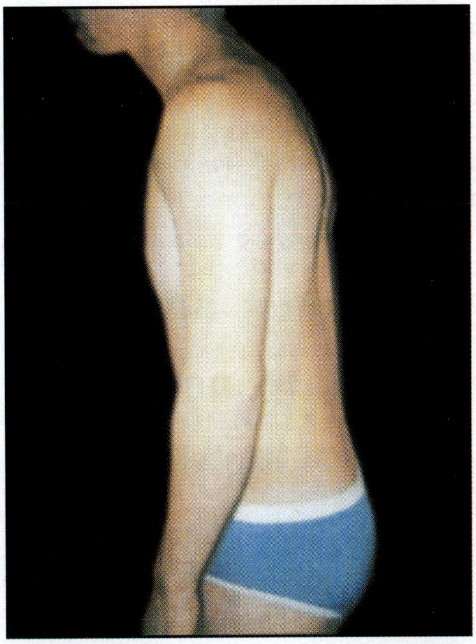

Fig. 34.8: Clinical presentation in a patient with disc slip

Remember

About disc disease

- It is due to ageing process.
- It passes through three stages.
- There are four types of disc prolapse .
- Disc prolapse is a complication of Stages I and II.
- Herniation can take place into the body or posteriorly into spinal canal.

CLINICAL FEATURES

Clinical features can be discussed under three headings:

Low backache Back pain is common in the second decade, disc disease and disc herniation in the third or fourth decade. *The usual history of lumbar disc herniation is of repetitive low back pain, radiating to the buttocks and decreased by rest.* Pain is increased by flexion episode, sitting, straining, sneezing, coughing, etc. Pain is decreased by rest and in semi-Fowler position.

Radiculopathy This refers to pain in the distribution of the sciatic nerve and is invariably due to disc herniation. This is called as sciatica. *The radicular pain from the nerve root compression due to herniated disc is evidenced by leg pain equal to or more than the back pain.* Pain usually begins in the lower back radiating to the sacroiliac regions, buttocks and thigh. The radicular pain usually extends below the knee.

Nerve root compression About 95 per cent of the disc prolapse takes place through the L_{4-5} region compressing the L_5 nerve root (Fig. 34.9). The other nerve roots commonly involved are L_4 and S_1 due to disc prolapse between L_{3-4} and L_5-S_1 respectively. Table 34.1 shows the various clinical manifestation following nerve root compression.

Remember one question test: Radicular pain

Between the knee and the ankle, where is the pain?

- Front → L_4
- Side → L_5
- Back → S_1

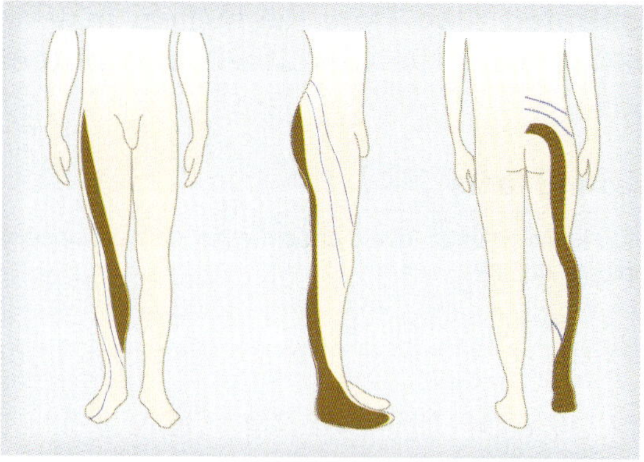

Fig. 34.9: Dermatomal pattern from above downwards belong to L_4 L_5 S_1 nerve roots respectively

EXAMINATION OF THE BACK (Table 34.2) *(Also See Section on Clinical Methods)*

1. *Inspection* Note any postural defects like scoliosis, lordosis or kyphosis
2. *Palpation* consists of:
   a. *Tenderness* Look for the following points:
      - Localised tender infiltrates of the skin and subcutaneous tissue.
      - Palpable tender induration of small intervertebral muscles.
      - Tenderness at the level of posterior articulation of the involved segment and pain on percussion of affected intervertebral space.
   b. *Movements* All the movements of the spine are tested.
3. *Evaluation of neurological system* The dermatomal and the myotomal distribution are carefully analysed (see Table 34.1) to detect the level of lesion.

Table 34.1: Nerve root compression

Disc prolapse between	*Pain*	*Radiation*	*Sensory loss*	*Motor loss*	*Reflexes loss*	**SLRT*
L_3 and L_4 L_4 nerve root is involved	Lumbar region	Along the antero-medial aspect of the thigh	Medial shin	Quadriceps	Knee jerk	Normal
L_4 L_5 95% disc prolapse occur here L_5 root involved	Lumbar region, groin, sacroiliac region	Lateral thigh, leg, dorsum of the foot and hallux	Hallux area	Extensor hallucis muscle	Medial hamstrings	Reduced
L_4 and S_1 S_1 root is involved	Same as above	Buttocks, posterior thigh, leg and lateral foot	Lateral foot	Gastrocnemius	Ankle jerk	Reduced

Easy way to remember

L_4 root involvement—remember '4' heads of quadriceps. Hence knee jerk lost (Fig. 34.10)

L_5 root involvement—remember '5' toes—Great toe and lateral 4 toes lose extension (Fig. 34.11)

S_1 root involvement—remember 'A' of tendo-Achilles. Hence, ankle jerk lost (Fig. 34.12)

*SLRT—straight leg raising test

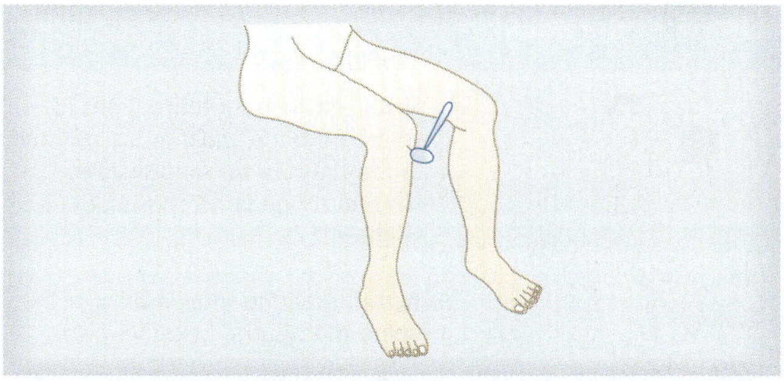

Fig. 34.10: Involvement of L_4 myotome (Patient is unable to extend the knee and loss of knee reflex)

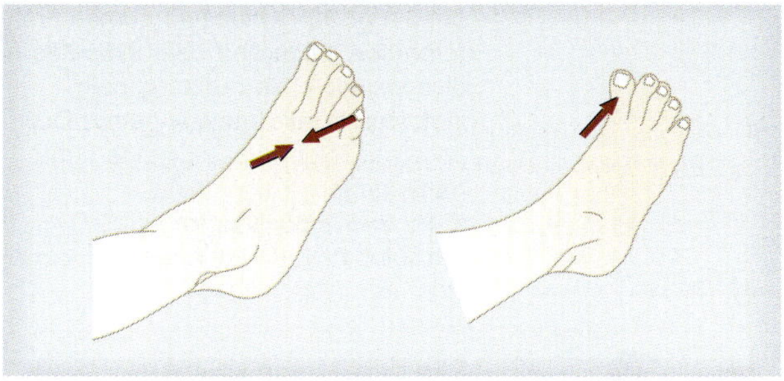

Fig. 34.11: Involvement of L_5 myotome, patient is unable to extend the toes

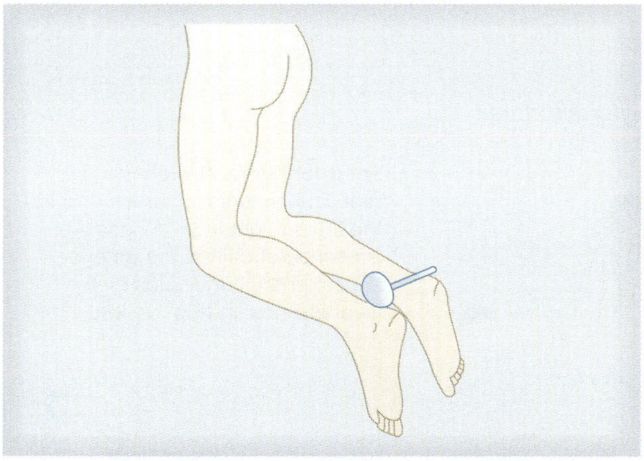

Fig. 34.12: S_1 myotome involvement loss of ankle jerk and plantarflexion

4. *Clinical tests* These tests are based on the stretching of sciatic nerve over the prolapsed disc:
   a. Forward bending to touch the toes.
   b. Sitting and alternatively extending one leg and then the other.
   c. *Slump test* Sitting bent forward and extending one leg and then the other.
   d. *Straight leg raising test (SLRT)* patient is in supine position, the examiner raises the leg straight one after the other. Up to 30° nerve is not put under stretch. Between 30 and 70° nerve comes into contact with the prolapsed disc and the patient complains of pain. Beyond 70° if the patient complains of pain, it is usually not due to disc prolapse but could be due to sacroiliac joint involvement.
   Modifications of SLRT
      - ***Lasègue's test*** Here, the hip is flexed, knee is flexed and the leg is slowly straightened.
      - ***Bückling's sign*** Perform an SLRT till the patient complains of pain. Now ask the patient to flex the knee. Pain decreases due to relief of tension on the nerve.
      - ***Sicard's test*** After doing SLRT, dorsiflex the great toe. This puts further tension on the sciatic nerve and the patient complains of pain.
      - ***Fajersztajn's test*** After doing SLRT, dorsiflex the foot. This tenses the sciatic nerve and the patient complains of pain.
   e. *Well leg raising test* Here, the patient is asked to perform SLRT of the normal limb. If the patient complains of pain on the affected side, then it is highly suggestive of disc prolapse and this is a pathognomonic test which has more relevance than the conventional SLRT.
   f. *Bilateral straight leg raising test* Here, patient is asked to raise both the legs simultaneously. This is a test for the sacroiliac joint rather than the spine. During the first 70°, stress is on the SI joint, over 70° stress is on the lumbar spine.
   g. *Femoral nerve stretch test (reverse SLRT).* Here, the patient is in prone position and is asked to lift the leg straight. This puts a stretch on the femoral nerve. If the patient complains of pain, it indicates a high level disc prolapse ($L_{1\text{-}2\text{-}3}$).

Remember

About SLRT

- SLRT exerts tension on the sciatic nerve as it passes over the prolapsed disc.
- In disc prolapse SLRT is positive usually between 30° and 70°.
- Many modifications of SLRT either exert more tension (Fajersztajn's test) or relieves tension on the sciatic nerve. (Bückling sign).
- Contralateral well leg raising test is more pathognomonic of disc prolapse than SLRT.
- Bilateral leg raising test has more relevance for SI joint pathology than back.
- Reverse leg raising test or femoral nerve stretch test is for detecting high lesion like L_1 root involvement.

Table 34.2: Clinical examination of the back

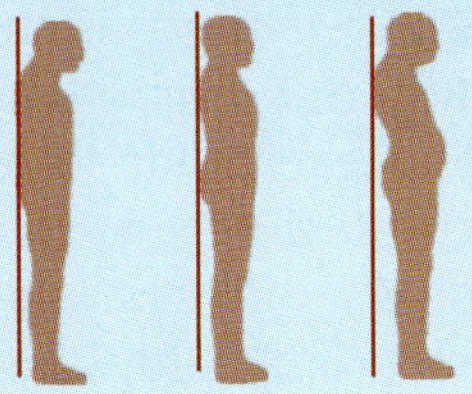

Fig. 34.13

Inspection With the patient in standing position look for postural abnormalities.
The figure from left to right depict thoracic hyperkyphosis, normal spine and exaggerated lumbar lordosis (Fig. 34.13).

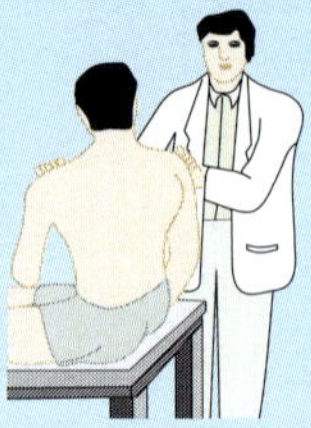

Fig. 34.17

4. **Rotation** Instruct the patient to rotate from the waist to the left and to the right as far as possible. Normal range is 45° per side (Fig. 34.17).

   Note: In all the movements of the spine the neutral position is 0°.

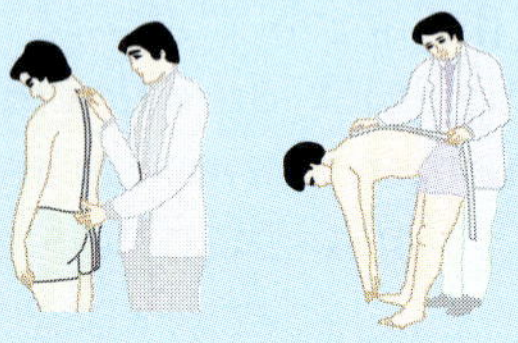

Fig. 34.14

Movements of the spine

1. **To test flexion**
   Instruct the patient to bend forwards as much as possible at the waist.
   Normal flexion is 80° or fingertips 3 to 4 inches from the floor (Fig. 34.14).

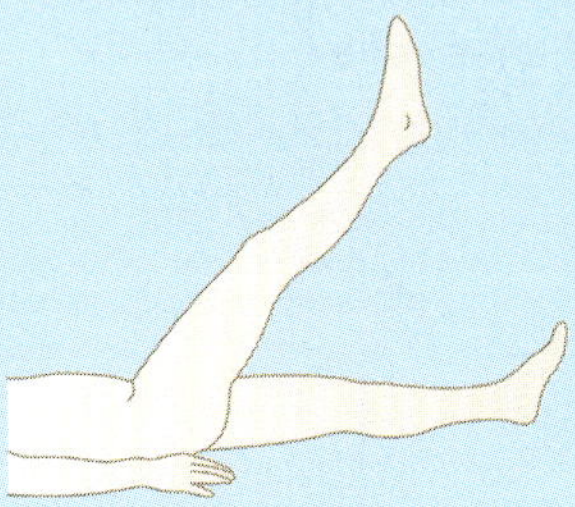

Fig. 34.18

SLRT With the patient in the supine position, raise his or her leg to the point of pain or 90° whichever comes first.
Inference: Localised pain indicates a disc lesion, while radiating pain indicates sciatic radiculopathy. Dull posterior thigh pain indicates tight hamstrings.
If the test is positive for sciatic radiculopathy, do Lasegue test, buckle sign, etc. (Fig. 34.18)

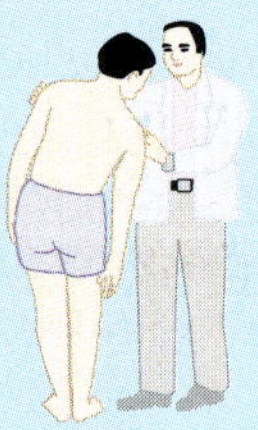

Fig. 34.15

2. **Lateral flexion**
   Instruct the patient to bend to the left and to the right as far as possible.
   Normal range is 35° on each side (Fig. 34.15).

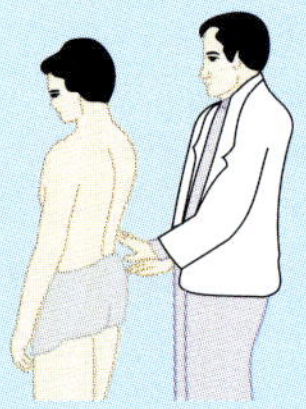

Fig. 34.19

Site of pain and sciatic radiculopathy in disc prolapse (Fig. 34.19). Elicit the tenderness over the spine as shown in this figure

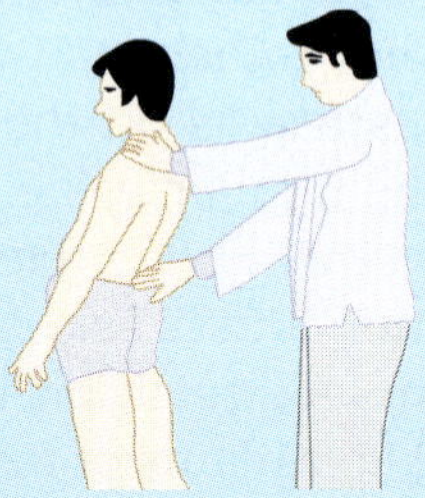

Fig. 34.16

3. **Extension**
   Instruct the patient to bend at the waist as far backward as possible. Normal range is 20 to 30° (Fig. 34.16).

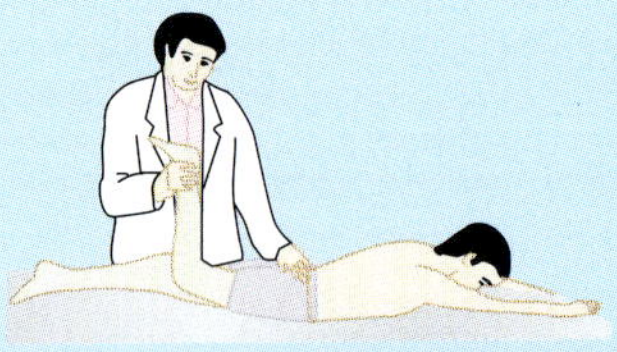

Fig. 34.20

Femoral nerve stretch test The patient is instructed to lift the leg straight in prone position. Presence of pain in the anterior aspect of thigh indicates high level disc lesion (Fig. 34.20).

Clinical facts

Diagnosis of the disc disease is a suspect if:

- Leg pain is minimal and back pain is predominant.
- If pain is bizarre or continuous.
- If the forward bending of the spine is normal.
- If the lumbar spine deviates to the opposite side.
- If tenderness is elicited over the midline.
- *Remember the hallmark of disc disease is repetitive low backache and buttock pain which is relieved by rest.*
- It is important to note that paraesthesiae and motor signs are seen in 96 per cent of cases of disc prolapse. Sensory signs are seen in 80 per cent. They are distributed along the involved nerve roots as explained earlier.

INVESTIGATIONS OF LOW BACKACHE

Radiography of the back is not very reliable as normal findings are observed in 7 to 46 per cent of the cases. Disc space is reduced in old cases; but in acute cases, it is maintained. Oblique view is recommended to rule out spondylolysis. It also helps to detect lumbar spondylosis (Fig. 34.21).

Myelography consists of injecting radiopaque dye (Myodil was used earlier now it is the water-soluble Iopamiro 300 which is being used) into the spinal

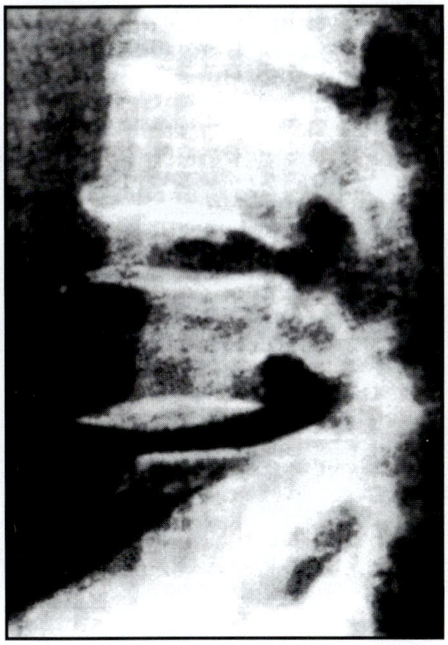

Fig. 34.21: Radiograph showing lumbar spondylosis

canal and taking radiographs of the back. It is helpful in detecting the intraspinal lesions, spinal stenosis and cases of previously operated (Fig. 34.22) backs. It is also indicated when the diagnosis is in doubt. It is an invasive procedure and is no longer performed. It is now replaced by noninvasive procedures like CT scan and MRI.

Remember

Diagnostic clues to detect high level disc lesion involving L_1 and L_2 nerve roots

- Pain in the groin or testicles
- Cauda equina lesion
- Positive femoral stretch test
- Atrophy of the involved limb
- 95% of the disc ruptures usually occur at L_4 L_5

CT scan It is a very useful noninvasive, painless outpatient procedure. It gives a cross-sectional study of the pathology. It, however, fails to detect intraspinal lesion, arachnoiditis and scar from disc herniation. It helps to detect the foraminal stenosis and the lateral disc prolapse (Fig. 34.23).

MRI This is also an extremely useful, painless, noninvasive outpatient procedure. It helps to detect the intraspinal lesion, helps to examine the entire spine and identifies degenerative disc (Figs 34.24). However, it is expensive and hence prohibitive.

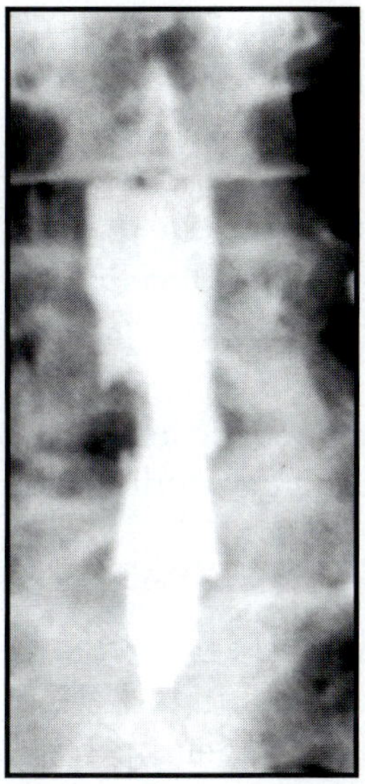

Fig. 34.22: Myelographic study of the lumbar spine

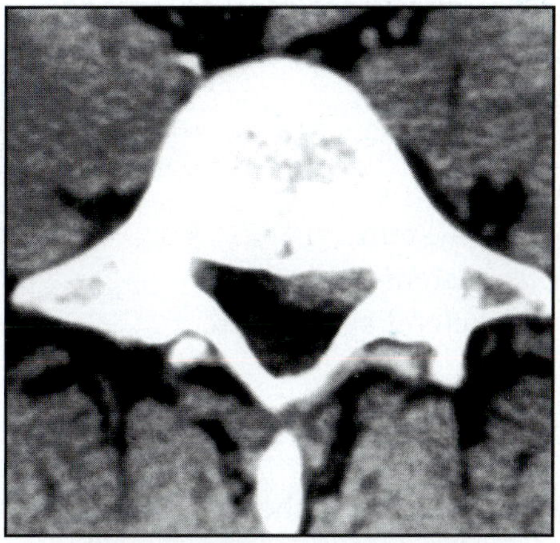

Fig. 34.23: CT scan showing posterolateral disc herniation

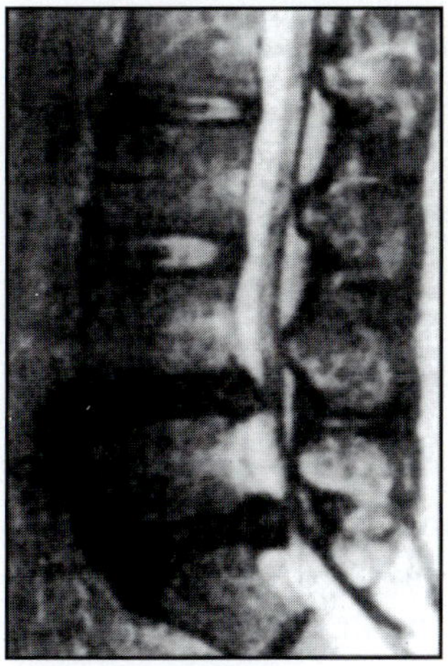

Fig. 34.24: MRI of lumbar spine showing bilateral disc prolapse

Section 4

Discography After identifying the disc correctly, through a needle, a radiopaque dye is injected into the space. This reproduces the pain experienced by the patient previously and is relieved by injecting Xylocaine. This confirms the diagnosis. It is a painful procedure and can introduce infection into the disc. Hence, it is less practised.

Other tests of diagnostic importance are *bone scans, EMG,* routine laboratory studies, injection studies, etc.

DIFFERENTIAL DIAGNOSIS

There are many causes for backache. The most common one being lumbar disc disease due to abnormal posture and ageing process. The differential diagnosis is as follows:

Extrinsic causes (unrelated to spine)

Diseases of the:

- Urogenital system
- Gastrointestinal system
- Vascular system
- Endocrine system
- Nervous system
- Musculoskeletal system, etc.

Intrinsic causes (related to spine)

Important causes

- Unstable spondylolisthesis
- Osteoporosis and compression of the vertebrae
- Marked loss of disc height at multiple levels
- Severe scoliosis.

Unimportant causes

- Lumbar spondylosis
- Mild discopathy
- Arthroses of the facet joints
- Disc calcification
- Spina bifida
- Schmorl's nodes
- Mild-to-moderate scoliosis.

Predominant cause of backache as already suggested is lumbar disc disease. Common diseases that mimick lumbar disc disease include ankylosing spondylitis, multiple myeloma, vascular insufficiency, arthritis of the hip joint, osteoporosis with stress fractures, extradural tumours, peripheral neuropathy, herpes zoster, etc.

Do you know the common diagnosis of low backache?

Well, here is a list:

- Common low backache (disc disease, muscle and ligament strain and sprain of the back)
- Myofascial pain
- Spondylosis
- Spondylolisthesis
- Facet syndrome
- Fibromyalgia
- Lumbar cord stenosis

Pitfalls: Only in 15% of the cases of low backaches, accurate diagnosis of a specific cause can be made.

TREATMENT OF LOW BACKACHE DUE TO LUMBAR DISC DISEASE

The principles of treating low backache due to lumbar disc disease are explained by **three R's**:

- **R**elieve pain in acute cases.
- **R**estore normal movements in chronic cases.
- **R**ecurrence is to be prevented.

The following are the treatment modalities in low backache.

Conservative therapy *Absolute bedrest is the best treatment for acute low backache.* Ice packs, nonsteroidal anti-inflammatory drugs (NSAIDs), muscle relaxants, antidepressants are recommended. Bucks extension skin traction and pelvic traction helps to relieve pain. As the pain decreases, isometric abdominal and lower extremity exercises are begun. Walking within limits of comfort is also encouraged. Sitting and riding in a car is discouraged. Back education and importance of proper posture is taught. Choice of exercises is based on the increase or decrease of pain by extension or flexion. *If pain decreases by extension, extension exercises are recommended. On the other hand, if the pain decreases by flexion, flexion exercises are recommended. Improvements in symptoms with extension is indication of a good prognosis with conservative care.* Lower extremity exercises increase the strength and relieve the stress on the back, but they may increase the lower extremity arthritis. Thus, the true benefit of such treatment may be in the promotion of good posture and body mechanics than strength.

Back braces or belts are recommended in acute stages. They are discarded as soon as symptoms decrease; otherwise, muscles become weak and hasten the degeneration.

See the pictorial display of proper postural habits and back exercises recommended for prevention of low backache (Tables 34.3 and 34.4).

Did you know?

Maximal load reduction on the disc with tight corsets is 20 to 30%.

Table 34.3: Proper postural habits (Figs. 34.25 to 34.30)

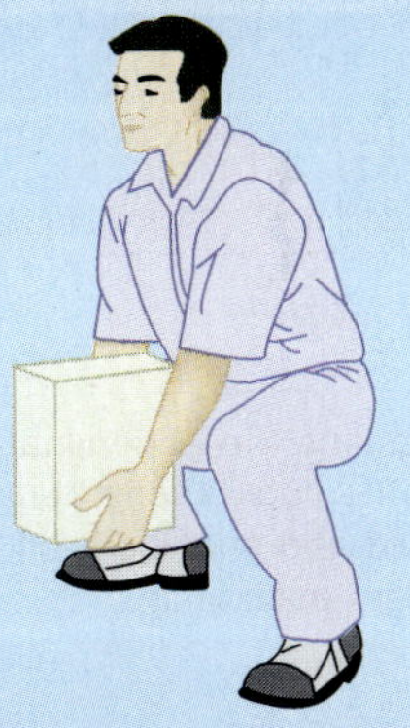

Fig. 34.25: *Lifting objects*—Bend at your knees and not at your waist. Hold the object you are lifting close to your body, not higher than your chest. It is easier to push rather than pull heavy objects, e.g. furniture, and keep the knees bent while pushing

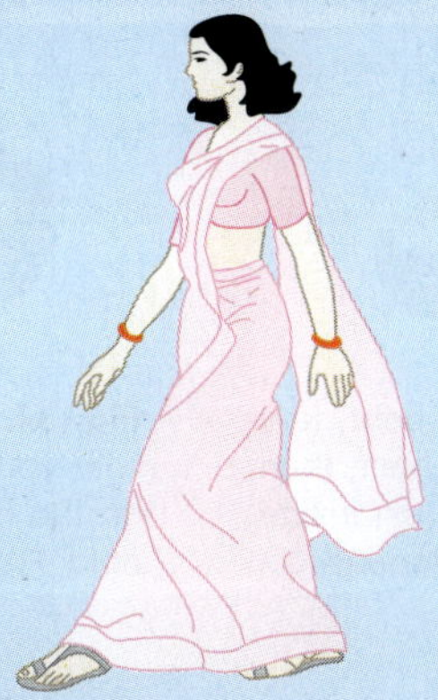

Fig. 34.26: *Walking*—Walk well with your head high, chin tucked in, toes pointing straight in front. Wear comfortable footwear. Take steps of a natural, comfortable length. Swing the arms naturally

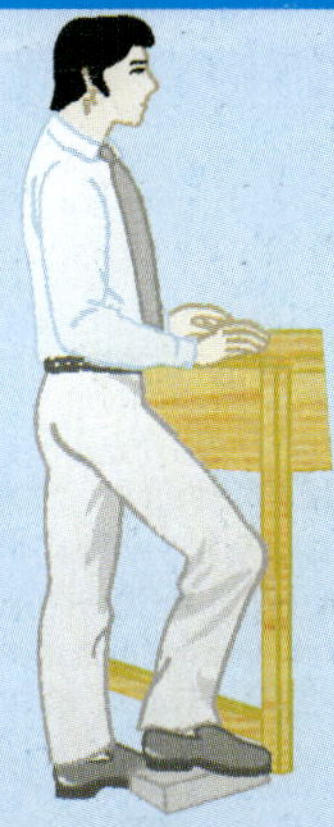

Fig. 34.27: *Standing*—Keep one foot in front and knees slightly bent while standing upright. If you have to stand for a long time, try keeping one foot higher than the other, on a low stool. Change your position often.

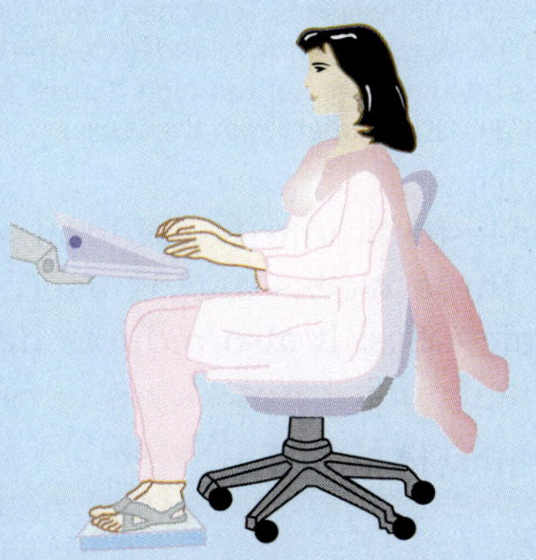

Fig. 34.28: *Sitting*—Ensure your back is firmly touching the back of the chair. Keep the knees slightly higher than the hips, e.g. by using something to prop up your feet. Sit close to your desk or table to avoid bending forward. Do not sit for too long. And when driving, move the front seat close to the steering wheel and both hands should be kept on the wheel.

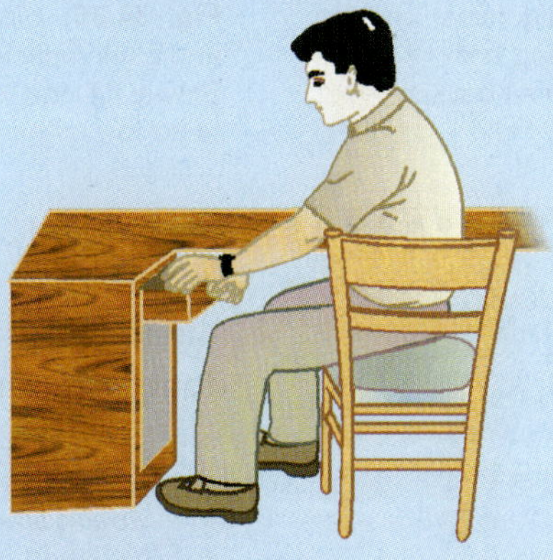

Fig. 34.29: *Turning and reaching out*— Do not twist your waist. Rather, turn by moving your feet. Keep the phone and such like objects within easy reach; do not strain to reach them. Stand on a stool to reach high objects.

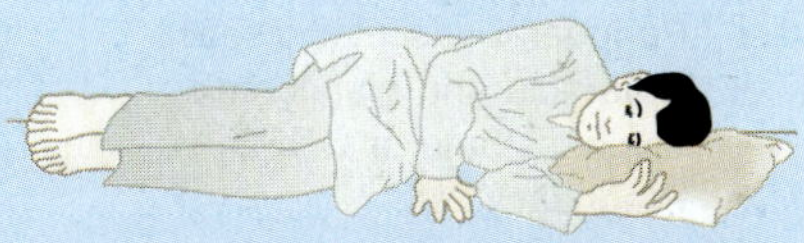

Fig. 34.30: *Sleeping*—If you sleep on your side, keep knees and lower body bent a little. On your back, put a pillow under your knees. Try not to sleep on your stomach—but if you must, put a pillow under your waist not under your head. Use a firm mattress—neither soft/ squashy nor very hard.

Table 34.4: Exercises for low backache (Figs. 34.31 to 34.36)

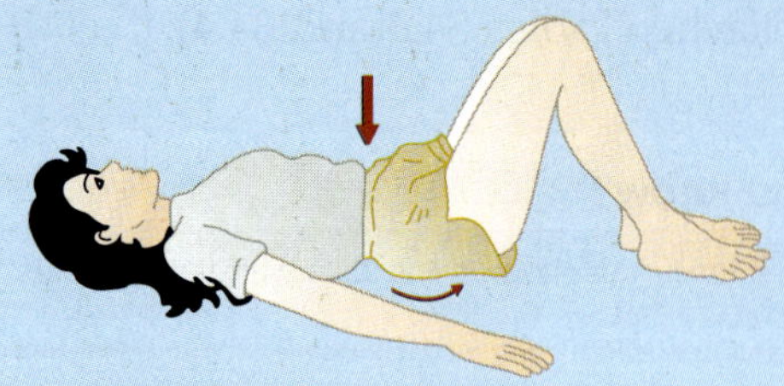

Fig. 34.31: *Pelvic tilt*—Makes abdominal muscles stronger. Lie on your back, legs bent, and feet flat on the floor with arms to your sides. Push your lower back against the floor—your hips will tilt up. Hold this position for a short while

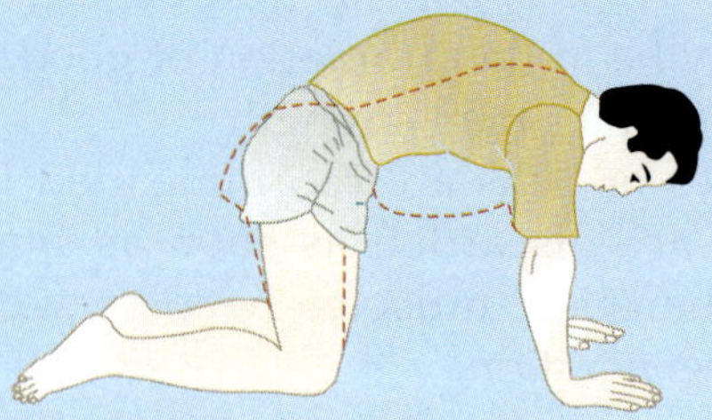

Fig. 34.34: *Cat and Camel*—Strengthens the back and abdominal muscles. Crouch on hands and knees. Keeping the head parallel to floor, arch your back and then let it gradually sag towards the floor by breathing out. Keep the arms straight

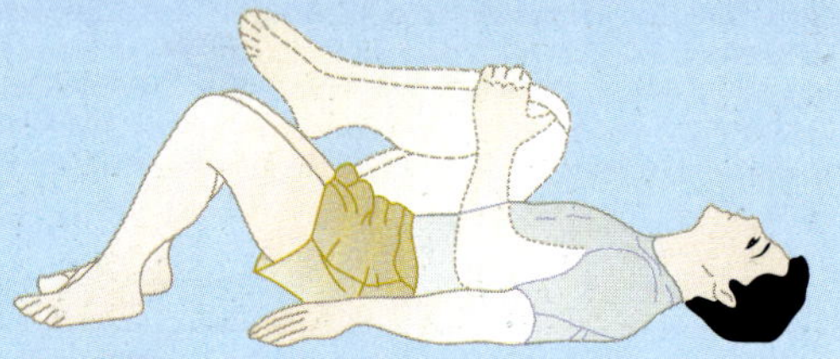

Fig. 34.32: *Knees to chest*—Lie on your back, knees bent, feet flat, arms to your sides. Raise first one knee to your chest, then the other, holding them with your hands as shown (or just inside your knee). Bring legs down one at a time and rest. Repeat

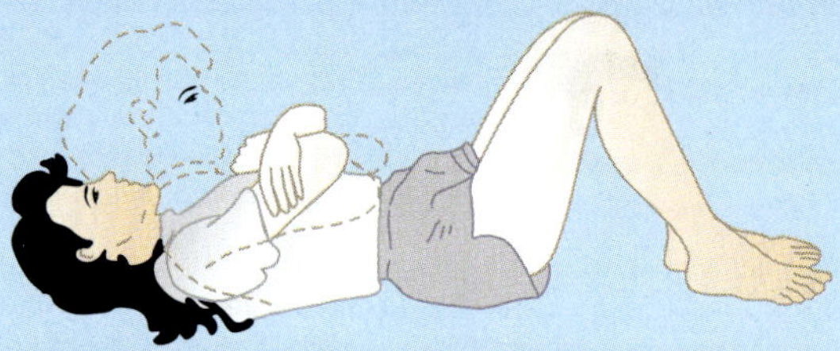

Fig. 34.35: *Semisit-up*—Strengthens the abdominal muscles. Lie with your back and feet flat on the floor, knees bent, arms folded on the chest. Lift only your head and shoulders off the floor and hold. Repeat, trying to hold longer each time

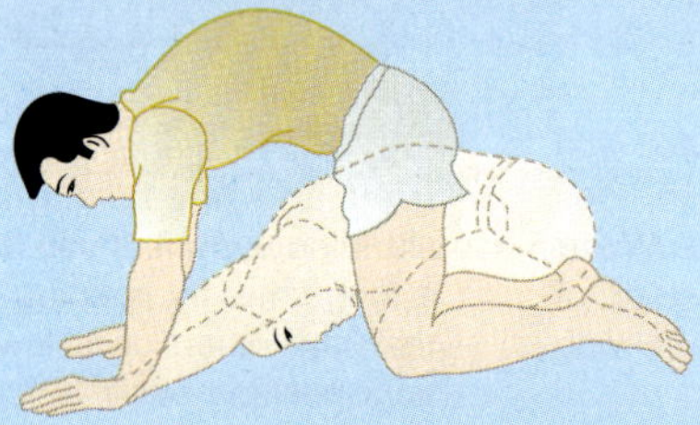

Fig. 34.33: *Trunk flex*—Stretches the back, abdominal and leg muscles. Crouch on the hands and knees. Bring chin in to the chest, and curve your back upwards. Gradually sit back on your heels, bringing the shoulders down to the floor. Hold

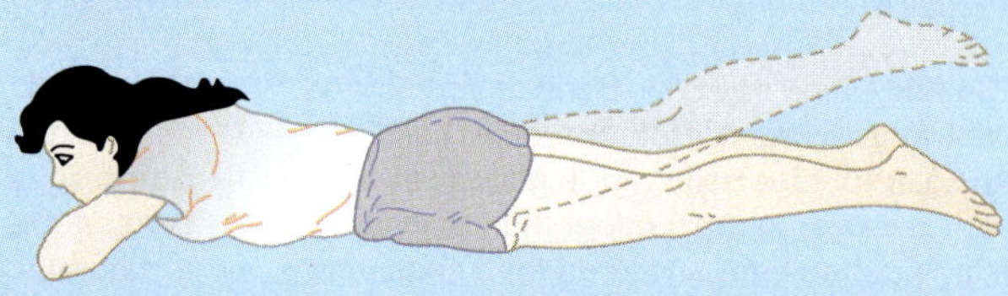

Fig. 34.36: *Hip stretch*—Strengthens and stretches hip, buttock and back muscles. Lie on the stomach, arms folded under the chin. Slowly lift one leg without bending, but not too high. Lower it and raise the other leg. Keep pelvis in contact with the floor

Remember

Contraindications to traction

- Hypertension
- Peripheral vascular disease
- Cataracts and glaucoma
- Labile asthma or COPD
- Pregnancy, etc.

How traction helps

- It relieves muscle spasm
- It may distract the facet joints
- It may distract the disc space

Epidural Steroids

Epidural steroids is a symptomatic method of treatment, and consists of injecting a long-acting steroid and a local anaesthetic into the epidural space. Its effect lasts for three weeks and is useful for subacute and chronic cases. It also reduces dependence on narcotics in chronic cases.

All about epidural steroid injection

- In vogue since 1950's.
- Effective in approximately 50% patients with low backache.
- It decreases inflammation and flushes out inflammatory proteins thereby reducing pain.
- It helps in better back rehabilitation.
- Maximum of three injections in a year with a two week gap is given.
- Adverse features include infection, dural puncture and arachnoiditis.
- It primarily decreases leg pain.
- After the injection, the patient is advised one day rest.

Note:
1. Each exercise is done one to five times twice daily.
2. The number of repetitions should be kept increasing to reach a minimum of ten repetitions twice daily.
3. Exercises are to be done slowly and smoothly.

How does exercise relieve low backache?

- Exercises pump the disc and increase water content.
- Relieves the muscle spasm and increase motion.
- Stretches and mobilises the facet joints.
- Repetitive motion helps the patient to overcome the fear of movement.
- Decreases the swelling around the nerves.

Surgery

Absolute indications
- Failed conservative management.
- Marked progressive weakness of muscles.
- Progressive neurological deficit.
- Cauda equina paralysis.

Relative indications
- Recurrent episodes of incapacitating sciatica.
- Pain unrelieved by complete rest from activity.

Principles of surgery The principle of surgery is to see that the pressure on the nerve root is relieved by removing the prolapsed disc. Dissection of muscles and bone removal should be kept at a minimum to prevent weakening of the spine.

Surgical Methods

1. *Laminectomy and disc excision* Earlier, this was the surgery of choice; but now, it is no longer resorted to as it makes the spine unstable.
2. *Hemilaminectomy* Here, part of the lamina is removed. It is considered by many as extended fenestration approach. If fenestration technique is properly done, hemilaminectomy is not necessary.
3. *Fenestration surgery* Here, the spine is approached unilaterally and the spine on the opposite side is not exposed. Here, only the contiguous margin of upper and lower laminae are removed and medial facetectomy is done. The disc is now excised. This procedure requires that the affected disc is correctly located by MRI and radiographic studies.
4. *Microscopic lumbar discectomy* (Fig. 34.37) Using an operating microscope, the disc can be excised through a very small incision (< 3.5 cm) with minimum damage to the structures and minimal blood loss. It is a technically demanding procedure and gives excellent results if done in properly indicated cases like a single level posterolateral disc prolapse. The patient can be discharged home within two days and he or she can return back to his or her normal work faster. In short, it can be described as a less invasive, less painful, more specific procedure giving maximum comforts to the patient. Dr PS Ramani calls it as "come today, go tomorrow" surgery!

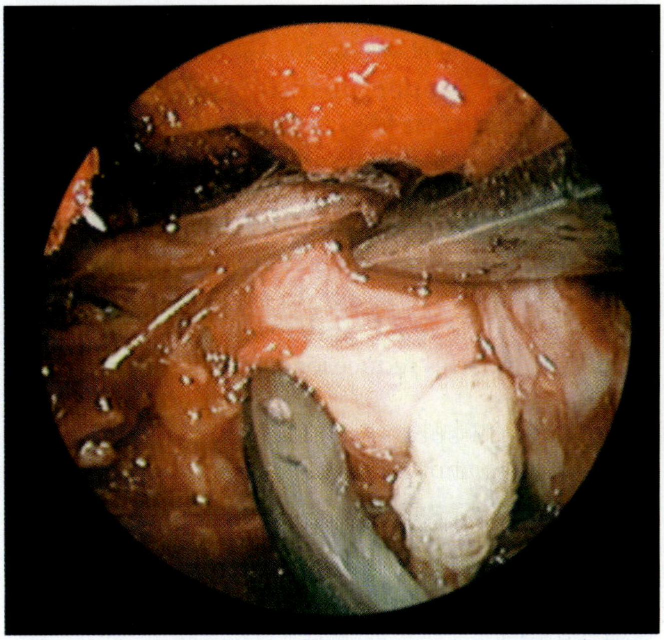

Fig. 34.37: Showing microscopic lumbar discectomy (MLD)

CHEMONUCLEOLYSIS

Indications are the same as for surgery. It is limited to lumbar spine. Drug used is chymopapain.

What is new in the treatment of low backache?

- MISS-(Minimally invasive spinal surgery) This consists of endoscopic spine surgery discectomy and was popularised by John Chiu.
- Laser discectomy
- Percutaneous discectomy (manual or automated)
- Total disc replacement (TDR): Total or partial disc replacement using a prosthetic disc nucleus for IVDP. It has a hydrogel core and is encased in a polyethylene jacket. It restores disc height and ensures normal range of mobility.

WAYS TO PREVENT RECURRENCE

This is the most important aspect of the management of backache. *Like in all other diseases, so in backache prevention is better than cure. Backache can be prevented to a large extent by observing the following measures:*

1. Adopting proper posture and creating an awareness that it is in the erect position that the back can withstand strain the best.
2. *Back education* Stress on the back is less when it is properly used during sitting, walking, etc. These proper habits have to be cultivated with practice.
3. *Back exercises* These aim to strengthen the abdominal, pelvic, back and thigh muscles. Strong healthy muscles reduce load on the discs and other structures.
4. *To avoid* all sports including the aerobic ones. Swimming and walking are encouraged.

Treatment plan of backache

1. **Conservative**	• Absolute bedrest • Traction • NSAIDs • Belts
2. **Epidural steroids**	• For subacute and chronic cases • Long-acting steroids + Local anaesthetics • Reduces dependence on narcotics • Effect lasts for 3 weeks
3. **Surgery**	• Done in proper indications • Open or microscopic or endoscopic lumbar discectomy
4. **Chemonucleolysis**	• Same indications as for surgery • Limited only to lumbar spine • Drug used is chymopapain
5. **Physiotherapy**	• Active and passive physiotherapy • Flexion or extension exercises
6. **Recurrence prevention**	• Back education • Proper postural habits • Back exercises • Avoid all sports

Remember

Consider serious causes of backache if any one of the following situations are encountered

- Pain in patients less than 10 years of age.
- First time backache in patients greater than 60 years.
- Unexplained weight loss.
- Chronic cough.
- Night pains.
- Intermenstrual bleeding.
- Altered bowel function.
- Altered bladder control.
- Visual disturbances and balance problems.

Remember the Do's and Don'ts

Do's

- Forward bent attitude.
- Body weight borne on the heels.
- Proper weight lifting as shown earlier.
- Sit with buttocks tucked under.
- While driving, push the seat forwards to raise the knees and decrease the lordosis.
- Flex the knees and hip when lying on the side.
- Turn to the side and then get up.

Dont's

- Sleep in the prone position.
- Rise from a sitting position suddenly.
- Bend over a washbasin.
- Wear high heels as pelvis is thrust forward and the spine bends backward.
- Use too high a chair.
- Use soft mattress which increases the lumbosacral extension. A firm mattress encourages lumbar spine to be straight.

Remember B's in backache

- **B**ad posture
- **B**edrest
- **B**elts
- **B**ack education
- **B**ack exercises
- **B**ed choice

APPROACH TO A PATIENT WITH LOW BACKACHE

Low backache is an extremely common malady afflicting the human race across the globe cutting the geographical boundaries, race, culture, etc. Eighty to ninety per cent of the human population will suffer from some form of backache, mild or severe in their lifetime. It is of interest to know the historical background regarding low back pain.

A quick historical review

- Backache and leg pain are known since beginning of history.
- Primitive culture called it a work of a demon.
- Greeks recognised the symptoms as disease.
- In the 18th century, Cotumis attributed pain to the sciatic nerve.
- In 1881, Lasegue test described a test to distinguish hip disease from sciatica (first described by Frost).
- Virchow Kocher, etc. described acute traumatic ruptures of the disc that resulted in death.

- Goldthwait in 1911 first attributed back pain to posterior displacement of disc.
- Dandy in 1929 first reported removal of a disc tumour from patients suffering from sciatica.
- Myelography was first described in 1922.
- Barr (1932) finally attributed the source of sciatica to the herniated lumbar disc.
- Barr (1934) suggested surgical treatment for disc excision.
- Layman Smith (1963) suggested enzymatic dissolution of disc.
- Kirkaldy-Willis opine ageing as the primary theory in disc disease.
- Nuchenson in 1964, White and Punjabi in 1982 described biomechanics of spine.
- Schnack in 1983 described clinical anatomy.

CAUSES OF BACKACHE

A variety of conditions related and unrelated to spine cause backache (see the box). The common causes of backache are:

Unaccustomed activities A sedentary person suddenly adopting an active form of life, etc.

Poor posture Improper posture during sitting, walking, standing, working places, enormous load on the back and results in backacke. This is by far the most common cause of low backache (Figs 34.38A to F).

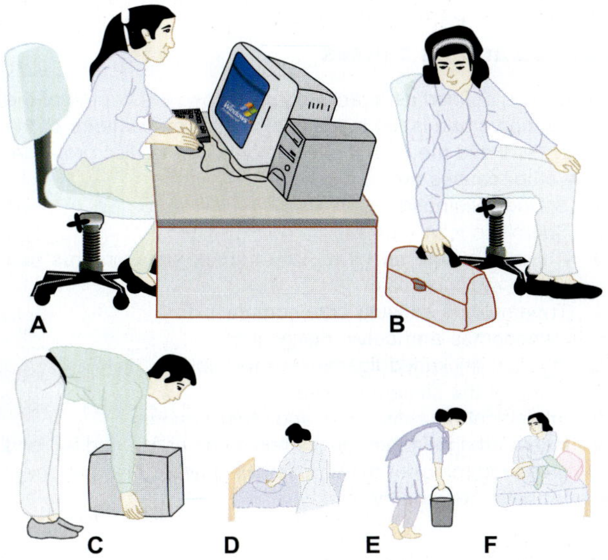

Figs 34.38A to F: Showing various common mechanisms of acute low backache: (A) Improper posture, (B) Sudden twist, (C) Faulty weightlifting, (D) Bending, (E) Sudden weightlifting, (F) Faulty sitting

Quick facts: causes of low backache (Fig. 34.39)

Common causes
- Back muscle sprain
- Prolapsed lumbar intervertebral disc
- Obesity
- Poor posture
- Facet joint arthritis
- Unaccustomed activities
- Occupational causes

Uncommon causes
1. *Congenital causes* (4 'S')
   - Scoliosis
   - Spondylolisthesis
   - Spina bifida
   - Spondylolysis
2. *Infective conditions*
   - Osteomyelitis
   - Tuberculosis
   - Brucellosis, etc.
3. *Traumatic causes*
   - Vertebral body injuries, posterior arch fractures
   - Muscle sprain/strain
   - Prolapsed disc
4. *Inflammatory causes*
   - Rheumatoid arthritis
   - Ankylosing spondylitis and other SSAs
5. *Neoplasms*
   - Benign—osteoid osteoma
   - Malignant—secondaries, multiple myeloma, etc.
6. *Metabolic causes*
   - Osteoporosis
   - Osteomalacia
7. *Degenerative conditions*
   - Osteoarthritis
   - Lumbar spondylosis
8. *Referred pain from*
   - Gynaecological diseases
   - Genitourinary diseases
   - Gastrointestinal conditions, etc.

Occupational backache Certain occupation places enormous stress on the back, e.g. garbage collectors, porters, etc.

Obesity Protruding abdomen places enormous strain on the back (see Fig. 34.2B).

Muscle strain In 80 per cent of the cases, backache is due to sprain of the back muscles during activity, sports, trauma, etc.

Prolapsed lumbar intervertebral disc This is the second most common cause for low back pain after muscle strain and ligament sprain. Discussed at great length in the previous section.

The facet joint osteoarthritis due to old age, repeated bending and twisting activities lead to arthritis of facet joints.

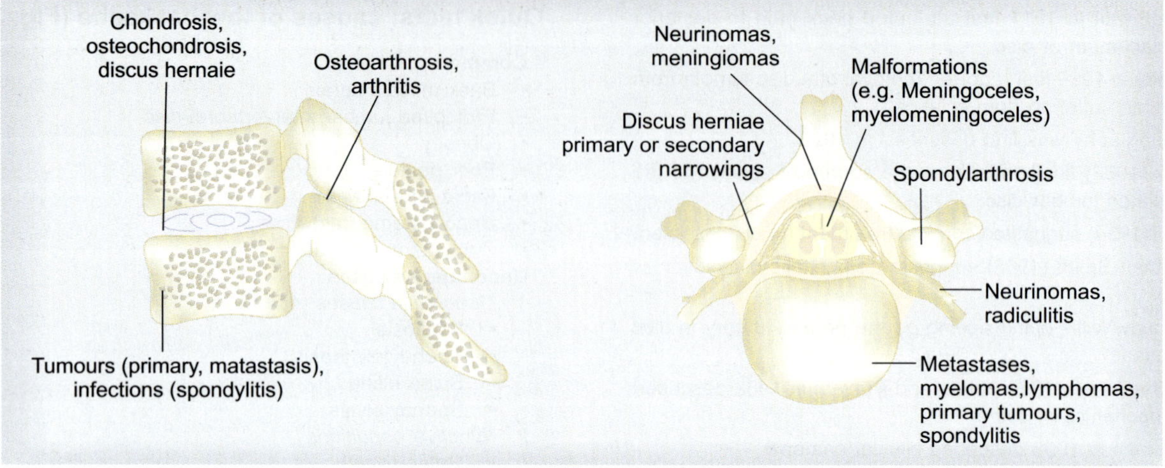

Fig. 34.39: Causes of uncommon lowbackaches and pathological processes of the spine, which can give rise to local spinal pain syndromes associated with painful muscle spasms

Spinal stenosis Spinal stenosis due to degenerative process is another common cause.

PRESENTING COMPLAINTS

Age Backache is more common in middle-aged and elderly people (usually degenerative). In young adults, it is due to trauma; and in children, it is usually due to organic lesions.

Age predilection and low backache

Age	Common causes
• < 20 years	Spondylolysis
• 20-40 years	Disc herniation
• > 40 years	Spondylosis
	Lumbar canal stenosis

Common to all age groups:
Ligament sprain/muscle strains.

Sex Osteoporosis, rheumatoid arthritis, etc. are more common in females. Ankylosing spondylitis, trauma, secondaries, etc. are more common in males.

Occupation People with sedentary jobs and heavy manual labourers are frequently prone for backache.

Pain

Over 90 per cent af the patients complain of pain in the back. The following points should be enquired:

Nature of pain Is it sudden (trauma) or gradual (spondylosis)? Was it preceded by weightlifting, sudden bending, etc? Is there remissions and exacerbations (disc disease) or is it continuous (tumours)? Is there history of night cries (e.g. TB spine)? Is it relieved by rest? Does it radiate to the lower limbs? etc.

Site Is the pain in the middle of the spine or paravertebral muscles? Is it in the dorsolumbar spine (trauma or tumour) or in the lumbar spine (disc disease)?

Sciatic pain Here, pain radiates along the course of the sciatic nerve (see causes for sciatica). Common cause is disc prolapse.

Sciatica and its causes

Sciatica is defined as a radiating pain along the course of the sciatic nerve and is felt in the back, buttocks, posterior of the thigh, legs and the foot. It is commonly due to disc prolapse. The other causes are:

1. Spondylolisthesis.
2. Sacroiliac joint arthritis.
3. Affliction of the nerve root by herpex simplex virus can cause radicular pain.
4. Tuberculoma causing cord compression.
5. Lymphomas and pelvic malignancy.
6. Incurled thickened ligamentum flavum.
7. Cysts of the sacral nerve root.
8. Intraspinal neurofibromas and other tumours.
9. Haemorrhage in the ependymoma can cause sudden and gross neurological deficit, mimicking acute disc prolapse.
10. Diabetic neuropathy, etc.

BIOCHEMICAL CAUSES

Recently, it has been suggested but not clearly demonstrated that blood pooling in various blood vessels surrounding the nerve roots may contribute to impaired nerve root formation and sciatica.

NEUROGENIC CLAUDICATION

This is a feature of spinal stenosis *(See p. 373).*

Neurological Symptoms

These consist of paraesthesia, muscle weakness, disturbance of sphincters, cauda equina syndrome, etc.

Facet Syndromes

Here, the patient complains of chronic backache, early morning stiffness, difficulty in getting out of bed, standing, sitting or climbing.

OTHER COMPLAINTS

There may be history of stiffness, pain in other joints (e.g. rheumatoid arthritis), constitutional symptoms (e.g. tuberculosis, malignancy, etc.), genitourinary complaints etc.

Physical Signs

Stance and gait Does the patient stand with a normal stance or has deformities like scoliosis, kyphosis, lordosis or pelvic tilt (see Fig. 34.13)? Is the gait normal or altered?

Spasm This is seen in acute painful conditions of the spine. The patient complains of pain in the paravertebral muscles and painful restriction of all the spine movements (see Fig. 34.8).

Movements There may be restriction of the spine movements due to the organic lesions affecting the back.

Swelling Swelling due to cold abscesses may be present.

Tenderness It may be present over the spinous process, in between the spinous processes, over muscles, ligaments, facet joints, etc.

NEUROLOGICAL EXAMINATION

This consists of examinations of the various dermatomes for sensations, myotomes for muscle power and reflexes (*ref. p.* 422).

SLRT and tension signs This is to know the effects of disc prolapse on the sciatic nerve (the tests are described on (*ref. p.* 423).

OTHER EXAMINATIONS

Other examinations include examinations of the adjacent joints, peripheral pulses, abdominal, rectal or paravaginal examinations.

INVESTIGATIONS

Blood tests These are useful in detecting metabolic, hormonal, infective and malignant conditions.

Radiology Routine plain radiographs of the lumbar spine is advised. Both anteroposterior and lateral views are usually required. Oblique views are helpful in detecting the fracture of pars. Though X-rays are not very helpful in detecting the disc prolapse, it is of value in diagnosing metabolic, degenerative, inflammatory, malignant conditions affecting the spine.

Myelography This procedure is not routinely used anymore because of its complications. However, it has a role in demonstrating blocks due to disc prolapse.

CT scan It is a noninvasive procedure and helps to identify the bone and soft tissue problems with greater accuracy.

MRI scan This is the gold standard in the investigations of the spine. It is noninvasive and is better than CT scan in diagnosing the bone and soft tissue problems around the spine. However, its high cost is prohibitive and is available only in major cities and centres.

TREATMENT

The underlying cause has to be detected and managed accordingly. The treatment for backache consists of drugs like NSAIDs, muscle relaxants, physiotherapy, traction, use of belts and corsets (Fig. 34.40). Proper postural habits, back exercises and back education go a long way in preventing the backache. Surgery is done for specific indications *(ref. p. 429).*

OTHER IMPORTANT CAUSES OF BACKACHE

- *Spinal stenosis* This is discussed at length in the Chapter on Regional Disorders of Spine *(ref. p. 372).*
- *Spondylolisthesis (ref. p. 368).*
- Tuberculosis of spine *(ref. p. 503).*

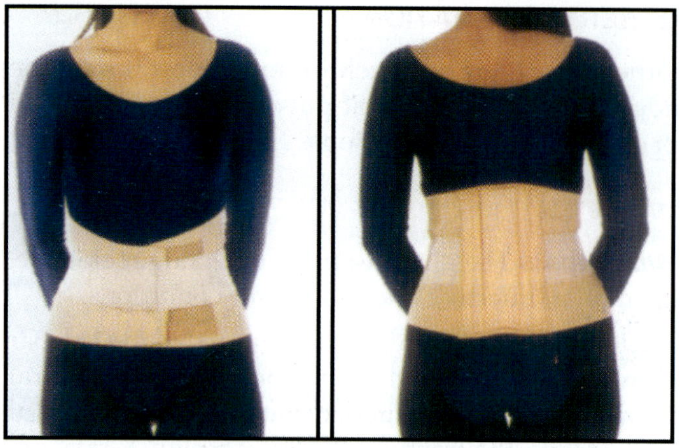

Fig. 34.40: Showing lumbar sacral belt application in LBA

- Spine injuries *(ref. p. 285).*
- Lumbar spondylosis *(ref. p. 552).*
- Osteomalacia *(ref. p. 479).*
- Osteoporosis *(ref. p. 481).*
- Ankylosing spondylitis *(ref. p. 538).*
- SI joint arthritis.
- Scoliosis *(ref. p. 362).*

BACKACHE IN SPECIAL SITUATIONS

BACKACHE IN CHILDREN (SCHOOL BAG SYNDROME)

It is indeed very pathetic that backache is no longer an unknown entity in children. Thanks to the practice of heavy school bags, the tender backs of children are subjected to untold misery.

Vital facts

Ideally, a child should not carry a bag of >10% of his or her body weight. But the scenario in present-day children's life is totally different.

Features

We can call this school bag related problems in a child as "school bag stress syndrome". Its features are:
- Pain in the shoulders, neck and back
- Tingling sensation in the arms, wrist and hands especially at night
- Head and neck are tilted to one side (postural imbalance)
- Frequent headaches
- An uncommon gait.

Prevention

Policy matter The school administrations and the government should devise strategies to lessen the burden of the books on the children. Providing lockers in the classrooms, reducing the number of books to be carried, giving less home work are some of the options. However, nothing seems to be happening over this front. Hence, the following improvisations can be tried:
- To use ergonomically designed school bags (Orthofix or orthogrip bags) (Fig. 34.41).
- These bags are easy on the shoulder and back
- They sit against the curve of the back
- They are provided with good padding for the bag straps, so that it does not burrow the skin (see box for safe school bag instructions).

Facts vital for school children (Safe School Bag Practice)

- Use an ergonomically designed school bag
- Use both straps to carry the bag
- The knapsack should have several compartments for equal weight distribution
- Heavy items are packed at the top so that weight is borne on the legs instead of the spine
- Both the straps should be worn across the shoulder and upper back to equalize the weight.

REPETITIVE STRESS INJURY (RSI)

Synonyms

- Occupational overuse syndrome (Scandinavia).
- Cumulative trauma disorder (USA).
- Work-related upper limb disorder (WHO).

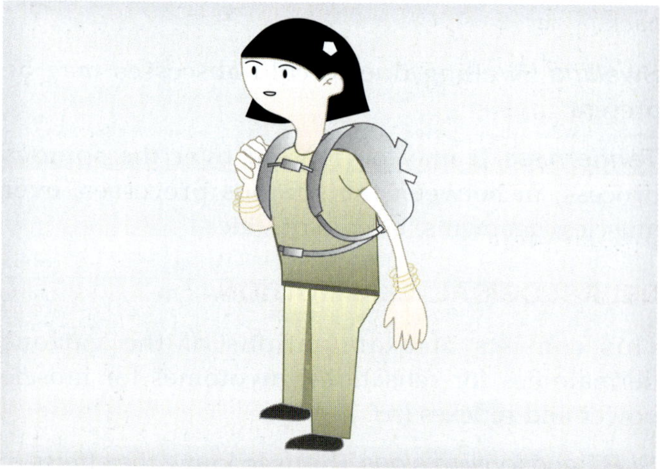

Fig. 34.41: School bag syndrome can be prevented by using Ergonomic school bags

Thanks to the computer boom in the not-so-distant past, software professionals were catapulated as cynosure of all eyes. However, this euphoria was short lived when they unsuspectingly became victims of a new computer related health hazard called the RSI. Of late, RSI is hogging all the limelight in the newspapers signifying its increased prevalence in the society. The moral of this story is that every sunny side has its darker shades too!

Definition

It is an overuse injury affecting the soft tissues (muscles, tendons and nerves) of the neck, shoulder, upper and lower back, arms and hands.

Note: In India, it is also called CRI (Computer Related Injury) and is due to improper computer use and improper postures.

Incidence

About 15 to 25% of all the computer users across the globe are affected by RSI.

Did you know?

RSI is not a new entity. It is present since centuries and was widely prevalent in:
- Musicians
- Butchers
- Assembly line centres
- Barbers
- Clerks, typists

However, it has seen a sudden boom thanks to the computer and call-centre cultures.

Who is at risk? Anyone who uses the computer for more than one hour every day is at risk and is seen in:
- Software engineers
- Bank employees
- Call centre staffs
- Children.

Presentation

RSI is infamous for a varied presentation stumping even with an experienced orthopaedician. Hence, a high degree of suspicion is required to diagnose this problem. The presentation could range from:
- Eyes — blurring of vision, watering of eyes, eye pain, etc.
- Head — headache, restlessness, etc.
- Neck pain
- Shoulder pain
- Arm pain
- Pain in the fingers
- Tingling and numbness
- Features suggestive of carpal tunnel syndrome, etc.
- Backache
- Foot pain, etc.

Stages

- *Stage I* Symptoms are seen only at work.
- *Stage II* Symptoms persist but disappear with rest.
- *Stage III* Symptoms are permanent.

Investigations

Routine investigations like laboratory tests, plain X-ray, CT scan, MRI, etc. are not of much importance in detecting RSI. The diagnosis is mainly clinical.

Treatment

RSI is easier to prevent than the arduous curative measure.

I. **Preventive measures:**
   - Adopting proper work habits
   - Adopting proper postures while working
   - Using ergonomically designed chairs
   - Taking 5 to 10 minutes break after every hour of work
   - Proper exercises every day
   - Avoiding too much of mental and physical pressures.

II. **Curative:** The curative measures are fortunately simple and consist of:
   - Drugs — NSAIDs, muscle relaxants etc
   - Physiotherapy — TENS, ultrasound, etc.
   - Exercises
   - Rehabilitation measures.

III. **Surgery:** Surgery is hardly required in an RSI patient.

BIBLIOGRAPHY

1. Anderson GBJ. Epidemiologic aspects of low back pain in industry. Spine 1981;6:53.
2. Arnaldi CC et al. Lumbar spinal stenosis and nerve root entrapment syndromes: definition and classification. Clin Orthop 1976;115:4.
3. Barr JS et al. Low back pain, and sciatica, results of treatment. J Bone Joint Surg 1951;33-A:633.
4. Basmajian JV. Therapeutic exercises. Baltimore: Williams and Wilkins Co, 1976;410-419.

5. Bell GR, Rothmann RH. The conservative treatment of sciatica. Spine 1984;9:54.
6. Bradford FK, Spurling RG. The intervertebral disk Ed2, Springfield, 1945, Charles C Thomas, Publisher.
7. Breig A, Troup JDG. Biomechanical consideration in the straight leg raising test. Spine 1979;4:242.
8. Canthen C. Lumbar spine surgery. Baltimore: Williams and Wilkins, 1983.
9. Christopher R Hyne. Ergonomics and back pain. Physio 1984;70:9.
10. Cover AB, Curwen IHM. Low back pain treated by manipulation. Br Med J 1955;19:705.
11. Cuikler JM et al. The use of epidural steroids in the treatment of lumbar radicular pain. J Bone and Joint Surg 1985;67-A:63.
12. Dankol DK, Pope MH, Lord J, Frymover JW. The relationship between work history, work environment and low back pain in men. Spine 1984;9:395.
13. Estridge MN, Routre SA, Johnson WG. The femoral stretching test: a valuable sign in diagnosing upper lumbar disc herniation. J Neurosurg 1982;57-813.
14. Ford LT, Goodman FG. X-ray studies of the lumbosacral spine. South Med J 1966;10-1123.
15. Frymoyer JW et al. Risk factors in low back pain: an epidemiological survey. J Bone Joint Surg 1983;65-A:213.
16. Goald HJ. Microlumbar discectomy: followup of 147 patients. Spine 1978;3:183.
17. Grieve GP. Mobilisation of the spine. New York: Churchill Livingstone 1975.
18. Harris R. Traction. In Litchy S (Ed): Massage, Manipulation and Traction. New Haven, Litch, 1960;223.
19. Hickling J. Spinal traction techniques. Physio 1972;58:58.
20. Hirschy JC, Leue WM, Berninger WH, Hamilton RH, Abbott GF: Ct of the lumbosacral spine: importance of the tomographic planes parallel to vertebral and plates. AJR 1981;136:47.
21. James AE, Jr Partain CL, Patton JA, et al. Current status of magnetic resonance imaging south. Med J 1985;78:580.
22. Judovich B. Lumbar traction therapy. JAMA 1955;159:549.
23. Kelsey JL et al. An epidemiologic study of lifting and twisting on the job and risk for acute prolapsed lumbar intervertebral disc. J Orthop Res 1984;2:61.
24. Kendall PH, Jenkins JM. Exercise for backache: a double blind controlled triale. Physio 1968;54:154.
25. Lidstrom A, Zachrisson M. Physical therapy on low back pain and sciatica. Scand J Rehab Med 1970;2:37.
26. Macnab I. Management of low back pain. In Abstrom JP (Jr), Editor. Current Practice in Orthopedic Surgery. St. Louis: CV Mosby Co 1973.
27. Macrae IF, Wright V. Measurement of back movement. Ann Rheum Dis 1969;28:584.
28. Macre IF, Wright V. Measurement of back movement. Ann Rheum Dis 1969;28:384.
29. McKenzie RA. Prophylaxis in recurrent low back pain. NZ Med J 1979;89:22.
30. Nachemson A. Advances in low back pain. Clin Orthop 1985;200:266.
31. Nachemson A. Physiotherapy for low back pain patients, a critical look. Scand J Rehab Med 1969;1:85.
32. Robinson JS. Sciatica and the lumbar disk syndrome: a historic perspective. South Med J 1983;76:232.
33. Rothman RH. The clinical syndrome of lumbar disc disease. Orthop Clin North Am 1971;2:463.
34. Steindler A, Luck JV. Differential diagnosis of pain low in the back: allocation of the source of pain by the procaine hydrochloride method. JAMA 1938;110(2):106.
35. Troup JDG. Straight leg raising (SLR) and the qualifying tests for increased root tension: their predictive value after back and sciatic pain. Spine 1981;6:526.
36. Wachemson AL. Prevention of chronic low back pain: the orthopaedic challenge for the 80's. Bull Hosp J Dis Orthop Inst 1981;44:1.
37. Weber H. Lumbar disc herniation: a controlled, perspective study with ten years of observation. Spine 1983;8:131.
38. White AA III, Gordon SL. Synopsis: Workshop on Idiopathic low back pain. Spine 1982;7:141.
39. Williams RW. Microlumbar discectomy: a conservative surgical approach to the virgin herniated lumbar disc. Spine 1978;3:175.

SECTION FIVE

GENERAL ORTHOPAEDICS

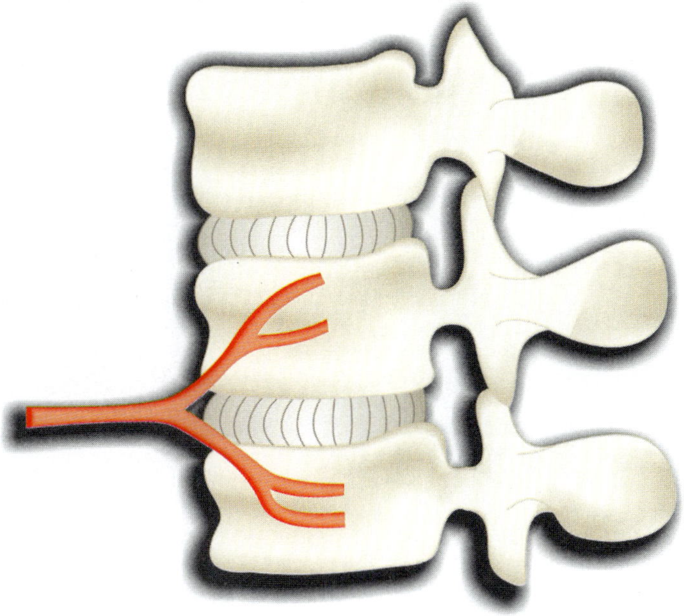

35

Congenital Disorders

INTRODUCTION

The following congenital disorders of interest are discussed in this chapter (Table 35.1).

Table 35.1: Congenital disorders

1. **Congenital disorders of trunk and upper extremity**
   - *Congenital torticollis*
   - Congenital elevation of scapula
   - Congenital pseudarthrosis of the clavicle
   - Congenital radioulnar synostosis
2. **Congenital disorders of hip and pelvis**
   - *Congenital dislocation of hip*
   - Coxa vara
3. **Congenital disorders of the lower limb**
   - Congenital dislocation of the knee
   - Congenital pseudarthrosis of the tibia
   - *Congenital talipes equinovarus (CTEV)*
4. **Congenital absence of part or all of long bones**
   - Radius
   - Tibia
   - Fibula

Note: The diseases *emboldened* are discussed in detail while the rest are merely mentioned.

Congenital disorders are defined as those *abnormalities of development that are present at the time of birth.* It is quite a common problem exceeded in frequency only by those of CNS and CVS systems.

Congenital disorders can be placed in three groups.

1. Those easily noticed by the mother, e.g. club-foot.
2. Those not readily noticed, e.g. congenital dislocation of hip (CDH).
3. Those clinically undetected but diagnosed radiologically, e.g. spondylolisthesis.

Congenital disorders are more prevalent in diabetic mothers, multiple pregnancies, older mothers, etc. Male and female have equal predilection.

Causes

The exact cause is not known. Most congenital disorders begin early in the life of the embryo when cell division is most active. Although a few congenital disorders may be due to uterine malposition, most are believed to be due to *genetic defects, environmental influences* or a combination of both.

Genetic factors Defects in the chromosomes of sperm and ovum result in specific disorders which follows Mendel's law.

Embryonic trauma Congenital disorders can also result from injury to the developing embryo at the time of differentiation of embryonic tissue into specific tissues by extraneous factors.

What is Teratogenesis?

Experimental production of congenital anomalies is teratogenesis. A teratogenic factor may be metabolic, hormonal, nutritional deficiency, chemicals, X-ray, trauma, infection, mechanical, thermal, anoxia, etc.

Duraiswamy could experimentally produce skeletal defects (Table 35.2) by using the above teratogenic factors.

Table 35.2: Congenital skeletal problems

Congenital skeletal problems
- Limb deficiency
  - Limb bud arrest
    - Terminal
    - Intercalary
  - Gross limb abnormality
- Limb deformities
  1. Upper limb and trunk
  2. Disorders of hip and pelvis
  3. Disorders of lower limbs

CONGENITAL DISORDERS OF UPPER LIMB

CONGENITAL TORTICOLLIS (WRYNECK)

Congenital torticollis is a condition where the sternocleidomastoid muscle of the neck undergoes contractures pulling it to the same side and turning the face to the opposite side (Fig. 35.1).

The exact cause of this condition is unknown; but hypothetically, it may be due to fibromatosis within the sternomastoid muscle.

Features

- Tumour palpable at birth or during the first two weeks of life.
- Common on the right side.
- May include the muscle diffusely but more often it is localised near the clavicular attachment of the muscle.
- It attains maximum size within 1 to 2 months, usually it diappears within a year.
- If it fails to disappear, then the muscle becomes permanently fibrotic and contracted and causes torticollis.

Aetiology

- Middle part of the sternomastoid is supplied by an end artery, which is a branch of the superior thyroid artery that gets blocked due to trauma, etc.
- Birth trauma—Breech delivery, improper application of forceps, etc. may cause injury to the sternomastoid muscle.

The above two reasons can result in sternocleidomastoid muscle ischaemia, necrosis and fibrosis later on.

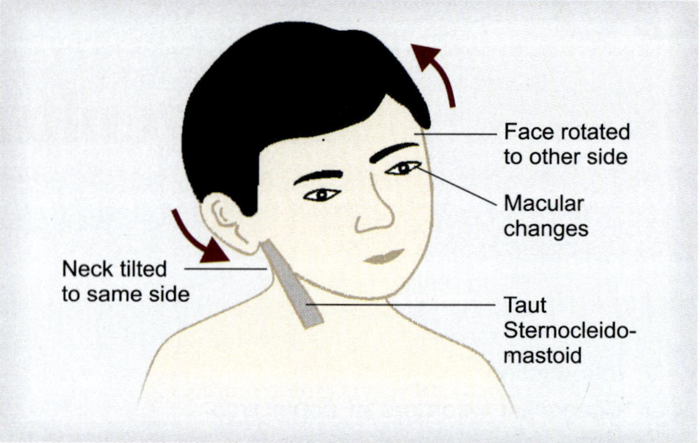

Fig. 35.1: Features of wryneck

Clinical Features

Deformity is the only complaint initially. Later, facial changes and macular problems in the retina may develop.

Deformities in congenital torticollis

- Primary
  - Tilt of the head to the same side
  - Taut sternomastoid
- Secondary
  - Facial appearance distorted
  - Macular changes in the retina

Treatment

Principles

- During infancy, conservative treatment consists of stretching of the sternomastoid by manipulation and physiotherapy. Excision is unjustified in infancy.
- Surgery is delayed till fibroma is well formed. The muscle may be released at one or both ends or the muscle may be excised as a whole.
- If the muscle is still contracted at the age of 1 year, it should be released.
- If wryneck is persistent for 1 year, it will not resolve spontaneously and needs to be interfered operatively.
- Exercise programme is successful:
  —when restriction of motion is less than 30°.
  —when there is no facial asymmetry.
- Nonoperative treatment after 1 year is rarely successful.

- Any permanent torticollis becomes worse during growth. Head is inclined towards the affected side, face is turned towards the opposite side, ipsilateral shoulder is elevated and the fronto-occipital diameter is increased.

Surgical Methods

The most commonly employed surgical method is subcutaneous tenotomy of the clavicular attachment of the sternomastoid muscle. This procedure is inaccurate and dangerous as there could be an injury to the external jugular vein and phrenic nerve. Hence release from its attachment on the mastoid process is also tried. Open tenotomy if done before the child is 1 year old, tethering of the scar takes place. If the surgery is done between 1 and 4 years of age, tilt of the head and facial asymmetry are corrected less satisfactorily. If done after 5 years of age, the secondary deformities are less corrected.

For older children or after failed operation, bipolar release of the muscle from both sides, Ferkel's modified bipolar release or Z-plasty of the muscle are tried.

[1]SPRENGEL'S DEFORMITY (Fig. 35.2A)

In this condition, scapula fails to descend down from its initial high position in the embryo. It is a tale of a disobedient scapula!

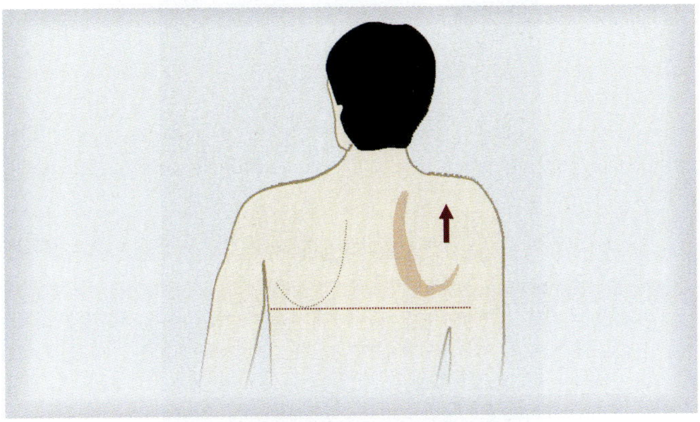

Fig. 35.2A: Showing congenital elevation of scapula (Sprengel's shoulder)

Here, the scapula lies more superiorly. It is hypoplastic and improperly shaped. It is associated with other congenital anomalies like cervical rib, etc.

Aetiology

This may be due to imperfect descent of the shoulder girdle by third month or a band of muscle from the skull to the scapula which has failed to grow.

Pathology

The pathological changes are seen in the bones and muscles. The scapula may be normal, broad or high and there could be other features like hemivertebra, wedging of vertebra, etc. Among the muscles, the trapezius may be absent, the rhomboids and levator scapulae are represented by a thin band.

Clinical Features

The scapula is high by 2 to 10 cm, the deformity is obvious, there is no functional impairment, all the shoulder girdle movements are normal, torticollis may be present in 10 per cent of the cases, crania bifida and spina bifida may also be present.

Cavendish's Gradings

- Group 1—Very mild
- Group 2—Mild, shoulder slightly unaligned
- Group 3—Moderate, shoulder high.
- Group 4—Severe, with superior angle of scapula near the occiput.

Treatment

For cases with mild deformity, no treatment is required and for severe cases, surgery is done after three years, and this consists of release of muscles from the scapula or transfer of origin of the trapezius muscle.

CLEIDOCRANIAL DYSOSTOSIS

For some mysterious reasons, clavicle chooses to remain absent either partially or wholly. It is a rare condition.

[1]**Otto Sprengel** (1852-1915), a German orthopaedic surgeon, described it in 1891.

Salient features

1. Aplasia of clavicles.
2. Exaggerated development of transverse diameter of cranium.
3. Delay in closure of clavicles.
4. Heredity.
5. Equal sex incidence.

Types

1. Where ends of the bones are normal, but a pseudarthritic gap is present in between.
2. Where there is a partial defect of one end, usually the acromial end.
3. Where the whole clavicle is absent.

Deformities of the clavicle is accompanied by variations in the following muscles: trapezius may be absent, pectoralis major may be maldeveloped, and other congenital malformations may be associated.

Aetiology

The exact cause is unknown, but the development of membranous bones may be affected during the first week of embryonic life due to various unknown factors.

Clinical Features

The patient is brought to the surgeon due to accidentally discovered trouble with the shoulder. Features of un-united fracture of the clavicle may be present. It may also present as complete absence of the clavicle. Tips of shoulder can be approximated to each other.

Treatment

Usually, it does not require any treatment, but if pain is present due to pressure of one or both ends, then removal of the part is indicated. As a rule, there is no disability or discomfort and abnormal mobility is not usually a hindrance.

CONGENITAL RADIOULNAR SYNOSTOSIS

I call this an unholy alliance of radius and ulna for their union causes unmitigated hardship to the sufferer.

Salient features

- Involves proximal ends of radius and ulna
- Bones fix the forearm in pronation
- Bilateral
- Familial tendency

Classification (Table 35.3)

Table 35.3: Classification of congenital radioulnar synostosis

Type I	*Type II*
• Medullary canals of the radius and ulna are joined together	• Radius is normal • Proximal end is dislocated either anteriorly or posteriorly
• Proximal ends of radius is malformed and fused to ulna for a distance of several cm	• Fusion to ulna is not as extensive as in type I
• Radius is longer and larger than ulna and the Shaft arches anteriorly	• Unilateral • Other deformities like syndactyly, etc. are present

Radiograph

Plain X-ray of the forearm including both elbow and wrist joints are essential to diagnose this condition (Fig. 35.2B).

Reasons for difficulty in treatment

1. Fascial tissues are short.
2. Interosseous membrane is narrow.
3. Supinator muscle is abnormal or absent.

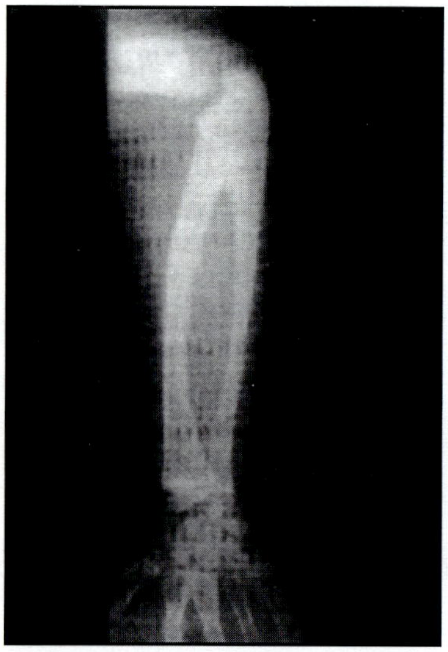

Fig. 35.2B: Radiograph showing congenital radioulnar synostosis

Treatment

Treatment is limited to osteotomy, to place the forearm in midprone position for better function.

Attempts to overcome the synostosis and give rotatory function to the forearm are doomed to failure because of the lack of properly functioning muscles. Fortunately, most patients are not disabled enough to justify an extensive operation.

MADELUNG'S DEFORMITY

It is an abnormality of the *palmar ulnar part of the distal radial epiphysis* in which progressive ulnar and volar tilt develops at the distal radial articular surface, resulting in dorsal subluxation of the distal ulna.

First described by Malgaigne in 1855 and later by [2]Madelung in 1878.

Though congenital, it is not obvious until late childhood and adolescence. It is a rare condition, incidence being only 1.7 per cent.

Causes

The causes could be autosomal dominant, dysplasic (diaphysial aclasis), genetic or idiopathic.

Acquired deformities distinguished by lack of appropriate physical findings, unilateral, less severe carpal deformities, and history of repetitive injury or stress.

Madelung's deformity consists of:
- Volar subluxation of hand.
- Prominence of distal ulna.
- Volar and ulnar angulation of distal radius (Fig. 35.3).

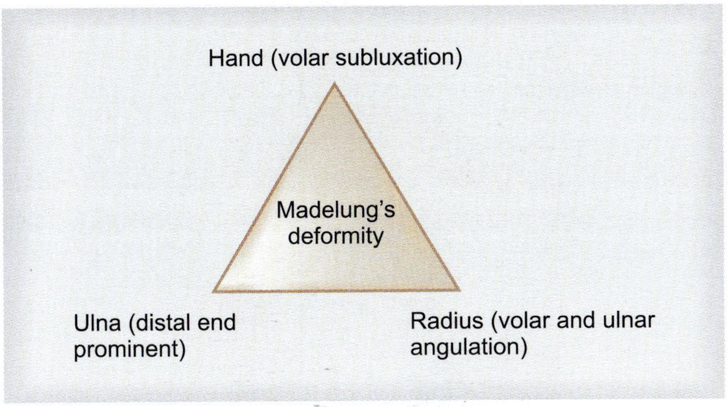

Fig. 35.3: Madelung's deformity

Other Features

This condition is commonly bilateral, girls are more affected. There is a positive family history, the deformity manifests in late childhood and adolescents with restricted wrist motion and minimal pain. As growth occurs, deformity worsens and the forearm is short.

Radiographic abnormalities are seen in radius, ulna and carpal bones. Radius is curved with its convexity dorsal and radial. Distal radial epiphysis is triangular in shape because of the failure of the growth in the ulnar and volar aspects of the epiphysis. Early closure of these aspects of epiphysis is frequent. Ulna is subluxated dorsally, its head is enlarged and the overall length of ulna is decreased. Carpus appears to have subluxated ulnarward and palmarwards into the distal radioulnar joint. Carpus appears wedge shaped with its apex proximal.

Treatment

Children with Madelung's deformity have minimal pain and excellent function. Hence, conservative treatment is given initially. Surgery is considered for severe deformity or persistent pain. In skeletally immature patients, distal radial osteotomy with ulnar shortening is (Milch resection) preferred. In skeletally mature patients, osteotomy and Darrach's procedure are done.

Deformity may recur after either procedure and range of motion of forearm usually does not improve after surgery.

CONGENITAL ABSENCE OF RADIUS (RADIAL CLUB-HAND)

Failure of the formation of the parts along the preaxial or radial borders of the upper extremity, deficient or absent thenar muscles, short or absent thumb, short or absent radius.

Quick facts
- One in one lakh birth.
- Incidence—4.7%.
- Bilateral in 50% of cases.
- Sexes equal.
- Right side more common.
- Complete absence more common than partial absence.
- Cause unknown/thalidomide/ genetic.

[2]**Otto Madelung** of Bonn. First described by Malgaigne in 1855 and later by Madelung in 1878.

Heikel's Classification

- Type I—Short distal radius
- Type II—Hypoplastic radius
- Type III—Partial absence of radius
- Type IV—Total absence of radius (most common).

Treatment

After birth, the deformity is corrected passively and splinted with a short arm plastic splint. Surgical correction, i.e. centralisation of hands is usually done at 3 to 6 months. Pollicisation is done at 9 to 12 months.

CONGENITAL DISLOCATION OF RADIUS (Fig. 35.4)

This is uncommon and is often confused with Monteggia fractures.

CONGENITAL DISORDERS OF LOWER LIMBS

DEVELOPMENTAL DYSPLASIA OF HIP (DDH) [Earlier Known as Congenital Dislocation of Hip (CDH)]

Definition Developmental dysplasia of hip is defined as partial or complete displacement of the femoral head from the acetabular cavity since birth.

Risk factors: (4 F's)
- Females
- First borns
- Familial
- Faulty intrauterine position (e.g. breech).

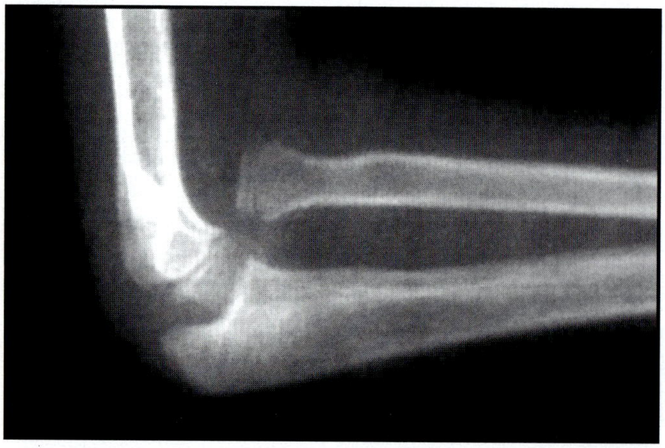

Fig. 35.4: Radiograph showing congenital dislocation of radius

Theories of Aetiology

1. *Genetic theory* Dysplastic trait is found in families.
2. *Hormonal theory* Hormone induced joint laxity.
3. *Mechanical theory* Faulty intrauterine positions particularly in the first born.
4. Primary acetabular dysplasia.

Remember

The incidences in DDH
- 1 per 1000 live birth.
- Left hip affected in 67% of cases.
- Family history present in 20%.
- Incidence of breech 30 to 50%.
- 1:3 cases are bilateral.
- Female preponderance.

Pathology

The following pathological changes are observed in DDH (Fig. 35.5) and the severity varies according to the stages of the disease.

Bone

Acetabulum There could be a primary acetabular dysplasia and the acetabulum is shallow. There could be a gap or groove at posterosuperior aspect. The triangular outer surface of ilium and acetabulum, are in the same line. Above the acetabulum, there is a depression containing the head of the femur.

Head of femur The dislocated head of femur at first appears normal, ossification is delayed, later head is flat on its posterior and medial aspect. Femoral head when present in the ilium is buffer or conical shaped.

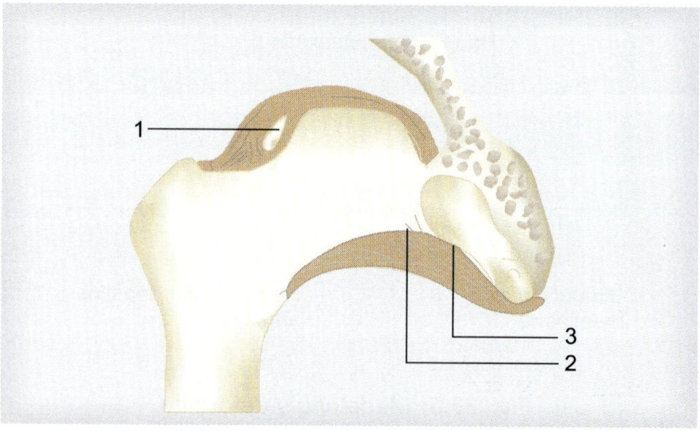

Fig. 35.5: Pathology in DDH: (1) elongated capsule, (2) stretched ligamentum teres, (3) fibrofatty tissue within the acetabulum

Neck of femur There could be shortening and anteversion.

Pelvis The pelvis is usually tilted forwards, it is small and atrophied. There is lordosis and it may be more vertical than normal.

Capsule The capsule could show *hour glass constriction,* one containing head and the other containing the acetabulum. Constriction is produced by iliopsoas and the ligamentum teres passes through this constriction and it is hypertrophied.

Muscles

Pelvifemoral group Adductors, sartorius, gracilis, rectus femoris, hamstrings, tensor fascia lata muscles. These muscles are shortened and they prevent reduction of the head.

Pelvitrochanteric group (obturators, quadratus femoris, Iliopsoas) These are elongated and the psoas forms an obstacle to reduction.

Gluteal muscles show little organic change but power is diminished.

Remember

Conditions due to packaging problems (i.e. decreased intrauterine space)

- DDH
- Torticollis
- Metatarsus adductus
- Increased type III collagen.

Stages of DDH (Fig. 35.6)

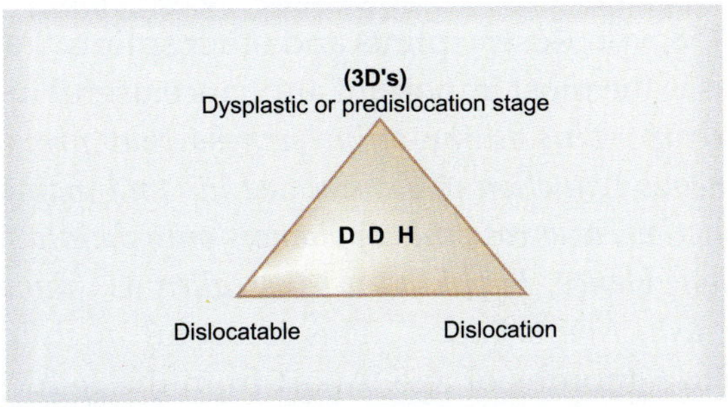

Fig. 35.6: Stages of developmental dysplasia of hip: (1) dysplastic stage, (2) dislocatable or subluxation stage, and (3) dislocation stage

Clinical Features

The clinical features vary in infants, children and adults (Table 35.4).

In infants First a thorough clinical examination is carried out to detect the presence of any other congenital anomalies. If the hip is dislocated, all features of dislocation are present. The gluteal and thigh folds are not symmetrical. The perineum is widened and abduction of the hip is decreased by 50 per cent while the internal rotation movement is increased. Radiographic examination in infants is of little value, but von Rosen's line (Fig. 35.7) is helpful in making an early radiological diagnosis in this age group.

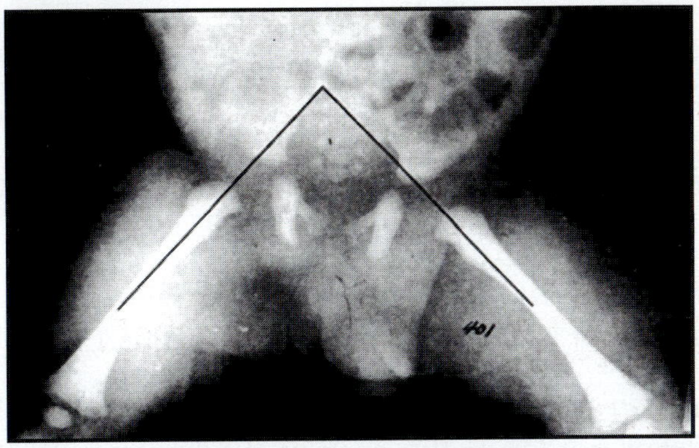

Fig. 35.7: Radiograph showing von Rosen's line

Table 35.4: Clinical features of DDH in various age groups at a glance

Infants	*Childhood and adolescents*	*Adults*
• Look for other anomalies. • If hip is dislocated all signs of dislocations present. • Thigh and gluteal folds asymmetric. • Perineum widened. • Abduction decreased by 50%. • Internal rotation increased. ***Tests*** 1. Galeazzi is sign positive. 2. Ortolani's sign of entry is positive. 3. Barlow's provocative test is positive (2,3 indicate reducible dislocation). 4. Delayed walking.	1. *Gait* Waddling/sailors 2. Lordosis 3. Deformity **Unilateral** shortening of leg **Bilateral** leg shortening with perineum wide, buttocks broad and flat 4. *Palpation* vascular sign of Narath is positive 5. *Movements* Abduction and lateral rotation are decreased 6. Telescopy is positive 7. *Measurements* Supratrochanteric shortening is present	• All the signs seen in adolescents • Pain in the hip • All the features of osteoarthritis hip

Children and adolescents Here, the patient shows a waddling or sailor's gait. There is an increased lumbar lordosis. The deformity frequently encountered in unilateral cases is shortening. In bilateral cases, both the lower limbs are short, perineum is wide, buttocks are broad and flat. Femoral artery is prominently felt. Abduction and lateral rotation movements of the hip are decreased. Telescopy and Trendelenburg tests are positive. Clinical tests of importance in infants are not of relevance in this age group (see Table 35.5).

Unlike in infants, radiographs of pelvis show important features in this age group (Fig. 35.8A). The following radiological parameters should be noted.

Perkin's line This is a vertical line drawn at the outer border of the acetabulum (see Fig. 35.15A).

Hilgenreiner's line This is a horizontal line drawn at the level of triradiate cartilage (see Fig. 35.15B).

Shenton's line This is a smooth curve formed by the inferior border of the neck of the femur with the superior margin of the obturator foramen. This line is broken in DDH (Fig. 35.8B).

Acetabular index Normal value is less than or equal to 30°.

CE angle of Wiberg The normal value is 15 to 30°.

The Hilgenreiner's line and the Perkin's line help to assess the position of the femoral head. Normally, the head lies in the lower and inner quadrant formed by these two lines. In DDH, the head lies in the upper and outer quadrant, the continuity of Shenton's line is broken in DDH (Fig. 35.8B). The acetabular index and the CE angle of Wiberg help to assess the acetabulum.

In adults DDH in adults shows all the features seen in adolescents. In addition, patient will have features of secondary osteoarthritis of the hip namely pain, stiffness, limp, crepitus, restricted movements, etc.

Treatment

The aim of treatment in DDH is to achieve and maintain an early concentric reduction to prevent future degenerative joint disease.

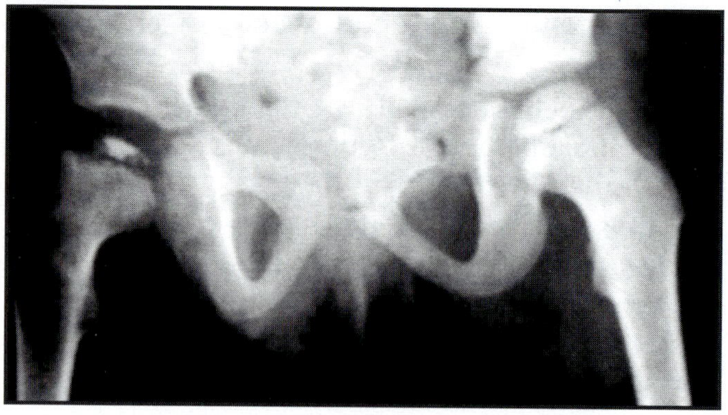

Fig. 35.8A: Radiograph showing congenital dislocation of hip

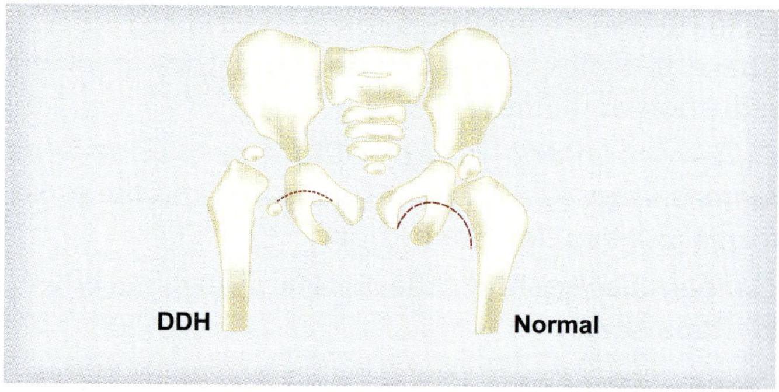

Fig. 35.8B: Shenton's line is broken in CDH

The methods to obtain reduction of the head into the acetabulum varies according to the age groups (see Table 35.6).

In infants Reduction can be obtained and maintained by Pavlik harness which was first described by Arnold Pavlik, in the former Czechoslovakia, in the year 1958, von Rosen splints and other splints. Pavlik harness is the most important appliance useful in this age group. *This is the only harness that promotes spontaneous reduction of a dislocated hip and maintains the reduction, whereas other appliances only maintain the reduction. Hence, Pavlik harness is called as "dynamic flexion abduction orthoses"*. This is useful in children less than 6 months of age. Apart from the reduction and the immobilisation, it allows active movements in all directions except extension and adduction. Nappies can be changed easily. The success rate of this harness is 85 to 95 per cent. However, as the age advances, soft tissue contractures develop along with secondary changes in the acetabulum, which bring down the success rate of Pavlik harness. Complications include osteonecrosis and failure of reduction (see Fig. 35.16).

Between 6 and 18 months As mentioned earlier, Pavlik harness has no role in the treatment of DDH in this age group. Here, the treatment of choice is gentle closed reduction and hip spica application (see Fig. 15.20). Open reduction is done if this method proves unsuccessful.

Remember

- Ortolani's test (is a test of entry) relocates a dislocated hip.
- Barlow's test (test of exit) dislocates a dislocatable hip.
- Both these tests lose their significance after infancy.

Between 18 and 36 months In this age group open reduction is the treatment of choice as closed reduction is often not successful. Open reduction is to be followed with either pelvic or femoral osteotomy to provide concentric reduction of the femoral head within the acetabulum.

Role of osteotomies Osteotomies are done for instability, failure of acetabular development or progressive head subluxation after reduction. They are done only if congruent reduction is possible, if there is satisfactory range of movements and if the femoral head has a reasonable sphericity.

The osteotomies could be femoral or pelvic and the choice is usually left to the surgeons, but there are some guiding principles.

Pelvic osteotomies are chosen if there is severe dysplasia and if radiographic changes are seen on the acetabular side. See Table 35.5 for different pelvic osteotomies.

Femoral osteotomies This is the procedure of choice if there are changes in the femoral head and if there is increase in anteversion of the neck.

3–8 years Here open reduction is followed either by femoral shortening or pelvic osteotomies.

8–18 years In this age group, open reduction is followed by femoral shortening or pelvic osteotomies. If osteoarthritis of the hip develops, total hip replacement is the surgery of choice. Arthrodesis of the hip is rarely done.

See Table 35.6 for the comparative study of the treatment regimen in various age groups in DDH.

Remember

Important radiological parameters in DDH

- < 6m: von Rosen's line (see Fig. 35.7).
- > 6m: Perkin's line, Shenton's line (see Fig. 35.8B), acetabular index and delayed ossification.

What is von Rosen's line?

This is a line which helps in the diagnosis of DDH radiologically in infants less than 6 months. It is an anteroposterior view of the pelvis taken with the lower limbs in full medial rotation and 45° abduction. When the hip is normal, upward prolongation of the long axis of the shaft of the femur points towards the lateral margin of the acetabulum and crosses the pelvis in the region of the sacroiliac joint. When the hip is dislocated upward, prolongation of this line points towards anterior iliac spine and crosses the midline in the lower lumbar region. This line is not useful after 6 months. Standard anteroposterior views are preferred in a child older than 6 months.

Innominate Osteotomy in DDH

Salter's osteotomy This is indicated in patients with instability after reduction or in persistent DDH between 18 months to 6 years. The procedure consists of using the symphysis pubis as a hinge, osteotomising the acetabulum to cover the head (see Fig. 35.17).

Pemberton's osteotomy It is indicated in paralytic dislocation and in postacetabular deficiency between 1 and 10 years. Here, the osteotomy is done through the acetabular roof using triradiate cartilage as the hinge.

Steel's osteotomy This is useful in older children when symphysis pubis and the triradiate cartilage are fused. This is a triple innominate osteotomy.

Shelf operation It is indicated in CDH with recurrence. Here, the acetabulum is extended laterally and anteriorly by bone graft (see Fig. 35.18).

Chiari's osteotomy This is a salvage procedure and is indicated in children older than 4 years. Here, the osteotomy is done through the ilium above the acetabulum and the distal fragment is pushed medially (see Fig. 35.19).

Table 35.5: Clinical tests in DDH

Clinical tests	*How to perform?*	*Inference*
[3]**Barlow's test** 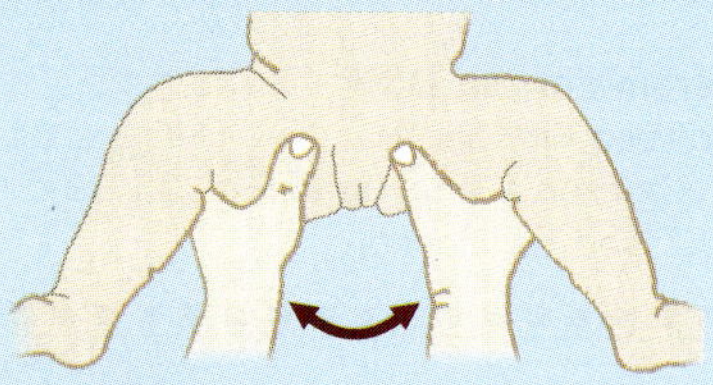 **Fig. 35.9**	This test is done within 2 to 3 days of birth. The infant is supine with the knees fully flexed and the hip at 90° of flexion. The hip is slowly abducted to 45° and the head is slowly pushed towards the acetabulum by the fingers.	This test is positive when the joint is dislocated and the femoral head returns to the acetabulum with a click or jerk. Reliable and useful up to 6 months after which the greater trochanter cannot be held with tip of the middle finger.
[4]**Ortolani's test** 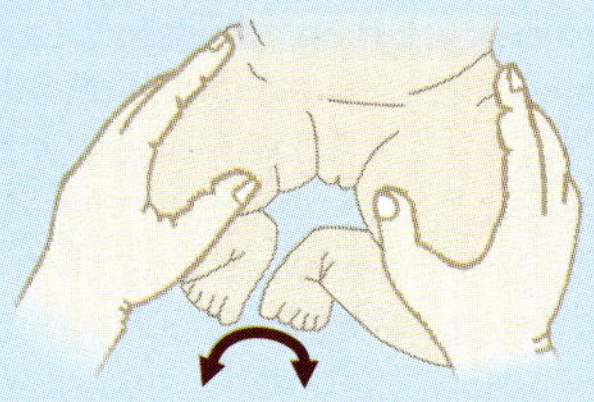 **Fig. 35.10**	This test is done between 3 and 9 months and is not satisfactory in a newborn. Here, the infant is supine, with the hip and knee flexed. The hip is slowly adducted and abducted to detect any reduction of the femoral head into the acetabulum.	This test indicates the reduction of the dislocated hip. *These two tests are generally reliable and should be performed as a screening tests in all cases of suspected CDH. They are misleading if abduction is restricted due to adduction contractures.*
Galeazzi or Allen's sign 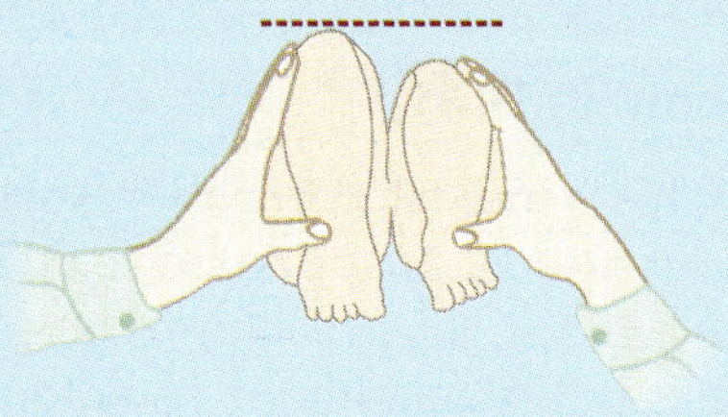 **Fig. 35.11**	The child is in supine position with both the hip and the knee in flexion. The level of both the knee joints are noted with reference to a horizontal line. This test is useful in assesing unilateral cases of CDH in children between 3 and 8 months.	Normally, both the knees should be at the same level. In DDH, the affected knee is seen beneath the horizontal line indicating femoral shortening. The shortening is in the supratrochanteric region and can be assessed by the Bryant's triangle.
Skin fold test of thigh 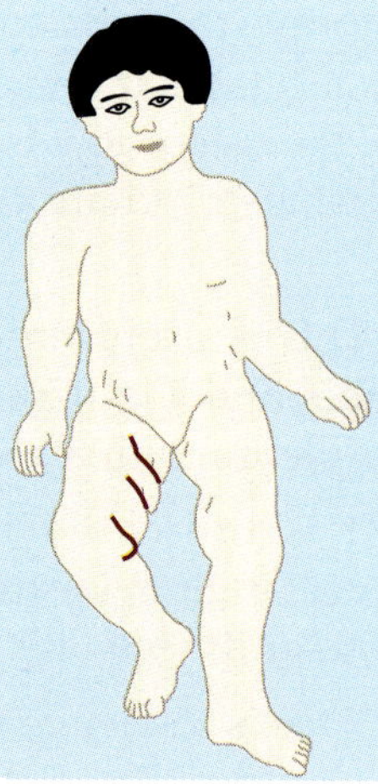 **Fig. 35.12**	The child is completely stripped and in the vertical position, the levels of the thigh folds studied.	Normally, the thigh folds are symmetrical in nature. In DDH, they are no longer symmetrical due to the shortening of the affected limb.

Contd...

[3]**Thomas Geoffrey Barlow** (1915-1975) Orthopaedic Surgeon, England.
[4]**Ortolani Marius** (1937), Orthopaedic Surgeon, Italy.

Contd...

Skin fold test of gluteal region 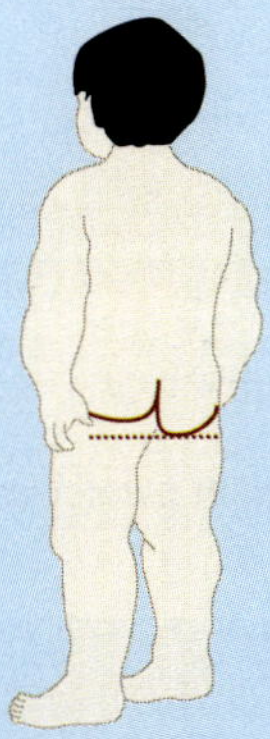 **Fig. 35.13**	The procedure is similar to the one performed above, but here the levels of the gluteal folds are noted.	Normally, the thigh folds are symmetrical in nature. In DDH they are no longer symmetrical due to the shortening of the affected limb.
[5]**Trendelenburg** test 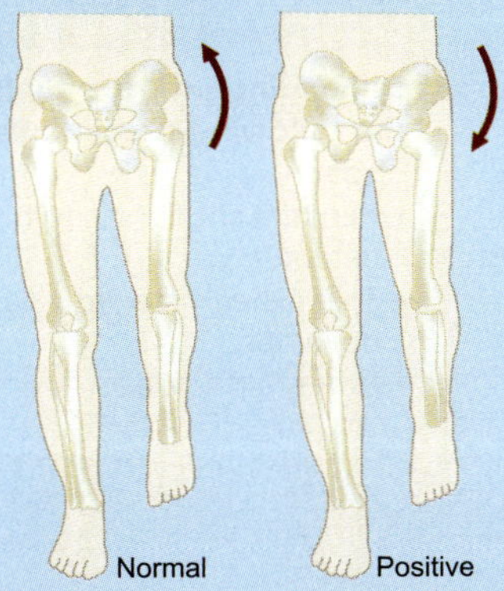 **Fig. 35.14:** Trendelenburg test	The patient is made to stand first on the normal limb and then on the affected limb. The contralateral leg is then raised from the ground.	When standing on the normal limb, the opposite hip is in a higher position, but when the patient or the child stands on the affected limb, the opposite pelvis drops indicating impairment of abductor mechanism due to DDH. This test cannot be performed in infants.

Radiographic Features and Treatment Methods in DDH (Figs 35.14 to 35.20)

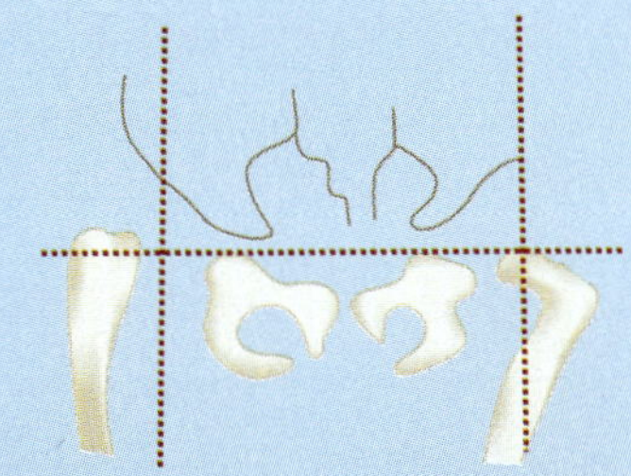

Fig. 35.15: X-ray Pelvis in DDH: (A) Perkin's line, (B) Hilgenreiner's line, (C) normal location of head, and (D) location of head in DDH

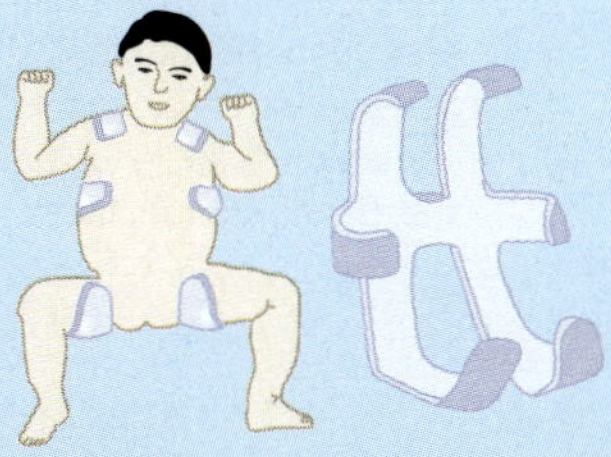

Fig. 35.16: Pavlik harness in DDH

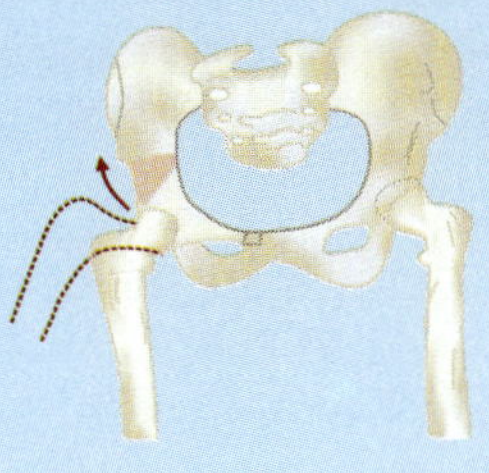

Fig. 35.17: Salter's osteotomy

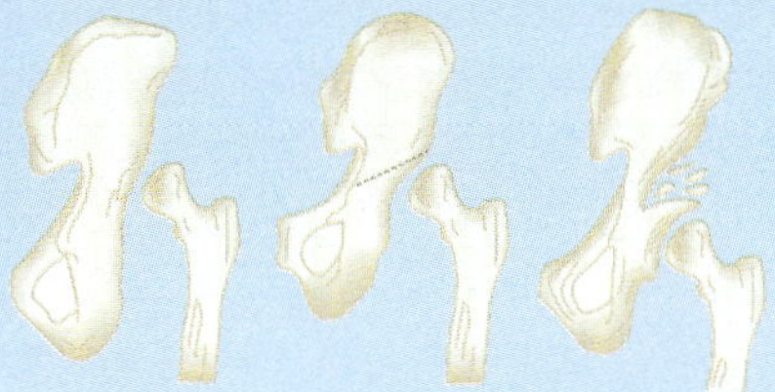

Fig. 35.18: Acetabular shelf operation

[5]**Trendelenburg Frederick** (Berlin). Professor of Surgery of Rostook, Bonn, Liepzig. He first described CDH in 1895.

Contd...

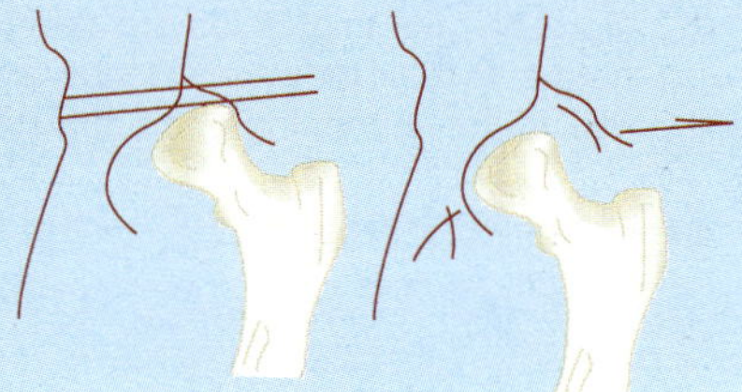

Fig. 35.19: Showing Chiari's osteotomy

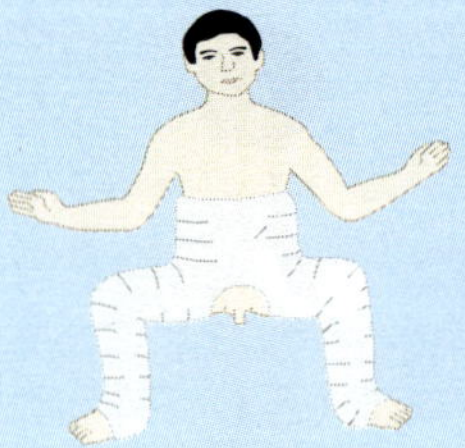

Fig. 35.20: DDH treated with plaster cast in frog leg position

Table 35.6: Treatment divided into five age groups

Newborn (6 months)	*6–18 months*	*Toddler (18–36 months)*	*Child (3–8 years)*	*Juvenile and young adults (8–18 years)*
Hold If need pull	*Pull and hold*	*Break and hold*	*Open and break*	*Open and replace*
• Pavlik harness and von Rosen splint are applied for 2 months. Later wean, by removing it 2 hours/day doubled every 2–4 weeks until device is worn in the night only. Night bracing is continued till X-rays are normal. *X-rays are taken at* 1 month 6 month 1 year intervals **If dislocation persists for 6 to 8 weeks, abandon this programme and institute** • **Traction** • **Closed reduction** • **Casting**	In this age group harness is not successful. The recommended regime as follows: • Preoperative traction • Adductor tenotomy • Closed reduction and arthrogram. • Hip spica after confirmation of stable reduction. Desired position of the hip joint is human position (i.e. 95° flexion and 40° abduction at the hip). • Open reduction in child less than 18 months is done when closed reduction fails by using the Bikini skin incision.	Here open reduction is combined with femoral or pelvic osteotomy or both and is the treatment of choice. ***Femoral osteotomy*** is tried first for untreated CDH and is useful in less than 8 years of age **Pelvic osteotomy** The following varieties are described • **Salter's** uses Symphysis pubis as the hinge. Useful between 18 months and 6 years • **Pemberton** Uses triradiate cartilage as the hinge. Useful between 1 and 10 years of age. • ***Steel*** (Triple innominate osteotomy) Useful in older children when symphysis pubis and triradiate cartilages are fused. • ***Shelf operations*** Here acetebulum is extended anteriorly, laterally and posteriorly. Useful in CDH which have recurred after reduction. • ***Chiari's oseotomy*** Here medial displacement of the distal fragment is done usually as a last resort. Useful in children over 4 years of age.	Here open reduction is the treatment of choice and is usually followed with femoral shortening (Klisic and Jankovic) and if necessary pelvic osteotomy.	**Depending on the situation, the following procedures are chosen** • Femoral shortening with pelvic osteotomy. • THR when osteoarthritis develops. • Rarely arthrodesis

CONGENITAL DISLOCATION OF KNEE

This is uncommon and three types are described:

1. *Traumatic developmental type* is the most common, due to malposition in uterus.
2. *A primary embryonic defect* is associated with other defects like spina bifida.
3. *Quadriceps contracture* or congenital absence or hypoplastic anterior cruciate ligament.

Three degrees

1. Congenital hyperextension.
2. Congenital hyperextension with anterior subluxation of tibia on femur.
3. Congenital hyperextension with anterior dislocation of tibia on femur usually associated with other skeletal abnormalities.

Pathology

Varies with severity but anterior capsule and quadriceps are contracted. There are always intra-articular adhesions, hypoplasia or absence of patella or lateral dislocation of patella, and hypoplastic vastus lateralis.

Treatment

Mild to moderate In these cases, *conservative methods* like Pavlik harness, serial casting and skeletal traction are the treatment of choice.

Severe In severe cases, surgery is indicated and is done by anteromedial approach. Surgery should be done before the child is 2 years of age. Two surgical methods are described:

Neibauer and King technique is a Z-plasty of quadriceps

Curtis and Fischer Quadriceps above patella is divided by inverted V-incision.

CONGENITAL PSEUDARTHROSIS OF TIBIA

Congenital pseudarthrosis of tibia is a rare condition (Fig. 35.21). It can also be seen in other long bones like femur.

Incidence

- Incidence is 1 in 2.5 lacs live births.
- In 50 to 90 per cent of cases neurofibroma is present.

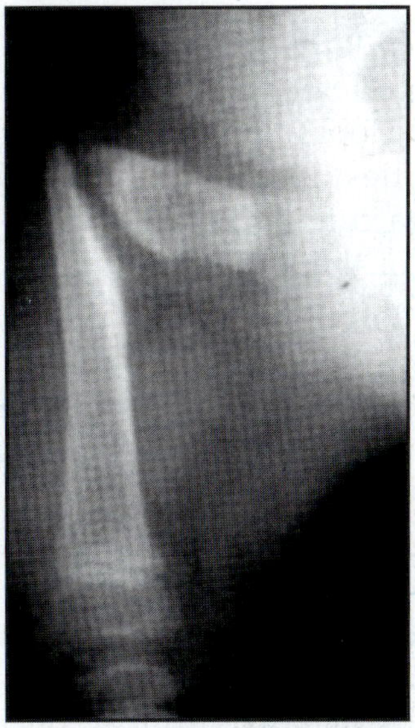

Fig. 35.21: Radiograph showing congenital pseudarthrosis of femur

Classification

[6]Boyd has classified this condition into six types and is the most accepted classification (Table 35.7).

Table 35.7: Boyd's classification

Type I	• Anterior bowing and a defect in the tibia is present at birth. • Other congenital anomalies are present.
Type II	• Pseudarthrosis with anterior bowing and an hour glass constriction of tibia present at birth. • Spontaneous fracture occurs before 2 years. • High risk tibia. • Most frequent type. • Associated with neurofibroma. • Poorest prognosis.
Type III	• Pseudarthrosis develops in a congenital cyst. • Recurrence of fracture is less frequent. • Good results.
Type IV	• Pseudarthrosis originates in a sclerotic segment of bone. • Medullary canal is obliterated. • An incomplete or stress fracture develops. • Prognosis good.
Type V	• Pseudarthrosis tibia is associated with dysplastic fibula. • Pseudarthrosis of fibula or tibia or both.
Type VI	• Pseudarthrosis occurs as an intraosseous neurofibroma. • Very rare condition.

[6]**Boyd HB** (1941) other contributions: (a) Classification of trochanteric fractures. (b) Described nonunion of long bones.

Clinical Features

In this condition, deformity is the chief complaint and the patient develops anterior bowing of the tibia of various severities. In a few cases, there could be pathological fractures.

Radiograph of the leg, AP and lateral views, are sufficient to make an accurate diagnosis.

Treatment

Principles

- It depends on the age and type.
- True pseudarthrosis will not unite with casting alone.
- Tibial cyst curettage and bone grafting is done in small lesions.
- Treatment is usually surgical, once a fracture develops.

Established Pseudarthrosis

1. *Boyd dual onlay graft* is the treatment of choice in patients with stress fractures.
2. *Osteotomy, intramedullary nailing, bone grafting and excision of thick tissue* is done for more established pseudarthrosis because retraction is common. Bracing is continued till skeletal maturity. Fairly good results. Causes of failure of union in some cases were attributed to distal location of the lateral pseudoarthrosis and the concomitant pseudoarthrosis.
3. *Macfarland's bone grafting* For anterior bowing with impending fracture, a single graft is placed posteriorly so as to span the pseudarthrosis.
4. *Sofield's multiple osteotomies with internal fixation by medullary nails* is useful when the distal fragment is too short to be held by a graft.
5. *Other treatment:*
   - *Pulsed EMF* This method has been tried and is found to be successful for fracture occurring through a cyst.
   - *Free vascularised fibular graft* This method has also been tried and the results are good.

CONGENITAL TALIPES EQUINOVARUS (CTEV)

One may pride in having flat foot, agile foot, nimble foot, but look at the tale of woes a club-foot presents to the unfortunate victim affected with this malady!

Interesting features of CTEV

Talipes It is a Latin word derived from *Talus* = ankle, *pes* = foot

Original meaning: A deformity that causes the patient to walk on the ankle.

Present-day meaning is any variety of club-foot.

Club-foot It is so called because severe untreated talipes equinovarus has a club-like appearance.

This is the most common congenital foot disorder. Incidence is 1.2/1000 live births. Males are more commonly affected than females.

How is congenital TEV different from acquired TEV (Table 35.8).

Types of CTEV (Aetiology)

1. **Osseous type**	Club-foot is associated with absence of tibia and fibula.
2. **Muscular type**	Arthrogryposis multiplex congenita or multiple congenital contractures.
3. **Neuropathic type**	Due to spina bifida, etc.
4. **Idiopathic type**	No apparent cause, commonest variety.

Table 35.8: Differences between CTEV and ATEV (Fig. 35.22)

CTEV	*ATEV*
1. Present since birth	1. Not present from birth
2. May be associated with spina bifida	2. May be due to polio, cerebral palsy, etc.
3. Bilateral	3. Usually unilateral
4. Skin, subcutaneous tissue, muscles are normal	4. Trophic changes in the skin, muscles are flaccid (LMN lesion) or spastic (UMN lesion)
5. Transverse crease is seen across the sole on the medial side	5. No transverse crease
6. Bones are normal in thickness	6. Bones are thinner than normal

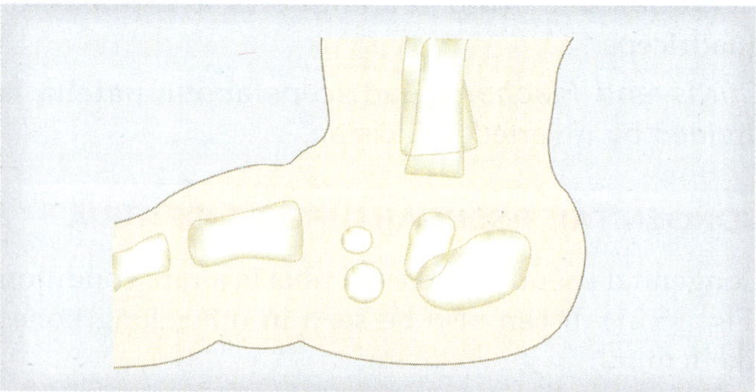

Fig. 35.22: In CTEV the talus is displaced medial and down

Idiopathic CTEV This is the most common type of CTEV one encounters in clinical practice. There is no apparent cause and various theories are proposed (Table 35.9).

Table 35.9: Theories of CTEV (Figs 35.23A to I)

Theories	*What do they say?*
1. **Turco's**	Medial displacement of navicular and calcaneus around the talus
2. **Brockman's**	Congenital atresia of the talonavicular joint
3. **Mc-Kay's**	Three-dimensional bony deformity of the subtalar complex
4. **Intrauterine**	Due to compression by malposition of foetus *in utero*
5. **Genetic**	General population 1:800 • In siblings 1:35 • In identical twins 1:3
6. **Germ plasm theory**	Primary germ plasm defect in talus with subsequent soft tissue changes.
7. **Soft tissue theory**	Primary soft tissue defect with secondary bony changes
8. **Prenatal muscle imbalance theory**	Weak pronators and overacting extensors and invertors

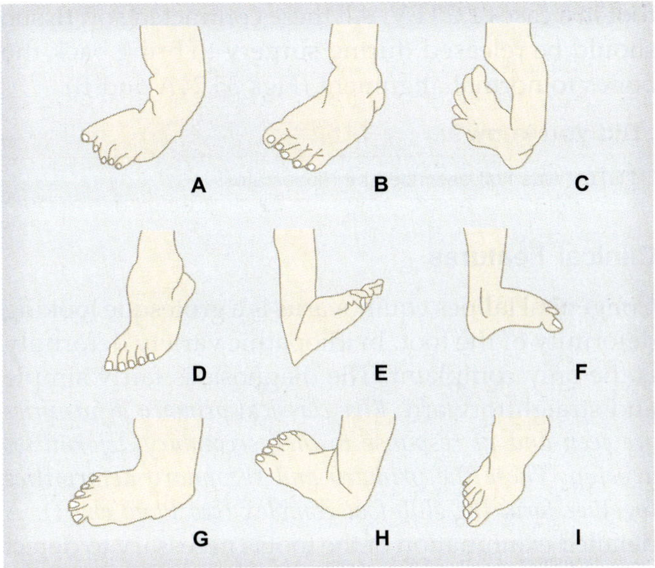

Figs 35.23A to I: Different varieties of foot deformities: (A) Varus, (B) Equinovarus, (C) Calcaneovarus, (D) Equinus, (E) calcaneus, (F) Cavus, (G) Valgus, (H) Calcaneovalgus, and (I) Equinovalgus

Pathology

The pathology in CTEV affects all the bones and joints of the foot with corresponding soft tissue contractures especially of the posteromedial structures. The primary problem usually lies in the bones with secondary soft tissue contractures. But sometimes the primary pathology may be in the surrounding soft tissues which brings about secondary changes in the bones; however, the latter event is rare. Table 35.10 shows the bony changes and also the structures involved in the posteromedial aspect of the ankle and

Table 35.10: Bony and soft tissue changes in CTEV

Bones and joints (bony)	*Muscles, capsules, ligaments (soft tissues)*
1. **Calcaneus** is in varus position 2. **Talus** displaced medial and plantarwards (Fig. 35.22) 3. **Navicular** medially displaced and rotated 4. **Cuboid** displaced medially and articulates with the non-articular surface of the calcaneus **(known as cuboid sign or locked cuboid)** 5. **Metatarsals** deviates medially at tarsometatarsal joints 6. **Talocalcaneal articulation** is a ball and socket joint. The anterior and middle articulation of the calcaneum forms the socket and the head of the talus forms the ball which is dislocation in CTEV 7. **Tibia** usually shows medial torsion, rarely lateral torsion *In short, all the above bones are displaced down and medial in a case of CTEV*	***Structures contracted on the medial side (3)*** *Rule of 3* **3 Muscles**: • AHL • TP • FHL **3 Ligaments**: • Deltoid • Spring • Plantar **3 Capsules of**: • Subtalar • Tarsal • Tarsometatarsal joints ***Structures contracted on the posterior side*** (2) *Rule of 2* **2 Muscles**: • Tibialis posterior • Tendo-Achilles **2 Ligaments**: • Talofibular • Calcaneofibular **2 Capsules**: • Ankle joint • Subtalar joint **Structures involved on the anterior side (1)** *Rule of 1* **1 Muscle**: • Tibialis anterior inserted abnormally **1 Ligament**: • Superior peroneal retinacula **1 Capsule**: • Calcaneocuboid, joint

Note: AHL → Abductor hallucis longus, TP → Tibialis posterior, FHL → Flexor hallucis longus foot in a case of CTEV. All these contracted soft tissue should be released during surgery to bring back the bones to normal alignment (Figs 35.24A and B).

Did you know?

CTEV was first described by Hippocrates.

Clinical Features

Congenital talipes equinovarus is a grotesque looking deformity of the foot. In idiopathic variety deformity is the only complaint. The diagnosis is fairly simple and straightforward. *Five classical primary deformities are seen and in response to this, secondary deformities develop. These the primary and secondary deformities together form the club-foot complex (see Flow chart).* A detailed examination of the foot is necessary to detect the full spectrum of deformities in CTEV.

With advancing age, the cosmetically unsightly club-foot (Fig. 35.25) starts posing functional problems like altered gait (stumbling gait) (Fig. 35.26), callosities, degeneration and arthritic changes in the ankle and foot joints. Correction is a must to restore normalcy.

In other varieties of CTEV, clinical features peculiar to the aetiological factors can be elicited.

Three clinical tests are of extreme importance in CTEV and are described below:

Dorsiflexion test In a newborn child, it is possible to dorsiflex the foot till its dorsal surface comes in contact with the anterior surface of the tibia. This is not possible in CTEV and this can be used as a screening test (Fig. 35.27).

Plumbline test This test helps to detect the tibial torsion. The child is made to sit on a table with both the lower limbs hanging from the edge. A line drawn from the centre of the patella to the tibial tubercle when extended down, should cut the foot at the first or second intermetatarsal space normally. This is called the plumbline. In CTEV, with medial rotation of the tibia, it cuts the fourth or fifth intermetatarsal space and vice versa in lateral rotation of the tibia (Fig. 35.28).

Scratch test This test is perfomed to detect muscle imbalance in an infant who cannot obey commands.

- *Medial scratch test* In a normal child, when the medial sole is scratched, the foot everts. This tests the peroneals.

Flow chart 35.1: Club-foot complex

Club-foot complex

Primary deformities ↓

1. Equinus
2. Varus
3. Cavus
4. Forefoot adduction
5. Internal tibial torsion

Late changes

1. Degeneration of joints
2. Fusion of joints

Secondary deformities ↓

1. Foot size is decreased to 50%
2. Medial border is concave, lateral border is convex
3. Forefoot is plantarflexed upon hindfoot
4. Skin is stretched over the dorsum of the foot
5. Callosities are present over the dorsum of the foot
6. Stumbling gait
7. Hypotrophic anterior tibial artery
8. Atrophy of muscles in anterior or posterior compartments of the leg

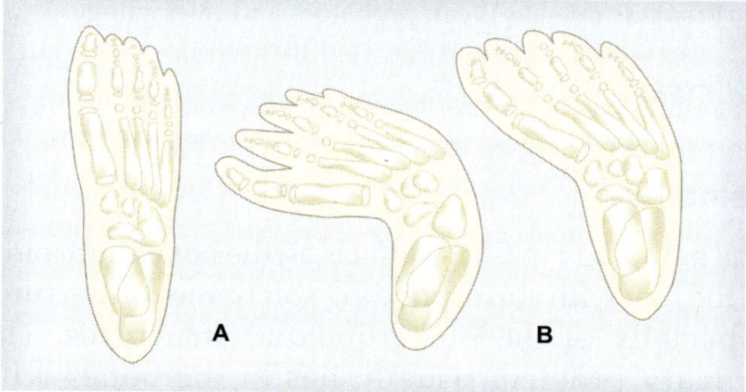

Figs 35.24A and B: Showing: (A) Normal foot, (B) Foot in CTEV

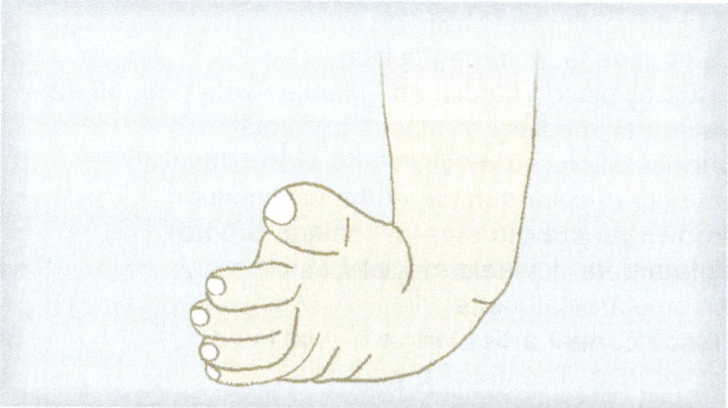

Fig. 35.25: Unilateral club-foot

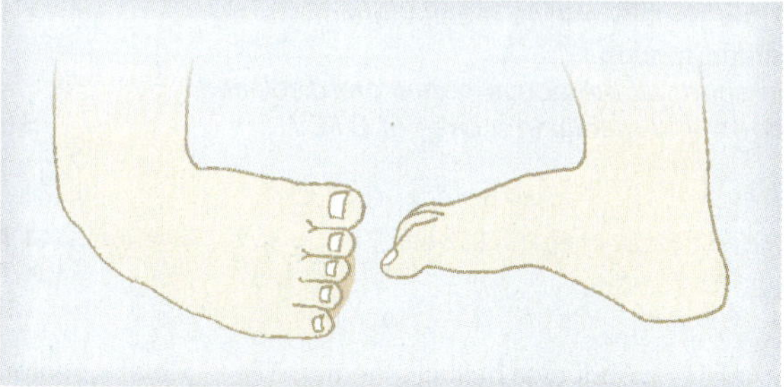

Fig. 35.26: Bilateral CTEV

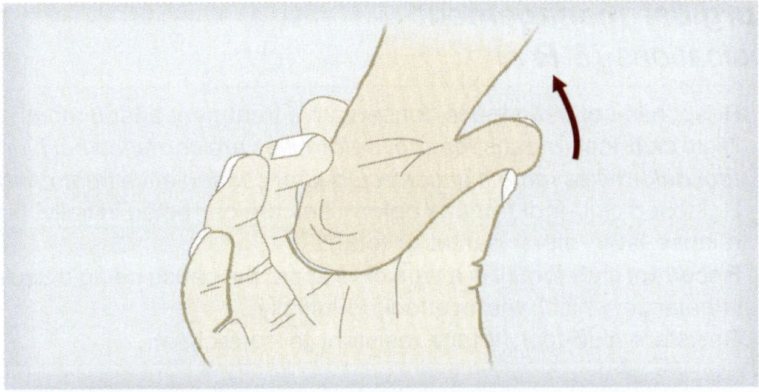

Fig. 35.27: Dorsiflexion test in a newborn

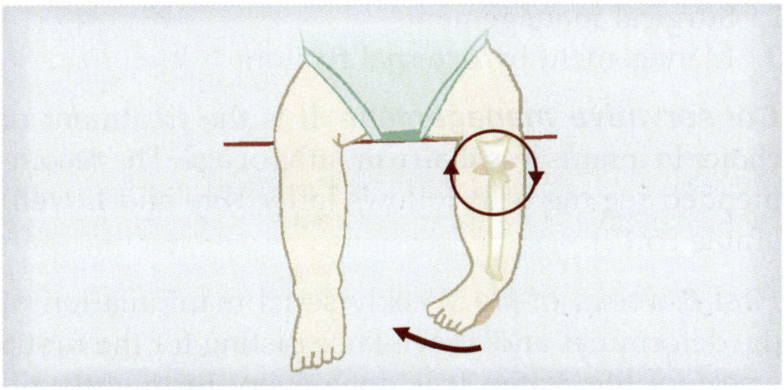

Fig. 35.28: Plumbine test to detect tibial torsion

- *Lateral scratch test* Here, when the lateral sole is scratched, the child inverts the foot. This tests the invertors.

Investigation

Since CTEV is a mechanical problem, laboratory investigations are less useful. Radiography is by far the most important investigation. It helps to know the exact angles of each deformity seen clinically in CTEV. In anteroposterior view, the angles formed between the long axis of the talus and the calcaneum, the talus and the metatarsals are evaluated. This helps to know the angle of varus and the forefoot adduction. In the lateral view, the angle formed between the talus and the tibia, and talus and calcaneum helps to know the extent of equinus and varus respectively (Table 35.11).

X-ray views are to be taken with feet in the stabilisation frames.

AP view is to be taken with tibia absolutely vertical.

Table 35.11: Showing various radiographic angles in CTEV

Anteroposterior	*Lateral*
1. **Talocalcaneal angle** is reduced (normal is 30–35°)	1. **Talocalcaneal angle** is reduced (normal is 25–50°)
Talocalcaneal Index = TC angle (AP view + TC angle lateral view) should be at least 40°, which is ↓ in CTEV. **The study of talocalcaneal angle on the radiographs indicates the extent of varus.**	
2. **Talometatarsal angle** This angle indicates extent of forefoot adduction Normal is 5 to 15° In CTEV it is 0° to negative	2. **Tibiocalcaneal angle** This angle indicates extent of equinus Normal is 5 to 15° It is negative in CTEV

Lateral view is the stress dorsiflexion view.

In children of older age group; anteroposterior and lateral standing radiographies are preferred.

Apart from giving the accurate estimate of the angle of the deformities, radiology helps in confirmation of the correction of the deformities by various treatment modalities. *It is a simple fact that all angles should be restored back to normal following treatment. Any residual uncorrected angle is a future pointer to relapse* (Figs 35.29A and B).

> **Remember**
> **Clinical tests in CTEV**
> - Scratch test
> - Dorsiflexion test
> - Plumbline test

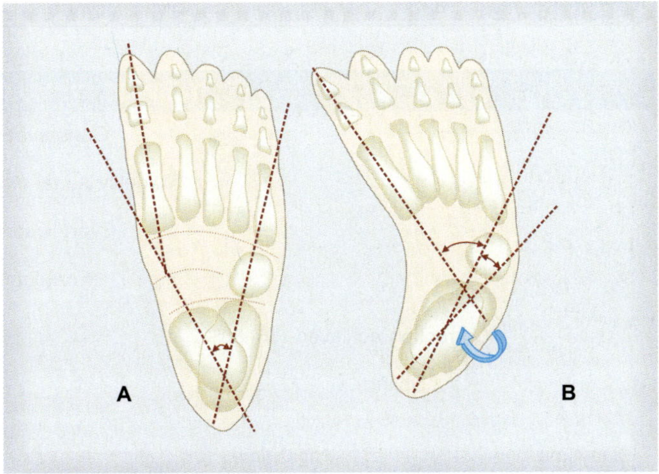

Figs 35.29A and B: Showing: (A) Talometatarsal angle, (B) Talocalcaneal angle

Management

Broadly speaking, CTEV can be managed by three methods.

1. Conservative management

2. Surgical management
3. Management by external fixators.

Conservative management It is the treatment of choice in infants less than 6 months of age. The recommended regime is as follows (after Kite and Lovell) (Table 35.12).

First 6 weeks of life Weekly serial manipulation of the deformities and above-knee casting for the first 6 weeks of life. Later, it is done every fortnightly till correction is achieved. Manipulation by mother is not usually sufficient (Fig. 35.30). Success rate of serial manipulation and casting ranges from 15 to 80 per cent. If correction is achieved in first 6 months of age, Phelp's brace is used during the daytime and Dennis Browne splint during the night time from 6 to 18 months to prevent recurrence. After 18 months, below-knee walking calipers are given up to 4 years of age. From 4 years to skeletal maturity, regular follow-up is advised.

Remember order of correction of deformity

The mnemonic ADVERB helps to remember the order of correction.

AD—Forefoot adduction is corrected first
V—Correction of heel varus next
E—Lastly correction of hindfoot equinus

RB—This order is followed to prevent **"Rocker Bottom Foot"** which develops if foot is dorsiflexed through hindfoot rather than midfoot.

Surgical management

*Indications (**5 R's**)*

- **R**esponse not obtained to conservative treatment after 6 months.
- **R**igid club-foot (means *forefoot deformities are corrected but hindfoot deformities remain uncorrected after conservative treatment).*
- **R**elapsed club-foot (means deformities are corrected initially, but relapse later, either partial or total).
- **R**ecurrent club-foot (it is a type of relapse, the cause being muscle imbalance which was overlooked initially).
- **R**esistant club-foot (totally resistant to correction).

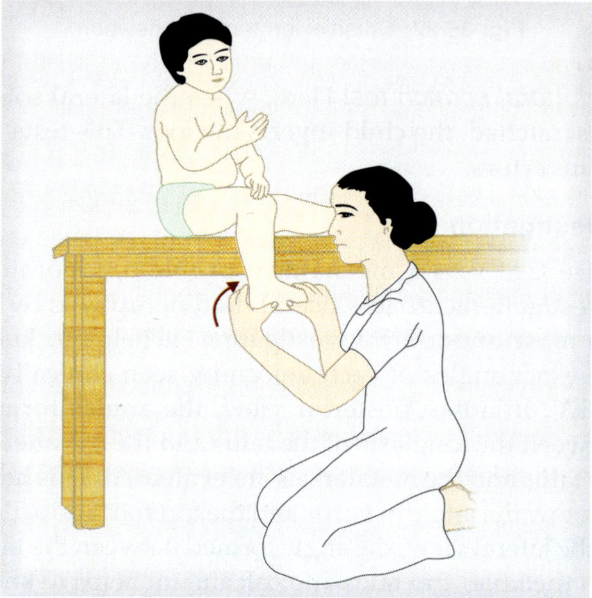

Fig. 35.30: Showing a mother manipulating her child's CTEV foot

Table 35.12: Modus operandi for CTEV

Conservative management
↓
Weekly serial manipulation and casting
↓
Every week for first 6 weeks
↓
Fortnightly till 6 months

- Correction achieved (15–80%)
  ↓
  Splint
  - Daytime (Phelp's brace)
  - Night time (Denis Browne splint)

  ↓
  For 6–18 months
  ↓
  > 18 months up to 4 years
  ↓
  Below-knee walking or CTEV shoes
  ↓
  Frequent follow-up every year till skeletal maturity
- Correction not achieved
  - Surgery
    - < 4 years: Soft tissue release
    - > 4 years: Soft tissue release + A bony procedure
  - External fixator
    - JESS
    - Ilizarov

Surgical Methods (Table 35.13)

Soft tissue procedures are advocated for children less than 4 years. Bony procedures are added later on. For mild CTEV with no severe internal rotation deformtiy of calcaneus, a one-stage posteromedial release of TURCO is preferred.

STRUCTURES RELEASED IN TURCO'S PROCEDURE (POSTEROMEDIAL RELEASE)

1. On the posterior side:
   a. Z-plasty of tendo-Achilles to lenghten it (Fig. 35.31).
   b. Posterior capsulotomy of the ankle and subtalar joints.
   c. Release of posterior talofibular and calcaneo-fibular ligaments.
2. On the medial side:
   a. Lengthening of the tibialis posterior, flexor hallucis longus and flexor digitorum longus muscle.
   b. Release of talonavicular ligament, spring ligament and the superficial part of deltoid ligament.

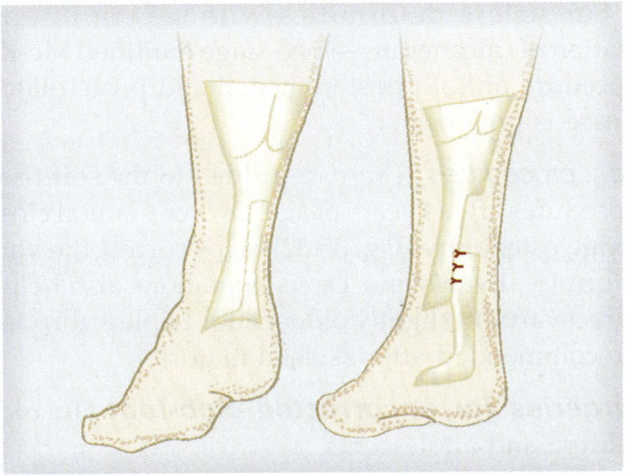

Fig. 35.31: Showing tendo-Achilles lengthening by Z-plasty for club-foot

   c. Release of interosseous talocalcaneal ligament, capsules of naviculocuneiform and first meta-tarso-cuneiform joints.
3. On the plantar side:
   a. Plantar fascia.
   b. Release of abductor hallucis and flexor digitorum brevis.

Table 35.13: Surgical treatment plan of CTEV

6 to 12 months (Turco's)	*12 to 36 months (McKay's)*	*1–5 years (Grey area)*	*Older child (untreated or treated with partial or total relapse)*
Cincinnati's incision is used Structures released are: **Medial** • TP/AHL/FHL/FDL muscles • Capsules of ST/Tarsal/TM joints Ligaments—deltoid/plantar/spring ligaments **Posterior** • Tendo-Achilles lengthening by Z-plasty (Fig. 35.31) • Postcapsulotomy of the ankle and subtalar joints • Calcaneofibular ligaments **Subtalar ligaments** • Talocalcaneal ligaments • Interosseous ligaments • Bifurcated Y-ligaments **Postoperative regimen** • Change cast at 2 weeks • Remove K-wire at 6 weeks • Long leg cast till 3 months • Phelp's brace or ankle foot orthoses for 6 to 9 months	Cincinnati's incision All the structures on the postero-medial side are released as in Turco. In addition, lateral structures released are: • Superior peroneal retinaculum • Inferior external retinaculum • Dorsal calcaneocuboid ligament • Origin of extensor digitorum brevis muscle	Treatment guidelines unclear	1. **Metatarsus adductus** > 5 years metatarsal osteotomy. 2. **Hind-foot varus** > 2–3 years modified McKay's procedure. **3–10 years** **Dwyer's** lateral closed wedge osteotomy of calcaneus is done. **Dillwyn Evan's** procedure—resection and arthrodesis of calcaneocuboid joint. **Davis procedure** wedge resection from the midtarsal area. **10–12 yr of age** Triple arthrodesis. 3. **Equinus** Mild—Tendo-Achilles lengthening and postcapsulotomy of ankle and subtalar joints is done. Sever-Lambrunidi's triple arthrodesis is done. 4. **All three deformities are present** over ten years triple arthrodesis is done. 5. **Ilizarov and Joshi's** external fixator frames useful in rigid, relapsed and untreated club-foot.

For severe deformities with severe internal rotation of calcaneum—a one-stage modified Mc-Kay procedure of both posteromedial and posterolateral release is preferred.

Bony procedures These are added to the soft tissue procedures after 4 years of age. Dwyer's lateral closed wedge osteotomy (Fig. 35.32) helps correct the varus deformity, Evan's and Davis operations also help to correct varus in slightly older child. Triple arthrodesis is recommended after skeletal maturity.

Surgeries for uncorrected club-foot In older children and adolescents

Triple arthrodesis (Figs. 35.33A and B) Indicated for children more than 10 years. It is functionally and cosmetically, superior. Lateral closed wedge osteotomy through subtalar and midtarsal joints is done to fuse all the three joints of the foot namely the subtalar, talonavicular and calcaneocuboid joints.

Talectomy It is a salvage procedure and is indicated for severe uncorrected club-foot. It is also indicated in those cases previously corrected and unsuccessful. For uncorrectable CTEV by any other procedure, talectomy is useful as a salvage procedure.

Surgery for recurrent club-foot (recurrence is due to muscle imbalance, here peroneals are weak and invertors are strong).

Garceaus method Transfer of tibialis anterior to middle cuneiform bone.

Modified Garceaus method Transfer of tibialis anterior to base of fifth metatarsal bone.

Surgery for correction of tibial torsion in club-foot (Sell's criteria) more than 15° torsion should be corrected by derotation osteotomy. Otherwise all deformities will recur due to the pressure of the caliper on the lateral border of the foot.

Caliper is used after the correction to maintain the correction of deformities obtained either by conservative or surgical measures.

Treatment by external fixators (Fig. 35.34) This is a recent concept in the management of CTEV and is reserved for difficult cases. There are two types of external fixator frames, one is designed by Ilizarov, a Russian orthopaedic surgeon. The second one is designed by an Indian orthopaedic surgeon, Dr. BB Joshi. This frame is known as Joshi's external stabilisation system popularly called as JESS.

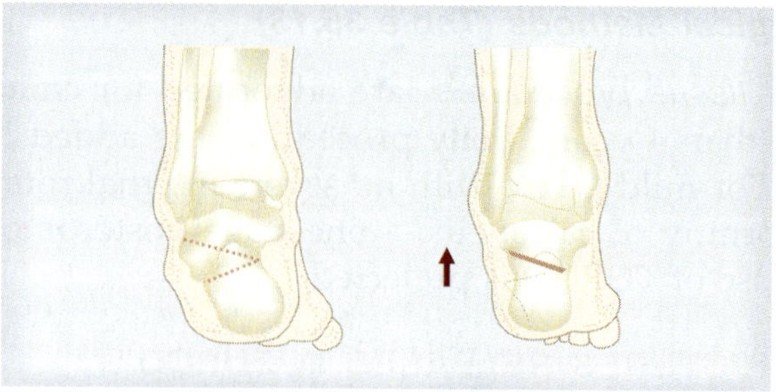

Fig. 35.32: Showing Dwyer's lateral closed wedge osteotomy

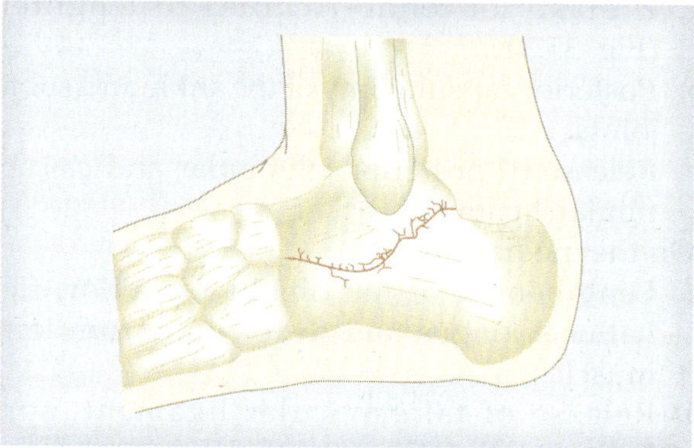

Fig. 35.33A: Showing triple arthrodesis in CTEV

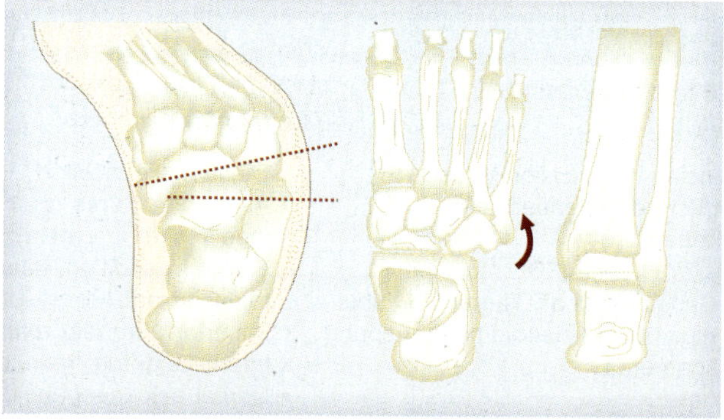

Fig. 35.33B: Showing triple arthrodesis in CTEV

When done in properly indicated cases, external fixator produces excellent results. It is a semi-invasive, bloodless surgery and can be done without a tourniquet. Though technically very demanding, it avoids all the complications of surgery and a postoperative scar. It is known to correct all the components of the deformities both bony and soft tissues. The rate of relapse or recurrence is compartively less; and even if it does occur, the options of surgery are always open.

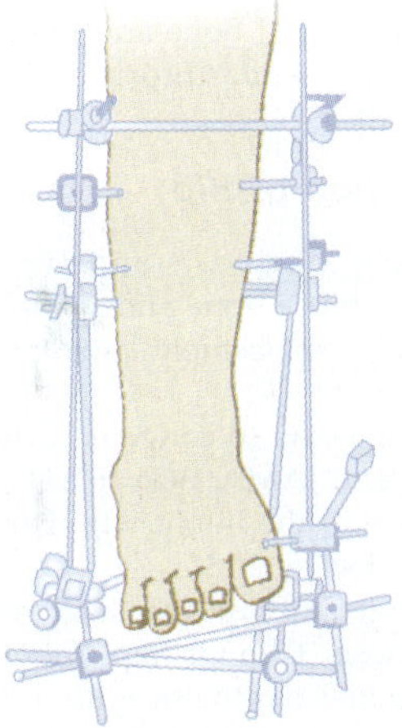

Fig. 35.34: External fixators (JESS)

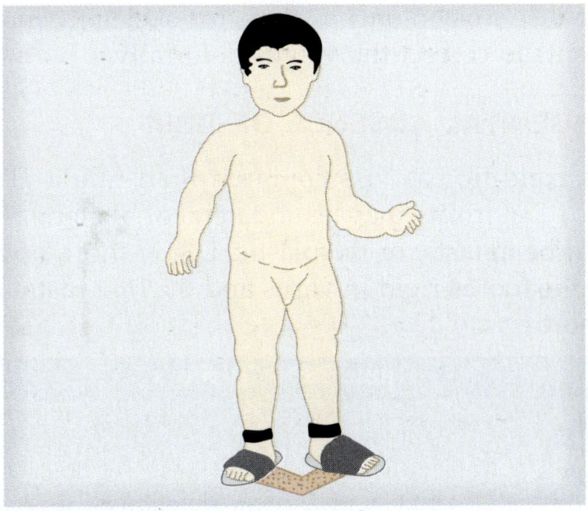

Fig. 35.35: Showing a Denis Browne splint

Remember

Three I's for relapse
- Improper and inadequate conservative treatment and also surgical release of contracted structures
- Imbalance of foot muscles if left uncorrected
- Internal torsion of tibia if overlooked

RETENTION OF CTEV CORRECTION

Whatever may be the methods of correction of CTEV whether conservative, surgical or by external fixators, retentions of the corrected deformities should be done by one of the following methods to prevent relapse:

a. Denis Browne splint—used usually during the night time (Fig. 35.35).
b. Phelp's brace—used mainly in the daytime.
c. Below-knee walking calipers.
d. CTEV shoes—these are mainly used when the child starts walking and up to 5 years of age (Fig. 35.36).

Quick facts

Do you know how does a CTEV shoe differ from an ordinary shoe?
1. It has a straight inner border which helps prevent forefoot adduction
2. It has an outer shoe raise and this helps prevent foot-inversion
3. There is no heel and this helps prevent equinus.

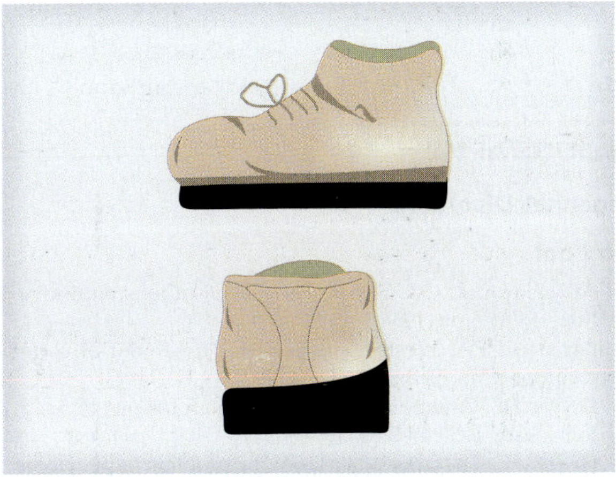

Fig. 35.36: Showing CTEV shoes

CONGENITAL ABSENCE OF FIBULA

Fibula is partially or completely absent more often than any other long bones of the body (Table 35.14).

Treatment

Type I Lengthening of the affected tibia and epiphyseal arrest of opposite limb is done.

Type II Presence of tight band in place of absent fibula should be excised.

Table 35.14: Coventry and Johnson's classification

Type I	*Type II*	*Type III*
• Fibula is partially absent • Unilateral • Leg is mildly or moderately short	• Unilateral absence of fibula • Anterior bowing of tibia • Equinovalgus foot • Ipsilateral femur is short	• Unilateral or bilateral • Associated with other severe anomalies • Prognosis is poorest

Wiltse's osteotomy is done for skeletally mature patients to correct the valgus deformity.

CONGENITAL ABSENCE OF TIBIA

This condition is less common than fibula (Table 35.15). Deformity may be unilateral or bilateral. Tibia could be aplastic or dysplastic. Leg is short, bowed, and the foot is rigid in varus and the first metatarsal is short.

Table 35.15: Types

Types	*Features*	*Treatment*
Type I	Total absence of tibia	Transfer of fibula
Type II	Distal tibial aplasia	Tibiofibular fusion
Type III	Distal tibial aplasia + Diastasis of inferior tibiofibular syndesmosis	• Calcaneofibular fusion • Disarticulation of ankle • Modified Boyd's amputation

BIBLIOGRAPHY

Congenital Disorders

Club Foot

1. Attenborough CG. Severe congenital talipes equinovarus. J Bone Joint Surg 1966;48-B:31.
2. Barenfeld PA, Wesley MS. Surgical treatment of congenital clubfoot. Clin Orthop 1972;84:79.
3. Dwyer FC. Osteotomy of the calcaneum for pes cavus. J Bone Joint Surg 1959;41-B:80.
4. Dwyer FC. The present status of the problem of pes cavus. Clin Orthop 1975;106:254.
5. Evans D. Relapsed club foot. J Bone and Joint Surg 1961;43-B:722.
6. Garceau GJ. Recurrent clubfoot. Bull Hosp Joint Dis 1954;15:143.
7. Kitc JH. Principles involved in treatment of club foot. J Bone and Joint Surg 1939;21:595.
8. McKay DW. New concept of and approach to clubfoot treatment. Section 111. Evaluation and results. J Paediatr Orthop 1983;3:141.
9. Turc VJ. Surgical correction of the resistant club foot: one stage posteromedial release with internal fixation: a preliminary report. J Bone and Joint Surg 1971;53-A:477.

Congenital Pseudarthrosis

10. Boyd HB, Sage FP. Congenital pseudarthrosis of the tibia. J Bone and Joint Surg 1958;40-A:1245.
11. Charnley J. Congenital pseudarthrosis of the tibia treated by an intramedullary nail. J Bone and Joint Surg 1956;38-A:283.
12. Wall JJ. Congenital pseudarthrosis of the clavicle. J Bone Joint Surg 1070;52-A:1003.

Congenital Dislocation of Hip

13. Barlow TG. Early diagnosis and treatment of congenital dislocation of the hip. J Bone and Joint Surg 1962;44-B:292.
14. Chiari K. Medial displacement osteotomy of the pelvis. Clin Orthop 1974;98:55.
15. Coleman SS. Diagnosis of congenital dysplasia of the hip in the newborn infant. JAMA 1956;162:548.
16. Colonna PC. Care of the infant with congenital dislocation of the hip. JAMA 1958;166:715.
17. Ortolani M. Congenital hip dysplasia in the light of early and very early diagnosis. Clin Orthop 1976;119-26.
18. Pavlik A. Functional treatment with a harness as a principle for the conservative treatment of congenital hip dislocation in infants. Z Orthop 1957;89:341.
19. Perkis G. Signs by which to diagnose congenital dislocation of the hip. Lancet 1928;1-648.
20. Salter RB. Specific guidelines in the application of the principle of innominate osteotomy. Orthop Clin North Am 1972;3:148.
21. von Rosen S. Diagnosis and treatment of congenital dislocation of the hip joint in the newborn. J Bone Joint Surg 1962;44-B:284.
22. Wagner H. Osteotomies for congenital hip dislocation. In the hip society. Proceedings of the fourth open scientific meeting of the hip society, 1976. St Louis: CV Mosby Co 1976.

Other Congenital Disorders

Congenital Wryneck

23. Chandler FA. Muscular torticollis. J Bone Joint Surg 1948;30-A:566.
24. Covertry MB, Harris L. Congenital muscular torticollis in infancy: some observations regarding treatment. J Bone Joint Surg 1959;41-A:515.
25. Kaplan EB. Anatomical pitfalls in the surgical treatment of torticollis. Bull Hosp Joint Dis 1954;15:154.

Congenital Elevation of Scapula

26. Cavenelish ME. Congenital elevation of the scapula. J Bone Joint Surg 1972;54-B:395.
27. Green WT. The surgical correction of congenital elevation of scapula. Personal Communication, 1962.

Congenital Radioulnar Synostosis

28. Cohn BNE. Congenital bilateral radioulnar synostosis. J Bone Joint Surg 1932;14:404.
29. Wilkic DPD. Congenital radioulnar synostosis. Br J Surg 1913-1914;1:366.

36 Developmental Disorders

INTRODUCTION

To understand the developmental disorders of bones, it is very essential to know the basic bone cell types and the method of ossification. The osteogenic or osteoprogenitor cells are the precursors of osteoblasts, chondroblasts and perhaps osteoclasts also. The osteogenic cells are found both in the periosteum and the endosteum.

The osteoblasts synthesise and secrete the organic intercellular substance called the osteoid tissue. The cells then get trapped within this substance in lacunae or cavity and the cells are now called as osteocytes. The intercellular substance so formed is a mixture of matrix with type-I collagen as its main constituent, inorganic salts consisting mainly of calcium in the form of hydroxyapatite [$Ca_{10}(PO_4)_6(OH)_2$] and water.

The osteoclasts are multinucleated giant cells which are concerned with bone resorption and hence takes part in bone remodelling. The chondrocytes are the cartilage forming cells.

Remember

Bone cell types

- Osteoprogenitor cell is a common precursor of osteoblasts, chondroblasts and osteoclasts.
- Osteoblasts are bone forming cells.
- Chondrocytes are cartilage forming cells.
- Osteocytes originate from osteoblasts.
- Osteoclasts are bone remodelling cells.

The process of the formation of organic intercellular substance by osteoblasts is known as ossification. This osteoid tissue rapidly gets mineralised in normal conditions.

BONE OSSIFICATION METHODS

In the intrauterine life, bone development starts as a condensation of mesenchymal cells. The gaps in these condensations are future areas of joint development. These mesenchymal cells differentiate into chondrocytes which form the cartilage. Thus, in embryonic life most of the skeleton is composed of cartilage. The chondrocytes so formed proliferate and secrete intercellular substance. After this, the chondrocytes mature and secrete alkaline phosphatase which initiates the process of calcification of the cartilaginous matrix. This calcified matrix impairs diffusion of nutrients resulting in death of the chondrocytes. This results in disintegration and dissolution of calcified matrix, paving way for the ingrowth of the highly vascular and cellular tissue. This brings in osteoblasts which surround the remnants of calcified cartilage and lay down new bone. Thus, the process of ossification begins. Two centres of ossification are formed, one in the diaphysis which extends to replace the entire diaphysis of the cartilage model with bone and the other in the epiphysis. The growth plate is a condensation of cartilage between these two centres of ossification. It contributes towards longitudinal growth of the bone till skeletal maturity after which it is replaced by bone.

This process of mesenchymal cells changing to chondroblasts which then become chondrocytes and form cartilage model of bone, which is later converted into bone by the action of osteoblasts is called as *endochondral ossification* and is typically seen in long bones.

When bone is formed directly from the mesenchyme, without intervening stages of cartilage formation, it is called *intramembranous ossification*. This type of ossification is seen in flat bones of the skull.

Remember

About bone development

- Mesenchymal cells convert into chondroblasts.
- Chondroblasts change to chondrocytes and forms the cartilage model of the entire skeletal system.
- This cartilage model is replaced by bone due to the action of osteoblasts. This process is known as endochondral ossification.
- Intramembranous ossification refers to a situation wherein the mesenchymal cells directly form bone without the intervening cartilage cells.
- Bone formed by the above two methods undergo constant remodelling.

Thus the bone so developed, either by intramembranous or endochondral ossification, is constantly being resorbed and reformed by the action of osteoclasts. This process is known as remodelling. Remodelling develops and preserves the structure and size of the bone apart from providing a mechanism for maintaining calcium ionic homeostasis in body fluids. Thus, bone is not a static tissue as it appears to be. Developmental disorders result if there is any defect in the growth process so far discussed.

Bone dysplasias are generalised disorders of skeleton due to disturbance of growth and development of either bone or the cartilages. There are structural defects in more than one system, with generalised malformations of bone. Genetics has a role in dysplasias, the inheritance being dominant, recessive, X-linked or multifactorial.

DIAGNOSTIC GUIDELINES

Developmental disorders have the following diagnostic guidelines in common.

History In the patients with developmental disorders usually there is a family history and are associated with multiple fractures.

Clinical Examination

Stature Many dysplastic patients are dwarfs (less than 1.25 m in height)

Three types of dwarfs are described

1. *Proportionate dwarfs* both trunk and limbs affected
   - Hurler's disease
   - Osteogenesis imperfecta
   - Hypophosphatemia.
2. Short limbed dwarfs with normal spine
   - Achondroplasia
   - Hypochondroplasia.
3. Short limbed dwarfs with considerable spine involvement
   - Spondyloepiphyseal dysplasia
   - Morquio's disease.

Increased joint laxity is seen in

1. Ehlers-Danlos syndrome
2. Marfan's syndrome
3. Morquio's disease
4. Osteogenesis imperfecta.

Distribution

1. Generalised in some, familial history is present.
2. Not generalised in the rest, affects only one side of the body or one limb, and is not familial.

Remember

Dysplasia hallmarks

- **History**
  - Familial
  - Multiple fractures
- **Examination**
  - Dwarfs (Three types:)
    1. Short limbed
    2. Short limbed with normal spine
    3. Short limbed with abnormal spine
  - Excessive joint laxity
- **Distribution**
  - Usually generalised
  - Rarely localised, e.g. melorheostosis

CLASSIFICATION OF DEVELOPMENTAL DISORDERS (Table 36.1)

Table 36.1: Classification (Aegster's)

Cartilaginous	*Bony*	*Miscellaneous*
Disturbed chondroid formation **Heterotropic chondroblastic proliferation** • Multiple exostosis • Enchondromatosis **Abnormal chondroblast maturation** • Achondroplasia • Metaphyseal dysostosis **Abnormal epiphyseal centre** • Multiple epiphyseal dysplasia • Spondyloepiphyseal dysplasia, etc. **Abnormal mucopolysaccharide metabolism** • Hurler's disease • Morquio's disease	*Disturbed osteoid formation* **Deficient osteoid formation** • Osteogenesis imperfecta **Increased osteoid formation** • Osteopetrosis • Osteopoikilosis **Abnormal osteoid production** • *Fibrous dysplasia* • Neurofibromatosis • Pseudarthrosis	• Cleidocranial dysostosis • Nail patella syndrome • Marfan's syndrome • Chromosomal abnormalities producing skeletal dysplasias

Role of Radiograph

It detects lesions even if missed clinically. It also helps to label the lesions as epiphysial, metaphyseal or diaphyseal and shows increase (e.g. osteopetrosis) or decrease (osteogenesis imperfecta) in the bone density.

Three films often suffice: AP view of the wrist and hands, pelvis and hips and lateral view of the spine.

ACHONDROPLASIA

Achondroplastic is melancholic at heart, as he weeps at his stature but gives the greatest gift to mankind that is laughter, as he dispells the gloom on the weary faces of the people, by his clowning antics at the circus!

Definition It is a defect in the enchondral ossification of the bone, with the membranous ossification being normal.

This is the most common type of dwarfism one encounters in clinical practice. The limbs are short and the head is big; because, along with the growth of the limbs, growth of the base of the skull is affected, but the membranous bones of the vault escape.

Clinical Features

The patient is a short-limbed dwarf (Figs 36.1A and B). The fingers are short and stumpy and do not reach below the upper one-third of the thigh as he stands.

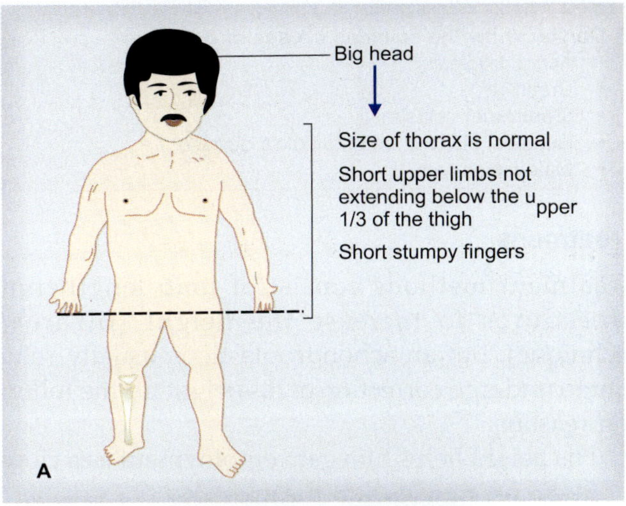

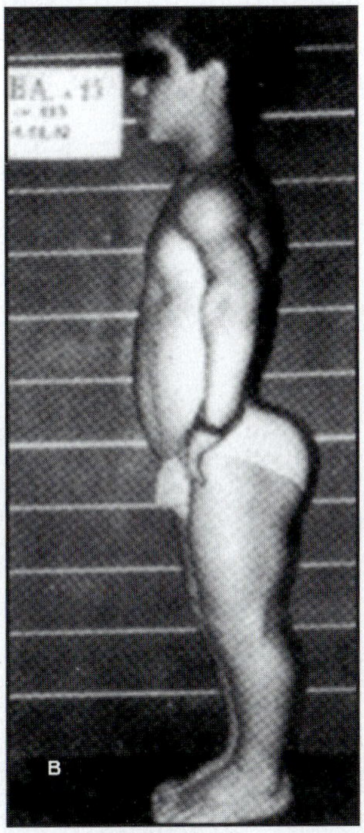

Figs 36.1A and B: Showing features of achondroplasia

The patient can kiss his toes with the knees straight. Head is large, nose is flattened, but the length of the trunk may be normal and occasionally may show kyphoscoliosis or lordosis. Cervical lordosis and increased lumbar lordosis develop in the later stages of the disease. The intelligence and sexual developments are normal.

X-ray findings Ilium is quadrilateral in shape and there is coxa vara (Fig. 36.2).

Quick facts

Do you know the common causes of dwarfism?
- Achondroplasia
- Cretinism
- Diaphyseal aclasia
- Hunter's, Hurler's and Morquio's disease
- Malnutrition, etc.

Treatment

Treatment methods consist of limb lengthening procedures to increase the height (Ilizarov's technique). But an achondroplastic is usually reluctant to undergo correction of his height for the following reasons:
- His height helps him gain employment as a clown in circus, movies and theatres.
- He is entitled for benefits offered to a handicapped person by the government and other agencies.
- Limb lengthening procedures are expensive and time consuming.

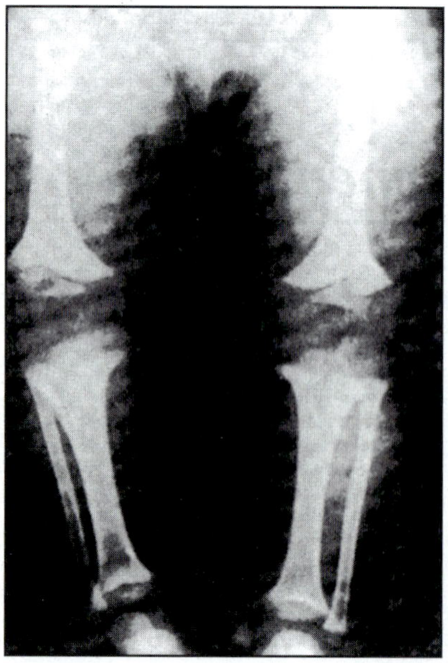

Fig. 36.2: Radiograph showing achondroplasia

Remember

About achondroplasia
- Failure of endochondral ossification
- Commonest type of dwarf
- Normal intelligence
- Usually employed as a clown
- Limb lengthening procedures help

OSTEOGENESIS IMPERFECTA

To be a blue eyed boy is great but to virtually have blue eyes is a misery. Read on the story of osteogenesis imperfecta to find out why?

Definition It is a hereditary condition characterised by *fragility of bones, deafness, blue sclera, laxity of joints and a tendency to improve with age.*

It is a disease of the mesodermal tissues with deposition of normal collagen in bone, skin, sclera and dentine.

Aetiology

The aetiological factors could be heredity, mendelian recessive—in prenatal cases, and mendelian dominant—in postnatal cases.

Pathogenesis and Pathology (Table 36.2)

Primary defect is failure of osteoblast formation during enchondral ossification, osteoid formation does not take place. Features of bones are:
- Periosteum is thick but the cambium layer is thin.
- Bone is short and thin and the epiphysis is bulbous.
- Cortex is thin and medullary contents are fatty and fibrous.

Table 36.2: Types of osteogenesis imperfecta

Clinical types	*Features*
I. Fetal or prenatal or congenital type	• Multiple fractures are present at birth. • In severe forms infants may be stillborn or die within a few weeks.
II. Infantile form	• Less severe. • Multiple fractures. • Skull is thin and globular.
III. Adolescent form	• Normal at birth. • Fractures due to trivial trauma in childhood.

- Bones break easily but heal well with abundant callus. Fracture is usually subperiosteal and heals by periosteal bone formation.
- Deformity results from bending and fractures.
- Vertebral bodies are biconcave.
- Scoliosis.
- Skull is thin and globular.

Classification (Falvo's)

Osteogenesis imperfecta tarda type I This type has presence of bowing at long bones.

Osteogenesis imperfecta tarda type II No bowing of long bones in this type.

Fractures may be present in both the types but rare in type II.

Clinical Features

The patient presents with blue sclera, dentinogenesis imperfecta and generalised osteoporosis (Fig. 36.3). Blue sclera is seen only in 92 per cent of cases, while the other two features are seen in almost all cases. Osteoporosis gives rise to bowing and multiple fractures. Fractures are usually due to trivial trauma but surprisingly heals well. Other features include: deafness due to otosclerosis, laxity of joints, dwarfism, broad skull, poorly calcified decidual teeth, but permanent teeth are normal and the blood chemistry is normal.

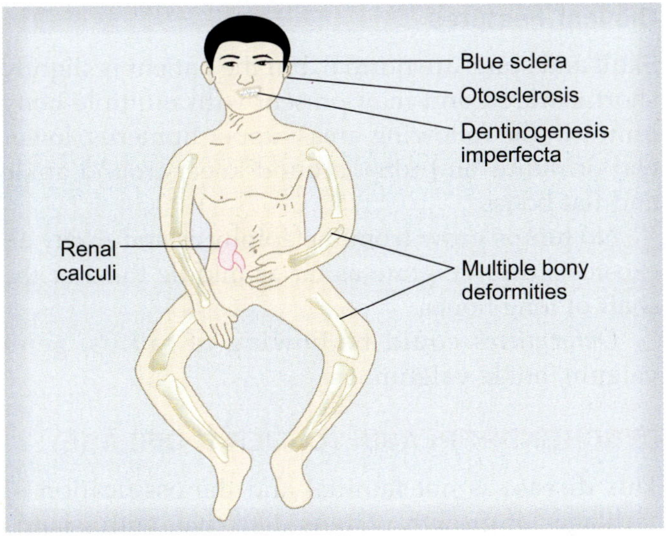

Fig. 36.3: Showing features of osteogenesis imperfecta

Remember

The mnemonic **BLOOD** in osteogenosis imperfecta

BL—Blue sclera

O—Otosclerosis

O—Osteoporosis

D—Dentinogenesis imperfecta.

Quick facts

Do you know the 4 O's responsible for easy fractures

- Osteoporosis
- Osteopetrosis
- Osteomalacia
- Osteogenesis imperfecta

Remember

3F's in osteogenosis imperfecta

- **F**ragile bones
- **F**ractures—multiple and frequent
- **F**etal variety is fatal

Radiological Types

1. **Thick bone type** (Fig. 36.4)
   - Seen only in congenital cases
   - Shafts of long bones are thicker than normal
2. **Thin bone type**
   - The long bones are thinner and ends are bulbous
   - Vertebral bones are thin and biconcave
   - Cortex is thin
3. **Osteogenesis imperfecta cystica**
   - Fracture unites promptly with large callus

Investigations

a. ***Laboratory tests*** There is no specific laboratory test for this disease. Prenatal determination of the

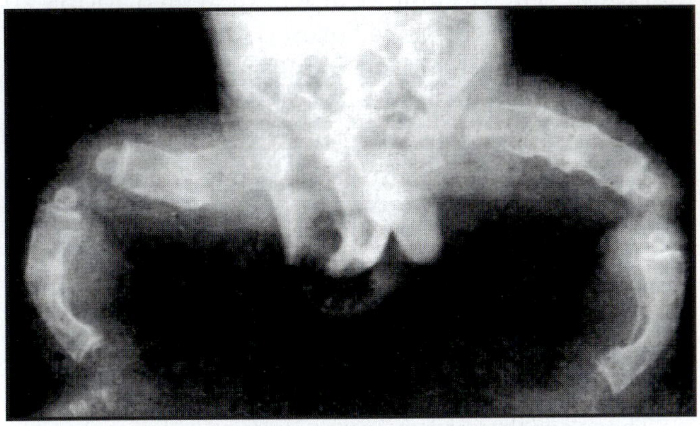

Fig. 36.4: Radiograph showing thick bone type of osteogenesis imperfecta

Section 5

probability of osteogenesis imperfecta on the fetus can be achieved by amniocentesis and estimation of *inorganic pyrophosphate.* This compound is elevated 3 to 4 times the normal value.

b. ***X-ray*** of the affected limbs helps to make a diagnosis.

Treatment

Principles

Protect the child till the tendency of the fracture lessens as age advances.

Administer vitamins, oestrogens and androgens.

Operate in infantile type as the tendency to fracture is much higher and hence the treatment of choice is multiple osteotomies with intramedullary nailing.

Surgical Methods

Sofield's method consists of multiple osteotomies and realignment and IM nail fixation. It is useful for long bones and is indicated for fresh fractures and correction of bowing. There is no growth disturbances in this technique.

Bailey and Duboy's Here, telescopic medullary rod is used which elongates as growth occurs.

William's Here, retrograde nailing is done by fixing an extension to the distal end of the rod and driving the nail through the heel

MUCOPOLYSACCHARIDE DISORDERS

The bone has two components—organic and inorganic. The organic component which forms 70 per cent of the bone is formed mainly by type-I collagen (90–95%) and the remaining 5 to 10 per cent is formed by the mucopolysaccharides which are protein polysaccharides. The principal mucopolysaccharide is chondroitin IV sulphate. Its role is not clear, but it appears to inhibit mineralisation of bone by strongly complexing with calcium ions.

In certain diseases, increased urinary excretion of polysaccharides results in loss of polysaccharides from bone and cartilage causing specific skeletal deformities.

These are the inborn errors of mucopolysaccharide metabolism.

MORQUIO-BRAILSFORD DISEASE

The following features are seen, normal development till five years, dwarfism is present, kyphosis is present, manubriosternal angle is more than 96° *(pathognomonic),* vertebra are too flat with a narrow tongue of bone projecting forwards *(platyspondyly),* hips are grossly distorted, genu valgum and varum are severe, marked ligamentous laxity, skull and mentality are normal. *Keratin sulphate is found in urine.*

HURLER'S (GARGOYLISM)

The features are coarse skin, wide set eyes with corneal opacity, bloated lips and eyelids, mental retardation, limb deformities are same as in Morquio's. There is no platyspondyly. *Dermatin sulphate and heparin sulphate are found in urine. Cardiopulmonary complications are common unlike in Morquio's.* These patients rarely survive into adults.

HUNTER'S DISEASE

Hunter's disease differs slightly from Hurler's, it is less severe and shows X-linked inheritance. All patients are males.

HEREDITARY MULTIPLE EXOSTOSIS (DIAPHYSEAL ACLASIA)

Diaphyseal aclasia is autosomal dominant and there is a failure of bone remodelling, excess of metaphysis is not resorbed, but forms irregular cartilage capped exostosis.

Clinical Features

Skull and spine are normal, but the patient is slightly short statured and may present with multiple bony lumps in the following areas: upper humerus, lower end of radius and ulna, around knee, around ankle and flat bones.

No lumps grow from the epiphysis and rarely an exostosis does migrate as far as middle third of the shaft of long bones.

Deformities could be bowing of radius, genu valgum, ankle valgum, etc.

DYSCHONDROPLASIA (OLLIER'S DISEASE)

This disease is not familial and the ossification of cartilages at growth plate is defective, with islands of unossified cartilage.

Clinical Features

It is typically unilateral and the affected limb is short and bent. There is valgus and varus at the knee and ankle. Relative shortening of the ulna with the radius curved and sometimes dislocated is often seen. Malignant change occurs in 1 per cent of the cases. Fingers and toes contain multiple enchondromas.

MAFFUCCI'S DISEASE

Dyschondroplasia and multiple haemangiomatas are seen in Maffucci's disease.

Radiology

Translucent islands or columns of cartilage are seen in the metaphysis. In addition, there are development of dense irregular spots, shaft is curved but normal, and metaphysis is mottled or streaky.

OSTEOPETROSIS

MARBLE BONE DISEASE, ALBERS-SCHÖNBERG'S DISEASE

Here, the bone looks excessively dense and structureless on the X-ray. Bone has a marble appearance but breaks easily as it is very brittle.

Note: Marble bone disease is due to functional deficiency of osteoclasts leading to failure of bone resorption.

Complications

It could be due to insufficient formation of bone marrow, and due to encroachment on cranial foramina which causes optic atrophy, deafness and facial palsy.

Pathology

There is continued new bone deposition on unresorbed calcified cartilage and there is failure of remodelling which starts at birth and continues throughout life. Bone is as hard as marble or as brittle as chalk and it is grey or white on section.

Aetiology

Aetiology is unknown, consanguinity has a role to play and it is inherited as simple mendelian recessive or dominant.

Clinical Features

The disease starts during gestation and is progressive till growth stops. The intensity varies, in mild type formation of dense bones occurs slowly, intermittently and incompletely. Malignant type occurs in consanguinous marriages. Bone is dense and brittle. Fractures are frequent and heal slowly. Anaemia, optic atrophy, facial palsy, deafness, hydrocephalus are the other features.

Radiology

Entire long bone may be dense or dense bone may alternate with normal bone. Metaphysis is club shaped. The skull density is maximum at base with a small pituitary fossa and sparing of maxilla and mandible.

Prognosis

Age at onset and severity determines the outcome. If it appears at birth, it is fatal by the end of two years.

Other Variants

1. Candle bones (melorheostasis, Leri's disease)
2. Spotted bones (osteopoikilosis)
3. Stripped bones (osteopathia striata).

EPIPHYSEAL DYSPLASIAS

Epiphyseal dysplasia multiplexa is the rarest in this group and is familial. Face, skull and spine are normal.

X-ray features Epiphysis appears late and close early, illformed, irregular and mottled, shape altered, deformity and stiffness results, and secondary osteoarthritis is common.

Epiphyseal dysplasia punctata is a variation of epiphyseal dysplasia multiplexa. It is more severe and is obvious at birth.

Conradi's disease The components are epiphyseal dysplasia, mental retardation, cataract, congenital heart disease and dwarfism. Mottling disappears with growth.

Epiphyseal dysplasia hemimelia affects epiphysis of ankle, knee and only one limb is involved. One-half of the epiphysis either medial or lateral is involved. The child presents because of limp or stiffness.

METAPHYSEAL DYSPLASIAS

Metaphyseal dysplasia (Pyle's disease) It is an autosomal recessive and there is a failure of remodelling of the metaphysis. Erlenmeyer flask deformities of distal femur and proximal tibia may develop. It may also be associated with genu valgum.

Craniometaphyseal dysplasia It is an autosomal dominant and is confused with Pyle's disease. There is metaphyseal widening, thickening of the skull and mandible.

Metaphyseal chondrodysplasia It is autosomal dominant, the metaphysis is irregular and cystic. Varus deformities of the hips and knees may be seen.

DIAPHYSEAL DYSPLASIA

Progressive diaphyseal dysplasia (Canuati's or Engleman's disease) This disease shows fusiform widening and sclerosis of shafts of long bones and skull. Femur, tibia, forearm bones are symmetrically affected. Cortical thickening is superficial, bone ends are normal, painful limbs, waddling gait, weakness, etc. are the other associated findings.

Craniodiaphyseal dysplasia shows expansion of long bone shafts and is associated with gross thickening of skull and face.

FIBROUS DYSPLASIA

Fibrous dysplasia is a rare disease with fibrous replacement of bones. It may be *monostotic or polyostotic*.

Aetiology

It is unknown, begins in childhood, progresses beyond puberty and has equal incidence in both sexes.

Pathology

Gross Bone is irregular and bent, long bones are shortened, pathological fractures heal readily, **shepherd crook deformity** is seen in upper femur and is the hallmark of this disease (Fig. 36.5) and base of skull becomes hyperostotic (shaft of femur bowed, varus neck).

Microscopy This shows dense collagen tissue, giant cells are sparse, and islands of cartilage are seen in only 10 per cent cases.

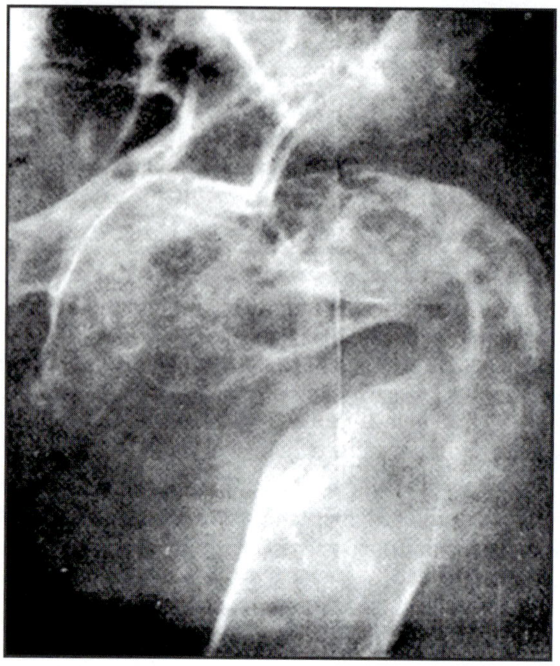

Fig. 36.5: Radiograph showing shepherd crook deformity in fibrous dysplasia

Clincal Features

Clinical features in early childhood is mild and asymptomatic. Onset is seen in less than 10 years of age. The patient may present with limp, pain, and fractures. Females have abnormal vaginal bleeding. Bending deformity and shortening of the bones are common features and lengthening is rare. *Shepherd crook deformity is quite characteristic*. There is asymmetry of head and face and local irregular brown patches if seen are associated with polyostotic types. Sexual precocity is typical in females.

ALBRIGHT'S SYNDROME

It is a unilateral polyostotic fibrous dysplasia with sexual precocity in females.

Laboratory Investigation

Serum calcium, phosphorus, alkaline phosphatase are normal. In severe cases, alkaline phosphatase may increase.

Radiology

Localised lesions are cystic, multilocular, and show ground glass appearance, pathological fracture may occur. Shepherd crook deformity and Harrison's grooves following rib fractures, intrapelvic protrusion of acetabulum, and hyperostosis at the base of the skull, are the other important features.

Treatment

Surgery is the treatment of choice in fibrous dysplasia and consists of:

	Problems	Preferred surgery
I.	Long bones fractures	Open reduction + Internal fixation + Bone grafting
II.	Cyst	Curettage + Bone grafting
III.	Coxa vara	Subtrochanteric osteotomy + Internal fixation + Bone grafting
IV.	Limb length discrepancy	• Epiphyseal arrest before skeletal maturity • Ilizarov's treatment
V.	Limb severely shortened and deformed	Amputation

Remember

4 S's in fibrous dysplasia

- **S**hepherd crook deformity
- **S**exual precocity in females
- **S**erum investigations are normal
- **S**urgery is the treatment of choice

NAIL-PATELLA SYNDROME (ONYCHO-OSTEODYSPLASIA)

The features are autosomal dominant gene, nails are hypoplastic, patella is unduly small or absent, radial head may subluxate laterally, bony excrescences develop on the lateral aspect of the ilium and there could be congenital nephropathy.

[1]MARFAN'S SYNDROME

It is autosomal dominant and there is a defect in elastin collagen. Ocular lens dislocation and aortic aneurysm are seen. The patient is tall with disproportionate legs. Chest deformities, scoliosis, long digits, generalised joint laxity, high arched palate and hernias may be seen.

Note: Marfan's syndrome was described by Marfan, a French paediatrician in 1896. *Abraham Lincoln was affected with Marfan's syndrome.*

[1]**Bernard Marfan** (1896) French Paediatrician

HOMOCYSTINURIA

It is autosomal recessive and the patient is prone to lens dislocation. Osteoporosis, widening of epiphysis and metaphysis, mental defect, stickiness of platelets are other associated features.

ACROCEPHALOSYNDACTYLY (APERT'S SYNDROME)

It is autosomal dominant. Head has a peculiar shape with high broad forehead *(tower shaped).* Flat occiput, bulging eyes, prominent jaws, and associated syndactyly of fingers and toes are other findings.

CARPENTER SYNDROME

Carpenter syndrome is Apert's syndrome with polydactyly.

CLEIDOCRANIAL DYSPLASIA

See Chapter on "Congenital disorders."

CONGENITAL NEUROFIBROMATOSIS

VON RECKLINGHAUSEN'S DISEASE

This disease targets the skeletal system with impunity. It is autosomal dominant and development of neurofibromas within ectodermal and mesodermal tissues takes place.

Clinical Features

Clinical features consist of skin lesions—*pigmented cafe-au-lait spots,* multiple neurofibromas which are derived from endoneurium and perineurium, etc.

Locations of the neurofibromas

1. *Subcutaneous* Tender painful palpable nodules.
2. *Subperiosteal* Periosteal reaction or a bone cyst.
3. *Endosteal* Bone cysts, pseudarthrosis, etc.
4. *Intraspinal* Dumb-bell shaped tumour, paraplegia never occurs.

Skeletal changes Incidence is about 30 to 50 per cent.

Long bones Show reduced growth rate, periosteal cysts, cortical cysts, osteoporosis, rarely increased density and multiple bone cysts, and congenital pseudarthrosis.

Spine Scoliosis is the most common skeletal lesion and there could be kyphosis or kyphoscoliosis. This disease is consistently associated with "cafe-au-lait spots" and elephantiasis due to diffuse hypertrophy of all soft tissues.

Less common lesions are head lesions, macrocranium, optic glioma, bilateral acoustic neuroma, cervical kyphosis, and vascular lesions.

Diagnostic criterion

Any two of the following:
- Positive family history
- Positive biopsy finding
- Minimum six "cafe-au-lait spots"
- Multiple subcutaneous neurofibromas
- Iris nodules called Lysch nodules

Radiology

X-ray features show kyphoscoliosis, lateral scalloping, pencil pointing of vertebral margins, and adjacent twisted *ribbon ribs* (characteristic).

Treatment

Complete excision is the only treatment and elephantiasis needs repeated resection. Scoliosis needs early correction and fusion. Painful spinal tumours require laminectomy and removal. Kyphosis needs anterior correction and spinal fusion. Anterolateral bowing of tibia should be protected against pathological fracture till skeletal maturity is reached. Surgical intervention is necessary if fracture occurs.

PAGET'S DISEASE

Paget's disease is seen after 40 years of age and is more common in males. There is impairment in the bone resorption and bone formation due to defective osteoclastic functions. As a result of this, bone gets thickened and bent more so the tibia. Bone is soft in the initial stages and dense later.

Clinical Features

The affected bones are thickened and bent. The patient complains of dull pain and deformities.

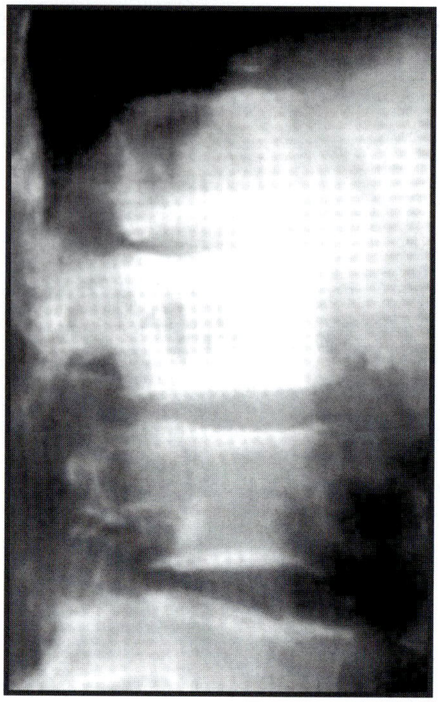

Fig. 36.6: Radiograph showing Paget's disease

Investigations

Laboratory investigation Serum alkaline phosphatase is increased.

Radiograph shows multiple lytic areas with intervening new bone formation (Fig. 36.6).

Treatment

It is essentially conservative and the drugs of choice are calcitonin or diphosphonate.

BIBLIOGRAPHY

1. Albright JA. Management overview of osteogenesis imperfecta. Clin Orthop 1981;159:80.
2. Albright JA. Systemic treatment of osteogenesis imperfecta. Clin Orthop 1981;159:88.
3. Bleck EE. Nonoperative treatment of osteogenesis imperfecta: orthotic and mobility management. Clin Orthop 1981;159:111.
4. Bailey JA. Orthopaedic aspects of achondroplasia. J Bone Joint Surg 1970;52:A;1285.
5. Goldberg MJ. Orthopedic aspects of bone dysplasias. Orthop Clin North Am 1976;7:445.
6. McKusick VA. Heritable disorders of connective tissue, 4th edn. St Louis: CV Mosby Co, 1972.

37

Metabolic Disorders

INTRODUCTION

Metabolic bone disease is largely a consequence of an upset in bone remodelling activity and/or mineralisation occurring at the periosteal, endosteal, haversian and trabecular surfaces. The cells involved in remodelling are derived from mesenchymal cells. From these cells arise multinucleated osteoclasts which resorb bone and osteoblasts which lay down osteoid and initiate mineralisation. Some osteoblasts persist as osteocytes and the remainder die.

Mineralisation of osteoid involves the deposition of calcium and phosphate as hydroxyapatite crystals (Fig. 37.1). These are situated at regular intervals along the collagen fibrils of the osteoid.

BONE FORMATION AND REMODELLING

Bone growth starts *in utero* and continues for nearly two decades. Normal bone is formed either *de novo,* by intramembranous ossification from osteoblasts or by endochondral ossification from pre-existing cartilaginous models. The long bones and the vertebrae increase in size by a combination of these two processes.

There is a constant remodelling in such a way that the net bone formation equals net bone resorption. The remodelling takes place by the cells on the periosteum, haversian, endosteal, and trabecular surfaces. This process begins during the fetal period, accelerates during infancy and continues throughout life.

Role of Calcium

The mineral in the bone serves a major structural role and remains metabolically stable under normal circumstances. The main mineral deposited on the organic matrix is calcium in the form of $Ca_{10} (PO_4)_6 (OH)_2$. It is deposited in either cortical or trabecular bone. It has a twin role of structural and metabolic importance.

CALCIUM METABOLISM

About 0.6 to 1.0 gm of calcium is ingested and equal amount is excreted every day.

Vitamin D, PTH, bile salts, calcitonin help in the absorption of calcium from the upper small intestine, while the oxalates, citrates, phosphates, phytic acids and fats impair absorption. Calcium so absorbed gets deposited mainly into the bone. The remaining is excreted through the kidney and intestine. Hormones regulate this calcium homeostasis (Fig. 37.2). Hormones which help calcium to get deposited into the bone are oestrogen, thyroxine, growth hormone and testosterone, while that which remove the calcium from bone are glucocorticoids, thyroid hormones, PTH and acidosis. Any upset in this delicate balance either results in increase or decrease in serum calcium. These homeostatic mechanisms normally maintain the ratio of calcium and phosphorus ions to 2.5:1 (Table 37.1). The calcium homeostasis and its regulation is displayed in the Figure 37.2 and Table 37.1.

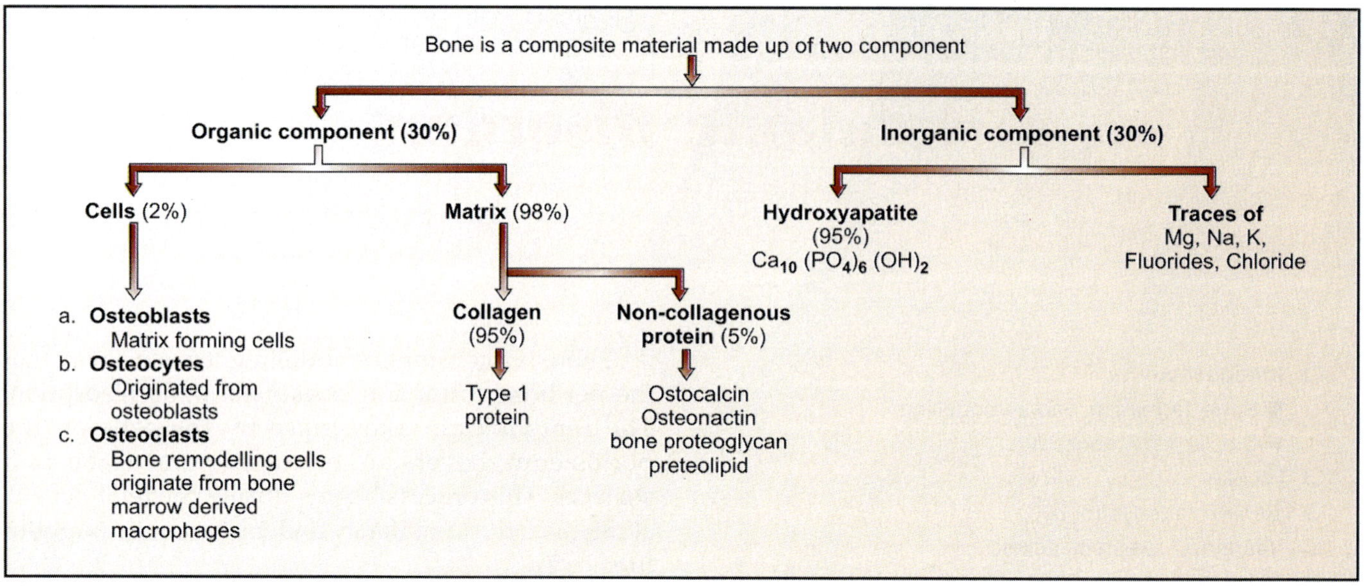

Fig. 37.1: Showing composition and structure of a bone

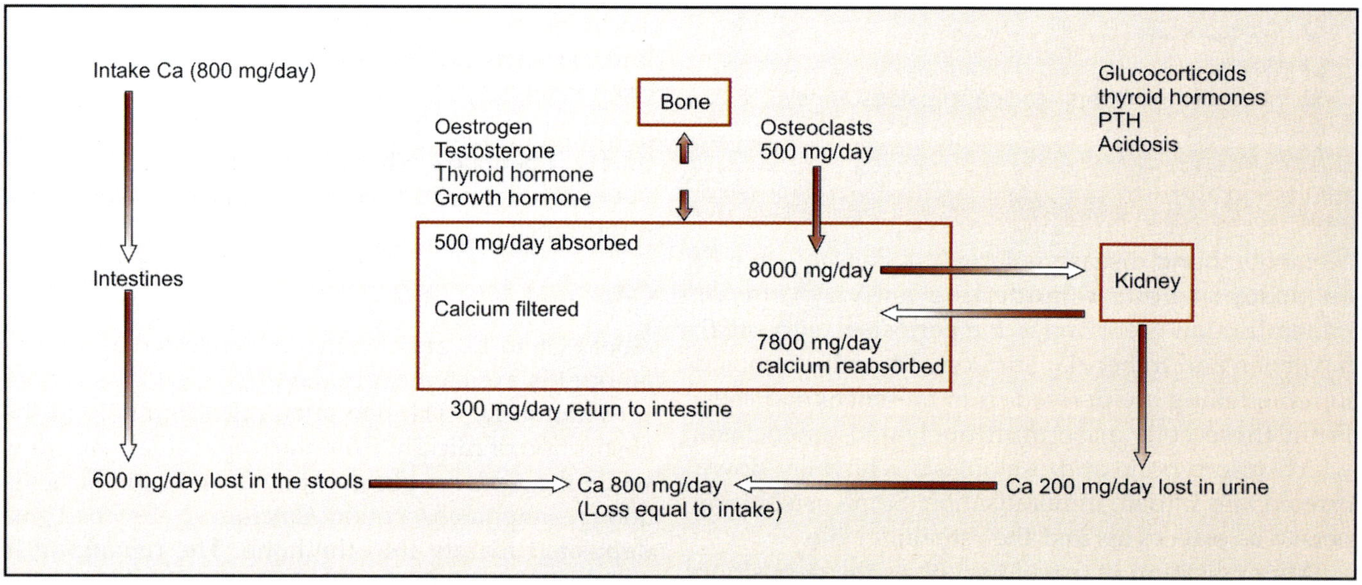

Fig. 37.2: Showing dynamics of bone homeostasis

Remember

About calcium

- Indispensable to life.
- Total calcium content of body is 1 kg.
- Only one gram is found in ECF and plasma.
- Remainder is in the skeleton.
- Normal requirement is 0.6 to 1.0 gm/day.
- Provides bone its hardness and strength.
- Helps in blood coagulation, neuromuscular excitability, enzyme actions, etc.
- Tetany is due to low calcium levels.
- Sulkowitch test for calcium in urine is important.

Remember

Important causes of hypercalcaemia

- Hyperparathyroidism
- Chronic renal insufficiency
- Rickets
- Osteomalacia
- Nephrosis
- Malabsorption syndrome
- Celiac disease
- Sprue

Important causes of hypocalcaemia

- Hypoparathyroidism
- Secondaries in the bone

Table 37.1: Regulation of calcium and phosphorus metabolism

Hormones	*PTH (Parathyroid)*	*1,25 $(OH)_2$ D (Kidney)*	*Calcitonin (Thyroid)*
Factors ↑	• ↓ Serum calcium	• ↑ PTH • ↓ Serum calcium • ↑ Phosphorus	• ↓ Serum calcium
Factors ↓	• ↑ Serum calcium • ↑ 1,25 $(OH)_2$ D	• ↓ PTH • ↑ Serum calcium • ↑ Phosphorus	• ↓ Serum calcium
Action on end organs			
• **Intestine**	• No direct effect • Acts indirectly on bowel by ↑ 1,25 $(OH)_2$ D	• Strongly stimulates intestinal absorption of calcium and phosphorus	
• **Kidney**	• Converts 25 (OH) D to 1,25 $(OH)_2$ D • ↑ Absorption of Ca • Promotes excretion of phosphorus		
• **Bone**	• Stimulates osteoclastic resorption of bone • Stimulates recruitment of pro-osteoclasts	• Strongly stimulates osteoclastic resorption of bone	• Inhibits osteoclastic resorption of bone
Net effect on calcium and phosphate in	• ↑ Serum calcium • ↓ Serum phosphate	• ↑ Serum calcium • ↑ Serum phosphate	• ↓ Serum calcium (transient)

Note: The skeletal system consists of 95% of calcium and 80% of phosphorus in the body

- Sarcoidosis
- Multiple myeloma
- Hyperproteinaemia
- Vitamin D intoxication
- Production of PTH like hormone by neoplasms of ovary, kidney, lung, etc.

Six important metabolic diseases are discussed in this Chapter:

1. Rickets
2. Renal osteodystrophy
3. Osteomalacia
4. Hyperparathyroidism
5. Osteoporosis
6. Conditions causing osteosclerosis.

RICKETS

Definition *It is a metabolic disease of childhood in which, the osteoid, the organic matrix of bone, fails to mineralise due to interference with calcification mechanism.* It is usually common between six months and two years.

Causes

Four main causes:

1. *Vitamin D deficiency:*
   - Reduced dietary intake*
   - Reduced amount of sunlight*
   - Pigmented skin.
2. *Malabsorption due to:*
   - Celiac disease
   - Hepatic osteodystrophy.
3. *Renal disease:*
   - Glomerular failure
   - Renal osteodystrophy.
4. *Antiepileptic drugs* favours formation of hepatic enzyme which prevents conversion of calciferol.

Remember

About Vitamin D

- Two principle vitamin Ds nutritionally useful are calciferol D_2 and cholecalciferol D_3.
- 1,25 dihydroxy vitamin D is formed in the kidney and is the active form.
- It aids in the absorption of calcium from the gut.
- It is necessary for calcium deposition in bone.
- Its lack upsets the calcification of cartilage and mineralisation of osteoid.

Metabolic abnormality in rickets

Vitamin D ↓ → ↓ 1,25 $(DH)_2$ → D_3 ↑ → ↓ Calcium absorption → Hypocalcaemia → ↓ PTH → Ca level ↑ → Bone resorption increased → Compensatory attempts to bone formation → ↑ Alkaline phosphatase → Negative Ca and P level

Ca level is increased by mobilisation of bone stock, increased intestinal absorption, decreased renal excretion and decreased phosphate absorption.

Quick facts

Do you know the daily requirements of calcium?

Adult	50 mg
Child	700 mg
Adolescent	1000–1300 mg
Pregnant women	1500 mg
Lactating women	2000 mg
Postmenopausal women	1500 mg
Major fracture	1500 mg

TYPES OF RICKETS

Fetal rickets This is commonly seen in osteomalacic mothers.

Infantile rickets (nutritional rickets) This is rare before 6 months and is the most common form of rickets, seen in 6 months to 3 years of life.

Late rickets or rachitis tarda This is a late onset rickets, familial, and it is a vitamin D-resistant rickets.

Quick facts

Varieties of rickets

Type I	This is due to dietary deficiency or defects in metabolism of vitamin D.
Type II	This is due to low serum phosphorus due to dietary phosphate deficiency or defective tubular resorption. *Type I dietary deficiency of vitamin D is the most common variety of rickets.*

Clinical Features

Symptoms Patient complains of bone pain during rest and excessive perspiration in upper half of the body (Fig. 37.3). He or she loathes to use the limb and the weakness of proximal muscles of the lower limbs produces waddling gait. There is evidence of catarrh of mucous membranes (recurrent diarrhoea, constipation, bronchitis). Irritability of CNS produces convulsions, laryngismus, spasmophilia, Chovstek's sign, opisthotonos, etc.

Signs

Deformities of Rickets (from head to toe)

Skull

- Broadened forehead
- Skull squared (caput quadratum)
- Frontal and parietal bossing—seen after the age of 6 months.
- Craniotabes is a ping-pong sensation on compressing the membranous bones of the skull.

Chest

- Pigeon chest due to prominent sternum.
- Narrow chest.
- Rickety rosary (enlargement of costochondral junction).
- Harrison's sulci due to diaphragmatic pull on the soft ribs.

Bones

- *Enlargement of the metaphyseal segments* of long bones like radius, tibia, costochondral junction, etc. seen in children between 6 and 9 months of age.

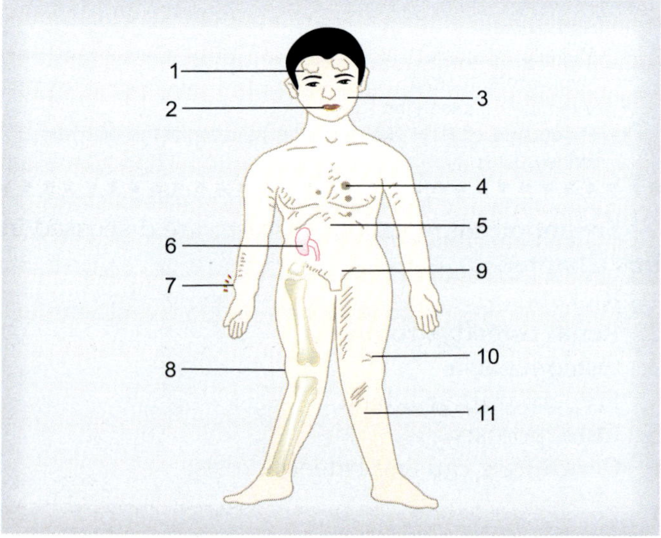

Fig. 37.3: Showing skeletal changes in rickets (1) Frontal bossing, (2) Dentition changes, (3) Chovstek's sign, (4) Rickety rosary and pigeon chest, (5) Malabsorption, (6) Aminoaciduria, (7) Expanded wrist, (8) Pelvis deformity, (9) Genu valgum, (10) Myopathy, (11) Skin changes

- *Vertebral columns* show exaggerated curvature.
- *Pelvis* is trefoil shaped.
- *Coxa vara*
- *Femur* is bent anteriorly and laterally.
- *Knock knee (genu valgum)*
- *Bowed tibia.*

Other Features

Other features encountered in rickets are wizened look, delayed dentition, prominent abdomen, separation of recti, pale and flabby skin, and incomplete fractures, etc.

Quick tests

How do renal rickets differ from nutritional rickets?

- Less osteoid formation and increased osteoclastic resorption of bone.
- Osteosclerosis is seen at the base of the skull.
- Slipped capital femoral epiphysis is more common.
- Delay in skeletal maturation.

Pathology

Bones of the skeletal system Bones are soft and porotic and bend easily. Epiphyseal line of 2 mm is normal but in rickets, it forms a wide irregular band. Metaphysis is broad and irregular.

Bony trabeculae are weak and continued stimulation makes the connective tissue hyperplastic, so that the extremity of bone appears mis-shaped and unmodelled.

These changes are most marked at the actively growing part of the bone and only affects the bone being deposited during the active phase of the disease. Bone formed before and after the active phase is normal.

Investigations

X-ray of the part Lovette and Jones radiological changes (Table 37.2).

Remember

Characteristic X-ray findings (Figs 37.4A and B)

- Delayed appearance of epiphysis and widening of the epiphyseal plates.
- Champagne glass appearance (widening and cupping of the distal ends of long bones) also called 'trumpeting'.
- Space between diaphysis and epiphysis is increased.
- Deformity and bowing of the ends of long bones.
- Thickened epiphysis.
- Decreased density of cortex (rarefaction).
- Trabecular pattern is course.

Table 37.2: Radiological changes in rickets

Stages	*Epiphysis*	*Metaphysis*	*Periosteum*	
Acute	*Cloudy*	*Splayed out*	*Thickened*	*Fractures of long bones*
II	• Mottled • Irregular • Ill-defined	• Ragged broad than normal	Thickening disappears	
III	• Shadow • Denser • Mottled	• Appearance of a dense line	No thickening	
IV		• Increased • Clearly defined Ca^+ (N)		

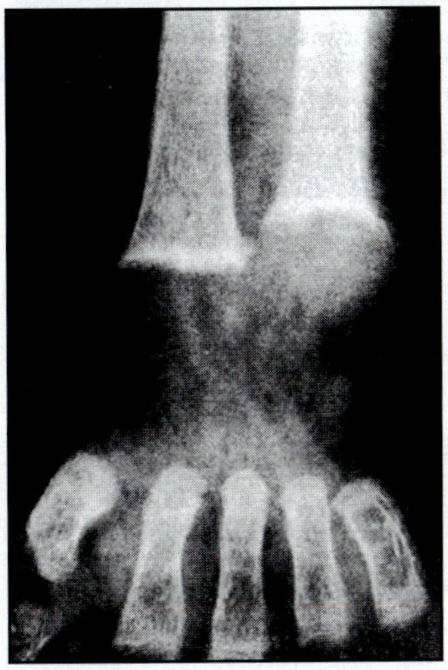

Fig. 37.4A: Radiograph showing metaphyseal cupping and irregularity of epipyseal plates seen in rickets

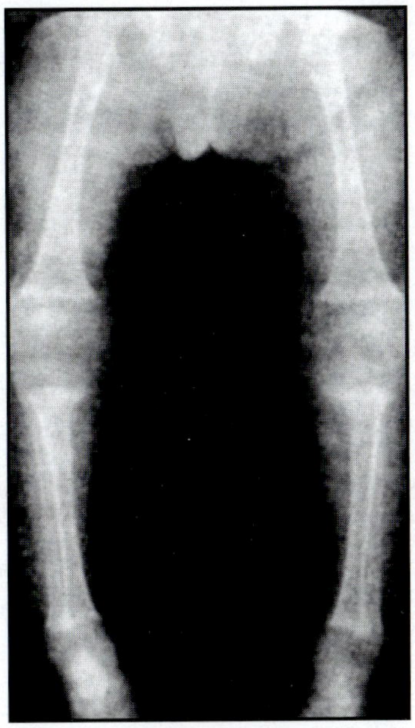

Fig. 37.4B: Radiograph showing features in rickets

Biochemistry

1. Calcium is normal or decreased (due to compensatory hyperparathyroidism).
2. Serum phosphorus is low.
3. Alkaline phosphatase is normal.
4. Urinary calcium is low (excretion less than 5 mg/kg/24 hr).

   Importance of biochemical values in this condition is their return to normal upon correct therapy.
5. Levels of 2, 5-hydroxyl D if low will indicate effectiveness of treatment.

Treatment

Medical treatment in the initial stages aims to bring about quick healing. A single oral dose of 6 lakh IU of vitamin D is given. A second same dose may be required after 3 to 4 weeks of treatment if no sclerotic (healing sign) change is seen on the radiograph at the metaphyseal side of the growth plate. A maintenance dose of 4,000 IU of vitamin D may be required if the child responds to the above treatment regimen.

Prevention of deformity can be done by absolute and strict bedrest, rickets splints, etc.

Treatment of Established Deformity

Correction by splints (Mermaid splint) This is mainly useful when the disease is active and the deformity is slight. It is very effective in children and in preventing deformities concerning the lower limbs. But it is slow and requires continual supervision.

Correction by osteotomy is indicated when deformity is near the joint and when the growth stops. It is done during III stage (Lovett's) (nonunion follows if done before).

Differential Diagnosis

Acute poliomyelitis, congenital syphilis, septic arthritis, infantile scurvy, etc.

RENAL OSTEODYSTROPHY

Renal osteodystrophy was first described by Lucas in 1883. In this condition, bone is diseased due to glomerular failure and renal tubular disease. Three forms are described:

1. Renal dwarfism
2. Renal pseudorickets
3. Renal osteitis fibrosa cystica.

Why is renal rickets a low-grade rickets?

Absorption of vitamin D and Ca from GIT is unimpaired. Hence osteoid tissue is being formed. So weight bearing deformities are not as pronounced as in rickets.

True florid phase of rickets is never seen. Shortness of stature is because enchondral ossification is affected at the growth plate.

Causes

At birth Congenital polycystic kidney and congenital hydronephrosis, etc.

Later Chronic glomerulonephritis, chronic interstitial nephritis, chronic pyelonephritis, and nephrosis due to heavy metal poisoning, etc.

Clinical Features

In renal rickets (Table 37.3) the clinical features could either be due to renal lesion *per se*, tubular defects (Table 37.4) or due to the growth disturbances and the resultant bony changes. Symptoms are present from early days of life. The child is normal for first few years before the symptoms start appearing. It is considered under three groups.

Parson's Radiological Features

1. *Atrophic type*
   - Epiphysis is broad and irregular.
   - Metaphysis is broad, uneven, and ragged.
   - Bone is osteoporotic and osteomalacic.
2. *Florid type*
   - Metaphysis has cup-shaped defect due to greater absence of calcium in the central axis of the bone than beneath the periosteum. It is broadened and there is subperiosteal new bone formation.
3. *Wooly stippled or Honeycomb type*
   - Metaphysis is grossly increased and irregularly honeycombed, stippled or wooly.
   - Bone is eaten away subperiosteally and has moth-eaten appearance.
   - Osteitis fibrosa may develop.

Table 37.3: Features in renal rickets

Those due to renal lesion	*Due to disturbance of growth*	*Bone changes*
• Thirst • Polydipsia • Polyuria • Urine – Low specific gravity – Output 1200–3700 ml/day – Albumin and Casts ++ • CVS symptoms of renal origin • Kidney failure: headache, GIT disturbances and drowsiness • Death due to uraemia	• Stunted growth • Body weight small • No malnutrition • Patient surviving beyond puberty shows infantilism and dwarfism • Mental development is normal up to puberty, thereafter mental sluggishness • Secondary sexual characters do not appear	• Genu valgum is the most common manifestation (Fig. 37.5). Age of onset is 11 to 14 years • Enlargement of epiphysis • Costochondral rosary • Bow legs, Harrison's sulci, etc. • May be associated with parathyroid hyperplasia.

Investigations

X-ray demonstrates calcification of kidneys, calculus formation, osteoporosis and osteitis fibrosa in the bone.

IVP demonstrates irregularities of renal pelvis and ureter.

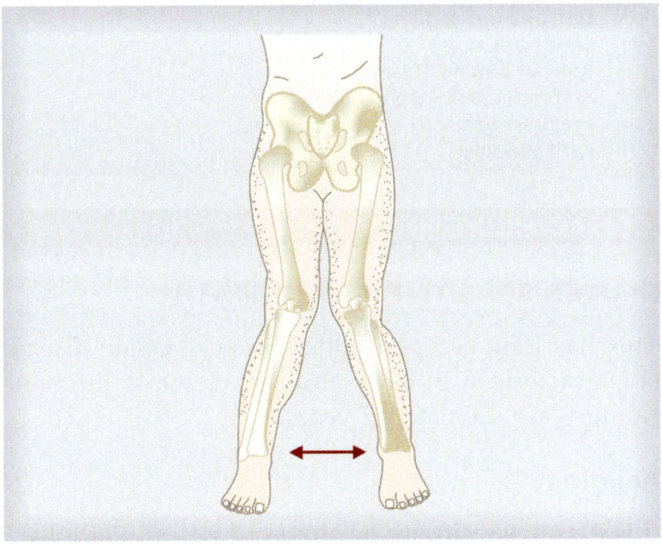

Fig. 37.5: Showing genu valgum deformity in renal rickets

Table 37.4: Tubular defects due to renal rickets

Kidney lesions

↓

Total renal insufficiency
- Found in congenital polycystic kidneys, chronic glomerulonephritis, focal nephritis

Main skeletal change is osteitis fibrosa

↓

PCT defect (Lignac-Fanconi syndrome)

Features
- Polydipsia, polyuria, anorexia, vomiting
- Rickets and dwarfism
- Children usually die before puberty
- Hyperphosphaturia, low serum phosphorus
- Normal calcium level
- Glucosuria and ketonuria.

Primary Lesions: *Impaired absorption of glucose and phosphates due to failure of phosphorylation*

- Abnormal deposition of crystals in the cornea, spleen and lymph nodes gives the syndrome the name **"Cystinosis"**

Treatment
- Massive doses of vitamin D

Tubular insufficiency

↓

DCT defect (Renal or Hypochloraemic acidosis)

Features
- Disturbance of potassium and creatinine secretion
- Failure to absorb water and secrete ammonia
- Excreting large amounts of urine containing Na, K, Ca.
- Loss of bicarbonate and retention of Ca
- Acid-base imbalance
- Osteitis fibrosa cystica picture

Treatment
- Excessive alkalinising salts like ammonium and calcium chloride
- Vitamin D in large doses

Note: Chronic renal failure causes rickets due to increased PTH level, acidosis and hypocalcaemia.

Treatment

Treat the underlying renal disease (e.g. removal of posturethral valve, etc.). Surgical intervention is done before puberty. Treatment is of little help in congenital polycystic kidney and renal hypoplasia. Good results are seen in hyperchloraemic renal acidosis and nephrocalcinosis. Organic acid with sodium citrate helps absorption of calcium from the intestines. Vitamin D in the form of OHD or 1,25

$(OH)_2$ is to be given in high doses (1 lakh IU). In active stages, weight bearing is prevented and use of splints is recommended. Avascular necrosis of femoral head may appear due to treatment with steroids. Haemodialysis or kidney transplant may help.

VITAMIN D-RESISTANT RICKETS

It develops due to failure of phosphate reabsorption from the kidney.

Clinical Features (Table 37.5)

The disease is familial and there is excessive faecal loss of calcium and defect in the formation of 1,25 $(OH)_2D$ by the kidney. Children tend to survive into adulthood exhibiting features of osteomalacia.

There is a prominent occipital protuberance and features of dolicocephaly (anteroposterior diameter increases but transverse diameter decreases). The patient has short stature and nose is saddle shaped.

Tackle Deformity

Tackle deformity (Fig. 37.6) is the hallmark of this disease (bow leg on one side and knock knee on the other). There is marked ligamentous instability.

Remember

The term vitamin D-resistant rickets refers to any condition that requires more than 1 lakh IU of vitamin D to produce healing.

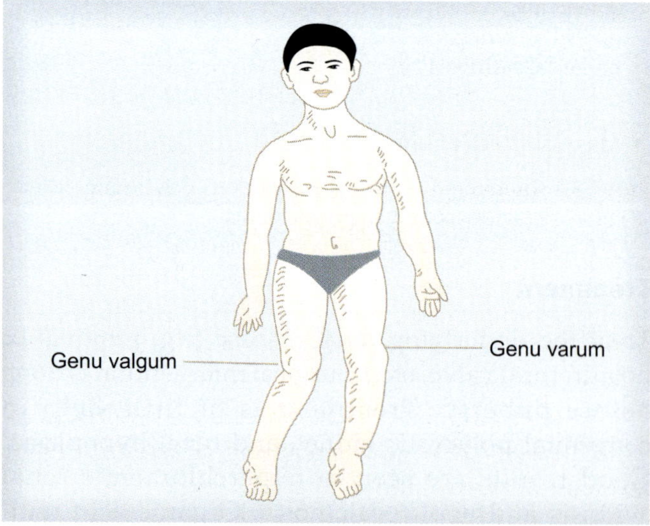

Fig. 37.6: Showing tackle deformity typical of vitamin D-resistant rickets

Table 37.5: Features of rickets: vitamin D-dependent and -resistant

	Vitamin D-dependent rickets	*Vitamin D-resistant rickets*
Onset	Acquired	Heredity
Muscle wasting	Present	Absent
Hypocalcaemic tetany	May occur	Present
Serum phosphorus	Always low, never returns to normal even after large doses of phosphorus	Low or normal, returns to normal with treatment
Growth	Becomes normal with treatment	Will not become normal with treatment. Patient remains dwarfed

Treatment

The aim of the treatment is to give doses of vitamin D (0.5-1.0 lakh IU/d) and to maintain Sulkowitch test at 1+ or 2+.

Prognosis

Complete cure of skeletal dystrophy may occur if the individual survives more than 16 to 17 years. Occurrence of bone deformity is a grave omen, average duration of life is less than two years if kidney is untreated.

Quick facts

A quick look at the late deformities seen with vitamin D-resistant rickets
- Genu varum/valgum
- Coxa vara
- Anterior bowing of femur
- Anterolatetal bowing of tibia
- Protrusio acetabuli
- Kyphoscoliosis

CELIAC RICKETS

GLUTEN-SENSITIVE ENTEROPATHY

This has long escaped notice because celiac disease is characterised in early childhood, while the bone changes are seen after 7 years.

Aetiology

It is due to sensitivity to gluten of wheat. Pathology is same as in vitamin D-resistant rickets.

Clinical Features

Onset is during infancy or early childhood. Patient presents with diarrhoea, anorexia, and irritability. Pale, foul, bulky stools may be absent but steatorrhoea may be seen. Retarded growth and development, wasting of proximal muscles, abdominal protuberance, iron deficiency anaemia, rickets, osteomalacic features are the other clinical findings.

Investigations

Duodenal biopsy shows loss of villi, and faecal examination shows in microscopical smears for fat (quantitative faecal fat normal up to 5 per cent of ingested fat).

Treatment

Conservative method consists of gluten-free diet, high potency vitamin D, calcium lactate injections, etc.

Quick tests Comparative blood picture in the four common varieties of rickets (Table 37.6).

Table 37.6: Types of rickets

Types of rickets	*Calcium*	*Phosphorus*	*Creatinine*	*Alkaline phosphatase*
1. Nutritional	Normal or low	Low	Normal	High
2. Vitamin D-resistant	Normal	Low	Normal	High
3. Renal	Normal or low	High	High	High
4. Hypophosphatasia	Normal or high	Normal	Normal or high	Very low

Note Hypophosphatasia is a genetically determined error of metabolism with low alkaline phosphatase activity and increased urinary excretion of phosphoryl ethanolamine.

OSTEOMALACIA

It is the adult counterpart of rickets and is characterised by failure of mineralisation and an excess of osteoid due to an interference with calcification mechanism. *The osteoid is increased at the cost of mineralised bone.*

Aetiology

1. Decreased vitamin D absorption from the intestine.
2. Derangement of vitamin D and phosphorus metabolism (hereditary or acquired).

Pathogenesis

It could be due to the following reasons:

1. Decreased *vitamin D metabolism* could be due to dietary malabsorption or disturbed metabolism.

Remember

Role of Vitamin D on

- Gut—Increase in calcium absorption.
- Bone—Increase in bone formation and mineralisation.
- Kidney—Decrease in phosphate reabsorption and increase in calcium reabsorption.

2. *Inorganic phosphate decreased* Hypophosphataemia impairs function of osteoblasts and thereby affects collagen synthesis and mineralisation. It could be due to renal disease, decreased PTH, or increased antacid (nonabsorbable).
3. *Chronic acidosis* due to renal disease adversely affects the calcium metabolism in the following ways:
   a. Bone mineral calcium is used up to buffer excess H^+ ions.
   b. Acidosis decreases calcium absorption.
   c. Causes hypophosphataemia and vitamin D-resistance.

Pathology

Increased osteoid (due to osteoblastic activity, and normal osteoclasis) is deposited in compact and cancellous bone (Figs 37.7A and B). This results in deformities because bone is soft thereby fractures occur easily but heals well.

Clinical Features

Symptoms The patient complains of generalised skeletal pain and muscle weakness. There may be acute pain due to fracture. Other symptoms related to causative factors like dietary, renal and GIT may be seen.

The following deformities are encountered; scoliosis, kyphosis, coxa vara, protrusio acetabuli, thighs and legs are bent, pelvis is trefoil, etc.

Radiographic features reveal generalised demineralisation, loss of transverse trabeculae, no subperi-

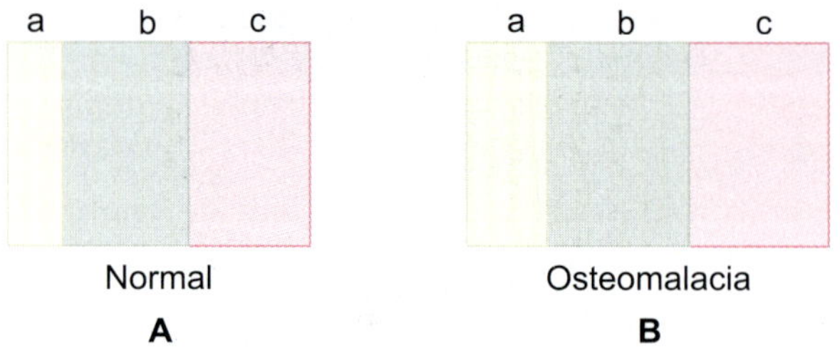

Figs 37.7A and B: Showing bony densities in osteomalacia (a) osteoid, (b) bone, and (c) marrow

osteal resorption of bone, etc. Presence of Looser's zones are quite characteristic of osteomalacia.

Remember

About looser's line

- **Looser's line** (Syn: Pseudofracture, Milkman's line) It is transverse, bilaterally symmetrical and incomplete.
- Fractures healed with defective callus.
- Sometimes only evidence of osteomalacia in treated cases.

Sites

- Axillary borders of scapula
- Ramus of pubis or ischium
- Neck of femur
- Ribs

They heal when osteomalacia is treated

Spine The bodies of spine are biconcave and are called "codfish spine".

Hip show protrusio acetabuli and triradiate pelvis.

Laboratory Investigation

The following changes are seen in the blood: serum calcium is normal or decreased, serum phosphatase is normal or decreased, alkaline phosphatase is slightly increased (rarely exceeds 200 IU), and serum PTH is increased.

Treatment

The following conservative regimen is recommended. Calcium is given at 0.5 to 3 gm/day, vitamin D 10,000 IU/day, high protein diet. The gastrointestinal tract errors are also corrected simultaneously.

HYPERPARATHYROIDISM

When parathyroid is on the rampage, it outbeats its big brother thyroid in ravaging the body but mercifully targets the skeletal system mainly unlike the all system effects of thyroid!

Parathyroid secretes parathyroid hormone, excessive secretion of which results in hyperparathyroidism. It may be *primary* or *secondary.*

PRIMARY HYPERPARATHYROIDISM (Osteitis Fibrosa Cystica, von Recklinghausen's Disease)

In the beginning of the chapter the role of parathormone has been highlighted. *The net result is it increases serum calcium and decreases serum phosphorus through its action on kidney, bone and intestines.*

Pathogenesis

Rise in the level of parathormone causes increased osteoclastic activity which resorbs the bone. Consequently, there is increased osteoblastic activity resulting in fibrous replacement of bone and consequent weakening.

Remember

About parathormone

- Secreted by principal or chief cells of parathyroid
- Maintains serum calcium level
- Lowers serum phosphorus level
- Increases diuresis of phosphorus
- Promotes renal and intestinal reabsorption of calcium
- Stimulates action of osteoclasts
- It will directly affect dissolution of bone
- Inhibits calcifying effect of vitamin D
- Increases solubility of calcium and phosphorus

Pathology

An adenoma in the parathyroid glands is usually seen.

Causes

Adenoma accounts for more than 90 per cent of the cases, carcinoma is rare and hyperplasia of the chief cells is seen in 6 per cent of the cases.

Clinical Features

This disease equally affects both sexes. It is common in middle-aged women. The patient complains of severe pain and tenderness over the back and lower limbs, generalised muscle weakness and hypotonia. Pathological fractures and delayed union may be seen. Deformities of limbs and spine are common features. Hyperphosphaturia, polyuria, polydipsia, renal calculi are some of the urinary complications.

Skeletal changes seen are diffuse bone resorption due to increased osteoclastic activity (Fig. 37.8), multiple deformities (because bone is soft due to replacement with fibrous tissue), pathological fractures, marrow fibrosis, brown tumour due to cavities filled with blood, multiple bone cysts, etc. Fracture healing is normal.

Radiology

Radiographic features show generalised rarefaction, trabeculae and cortex are thin, cysts and bending deformities, diffuse osteoporosis of skull, pin head stippling of skull also called salt and pepper appearance, vertebrae are porotic and indented by discs, demineralisation of mandible, disappearance of lamina dura in the tooth.

Laboratory Investigation

Increased calcium levels in the serum, decreased phosphorus levels in the serum, hypercalciuria, hyperphosphaturia and increased alkaline phosphatase are some of the important laboratory findings.

Treatment

Medical treatment consists of providing large doses of calcium, phosphorus and vitamin D. Treatment of choice is parathyroidectomy. For hyperplasia, three glands and a portion of the fourth are removed. Preoperative calcium is avoided.

Orthopaedic management consists of support by splints and corrective osteotomies for bony deformities.

Differential Diagnosis

- Secondary hyperparathyroidism
- Osteomalacia
- Osteoporosis
- Sarcoidosis
- Vitamin D intoxication.

SECONDARY HYPERPARATHYROIDISM

Normal kidneys eliminate phosphorus easily. When kidney is diseased, phosphorus is not excreted. Increased levels of phosphorus in serum results in increased calcium and phosphorus levels in the serum and the excess is deposited in the tissues. This is the pathogenesis in secondary hyperparathyroidism and is seen in certain diseases of the kidney.

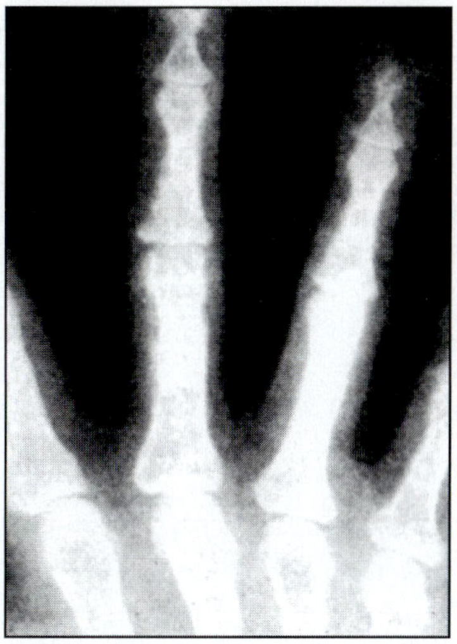

Fig. 37.8: Radiograph showing extensive subperiosteal resorption of bone in hyperparathyroidism

Eventual result is renal rickets in a child and renal osteomalacia in adults. This is high phosphorus rickets compared to normal or low phosphorus rickets in vitamin D deficiency.

OSTEOPOROSIS (Table 37.7)

Definition *It is a generic term referring to a state of decreased mass per unit volume of a normally mineralised bone due to loss of bone proteins.*

Remember

About osteoporosis

It is the most common skeletal disorder in the world, next only to arthritis. In osteoporosis there is a long latent period before clinical symptoms develop. Most prevalent complications are fractures of vertebral bodies, ribs, proximal femur, humerus, distal radius with minimal trauma.

Most common cause is involutional bone loss in perimenopausal age group.

Causes

1. *Disuse*
   - Prolonged bedrest or inactivity
   - Prolonged casting or splinting
   - Paralysis, space travel, etc.
2. *Diet*
   - Calcium, protein, vitamin C low in the diet
   - Chronic alcoholism
   - Anorexia nervosa.

Table 37.7: Showing the types of osteoporosis

Classification		
Epidemiological factor	**Type I (Postmenopausal)**	**Type II Age related**
Age	55-75 years	70 years (Female) 50 years (Male)
Sex (Female : Male)	6:1	2:1
Bone metabolism		
• Pathogenesis	- Osteoclast activity	- Osteoblastic activity
• Net bone loss	Mainly trabecular.	Cortical and trabecular
• Rate of bone loss	Rapid/short duration	Slow/long duration
• Bone density	2 SD below normal	Low or normal
Clinical signs		
Sites	Pain and stress fracture of Vertebra (rush) Distal forearm	Pain and stress fracture of Vertebra (multiple wedge) Proximal hip and tibia.
Other sites	Hip (intracapsular) Tooth loss	Hip (extracapsular) Dorsal kyphosis
Laboratory values		
• Serum calcium	N	N
• Serum phosphorus	N	N
• Alk phosphatase	N	N
• Urine calcium	↑	N
• PTH function	↓	↑
• Renal conversion of 25 $(OH)_2$ D to 1,25 (OH)D	Secondary ↓ due to ↓ PTH	Primary ↓ due to ↓ responsiveness
• GIT Calcium absorption	↓	
Prevention		
• **High Risk patients**	Oestrogen, calcitonin and calcium supplementation; adequate vitamin D is given; Adequate weight bearing activity; minimisation of associated risk factors are recommended.	Calcium supplementation, Adequate vitamin D, Adequate weight bearing activity and Minimisation of risk factors.

3. *Drugs* whose prolonged use causes osteoporosis are heparin, methotrexate, ethanol, glucocorticoids, etc.
4. *Idiopathic* variety is seen in adolescent and middle-aged male population.
5. *Genetic* role is seen in osteogenesis imperfecta.
6. *Chronic illness* like rheumatoid arthritis, cirrhosis, sarcoidosis, renal tubular acidosis, etc.
7. *Neoplasms* like bone marrow tumours (myeloma, lymphoma, leukaemia).
8. *Endocrine abnormalities* Hyperparathyroidism, increased levels of glucocorticoids, oestrogens, etc.

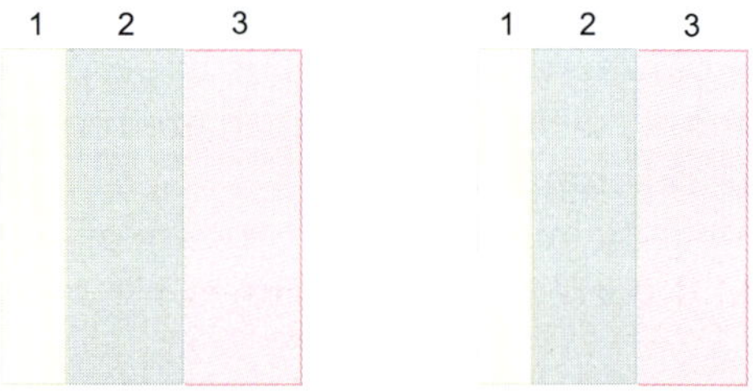

Fig. 37.9: Showing bone density on osteoporosis (1) osteoid, (2) bone, and (3) marrow

Remember

In osteoporosis

- Decreased density is due to deficiency of protein matrix in which calcium is laid down (Figs 37.9 and 37.10)
- Here rate of bone resorption is greater than bone formation
- Most commonly it is due to ageing process
- But the most common cause is involutional bone loss in perimenopausal women

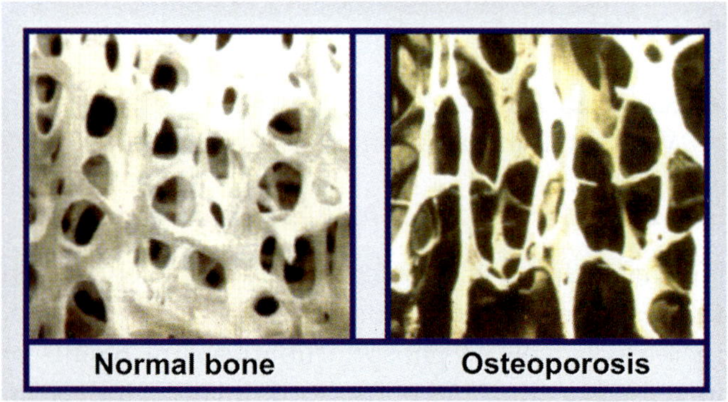

Fig. 37.10: Showing trabecular pattern in osteoporosis

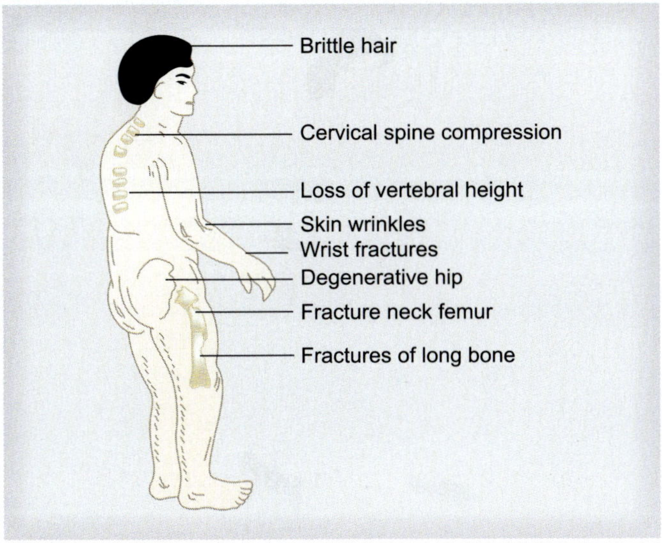

Fig. 37.11: Showing features of osteoporosis

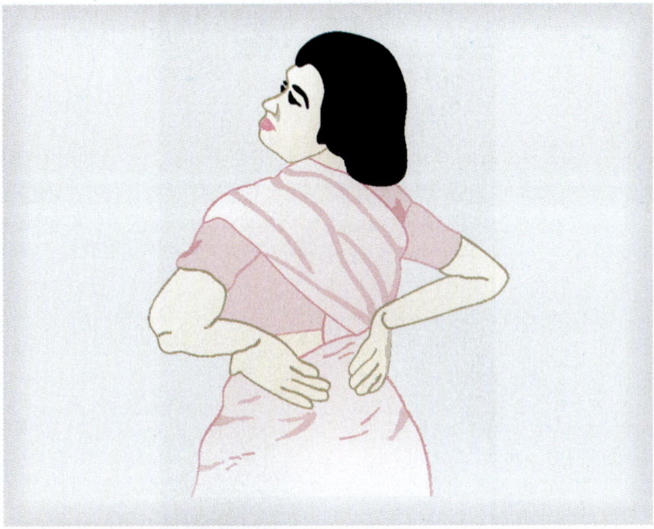

Fig. 37.12A: Backache is the most common presentation in osteoporosis

Clinical Features (Fig. 37.11)

Early symptoms The patient complains of acute pain in middle or low thoracic or high lumbar region (Fig. 37.12A). Sudden movement, sitting, sneezing, cough, etc. increases pain. It is relieved by rest.

Most common symptom of osteoporosis is back pain secondary to vertebral compression. However, in some cases, fractures of axial skeleton may be seen with trivial trauma. Round type of gibbus due to compression of thoracic vertebrae is commonly seen (Fig. 37.12B).

Investigation

1. *Radiology* Changes seen in the spine are:
   a. Loss of vertebral height due to symmetric transverse compression.
   b. Biconcave central compression (codfish spine) due to the pressure of the bulging disc into the bodies.
   c. Anterior wedge compression (Fig. 37.13).

   Other bones
   a. Ground glass appearance due to generalised rarefaction.
   b. *Singh's index* This is the grading of the trabecular pattern of the neck of femur from 1 to 6 (see Fig. 17.12B).
   c. Metacarpal index, etc.
   d. Pathological fractures.

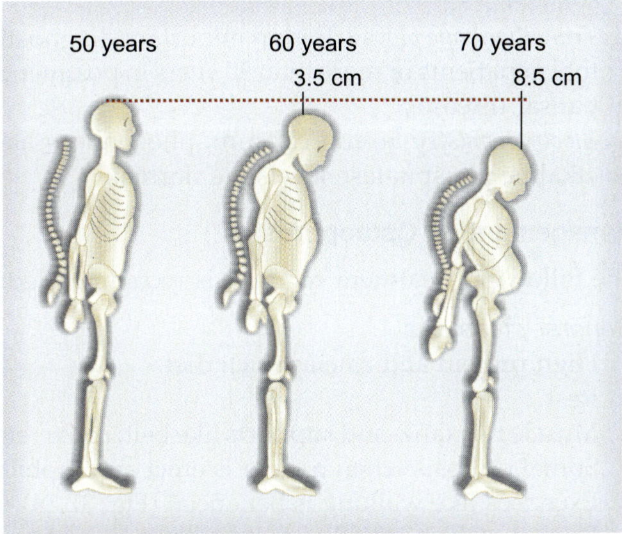

Fig. 37.12B: Showing progressive loss of height due to osteoporosis

2. Techniques for bone mass measurement—densitometry.
   a. Single photon absorptiometry is used to assess the amount of cortical bone mineral in appendicular skeleton.
   b. Mineral status of axial skeleton is assessed by dual photon absorptiometry and quantitative CT scan.
3. Total body neutron activation analysis to determine calcium content of the entire body.

Section 5

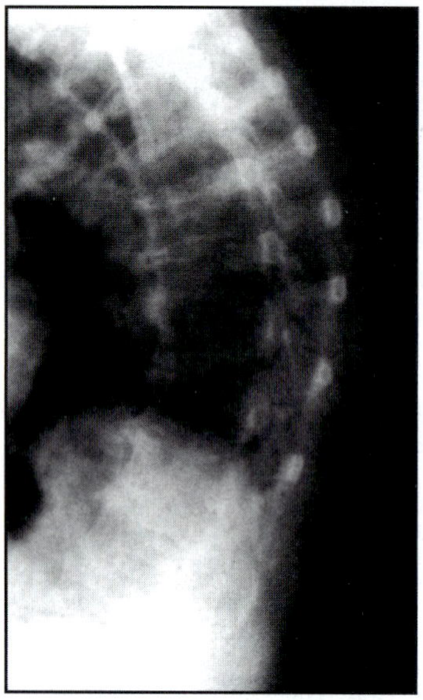

Fig. 37.13: Radiograph showing kyphotic deformity in osteoporosis

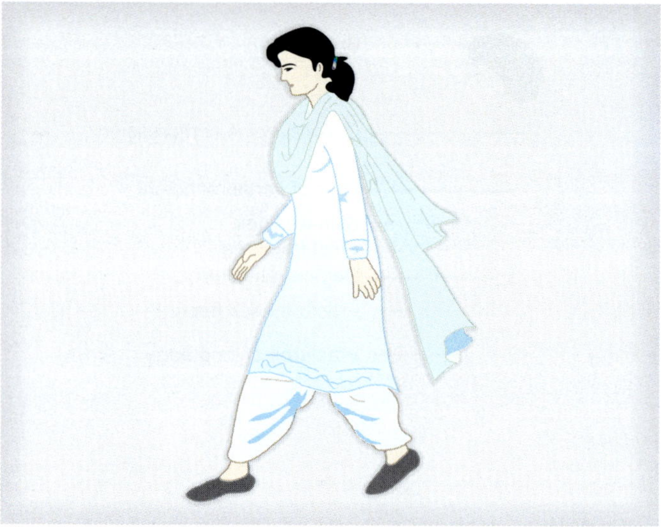

Fig. 37.14: Regular exercises like walking is of great help in elderly patients suffering from osteoporosis

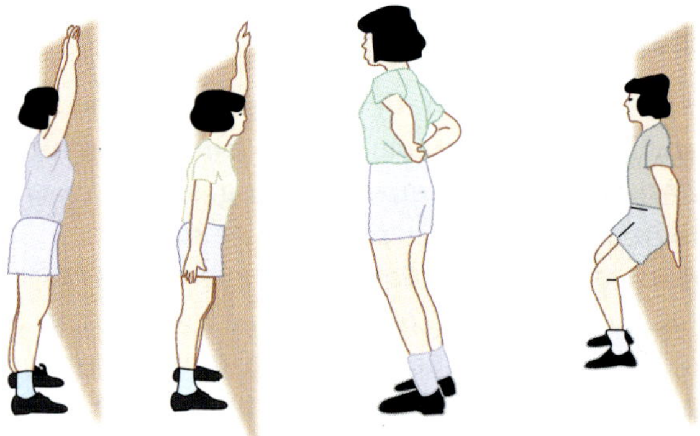

Figs 37.15A to C: Showing various posture correction exercises in osteoporosis patient (A) Wall arching, (B) Back bending, (C) Wall sliding exercises

4. *Transiliac bone biopsy* It is an important diagnostic tool in patients of more than 50 years in postmenopausal diseases.
5. *Blood chemistry* Serum calcium, phosphorus and alkaline phosphatase levels are normal.

Management of Osteoporosis

The following treatment regimen is recommended:

General measures

- High protein and calcium rich diet.
- Rest.
- Muscle relaxants and supports like belt, collar, etc.
- Spinal orthosis when patient is erect and mobile.
- Exercises like walking is beneficial (Fig. 37.14).
- Posture exercise: Wall arch, back bending and wall sliding postural exercises help to improve posture and overcome hunched back (Figs 37.15A to C).

Drug Therapy in Osteoporosis

Drugs form the mainstay of treatment of osteoporosis. The various combinations suggested are as confusing as the disease. However, an effort is made here to provide a simplistic analysis of the drugs commonly used in osteoporosis.

Hormone Replacement Therapy

The role of oestrogen and progestogens in preventing and treating osteoporosis has been well documented. Oestrogens are the most effective treatment for osteoporosis in perimenopausal and early menopausal women. Oestrogens dose is 0.625 mg daily or 0.3 mg if combined with calcium. HRT is known to reduce the rate of fractures by 75 per cent in the oestrogen group. Birth control pills are also known to prevent osteoporosis. The role of progesterone is still not well documented.

Biphosphonates

These drugs inhibit the action of the osteoclast bone cells, which are responsible for removing the bone mass by binding themselves to the inner linings of the bones. The dose of alendronate is 10 mg/day.

Etidronate is another commonly used biphosphonate. Tiludronate, risedronate, and ibandronate are some of the newer drugs.

Calcitonin

Salmon calcitonin has been used for treating osteoporosis. Calcitonin can be given in the form of injections (Dose 50–100 IU/day) or in the form of nasal spray (dose 200 IU). It is used for the treatment of osteoporosis in women who are at least five years postmenopausal and in some cases of men. It is known to slow down bone loss as it is a powerful inhibitor of osteoclastic activity, increase bone density and reduce the risk of fractures. It is also known to reduce the pain.

Alfacalcidol

This is a synthetic analogue of calcitriol, an active metabolite of vitamin D. It changes to calcitriol in the liver. It decreases bone resorption, increases bone mineralization and formation. It also reduces the rate of fractures and improves the bone quality. Recommended dose is 0.5 mcg/day. It is sometimes given along with calcium.

Role of Fluorides in the Treatment of Osteoporosis

Fluorides are known to increase the bone mass. Lower dose of 25 mg slow release fluorides twice daily along with 400 mg of calcium twice daily is recommended. The side effects are gastrointestinal upsets and increased risk of cortical bone fractures.

A Quick recap of the drugs used in osteoporosis:

- Calcium and vitamin D
- HRT
- Biphosphonates
- Calcitonin
- Alfacalcidol
- Fluorides
- SERMS
- Phytoestrogens
- Painkillers
- Anxioilytics and antidepressants

Drug Options in the Treatment of Osteoporosis

Treatment of osteoporosis with the drugs is as confusing as the disease itself. Many drugs are now available in the market with many permutations and combinations. Though the initial choice of the drugs depends on various factors like sex, age, presence or absence of uterus in women, tolerability, etc.; most of the times, it is the treating physician who makes the choice based on his experience. An effort is made here to present the more appropriate of the drug options in the order of preference.

Common Preference

Calcium supplements in the dose of 1000 to 1500 mg/day and vitamin D analogue (0.25 mg BD or vitamin D in the dose of 600–2800 IU/day).

First Preference

Perimenopausal and early postmenopausal (first 5 years) oestrogen replacement therapy (0.625 mg/day).

Second Preference

For the next ten years, SERMS (e.g., Raloxofene). They are known to decrease the oestrogen's dreaded side effects (like causing increased incidence of uterine or breast cancers), while maintaining their beneficial effects (like increasing bone mineral density), decreasing menopausal symptoms, cardioprotective activity, etc. SERMS are known to act by selectively blocking certain oestrogen receptor sites, hence their name.

Third Preference

Alendronate (10 mg/day). This is preferred next due to its proven efficacy in decreasing the hip fractures.

Fourth Preference

Calcitonin 200 IU puff/day intranasal or 100 IU subcutaneously. This is found to be very effective to reduce the pain due to crush fractures of the vertebra.

Fifth Preference

Combination of the above drugs.

However, despite of the several options, the final choice is of the treating physician, weighing all the necessary factors.

Drugs preferences in osteoporosis in order of importance

- In all age groups: Calcium and vitamin D
- Perimenopausal and early menopause: HRT
- Next 10 years: SERMS
- After 65 years preferably: Alendronate
- For severe pain due to vertebral fractures: Calcitonin
- Combination of the above drugs

Note: Choice of the drugs varies according to the treating physicians. This is only a guideline and can be tailor-made to suit the individual patient.

Metabolic disorders at a glance

Rickets	• Organic bone matrix fails to get mineralised. • *Nutritional rickets is the most common variety* • Characteristic rachitic features • Genu valgum is the most common deformity
Osteomalacia	• Adult counterpart of rickets • Here excess osteoid is not mineralised • *Looser's line is the hallmark of this disease*
Renal rickets	• A low-grade rickets • Defect could be in PCT or DCT • Growth is stunted and dwarfism is a feature • *Genu valgum is the most common deformity and manifests late at 11 to 14 years* • Treating underlying renal disease is important
Vitamin D-resistant rickets	• Defined as any rickets requiring more than 1 lakh IU of vitamin D • It is due to failure of phosphate reabsorption from kidney • There is defect in the formation of 1, 25 dihydroxyl vitamin D by kidney • *Tackle deformity is the hallmark*
Hyperparathyroidism	• Excess PTH stimulates action of osteoclasts • Bone resorbed resulting in multiple cavities • Brown tumour is characteristic • *Pin head stippling and absence of lamina dura is the hallmark*
Osteoporosis	• Commonest skeletal disorder in the world next to arthritis • It is age related and postmenopausal • Pathological fractures are very common • *The disease is due to loss of bone proteins*

SCURVY

Definition It is a nutritional disorder caused by deficiency of vitamin C and is characterised clinically by a generalised haemorrhagic tendency.

The severe form of disease is rare and mild varieties are more common. Deficiency targets the cells of skeletal system more often.

Aetiology

- Most frequent between 5 and 10 months in artificially fed infants.
- Vitamin C-deficient diet.
- When seen with rickets, it is called Barton's disease.

Pathology

Cohesive property of the matrix of connective tissue and endothelium is impaired resulting in capillary haemorrhage. Gum bleeding is seen. Within the bone, subperiosteal haemorrhage is characteristic. Haemorrhage within the metaphysis interferes with ingrowth of osteoblastic tissue. Thus ossification is disturbed. This weakens the bone leading to separation of epiphyseo-metaphyseal junction. Bleeding throughout the marrow results in it being replaced by fibrous tissue causing secondary anaemia. *Thus, in scurvy osteogenesis is affected while osteoclasts continue normal function.*

Clinical Features

The affected child is restlesss, pale and febrile. The affected limb is swollen, tender, painful, muscles are in spasm and the child loathes to use the limb. This voluntary immobilisation of the extremities is called *pseudoparalysis*. The gums display a bluish, spongy swelling, especially around the upper central incisor teeth. Brittle and loose teeth, ecchymosis beneath the skin, haematemesis, haematuria, anaemia, weight loss, anorexia, etc. are the other features. Sometimes even death supervenes.

The lower femur, the upper tibia and the upper humerus are favoured sites for epiphyseal fracture separation. Costochondral separation are typical. Mild forms of scurvy are more common. In adults, pain and tenderness over the bone and fracture with mild trauma is suggestive.

Did you know?

The combination of rickets and scurvy is known as Barton's disease.

Investigation

Blood ascorbic acid level is normal and is around 0.5 mg/dl (N = 1 gm/dl). Anaemia is common.

Radiology

- Characteristic lines (see box) are seen.
- Ground glass appearance of the bone.
- Subperiosteal fractures are seen.
- Epiphyseal fracture separation, etc. results.

Differential Diagnosis

1. Rickets
2. Osteomalacia
3. Osteogenesis imperfecta
4. Acute poliomyelitis
5. Septic arthritis, etc.

Treatment

Treatment is essentially conservative and consists of supplementing vitamin C in the diet and also encouraging the child to take foods rich in other vitamins. The painful joints and the fractures needs to be immobilised with plaster splints.

Remember

The radiological lines in scurvy (Fig. 37.16)

- *White line of Frankel*—dense line between epiphysis and metaphysis
- *Scurvy line*—dense line within the metaphysis
- *Winberger's line*—dense line within the epiphysis
- *Pelkan spur*—a bone spur from the lateral border of the metaphyisis

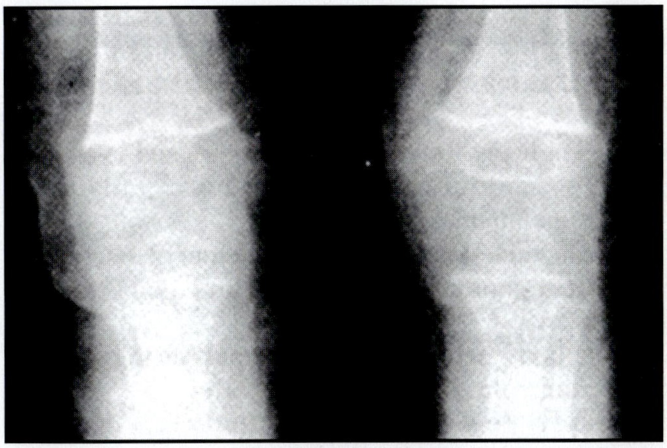

Fig. 37.16: Radiographs showing lines in scurvy: white line of Frankel and Winberger's line

METABOLIC DISORDERS LEADING TO OSTEOSCLEROSIS

Important diseases which cause osteosclerosis are fluorosis, secondaries from prostate, osteopetrosis, Paget's disease, renal osteodystrophy, etc. of these fluorosis is of pubic health importance.

FLUOROSIS

Fluorosis is a pubic health problem in our country in states like Andhra Pradesh, Tamil Nadu, etc. It results when the fluoride content of drinking water exceeds 1 PPM. As a result, excess calcium gets deposited in bone and soft tissues.

Clinical Features

Fluorosis first starts as mottling of the enamel of the upper incisors. Dental fluorosis results in the destruction of the tooth and ultimately its loss.

In the skeletal system, spine is more commonly affected. The posterior longitudinal ligament is thickened and may compress the cord. This may lead to spastic paraparesis.

Investigations

Laboratory tests reveal high fluoride levels in blood and urine. Radiographs show calcification at posterior longitudinal ligament in spine and intraosseous membrane in the leg and forearm. Pelvis, spine and other bones show increased density. Bone biopsy clinches the diagnosis.

Treatment

The patient is encouraged to drink defluorinated water. Preventing the disease by defluorination of drinking water is by far the best measure to tackle this menacing problem.

BIBLIOGRAPHY

1. Cartis JA, Kool SW, Fraser D, Greenbery ML. Nutritional rickets in vegetarian children. Can Med Assoc J 1983;128:150.
2. Doppelt SH. Vitamin D, rickets and osteomalacia. Clin Orthop Clin North Am 1984;15:671.
3. Klein KL, Maxwell MH. Renal osteodystrophy. Orthop Clin North Am 1984;15:687.
4. Lavinger RD. Rickets (grand round series). Pediatrics 66:365, 1980.

38

Osteomyelitis

INTRODUCTION

Osteomyelitis is one of the most difficult and challenging problems encountered in orthopaedics. From the life-threatening acute osteomyelitis to the disabling chronic osteomyelitis (Figs 38.1A and B), it frustrates and thwarts the best efforts of orthopaedic surgeons. The ravaging effects of osteomyelitis on a bone and its neighbouring joints is a tale of dismay and gloom.

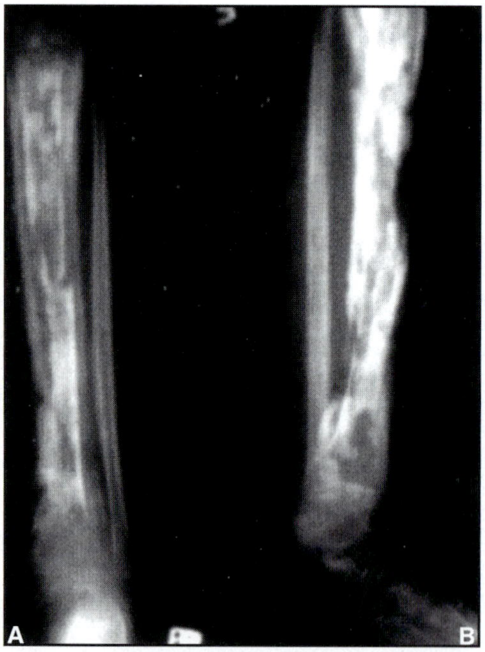

Figs 38.1A and B: Radiographs showing (A) Acute osteomyelitis of femur showing periosteal reaction, and (B) chronic osteomyelitis with diaphyseal sequestrum of tibia

It has been our common clinical experience that the incidence of acute osteomyelitis is definitely on the wane and the incidence of chronic osteomyelitis is on the rise. This is primarily because of the rise in road traffic accidents (RTAs) leaving a bizarre of compound and complex fractures which are the major cause of infection in bone. This is followed next with the rise in infection rate following surgeries on bones and joints. The fall in the incidence of acute osteomyelitis could probably be explained to the frequent and early use of antibiotics in patients presenting with fever. The fall in mortality rate due to acute osteomyelitis is a welcome trend but equally worrying is the high incidence of chronic osteomyelitis which is a disturbing trend. The fall in mortality rate is compensated by the rise in morbidity rates while the ideal thing would be a fall in both the rates.

Definition Osteomyelitis is defined as a suppurative process of the bone caused by pyogenic organisms or simply a pyogenic infection of the cancellous portion of the bone.

Classification

Three types are described based on duration of symptoms, route of spread of infection and host response (Table 38.1).

Table 38.1: Classification of osteomyelitis

Duration	*Route of spread Waldogel's*	*Host response*
1. Acute (<2 weeks)	1. Haematogenous (most common)	1. Pyogenic
2. Subacute (2–3 weeks)		2. Non-pyogenic
3. Chronic (>3 weeks)	2. Direct	
4. Residual	3. Contiguity	

Haematogenous spread with primary infection being elsewhere like tonsillitis, ASOM, pyoderma, etc. is the common mode of spread. Spread from neighbouring infective sites like septic arthritis and direct inoculation of infecting organisms by way of penetrating wounds, punctured wounds, trauma, etc. come second.

ACUTE OSTEOMYELITIS

Aetiology

The aetiological factors causing osteomyelitis can be best understood if discussed under the following heads (Fig. 38.2).

Agent Factors

The following myriad of incriminating organisms are responsible for its causation:

1. *"S" series organisms* ("S" denotes severe osteomyelitis and those organisms causing it start with the letter "S")
   - *Staphylococcus aureus (60–85%)* This is the most common organism causing acute osteomyelitis.
   - *Streptococcus haemolyticus (8–10%)*
   - *Salmonella* osteomyelitis is relatively rare and presents an interesting picture as most of its features start with "S" .
     - —Several bones involved
     - —Symmetrical involvement of bones
     - —Severe osteomyelitis
     - —Spine may be involved
     - —Sickle cell anaemia present
     - —Stool culture may be positive.
2. *P-series organisms* (their mode of entry is through punctured wounds)
   - *Pseudomonas*
   - *Pneumococcus.*

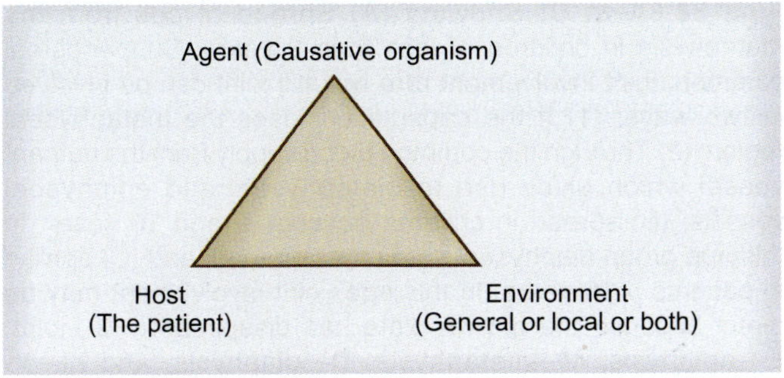

Fig. 38.2: Aetiological factors causing osteomyelitis

3. *C-series* (C denotes compound fractures)
   - *Clostridium welchii*
   - Coliforms *(E.coli).*
4. *B-series*
   - *Brucella bacillus.*
5. *H-series*
   - *Haemophilus influenzae* (7 months to 4 years) This is known to cause osteomyelitis in the age group of 7 months to 4 years.
6. *T-series*
   - *Treponema pallidum* (syphilitic osteomyelitis)
   - Tubercle bacillus (*Mycobacterium*).
7. *Fungal osteomyelitis (ABC)*
   - Actinomycosis
   - Blastomycosis
   - Cryptococcosis and coccidiodomycosis

   These usually cause chronic osteomyelitis.

Host Factors

Age

In children the incidence is 88 per cent (because more prone for injury and to fall).

In adults 12 per cent.

Hence, it is predominantly a disease of childhood.

Sex Male preponderance (? more playful).

Economic status Low socioeconomic groups are more susceptible.

Quick facts

General factors	Local factors
• Anaemia	(Responsible for localisation of infection at metaphysis, especially in children)
• Debility	• Hair pin bend vessels
• Infection	• Metaphyseal haemorrhage
• Poor nutrition	• Defective phagocytosis
• Poor immune status	• Rapid growth at metaphysis
	• Necrotic tissue acts as a culture media
	• Anoxia
	• Vasospasm

Environmental Factors

General factors All the above-mentioned general factors bring down the resistance of the patient thereby making them susceptible for infection.

Local factors are extremely important in localising the infection to the metaphysis.

Hair pin bend of the metaphyseal vessels (Fig. 38.3) This slows down the circulation for a moment which is sufficient for the organisms to escape out.

Metaphyseal haemorrhage results from the bleeding due to microscopic trauma. The blood clot so accumulated acts as an excellent culture media for the escaped organisms to grow.

Defective phagocytosis WBCs here are busy removing the debris of the decalcification due to growth process. So their function of eliminating the offending organism is slightly impaired.

Rapid growth at the metaphysis makes the cells more susceptible to the action of bacterial toxins as the cells are immature.

Vasospasm Though protective as it arrests further bleeding from the traumatised vessels, it also causes anoxia and failure of antibiotics and other defence cells from reaching the area.

Anoxia due to vasospasm, it helps the bacteria grow.

Thus, acute osteomyelitis develops as a result of the combination of agent, host and environment factors.

Pathophysiology

The infection results in the formation of abscess at the region of metaphysis. The pus so formed finds its way out through the *area of least resistance*. In children less than 2 years (Figs 38.4A to C), periosteum is loosely attached to the cortex and hence forms a potentially weak point. The subperiosteal abscess so developed will either spread through the soft tissues and drain to the outside by forming a sinus breaking the skin or it will percolate down towards the diaphysis between the periosteum and the cortex and enter the shaft through the widened haversian pores due to anoxia. Spread to the joint is limited by the growth plate. Between 2 and 16 years, periosteum is firmly attached to the cortex, and with the growth plate still present, the pus has to spread towards the diaphysis at a slow pace. Above 16 years, the growth plate has disappeared, the periosteum is firmly adherent, and the pus spreads towards the diaphysis very slowly (Figs 38.5 and 38.6).

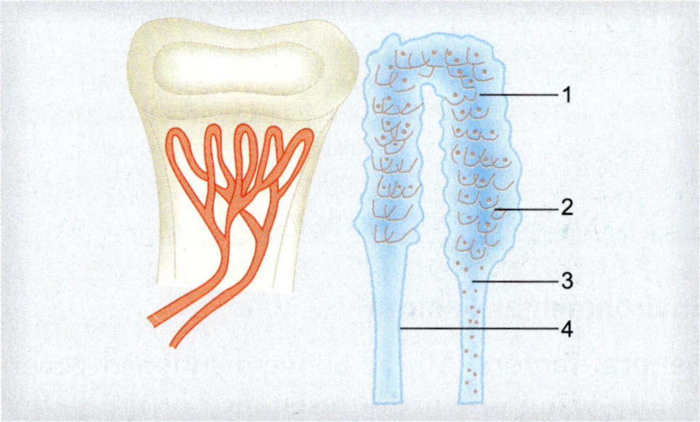

Fig. 38.3: Showing microanatomy of the hair pin bend vessels: (1) thrombosed vessel, (2) bacterial colonies, (3) artery, and (4) vein

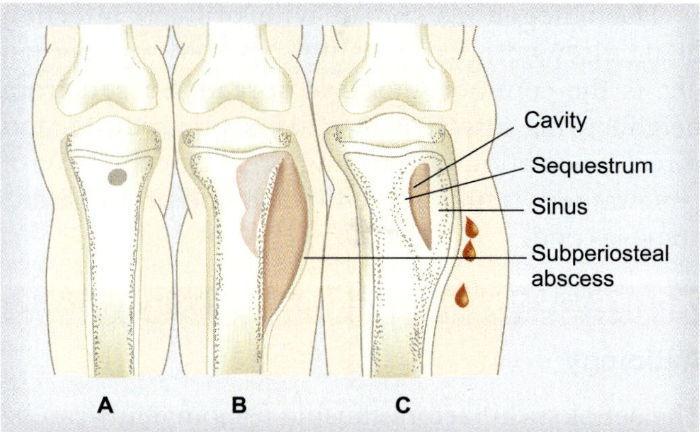

Figs 38.4A to C: Showing pathological events in acute osteomyelitis in < 2 years (A) Beginning of the infection in the metaphysis, (B) Formation of a subperiosteal abscess, (C) Formation of a discharging sinus and sequestrum

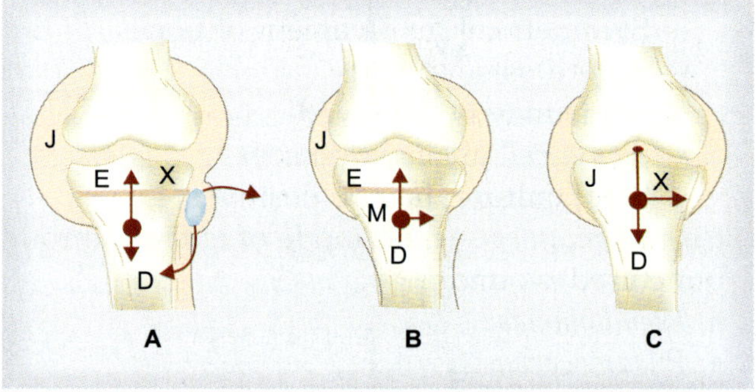

Figs 38.5A to C: Showing (A) Spread of pus from the metaphysis in children of less than 2 years. Subperiosteal common, joint involvement rare but still joint can be involved in two ways: (1) If the capsule encloses the metaphyseal region, (2) Through the common blood supply from the nutrient vessel which gives rise to metaphyseal and epiphyseal vessels; (B) spread in children between 2 and 16 years. In this age group diaphyseal spread is common; and (C) spread in patients > 16 years. In this age, joint involvement may be direct because the growth plate has disappeared (J—joint, E—epiphysis, M—metaphysis, D—diaphysis, and X—no spread)

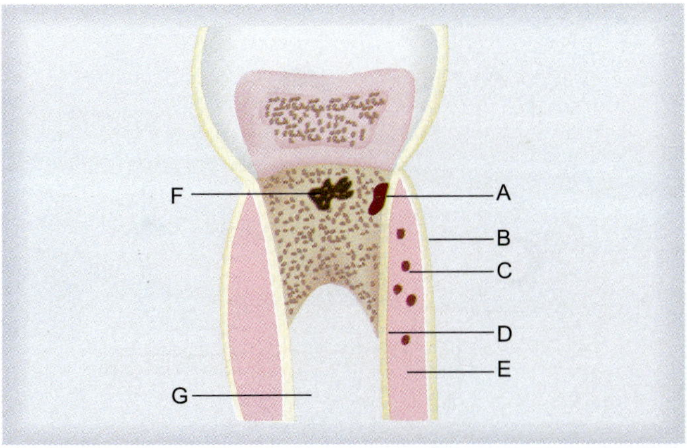

Fig. 38.6: Showing entire spectrum of pathological changes in osteomyelitis: (A) sequestrum, (B) periosteum, (C) pus, (D) cortex, (E) involucrum, (F) bone abscess, and (G) medullary cavity

Quick facts: Spread in acute osteomyelitis

< 2 years	2–16 years	> 16 years
• Subperiosteal (common) • Diaphysis (rare) • Joint space (rare)	• Subperiosteal (rare) • Diaphysis (common but slow)	• Diaphysis (common but very slow) • Joint space involved • Extraperiosteal (rare)

Clinical Features

Acute osteomyelitis is a clinical catastrophe. It presents in the following manner:

Fever This is the most common presenting symptom. The child usually has very high fever and is associated with profuse sweating, chills and rigours. Sometimes the presentation is so acute that the child may be in shock and unconscious.

Swelling This usually follows the fever and may affect the ends of long bones. The swelling may be acutely painful and the skin may appear red.

Limitation of movement The child may not move the joint near the affected bone due to pain and swelling. In fact, the child may lie still without moving the joint and this is sometimes called a state of pseudoparalysis.

Clinical Signs (Table 38.2)

General features of anaemia, dehydration, pyrexia, *pulse rate, shock and toxicity may be present.

Local features The local swelling may show increased temperature, may be tender to touch, and the skin is

Table 38.2: Clinical facts

	General	*Local*
Symptoms	• Fever (95%) • Sweating • Chills and rigours • Patient is usually in shock	• Local swelling (80%) • Limitation of movement (50%)
Signs	• Increased temperature • Increased pulse rate • Anaemia (?) • Signs of dehydration and shock	• Tenderness (80%) • Local erythema (50%) • Raised temperature (50%) • Fluctuation present (20%) • Effusion (10%) • Decreased movements (50%)

stretched. Movements of the neighbouring joints are decreased and there may be effusion in them too.

Investigations

The investigations of acute and chronic osteomyelitis is compared for easy remembrance and understanding (Tabe 38.3). In general, in acute osteomyelitis, laboratory investigations and bone scan are more useful while radiology is of much help in chronic osteomyelitis.

Management

Acute osteomyelitis is an orthopaedic emergency which needs in patient admission. The management can be discussed as general and local.

General management Conservative management is the mainstay of treatment (Fig. 38.7).

The mnemonic *RESTS* sums up the conservative line of treatment:

Rest in bed, protect affected part with splints to alleviate pain and spasm.

Elevation of the part, warm and moist packs to reduce the swelling.

Systemic treatment—blood transfusions, intravenous fluids to correct shock and hypovolaemia.

Treatment—with antibiotics discussed below helps to reduce toxicity.

Surgery—properly indicated and timed to prevent complications.

Table 38.3: Investigations in osteomyelitis

General	*Acute osteomyelitis*	*Chronic osteomyelitis*
Haemoglobin (%) ESR WBCs	Normal or decreased Normal or increased Neutrophils increased	Decreased Increased Lymphocytes are increased
X-rays	**< 48 hours** Few changes • Rarefaction is the earliest sign • Loss of demarcation of line between subcutaneouas shadows and muscles • Appearance of transverse lines of increased densities outward from the muscles **> 2 weeks** Periosteal new bone formation is seen • Rarefaction	• **Sequestrum** identified by the denser X-ray shadow. The density is because of the the impermeability for the X-rays. • **Involucrum** (new bone surrounding the sequestra) • Cloacae (holes through which sequestra is released) • **Irregular bone thickening** • ? Pathological fracture
Bone scan (Technetium 99m, GA-67, Indium-111-labelled leucocytes)	• Confirms diagnosis as early as 24–48 hr after the onset in 90–95% of cases in early stages • Focal area of early uptake • But it cannot distinguish a tumour from infection (non-specific)	• Useful in detecting sequestrum
Blood culture (taken at three different times at least two hours apart)	Positive in 60%	—
Gram's staining (aspirate from infected bones)	Helps choose the appropriate antibiotics	—
Sinograms		• Methylene blue • Radiopaque dyes to identify sinus tract before doing sequestrectomy
Cement beads (see Fig. 38.8)	—	• To identify avascular bone from vascular bone

Note: In acute osteomyelitis bone scan helps in early diagnosis with almost 100% accuracy. X-ray has its limitation. Chronic osteomyelitis can reasonably be diagnosed well on X-rays.

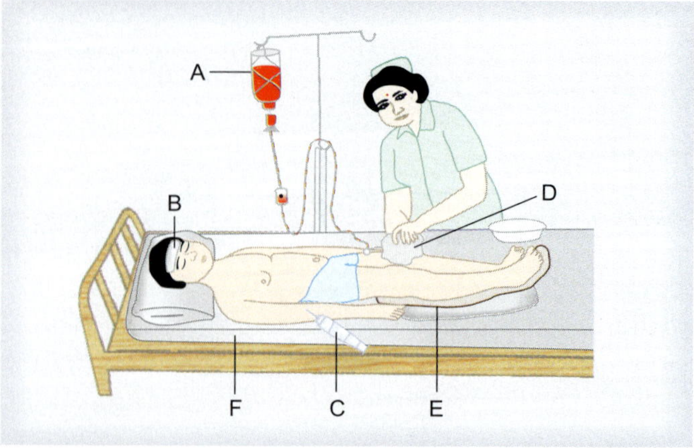

Fig. 38.7: Showing principles of treatment in acute osteomyelitis: (A) IV fluids and blood transfusion, (B) tepid sponging, (C) intravenous antibiotics, (D) cryotherapy, (E) splints and elevation of the affected part, (F) rest in bed and hospitalisation

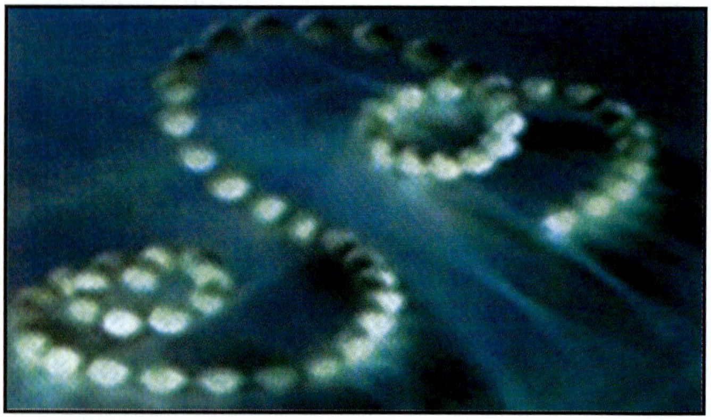

Fig. 38.8: Cement beads in chronic osteomyelitis

Principles of antibiotic therapy This is the mainstay of treatment in acute osteomyelitis. Lack of understanding of the correct principles of antibiotic therapy in acute osteomyelitis leaves a sequela in the form of chronic osteomyelitis. This underlines the importance of correct antibiotic therapy (all **A's**).

Appropriate drug—usually the drug chosen is a broad-spectrum bactericidal agent.

Appropriate route—intravenous for the first 2 weeks and oral for the next 4 weeks.

Appropriate dose—of the drug depending on the body weight of the patient.

Appropriate time to stop—when the disease is eradicated, controlled or resistance or side effects to the drugs develops.

Appropriate adjunctive measures—a combination of ampicillin and cloxacillin are found to be very effective though penicillin G is still the drug of first choice in our country. Fusidic acid is preferred in the Western countries.

Current trends in antibiotic therapy This consists of a short course of intravenous antibiotics for a period of 2 weeks, followed by oral antibiotics for further 4 weeks. Proper monitoring of the serum antibiotic level is very much essential to obtain good results.

Nade's principles for acute osteomyelitis aptly sums up the action of antibiotic therapy

1. An appropriate antibiotic is effective before pus forms.
2. Antibiotic cannot sterilise avascular tissue.
3. Antibiotic prevents reformation of pus once removed.
4. Pus removal restores continuity between periosteum and cortex which restores blood flow.
5. Antibiotics should be continued after surgery.

Local management The focus here is on well-timed surgery if any one of the following indications are present.

Nade's indications for surgery

- Abscess formation.
- Severely ill and moribund child.
- Failure to respond to intravenous antibiotics for more than 48 hours.

Antibiotics therapy in osteomyelitis

- Penicillins
- B-lactamase inhibitors
- Cephalosporins
- Ciprofloxacin
  — Parenteral IV antibiotics for 4–6 weeks.
  — Oral antibiotics for 2–4 weeks.

Local antibiotics: Antibiotics impregnated with cement beads provide high dose of antibiotics locally.

Surgical Methods

Depending upon the situation any one of the following surgical methods could be employed:

1. *Aspiration* It helps in decompresssion and the material so obtained may be used to identify the organism and also check for antibiotic sensitivity.
2. *Incision and drainage* helps to drain the subcutaneous abscess.
3. *Multiple drill holes* If the abscess is subperiosteal, this technique helps to drain the pus by making multiple holes in the cortex.
4. *Small bone window* If the multiple drill holes do not drain the pus, a small window of bone is removed from the cortex and the pus is evacuated.

Differential Diagnosis

Acute septic arthritis Here the infection is in the joint, in osteomyelitis it is in the bone near the joint. Hence, joint movements are severely restricted and more painful in acute septic arthritis.

Scurvy Features of pseudoparalysis, bleeding gums, tender limbs, etc. are the features.

Acute anterior poliomyelitis Here pain and tenderness are spread throughout the muscle mass, whereas in osteomyelitis tenderness is greatest on direct pressure over the bone.

Cellulitis It is difficult to differentiate from acute osteomyelitis, however, cellulitis has no edge, no fluctuation, no pus and no limits.

Other Differential Diagnosis

Erysipelas, erythema nodosum, Ewing's sarcoma, sickle cell anaemia, etc.

Complications (seen in 5% of the cases)

1. Septicaemia and pyaemia are the common general complications.
2. Septic arthritis due to extension of the neighbouring foci of infection into the joint.
3. Chronic osteomyelitis develops due to improper and inadequate treatment. The incidence rate is 5 to 10 per cent.
4. Pathological fractures and growth disturbances are relatively rare.
5. Recurrence rate in acute osteomyelitis:
   - Metatarsals more than 50 per cent.
   - Around the knee more than 25 per cent.
   - Due to late diagnosis more than 25 per cent.
6. Mortality rate is less than 2 per cent due to early antibiotic therapy.

Prognosis

The following are the bad prognostic factors:

- *Age* if children.
- *Agent* if *Staph. aureus.*
- *Site* if nearer to trunk.

Course

- Ninety per cent resolve due to early diagnosis and effective antibiotic therapy.
- Eight per cent show morbidity.
- Two per cent have mortality.

Characteristic points in acute osteomyelitis

- Disease is common in children.
- *Staphylococcus aureus* is the common organism.
- Metaphysis is involved.
- Fever is the common presenting symptom.
- Bone scan helps in early diagnosis.
- Conservative management is the mainstay of treatment. and ninety per cent resolve.

Note: Acute osteomyelitis in epiphysis is taken to be caused by *Staphylococcus aureus* unless proved otherwise.

SUBACUTE OSTEOMYELITIS

Subacute osteomyelitis is caused by *Staphylococcus aureus*. The patient complains of pain without constitutional symptoms. Temperature may be increased or normal. It is not detected until at least two weeks has elapsed. Blood culture is positive in only 60 per cent of the cases, and WBC and ESR are raised in only 50 per cent of the cases.

Subacute osteomyelitis is due to:

- Increased host resistance.
- Lowered bacterial resistance.
- If antibiotics are administerd before symptoms appear.

CHRONIC OSTEOMYELITIS

Any osteomyelitis lasting for more than three weeks is termed as chronic. Chronic osteomyelitis can arise from any one of the following ways:

- Sequelae of acute osteomyelitis (5–10%)
- Following compound fractures
- Following surgery on bones and joints
- Chronic from the beginning (e.g. tuberculosis, syphilis, Brodie's abscess)
- Anaerobic organisms (sclerosing osteomyelitis of Garre)
- Fungal osteomyelitis.

Quick facts

Salient features in chronic osteomyelitis

- Systemic symptoms would have disappeared.
- One or more foci in the bone containing pus, sequestra or draining sinuses, etc.
- Acute exacerbation is due to trauma, lowered resistance, etc.

Clinical Features

Symptoms are very few. Fever, pain, swelling are seen in acute exacerbation of chronic osteomyelitis.

Signs (Fig. 38.9)

Irregular thickening of bone develops due to unequal pace of destruction of bone and new bone formation. This is a characteristic feature of chronic osteomyelitis.

Sinuses are usually multiple and are fixed to the underlying bone. The presence of sinuses indicates unabsorbed sequestra, unobliterated cavities and presence of anaerobic organisms. They are immobile and adherent to the bone.

Note: History of discharge of tiny bony spicules through the sinus, clinches the diagnosis of chronic osteomyelitis with certainty.

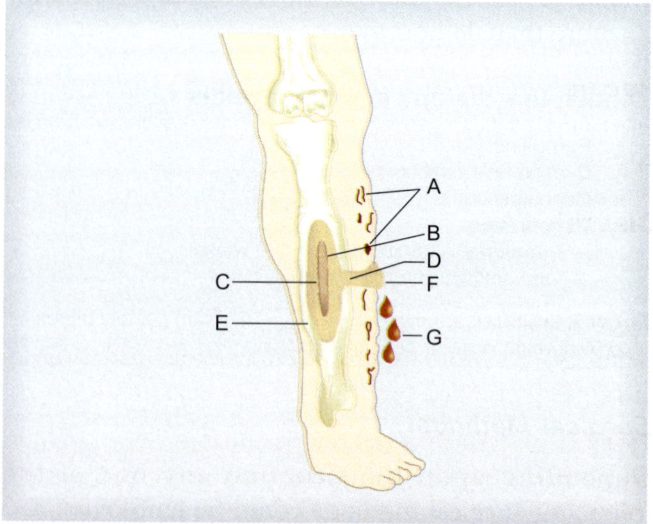

Fig. 38.9: Showing features in chronic osteomyelitis: (A) multiple scars and sinuses, (B) sequestrum, (C) cavity, (D) sinus tract, (E) irregular thickening of bone, (F) sprouting granulation tissue, (G) discharge of bony spicules and pus

Scars and muscle contractures develop due to the spread of infection from the bones to the muscles and the consequent fibrosis.

Shortening or lengthening of the bones may occur due to the affection or stimulation of the growing epiphysis respectively.

Deformities and decreased movements develop due to scars and contractures.

Pathological fractures may occur either due to chronic osteomyelitis which weakens the bone or due to extensive debridement during surgery which leaves a thin layer of bone.

Note: Sequestra It is a dead bone within a living bone and is defined as an infected granulation tissue. The inflammatory foci is surrounded by sclerotic bone supplied with blood and covered by periosteum, scarred muscle and subcutaneous tissues.

Quick facts: Sequestra

Disease	Type of sequestra
TB Osteomyelitis	→ Sandy/feathery
Actinomycosis	→ Black
Pin tract infection	→ Ring
Chronic osteomyelitis in children	→ Diaphyseal

Investigations

Sequestra can be identified by X-ray, tomography, sinogram, CT scan, gallium-67 and indium-111-labelled leucocyte scan, etc. X-ray changes have been enumerated in Table 38.3.

Classification

As suggested by Cierney and Mader (Fig. 38.10):

Type I *Medullary osteomyelitis* This is due to haematogenically infected compound fracture or infected intramedullary nails.

Type II *Surface osteomyelitis* Limited to the surface of the bone exposed due to inadequate soft tissue coverage.

Type III *Localised with full thickness cortical* separation, and is usually common in infected non-union.

Type IV *Diffuse* Entire bone is involved.

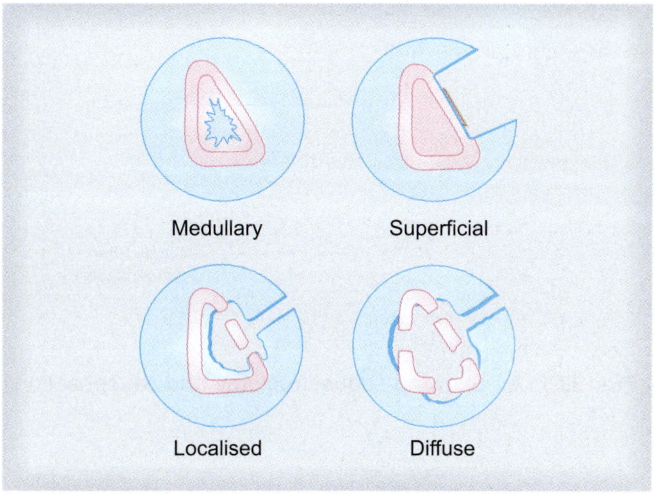

Fig. 38.10: Showing Cierney and Mader's classification

Management of Chronic Osteomyelitis

Goal Eradication of the infection by achieving a viable and vascular environment. This can be done by radical debridement by way of sequestrectomy and resection of scarred and infected bone and soft tissue. Appropriate antibiotic is also required. Finally, reconstruction of both the bone and soft tissue defects may be needed.

Principles of treatment As is evident from the goal, surgery is the treatment of choice.

1. *Surgery* is to be undertaken only when fever and infection has subsided, living bone can be distinguished from the dead bone and when involucrum appears sufficient to maintain length and contour of the bone after excision of any large sequestra.
2. Secondary infection is almost always present. When surgery is indicated, culture is done and antibiotics started at least four days before surgery and is continued for two weeks.
3. When acute exacerbation fails to respond to conservative treatment, incision and drainage have to be done.

Surgery Methods

Sequestrectomy and saucerisation (Figs 38.11A and B) Sequestrum is identified on the X-ray as it is more dense and lies free in the cavity. It takes 2 to 3 months before it is isolated, separated and easily seen on the X-ray and only then sequestrectomy is

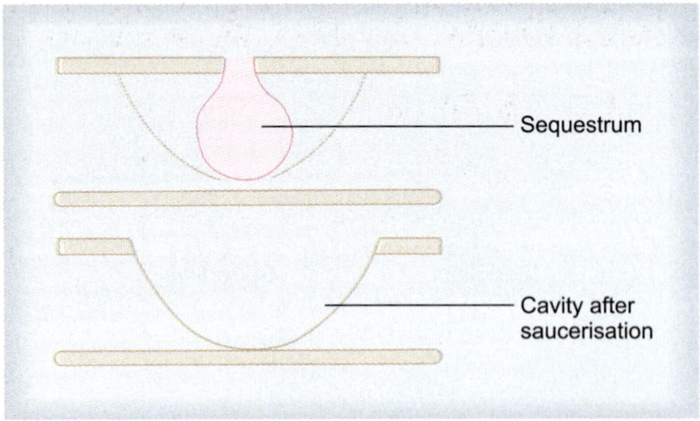

Fig. 38.11A: Showing sequestrectomy and saucerisation

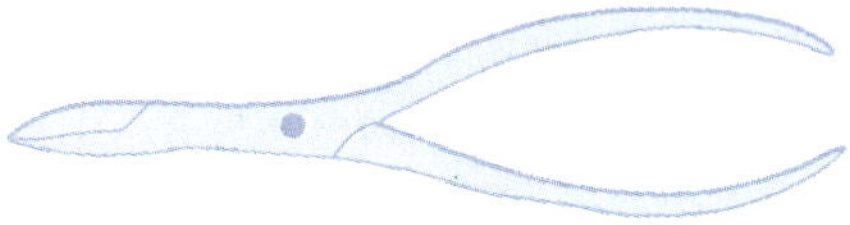

Fig. 38.11B: Showing sequestrum forceps (19 cm) straight/angular

planned. All the sinus tracts are injected with methylene blue 24 hours before surgery. By making multiple drill holes, the cortex is removed in a rectangular fashion. Sequestrectomy is done next. The cavity is curetted till fresh bleeding occurs and the deep shape of the cavity is converted into a shallow cavity.

Note: Sequestrectomy usually leaves a deep cavity beneath which is potentially a dead space favouring collection of pus and other debris. To prevent this from happening, the deep cavity is made shallow for effective drainage of the collected materials.

After sequestrectomy, there is a huge gap in the bone and there are four basic methods of immediate biological management of dead space so left:

1. Local closure if the space left is very small.
2. Myoplasty for slightly larger space, surrounding muscles can be packed into the cavity.
3. Cancellous bone grafts for a space less than 2.5 cm.
4. Free vascularised bone graft for larger areas.

Other Methods of Treatment

1. Papineau et al described an open grafting technique for chronic osteomyelitis. The operation is divided into three stages:
   Stage I Radical excision of all the infected tisssue.
   Stage II Cancellous autogenous bone grafting.
   Stage III Wound coverage by skin grafting and other techniques.
2. Hyperbaric oxygen therapy.
3. Closed suction drainage (Fig. 38.12): After sequestrectomy, the wound is closed over a suction drain. Through an inlet tube, an irrigation fluid consisting of saline, antibiotics and detergent is pushed into the medullary cavity and drained out through an outlet tube to which a slow suction is applied. This enables the wound to be continuously bathed in this antibiotic solution.
4. Amputation is done rarely in the following circumstances: If the patient's life is endangerd by infection or in extensive infection. Lots of circumspection should be used while deciding upon amputation for chronic osteomyelitis. It should be the last choice and not the first. I would like to recall about a patient who had a very bad chronic osteomyelitis following compound fracture of both bones of left leg and was treated with debridement and internal fixation with a medullary nail which also got infected and compounded his problems. He was suggested to undergo a below-knee amputation as he had a very wide open sinus draining pus for over 3 years. He approached me with a plea to save his limb. Implant was removed, radical debridement was done, a myocutaneous flap was fashioned to close the wound and the patient was treated with appropriate antibiotics. The results were excellent. Hence, I feel, not to give room for desperation in bad cases of chronic osteomyelitis, but still try to

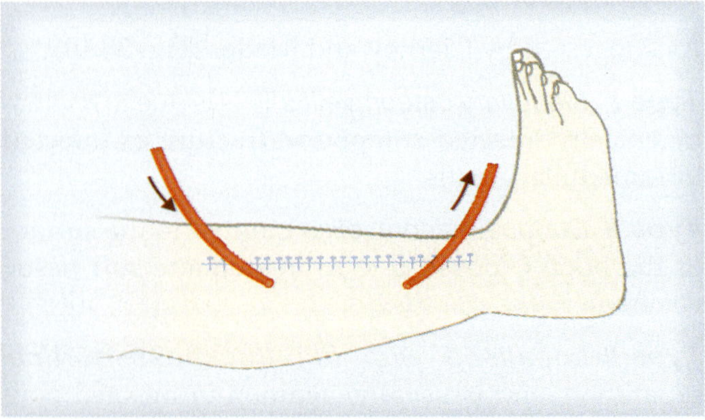

Fig. 38.12: Closed continuous suction irrigation system for chronic osteomyelitis

manage it by conventional methods which is often successful.

5. Ilizarov's method: It has been found to be a very effective method of managing chronic osteomyelitis of late. Though technically very demanding, if planned and executed properly, it gives very good results in bad cases of chronic osteomyelitis.
6. Excision of bones can be done, if smaller bones are involved like phalanges, carpal bones, etc.

Complications

1. *Most common complications* Pathological fracture is by far the most common complication. The incidence is 5 to 10 per cent. It requires Papineau treatment comprising thorough debridement, grafting and stabilisation of fracture fragments by external fixators.
2. *Common complications*
   a. *Acute exacerbation* of existing chronic disease initiated by a change in bacterial flora or by decrease in the general resistance of the patient which flares up the dormant infection.
   b. *Growth disturbances* Usually, the growth is not affected (64%); more commonly, shortening may be seen (64%) due to the arrest of the growth plate by the neighbouring infection and very rarely there may be stimulation of the growth plate resulting in lengthening (5%) of bones.
   c. *Deformities* develop due to soft tissue, muscle and joint contractures and also due to growth plate disturbances.
3. *Rare complications*
   a. *Amyloidosis* due to long-standing infection.
   b. *Epithelioma* of the sinus tract due to chronic discharging sinus which induces metaplasia and formation of squamous cell carcinoma (incidence < 1%).

Residual Osteomyelitis

In residual osteomyelitis there is complete absence of signs and symptoms. There are no draining sinuses. There is soft tissue scarring, skin is fixed to the bone and the underlying bone is sclerotic.

OSTEOMYELITIS OF SPECIAL IMPORTANCE

[1]BRODIE'S ABSCESS

Brodie's abscess is a localised form of chronic osteomyelitis, involves metaphyseal and epiphyseal area, and is common in young adults. The patient complains of intermittent pain of long duration and local tenderness. Causative organism is low virulence *Staph. aureus* in 50 per cent of the cases.

Investigation

Radiograph shows varied appearance. Usually, a cavity is seen at the metaphysioepiphyseal junction. Frequently requires biopsy for diagnosis.

Treatment

Treatment consists of appropriate antibiotics, curettage and bone grafting, and the wound is loosely closed over a drain.

SCLEROTIC OSTEOMYELITIS OF GARRE

- It is a chronic or subacute form of osteomyelitis.
- It usually affects the subperiosteal region of the bone.
- Bone is thickened.
- Affects children and young adults.
- The cause is unknown, but it could be due to low-grade anaerobic infection.
- A secondary infection may occur at a distant site. This is a chronic or subacute form of chronic osteomyelitis. It is common in children and young adults. It usually affects the superiosteal region and the bone is thickened. Though the exact cause is not known, it could be due to low-grade anaerobic infection. A secondary infection may occur at a distant site.

Clinical Features

The patient may complain of intermittent pain, swelling, tenderness and low-grade fever, etc.

Investigations

Radiographs show expanded bone with generalised sclerosis.

[1]**Sir Benjamin Brodie** (1783-1862), London

ESR is usually raised.

Biopsy is definitive and confirmatory.

Treatment

Treatment consists of fenestration of sclerotic bone and appropriate antibiotics should be given.

TUBERCULAR OSTEOMYELITIS

Treatment discussed in Chapter on Tuberculosis of Bones and Joints.

BIBLIOGRAPHY

1. Blockey NJ, Watson JT. Acute osteomyelitis in children. J Bone Joint Surg 1970;52-B:77.
2. Cole WG, Dalziel RE, Leitl S. Treatment of acute osteomyelitis in childhood. J Bone Joint Surg 1982;64-B:218.
3. Jackson MA, Nelson JD. Etiology and medical management of acute suppurative bone and joint infections in pediatric patients. J Pediatr Orthop 1982;2:313.
4. Learmonth ID, Dall G, Pallock DJ. Acute osteomyelitis and septic arthritis in children: a simple approach to treatment. S Afr Med J 1984;65:117.
5. Orr HW. The treatment of acute osteomyelitis by drainage and rest. J Bone Joint Surg 1927;9:733.
6. Trueta J. Acute haematogenous osteomyelitis: its pathology and treatment. Bull Hosp Joint Dis 1993;145.

39

Skeletal Tuberculosis

INTRODUCTION

Though ubiquitous in distribution, tuberculosis has firmly entrenched itself with the Third World, thanks to the illiteracy, poverty, poor hygienic conditions and a host of other favourable factors. India is infamous for hosting nearly one-fifth of the thirty million people suffering from tuberculosis throughout the world. Though largely preventable, tuberculosis can be successfully combated by an effective chemotherapy. The bugbears of treatment being its long duration, poor patient compliance, emergence of drug resistance and others. Skeletal tuberculosis mercifully is not as common as pulmonary tuberculosis and accounts for only 1 to 3 per cent of the cases.

Tuberculosis, being mainly the disease of Third World, it is no wonder that India has produced pioneers like Dr Tuli, Dr Kumar, Dr Shanmugasundaram and others whose work on skeletal tuberculosis has been acknowledged worldwide.

HISTORY

- Hippocrates (460–370 BC) was the first to suggest the relationship between pulmonary disease and spinal deformity.
- Percival Pott (1714–1788) described the "gibbus" deformity and its sequelae. He did not describe the disease or its tuberculous nature.
- Laennec (1781–1826) described the basic microscopic lesion, ***the tubercle.***
- Drugs Streptomycin was first used in 1947, PAS in 1949 and INH in 1952.

Note: TB is one of the oldest diseases afflicting mankind. It has been found in Egyptian mummies dating back to 3400 BC.

Skeletal tuberculosis is always *secondary*, the primary foci being either in the lungs, lymph nodes or gastrointestinal tract. The incidence of bone and joint tuberculosis is 2 to 3 per cent. Fifty per cent of these cases are found in the vertebral column. The other major areas affected in order of predilection are hip, knee, foot, elbow, hand, shoulder, and others.

Skeletal tuberculosis occurs mostly in the first three decades of life but no age is immune.

Aetiology

1. *TB bacillus*
   a. Human (more common) *Mycobacterium tuberculosis*.
   b. Bovine (rare) *M. bovine.*
2. *Route* Always secondary, may spread to the bone through:
   a. Blood, e.g. through Batson's plexus in tuberculosis of spine
   b. Lymphatic spread
   c. Direct.
3. *Precipitating factors*
   a. General factors like anaemia, debility, etc. help precipitate the infection.
   b. Local factors like trauma, etc. localise the problem to the bone.
4. *Local trauma* causes vascular stasis and intraosseus haemorrhage.

How does osteoarticular tubercular lesion develop?

Primary focus
May be active or quiescent (lungs, tonsils, mediastinum, mesentery, etc.)
↓
Bacillaemia
↓
Through the arteries and veins (e.g. Batson's plexus in the spine)
↓
Reach the skeletal system
↓
Tubercle develops

Vital facts:

Did you know?
A minimum gap of 2 to 3 years is required between the primary and skeletal TB.

Pathology

Following injury, the vessels rupture and there is haemorrhage. The tubercle bacilli present in the circulation settle and proliferate in the blood clot so formed. A tubercle follicle is formed and it consists of lymphocytes, giant cells and endothelial cells. Small such tubercle follicles coalesce to form a larger follicle which undergoes caseation at the centre and fibrosis at the periphery. The caseation at the centre of the shaft breaks down forming pus. It spreads towards the subperiosteal region, breaks the periosteum and tracks along the lines of least resistance. It reaches the skin and forms the cold abscess (not warm). Later on, it breaches the skin forming the sinus.

Changes in the marrow In the early stages there is increase in the polymorphs. In the later stages it is replaced by lymphocytes. The marrow is slowly surrounded by fat cells and is replaced by fibrous tissue.

Lamellae There may be osteoporosis due to the action of osteoclasts or due to metaplasia. Osteosclerosis may also be seen.

Periosteum Increased vascularity in the periosteum leads to new bone formation and the consequent subperiosteal thickening.

Clinical Features

Clinical features are best summed up by the diagnostic triad (Fig. 39.1)

Monoarticular The patient usually complains of pain in one joint which is dull aching and chronic in nature. He or she may give history of night cries which is due to the rubbing of inflamed articular surfaces against each other due to the release of muscular spasm at rest. The joint movements are decreased in all directions, initially due to muscle spasm and later due to arthritis. *The wasting of the limb muscles is gross and is out of proportion.* Regional lymph nodes may be enlarged.

Constitutional symptoms This is present in approximately 20 per cent of the cases. It consists of low-grade fever, lassitude in the afternoon, loss of appetite and weight, night sweats, anaemia, tachycardia and evening rise of temperature.

Investigations

General investigations These consists of haemoglobin estimation, total and differential count, raised ESR, urine routine tests, etc.

Other investigations

1. *Positive evidence of the disease*
   a. Identification of organism on culture from the joint, histology, etc.
   b. Reproduction of disease by inoculating guinea pigs.
2. *ZN stain* for acid-fast bacilli in aspirate or excised tissue.
3. *Guinea pig test*
4. *Mantoux test* is significant only in the first 3 to 4 years of life, adults are usually positive. Negative test does not rule out tuberculosis.

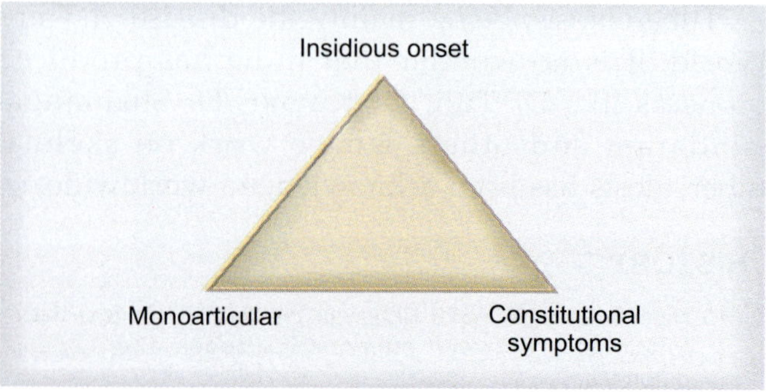

Fig. 39.1: Showing diagnostic triad of skeletal tuberculosis

5. *X-ray*
   - No typical finding for tuberculosis.
   - Earliest sign is decalcification of bones (rarefaction).
   - Late signs are joint destruction.
6. *Biopsy* of regional lymph nodes may show "tubercles".
7. *Exploratory arthrotomy* is the certain way of ascertaining diagnosis. The tissue may be cultured or may be injected into a guinea pig.

Principles of Treatment

1. *General treatment* This includes rich protein diet, haematinics, adequate exposure to sunshine, etc. The general treatment aims at building up the general resistance of the patient.
2. *Chemotherapy* is the mainstay of treatment and is discussed in detail below.
3. *Local treatment* aims to prevent, correct, or decrease the defomities. If the disease is osseous, aim at ankylosis in functional position by immobilisation. If the disease is synovial, aim at mobility by traction.
4. *Operative treatment* consists of partial capsulectomy, synovectomy, osteotomy, curettage, arthrodesis, etc. depending on the stage of tuberculosis.
5. *Treatment of tubercular abscess* Conservative treatment is recommended in most of the cases. Aspiration is done if the abscess is tense.

Chemotherapy (Table 39.1)

Drugs used for the treatment of tuberculosis are grouped as follows.

First line of drugs These have the greatest level of efficiency and have an acceptable degree of toxicity.

The following are the first line of drugs used in tuberculosis (mnemonic **PRISE**).

P—Pyrazinamide
R—Rifampicin
I—INH
S—Streptomycin
E—Ethambutol.

Second line of drugs These are useful if the patient develops resistance to the first line of drugs (mnemonic **CAKECA**).

C—Capriomycin
A—Amikacin
K—Kanamycin
E—Ethionamide
C—Cycloserine
A—Aminosalicylic acid (PAS).

The second line of drugs are used only for treatment of the diseases caused by resistant microorganisms or by non-TB mycobacteriae. All drugs are given parenterally and are potentially ototoxic and nephrotoxic. Hence, no two drugs from this group should be used simultaneously. These are not used with streptomycin for the same reasons.

Chemotherapy regimes

1. *Nine-month regime* Nine months of rifampicin and INH are effective for all forms of disease.
2. *Six-month regime*

   First two months, INH + Rifampicin + Pyrazinamide

   Next four months, INH + Rifampicin

   When the primary resistance to INH is high, therapy is usually initiated with four first line drugs.
3. *Third regime* Here three to four drugs are used in the first 4 months, two to three drugs in the second 4 months, one or two drugs in the third 4 months and one drug (i.e. INH) in the last three to four months of treatment.

Current Trends of Chemotherapy in Musculoskeletal TB

- INH is the most potent anti-TB drug currently available
- 4-Drug therapy is the recommended regime and consists of Rifampicin, INH, Pyrazinamide and Ethambutol. After 3 months, Ethambutol is withdrawn and three-drug regime is further continued for nine months. Later, only Rifampicin and INH are continued for a further six months. The total duration is thus 18 months.
- 10 mg Pyridoxine is given simultaneously to prevent peripheral neuropathy due to INH.

Know Tuli's 16-month chemotherapy regime:

- Rifampicin, INH, and Ethambutol for first 4 months
- Pyrazinamide replaces Rifampicin in the second 4 months
- In the next four months, Rifampicin is given with INH
- In the last four months, INH is the only drug.

Table 39.1: Chemotherapeutic drugs in skeletal tuberculosis

	Drugs	Antibacterial activity	Mechanism	Absorption	Chemistry	Dose	Untoward effects
1.	INH (primary drug for chemotherapy of tuberculosis)	Bacteriostatic for resting bacilli	Inhibits biosynthesis of mycolic acid, a constituent of the cell walls	Gets rapidly absorbed, diffuses into all body fluids and cells, penetrates the caseous material	Hydroxide of Isonicotinic acids	• Adults 5 mg/kg body wt • Children 10–20 mg/kg body wt	• Rash 2% • Fever 1.2% • Jaundice 0.6% • Peripheral neuritis 0.2%
2.	R-cin (Rifampicin)	Inhibits most of gram +ve, gram -ve, and myco TB, bactericidal	Inhibits RNA synthesis	Peak action in 2–4 hr	Semisynthetic derivative of Rifampicin	10 mg/kg	• Hepatitis • Orange colour to urine, etc. Well tolerated
3.	Ethambutol	Bacteriostatic, suppresses growth of most INH and SM-resistant TB bacilli	Inhibits incorporation of mycolic acids	Absorbed well from GIT		15 mg/kg (not used in children < 5 yr)	• Optic neuritis • Urate conc. increase in blood
4.	Streptomycin	It usually suppresses growth of most INH-resistant TB bacilli	Acts only on extracellular microbes			20–35 mg/kg	• 8.2% incidence, Involves auditory and vestibular actions of 8th cranial nerve
5.	Pyrazinamide			Well absorbed	Synthetic analogue of Nicotinamide	20–35 mg/kg	Injury to liver hepatitis
6.	Ethionamide	Suppressor	Inhibits acetylation of INH	Rapid and well absorbed		250 mg/BD 15–20 mg/kg	Metallic taste hepatitis
7.	PAS	Suppressor	Inhibits PABA	Readily absorbed	Structural analogue of PABA	Daily dose of 14–16 gm	Epigastric pain Nausea, anorexia
8.	Cycloserine			Rapidly absorbed		15–20 mg/kg	CNS toxicity
9.	Kanamycin				Aminoglycoside	1 gm/day	Ototoxic/ nephrotoxic
10.	Capreomycin					15–30 mg/kg	
11.	Amikacin						

GENERAL PRINCIPLES OF CHEMOTHERAPY IN TUBERCULOSIS

- Most patients are now treated in ambulatory setting.
- Prolonged bedrest is not necessary.
- The patient is seen at frequent intervals.
- To prevent emergence of drug resistance, treatment must include at least two drugs.
- Standard 6 month regimen preferred for adults and children.
  - — Rifampicin—first 2 months.
  - — INH and pyrazinamide—next four months.

    or
  - — INH + Rifampicin—for nine months equally effective.
- Ethambutol is added to the initial treatment for patients when resistance to INH is suspected.
- Treatment is to be continued for at least six months and after three negative cultures have been obtained.
- If INH and RMP cannot be used, treatment is continued for eighteen months.
- Certain patients should receive initially four drugs to ensure that the microorganisms will be susceptible to at least two drugs.
  - — Rifampicin, INH and pyrazinamide (4th drug either ethambutol or streptomycin).
- Ninety per cent of the cases who receive optimal treatment will have negative culture within three to six months.

- Cultures that remain positive after six months indicate emergence of drug resistance and an alternative therapeutic programme is then considered.
- The drugs should be continued for an average of twelve months.
- INH must be part of any multidrug therapy.
- In patients on multidrug therapy with neural complications, pyrazinamide should be used for three months.
- Middle path regime was first described in the year 1975 by Tuli and Kumar.

Prognosis

- Ninety-five per cent of uncomplicated cases of tuberculosis spine heal by conservative regimen.
- In patients with neural complications 50 per cent recover with drugs and rest alone, while the other 50 per cent recover after surgery.
- After surgery, 70 per cent recover completely 15 per cent show useful partial recovery, and 15 per cent show negligible recovery.

Vital facts:

The onset of recovery after initiation of chemotherapy may take as long as three months.

Quick facts: skeletal tuberculosis (general)

- Incidence is 2 to 3 per cent
- Usually monoarticular
- Always secondary
- Spine is affected commonly
- Only 20 per cent show constitutional symptoms
- Cold abscess is a feature
- Chemotherapy is the mainstay of treatment.

TUBERCULOSIS SPINE

(Known after Sir Percival Pott)

This is the most common form of skeletal tuberculosis constituting about 50 per cent of all cases.

Regional distribution

1. Cervical—12 per cent
2. Cervicodorsal—5 per cent
3. Dorsal—42 per cent
4. Dorsolumbar—12 per cent
5. Lumbar—26 per cent
6. Lumbosacral—3 per cent

As is evident from the above data, spinal tuberculosis commonly affects the lower thoracic and lumbar vertebra accounting for nearly 80 per cent of the cases. The reasons cited for this area of predilection are:

1. Large amounts of spongy tissues within the vertebral body.
2. Degree of weight bearing which is comparatively more.
3. More vertebral mobility is seen here.

Sites of Involvement within the Vertebra

It is observed that spinal tuberculosis could start in any of the part (Fig. 39.2) of the vertebra (95% anterior; 5% posterior elements).

1. **Central** Less common. This is known to produce central or *concertina* collapse of the vertebra.
2. **Metaphyseal or intervertebral space (98%)** This is the most common area of involvement and is not without reason. Embryological development explains the reasons for this.

   Lower half of one vertebra and upper half of the adjacent vertebra with the intervening disc all develop from one sclerotome, which has a common source of blood supply (Fig. 39.3). Hence, bacillaemia involves this embryological section more often.
3. **Anterior or periosteal** Here, anterior surface of vertebral body is involved and it may give rise to anterior wedge compression of the vertebra.
4. **Appendiceal** Occasionally, transverse process and rarely vertebral arch are affected.
5. **True tubercular arthritis** Seen in the atlantoaxial and at atlanto-occipital joints.

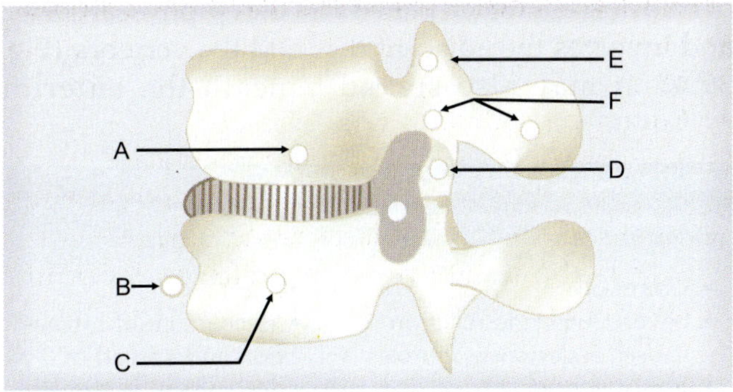

Fig. 39.2: Showing sites of involvement TB spine: (A) metaphyseal, (B) anterior, (C) central, (D) true arthritis, (E) appendiceal, and (F) posterior spinal elements

Section 5

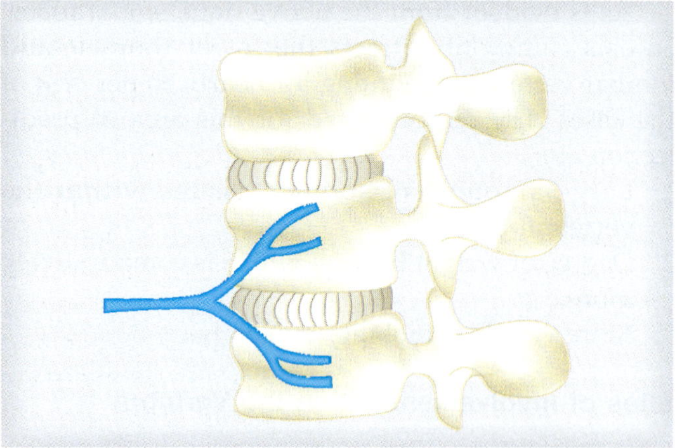

Fig. 39.3: Showing blood supply of vertebrae

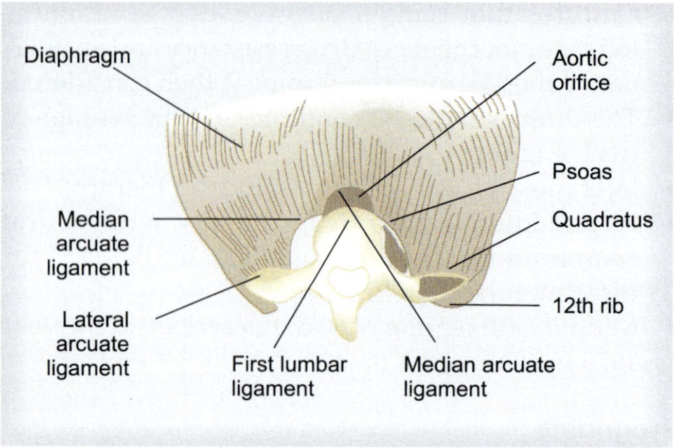

Fig. 39.4: Showing spread of the cold abscess through the diaphragmatic orifices

Sequences of Pathological Events

As mentioned earlier, due to primary foci in the lungs, lymph nodes or abdomen, bacillaemia develops and the organisms reach the spine through the Batson's plexus.

Tuberculous endarteritis which develops following the infection results in marrow devitalisation. Later on, the tubercular follicle develops. Lamellae are destroyed due to hyperaemia causing osteoporosis. As a result of this, the vertebral body gets easily compressed. In the thoracic vertebrae, because of the normal kyphotic curve, anterior wedge compression is more common. In the lordotic cervical and lumbar vertebra, wedging is minimal.

Two types of vertebral reactions are commonly encountered in skeletal tuberculosis (Table 39.2).

This non-pyogenic infection results in formation of cold abscess which penetrates the epiphyseal cortex and involves the adjacent disc and the vertebra (Fig. 39.4). It may also spread beneath the anterior longitudinal ligament and reach the neighbouring vertebra. When it spreads posteriorly, it may cause pressure on the spinal cord which is more common in the thoracic area as the spinal canal is small here. The posterior longitudinal ligament limits the spread of sequestra and bone fragments into the joints (Fig. 39.5). Sometimes the cold abscess may penetrate the anterior longitudinal ligament and migrate along the *lines of least resistance*—Figure 39.4 (i.e. along the fascial planes, blood vessels, nerves).

Note: Cold abscess consists of serum, WBCs, caseous material, granulation tissue and tubercle bacilli.

Table 39.2: Types of vertebral reactions

Exudative reaction	*Caseative reaction*
• Common • Severe hypergic reaction causes severe osteoporosis • Rapid spread • Abscess is formed frequently • Constitutional symptoms are pronounced	• Rarer • Mechanism of formation and spread of destruction is similar to exudative type but is slower.

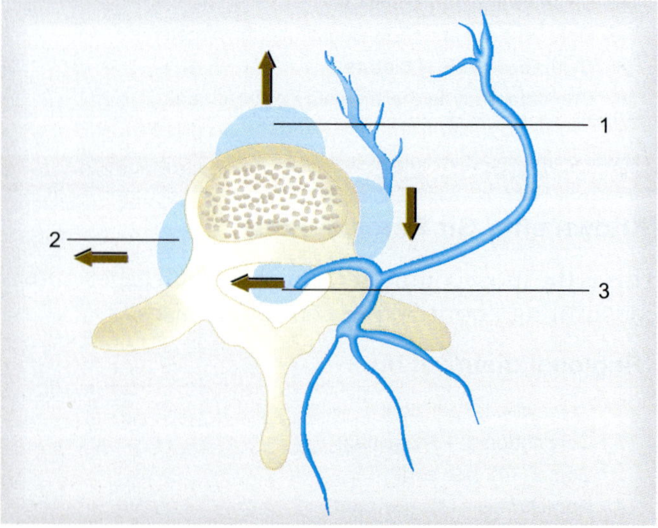

Fig. 39.5: Showing spread of cold abscess: (1) anteriorly, (2) laterally, and (3) forwards spinal canal

Clinical Features

Tuberculosis of spine is usually insidious in onset although sometimes it may present acutely. The constitutional symptoms almost always antedate local spinal involvement. Weakness, anorexia, night sweats and cries, evening or afternoon rise of temperature, loss of appetite and weight are some of those.

The patient may complain of back pain which is localised over the site of vertebral involvement or is referred depending on the specific nerve root irritation. Thus, if cervical roots are involved, pain radiates to the arm; if dorsal roots are involved, the patient complains of girdle pain; if lumbar nerve roots are involved; patient complains of radiating pain to the groin; and if sacral roots are involved, the patient complains of sciatica.

Back stiffness is another common earliest complaint given by the patient. The patient is unable to bend and pick up the objects on the ground. The patient may give history of night cries. If the patient complains of stiffness, weakness, awkwardness of lower extremities, it heralds the onset of paraplegia.

Physical Findings

The patient has a very protective attitude and has a very cautious and careful gait. The muscle spasm straightens out the spine. The spinous process of the involved vertebra is tender to percuss and when an attempt is made to rotate the vertebra. Back movements are decreased in all directions, especially forward, flexion. There is pronounced wasting of the back muscles. The clinical attitude of the patient varies according to the region involved (see box). Cold abscess may be seen as paravertebral swelling or in areas already described. The patient may develop or present with neurological complications like spastic or flaccid paraplegia. Of the various deformities of spine due to tuberculosis, *kyphotic* deformity is the most common and is seen in over 95 per cent of the cases (Fig. 39.7).

General examination reveals signs of anaemia, debility, involvement of lungs, lymph nodes, etc.

Spread of cold abscess (Fig. 39.6)

Cervical region
1. Behind the prevertebral fascia
2. Posterior edge of sternomastoid
3. Retropharyngeal space
4. Mediastinum, from here it may gravitate towards
   - Trachea
   - Oesophagus
   - Pleural cavity

Thoracic region (Fig. 39.6)
1. May press the spinal cord posteriorly causing paraplegia
2. May spread laterally towards the extrapleural space causing effusion
3. It may penetrate the ALL and may lie in the mediastinum
4. It may remain prevertebral (i.e. in post-mediastinum) or from here it may spread to
   - Through the lateral aortic ligament and quadratus lumborum
     ↓ Remains behind the kidney
     or
     Extends along the nerves related to the bed of kidney
     ↓ Along the 12th, ilioinguinal, and iliohypogastric nerves
     ↓ And presents on anterior abdominal wall
   - Through the medial aortic ligament
     ↓ Enters the psoas sheath
     ↓ Reaches the lesser trochanter where psoas gets inserted
   - Through median aortic ligament
     ↓ Forms a lumbar abscess

Lumbar region
1. Psoas sheath
2. Iliac crest
3. Along the femoral vessels to the femoral triangle
4. Along the gluteal vessels to gluteal region
5. Rarely to the iliac crest
6. May present in the Petit's triangle

Note: Cold abscess is called "cold" because it is not associated with features, like redness, heat, etc. as in pyogenic abscess

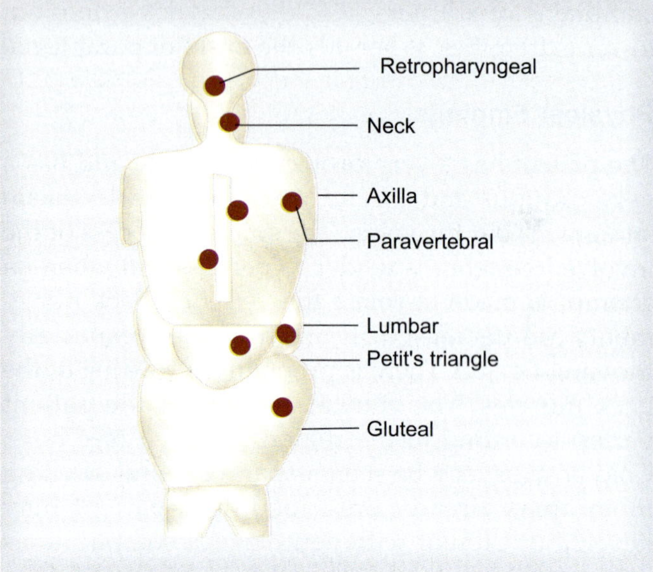

Fig. 39.6: Showing the sites of cold abscess in TB spine

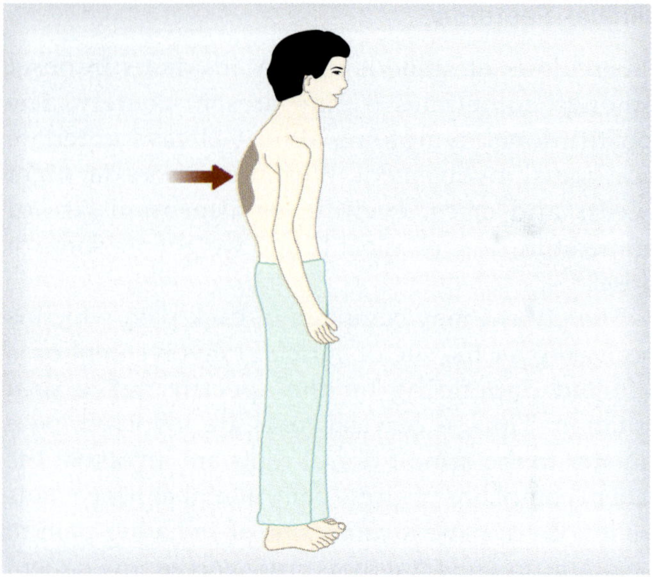

Fig. 39.7: Showing kyphotic deformity in tuberculosis of spine

Quick facts: Typical attitudes in skeletal TB

- Upper cervical → Wryneck
- Lower cervical → Military position
- Lower thoracic → Alderman's gait
- Upper lumbar → Prominent abdomen
- Lower lumbar → Increased lordosis

Quick facts: Spine irregularities in skeletal TB

a. Kyphosis (95%)
b. Scoliosis (5%)
c. Lordosis
d. Boarding
e. Paravertebral thickening.

Other features

- Muscle spasm
- Wasting of all spinal muscles
- Spastic or flaccid paraplegia (20%)
- Cold abscess (20%)
- Sinuses (13%)
- Complications of skeletal TB.

Investigations

Laboratory tests These tests show anaemia, lymphocytosis, hypoproteinaemia, mild increase in ESR, etc. Mantoux test is helpful, especially in children below 2 to 3 years but is not diagnostic.

The importance of general tests lies in indicating chronic disease.

Radiographs X-ray of the affected vertebrae is a very important diagnostic test and it is observed that the average number of affected vertebra are usually three. The following changes are seen on the X-ray:

Earliest change This consists of disc space narrowing and subsequent loss of disc space in the common paradiscal lesions. The bones look rarefied and osteopenic (about 40 per cent of calcium loss must take place to show a radiolucent sign on the X-ray).

Late changes This includes anterior wedge compression in anterior vertebral involvement, central vertebral body collapse also called as "concertina collapse" (Fig. 39.8) in central involvement, destruction of the posterior elements in the posterior affection, etc.

Soft tissue swelling and its calcification are highly predictable of tuberculosis. In the healing stages, the vertebral body and the posterior elements may appear more dense due to sclerosis.

Paravertebral shadow If seen on the X-ray indicates cold abscess (Figs 39.9A and B).

1. *Cervical region* In between the vertebral bodies and pharynx (retropharyngeal).
2. *Upper thoracic* V-shaped shadow and widened mediastinum.
3. *Below fourth thoracic vertebra* fusiform or birdnest shadow appearance.

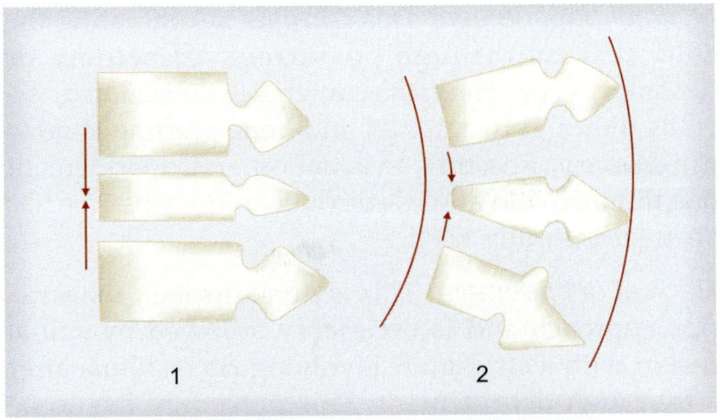

Fig. 39.8: Showing (1) concertina collapse, and (2) anterior wedge compression

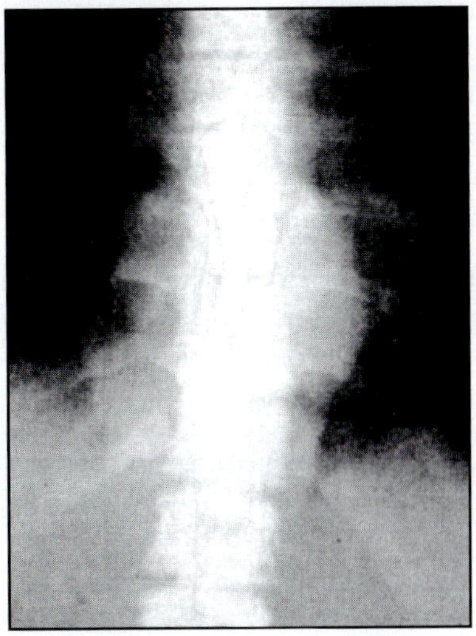

Fig. 39.9A: Showing tense paravertebral abscess in tuberculosis of lower dorsal spine

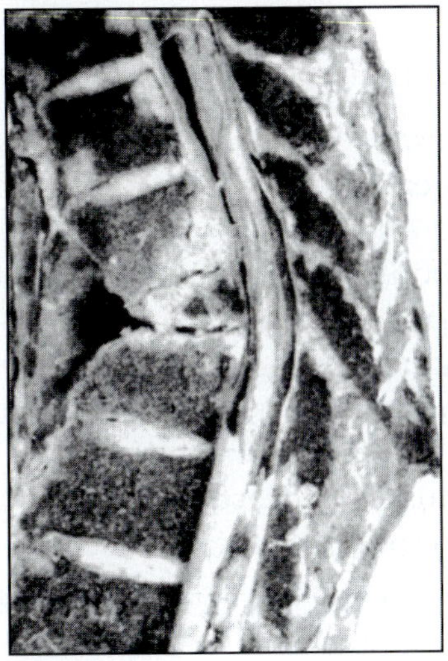

Fig. 39.9B: Showing a specimen of tuberculosis spine

4. *Psoas abscess* unilateral or bilateral widening of psoas shadows in the lumbar region.
5. *Aneurysmal phenomenon* tense thoracic vertebral abscess showing a scalloping effect variety.

Note: The most common is paradiscal, rarest is appendiceal involvement in spinal tuberculosis.

CT scan Identifies paravertebral soft tissue swelling more readily than X-rays. It helps to assess the degree of neural compromise and helps in better evaluation of the pathologic process. Some prefer CT to X-ray to determine the clinical progress. Findings are similar to X-rays.

Note: The only detectable abnormality on plain X-ray and CT scan specifically related to tuberculosis is *fine calcification in the paravertebral soft tissue shadow.*

MRI It helps in further delineation of the disease and helps to detect the cord compression. It does not eliminate the need for biopsy. It is 94 per cent accurate (Figs 39.10A and B). Small calcifications seen on X-rays are not seen on MRI.

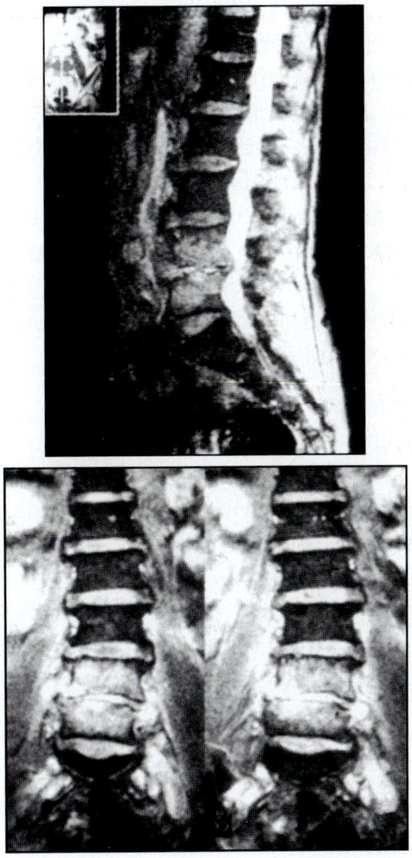

Figs 39.10A and B: Magnetic resonance imaging (MRI) of lumbar spine showing tubercular lesion of L_4 and L_5 vertebra

Gallium scanning is useful in disseminated TB.

Biopsy No one diagnostic test is 100 per cent accurate for definitive diagnosis. Hence, diagnosis is dependent on culture of the organism and requires biopsy by percutaneous technique with CT control.

Ultrasound is useful to detect size of cold abscess in lumbar vertebral disease.

CT scan and MRI are also helpful in detecting tubercular affection of posterior spinal elements, craniovertebral and craniodorsal region, sacrum and sacroiliac region.

Treatment

Definitive diagnosis by biopsy and culture is a must before starting the treatment, because of the toxicity of the chemotherapeutic regime and length of the treatment required.

Non-operative and operative methods evaluated by the Medical Research Council working party are as follows:

- Radical surgery performed under chemotherapeutic coverage gives better results with regard to deformity correction, development of paralysis and resolution.
- Chemotherapy with long-term bedrest with or without cast is ineffective.
- When facilities for radical surgery are not available *ambulatory chemotherapy* is the treatment of choice. **Chemotherapy** controls 90 per cent of tuberculosis spine as already mentioned and has been discussed in great detail (*ref. p. 501*).

Indications for surgery

- Neurologic symptoms.
- Kyphosis with several vertebral involvement, severe kyphosis, progressive kyphosis, etc.
- Resistance to chemotherapy.
- Recurrence of disease.
- Cord compression.
- Progressive impairment of pulmonary function.
- Spinal instability.

Surgical procedures The following surgical procedures are described.

Aspiration This technique is useful to aspirate the contents of a cold abscess through a thick bored needle. The needle should be inserted below the abscess so as to enable the gravity to help drain the contents.

Minimal debridement This consists of evaluating the cold abscess through costotransversectomy or decompression. Here, the contents are evacuated, the walls thoroughly curetted and bone grafting is done if necessary. Recently, evacuation and debridement of a thoracic cold abscess through a thoracoscope has been successfully tried.

Radical debridement This is done through the anterior approach and is invariably followed by spinal fusion with a strut graft involving rib or fibula after a thorough debridement. This procedure has to be done before abscess or neurological complications develop. Fusion could be anterior or posterior; but in the former, normal anterior compressive forces are brought into play resulting in a high rate of successful bony fusion. Progression of disease and pseudarthrosis are common in posterior fusion. The only indication for posterior fusion is to add support for the disease at cervicothoracic or dorsolumbar regions.

Objectives of surgery Surgery helps to excise the infected tissue, decompress the intraspinal neural elements, reduce the spinal instability and provide stability by spine fusion techniques.

Complications of tuberculosis spine

1. Paraplegia
2. Cold abscess
3. Sinuses
4. Secondary infection
5. Amyloid disease
6. Fatality

MIDDLE PATH REGIME

Tuli and Kumar advocated triple drug therapy without surgery. In their series operative treatment was reserved for patients:

1. Not responding favourably to drug therapy after six months of treatment.
2. Recrudescence of the disease.
3. Patients with neural complications.

Operative treatment is combined with six to twelve months of bedrest, followed by eighteen to twenty-four months of spinal bracing.

Did you know?

Tuli's middle path regime is the most widely accepted protocol for the management of spinal TB.

TB SPINE WITH PARAPLEGIA

The incidence of this complication is 10 to 30 per cent and it is most often associated with tuberculosis of the dorsal spine.

The following are the reasons cited for this:

- TB is more common in dorsal spine.
- Spinal cord terminates below L_1.
- Spinal cord is smallest in this region.
- Normal curve of the thoracic spine encourages marked kyphosis.
- Anterior longitudinal ligament in the dorsal region loosely confines the abscess.

Pathology

Paraplegia could result due to inflammatory causes, mechanical causes, intrinsic causes and due to spinal tumour disease (Table 39.3).

Table 39.3: Causes of paraplegia

Inflammatory causes	*Mechanical causes*	*Intrinsic causes*	*Spinal tumour disease*
• Oedema • Granulation tissue • Abscess • Caseous tissue This is the most common cause	• Tubercular debris • Sequestra • Stenosis of vertebral canal • Internal gibbus	• Prolonged stretching • Infective endocarditis • Pathological dislocation • Tuberculosis meningomyelitis • Syringomyelia	• Extradural granuloma • Tuberculoma • Peridural fibrosis

Classification

Seddon's Classification

1. Early onset paraplegia is associated with active disease. It is seen within two years of onset of the disease.
2. Late onset paraplegia is associated with healed disease. It is seen after two years after the onset of disease.

Clinical Features

Rarely paraplegia may be the presenting symptom. Late onset paraplegia may be associated with clumsiness, twitching, increased reflexes, clonus, positive Babinski's sign, etc. Motor functions are usually affected first. The paralysis usually follows the following stages in order of severity—muscle weakness, spasticity, incoordination, paraplegia in extension, flexor spasms, paraplegia in flexion (severe form), and flaccid paraplegia lastly (see Box).

Kumar's grading of paraplegia

Grade I	Negligible, patient is unaware, physician detects ankle clonus, and upgoing plantar.
Grade II	Mild, patient aware but walks with support.
Grade III	Moderate, non-ambulatory, paralysis in extension. Sensory deficit < 50 per cent.
Grade IV	Severe grade III + severe paraplegia + sensory deficit more than 50 per cent.

Clonus is the first most prominent early sign of Pott's disease. Sense of position and vibration are the last to disappear.

Rarely paraplegia may develop suddenly due to:

1. Thromboembolism
2. Pathological dislocation
3. Rapid accumulation of infected material.

Principles of Treatment

Three schools of thought are described for management of paraplegia due to tuberculosis.

Bosworth Immobilisation and early posterior arthrodesis.

Hodgson radical anterior decompression and arthrodesis.

[36]***Tuli and Kumar's*** Middle path regime. As mentioned earlier, this is the most widely accepted treatment regimen for spinal TB (see box)

What is the protocol in the middle path regime?

- Admission, rest in bed or plaster of Paris cast.
- Chemotherapy.
- X-ray and ESR once in three months.
- Gradual mobilisation in the absence of neurological complications.
- Spinal braces—18 months to 2 years.
- Abscesses are aspirated or drained.
- Sinuses heal within 6 to 12 weeks.
- If no neural complications develop; if response is obtained within 3 to 4 weeks of triple drug therapy, surgery is unnecessary.
- Excisional surgery for posterior spinal disease.
- Operative debridement for patients who do not show arrest of disease after 3 to 6 months of chemotherapy.

[36]**SM Tuli** (1975) Varanasi

Treatment of Pott's Paraplegia

The following measures are adopted in the treatment of Pott's paraplegia.

Conservative treatment Chemotherapy is the mainstay of this method and has already been described. Immobilisation of the spine to provide rest and thereby promote healing is done by traction (in cervical region) plaster cast or brace (in dorsal region), etc. Management of bed sores, bladder and bowel management is done as already discussed in the management of spinal injury. Physiotherapy and occupational therapy helps in the treatment of the paralysed lower limbs.

Surgical treatment The incidence of surgery has considerably decreased as chemotherapy is found to be successful in treating Pott's paraplegia. Only 5 per cent of the cases require surgery in uncomplicated cases and 60 per cent of the cases with neurological deficits require surgery.

Main indications for surgery

- Failed conservative treatment: If the patient does not respond to conservative treatment even after 3 to 6 months.
- In doubtful diagnosis.
- Fusion for mechanical instability by some grafts, implants, etc. either by the anterior or posterior approach.
- Recurrence of the disease after treatment.
- In rapid onset paraplegia.
- In disease secondary to cervical disease and cauda equina paralysis.

Other indications

- Recurrent paraplegia.
- Painful paraplegia—due to root compression, etc.
- Posterior spinal disease—involving the posterior elements of the vertebra.
- Spinal tumour syndrome resulting in cord compression.
- Rapid onset paraplegia due to thrombosis, trauma, etc.
- Severe paraplegia.
- Secondary to cervical disease and cauda equina paralysis.

Surgical Techniques

Costotransversectomy This is indicated for a tense paravertebral abscess. As the name suggests, excision of the transverse process of the affected vertebra and about an inch of the adjacent rib to facilitate the drainage of abscess is done (Fig. 39.11). If pus is yielded under pressure, one has to wait up to six weeks for improvement. If no improvement occurs, anterolateral decompression is done.

Anterolateral decompression (ALD) The structures removed in this procedure are posterior part of the rib, transverse process, pedicle and part of the vertebral body anterior to the cord (Fig. 39.12). This is the surgery of choice for Pott's paraplegia. It helps to effectively remove the solid and liquid debris. ALD is done through an extrapleural mediastinal approach. Bone graft may be inserted if needed (Fig. 39.13).

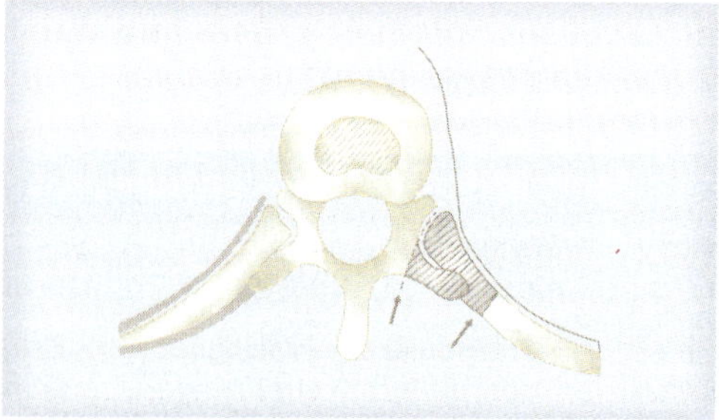

Fig. 39.11: Showing structures removed in costotransversectomy

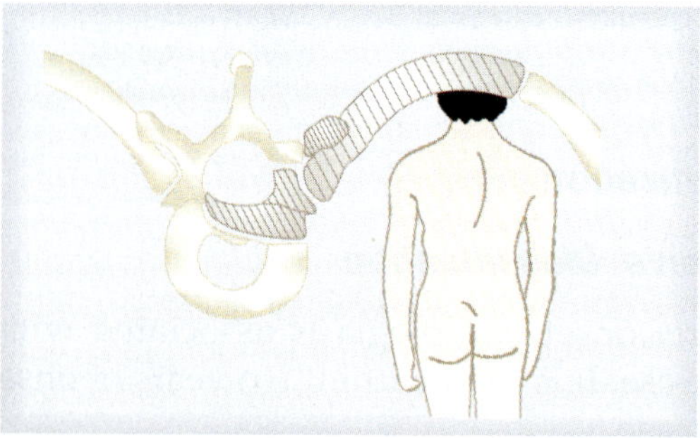

Fig. 39.12: Showing structures removed in ALD

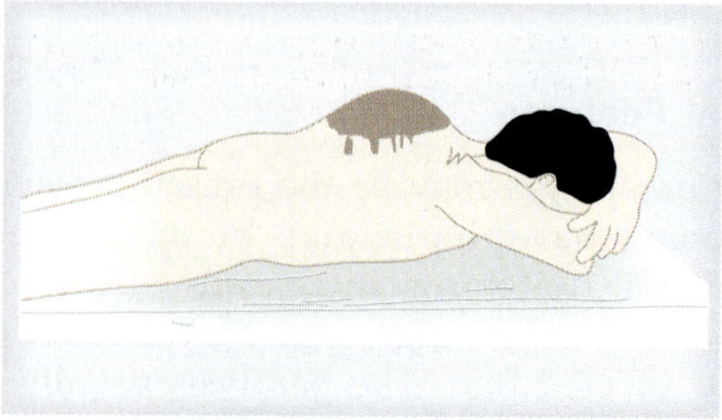

Fig. 39.13: Showing approach for ALD and costotransversectomy

Anterior decompression This is technically more demanding. Here, the affected vertebra is approached through a transplerual or transperitoneal route, diseased tissue is curetted and a bone graft is inserted.

Laminectomy In Pott's paraplegia, anterior part of the cord is predominantly affected and laminectomy does not decompress this part of the cord. Moreover, it makes the spine unstable as it removes the healthy areas of the vertebrae. Hence, this procedure is not commonly recommended.

If arthrodesis of the spine is required after the above procedures, anterior arthrodesis is normally preferred. Posterior spinal arthrodesis has limited value and is usually done to stabilise the cranio-vertebral region. Paralysis secondary to cervical disease is treated by either laminectomy and posterior arthrodesis or radical debridement and anterior arthrodesis. Severe cauda equina paralysis requires lumbar transversectomy.

Prognosis in paraplegia is better in:
- Central cord involvement.
- Early onset paraplegia.
- If general conditions are good.

Cold abscess is another complication. It can present as one of the **three P's**:
- **P**alpable tumour in neck, back, thigh, etc.
- **P**ressure symptoms on the cord.
- **P**resent on radiographs of spine (*refer p. 506*).

Treatment

Early aseptic evacuation is indicated. Aspiration if the contents are very fluid, but majority require open surgery for evacuation, e.g. costotransversectomy for tense paravertebral abscess, ALD for less than tense paravertebral abscess.

TUBERCULOSIS OF THE HIP JOINT

Tuberculosis of the hip joint is ranked next to spinal tuberculosis (10:7) and it constitutes 15 per cent of all osteoarticular tuberculosis. It is always secondary. The initial focus of infection could be either in the: (i) acetabular roof, (ii) epiphysis, (iii) metaphyseal region, (iv) greater trochanter, (v) synovial membrane (rare), and (vi) trochanteric bursae (Fig. 39.14).

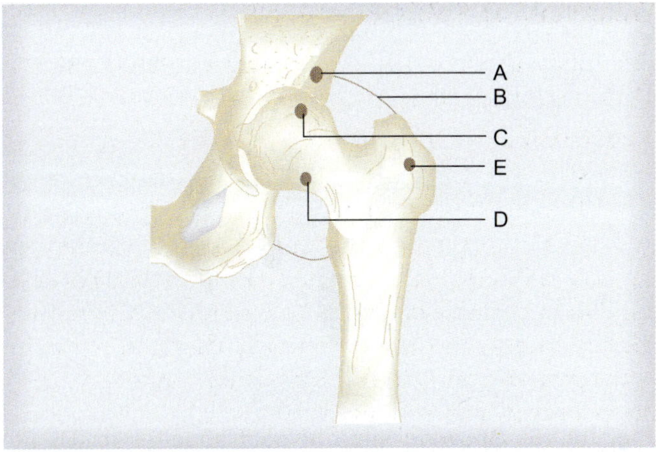

Fig. 39.14: Showing sites of common tubercular infection of the hip, A—acetabular roof, B—synovium, C—epiphysis, D—metaphysis, and E—greater trochanter

Pathogenesis

Tuberculosis elsewhere like lungs, tonsils, GIT, etc. spreads through the haematogenous route, the tubercular infection develops in any one of the six sites already mentioned. Synovial membrane is the one most commonly affected. Here, the tubercle formation causes synovial hypertrophy resulting in pannus formation. This pannus destroys the articular cartilage resulting in the development of fibrous ankylosis of the hip. Bony ankylosis rarely develops.

Microscopy shows tubercle formation, giant cells and lymphocytes. Upper end of the femur is intracapsular and the joint gets rapidly involved. On the contrary, the joint involvement in acetabular lesions is rare.

The smaller tubercles coalesce, undergo caseation and forms a cold abscess. This cold abscess tracks down along the areas of least resistance and may point in any one of following sites: (i) femoral triangle, (ii) inguinal region, (iii) medial side of the thigh, (iv) greater trochanter, (v) gluteal region, (vi) ischio-rectal fossa, (vii) lateral and posterior aspect of the thigh, and (vii) pelvis (Fig. 39.15).

Clinical Features

Tuberculosis of hip is common in the first three decades of life. The patient usually presents with painful limp and is the most common earliest symptom. He or she has an antalgic gait with a short stance phase. Pain is maximum towards the end of

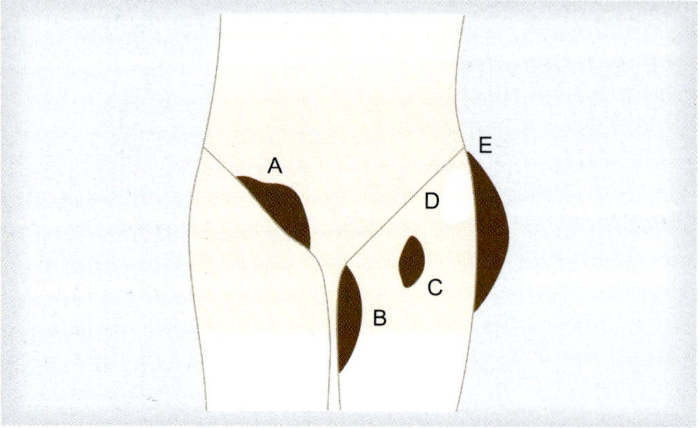

Fig. 39.15: Showing sites of cold abscess in TB hip (A) inguinal region, (B) medial side of thigh, (C) femoral triangle, (D) gluteal region, and (E) lateral aspect of thigh

the day and there is a history of night cries. There is marked wasting of the thigh and gluteal muscles. There may be presence of scars and sinuses. About 8 per cent of the patients may develop cold abscess in the regions shown in the figure above and 10 per cent may show pathological subluxation. Tenderness can be elicited by direct pressure in the femoral triangle or by bitrochanteric compression. The attitude differs depending upon the stage of the disease which is discussed later. The following deformities may develop in tuberculosis hip:

1. *Flexion deformity* In the initial stages of the disease, patient keeps the hip in flexion as this is the position of ease and of maximum joint capacity. Soft tissue contractures convert this into a fixed flexion deformity (FFD) making locomotion impossible. *In an effort to bring the limb on the ground and to make locomotion possible, the lumbar spine undergoes exaggerated lordosis and thus conceals the fixed flexion deformity.*

   The patient can lie down straight on the bed in the face of this fixed flexion deformity because of the exaggerated lordosis. This is confirmed by the easy passage of the examiner's hand between the bed and the back of the patient. Normally, this is not possible. In order to reveal this FFD, Thomas test is carried out. The unaffected hip of the patient is flexed over the abdomen till the lumbar lordotic curve disappears. The affected hip then assumes a position of flexion and the degree of FFD is calculated by the angle formed between the thigh and the bed.

2. *Adduction deformity* Soft tissue contractures convert the adduction position adapted by the patient due to the spasm of the adductor muscles following damage to the articular cartilage, to one of the fixed adduction deformities. *The limb is now brought to the ground by the elevation of the pelvis as evidenced by the anterior superior iliac spine being at a higher level on the affected site. There is scoliosis of the spine away from the deformity.*

   The adduction deformtiy can be revealed by squaring the pelvis. This is done by adducting the affected limb till both the anterior superior iliac spines lie in the same straight line. The angle formed between the vertical and the adducted limb is the angle of fixed adduction deformity.

3. *Abduction deformity* In the initial phases of the disease, because of the increase in the joint space due to effusion, the limb assumes a position of flexion, abduction and external rotation. If fixed in this position by soft tissue contractures, the patient develops a fixed abduction deformity. *The limb is then brought to the ground by the downward tilt of the pelvis as evidenced by anterior superior iliac spine (ASIS) lying at a lower level with the corresponding scoliosis of the spine towards the affected side.*

   The fixed abduction deformity can be revealed by abducting the affected limb till both the anterior superior iliac spine lie in the same level. The angle formed between the vertical and the abducted limb is the angle of fixed abduction deformity.

Limb length discrepancy In the initial stages, there may be apparent lengthening; but in the advanced stages, the patient develops shortening.

Stages of tuberculosis hip The following stages are described in tuberculosis hip.

- *Stage I* (*Stage of synovitis*) Here, the disease is synovial with the patient assuming flexed, abducted and external rotated position of the limb. There is *apparent* lengthening. There is no real shortening and the extremes of movements are decreased and painful (here apparent length more than true length).
- *Stage II* (*Stage of early arthritis*) The local signs are exaggerated. The spasms of the adductors and flexors result in fexion, adduction and internal rotation of the affected limb. There is apparent

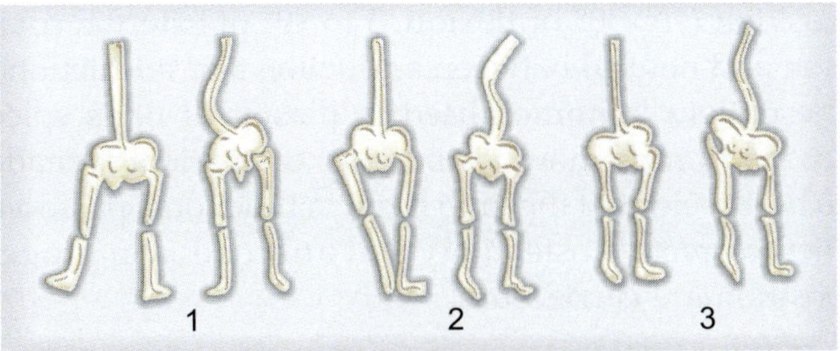

Fig. 39.16A: Showing stages of tuberculosis hip: (1) stage of synovitis, (2) stage of early arthritis, and (3) stage of advanced arthritis

shortening, significant muscle wasting and hip movements are decreased in all directions. True shortening may be less than 1 cm (here apparent length less than true length).

- *Stage III (Advanced arthritis)* The flexion, adduction, internal rotation deformity found in Stage II are exaggerated. There is a true shortening with considerable restriction of hip movements and muscle wasting. There is gross destruction of the articular cartilage of the head of the femur and acetabulum (apparent length is less than true length) (Figs 39.16A and B).
- *Stage IV (Advanced arthritis with subluxation of dislocation)* Migrating acetabulum, frank pathological posterior dislocation, mortar and pestle hip, protrusio acetabuli are the features in this stage.

The Trendelenburg test is positive in all the above stages.

Investigations

Laboratory tests These tests show anaemia, lymphocytosis, increased ESR, etc.

Radiograph of the hip In the early stages, the radiographs show rarefaction of the bones; and in advanced stages, there may be reduction in the joint space. Depending upon the radiological features, Shanmugasundaram has described seven types of tuberculosis hip in advanced stages of arthritis (Figs 39.17A to E).

- *Normal appearance* Here the hip almost looks normal but for some rarefaction.
- *Travelling or wandering acetabulum* Here, because of the destruction of the joint due to arthritis and due to the muscle spasm, the head of the femur comes to lie in the region of the ilium.

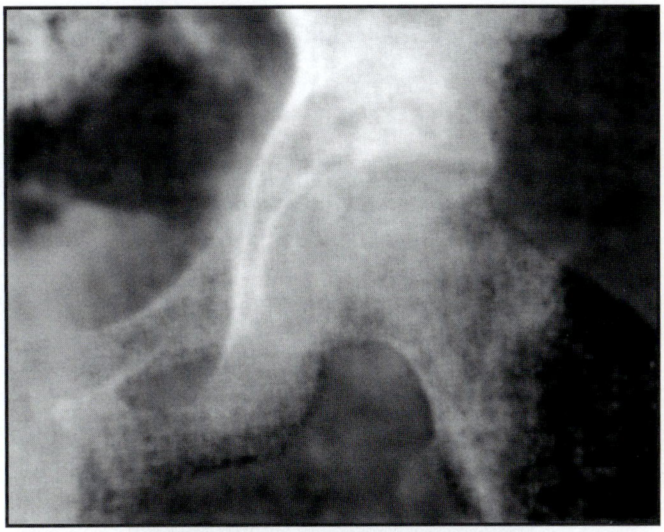

Fig. 39.16B: Radiograph showing advanced stage of TB hip, sequestra seen in the acetabulum

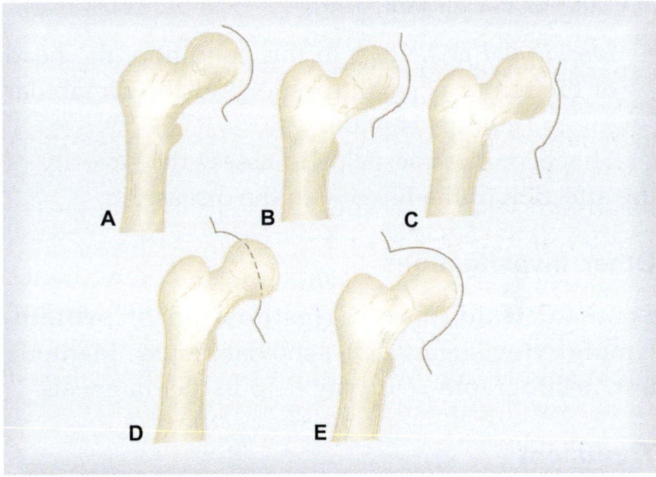

Figs 39.17A and E: Showing Shanmugasundaram's radiological types of TB hip: (A) Normal type, (B) Travelling acetabulum, (C) Dislocated type, (D) Protrusio acetabuli, and (E) Mortar and pestle

- *Dislocated hip* In this condition, there is pathological dislocation of the hip joint.
- *Perthes' type* Here, the head of the femur is dense and there could be collapse.
- *Atrophic type* Here, the head of the femur is small and atrophic.
- *Protrusio acetabuli type* Here, there is gross reduction of the joint space and head of the femur threatens to protrude through the acetabulum into the pelvic cavity (Fig. 39.18).

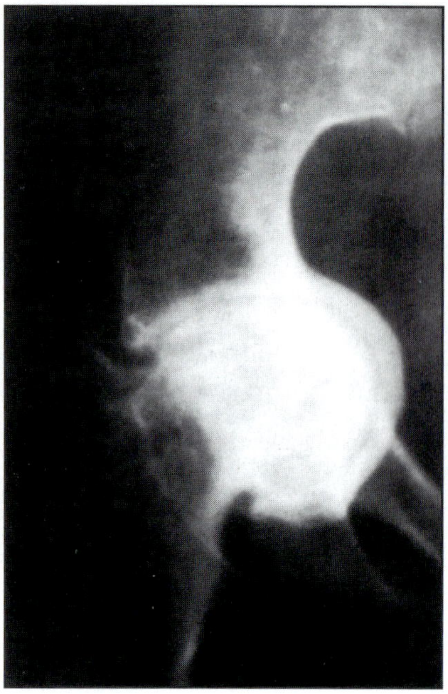

Fig. 39.18: Radiograph showing protrusio acetabuli

- *Mortar and pestle type* In this condition, the head of the femur is small (pestle) and the acetabular cavity (mortar) is wide.

This classification helps to assess the severity of the affection of the hip due to the disease.

Other Investigations

Synovial fluid analysis (estimation of protein, lymphocytes, sugar, etc.), synovial biopsy, Mantoux test, arthrography, etc. may help in the diagnosis.

Treatment

Early stages (synovitis and early arthritis) The patient is put on chemotherapy and traction. Traction reduces the muscle spasm, prevents or corrects the deformity and maintains the joint space. If favourable clinical response is obtained, hip is gradually mobilised. If the disease is not responding favourably, then synovectomy and arthrotomy are carried out in the synovitis stage. Synovectomy and thorough joint debridement is done in cases of early arthritis.

Late stages (stage of advanced arthritis) The end result of this stage is fibrous ankylosis and the patient is put on chemotherapy and traction. Once gross ankylosis is accepted and if the limb is in proper position (10°-30° of flexion, 5 to 10° of external rotation and neutral between adduction and adduction), the patient is immobilised in plaster of Paris spica for six to nine months and later the patient is made to bear weight. If the limb is not in functional position, then corrective osteotomy and arthrodesis in proper position are carried out.

Surgical Treatment in Tuberculosis Hip

Synovectomy and arthrotomy This is done in synovitis stage when the disease is not responding favourably to conservative treatment. Partial synovectomy and joint drainage and lavage are done.

Synovectomy and joint debridement This is preferred in early arthritis. The joint is exposed through the posterior approach. Thorough debridement of the joint is done by evacuation and the walls are curetted and washed.

Osteotomy This is an upper femoral corrective osteotomy and is indicated in sound ankylosis in bad position in flexion adduction contractures. This helps to correct the deformity and change the line of weight bearing.

Displacement osteotomy is done in fibrous ankylosis with gross deformity.

Arthrodesis This is indicated in adults with painful fibrous ankylosis with active or healed disease. This procedure converts a painful hip to painless stable hip. The procedure could either be intra-articular or extra-articular or both.

Arthroplasty Stiff hip is a gross disability and is particularly not acceptable by Indian patients because they cannot use the Indian toilet. Here, girdle stone excision arthroplasty (Fig. 39.19) is preferred and it can be done in active or healed disease after the growth stops. This gives a mobile painless hip joint apart from controlling the infection and correcting the deformity. However, it leaves the hip unstable.

Total hip replacement is rarely done in tuberculosis hip. It is suggested after 10 years after the last evidence of active infection.

Amniotic arthroplasty has been tried in tuberculosis hip. But the results are far from satisfactory.

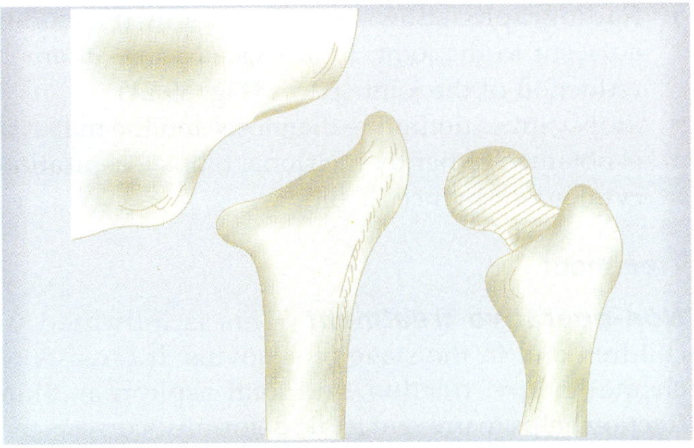

Fig. 39.19: Showing girdlestone excision arthroplasty

Quick facts: Early stages (TB Hip)

SYNOVITIS AND EARLY ARTHRITIS

Triple drug therapy and traction
↓
Favourable clinical response
↓
Continue same treatment
↓
Hip mobilisation
↓
Ambulation after 4 to 6 months
↓
Non-weight bearing first 12 weeks
↓
Partial weight bearing for next 12 weeks
↓
Discard crutches after unprotected weight bearing after 18 to 24 months

ADVANCED ARTHRITIS (treatment plan)
(Articular cartilage involved)

- Traction
- Chemotherapy

Once gross ankylosis is accepted

If in proper position	If in bad position
↓	↓
POP cast for 6 to 9 months	Corrective osteotomy and/or arthrodesis
↓	↓
Partial weight bearing after 6 months calipers and crutches for nearly 2 years	Partial weight bearing after 6 months of calipers and crutches for nearly 2 years.

Treatment facts: Tuberculosis hip

- Chemotherapy
- Traction—skin or Thomas splint
- If disease is synovial, aim at mobility
- If articular cartilage is involved, aim at arthrodesis in functional position.

Quick facts: Tuberculosis hip

- Second in frequency in skeletal tuberculosis
- Limp is the earliest symptom
- Three classical deformities
- Passes through four pathological stages
- Fibrous ankylosis is the end result.

TUBERCULOSIS OF THE KNEE

This is the third common site for skeletal tuberculosis. Incidence is 10 per cent. It is also always secondary and may start in any one of the following sites in the knee joint.

Sites

1. Synovium (common).
2. Subchondral bone (of distal femur, proximal tibia or patella).
3. Juxta-articular osseous foci.

The infection so developed results in tubercle formation and the synovium undergoes hypertrophy forming a pannus which destroys the articular cartilage of the joint and results in fibrous ankylosis.

Remember

Five classical deformities in TB knee

1. Flexion
2. Posterior subluxation
3. Lateral subluxation
4. Lateral rotation
5. Abduction of tibia

The above deformities are due to spasm and contractures of the hamstring muscles.

Clinical Features

The disease is insidious in onset, showing systemic and local features of tuberculosis. The joint shows effusion and evidence of synovial hypertrophy. The swelling is white in colour. There is tenderness along the joint line and synovial reflections. During the synovial stage, the movements are reduced and painful. In the arthritis stage (Figs 39.20A to C), the

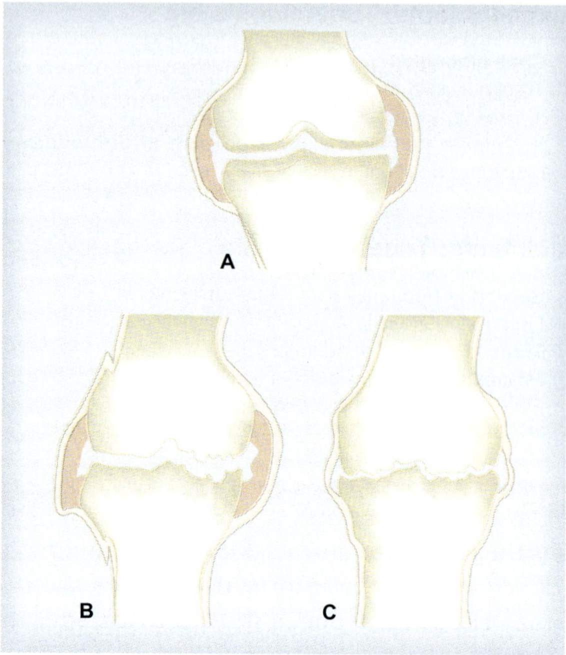

Figs 39.20A to C: Showing stages of TB knee: (A) synovitis, (B) early arthritis, and (C) advanced arthritis fibrous ankylosis

joint movements are grossly restricted with painful spasm. There is gross quadriceps atrophy and lymphadenopathy. In the growing child, transient limb lengthening may be seen due to juxta-epiphyseal hyperaemia.

In advanced stages of the disease, triple deformity (actually it is quadruple deformity) is seen (see box). The pathomechanics of the development of this deformity is interesting:

- To accommodate for the increased swelling due to synovitis, the knee joint assumes the flexion attitude as it is the position of ease and maximum capacity
- External rotation deformity develops as the patient keeps the lower limb externally rotated from the hip
- In this position, gravity assisted ITB contracture subluxates the tibiofibular joint
- Next due to the action of the biceps femoris and ITB, the tibiofibular joint rotates externally
- The above deforming forces further pull the leg into valgus.

Investigations

- General investigations reveal the chronicity of the infection.
- Radiographs show osteoporosis in the bones adjacent to the joint. In advanced stages there is reduction of the joint spaces (Fig. 39.21).
- Biopsy gives definitive diagnosis and the material is obtained either by incisional biopsy, aspiration cytology or by needle biopsy.

Treatment

Non-operative treatment This is indicated in children and in the stage of synovitis. It consists of chemotherapy, traction, and joint aspiration. Skin traction helps to prevent triple deformity, corrects the deformities and to keep the joint surfaces distracted.

Surgical treatment

- In the synovial stage, if the disease is not responding favourably, arthrotomy and partial synovectomy are done.
- In the stage of early arthritis synovectomy, joint debridement and curettage of the juxta-articular foci are carried out.
- In advanced arthritis, arthrodesis is the treatment of choice and the indications being, advanced tuberculosis, triple deformity, gross instability and painful ankylosis after earlier synovectomy.

Supracondylar osteotomy is preferred in varus or valgus deformity. Arthroplasty is also being tried without much success.

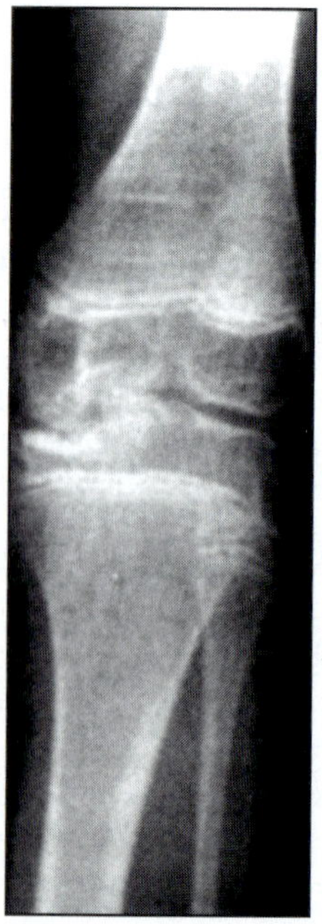

Fig. 39.21: Radiograph showing tuberculosis of the knee

Quick facts: Treatment of tuberculosis knee

Synovitis
- Chemotherapy
- Traction
- Joint aspiration

When active symptoms decrease
- Active and assisted exercises
- Crutch walking after 12 weeks for 6 to 12 months
- Protected weight bearing for 18 to 24 months
- If disease is not responding favourably, arthrotomy and synovectomy done

Early arthritis
- Synovectomy
- Joint debridement
- Curettage of juxta-articular foci

Postoperative regimen
- Drug therapy
- Traction
- Exercises
- Suitable braces

Advanced arthritis

Arthrodesis (advantages)
- Stable knee
- Disease foci eliminated
- Corrects deformity
- Painless knee

Charnley's compression arthrodesis
- Diseased tissue clearance
- Compression pin removed at 4 weeks
- Patient is encouraged to walk after 4 weeks

Role of supracondylar osteotomy This is indicated in the following situations—where the disease has healed with painless range of movements in an unacceptable position and in valgus or varus deformity.

TUBERCULOSIS OF THE SHOULDER

This is quite uncommon and accounts for only 2 per cent of the cases. It is more common in adults. Incidence of concomittant pulmonary tuberculosis is high. The tuberculosis of the shoulder could start in any one of the following sites:

1. Synovium
2. Glenoid
3. Head of humerus.

Pathology

Same as in other forms of skeletal tuberculosis.

Clinical Features

Tuberculosis of the shoulder rarely presents at the stage of synovitis. Abduction and external rotation movements of the shoulder are grossly decreased. There is wasting of the deltoid and supraspinatus muscles. *Common variety is dry type and is called as caries sicca since there is no effusion into the joint.*

Cold abscess formed could present at:

1. Supraspinous fossa
2. Deltoid
3. Biceps.

Late stages In the late stages, destruction of the upper end of humerus and glenoid cavity are seen. Fibrous ankylosis is the end result.

Radiology

Radiographs show generalised rarefaction, articular cartilage erosion, cavities in the head of the humerus and little periosteal reaction. In the advanced cases, there is inferior subluxation of the humeral head (Fig. 39.22).

Treatment

Treatment is essentially as in other forms of tuberculosis. Chemotherapy is the mainstay of treatment. The shoulder is immobilised in saluting position (70 to 90° in abduction and 30° in flexion) to encourage ankylosis in functional position. The

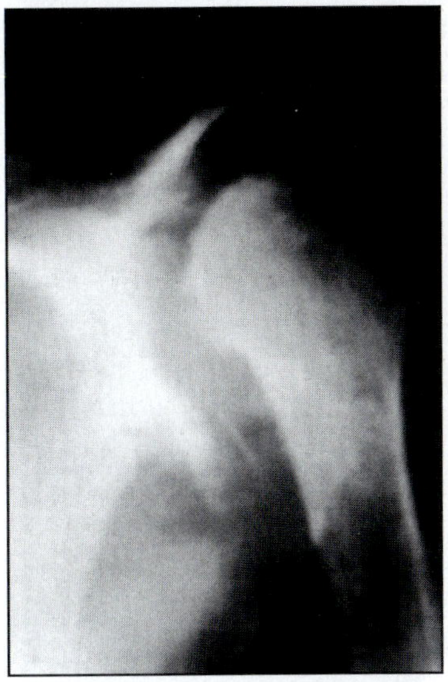

Fig. 39.22: Radiograph showing tuberculosis of the shoulder

shoulder is put in abduction frame after 3 months. As a rule, sufficient compensatory movements develop at the scapulothoracic joint. Generally, a sound fibrous ankylosis develops and since this is a non-weight bearing joint, a sound fibrous joint is acceptable.

Indications for arthrodesis are painful ankylosis, uncontrolled disease, recurrence, etc.

TUBERCULOSIS OF THE ANKLE

This is very uncommon, and the incidence is only 5 per cent. Sites of involvement could be:

1. Synovium
2. Distal end of tibia
3. Malleoli
4. Talus
5. Rarely calcaneum.

Clinical Features

Pain in the region of the ankle, limp, swelling over and front of the joint, malleoli and tendo-Achilles. Ankle joint is held in plantar flexion. In the late cases, there is pathological anterior dislocation of the ankle joint. Ankle movements are decreased. There is gross wasting of calf muscles, and evidence of sinus formation.

Radiology

Radiographs in the early stages show marked osteoporosis of the ankle bones and in late stages there is destruction of ankle joint (Fig. 39.23).

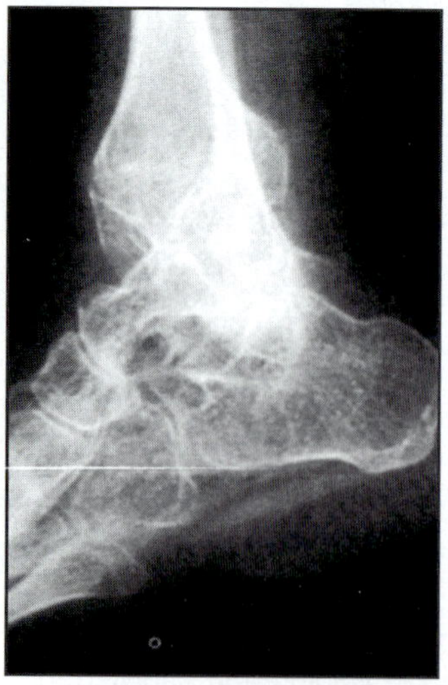

Fig. 39.23: Radiograph showing tuberculosis of the ankle

Treatment

Aim Here, the aim is to achieve painless ankylosis in neutral position of the ankle. This is achieved by observing the following principles. Chemotherapy is as already discussed, immobilisation in below-knee plaster cast in neutral position, crutch walking for first 8 to 12 weeks with plaster on and after 6 months below-knee caliper is worn for 2 years.

Surgery

Indications

1. When the conservative treatment fails.
2. When the diagnosis is in doubt.

Methods

1. Synovectomy and joint debridement during the stages of synovitis and early arthritis.
2. Arthrodesis for advanced and persistent disease.

TUBERCULAR OSTEOMYELITIS

Here, the onset of tuberculosis foci is within the bone. Because of deficient anastomosis of the osseous arteries in the childhood, thrombosis caused by tubercular pathology may lead to sequestration of a major part of the diaphysis.

TUBERCULAR OSTEOMYELITIS WITHOUT JOINT INVOLVEMENT

This can occur in any of the long tubular bones and the incidence is 2 to 3 per cent and 7 per cent occurs at multiple sites.

Clinical Features

The patient complains of pain in the affected bone. Swelling is warm and tender. There may be cold abscess or sinus formation or ulcer may be present. Enlargement of regional lymph nodes are seen.

Radiology

Radiographs of anteroposterior and lateral views of the affected part show irregular cavities, little sclerosis (honeycomb appearance), and soft tissue swelling.

SPINA VENTOSA TYPE

In these cavities contain soft feathery sequestra. Subperiosteal new bone formation is present. If it is complicated by sinus or secondary infection, intense reactive sclerosis, sequestra and pathological fractures are seen.

Tuberculosis of long tubular bones The incidence is 3 per cent and occurs in metaphysiodiaphyseal junction. It may also start as a diaphyseal lesion.

Disseminated skeletal This is very rare with 7 per cent incidence only. It may be due to haematogenous spread or may be due to repeated impregnations at different sites. Rarely, it may present as multiple cystic lesions called as *osteitis tuberculosa multiplex cystioides.*

Treatment Chemotherapy is the mainstay of treatment and radiographs are taken once in 6 months (Fig 39.24).

Tuberculosis of short tubular bones This involves metacarpals and metatarsals. In phalanges it is uncommon after the age of 5 years. This is called tuberculosis dactylitis (Fig. 39.25). *Hand is more frequently involved than foot.* Due to lavish blood flow through a large nutrient artery entering almost in the middle of the bone.

- The first inoculum of infection is lodged in the centre of marrow cavity, which leads to a spindle-shaped expansion of bone called *spina ventosa.*

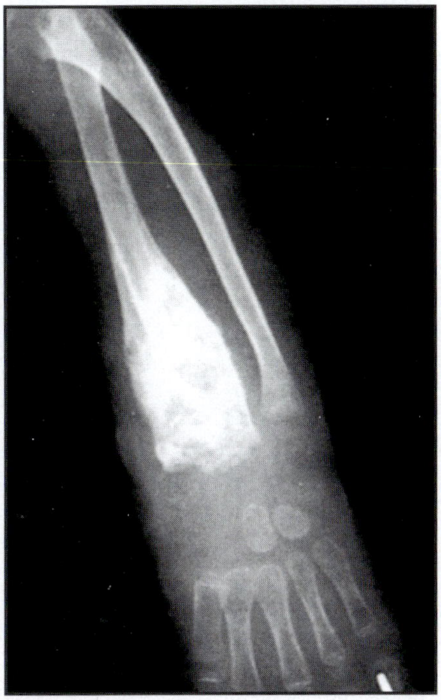

Fig. 39.24: Radiograph showing TB distal third of radius

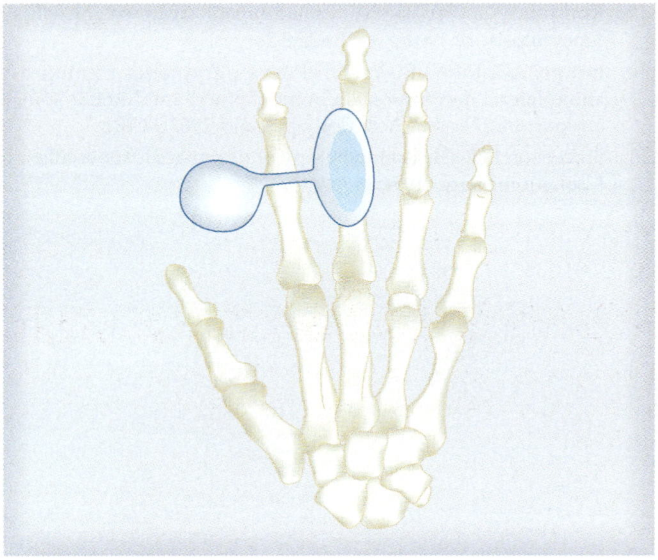

Fig. 39.25: Showing tubercular dactylitis

- There is subperioseal new bone formation, abscesses and sinus formation are also seen.
- Secondary infection causes further thickening of the bones.

Radiographs Features are lytic lesions in the middle of the bone, subperiosteal new bone formation is present, soft cork-like sequestra and spina ventosa honeycomb type.

Treatment

Chemotherapy is the mainstay of treatment and has been already discussed *(p. 501).*

BIBLIOGRAPHY

1. Ahm BH. Treatment of Pott's paraplegia. Acta Orthop Scand 1968;39:145.
2. Allen AR, Stenson AW. The results of combined drug therapy and early fusion in bone tuberculosis. J Bone tuberculosis, J Bone Joint Surg 1957;39-A:32.
3. Bickel WH. Tuberculosis of bones and joints. Mayo Clin Proc 1953;28:370.
4. Bosworth DM. Treatment of tuberculosis of bone and joint. Bull NY Acad Med 1959;35:167.
5. Freidman B. Chemotherapy of tuberculosis of the spine. J Bone Joint Surg 1996;48-A:451.
6. Goel MK. Treatment of Pott's paraplegia by operation. J Bone Joint Surg 1967;49-B:674.
7. Hodgson AR, Skiness OK, Leong CY. The pathogenesis of Pott's paraplegia. J Bone Joint Surg 1967;49-A:1147.
8. Hodgson AR, Stock FE. Anterior spine fusion for the treatment of tuberculosis of the spine: the operative findings and results of treatment of the first one hundred cases.

9. Konstam PG, Blevosky A. The ambulant treatment of spinal tuberculosis. Br J Surg 1961-63;50:26.
10. Longenskiold A, Riska EB. Pott's paraplegia treated by anterolateral decompression in the thoracic and lumbar spine: a report of 27 cases. Acta Orthop Scand 1967;38:181.
11. Stevenson FH. The chemotherapy of orthopaedic tuberculosis. J Bone Joint Surg 1954;36-B:5.
12. Tuli SM. Results of treatment of spinal tuberculosis by middle path regime. J Bone and Joint Surg 1975;57-B:13.
13. Tuli M, Srivastava TP, Verma BP, Sinha GP. Tuberculosis of spine. Acta Orthop Scand 1967;38:445.
14. Wilkinson MC. The treatment of tuberculosis of the spine by evacuation of of the paravertebral abscess and curettage of the vertebral bodies. J Bone and Joint Surg 1955;37-B:382.

40

Disorders of Joints (Arthritis)

- ❑ Introduction
- ❑ Infective arthritis
- ❑ Gonococcal arthritis
- ❑ Syphilis of joints
- ❑ Neuropathic joints
- ❑ Haemophilic arthritis

INTRODUCTION

Arthritis is a non-specific term denoting acute or chronic inflammation of the joint. Clinically, arthritis falls into the following groups:

1. *Osteoarthritis*
   - Primary
   - Secondary
2. *Rheumatoid arthritis*
   - Adult
   - Juvenile
3. *Infective arthritis*
   - Acute
   - Chronic
4. *Metabolic arthritis*
   - Gout
   - Pseudogout
5. *Non-specific monoarthritis*
6. *Neuropathic joint disorders*, e.g. Charcot's
7. *Special forms*:
   - Haemophilic arthritis
   - Psoriatic arthritis
   - Psychogenic arthritis.

Nearly ten per cent of the population suffer from one form of the arthritis or the other.

INFECTIVE ARTHRITIS

PYOGENIC INFECTION OF JOINT OR SEPTIC ARTHRITIS

Definition Septic arthritis is defined as a bacterial infection of the joint which causes an intense inflammatory reaction with migration of polymorphonuclear leucocytes and subsequent release of proteolytic enzymes. This could lead to destruction of the articular cartilage and later the joint.

Do you know?

Newer definition of septic arthritis
A positive synovial fluid culture or a synovial fluid WBCs count of greater than 50,000 with 75% polymorphic neutrophils and a negative lyme titre.

Causative organisms The most common offending organisms are *Staphylococcus aureus* (50%), *Streptococcus* (20%), *Pneumococcus* (10%), *Gonococcus*, *E. coli*, etc. *H. influenzae* is very common in children less than 2 years. *Blood culture is positive only in 60 per cent of cases.*

Routes of entry for organisms: 5 P's
Primary focus is in RS, GIT, etc.
Pyogenic osteomyelitis
Punctured wounds
Pneumonia, typhoid, etc.
Primary focus within the joint, absent in few.

Predisposing factors The following act as predisposing factors—trauma, diabetes, steroid therapy, malignancy, etc.

Sites of involvement of the joint

In adults

- Knee (53%)
- Hip (20%)

- Elbow (17%)
- Shoulder (10%)

In children
- Knee (39%)
- Hip (32%)

Remember

Ninety per cent of cases of septic arthritis are monoarticular and ten per cent are polyarticular.

Pathology

The following pathological events take place:
1. *Exudation into joint* This could be serous, sero-fibrinous or purulent depending upon the severity of infection.
2. *Destruction of articular cartilage* by plasmin, cathepsin, prostaglandins, etc.
3. *Capsules*, ligaments are destroyed by pus.

Clinical Features

Septic arthritis usually presents as monoarticular affection in 90 per cent and polyarticular in 10 per cent of cases and fever is seen in only 50 per cent of the cases. Limp is a common complaint (Fig. 40.1). The severity of clinical manifestation depends upon the severity of disease (Table 40.1).

Table 40.1: Types of septic arthritis

Serous	*Serofibrinous*	*Purulent*
• Pain is less • Movements of the joint ↓ • Local temperature ↑ • Flexion deformity	• Tenderness +ve • Fever +ve • Night pains +ve	• Patient is very ill • Pain +ve • Wasting +ve • Temperature ↑

Note: Nearly one-third of patients affected with bacterial arthritis suffer loss of joint function.

Investigations

Joint aspirate and synovial fluid analysis This is the most accurate diagnostic tool for septic arthritis. The synovial fluid is tested for cells, sugars and proteins. Gram staining is positive in 60 per cent of the cases for gram-positive cocci.

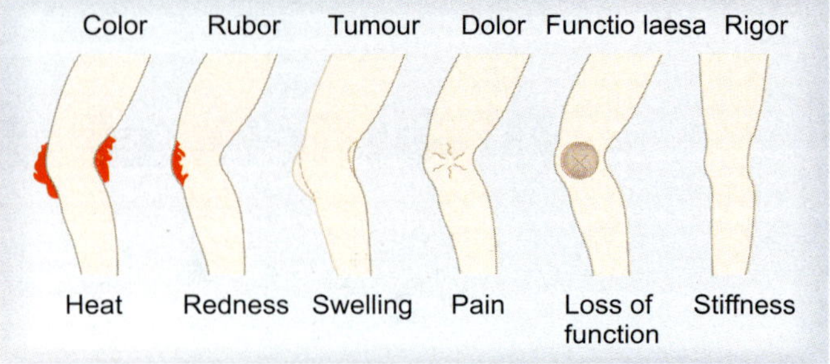

Fig. 40.1: Showing the cardinal signs of inflammation

Laboratory investigations WBCs (polymorphs) are raised to 50,000 to 1,00,000 (80% of cases), ESR increased more than 20 mm/hr (in 50% of cases), Hb percentage decreases. Blood culture is positive in 35 to 50 per cent of the cases. CRP should be done within 24 hours of presentation.

The importance of C-reactive protein (negative predictor)

If the CRP is <10 mg/dl, the probability that the patient does not have septic arthritis is 87%.

Radiology

Early stages The earliest findings in the radiographs are soft tissue swelling and periarticular osteoporosis.
Late stages In the later stages, cartilage destruction, loss of joint space, necrosis of bone, epiphyseal disturbances, fibrous ankylosis, and bony ankylosis (Figs 40.2A to C) may be seen.

Treatment

1. *Arthrotomy or joint drainage* The joint is aspirated first, if pus is present, open arthrotomy is indicated. The pus is cultured and is subjected to Gram staining. Appropriate antibiotics are then chosen and are given intravenously before surgical drainage. Antibiotics are used for a minimum period of 2 to 4 weeks.
2. *Immobilisation* of the joints by using plaster of Paris splints in functional position reduces pain.
3. *Radical treatment* is reserved for all except, for very early cases, which do not respond rapidly within 24 hours to antibiotics and immobilisation.
4. If cartilage is destroyed, aim for ankylosis in functional position by plaster casts.

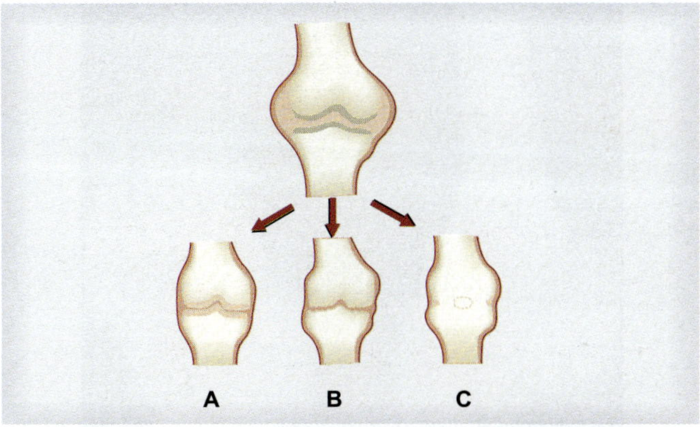

Figs 40.2A to C: Stages of septic arthritis (A) Synovitis (B) Arthritis, and (C) Bony ankylosis

Complications

1. Joint destruction (Fig. 40.2B).
2. Pathological dislocation.
3. Osteoarthritis in later years.
4. Ankylosis—fibrous or bony (Fig. 40.2C).
5. Acute osteomyelitis.
6. Amyloidosis very rarely develops.
7. Septicaemia, pyaemia, etc.

Remember

Tom Smith arthritis is a septic arthritis of the hip joint seen in infants.

Quick facts

- Sites of septic arthritis in parenteral drug abusers:
  1. Sacroiliac joint
  2. Sternal articulations
  3. Pubic symphysis
- Organisms responsible are:
  1. *Staphylococcus aureus*
  2. *Pseudomonas aeruginosa*
  3. *Serratia marcescens*
- In sickle cell anaemia, *Salmonella* is the organism causing septic arthritis
- In nail pricks *Pseudomonas aeruginosa* is the organism The most common site is the second metatarsophalangeal joint

GONOCOCCAL ARTHRITIS

The incidence of gonococcal arthritis is less than one per cent and it is familiarly known as a three weeks infection. The male to female ratio is 5:1 and the age of predeliction is between 20 and 30 years.

It usually results due to lack of treatment for gonorrhoea. Forty per cent of the cases are monoarticular, knee being the most common.

Pathology

Gonococcal arthritis can present as acute, subacute and chronic. The important pathological features are synovitis, effusion, cartilage erosion, and destruction of cartilage.

Clinical Features

Gonococcal arthritis is usually sudden in onset. The patient presents with chills, fever, pain and swelling of the joint. On examination, there is raised temperature and tenderness. There may be history of urethral discharge. The disease may become chronic due to inadequate and improper treatment.

Treatment

The treatment methods consist of local measures like splints, chemotherapy by intravenous penicillin G, rest to the part, aspiration with a thick bored needle and arthrotomy to clear the joint debris.

SYPHILIS OF JOINTS

The incidence of syphilis of the joints is definitely on the decline due to the early use of antibiotics. Syphilitic arthritis is caused by *Treponema pallidum* and can be classified as follows (Table 40.2).

Investigations

1. Wassermann's test is positive.
2. *Treponema pallidum* immobilisation test is positive.
3. Joint fluid aspiration and synovial fluid analysis—for cell, sugar, protein, etc.

Treatment

Antisyphilitic treatment is done but, it is often not successful.

Table 40.2: Showing classification of syphilitic arthritis

Congenital	*Acquired*
1. **Parrot's syphilitic joint** *Features* • Epiphysitis • Effusion • Separation of epiphysis 2. **Clutton's joints** *Features* • Symmetrical • Hydrarthrosis • Painless • 8 to 16 years of age	**Early** a. Arthralgia • Secondary stage of syphilis • Nocturnal pain is present • Spasm of muscles b. Hydrarthrosis • Serous synovitis • Symmetrical involvement c. Gummatous arthritis • Synovial form • Osseous form usually affects the knee, resembles osteoarthritis, painless polyarthritis, etc. d. Charcot's joint is a neuropathic joint

NEUROPATHIC JOINTS ([1]CHARCOT'S)

This causes extensive destruction of the joint as it is painless. The following are some of the important causes of neuropathic joints.

1. Syringomyelia (25%)
2. Tabes dorsalis (4–10%)
3. Syphilis
4. Rheumatoid arthritis
5. Intra-articular steroids
6. Traumatic division of sciatic nerve
7. Chronic liver disease
8. Prolonged administration of drugs like indomethacin, etc.

Sites Knee, ankle, hip, elbow, shoulder, wrist and intervertebral joints in that order. It is rare before 40 years.

Pathology

The following are the pathological changes seen in the joint—gross destruction of the joint, the capsules are thickened, osteophyte formation is seen, joint cavity is distorted and the loose bodies are present.

Pathological stages (Brailford's stages)

1. Stage of hydrarthrosis
2. Stage of atrophy
3. Stage of hypertrophy.

Clinical Features

In this condition premonitory signs are rare, onset is usually sudden and unexpected. Gross swelling and lax joint are commonly seen.

In the later stages of the disease, the following features are seen—lax joints, *striking absence of pain*, joint becomes flail and there is a diffuse erythema around the joints.

Radiograph

Gross destruction of the joints is cleary visualised in plain X-rays (Fig. 40.3).

Treatment

The treatment of choice is Charnley's compression arthrodesis but efficient bracing still has a major role to play (Figs 40.4A and B).

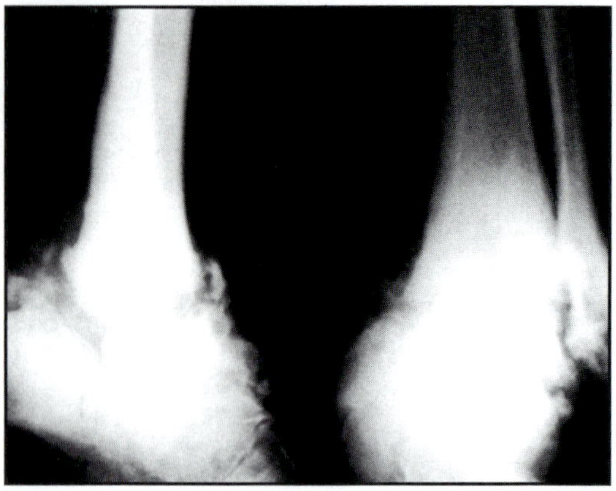

Fig. 40.3: Radiograph showing neuropathic ankle joint

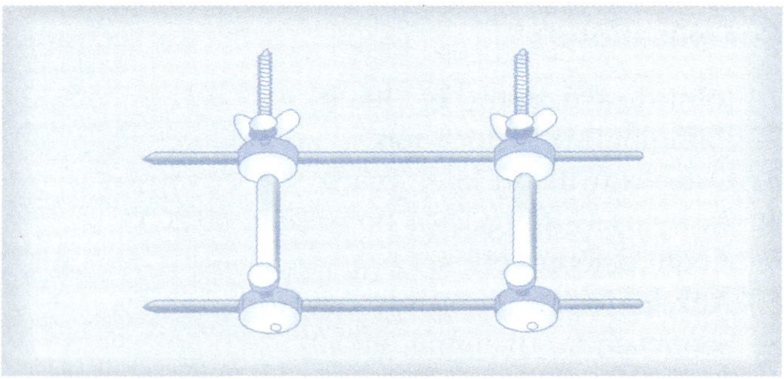

Fig. 40.4A: Showing Charnley's compression clamp with 2 pins

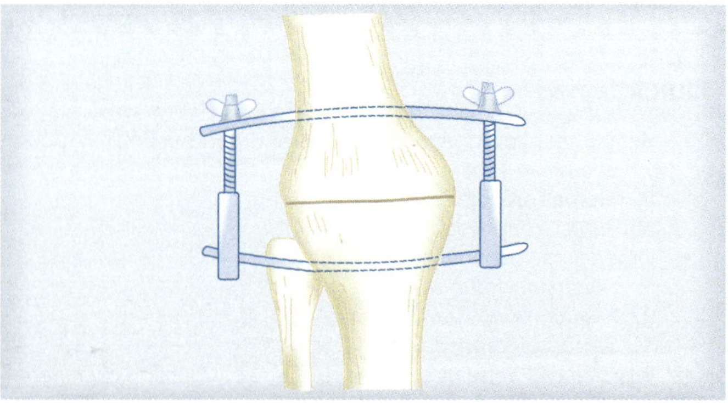

Fig. 40.4B: Showing Charnley's compression arthrodesis

HAEMOPHILIC ARTHRITIS

BLEEDER'S JOINTS

Definition It is a hereditary coagulative disorder characterised by haemorrhages, which is spontaneous and is due to trivial trauma. It is X-linked, carried by female, manifest in male, cause being *prolonged clott-*

[1]**Jean Martin Charcot** (1825-1893) of Paris. He first distinguished between gout and rheumatoid arthritis and Charcot's joints.

ing time. Table 40.3 shows different types of haemophilia.

Incidence is 3 to 4 per one lakh population.

Severity of factor VIII deficiency and the clinical effects is shown in Table 40.4.

Table 40.3: Types of haemophilia

Haemophilia A	80 per cent cases due to ↓ factor VIII
Haemophilia B	15% due to ↓ factor IX (Christmas disease)
Haemophilia C	Both male and female affected. Autosomal dominant
von Willebrand's disease	Both platelets and factor VIII are deficient

Table 40.4: Deficiency of factor VIII and its effects

< 1%	Severe bleeding
< 5%	Gross bleeding with minor trauma
< 5-25%	Severe bleeding after trauma or surgery
< 25-50%	Bleeding after excessive trauma or injury

Pathology

The defective blood interacts with the synovial fluid and causes irritation to the synovial membrane. Due to the proliferation of the macrophages, there is synovial hyperplasia and pannus formation which ultimately causes destruction of the articular cartilage of the joint (Figs 40.5A to C).

Clinical Features

Bleeding is spontaneous and is usually due to trivial trauma. Acute haemarthrosis occurs within hours. The joint is warm, tender and flexion attitude develops. Acute phase lasts for a few weeks. With each attack joint movement decreases, fixed flexion deformity occurs, degenerative arthritis sets in and results in fibrous ankylosis. There is gross muscle atrophy.

Investigations

Plain X-ray: Based on the radiological findings, haemophilia arthritis can be graded into three stages (Table 40.5).

MRI: This gives more information both about the soft tissues and bones of the joints than the conventional radiographs.

Table 40.5: Radiological stages in haemophilia

Early stage	*Intermediate stage*	*End stage*
• Distended synovium • No para-articular skeletal abnormality	• Persistent boggy swelling • Osteoporosis of the epiphysis • Joint interval is normal • Subchondral cysts are present • Squaring of the patella • Intercondylar notch of femur and trochlear notch of ulna widened	• Joint disorganised • Subchondral cysts are large • Fibrous ankylosis is present

Laboratory Tests

The classical feature of this disease is: bleeding time is normal, but the clotting time is prolonged.

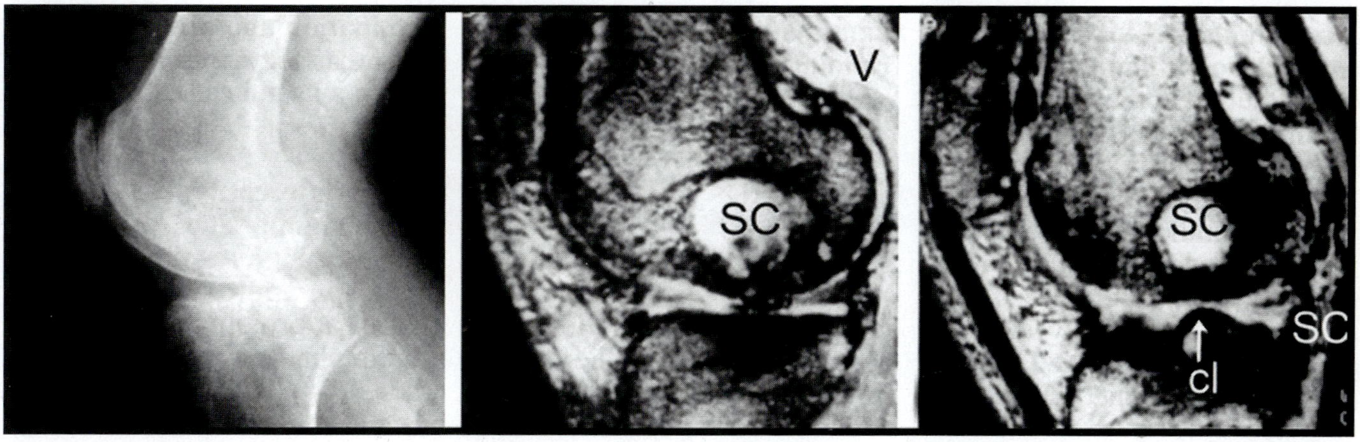

Figs 40.5A to C: Showing haemophilic arthritis of the knee: (A) Radiograph, (B and C) MRI

Section 5

Prothrombin time and other routine laboratory investigations need to be done.

Treatment

This varies according to the stages of the disease.

Acute stage

a . For injuries of less than four hours, the patient is treated on OPD basis. Factor VIII is replaced and is discharged home on the same day.

b. For injuries more than four hours, factor VIII is replaced, joint is aspirated with a thick bored needle and immobilised with splints.

If resolution	Recurrence
Occurs • Patient is mobilised • Caliper wear is suggested	• Factor replacement is done • Immobilisation is carried out • Aspiration is done

Late cases Treated as in patient, trial aspiration is done, prolonged immobilisation, factor VIII is replaced and later mobilisation, caliper and splints are recommended.

Chronic haemarthropathy

1. *For recent contractures*: Plaster immobilisation, dynamic traction and physiotherapy.
2. *For postsubluxation of tibia*: Dynamic traction.
3. *For painful unstable joints*: Orthotic splintage.
4. *Surgery* is indicated for painful, stiff joints, stiff contractures, and recurrent bleeding into the joint.

Surgical methods These include synovectomy and internal fixations for fracture nonunion. Supracondylar osteotomy for severe flexion contractures of knee, arthrodesis for severely disorganised joints, total hip replacement for pain in the hip in advanced stages and tendo-Achilles lengthening for tendo-Achilles contractures, etc.

41

Rheumatic Diseases

INTRODUCTION

There is a tendency among the students and most of the clinicians to label all cases of polyarthralgia as rheumatoid arthritis. Though there is no dispute about the fact that the most common cause of polyarthritis is rheumatoid, yet not all cases of polyarthritis is rheumatoid. There are a plethora of conditions with this presentation. Rheumatoid and its variants are infamous in creating diagnotic dilemmas. Difficult to diagnose and difficult to treat, it is indeed a problem which presents a nightmarish experience both to the doctor and the patient.

We are all familiar with the saying regarding rheumatic fever, "It licks the joint but bites the heart."Contrarily, it can be said of rheumatoid arthritis, "It bites the joints, licks all other systems of the body and barks at the treating physicians!"

A chronic scourge which writes the obituary of the joints, especially those of hands and feet, rheumatoid arthritis is a problem which needs to be understood *in toto* to successfully combat it and keep it subdued and improve the quality of those unfortunate victims afflicted by this malady.

The rheumatic diseases embrace an amazing array of hereditary and acquired disorders with a wide variety of clinical features. As per the present understanding, rheumatic disorders can be classified under three broad headings.

CLASSIFICATION

Diffuse systemic

- Rheumatoid arthritis
- Seronegative spondyloarthritis
- Systemic lupus erythematosus (SLE)
- Polymyositis
- Scleroderma.

Localised articular

- Osteoarthritis
- Crystal-induced arthritis
- Traumatic arthritis.

Non-articular

- Fibromyalgia
- Low back pain
- Tenosynovitis.

RHEUMATOID ARTHRITIS

Definition Rheumatoid arthritis is the ***most common*** inflammatory disease of the joints. It is a systemic disease of young and middle-aged adults characterised by proliferative and destructive changes in synovial membrane, periarticular structures, skeletal muscles and perineural sheaths. Eventually, joints are destroyed, fibrosed or ankylosed. *It is a widespread vasculitis of the small arterioles.*

Incidence is 3 per cent.

Sex Eighty per cent affected are women; Male:Female ratio is 1:3

Age No age is exempt, mean age is 40 years.

Aetiology

The exact cause is unknown, but malfunction of the cellular and humoral arms of the immune system are cited as the probable cause.

Current hypothesis An initiating antigen triggers an aberrant response, which becomes self-perpetuating long after the offending antigen has been cleared.

Antigenic agents Which probably act as predisposing factors are viruses: rubella, Epstein-Barr, etc. genetic (common in people with HLA DR_4 60%), psychological stress, allergic factors, endocrine factors and metabolic factors.

Pathogenic Spectrum (Fig. 41.1)

Against unknown exciting antigenic agents rheumatoid factors are elaborated. Rheumatoid factors are synthesised in rheumatoid synovial tissue and are mainly IgM in 70 to 90 per cent of cases. In the remainder 10 to 30 per cent, it could be IgG, IgA or IgE. This rheumatoid factor along with IgG triggers off a compliment cascade. The WBCs engulf this immune complex and elaborate lysosomes. Neutrophils release procollagenase which is converted into an active collagenase by the synovial fluid. This splits the collagen of the articular cartilage. The neutral proteases complete the degradation of the collagen fibrils.

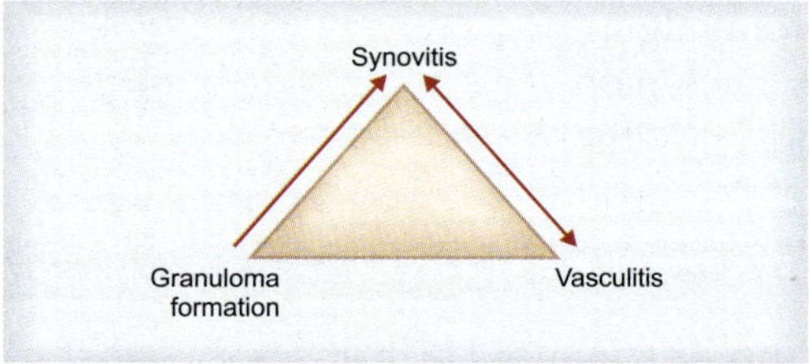

Fig. 41.1: Rheumatoid arthritis = Synovitis + Vasculitis + Granuloma

Pathology

As explained earlier, due to the synthesis of auto-antibodies, against unknown antigenic agents in the synovium, primary synovitis sets in (Fig. 41.2). This primary synovitis gives rise to pannus, which in turn forms the villus. This villus migrates towards the joint causing its destruction and ankylosis, fibrous in the early stages followed by bony ankylosis in the late stages.

Microscopy It reveals rheumatoid units which is an area of fibrinoid necrosis surrounded by fibroblasts arranged radially and it is surrounded by a fibrous capsule. This rheumatoid unit is found in the muscle, vessels, nerves, synovium, etc. Vasculitis is widespread, and commonly affects the arterioles. Muscles show nodular polymyositis. Subcutaneous nodules

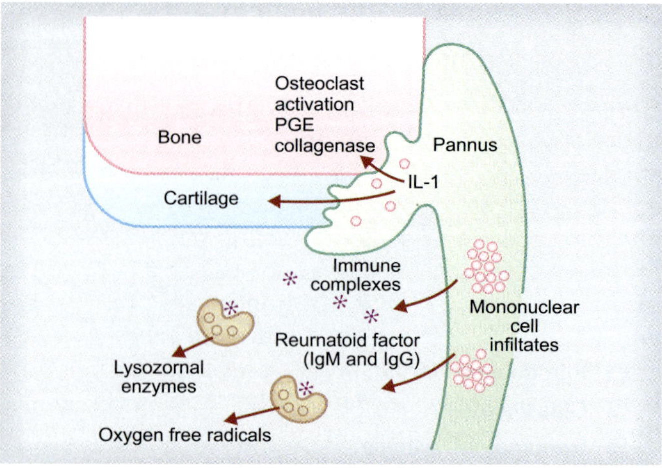

Fig. 41.2: Pathogenesis in rheumatoid arthritis

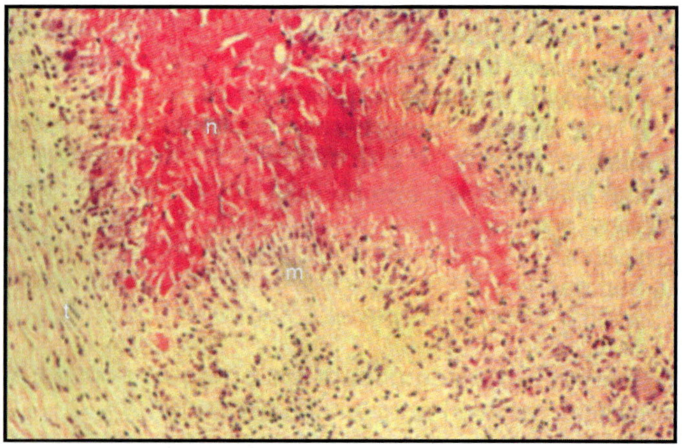

Fig. 41.3: Microscopic features of rheumatoid arthritis subcutaneous nodule

(Fig. 41.3) are made up of central necrotic area, palisade formation by mononuclear cells, round cell infiltration and fibrous capsule. Lymph nodes show hyperplasia. Nerves show perineural necrosis or fibrosis and heart rarely shows changes unlike in rheumatic fever.

Recent diagnostic criteria for rheumatoid arthritis

According to the American College of Rheumatology in 1987 revised criteria at least 4 out of 7 criteria should be fulfilled to make a diagnosis of rheumatoid arthritis.

- Morning stiffness for minimum one hour every day, at least for six weeks.
- Arthritis or swelling of 3 or more joints for > 6 weeks.
- Arthritis or swelling of hand joints (wrist, metacarpal) for more than 6 weeks.
- Symmetrical swelling (arthritis of same joint areas) more than 6 weeks.
- Serum rheumatoid factor present.
- Radiographic features of RA.
- Rheumatoid nodules.

Clinical Features in Rheumatoid Arthritis

Rheumatoid arthritis usually presents in three forms:

Classical presentation In this group, the patient is usually a woman in her mid-30s. Pain, swelling, stiffness of the small joints of hands and feet are the common presenting complaints. The patient also gives history of weight loss, lethargy and depression. Joint swelling could be symmetrical and the patient presents with deformities of bones and joints in the late stages. *The patient gives history of remissions and exacerbation of symptoms with seasonal variations.* This is a very classical complaint in the absence of which diagnosis of rheumatoid arthritis should be carefully made. Symptoms fluctuate from day to day.

Other presentations This consists of palindromic presentation involving one or two joints, systemic presentation—usually seen in middle-aged men presenting with pleurisy, pericarditis, etc. It mimicks malignancy. It may present as polymyalgia particularly in elderly patients. It may present as monoarthritic swelling. Sometimes the presentation may be very explosive unlike the usual chronic presentation.

Extra-articular features Two or more features are present in 75 per cent of the cases. Rheumatoid factor is invariably present and indicates a bad prognosis.

1. Subcutaneous nodules are present in 25 per cent of the cases. It is seen over the elbow, sacrum and occiput. Nodules may also be present in lungs, eye, hearts, etc. When present over flexor tendon, it may cause trigger finger.
2. Widespread vasculitis.
3. Blood abnormalities commonly encountered in rheumatoid arthritis are chronic anaemia, iron deficiency anaemia, vitamin B_{12} and folate deficiency, leucocytopenia, thrombocytosis and marrow hypoplasia.
4. Osteoporosis could be generalised or localised in bones around the joints.
5. Eye changes seen in rheumatoid arthritis are keratoconjunctivitis sicca or Sjögren's syndrome, episcleritis (common), scleritis (serious problem), secondary glaucoma and scleromalacia perforans.
6. Lung affections in rheumatoid arthritis are pleurisy, pleural effusion, Caplan's syndrome (RA + pneumoconiosis involving the upper lobes) and fibrosing alveolitis in 2 per cent.
7. Heart affections in rheumatoid arthritis are pericardial friction (10%), pericardial effusion (30%), arrhythmias and heart block.
8. Neuromuscular system involvement includes carpal tunnel syndrome, mononeuritis multiplex, muscle wasting, subluxation of C_1 and C_2, etc.
9. Reticuloendothelial system affections include splenomegaly (5%), Felty's syndrome in 1% (RA+ splenomegaly + Neutropenia), generalised lymphadenopathy and painless pitting oedema of the feet and ankles.

ORTHOPAEDIC DEFORMITIES IN RHEUMATOID ARTHRITIS

Rheumatoid arthritis can affect any joint in the body. *It involves the peripheral joints more often and very rarely affects the larger joints.* Of particular importance are the affection of the temporomandibular joint and atlantoaxial joint which can prove lethal due to the cord compression (Fig. 41.4). Figure shows frequency of invovlement of various joints in rheumatoid arthritis.

Quick facts

Joints involved in rheumatoid arthritis

- Metacarpophalangeal and interphalangeal joints of the hand.
- Shoulder elbow and wrists.
- Hip, knee and ankle.

Others: Temporomandibular joint, atlantoaxial joints and facet joints of the cervical spine.

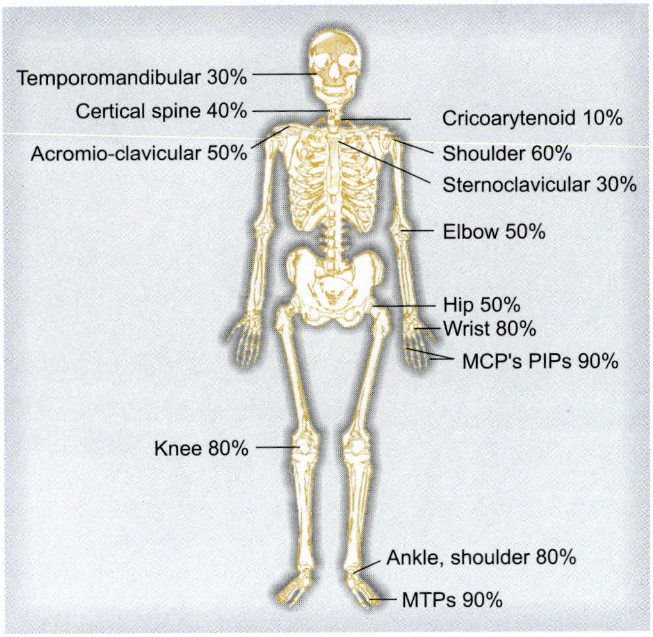

Fig. 41.4: Showing frequency of involvement of different joint sites in established RA

Section 5

Orthopaedic deformities of the hand (rheumatoid hand) The following are some of the very common deformities seen in the hand (Figs 41.5A to C).

a. *Symmetrical peripheral joint swelling* of metacarpophalangeal and interphalangeal joints (Fig. 41.5A).
b. *Ulnar deviation* of the hand is due to rupture of the collateral ligaments at the metacarpophalangeal joints which enables the extensor tendons to slip from their grooves towards the ulnar side (Figs 41.6A and B).
c. *Boutonniere's deformity* is due to the rupture of central extensor expansion of the fingers resulting in flexion at the PIP joint (see Fig. 41.5C).
d. *Swan neck deformity* is due to the rupture of the volar plate of the PIP joints which enables the tendons to slip towards the dorsal side. This is also known as *intrinsic plus deformity*. Here there is hyperextension of the PIP joint and flexion of the DIP joints.
e. *Trigger fingers and trigger thumb are* due to nodules over the tendons.
f. Z-deformity of the thumb.
g. Subluxation and dislocation of metacarpophalangeal joints.

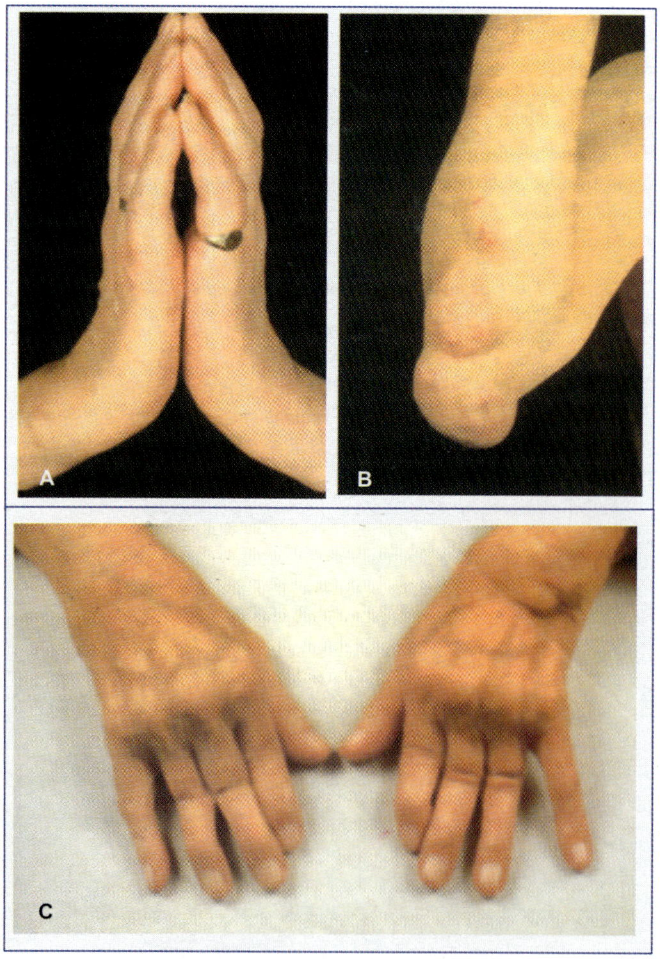

Figs 41.5A to C: Showing rheumatic features of the hand and the elbow

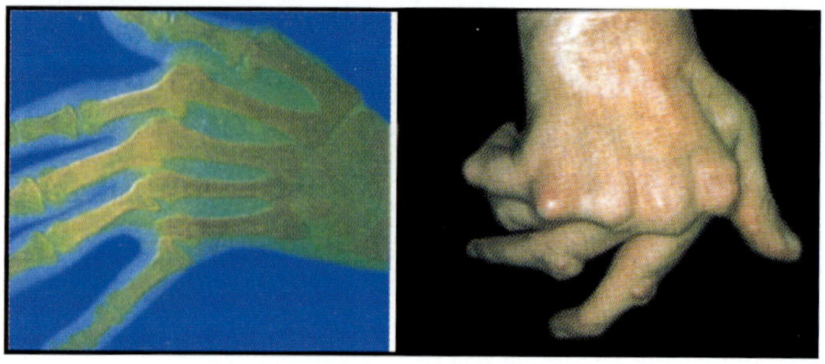

Figs 41.6A and B: Showing rheumatoid hand

Rheumatoid foot It affects the forefoot, midfoot and hindfoot. In the forefoot, the patient may develop hallux valgus deformity of the great toe, claw toes, callosity over the dorsum and the sole, widening of the forefoot, etc. The heel may show valgus deformity.

Ninety per cent of patients with rheumatoid arthritis of long-standing duration have foot deformities. Forefoot is more commonly affected than the hindfoot (Also see box).

Vital facts: About foot deformities in rheumatoid arthritis:

- Callosity under PIP joint
- Plantar callosity
- Atrophy of plantar metatarsal fat pad
- Prominent metatarsal head
- Excessive plantar tilt of metatarsals
- Claw toes
- Hammer toes
- Rheumatoid nodules
- Calcaneal erosions
- Achilles tendinitis
- Flattening of longitudinal arch
- Bunion
- Hallux valgus
- Overriding of second and third toes
- Splaying of forefoot due to divergent metatarsals.

Section 5

Other joints In the knee initially there is a gross soft tissue swelling due to synovitis; and in the later stages, the patient may develop fibrous ankylosis or bony ankylosis due to widespread destruction of the articular cartilage by the pannus. Similarly, other major joints of the body like the hip, ankle, shoulder, elbow could be involved.

Do you know the frequency of joint involvement in rheumatoid arthritis? (see Fig. 41.14)

- MCP/MTP/PIP joints — 90%
- Knee, ankle and wrist — 80%
- Shoulder — 60%
- Hip, elbow, acromion — 50%
- Cervical spine — 40%
- Temporomandibular and sternomastoid joints — 30%
- Cricoarytenoid joint — 10%

Note: Characteristically distal interphalangeal joint and sacroiliac joint are not involved in rheumatoid arthritis.

Investigation

Laboratory Hb percentage is low and shows normochromic, hypochromic anaemia. WBCs are decreased or normal, there is increased lymphocytes and the ESR is raised.

Serological tests

Basis Rheumatoid patient's serum contains RA factor which in the presence of γ-globulin agglutinates certain strains of streptococci sensitised by sheep cells and latex particles.

a. *Latex fixation test* Unknown serum + 7-globulin latex suspension

Agglutination
↓
- ↓ +ve when serum has abundant RAF
- ↓ If -ve, do more sensitive test as there is less rheumatoid arthritis factor in the serum

b. *Inhibition test* This test uses the characteristics of euglobulin from unknown serum. Euglobulin from normal serum neutralises the rheumatoid factor thereby inhibiting agglutination.

Euglobulin from rheumatoid serum have no effect on the rheumatoid factor and agglutination occurs. *This is the most sensitive test*. Positive even when rheumatoid arthritis factor is present in minute amounts.

RA serum of known high agglutinating activity
+
Unknown euglobulin
+
Standard 7- globulin latex suspension.
Agglutination's occurs
↓
Unknown serum → -ve latex test
→ +ve inhibition test
↓
- ↓ RA
- ↓ SLE (LE cell phenomenon)

Remember

RA factor is found in:

- 75 per cent of rheumatoid arthritis cases
- 10 per cent in healthy elderly people
- 10 per cent in malaria, etc.

Radiological Features of Rheumatoid Arthritis (Fig. 41.7)

- Soft tissue swelling.
- Juxta-articular osteoporosis.
- Erosion of joint margins.
- Joint spaces are decreased.
- Deformities.
- Atlantoaxial subluxation.
- Subchondral erosions and cyst formation.
- Fibrous and bony ankylosis develop in the late stages.

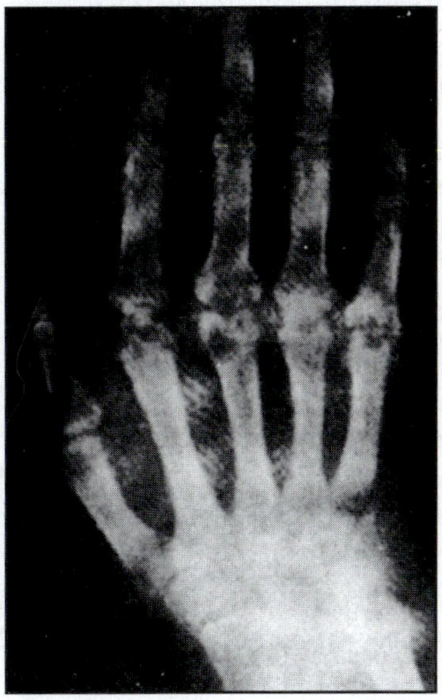

Fig. 41.7: Radiograph showing features of rheumatoid arthritis

Other common abnormalities These include increased C-reactive protein (CRP), increased alkaline phosphatase, increased platelets, and decreased serum albumin.

Synovial fluid analysis This is not performed routinely for diagnostic purposes but performed to exclude other causes of inflammation such as infection.

Synovial fluid in RA is typically yellow, watery and turbid due to high WBC and has a low sugar content.

MRI This gives valuable information about the various soft tissue damages in rheumatoid with far more greater accuracy (Fig. 41.8).

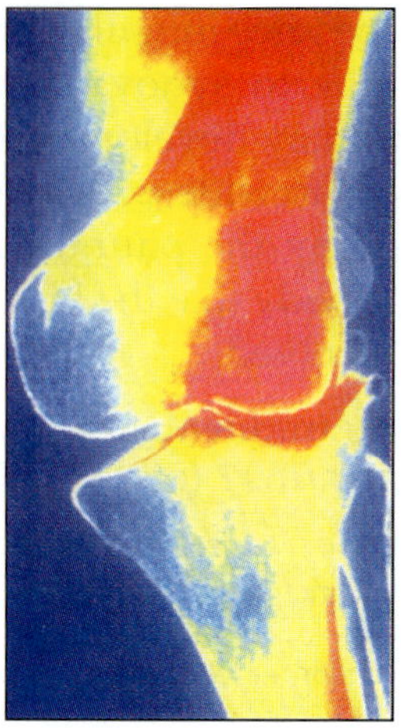

Fig. 41.8: MRI rheumatoid knee

Differential Diagnosis

Differential diagnosis of rheumatoid arthritis with various other conditions is shown in Table 41.1. However, for the differential diagnosis of rheumatoid arthritis with the all important osteoarthritis (see Table 41.2).

Quick facts of rheumatoid arthritis

- Most common chronic inflammatory disorder.
- 80 per cent in women.
- Exact cause is not known.
- Rheumatoid unit is present.
- History of remissions and exacerbations present.
- Symmetrical peripheral joint involvement.
- Rheumatoid arthritis factor is +ve in 70 per cent.
- Inhibition test is most sensitive.
- Extra-articular features are seen in 75 per cent.

Table 41.1: Differential diagnosis of rheumatoid arthritis

Early disease	*Established disease*
Common	*Common*
• Viral arthropathy	• Psoriatic arthritis
• Polymyalgia	• Erosive osteoarthritis
• Infection	• Chronic pyrophosphate disease
• Prodrome of hepatitis	• Chronic tophaceous gout
• Hypoparathyroidism	• SLE
	• Reiter's syndrome
	• Ankylosing spondylitis
Rare	*Rare*
• Sarcoidosis	• Amyloid arthropathy
• Acute leukaemia	• Multicentric reticulohistiocytosis
• Coeliac disease	
• Eosinophilic fascitis	

Management (Fig. 41.9)

Aims of treatment

1. To keep inflammatory process at a minimum, thereby, preserving joint motion, maintaining healthy muscles and preventing secondary joint stiffness and deformity.
2. To keep constitutional symptoms at a minimum.
3. The possible deformities are anticipated and prevented by appropriate splinting.
4. *Finally, surgical measures to correct the deformities, eliminate pain and provide stability are undertaken.*

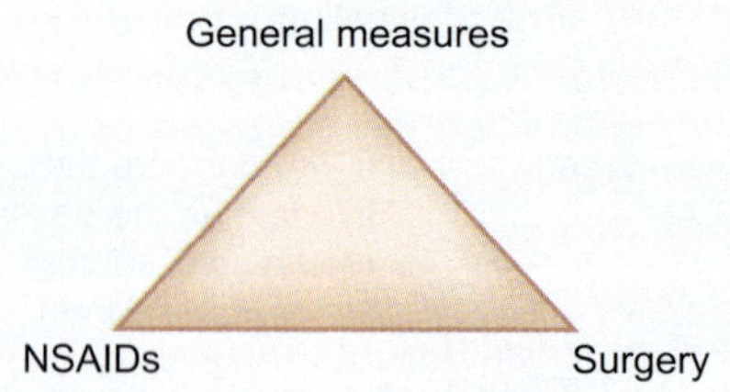

Fig. 41.9: Showing treatment triad for rheumatoid arthritis

General measures *It aims at improving the general condition of the patient and to keep the joints properly splinted in functional position to guard against the ensuing ankylosis.*

- Rest in bed.
- Good diet, rich in proteins and minerals.
- Transfusion and haematinics to correct the anaemia.
- Hormones combination of oestrogen and androgen to improve the bone stock.
- Removal of infective foci.

Splinting in the functional position helps in the event that ankylosis ensues. The splint is removed daily. Hot packs are given or the patient is placed in Hubbard tank at (92.6–102°F) and the joints are put into full range of motion.

While the joints are immobilised, muscle setting excercises are advocated. After removal of the splints, resistance exercises are begun.

Splints These are known to serve three main functions:

- Rest and relief of pain *(rest splints).*
- Prevention and correction of deformity *(corrective splints).*
- Fixation of damaged joint in a good functional position *(fixation splints).*

Drug Therapy

Three classes of drugs are used regularly.

- Analgesics
- Anti-inflammatory drugs
- Disease modifying drugs.

Steroids especially intra-articular injections have an important role.

No treatment is ideal and it is important to assess the patient's response so that the most effective regimen is adopted.

> **Commonly used methods of assessment** include; duration of early morning stiffness, number of tender swollen joints. Functional assessment, questionairres, ESR, radiographs, etc.

First Line of Drugs: NSAIDs

These are aspirin/ibuprofen/ketoprofen/diclofenac sodium naproxen/piroxicam, etc. They are the major pharmaceutical agents for pain relief in rheumatic diseases. About 20 per cent of patients admitted to the hospital are taking NSAIDs. Though useful, they have significant side effects.

Aspirin is the *drug of first choice;* but because of its undesirable side effects, other NSAIDs are chosen. But since the latter are more expensive, aspirin still remains the first choice drug.

Mechanism of action of NSAIDs They have an inhibitory action on the following pain mediating agents:

- Prostaglandin synthesis
- Leucotriene synthesis
- Lymphocyte activation
- Oxygen radical generation
- Cytokine production, etc.

Practical prescribing of NSAIDs There is no ideal NSAID. It is important to become familiar with a few of these drugs and to find the most appropriate NSAID for one particular patient. *If possible NSAIDs should be prescribed twice daily regimen, with a flexible dose to cover the main period of pain.* Initially, clinicians should prescribe NSAIDs with which they are familiar and not necessarily the latest drug.

Only one NSAID should be prescribed at one time and if the patient has not responded to an adequate dose within 2 to 3 weeks, an alternative NSAID should be given.

It is important to justify the use of NSAID, both in the short- and long-term. Other methods of pain relief should always be considered, such as exercises, heat and cold hydrotherapy.

> **Quick facts of NSAIDs**
>
> - Drugs of first choice
> - Aspirin still remains as the first choice
> - There is no ideal NSAIDs
> - Prescribe NSAID with which clinician is familiar
> - Ideal is twice daily regimen
> - Only one NSAID at a time
> - To be tried for a minimum of 2 to 3 weeks
> - NSAIDs provide only symptomatic relief.

NSAIDs provide only symptomatic relief. Most patients require daily treatment. These drugs probably do not have any influence on the disease process and may, therefore, be regarded as a background therapy with a variable daily dose according to symptoms.

Second Line of Drugs

Second line of drugs are used only if an adequate trial of first line drugs have failed to relieve symptoms satisfactorily or if there is radiological evidence of progressive disease. Second line drugs are alternatively known as *disease-modifying antirheumatic drugs (DMARD)* and are slow acting drugs. It would seem that they have influence on the underlying disease process, and may take several weeks or months to exert this effect.

To get maximum benefit, second line drug therapy should be contiued for *at least 6 months;* and in order to sustain the benefit, it needs to be continued indefinitely. They are all toxic.

When second line therapy is introduced, *symptomatic NSAIDs need to be continued in parallel.* If the response to the second line drug is good, the dose of NSAID can be reduced.

Commonly prescribed drugs include

- Injectable gold and oral gold (sodium aurothiomalate).

- Penicillamine
- Sulphasalazine
- Antimalarial drugs (e.g. chloroquine)
- Dapsone and levamisole.

The choice of the drug to be given first will depend on the experience of the prescriber and on the facilities available for monitoring. There is little evidence to suggest which drug should be prescribed first.

If after 6 months of adequate therapy, no response has been observed, an alternative drug may be tried.

At the end of a year of the treatment, 65 per cent would have improved, 35 per cent will have had to stop therapy because of toxicity or lack of therapeutic effect.

Antimalarial drugs They do not require intensive blood monitoring and if these facilities are limited, chloroquine or hydroxy chloroquine can be particularly used.

Other agents known to have second line drug effect include levamisole and dapsone. Levamisole is not freely available in some countries and its toxicity seems to be greater than that of gold and penicillamine. Dapsone has a high toxicity.

Indications of second line drugs *The ideal patient for a second line drug is one who has active synovitis with generalised inflammation in many joints, who is taking the recommended dose of the NSAID which is not producing relief of symptoms.*

Quick facts of second line drugs

- Used only if first line fails.
- Known as DMARD.
- To be continued for at least 6 months.
- Parallel NSAID is to be used.
- Choice of drugs is based on clinicians' experience.
- Antimalarial drugs are used if proper blood monitoring is not available.
- All drugs are toxic.

Third Line Drugs

Azathioprim, cyclophosphamide and chlorambucil can exert a second line effect in patients with rheumatoid arthritis. However, these drugs are considered under third line drugs because in addition to the toxicity which may arise acutely during their use, *there is also anxiety about late toxicity.* This late toxicity which may occur after prolonged therapy is an additional hazard for patients who are suffering from what is essentially a non-fatal condition. These drugs have, therefore, to be treated with respect though in selected cases they may be of benefit.

Corticosteroids Cyclosporin has been tried in patients with rheumatoid arthritis. The fact that it does not affect WBC is a theoretical advantage in patients with Felty's syndrome. Anxieties about long-term nephrotoxicity limit the use of cyclosporins to research programmes.

Newer Drugs for Rheumatoid Arthritis

- Tumour Necrosis Factor (INF α-blockers)

For example:

a. Etanarcept (25 mg/subcutaneous, twice a week)
b. Infliximab (2 mg/kg at 0,6,8 and weekly. IV infusions combined with oral methotrexate).
c. Interleukin-1-receptor antagonist (IL-IRA) Dose—100 mg/day by subcutaneous injection.

Indications

Failure of at least two standard DMARD drugs one of which is always methotrexate despite adequate trials (i.e. 6 months).

- Leflunomide (Immunomodulatory Drug)
  Indicated dose is 100 mg/day for 3 days then 20 mg/day.

LOCAL STEROIDS

Role of local corticosteroid treatment is considered when the rheumatoid arthritis affects one or two joints. It is also indicated in tendinitis, capsular or ligament involvement, carpal tunnel and compression syndromes. It is given weekly in acute cases and three monthly in chronic. *If two injections are ineffective, the treatment is discontinued.*

Surgical procedures in rheumatology Aim of surgery in rheumatoid arthritis is to:

- Relieve pain.
- Correct the deformity of the joints.
- Reduce joint instability.
- Improve the range of movements of the joints.

Surgical advice should be sought only when the disease is *clearly progressive and conservative measures are failing*, but before the patient starts to lose a significant amount of bone stock. If surgery is delayed, more bone is lost, the soft tissue deteriorates and the deformity increases.

Preoperative considerations Before surgery for rheumatoid disease, a number of specific points should be checked. Related conditions such as diabetes, hypertension and anaemia should be adequately treated and:

- Steroid dosage should be reduced.

- There should be no active infection.
- A radiograph of the cervical spine should be obtained to exclude instability.

Modus operandi of surgical procedures in rheumatoid arthritis

Synovectomy	• Failed chemotherapy • Joint destruction should be minimal • Useful in knee/ankle
Osteotomy	• Less than 60 years of age • When joint is partially damaged • Commonly done at hip (Intertrochanteric osteotomy and abduction osteotomy)
Arthrodesis	• Long-term relief • Reserved for peripheral joints where arthroplasty results in pain • Causes secondary osteoarthritis in bigger joints
Arthroplasty	• Advanced stages in hip and knee

Surgical Methods

Synovectomy It may be indicated in patients with rheumatoid arthritis if joint destruction is minimal and if the main cause of pain and swelling is synovitis, which is resistant to medication and physiotherapy. Synovectomy is usually carried out over the knee and ankle, in the elbow with radial head excision if necessary. In the wrist, dorsal synovectomy and resection of the distal end of the ulna can prevent attrition and rupture of extensor tendons. *Synovectomy has to be virtually complete to avoid regrowth with recurrence of symptoms.*

Osteotomy This should be considered in patients under the age of 60 years with osteoarthritis of the hip or knee due to rheumatoid arthritis. *Osteotomy has the advantage of relieving pain without sacrificing the joint surfaces which have only been partially damaged.*

At the hip, intertrochanteric osteotomy which contains the femoral head within the acetabulum is preferred. At the knee, abduction osteotomy is preferred.

Arthrodesis of the joint gives excellent long-term pain relief. But the stress may cause secondary OA in the adjacent joints unless they are able to compensate for the loss of movement. Lack of movement after fusion of the wrist can be absorbed at the elbow and shoulder without significant functional impairment, but fusion of the hip puts considerable strain on the spine and the knee.

Arthrodesis, therefore, tends to be preserved for peripheral joints, such as the wrist, ankle, and IP joints of the hands and feet where the functional loss is less disabling and arthroplasty is less reliable.

Arthroplasties of the hip, knee (Figs 41.10A and B), ankle, shoulder, elbow, wrist, and hand is indicated in advanced diseases causing severe pain and incapacitating disability due to stiffness and instability.

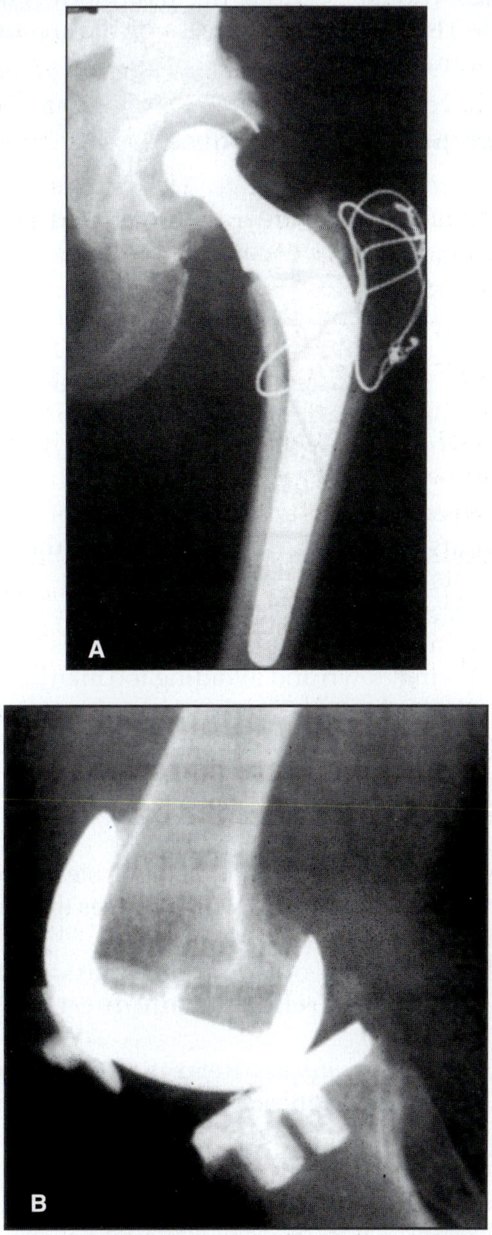

Figs 41.10A and B: Radiographs showing: (A)Total hip replacement and (B) Total knee replacement for rheumatoid arthritis of the hip and knee

Self-management Techniques for Rheumatoid and Other Forms of Arthritis

Self-management is the most important aspect of the treatment of rheumatoid and other forms of arthritis. People practicing self-management techniques tend to experience less pain and are more active than those who do not practice self-management. In this management, the patient is made aware of the disease and the rationale behind the treatment. They are made to realise that the success of the treatment is their ultimate responsibility.

The Ten Self-help Techniques

1. *Positive mental attitude*: The patient is told to focus on things other than pain and their own body. They are encouraged to think positively (Fig. 41.11).
2. *Regular medication*: The patient is told the value of regular and correct medication (Fig. 41.12).
3. *Regular exercises*: The patient should follow a regular and appropriate exercise programme, most suited for themselves (Fig. 41.13).
4. *Use of joints*: The patient is told the value of correct posture and the methods of using the joints wisely to reduce stress on the painful joints (Fig. 41.14).
5. *Energy conservation*: Patients are instructed to listen to the body's "inner signals" for rest. Slowing down and avoiding too many activities reduces the stress and strain on the joints.
6. *Assistive devices*: Devices like splints, braces and walking sticks can help stabilise the joints, provide strength and reduce pain and inflammation (Fig. 41.16).
7. *Adequate sleep*: A good adequate sleep provides rest to the ailing joints and reduces the pain and swelling (Fig. 41.17).
8. *Massage*: A good moderate massage brings warmth and relieves pain due to arthritis (Fig. 41.18).
9. *Relaxation techniques*: Relaxation techniques like yoga, meditation, etc. help to relax the muscles, mind and controls respiration, heart rate, blood pressure. This helps in the control of pain (Fig. 41.19).
10. *Modification in the daily activities*
    - Using Western toilets (Fig. 41.20)
    - Bath aids and railings
    - Long handle broomstick and mop to clean the floors (see Fig. 41.15)

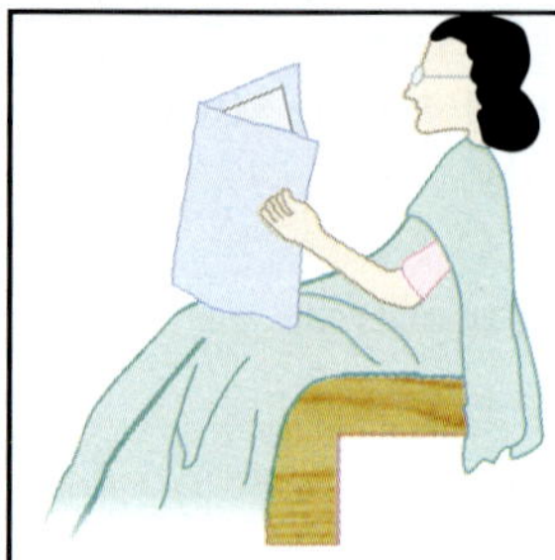
Fig. 41.11

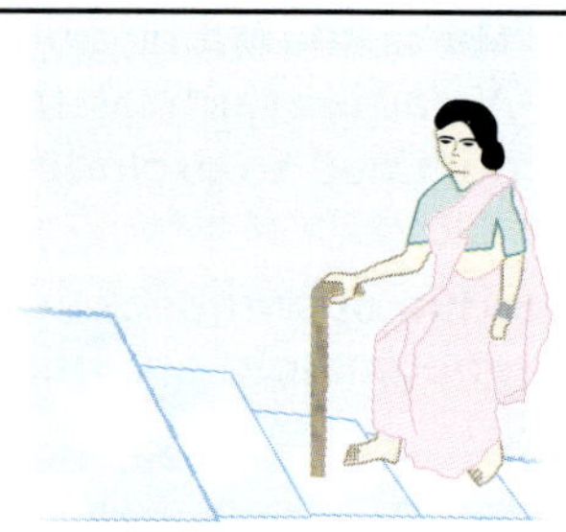
Fig. 41.16

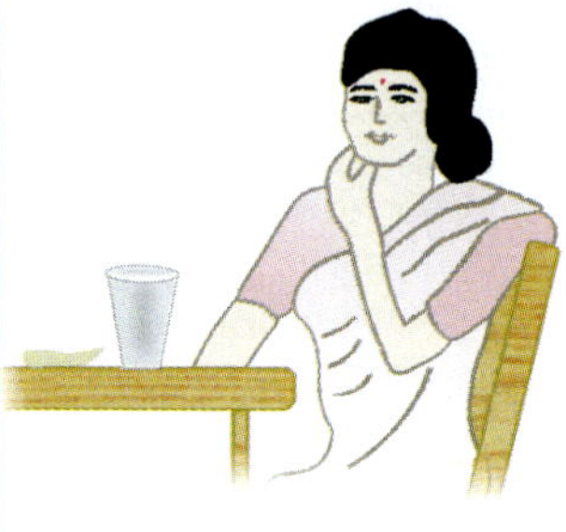
Fig. 41.12

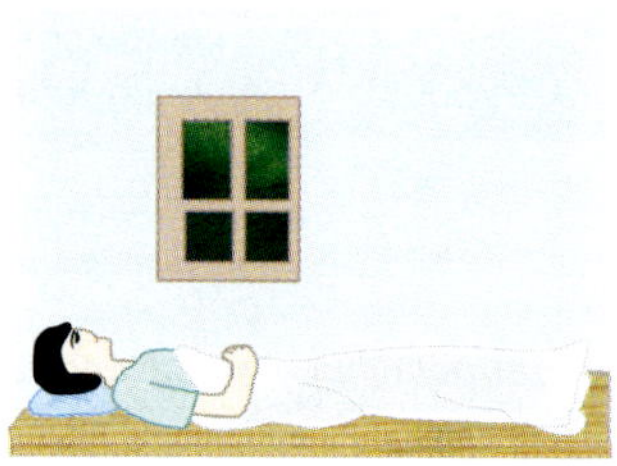
Fig. 41.17

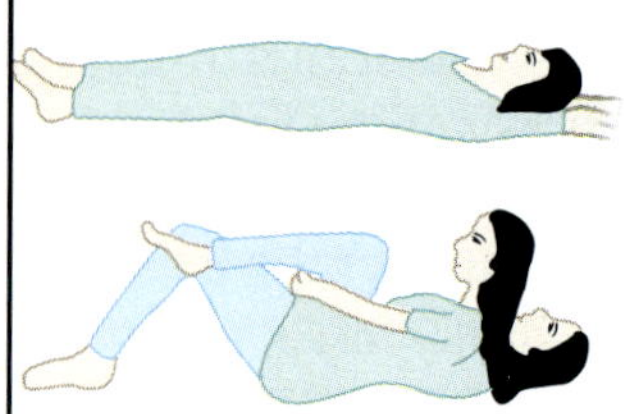
Fig. 41.13

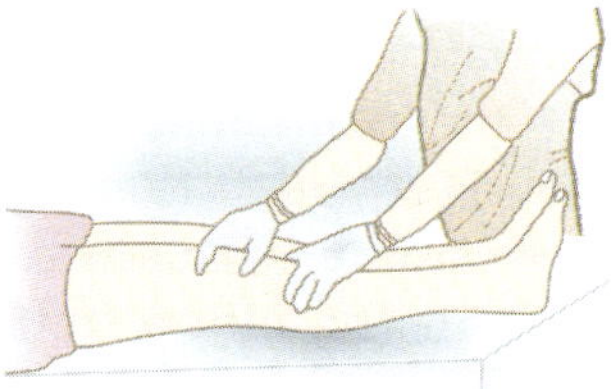
Fig. 41.18

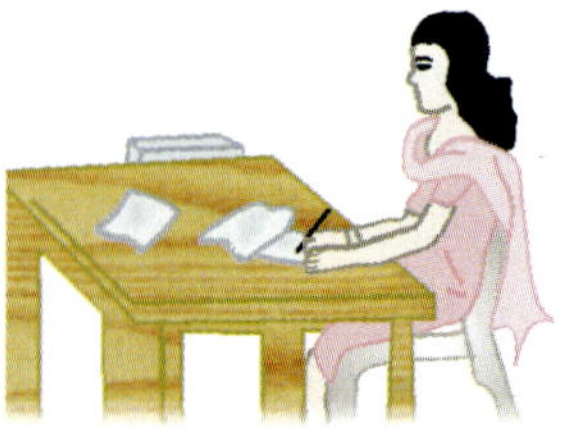
Fig. 41.14

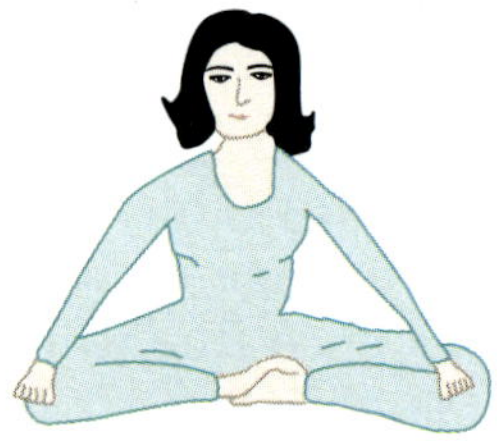
Fig. 41.19

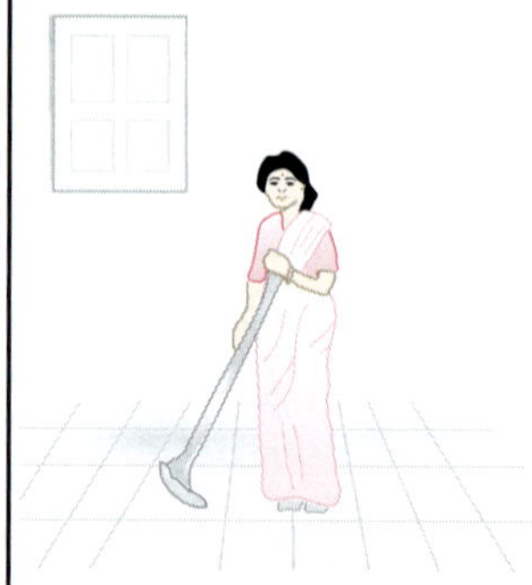
Fig. 41.15

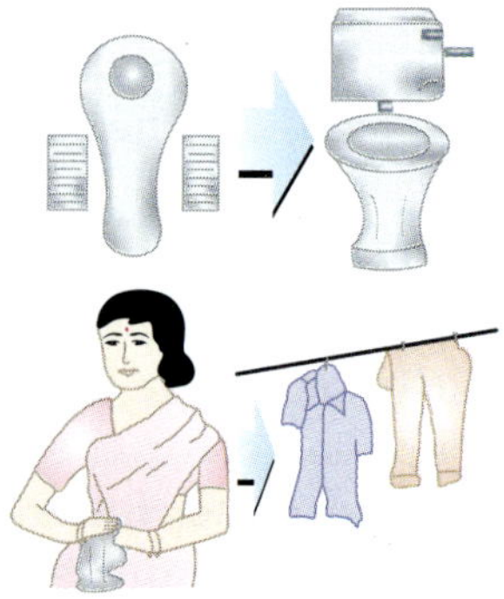
Fig. 41.20

Figs 41.11 to 41.20: Self-management techniques in the treatment of rheumatoid arthritis

Table 41.2: Showing the differences between rheumatoid arthritis and osteoarthritis

Rheumatoid arthritis	*Osteoarthritis*
• It is an autoimmune disease and often strikes in the prime of life. • It is usually seen between the ages of 25 and 50 years of age but can also occur in children and infancy. • It affects joints on both sides of the body and has a bilateral presentation. • It causes redness, warmth and swelling of the joints. • It affects many joints usually small joints of the hands and feet, and may affect the elbow, shoulders, wrist, hip, knee and ankles. • It can affect the entire system, with general feeling of sickness and fatigue, as well as weight loss. • There is history of prolonged morning stiffness. • It causes major fatigue.	• It is an age-related disease due to wear and tear of the cartilage. • It usually affects people after 40 years of age. • It usually affects isolated joints, or joints on only one side of the body at first. • It usually does not cause redness and warmth of the joints. It most commonly affects weight bearing joints or joints that are overused (e.g. knees and hip). • Discomfort is usually related to the affected joint. • Brief morning stiffness. • It rarely causes fatigue.

- Use of walking sticks while walking, climbing, etc.
- High chairs
- Avoid squatting on the ground for food, etc. Use of dining table and chairs are recommended
- To avoid squeezing clothes after washing and just rinsing them dry (see Fig. 41.20)
- To avoid walking on hard and uneven and rough surfaces
- To sleep on a hard surface.

SERONEGATIVE SPONDYLOARTHROPATHIES

Introduction

Seronegative spondyloarthropathies (SSA) group is gradually emerging as a new entity. These disorders are labelled as *seronegative* to indicate that they have in common the *absence of the rheumatoid factor*. The term spondyloarthropathies is used because in many cases there is involvement of the *spine and sacroiliac joints*. Hence, SSA can be defined as an *acute or chronic condition with characteristic involvement of axial joints, absence of RA factor and HLA abnormality*.

The clinical entities which appear to justify inclusions in the SSA group are as follows:

- Ankylosing spondylitis
- Reiter's disease
- Psoriatic arthritis
- Ulcerative colitis
- Crohn's disease
- Whipple's disease
- Behçet's syndrome

(Ulcerative colitis, Crohn's disease, Whipple's disease and Behçet's syndrome: Enteropathic arthritis)

Aetiology

The exact pathogenic mechanisms involved are not known. However, genetic factors appear to play an important role. The most complete evidence for familial aggregation is that for ankylosing spondylitis. The children of a person with HLA-B_{27} have a 50 per cent chance of carrying the same antigen.

There are some postulations regarding the possible mechanism for the association of HLA-B_{27} and SSA.

- HLA-B_{27} is a marker for immune response gene that determines susceptibility to an environmental trigger.
- HLA-B_{27} may act as a receptor site for an infective-agent.
- It may induce tolerance to foreign antigen with which it cross-reacts.

Salmonella, Shigella, Chlamydia, Yersinia and other micro-organisms are implicated in the pathogenesis of this group of arthritis.

Signs and Symptoms

The clinical manifestations include *articular* as well as *extra-articular* features.

Articular features These include low back pain due to progressive sacroiliitis and spondylitis. The patient complains of morning stiffness and decreasing lumbar lordosis.

Diffuse swelling of fingers and toes may occur due to small joint synovitis and tenosynovitis. The manifestation is referred to as *sausage digit*. Enthesopathy, i.e. pain at the site of insertion of ligaments and tendons can occur at Achilles tendon, plantar fascia and ischial tuberosities.

Extra-articular features These features include skin lesions such as *psoriasis, pitting of nails*, and penile ulcers, eye lesions like conjunctivitis, bowel disorders and genitourinary disturbances such as *dysuria* and *urethral discharge*.

Diagnosis

Radiological diagnosis *forms one of the proven diagnostic techniques in diagnosing SSA*. Radiological study of the affected joints will show *punched-out areas* exceeding deep into the subchondral bone.

CAT scan is also a very useful method that helps in the diagnosis. *It is indicated when plain X-rays are normal*. Early changes of sclerosis and bone erosion which are not visible on a plain X-ray, can be clearly demonstrated on CAT scan.

HLA-B$_{27}$ shows a strong association with SSA. Its presence adds weight to the diagnosis of these conditions. The frequency of its occurrence with SSA ranges between 16 and 100 per cent. In ankylosing spondylitis the frequency of its occurrence is as high as 85 to 90 per cent, while in Behçet's syndrome it is as low as 16 per cent. *In all patients of SSA, the RA factor is uniformly negative.*

One of the diagnostic pitfalls encountered is a mistaken diagnosis of RA. Hence, at the very outset, it is essential to differentiate between these two conditions (Table 41.3).

Table 41.3: Showing the difference between SSA and RA

	SSA	*RA*
Age	Young usually less than 40 years	Any age group
Sex	Predominantly male	Predominantly females
Symmetry	Usually asymmetrical	Usually symmetrical
Number of joints involved	Oligoarticular	Polyarticular
Spine involvement	Common	Only cervical spine
Enthesopathy	Typical	Not a feature
RA factor	Typically -ve	Typically +ve
HLA-B$_{27}$	+ ve in high percentage	-ve in normal population

ANKYLOSING SPONDYLITIS (SYN: MARIE-STRUMPELL DISEASE)

Definition This is a chronic progressive inflammatory disease of the sacroiliac joints and the axial skeleton.

Causes

Causes are unknown. It is found to be strongly associated with HLA-B$_{27}$ genetic marker (about 85 per cent).

The infective triggers are certain gram-negative organisms more so *Klebsiella*.

Age/sex Common in young male adults (M:F = 10:1).

Pathology

The initial inflammation of the joints is followed by synovitis, arthritis, cartilage destruction, fibrous and later bony ankylosis. The joints commonly affected are SI joints, spine, hip, knee and manubrium sterni.

Clinical Features

The patient usually complains of early morning stiffness and pain in the back. On examination patient has a stiff spine. Tests for sacroiliac joint involvement are positive (Figs 41.21 to 41.23). Cervical spine involvement is tested by asking the patient to touch the wall with the back of the head without raising his or her chin (Fleche's test). If the chest expansion is less than 5 cm, involvement of thoracic spine is suspected (Fig. 41.24). Gradually, a progressive kyphotic deformity of the entire spine develops (Fig. 41.25).

Diagnostic criteria for ankylosing spondylitis

- Insidious onset
- Age < 40 years
- Persistence for > 3 months
- Morning stiffness
- Improvement with exercise

Extra-articular manifestations These include acute iritis (25%), pericarditis, aortic incompetence, subluxation of atlantoaxial joints, apical lobe fibrosis, generalised osteoporosis, etc.

Differential Diagnosis

For differentiatial diagnosis of various types of SSA, see Table 41.4. For differences between ankylosing

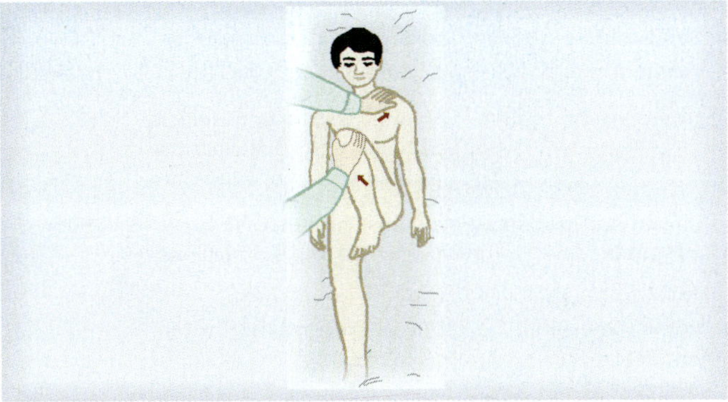

Fig. 41.21: Sacroiliac joint involvement: Pump handle test

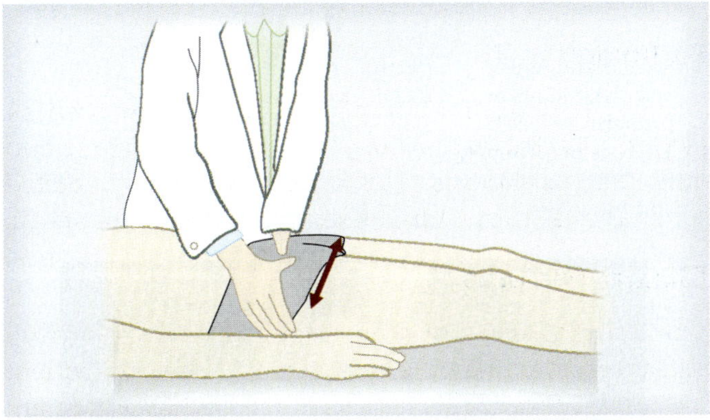

Fig. 41.22: Sacroiliac joint involvement: tested by the pelvic compression test

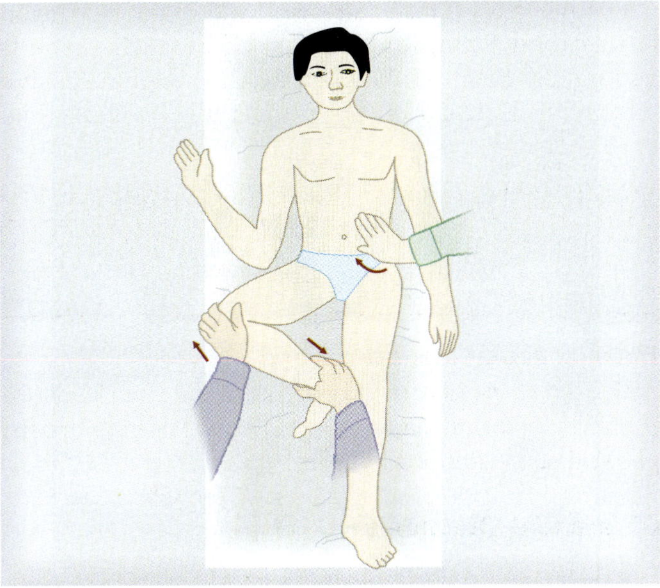

Fig. 41.23: Showing sacroiliac joint involvement: Fabre test

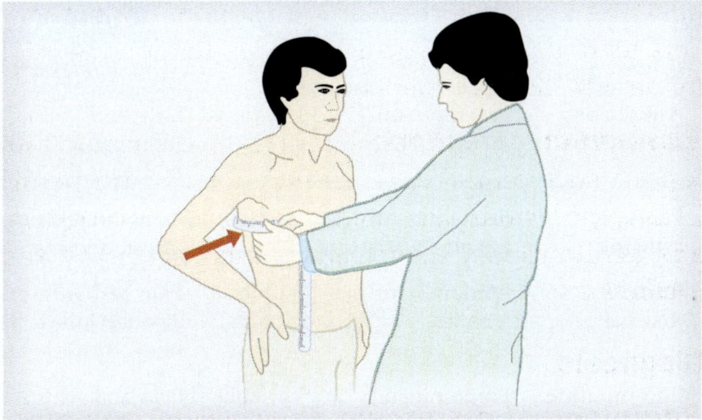

Fig. 41.24: Assessment of chest expansion in ankylosing spondylitis

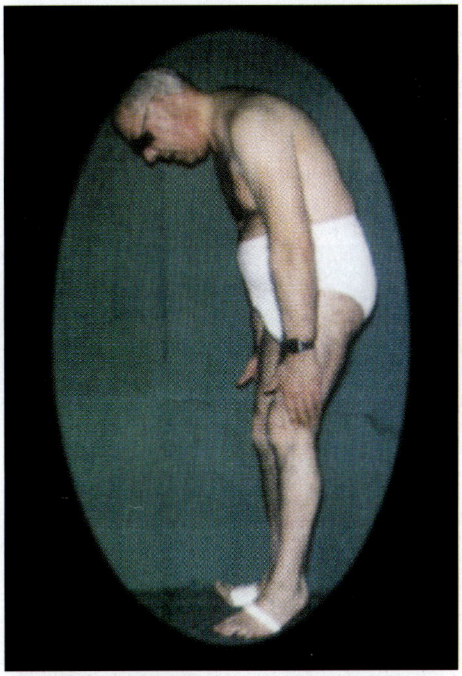

Fig. 41.25: This is how an ankylosing spondylitis patient looks

spondylitis and backache due to other causes, see Table 41.5.

Investigations

Radiographs of SI joint show haziness, subchondral erosions, sclerosis (Fig. 41.26A) widening of SI joint, etc.

Radiographs of spine show squaring of vertebra, loss of lumbar lordosis, calcification of anterior longitudinal ligament bridging osteophytes, bamboo spine (Fig. 41.26B), etc.

Table 41.4: Differential diagnosis SSA

Disease	*Sex and age*	*Onset*	*Signs and symptoms*	*Joints involved*	*Extra-articular lesions*	*HLA-B_{27}*
Ankylosing spondylitis	Predominantly males < 40 years	Insidious	Low back pain, morning stiffness and pain > 3 months	Intervertebral joints	Uveitis, conduction defects in heart, CNS disturbances, pulmonary complications	94%
Psoriatic arthritis	Predominantly females > 50 years	Variable	Pain and stiffness on affected joints	Distal and proximal IP joints	Uveitis, conjunctivitis, urethritis, and skin lesions	100%
Reiter's disease	Predominantly females. 16–35 years	Sudden	Pain and stiffness of affected joints, diarrhoea, dysuria, etc.	Weight bearing joints (knee and ankle)	Conjunctivitis, uveitis, buccal erosions, urethritis	83%
Enteropathic arthropathies (Crohn's disease, ulcerative colitis, Whipple's disease)	Predominantly males. Age group is not clear	Variable	Pain and stiffness of the affected joints, weight loss, diarrhoea, abdominal pain	Knee, ankle (most common), shoulder wrist, elbow also involved	Aphthous ulcers, uveitis, erythema nodosum	50%
Behçet's syndrome	Predominantly males. 15–40 years	Variable	Pain and stiffness of affected joints.	Knee, hand, ankle and wrist joints are primarily affected. There is involvement of elbow, shoulder and hip joints	Painful oral ulcers, genital ulcers, ocular lesions, skin lesions.	16%

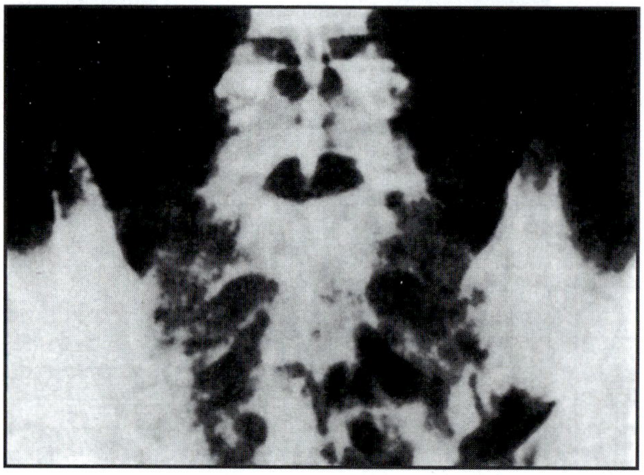

Fig. 41.26A: Radiograph showing sacroiliac joint sclerosis in ankylosing spondylitis

Table 41.5: Differential diagnosis of ankylosing spondylitis with other causes of backache

	Ankylosing spondylitis	*Backache due to other causes*
Morning stiffness	Present	Nil or minimal
Effect of inactivity	Aggravates pain and stiffness	Relieves pain
Effect of physical activity	Relieves pain	Aggravates pain

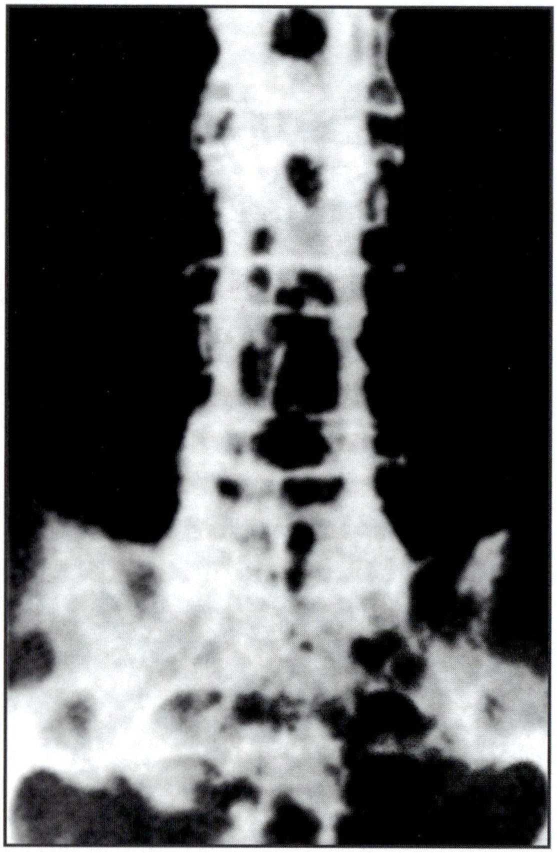

Fig. 41.26B: Radiograph showing bamboo spine in ankylosing spondylitis

Other investigations This consists of CT scan, MRI, bone scan, etc.

Laboratory investigations HLA-B_{27} is raised in 95%, raised ESR is seen in 50% and serum IgA is significantly increased.

Treatment

1. *General measures* This is extremely important and consists of the following measures:
   - Patient education
   - Family education
   - Genetic counselling
   - Avoid smoking
   - Regular exercises, especially swimming is of tremendous help
   - Physiotherapy and joint exercises
   - Occupational therapy.
2. *Conservative treatment* This consists of rest, NSAIDs (indomethacin), physiotherapy, back exercises, etc. Radiotherapy may also help.
3. *Surgical treatment* consists of spinal osteotomy to correct spine deformity, total hip replacement and total knee replacement for hip and knee joint ankylosis.

What is new in the treatment of ankylosing spondylitis?

Tumour necrosis factor antagonist Etanercept (Enbrel) 25 mg twice weekly is being tried with successful results.

FIBROMYALGIA

Introduction

This is a condition where pain is characteristically described as "Charley horses" scattered all over the body. It falls in the gambit of muscular endurance disorders with a widespread musculoskeletal pain involving all the four quadrants of the body namely the right, left, above and below the waist (Fig. 41.27).

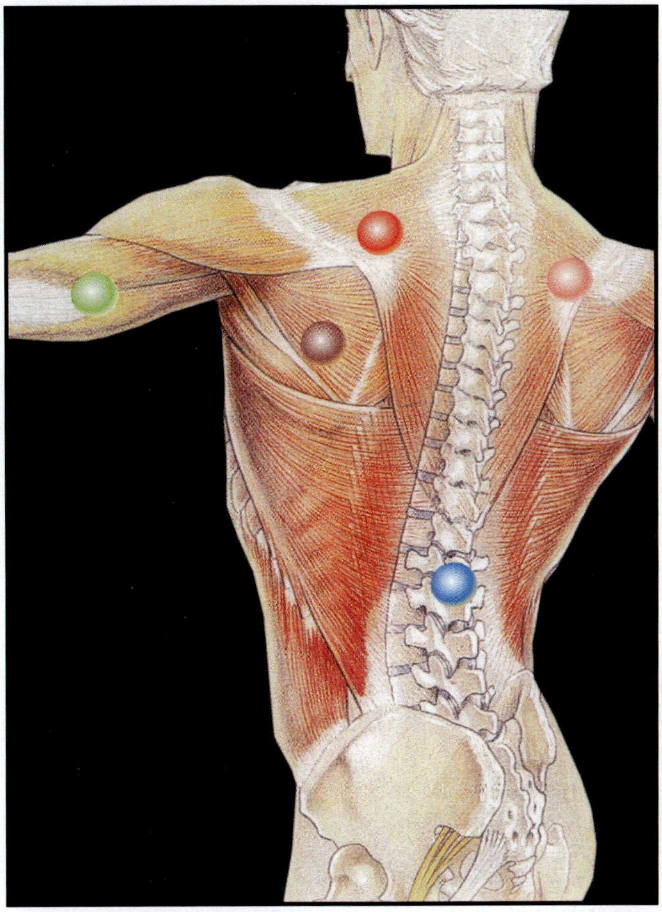

Fig. 41.27: Showing the sites of tenderness in fibromyalgia

Incidence

After osteoarthritis, this is the most common rheumatological disorder. The overall incidence is 2 to 5 per cent with women suffering 8 to 10 times more than man.

Causative Factors

- In 5 to 10 per cent, it could be hereditary.
- In a majority, any condition that lowers the endurance of the muscles can trigger this condition. Notorious among them are sleep disorders (Loss of Stage IV delta wave sleep), trauma, connective tissue disorders, infections, etc.

Clinical Features

- Pain: Its features include widespread gnawing pains, with increased activity, stress or poor sleep.
- Fatigue, stiffness, arthralgia, headache, chest and abdominal pains, etc. are some of the other complaints.

Diagnostic Criteria

- Widespread pain for at least three months in all the four quadrants of the body
- Pain should be elicited in at least 11/18 established tender points when a digital pressure of 4 kg is applied (Fig. 41.28).

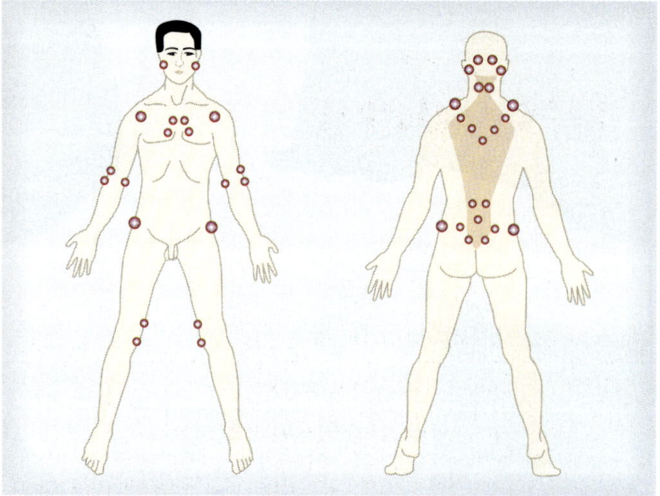

Fig. 41.28: Most common localisation of tender points in fibromyalgia. Adapted from Mau (circles) and Moll (shadowed area)

Treatment

A multidisciplinary approach seems to be an effective strategy in tackling this troublesome condition namely:

- *Initial phase*: Treat the underlying cause like sleep disorders, infection, connective tissue disorders, etc.
- *Second phase*: Myofascial release, massage and physical therapy are used to relieve the pain at the tender areas
- *Final phase:* Aerobic exercises are advocated to improve the muscle endurance.

Alternative Therapies

- *Diet therapy*: A diet rich in protein, amino acids and minerals are recommended.
- *Injection therapy*: A trigger point injection into the tender area with dry needling or injection, normal saline, local anaesthetic and steroid injection helps.
- *Physiotherapy*: Ultrasound, SWD, TENS, manipulations and massage are useful adjunctive measures.
- *Acupressure*: Stimulating the reflex points and specific points helps to lower the pain.

BIBLIOGRAPHY

1. Cach JE. Cash's Textbook of Orthopaedics and Rheumatology for Physiotherapists, Downe, DA (Ed). London, Boston, Faber and Faber, 1984.
2. Cooper NJ, Mageford M, et al. Secondary Health Service Care and second line drugs, costs of early inflammatory in Nortflok, UK.J Rheumatoid 2000:27:2115-2122.
3. Goldberg VM. Surgery for rheumatoid disease: Part 2: Early management of the rheumatoid joint. In American Academy of Orthopaedic Surgeons. Instructional Course Lectures. Vol. 33, St Louis, 1984, The CV Mosby Co.
4. Hill DF, Holbrook WP. Prevention and treatment of deformities in rheumatoid arthritis. JAMA 1950;142:718.
5. Imaging in rheumatology. Medicine International 75,3100.
6. Neustadt DH. HLA antigens in rheumatic diseases. Orthop Rev 1977;6:19.
7. Non-steroidal anti-inflammatory drugs. Medicine International 75,3105.
8. Principles of the examination of a patient with rheumatic disease. Medicine International 74,3085.
9. Snne DA. Surgery for rheumatoid arthritis; timing and techniques: general and medical aspects. J Bone and Joint Surg 1968;50-A:576.
10. Verdeck WN, McBeath AA. Knee synvectomy for rheumatoid arthritis. Clin Orthop 1978;134:168.
11. Wynn Perry CB. Rehabilitation of the Hand, 4th edn. London: Butterworths.

42

Degenerative Disorders

- ❑ Osteoarthritis of the knee
- ❑ Osteoarthritis hip
- ❑ Osteoarthritis of other regions
- ❑ Crystalline arthropathies
  - ■ Monosodium urate arthropathy (Gout)
  - ■ Pseudogout (CPPD)

OSTEOARTHRITIS OF THE KNEE

Definition It is defined as a degenerative, non-inflammatory joint disease characterised by destruction of articular cartilage and formation of new bone at the joint surfaces and margins.

The term osteoarthritis was coined by John spendon. However, it is a misnomer and the right term is osteoarthrosis or degenerative joint disease. It could be primary or secondary and the former is more common.

PRIMARY OSTEOARTHRITIS OF THE KNEE (ALSO CALLED IDIOPATHIC)

Aetiological causes for primary osteoarthritis Though exact cause is not known, the following factors are suspected to play an important role in the causation of primary osteoarthritis—obesity, genetics and heredity, occupation involving prolonged standing, sports, multiple endocrinal disorders and multiple metabolic disorders (Fig. 42.1).

Note: Genetic tendency in OA knee is twice as strong as OA hip.

Features

- It commonly affects the knee joint.
- All races are susceptible.
- Common in older age groups.
- Eighty per cent of people are affected by 40 years, but only 40 per cent show symptoms.
- It causes varus deformity of the knee in the late stages (Fig. 42.2).
- More than 50% have bilateral OA knee.

Quick facts: Osteoarthritis

1. *Who is prone to get osteoarthritis?*
   - Middle-aged patients
   - Women have a greater tendency than men
   - One in three people over 60 years are affected and more than three in four persons over the age of seventy show some radiographic evidence of the condition
   - Very rarely it can be seen in younger people.
2. *What are the typical symptoms of osteoarthritis?*
   - Pain
   - Early morning stiffness
   - Restricted range of joint movements
   - Swelling of the joints.
3. *What joints are usually affected?*
   - Weight bearing joints like hip, knee, ankle, etc.
   - Spine
   - Fingers.
4. *What causes osteoarthritis?*
   - Age more than 40 years
   - Female
   - Hereditary conditions
   - Previous joint injuries
   - Obesity
   - Diseases of the joints
   - Poor posture
   - Occupational stress and strain
   - A combination of the above factors.

   Note: The only factor which can be modified is obesity.
5. *How to make a diagnosis?*
   - Physical examination
   - Symptomatology
   - Radiography
   - Blood tests
   - CT scan and MRI.

Sequence of pathological events in osteoarthritis The disease process usually begins in the anteromedial compartment of the knee joint.

Fibrillation due to loss of water of the weight bearing articular cartilage is seen in early stages of the disease followed by complete loss of articular cartilage. This puts enormous pressure on the underlying bone which causes sclerosis and later eburnation. Cysts may develop in the subchondral area due to microfractures that degenerate. New bone formation takes place and results in osteophyte formation (Figs 42.3A and B).

Note: OA is characterised by architectural deterioration of articular cartilage and formation of new bone at the joint surfaces.

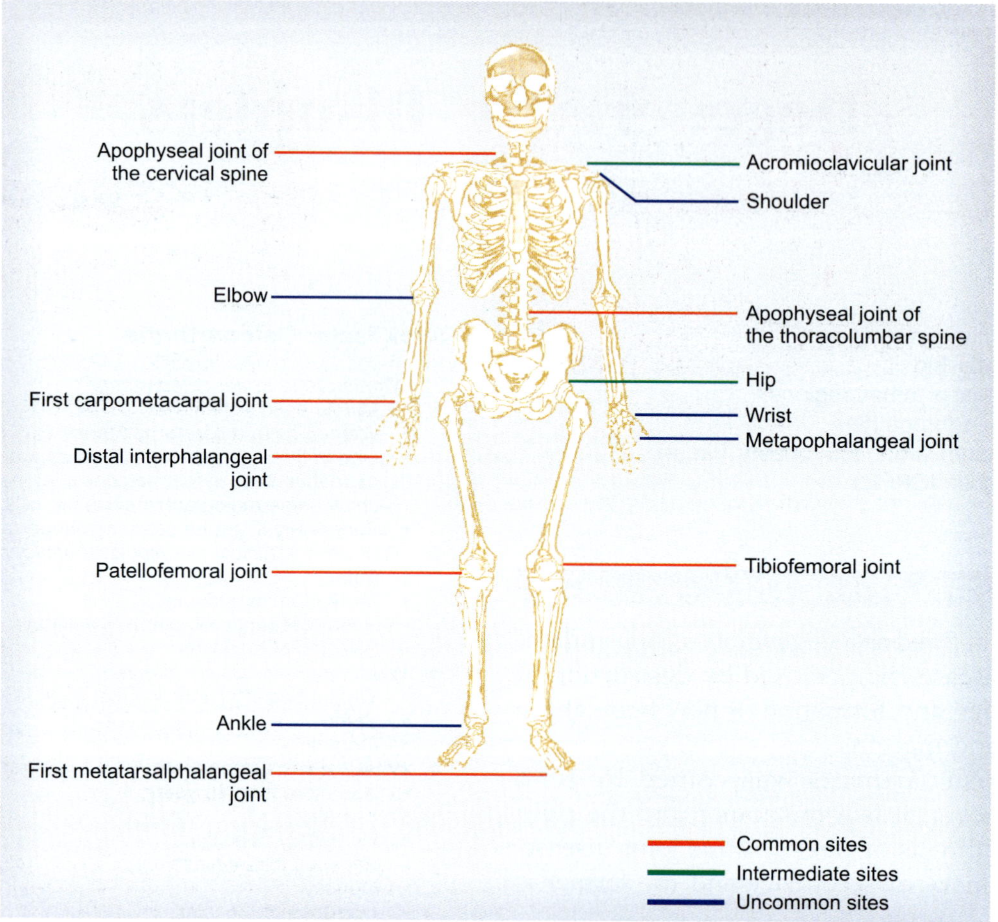

Fig. 42.1: Sites of primary osteoarthritis

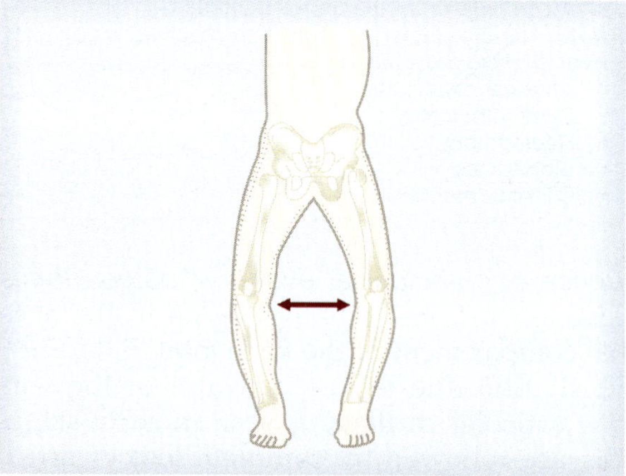

Fig. 42.2: Showing genu varum deformity in advanced osteoarthritis of knee

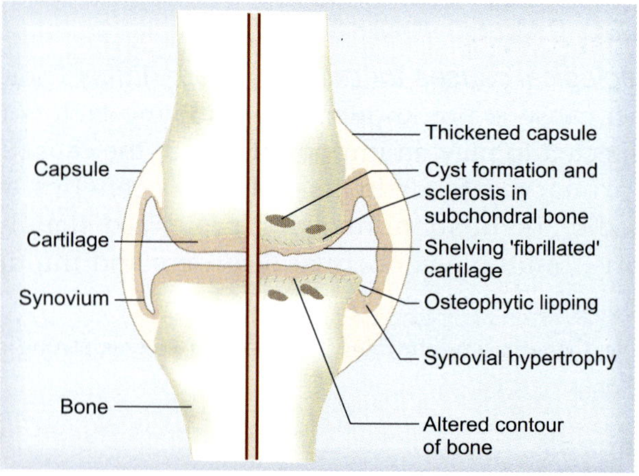

Fig. 42.3A: Pathological features of osteoarthritis knee

Clinical Features

Predominant symptom is pain which decreases on walking. The pain is poorly localised and is dull aching in nature. The patient has mild swelling of the knee joint and complains of early morning stiffness. Minimal tenderness and coarse crepitus can be elicited. If there are loose bodies in a joint, the patient gives history of locking or giving way. Terminal movements of the knee are restricted (Fig. 42.4). The patient complains of early morning stiffness

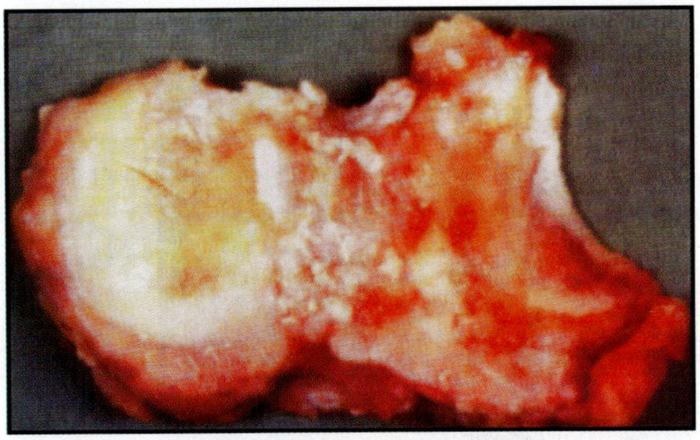

Fig. 42.3B: Pathological specimen showing destruction of articular cartilage in OA knee

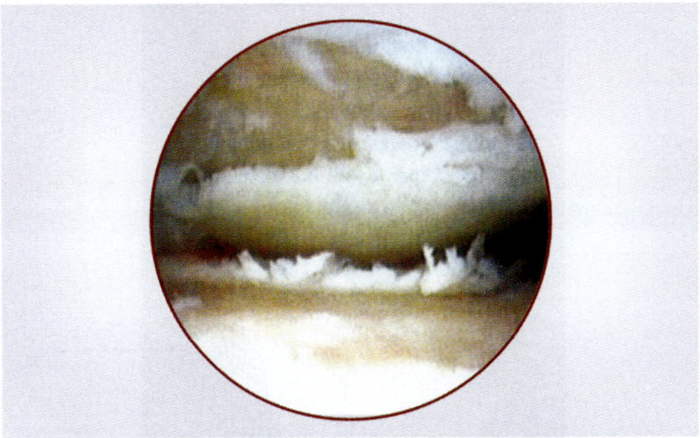

Fig. 42.3C: Arthroscopic view of degenerated cartilage in OA knee

which subsides over the day after some activity. Genu varum deformity may be seen in very advanced cases. Minimal effusion may be present. In some cases, osteophytes may be palpable.

Do you know the sources of pain in OA knee?

Well, it could be from

- Inflamed synovium
- Microfracture of subchondral bone
- Periosteum stretching by osteophytes
- Venous congestion in intraosseous compartment
- Joint distension
- Muscle spasm
- Bursal inflammations
- Affered joint mechanics
- Mental depression.

Investigations

Laboratory investigations are usually within normal limits. *Radiological examination* of the knee joint is the most important diagnostic tool. The following are the radiological features seen in osteoarthritis (Fig. 42.5) of the knee.

- Loss of joint space (due to destruction of articular cartilage).
- Sclerosis (due to increase cellularity and bone deposition).
- Subchondral cysts (due to synovial fluid intrusion into the bone).
- Osteophytes (due to revascularisation of remaining cartilage and capsular traction).
- Bony collapse (due to compression of weakened bone).
- Loose bodies (due to fragmentation of osteochondral surface).
- Deformity and malalignment (due to destruction of capsules and ligaments).

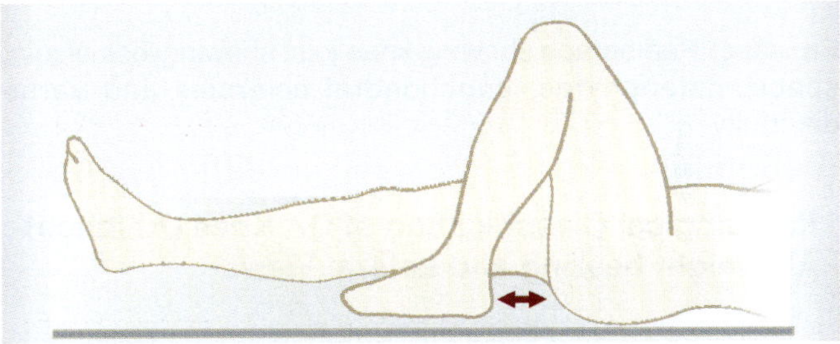

Fig. 42.4: Showing loss of terminal flexion in osteoarthritis knee

Quick facts: About complaints in OA knee

- Pain limits walking distance and capacity to work
- Limp
- Difficulty to kneel, get up from the chairs, getting in and out of the car
- Descend and ascend the stairs
- Limits capacity to work, even housework.

Examination of the Patient in OA knee

Standing

↓

From front → Deformity (Knock knee—Uncommon, Bow leg—Common)
- *Early stages* → Correctible by Manual stress (Indicates unilateral OA)
- *Late stages* → Not correctible (Bilateral) TKR needed

From the sides → Knee will not straighten fully (due to fibrous and capsular contractures)

Pitfalls of X-rays in OA Knee

- Not reliable in about 15% of the cases
- Weight bearing AP and lateral views are desired
- Only 40% of the people with severe X-ray changes experience pain.

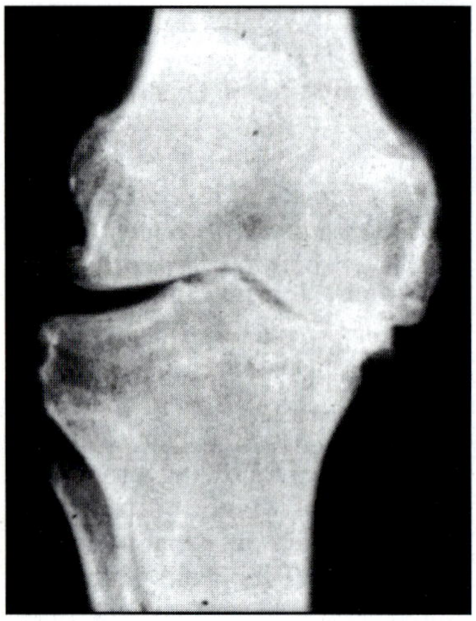

Fig. 42.5: Radiograph showing knee joint showing loss of joint space, osteophytes, subchondral sclerosis and varus deformity

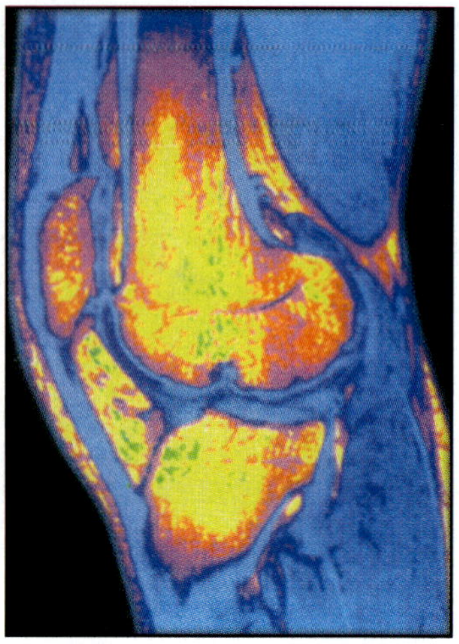

Fig. 42.6: MRI OA knee

Radiological Classification of OA Knee (Ahlbach) AP weight bearing and Lateral Views

Type I	—	Joint space narrowing.
Type II	—	Total loss of joint space
Type III	—	< 5 mm tibial erosion but posterior part of the plateau intact.
Type IV	—	> 5 mm tibial erosion and erosion of posterior plateau
Type V	—	Subluxation.

Note: Grades IV and V: TKR is the line of treatment.

Other Investigations

- Arthroscopic examination (see Fig. 42.3C)
- Synovial fluid analysis shows non-inflammatory picture. Bone scan shows increased uptake of technetium-99m, MRI and CT scan also helps to diagnose, subchondral cysts, osteophytes, etc. (Fig. 42.6).

Treatment

Aims of Treatment of OA Knee

It can be best illustrated by 4R's:

- Relieve pain
- Restore function
- Reduce disability if any by
- Rehabilitation.

Conservative methods This forms the mainstay of management in osteoarthritis of the knee. About 50 per cent of patients respond to conservative treatment which consists of the following measures (Fig. 42.7).

What is new in OA knee?

Viscosuplementation: (Intra-articular hyaluronan therapy) This procedure consists of removal of pathologic osteoarthritic synovial fluid and replacement of hyaluronan based products that restore the molecular weight and concentration of hyaluronan to normal values that is reduced in OA knee. Hyaluronan helps in joint lubrication, buffers load transmission, imparts anti-inflammatory properties to synovial fluid.

Indications for Intra-Articular Hyaluronic Acid Injection

- Failed conservative treatment
- If there are major risk factors for surgery
- Failed intra-articular steroid injections
- Advanced osteoarthritis.

By combining steroid injection with joint lavage, OA patients get more effective pain relief than with either therapy alone and pain could reduce for as long as 24 weeks.

Surgery

Indications for surgery

1. Pain refractory to conservative measures.
2. History of frequent locking episodes.
3. Haemarthrosis due to loose bodies or osteochondral fractures.
4. Deformity, usually genu varum.
5. Joint instability.
6. Progressive limitation of knee motion.

Surgical Methods

1. *Excision of osteophytes* is rarely done alone.
2. *Excision of loose bodies, meniscectomy, synovectomy*, and *reconstruction or joint debridement* are best done by arthroscopy.

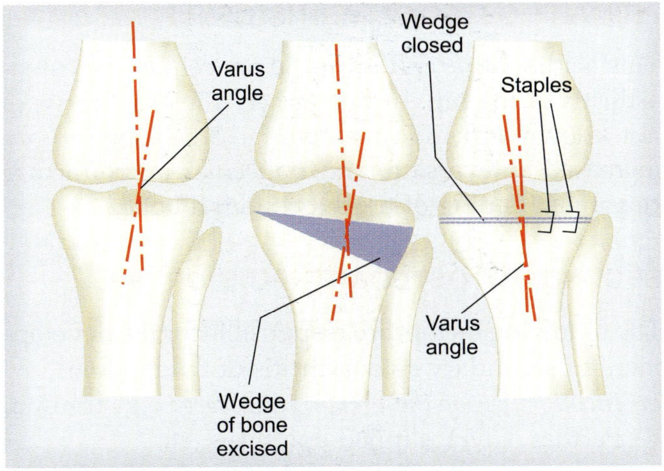

Fig. 42.7: Showing valgus high tibial osteotomy

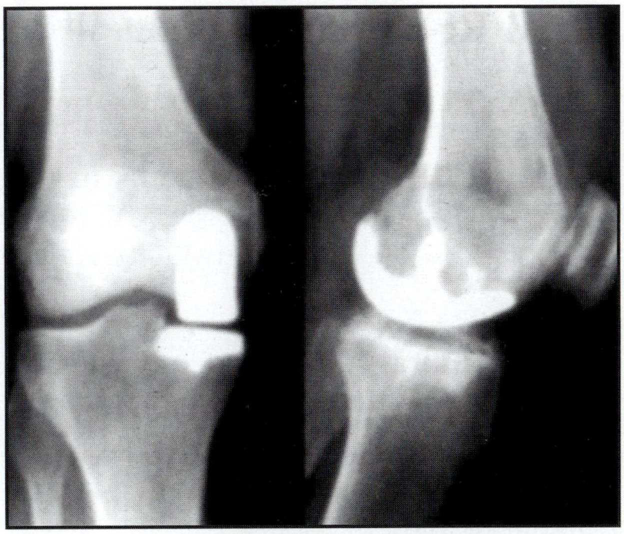

Fig. 42.8: Radiographs showing unicondylar knee replacement

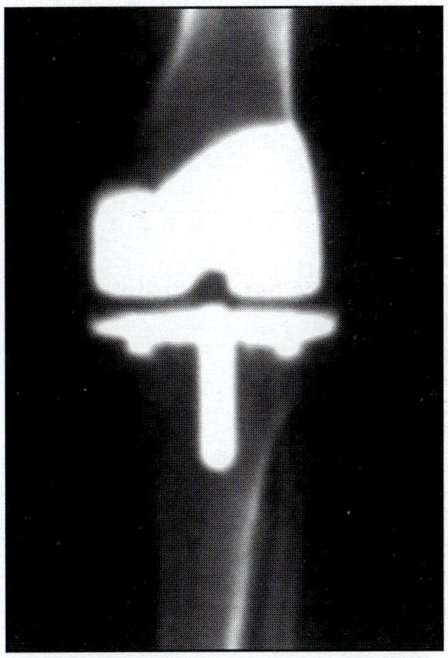

Fig. 42.9: Radiograph showing total knee replacement

3. *Proximal tibial osteotomy (Slocum's)* Indicated for unicompartmental osteoarthritis of knee with pain and also to correct varus (less than 15°) or valgus deformity (less than 12°). Pain is decreased in 80 per cent of the cases following surgery as osteotomy changes the line of weight bearing and brings the more normal surface to carry out the function of load transmission (Fig. 42.7). Mean failure rate is 40 per cent at 4 years.
4. *Distal femoral osteotomy* is indicated when varus or valgus deformity of the knee is more than 12 to 15°.
5. *Chondral resurfacing procedure*
   a. *Autologous chondrocyte grafting*: Autologous chondrocytes from the patient's knee are cultured for two weeks, re-inserted under a patch of periosteum.
   b. *Mosaic plasty*: Spare autologous hyaline cartilage from other areas of knee are inserted into the defect.
6. *Arthroscopic debridement* This is a successful palliative, temporising treatment of OA knee.
7. *Total knee arthroplasty* This is indicated when both the compartments of the knee joint are destroyed or if valgus or varus deformity is more than 15°. It is also indicated in failed conservative treatment (Figs 42.8 and 42.9).

Limitations of TKR

- Only 1 in 6 gain normal knee function after TKR, and the rest have residual symptoms
- Full flexion not regained
- Anterior wound prevents kneeling.

8. *Arthrodesis* is indicated less commonly than arthroplasty. If the patient is young and involved in heavy occupation, arthrodesis is indicated to give him a stable and strong knee. However, arthrodesis results in a stiff knee which is a severe disability.
9. *Patellectomy* It is rarely done except as a last resort. Contemplated in osteoarthritis present for several years.
10. *UKA (Unicompartmental Knee Arthroplasty)* This is again regaining its popularity over tibial osteotomy in treating unicompartmental OA, as it helps in early postoperative rehabilitation.

Macquet's HTO (High Tibial Osteotomy) This is another useful procedure.

Did you know?
It was Steindler who described osteotomy for OA knee in 1940.

SECONDARY OSTEOARTHRITIS OF KNEE

The causes for secondary osteoarthritis of the knee are as follows:

1. Obesity.
2. Valgus and varus deformities of the knee.
3. Intra-articular fractures of the knee, etc.
4. Rheumatoid arthritis, infection, trauma, TB, etc.
5. Hyperparathyroidism.
6. Haemophilia.
7. Syringomyelia.
8. Neurological disease like diabetes.
9. Overuse of intra-articular steroid therapy.

   It is generally observed that secondary osteoarthritis occurs in the younger age groups and is more severe than the primary. Apart from all the features of osteoarthrits, secondary osteoarthritis has the features of the corresponding aetiological condition.

Remember

Major complications of osteoarthritis of knee

- Joint deformities
- Subluxation
- Ankylosis
- Intra-articular loose bodies.

Remember

O's in osteoarthritis of the knee

- **O**besity
- **O**ccupation
- **O**ver 40 years of age
- **O**ther predisposing joint diseases
- **O**steophytes main characteristic feature of osteoarthritis
- **O**utward deviation of knee
- **O**steotomy required to correct bone deformities.

OSTEOARTHRITIS HIP

(FAMILIARLY CALLED AS MALUM COXA SENILIS)

This is second in frequency to knee joint, and it could be primary or secondary.

PRIMARY OSTEOARTHRITIS OF HIP

This is idiopathic and forms 50 per cent of the osteoarthritis of the hip. In this variety the exact cause is not known and the causative factors suspected are increased anteversion, and trabecular microfracture causing stiffening of the subchondral bone.

SECONDARY OSTEOARTHRITIS OF HIP

The following factors are responsible for the development of secondary osteoarthritis of the hip joint.

1. *Incongruity of the articular surface,* e.g. trauma, Perthes, CDH, slipped epiphysis, etc.
2. *Instability of the hip,* e.g. subluxation .
3. *Concentration of pressure load,* e.g. coxa vara, anteversion.
4. *Direct injury,* e.g. infection, trauma, etc.
5. *Constitutional causes,* e.g. obesity, hyperthyroidism, etc.
6. Bone diseases like AVN, rheumatoid arthritis, etc.

Remember

About secondary osteoarthritis

- Progress is relentless.
- Occurs in younger age group.
- Non-surgical treatment is futile.
- If surgery is prolonged for long, the optimal time for surgery is missed.

Pathology

The changes in the articular cartilage vary from fibrillation to complete destruction depending on the severity of osteoarthritis. The synovium is thick and congested. The subchondral bone shows sclerosis and cyst formation. The capsule is thick and fibrosed. New bone growth results in osteophyte formation in areas not under pressure.

Clinical Features

In osteoarthritis of the hip joint, the patient is asymptomatic in the early stages, later patient may complain of slight pain lasting for 1 to 2 days. Stiffness of the hip, muscle spasm, limp, restriction of terminal hip movements are the other complaints. As the disease advances, pain decreases, but the hip becomes more and more stiff. A mild flexion, adduction and external rotation deformity may be seen.

Radiology

Primary osteoarthritis In the early stages no changes are seen. In the later stages joint space is reduced, subchondral sclerosis, cysts, osteophytes, etc. may be seen (Fig. 42.10).

Secondary osteoarthritis Apart from features of osteoarthritis, features of the predisposing causes are also seen.

Treatment

Conservative measures consists of rest, heat, NSAIDs, muscle relaxant, massage, traction, manipulation, intra-articular steroids, etc.

Surgical Careful selection of the cases are done. Primary aim of surgery is relief of pain, while secondary aim is to restore movements, increase stability and deformity correction.

In the early stages of the disease when a fair amount of hip movements are still present, osteotomy helps.

Choice of osteotomy

Pauwell's varus osteotomy It is done if osteoarthritis is due to coxa valga.

Valgus osteotomy This is more common and is done in adduction deformity of the hip.

Displacement osteotomy (Mc Murray's) This is indicated in severe osteoarthritis of hip with large osteophytes.

Osteotomy (Figs 42.11A and B) helps by changing the line of weight bearing and bringing the normal surface into the line of weight transmission.

In the late stages of osteoarthritis, in elderly and in restriction of flexion less than 70°, osteotomy is of no value. The choice is then between cup arthroplasty, arthrodesis, hemireplacement arthroplasty and total hip replacement (Figs 42.12 and 42.13).

OTHER USEFUL APPROACHES IN THE MANAGEMENT OF OSTEOARTHRITIS OF HIP AND KNEE JOINTS

Simple changes around the home and daily activities causes dramatic improvement in the sympto-

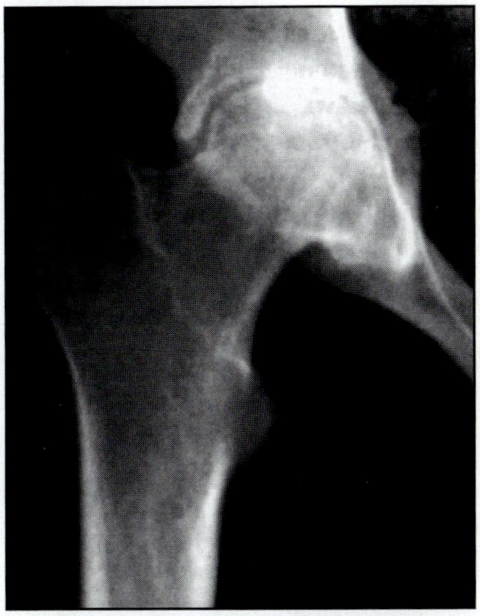

Fig. 42.10: Radiograph showing osteoarthritis of hip

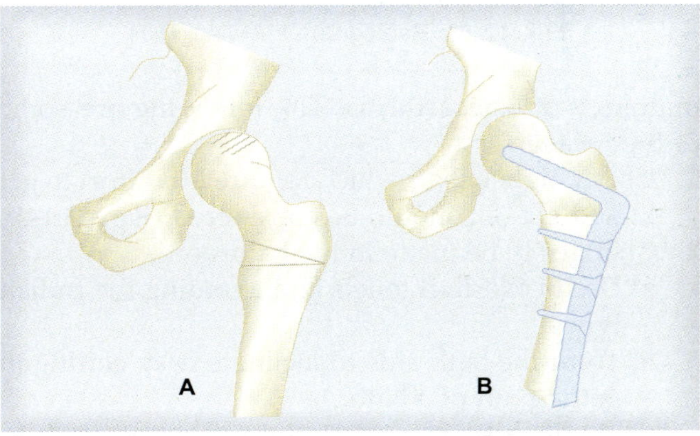

Figs 42.11A and B: Showing osteotomy for hip in osteoarthritis: (A) Before operation, (B) After operation

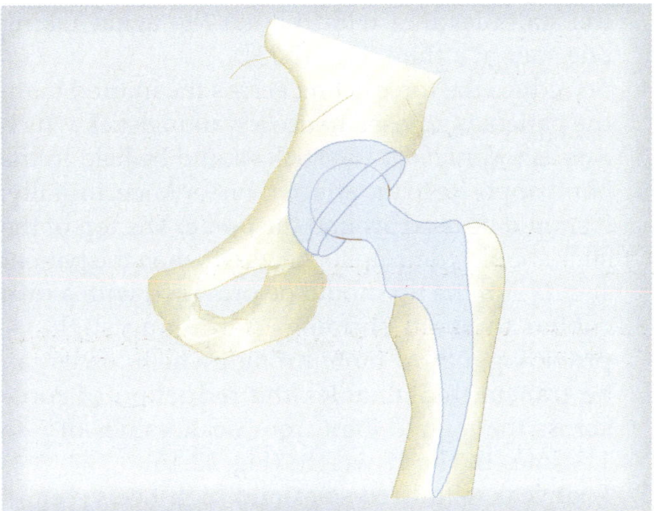

Fig. 42.12: Showing total hip replacement for osteoarthritis of hip

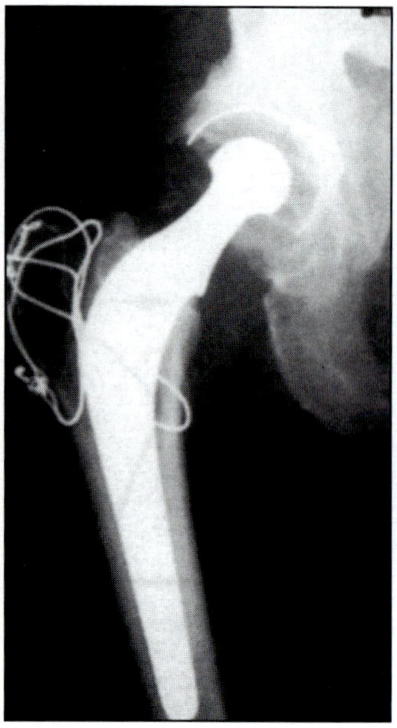

Fig. 42.13: Radiograph showing THR

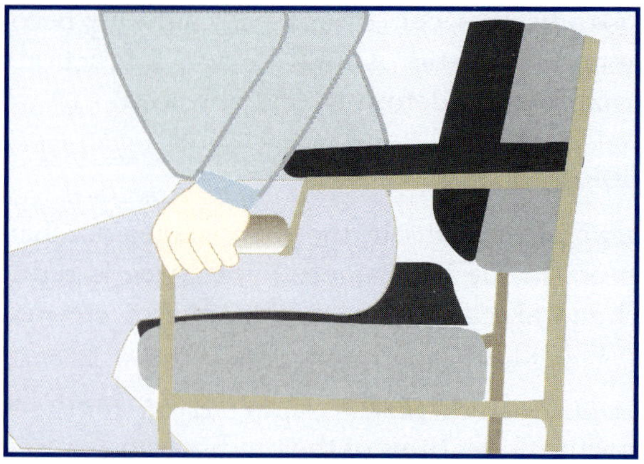

Fig. 42.14

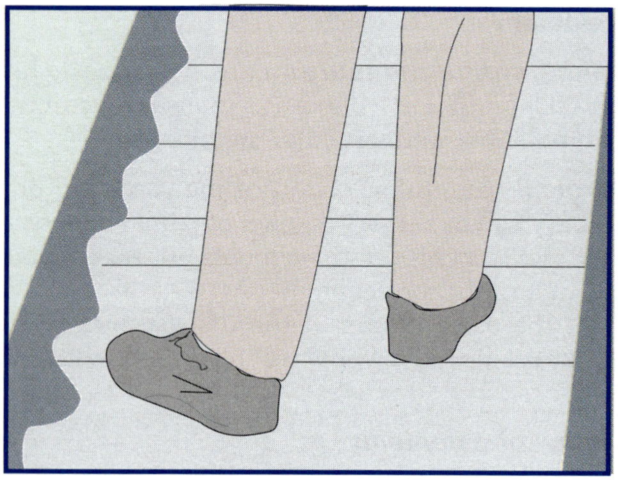

Fig. 42.15

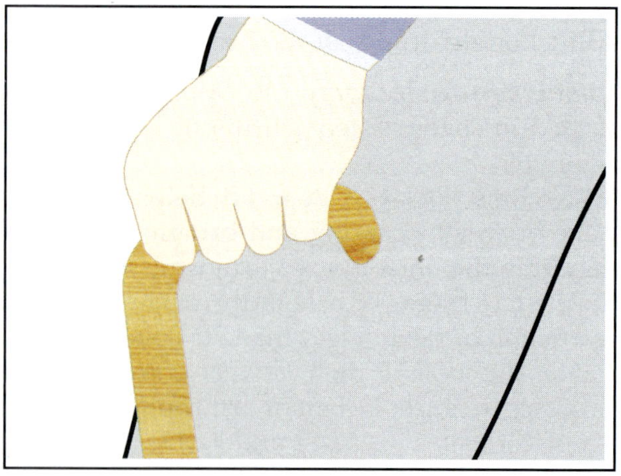

Fig. 42.16

Figs 42.14 to 16: Showing modification of living habits in the management of osteoarthritis of hip and knee: (14) Higher chairs, less effort, (15) Stairs often present a problem, and (16) Walking sticks of the right height

matology of osteoarthritis. The following are some of the measures:

1. Use of higher chair which require less effort to get in and get out should be considered (Fig. 42.14).
2. Changes to be made in the bathroom:
   - Use of Western toilets and avoiding the Indian types.
   - To fit the bath aids to facilitate easy getting in getting out of a bath.
   - To fit railings next to the toilet and bath to facilitate ease of movement.
3. Patients are advised to *climb* the stairs leading the *good leg* taking one stair at a time and to *descend* the stairs leading with the *bad leg,* again taking one stair at a time (Fig. 42.15).
4. To reduce the force acting across the injured joint, the patient is advised to use a walking stick which acts as a *third limb.* The stick should be held in the hand opposite to the affected hip or knee. Initially, it should be used around the home. The top of the stick should come up to the wrist when the patient stands and the tip should be provided with a firm rubber to avoid slipping. A walking stick, by providing a third limb through which forces can be transmitted, enables the reduction of force across the injured joint from peak values of 5 to 1.5 times the body weight (Fig. 42.16).
5. Footwear with hard soles and high heels should be avoided.

6. Cars with raised platforms and seats which facilitate easy getting in and getting out should be used.
7. If the patients are overweight, reduction in the weight helps to reduce the load on the joints.
8. General advice when standing:
   - Keep as upright as possible as this helps to put equal weight on both the legs.
   - Avoid sitting on a low or soft chair.
   - Avoid curling up in bed.
   - To stretch the front of the thigh and hip, lie on the stomach at least once a day for five minutes to thirty minutes.
   - To use a walking stick when walking inside or outside the house (cane reduces load by 40–50%).
   - To avoid uneven and rough ground or surfaces while walking.
   - To wear comfortable footwears.

ROLE OF EXERCISES IN THE MANAGEMENT OF OSTEOARTHRITIS OF THE HIP AND KNEE

Exercises from the mainstay of the patients own contribution in the treatment of osteoarthritis of the hip and knee.

Quick facts

Aims of the exercises in osteoarthritis hip and knee
- To increase the range of movements.
- To increase stability and shock absorption.
- To prevent deformity.
- To improve posture.
- To reduce pain and stiffness.

Rules of the exercises

- Build up the exercises gradually.
- Avoid rough ground while exercising.
- To take warm baths before starting the exercises.
- To perform the exercises 20 times each twice a day and later four times a day.

Types of Exercises in Osteoarthritis of Hip

Exercises Lying on the Back (Figs 42.17A to D)

1. *Pelvic tilt* Tighten the thigh and buttock muscles, pushing the knees flat, hold for a count of five and relax (Fig. 42.17A).
2. *Pelvic lift* Bend both the knees up, push on the feet and lift, hold for a count of five and relax (Fig. 42.17B).
3. *Leg stretch* Push one leg along the floor as though you are trying to make it longer than the other. Hold for a count of five and then repeat with the other leg (Fig. 42.17C).

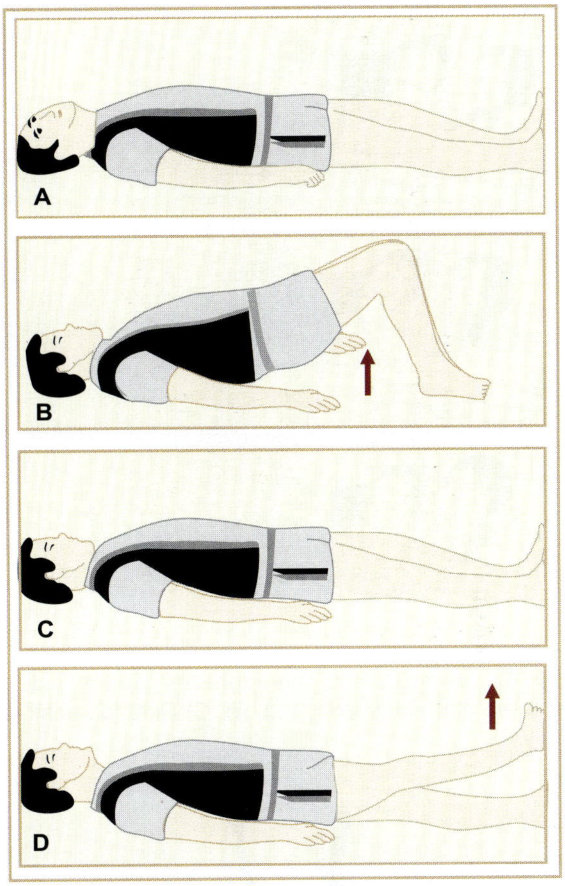

Figs 42.17A to D: Showing exercises on lying back: (A) Pelvic tilt, (B) Pelvic lift, (C) Leg stretch, and (D) Alternate leg raising

4. *Alternate leg raising* Keeping the knees straight, lift alternate legs six inches from the ground (Fig. 42.17D).

Exercises Lying on your Side, with the Painful Hip up (Figs 42.18A to C)

1. *Side leg raising* Keep the top leg straight and lift it up as high as possible, hold for a count of five and relax (Figs 42.18B and C).
2. *Knee and hip flexion* Bend the hip and knee of the top leg forwards, and hold for a count of five. Then straighten the leg and stretch backwards as far as it will go, hold for a count of five, then relax (Fig. 42.18A).

Exercises in Sitting Posture (Figs 42.19A and B)

1. *Knees together, feet apart* Keep the knees together and move the feet apart, hold for a count of five then relax (Fig. 42.19A).
2. *Feet together, knees apart* Keep the ankles together and move the knees apart, then relax (Fig. 42.19B).

Section 5

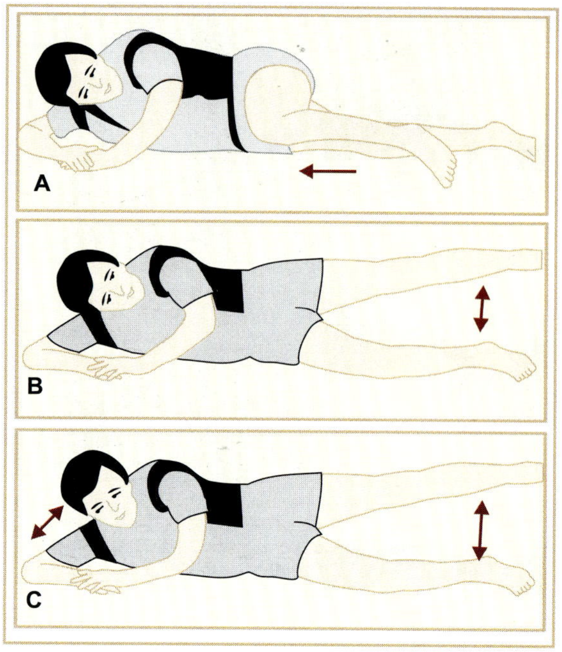

Figs 42.18A to C: Showing Exercises lying on side: (A) Knee and hip flexion, and, (B, C) Side leg raising

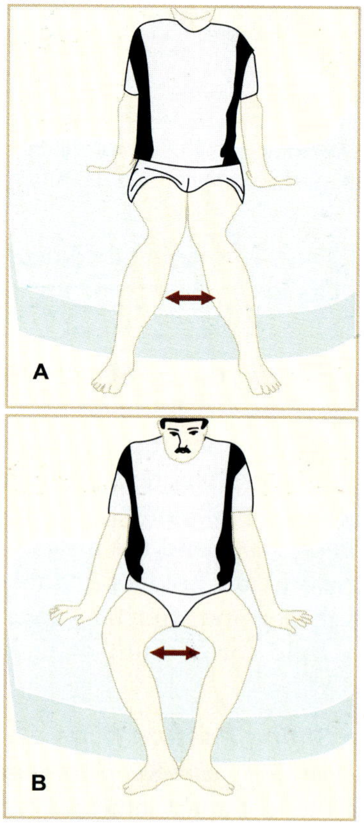

Figs 42.19A and B: Showing exercises while sitting: (A) Knees together, feet apart, and (B) Feet together, knees apart

Exercises in Standing Posture (Figs 42.20A and B)

1. *Standing leg swing* Hold into a table or chair with one hand, swing one leg forward and backward. Try to get the backwards swing as wide as possible (Fig. 42.20A).
2. *Standing side leg swing* Hold on to a chair with both hands. Swing bad leg out as far as it will go and then in. The outward swing is the hardest part and the leg should be allowed to fall back under muscular control (Fig. 42.20B).

OSTEOARTHRITIS OF OTHER REGIONS

Osteoarthritis spine (cervical and lumbar spondylosis) It is usually seen in the elderly age group and the patient presents with low backache. Osteophytes may compress the nerve roots at their exit at the intervertebral foramen and may cause neurological disturbances. Conservative treatment usually helps, but surgery may be required for prolonged pain and neurological deficits (Figs 42.21A and B).

Osteoarthritis of the small joints Osteoarthritis may affect the peripheral joints of the hand and foot. It may cause ankylosis at an increased rate in these joints (Fig. 42.22 and 23).

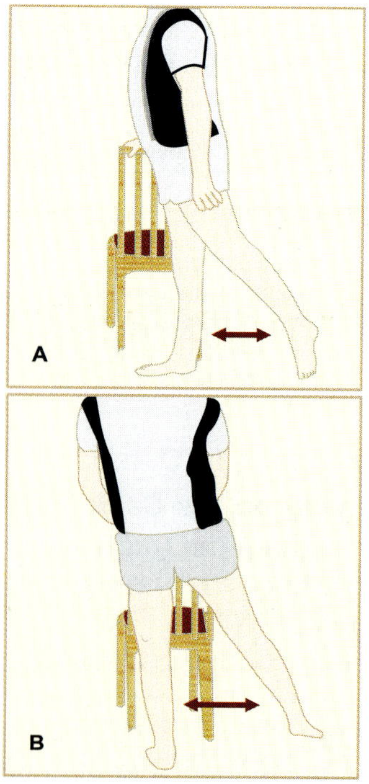

Figs 42.20A and B: Showing in standing: (A) Standing swing, and (B) Standing side leg swing

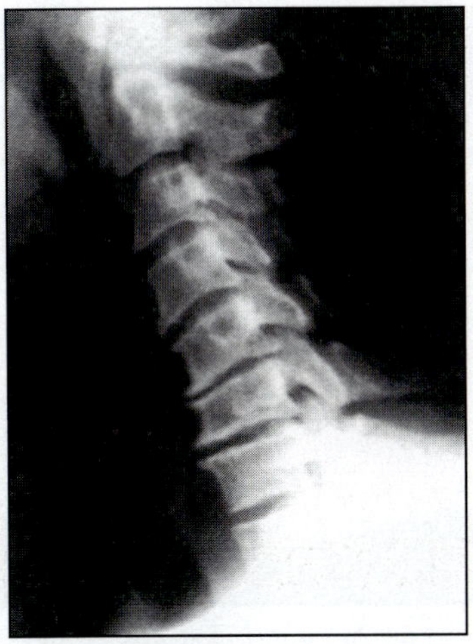

Fig. 42.21A: Radiograph showing cervical spondylosis

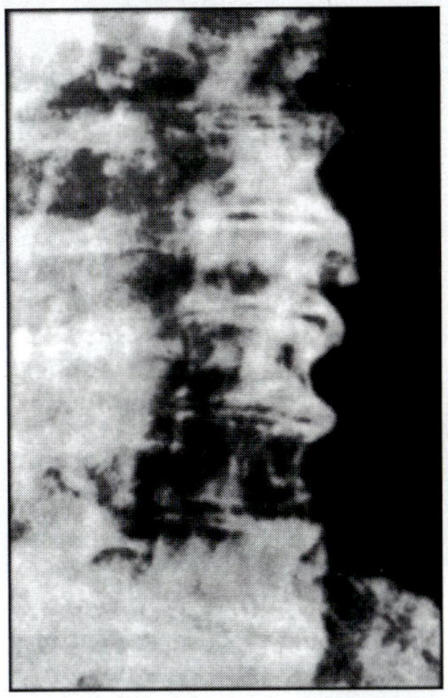

Fig. 42.21B: Radiograph showing narrowing of disc space and osteophyte formation in lumbar spondylosis

Remember in osteoarthritis of small joints

- Heberden's node—osteophytes around distal interphalangeal joints of the hand.
- Bouchard's node—osteophytes along proximal interphalangeal joints (Fig. 42.23).
- Mucinous cysts—cysts containing degenerative myxomatous fibrous tissue at the distal or proximal interphalangeal joints.
- Bunion is a combination of osteoarthritis and valgus angulation of the first metatarsophalangeal joint of foot.
- Erosive osteoarthritis: It is a hereditary severe osteoarthritis involving distal and proximal interphalangeal joints. Joint deformities and ankylosis result more often.
- Osteoarthritis of the first carpometacarpal joint of the thumb—seen in women more than 50 years (Fig. 42.22). They complain of pain and loss of grip.
- Osteoarthritis of the wrist—seen in Kienbock's disease, trauma, gout, nonunion scaphoid, etc.
- Osteoarthritis of the acromioclavicular joint—this is quite common.

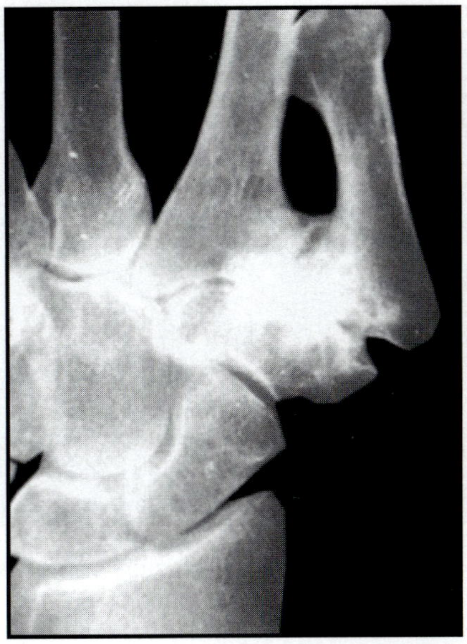

Fig. 42.22: Radiograph showing carpometacarpal joint of the thumb: loss of joint space and sclerosis

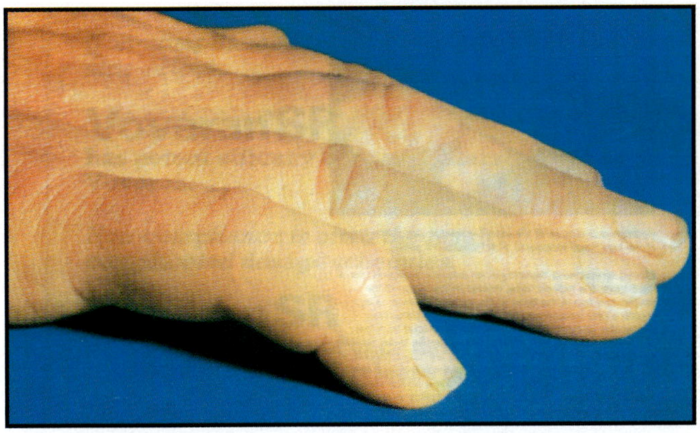

Fig. 42.23: Clinical photograph of OA hand

CRYSTALLINE ARTHROPATHIES

This group includes two interesting clinical entities:

1. Monosodium urate arthropathies (gout) (Fig. 42.24).
2. Calcium pyrophosphate deposition disease (CPPD).

MONOSODIUM URATE ARTHROPATHY (GOUT)

This is known as *gout* and may manifest itself as *acute* or *chronic*.

Sites It is usually monoarticular and the first metatarsophalangeal joint is the most common site of involvement (75%). Ankle, knee, wrist, fingers and

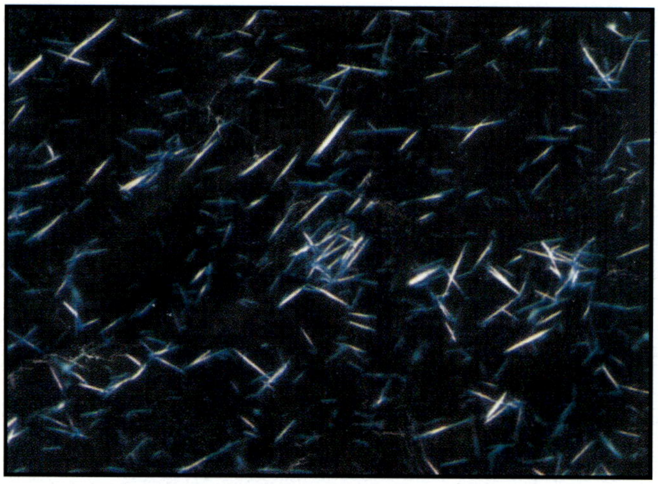

Fig. 42.24: Monosodium urate crystals viewed through a polarising microscope

elbow are other joints affected (Figs 42.25A and B). *Distal and lower extremity joints are involved more often.*

Role of hyperuricaemia Gout is usually associated with hyperuricaemia and may be associated with hypertension, obesity and atherosclerosis.

Did you know?

Gout is a disease of

- Affluence
- Alcoholism
- Obesity
- Old age
- Diuretic treatment

Incidence It is about 0.3/1000 population.

Age Men — After mid-twenties.
Women — After menopause.

Clinical Features

It has an abrupt onset. The patient may complain of pain, swelling, tenderness and increased temperature of the first metatarsophalangeal joint. Frequent gouty attacks disturb the sleep. Sometimes the inflammation is so gross that it may resemble cellulitis. Attacks are provoked by surgery, trauma, etc. Mild attacks resolve spontaneously within two days, more severe attacks may last for 7 to 10 days.

Gout has two extremes. At one end is obese alcoholic with family history of gout and no tophi while at the other extreme is a old, frail, taking thiazide diuretics and with tophi.

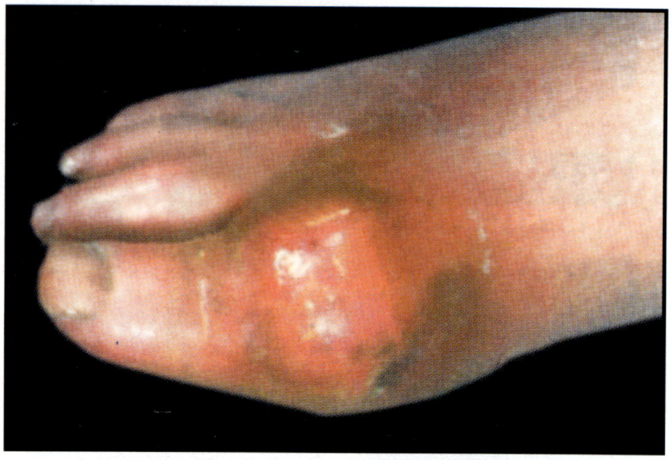

Fig. 42.25A: Showing features of acute gout

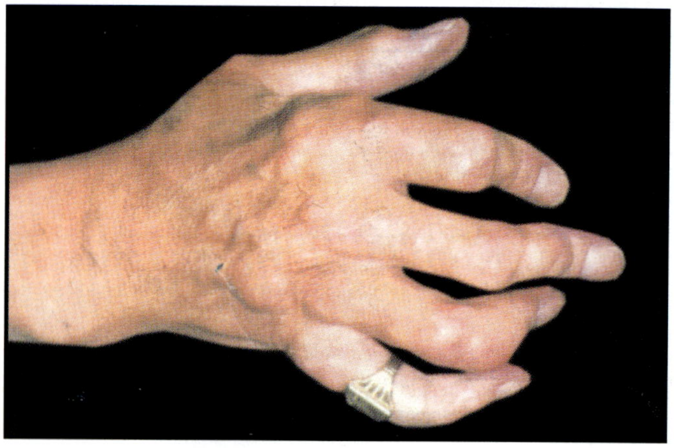

Fig. 42.25B: Showing features of chronic gout

TOPHI

These are deposits of monosodium urate crystals over pinnae, elbows Achilles tendon, distal IP joints is elderly patients.

Investigations

Laboratory investigations show leucocytosis and ESR is increased. Synovial fluid study is done under polarised microscopy for the presence of monosodium urate crystals. *This is the most important diagnostic method* (Fig. 42.24). Raised SUA level may be found.

Radiology

It is usally normal but may provide a helpful clue to detect chondrocalcinosis.

Treatment

Conservative method is the mainstay of treatment. The following measures are recommended: Indomethacin 75 to 100 mg oral initially. Later, it is given as 50 mg every 6 hours. As the attack subsides the drug may be tapered off. Intra-articular steroid also helps. Recurrent gouty arthritic attacks can be prevented by prophylaxis with colchicine (0.5 mg BD) or indomethacin (25 to 50 mg every day). When the above two drugs do not help, Allopurinol is indicated on a long-term basis.

Remember the Diagnostic Features of Gout

Attacks (4R's)

- **R**apid onset
- **R**ecurrent
- **R**arely seen > 10 days
- **R**emissions

Joints (Remember the Mnemonic FRAME)

- **F**irst MTP joint involved
- **R**ed hot joint
- **A**rticular involvement usually single
- **M**any urate crystals within neutrophils is joint fluid
- **E**xtreme pain.

Non-Articular features

- Hyperuricaemia
- Tophi (in elderly).

Remember

The drugs used in the prevention and treatment of gout:

- Indomethacin
- Colchicine } Prevention
- Allopurinol }
- Steroids.

Aspiration of the affected joint and intra-articular steroid injection terminates as acute attack of gout.

PSEUDOGOUT (CPPD)

Pseudogout is due to deposition of calcium pyrophosphate in the joints. Larger joints are more affected and 50 per cent involve the knee joints unlike in gout (Fig. 42.26). Other areas commonly involved are elbows, wrists, ankles, shoulder and hip. Synovial fluid study under polarised microscopy reveals CPP crystals. The disease is not as severe as gout and is much rarer.

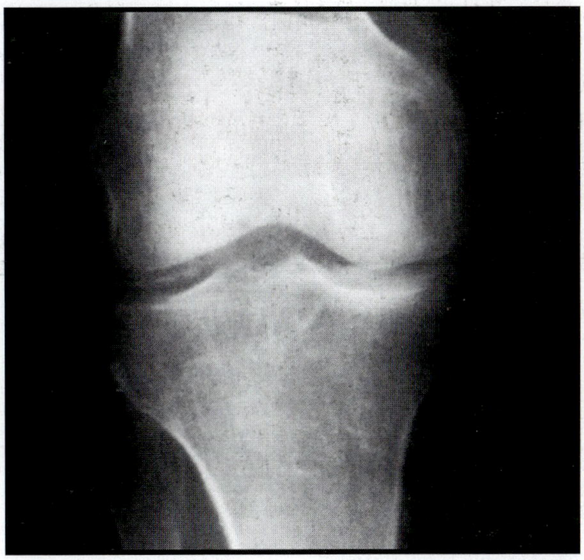

Fig. 42.26: Radiograph showing pseudogout in knee joint

BIBLIOGRAPHY

1. Ahlbach S. OA knee, a radiologic investigation. Acta Radiology 1968. Suppl;277;7-72.
2. Appel H, Friberg S. The effect of high tibial osteotomy on pain of osteoarthritis of the knee joint. Acta Orthop Scand 1972;43:558.
3. Bomboelli R. Osteoarthritis of the hip, 2nd edn. Berlin: Springer Verlag, 1983.
4. Broughton NS, Newman JH, Baily RA. Unicompartmental replacement and high TO for OA knee. JBJS, 1986;68-B:447-512.
5. Bryan RS. In Abstrom, JP Jr (Ed): Management of arthritis of the knee joint. Current Vol 5, St Louis: CV Mosby Co, 1973.
6. Chamberlain MA, Care G, Harfield B. Physiotherapy in osteoarthritis of knee. Annls Rh Disc 23:389.
7. Harrison MHM, Schajowicz, Traueta J. Osteoarthritis of hip; a study of the nature and evolution of the disease. J Bone Joint Surg 1953;35-B:598.
8. K Wayne Marshal. Current Opinion Rheumatology, Sept 2000.
9. Leach RE, Baungard S, Broom J. Obestiy: its relationship to osteoarthritis of the knee. Clin Orthop 1973;93:271.
10. Parish LC. A historical approach to nomenclature of rheumatoid arthritis. Arthritis Rheum 1963;6:136-58.
11. Pridie KH. A method of re-surfacing osteoarthritis knee joint. J Bone Joint Surg 1959;41-B:618.
12. Riggins RS, Kraus JP, Lipscomb PR. Osteoarthritis of the hip, a survey of treatments. Clin Orthop 1975;106:56.
13. Rodis EL. Osteoarthritis, what is known about prevention. Clin Orthop 1987;222:60.
14. Sheila C O Reilly, American Rheumatic Association, Jan 1999.
15. Steven E Harwim. Arthroscopy, March 1999.

43

Neuromuscular Disorders

- Cerebral palsy
- Poliomyelitis
- Arthrogryposis multiplex congenita
- Leprosy in orthopaedics
- Muscular dystrophies
- Neural tube defects

CEREBRAL PALSY (SYN: STATIC ENCEPHALOPATHY)

Definition This is a disorder of movement and posture caused by a non-progressive lesion in the immature brain, leading to global dysfunction.

Lesions In cerebral palsy the lesion could be either in the brain or the upper cervical cord, and the lesion is static.

Incidence is 0.6-5.9/1000 livebirth.

Classification

This is depicted in Table 43.1.

Table 43.1: Classification of cerebral palsy

Based on clinical types (Minear's)	*Based on severity*
1. Spastic (65%) (Commonest type) 2. Dyskinesia (25%) The following varieties are described Athetosis Tremor Choreiform Dystonia Rigidity 3. Ataxia 4. Mixed	1. Mild (25%) Independent in daily activities. 2. Moderate (50%) Needs help in daily activities and ambulation. 3. Severe Patient is bedridden and has a wheelchair existence.

Lesions in the brain In cerebral palsy the lesions in the brain can occur in the following four areas:

1. Cerebral cortex (spastic type)
2. Midbrain (dyskinesia)
3. Cerebellum (ataxic)
4. Widespread brain involvemenrt (rigidity and mixed).

Causes

In cerebral palsy the causes are different in prenatal, natal, postnatal and perinatal period and are listed as in Table 43.2.

Table 43.2: Causes of cerebral palsy

Prenatal	*Natal*	*Postnatal*	*Perinatal (0-7) days*
• Rubella infection • Fetal anoxia • Maternal diabetes	• Birth trauma • Anoxia • Prematurity	• Trauma • Encephalitis • Meningitis	• Most lesions causing CP occur during this period

Clinical Features

This depends on the location of lesions in the brain. Single muscle involvement is rare as in polio and entire portion of the body supplied by that area of brain is involved, the patients show delayed milestones and primitive reflexes are usually preserved.

Other clinical features depend on the geographic distribution of cerebral palsy and the asssociated handicapping situations (Table 43.3).

Orthopaedic Deformities

The following are the common orthopaedic deformities encountered in cerebral palsy.

Table 43.3: Clinical features of cerebral palsy

Geographic distribution of cerebral palsy	*Associated handicapping conditions*
1. Monoplegia (0.3%)	1. Sensory deficit in hand (50–60%)
2. Hemiplegia (50%)	2. Speech problems
3. Paraplegia (21%)	3. Mental retardation
4. Triplegia (3.1%)	4. Deafness
5. Quadriplegia (25%)	5. Visual defects
6. Diplegia	6. Seizures
7. Double hemiplegia	7. Perceptual problems
8. Tetraplegia	8. Emotional problems—most important
9. Total body involvement	9. Scoliosis

Note: Spasticity is a very common finding and its prominent features are hypertoncity, limp, contractures and hip dislocations.

Upper limb

1. Pronation contracture of the forearm.
2. Flexion deformities of the wrist and fingers.
3. Thumb in palm deformity.
4. Swan neck deformity.
5. Shoulder adduction and internal rotation deformity.

Lower limb

1. Adduction deformity (most common).
2. Flexion and internal rotation deformity.
3. Dysplastic and subluxated hip.
4. Dislocated hip.
5. Pelvic obliquity.

Spine

1. Scoliosis
2. Kyphoscoliosis.

Knee

1. Genu recurvatum
2. Genu valgum
3. Patella alta
4. Subluxation or dislocation of patella.
5. Knee flexion contracture—Figure 43.1 (most common).

Foot

1. Equinus deformity (Fig. 43.1)
2. Varus or valgus (Fig. 43.2)
3. Talipes equinovarus (Fig. 43.3)
4. Calcaneus deformity

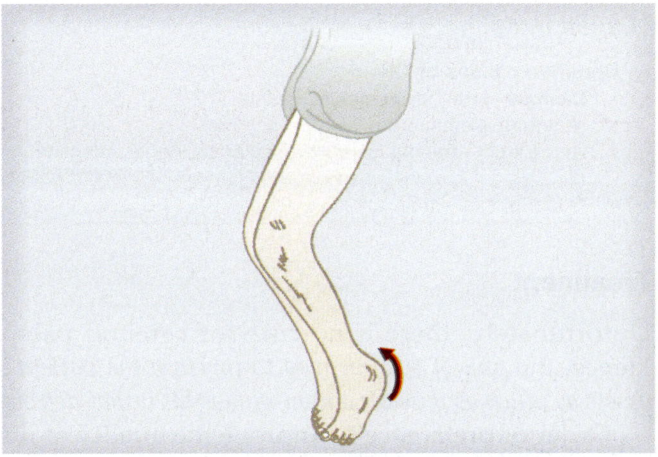

Fig. 43.1: Showing spastic contracture of the hip, knee and foot in cerebral palsy

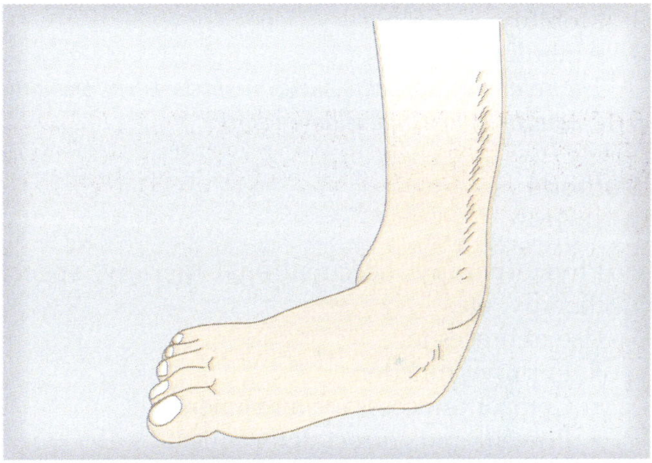

Fig. 43.2: Showing spastic equinovalgus

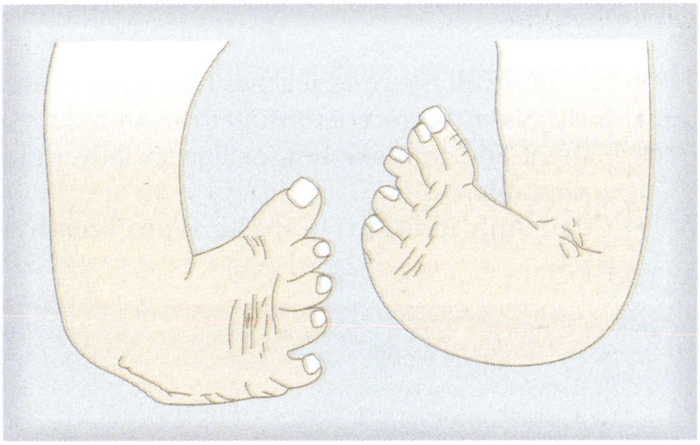

Fig. 43.3: Showing spastic equinovarus

5. Talipes cavus
6. Hallux valgus
7. Claw toes.

Section 5

Quick facts

Common causes of CP
- Diplegia—seen in premature infants
- Athetoid—kernicterus
- Hemiplegia—trauma, cerebrovascular accidents, infection, etc.
- Quadriplagia—brain anoxia.

Treatment

Unfortunately, there is no cure for cerebral palsy. Hence, the *aim of treatment is to increase the patient's assets as much as possible and minimise his or her defects.*

Order of preference to improve the quality of life in cerebral palsy is as follows:
1. Education and communication is the first priority.
2. Activities of daily life.
3. Mobility
4. Ambulation.

The role of orthopaedic surgeon starts when the child is 12 months of age and seldom before.

Methods

1. Motor age test.
2. Physiotherapy, occcupational therapy, speech therapy, etc.
3. Use of braces to:
   - Improve function.
   - Control unnecessary movements.
   - Prevent and correct deformities.
4. Drug therapy: The role of drug therapy is disappointing. Muscle relaxants, antiepileptics may have a role.
5. Surgery:
   - Not done till the child reaches five years of age.
   - Indicated to correct deformity in an ambulatory patient and to make him or her socially more acceptable.
   - Commonly indicated in spastic type of cerebral palsy.

Aim of surgery in cerebral palsy is
1. To correct the deformity.
2. To balance the muscle power.
3. To stabilise uncontrollable joints.

Choice of Surgery

1. *Operation on nervous system:*
   - Sympathectomy, rhizotomy (see box) (anterior or posterior).
2. *Operation on muscles and tendons:*
   - Tenotomy, tendon lengthening and tendon transfers.
   - Myotomy and muscle transposition.
3. *Operation on bones and joints:*
   - Bone lengthening or bone shortening to equalise the limb lengths.
   - Osteotomies to correct knock knee, and other bone deformities.
   - Arthrodesis of wrist, hip and foot to correct deformity, provide stability and to improve functions.

Vital facts: About Rhizotomy

- Popularised by Warwick Peacock of USA in 1980.
- This procedure consists of a selective severing of the distal rootlets of the cauda equina.
- Ideal patient is a spastic diplegic child at 3 to 8 years of age and who is quite ambulatory.
- This technique decreases the spastic tone without impairing sensation.

Pitfalls: It has no effect on shortened and contracted muscles and it is here that the orthopaedic surgery helps.

Prognosis in Cerebral Palsy

- There is no permanent cure.
- Athetoid child is more intelligent than spastic child.
- Twenty-five per cent go to schools.
- Twenty-five per cent are mentally retarded.
- Twenty-five per cent are not educable.
- All hemiplegics will walk (by 12 to 16 months).
- Most diplegics will walk (by 4 years).
- Quadriplegics and total body involvement will never walk but can be propped sitters.

POLIOMYELITIS

Definition This is a viral infection of the anterior horn cell of the spinal cord or nerve cells of brainstem, resulting in temporary or permanent paralysis. Common in children, often attacks young adults.

VIRUSES

The following Picorna group of viruses are known to cause poliomyelitis:
1. Brunhilde (type I)
2. Leon (type II)
3. Lansing (type III).

Pathogenesis

The virus is transmitted through the faeco-oral route and enters the nervous tissue and destroys the anterior horn nerve cells as a result of which the peripheral nerve degenerates resulting in muscle and tendon atrophy (Fig. 43.4). The bones become small, the joint capsules and ligaments become lax as there is no protection by the healthy muscles. All these results in development of various deformities.

Clinical Features

Polio usually affects children less than 12 months. There is a mild episode of fever, headache and diarrhoea. On examination, there could be mild neck stiffness and the child may find it difficult to move the affected limb (pre-paralytic). The lower limbs are more commonly affected and the paralysis could be partial or total (paralytic stage).

The paralysis of the muscles whether spinal (75%) or bulbar (25%) usually lasts till two months. Then there may or may be not be recovery for a period of two years. Any residual paralysis after two years of affection is permanent with no chance of recovery. Bulbar poliomyelitis is rare and affects the respiratory muscles. It may be fatal.

Quick facts

Features of paralysis due to polio

- Lower limb is more commonly affected than the upper limbs.
- The involvement is asymmetric.
- Though incomplete most of the times quadriceps are more often affected.
- Tibialis anterior is most often completely paralysed.
- The sensory system is not affected.
- In the residual stages (postpolio residual stages) the common deformities are (Fig. 43.5)
  a. Hip—Flexion, abduction and external rotation
  b. Knee—Flexion, triple deformity and genu valgum
  c. Foot —Talipes equinovarus

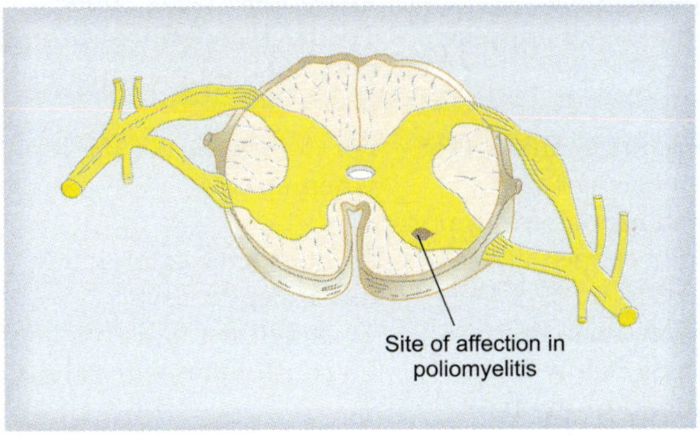

Fig. 43.4: Anterior horn cells are affected in poliomyelitis

Stages and their corresponding clinical features

← Preparalytic →|← Paralytic →

- **2 Weeks** (Incubation)
- **2 days** (Onset)
  - Headache
  - Fever
  - Malaise
  - Neck stiffness present
- **2 months** (Greatest paralysis)
  - **Spinal** (75%)
    - Involves neck, trunk and extremities
    - Lower limbs affected twice (Fig. 43.5)
  - **Bulbar** (25%)
    - Cranial nuclei affected
    - Nasal intonation
    - Difficulty in swallowing, etc.
- **2 years** (Recovery) Complete or none
- **> 2 years** (Residual)
  - Permanent
  - Mild-to-severe paralysis of trunk and all the 4 limbs

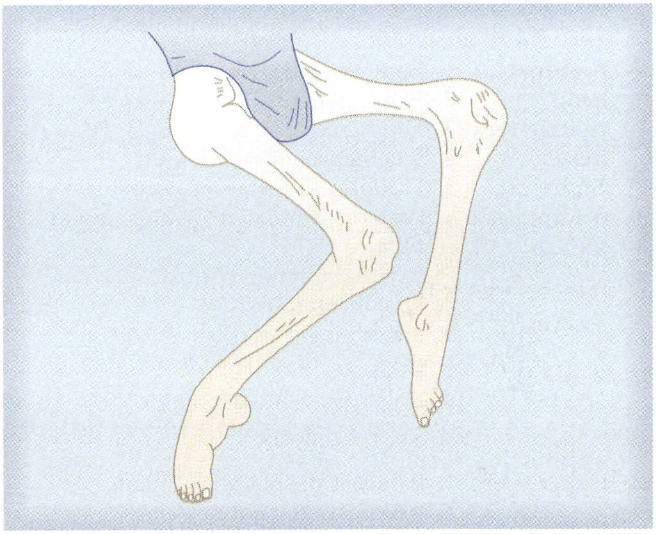

Fig. 43.5: Showing lower limb deformities in poliomyelitis

Orthopaedic Deformities

Orthopaedic deformities encountered in poliomyelitis are listed in Table 43.4.

Differential Diagnosis

Poliomyelitis has to be differentiated in the acute stages from:

a. Pyogenic meningitis
b. Guillain-Barré syndrome
c. Postdiphtheritic paralysis
d. Acute osteomyelitis
e. Scurvy.

Table 43.4: Common orthopaedic deformities encountered in poliomyelitis

I. **Foot and ankle**	1. Claw toes 2. Claw foot 3. Talipes equinus 4. Talipes equinovalgus 5. Flail foot 6. Pes cavus 7. Dorsal bunion 8. Talipes equinovarus 9. Talipes calcaneovalgus
II. **Knee**	1. Flexion contracture of the knee 2. Quadriceps paralysis 3. Genu recurvatum 4. Flail knee
III. **Hip**	1. Flexion abduction contractures of the hip 2. Paralysis of gluteus medius, maximus 3. Paralytic dislocation of hip
IV. **Iliotibial band contractures** (results in 9 classical deformities)	1. Lumbar scoliosis 2. Pelvic obliquity 3. Hip flexed and abducted 4. External rotation of femur 5. Flexion and valgus of knee 6. Posterior and lateral subluxaion of tibia 7. External rotation of tibia 8. Foot in equinus 9. Shortening
V. **Spine**	1. Kyphosis 2. Scoliosis 3. Kyphoscoliosis
VI. **Upper limbs**	1. Paralysis of shoulder, elbow, forearm and hand muscles

In the late stages from:
a. Cerebral palsy
b. Spina bifida
c. Myopathies
d. Muscular dystrophies, etc.

Treatment

Broad principles of the treatment

1. To prevent deformities from developing.
2. To assist returning of muscle power by graduated exercises.
3. To reduce disability by appropriate appliance or by operations on joints and muscles.

Treatment Methods

Early stages During the stages of onset, maximum paralysis and the stages of recovery the following treatment is recommended, the child is admitted into the hospital, and supportive treatment is given. The child is put on a ventilator support if there is respiratory paralysis due to bulbar polio. Warm and moist packs are given to the joints and all intramuscular injections are avoided during this phase. The affected joints are immobilised by plaster splints in functional positions.

Recovery stages In this stage the joints are properly splinted through various appliances (Table 43.5) to prevent or correct the deformities.

Quick facts: Conservative treatment

1. Stage of onset	• Bedrest
2. Stage of greatest paralysis	• Splints • Artificial respiration, etc.
3. Stage of recovery	• Physiotherapy • Walking aid • Crutches, etc
4. Stage of residual paralysis	• Can be corrected by provision of suitable Orthotic appliances or by operation

Role of Appliances (Fig. 43.6)

The purpose of external appliances is to support joints that have lost their normal control. They are more often required for lower limbs rather than upper limbs. The commonly prescribed appliances in Table 43.5.

Table 43.5: External appliances in poliomyelitis

1. Spinal brace	To support weak spine
2. Abdominal support	To check abdominal protrusion when abdominal muscles are weak
3. Hip, knee, ankle, foot orthosis with or without pelvic support	For deformities of the hip, when ankle
4. Knee caliper	To hold knee extended in quadriceps palsy
5. Below knee brace	To stabilise a flail ankle or foot
6. Single below knee (lateral or medial)	To control varus or valgus
7. Drop foot appliance	For mobile equinus deformity

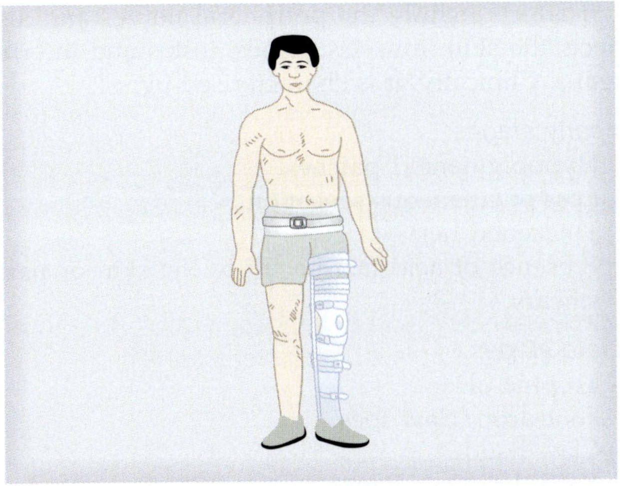

Fig. 43.6: Showing an above knee caliper (KAFO) in a polio patient

Stage of post polio residual paralysis During this stage, the role of orthopaedic surgeon is predominant and surgery is the treatment of choice.

Goals of surgery

1. To obtain muscle balance.
2. To prevent or correct soft tissue contractures.
3. To prevent or correct bony deformities.

Surgical methods

1. *Soft tissue release* for soft tissue contactures, e.g.
   i. *Soutter's release* Structures arising from anterior superior iliac spine are released for hip contractures.
   ii. *Ober-Yount's procedure* Consists of sectioning the iliotibial band (ITB) contractures.
   iii. *Tendo-Achilles* lengthening for equinus deformity of the foot.
   iv. *Steindler's release* of plantar fascia for cavus foot.
2. *Tendon transfers* This is indicated when dynamic muscle imbalance produces deformity requiring brace protection.

   Aims of tendon transfers
   - To replace the function of a paralysed muscle.
   - To remove the deforming force.
   - To provide stability by improving the muscle balance.

   Tendon transfers are not limited to any age group.
3. *Arthrodesis* This is done to:
   - Stabilise a flail joint.
   - Eliminate the need for brace and to improve function.
   - For permanent method of joint stabilisation.
4. *Osteotomies* to correct deformities like genu valgum, etc.
5. Ilizarov's technique for leg length equalisation and deformity corrections.

ARTHROGRYPOSIS MULTIPLEX CONGENITA

[SYNONYMS: MULTIPLE CONGENITAL CONTRACTURES (MCC)]

In the year 1841, Otto first described AMC. Swinyard and Beck gave the name MCC. AMC is a non-progressive syndrome characterised by:

1. Rigid and deformed joints.
2. Muscle absence or atrophy.
3. Cylindrical or ellipsoid joints with skin crease loss and subcutaneous atrophy.
4. Contractures of capsules and periarticular structures.
5. Dislocation of joints like hip and knee.
6. Normal mentality and intact sensation.

Causes

Intrauterine immobilisation of joints at various stages of development is due to:

- Myopathic cause seen in 10 per cent of cases. Autosomal recesssive.
- Neurogenic cause is due to reduced number or improper organisation of anterior horn cells, peripheral nerves and motor end plates, weakness of muscles, etc.
- Mechanical causes like breech, twins, oligohydramnios amniotic bands, etc. which reduce the intrauterine space.

Classification (Sharrard, Brown and Robson)

Eight types Two upper limb and six lower limb deformities are encountered.

Common variety is quadriplegic type (Fig. 43.7). Scoliosis is associated in 20 per cent of the cases of AMC, webbing of the knees is seen in some.

Common Orthopaedic Deformities in AMC

a. *Foot* Planovalgus and equinovarus.
b. *Knee* Flexion contracture and fixed in extension.

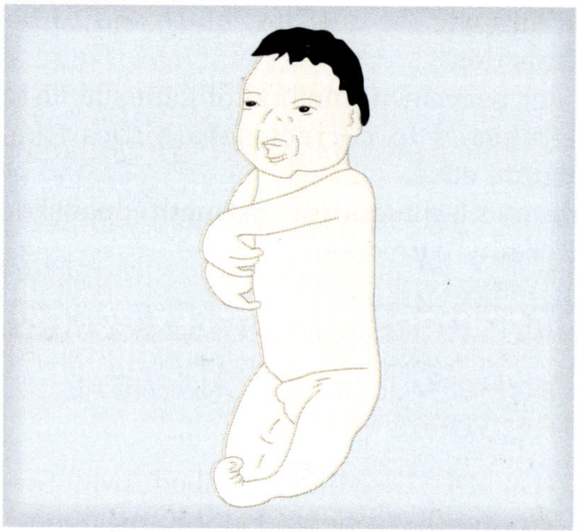

Fig. 43.7: Quadriplegic type is the most common variety of arthrogryposis multiplex congenita (AMC)

c. *Hip* Extension, abduction, external rotation.
d. *Shoulder* Medial rotation of shoulder.
e. *Elbow and wrist* Flexed.

Investigations

1. Muscle biopsy.
2. Electromyography.
3. Nerve conduction studies.
4. Radiograph for scoliosis, dislocation, etc.
5. Chromosomal studies.

Treatment

The treatment consists of passive stretching exercises, serial splinting of the limbs and surgical correction.

Principles of orthopaedic treatment

1. Muscle balance is to be restored if tendons are available for transfers.
2. Recurrence is the rule due to tough inelastic capsule and soft tissues.
3. Tenotomies should be accompanied by capsulotomy and capsulectomy.
4. Osteotomies are to be carried out once skeletal growth is over, otherwise recurrence occurs.
5. Maximum correction is to be obtained during the initial surgery. There is no role of wedging, etc.

LEPROSY IN ORTHOPAEDICS

Leprosy is a chronic infectious disease caused by *Mycobacterium leprae.*

It affects mainly the peripheral nerves and also affects the skin, muscles, bones, testes and internal organs. Clinically, it is characterised by:

In early stages

- Hypopigmented patches.
- Loss of cutaneous sensation.
- Thickened nerves.
- Presence of acid-fast bacilli in the skin or nasal smears.

In late stages

- Trophic ulcers.
- Foot-drop/claw toes.
- Claw hand.
- Nasal bridge collapse.
- Loss of fingers or toes.

National Leprosy Eradication Programme

It was launched in 1983, with the goal of arresting the disease by the turn of century based on multidrug therapy.

Problem of leprosy in India
- Four million cases.
- Prevalence rate—5.7/1000.
- Fifteen to twenty per cent cases of population are multibacillary.
- Twenty per cent result in deformities.

Classification

Three classifications are proposed as given in Table 43.6.

Investigations

1. Bacteriological examination of material obtained from the skin or nasal smears.
2. Foot pad culture of mice is 10 times more sensitive than the skin slit smears.
3. Histamine test.
4. Biopsy.
5. Immunological tests.

Tests fot detecting CMI

- Lepromin test
- Lymphocyte transformation test.

Tests for detecting humoral antibodies

- ELISA test, etc.

Table 43.6: Classification

Indian	*Madrid*	*Ridley and joppling*
Indeterminate	Indeterminate	Tuberculoid
Tuberculoid	Borderline	Borderline tuberculoid
Lepromatous	Tuberculoid	Lepromatous
Borderline	Lepromatous	Borderline both
Neuritic		Lepromatous

Treatment

Primary prevention by vaccine is not possible, so leprosy control is based on effective chemotherapy in Table 43.7.

Table 43.7: Drug treatment in leprosy

Multibacillary	*Paucibacillary*
Ripampicin 600 mg/month	R-cin 600 mg/month for 6 months
Dapsone 100 mg/day	+
Clofazimine 300 mg/month	Dapsone 100 mg/day for 6 months

If Clofazimine is not acceptable, Ethionamide—250 to 375 mg/day.

Duration of treatment is at least for two years till smear is negative.

BCG vaccine showed a high degree of protection in 80 per cent and 30 per cent in some cases.

ORTHOPAEDIC AFFECTIONS IN LEPROSY

Ankle and foot Every kind of deformity is seen in the foot. Deformity is gross, because patient continues to use the foot due to loss of sensations. Ankle is rarely affected in this disease (Table 43.8).

In leprosy, due to loss of sensation, there is absence of warning pain as a result of which, there is injury. Secondary infection following the injury is common.

Classification of Foot Deformities in Leprosy (Table 43.8)

Table 43.8: Classification of foot deformities in leprosy

Forefoot	*Midfoot*	*Hindfoot*
• Plantar ulcers • Toe deformities • Chronic osteo-myelitis of metatarsals • MTP joints destruction	• Aseptic necrosis of talus, etc. • Infective arthritis and osteomyelitis • Degenerative arthrolysis • Proliferative ankylosing arthropathy	• Chronic osteomyelitis of calcaneum • Plantar ulcers • Calcaneal spur • Gross destruction

FOOT-DROP

This is one of the very common complication encountered in leprosy. It is seen in 2 per cent of the cases.

- Common peroneal nerve is more commonly involved.
- Usually, it is completely damaged, sometimes only deep peroneal or superficial branch is involved.
- Occasionally, only external hallucis longus muscle is involved.

Consequence of Paralysis

- Foot-drop, drop toes, inversion and plantar flexion of the foot is decreased.
- High stepping gait.
- Instability of gait.
- Deformity due to contractures of tendocalcaneus and capsules of subtalar and ankle joints.
- Fixed equinovarus deformity.
- Destruction of foot.

Treatment

- For recent or incomplete drop foot: toe raising spring, physiotherapy, short wave diathermy, ultrasound, local steroids, etc. are the recommended forms of treatment.
- If more than one year after affection or if the lesion is complete, surgical correction is needed.

Before the surgical correction, ensure the following:

- Non-involvement of medial plantar nerve.
- No contractures of tendo-Achilles.
- At least 20° of dorsiflexion should be present. Tendo-Achilles shortening requires physiotherapy in the early stages and in the later stages tendo-Achilles lengthening.

Surgical Methods for Foot Drop

a. When there is no contracture and if the foot is mobile, tibialis posterior transfer is indicated.
b. Triple arthrodesis of Lambrunidi for fixed equinovarus deformity of the foot.

PLANTAR ULCERS

This is the other important foot complication in leprosy. It is also known as trophic ulcers due to neurological deficit. It has a spontaneous onset, it is painless, persists, and recurs. Healing process is not defective. Recurrent ulceration causes progressve destruction of the skeleton.

Sites Plantar ulcers are commonly seen over the ball of feet, especially the first metatarsal, and heel.

Treatment

Aim of treatment

- *To get the ulcer healed.*
- *To prevent its recurrence.*

Treatment methods Various methods of treating the plantar ulcers are mentioned in Table 43.9.

Table 43.9: Treatment plan in plantar ulcers

I. **To heal the ulcer** ***Principles*** *Provide rest* *Control infection* *Promote healing* **State of ulcer** 1. If acute • Rest, elevation • Eusol applications • Antibiotics • Incision and drainage • Dressing 2. If chronic: • Rest • Below knee caliper • Below knee plaster cast 3. Complicated ulcer: When it spreads to deeper structures like bone, joints, tendon, etc. • Ulcer debridement • Once infection is controlled treat it later as chronic ulcer as mentioned above. • Protective footwear later	**II. To Prevent Recurrence** **1. Non-surgical measures** • Healthy instructions • Protective foot wear – To protect skin from injury— use tough outer sole – To reduce stress of walking— use MCR in sole – To relieve vulnerable sites from pressure modification of foot-wear or use orthosis **Methods to relieve pressure** —Metatarsal bar (20%) —Arch support (30%) —Moulded insole (40%) —PTB cast rest **2. Surgical measures** Supplements and not substitutes for non-surgical measures. **Methods** • Scar excision • Osteotomies • Arthrodesis • Resection, etc. depending on indications

Note: MCR—microcellular rubber

AFFECTIONS OF THE HAND IN LEPROSY

The following are the common hand deformities encountered in leprosy.

1. *Ulnar claw hand* is due to affection of ulnar nerve at the elbow.
2. *Total claw hand* is due to the affection of ulnar nerve at the elbow and median nerve at the wrist (Fig. 43.8).
3. *Triple nerve palsy* the following nerves are affected:
   - Ulnar nerve at the elbow.
   - Median nerve at the wrist.
   - Radial nerve at the spiral groove.

Surgery for Hand

a. *Brand's many tailed tendon transfer operation (EF_4T)* Developed by Paul Brand at the Christian Medical College, Vellore, Tamil Nadu (India).

   Extensor carpi radialis longus is released from its insertion and brought into the flexor aspect of the forearm. Free graft from palmaris longus tendon is taken and is split into four strips which are then attached to the extensor expansion of the respective fingers (EF_4T).

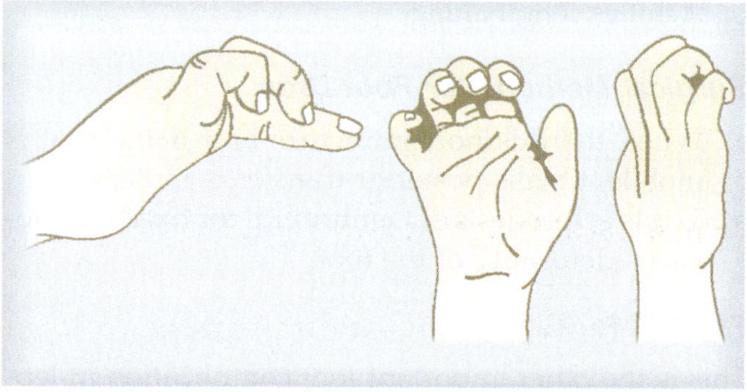

Fig. 43.8: Showing claw hand deformity in leprosy

b. *Restoration for opponens palsy* Flexor digitorum superficialis is detached from its insertion rooted through the palm and attached to the lateral margin of the extensor expansion.
c. *Ulnar claw hand* S. Bunnel's operation (refer Chapter on Peripheral Nerve Injuries).
d. *Triple nerve palsy* This is difficult to correct surgically.

MUSCULAR DYSTROPHIES

These are difficult problems to treat and the cause is usually not known.

Classification

This is as shown in Table 43.10.

Table 43.10: Classification of muscular dystrophies

Sex linked recessive	*Autosomal dominant*	*Autosomal recessive*
1. Duchenne's	1. Facioscapulohumoral	1. Limb girdle
2. Becker's	2. Scapuloperoneal	2. Childhood variety
3. Emery and Dreifus	3. Distal	3. Congenital dystrophy
	4. Occulopharyngeal	4. Limited to quadriceps

[1]DUCHENNE MUSCULAR DYSTROPHY

This is the most common type of muscular dystrophy encountered in clinical practice.

Clinical Features

This consists of delayed walking, abnormal gait and multiple falls (in less than 3 years child). Gower's sign is positive, hypertrophy of calf muscles, waddling gait, increased lumbar lordosis, weakness of shoulder muscles around 5 to 6 years, serrati, pectorals, deltoid, latissimus dorsi, biceps, triceps and brachialis muscles are weak. In lower limbs weakness of hip flexors, evertors of feet, tibialis anterior are seen, ocular, pharyngeal and masticatory muscles are never involved. Knee jerk is absent earlier than ankle jerk. Tendo-Achilles contractures appear first, later hamstrings, hip flexors and elbow follow. Intellectual impairment is present. Death below 16 years is due to respiratory infection or cardiac failure.

Investigations

- Serum glutamic oxaloacetic transminase (SGOT), serum glutamate pyruvate transaminase (SGPT), lactate dehydrogenase$_5$ (LDH$_5$) aldolase and creatinine phosphokinate (CPK) levels are raised.
- Muscle biopsy and electromyography (EMG) helps.
- Electrocardiogram (ECG) shows biventricular hypertrophy.

FACIOSCAPULOHUMERAL MUSCULAR DYSTROPHY

This is seen in second decade of life and the fascial musculature is involved early. The patient complains of inability to close the eyes, slurred speech, etc. Elevation of the scapula on abduction is characteristic. In the upper limbs deltoid and wrist flexors are spared. In the lower limbs anterior tibial muscle is involved earlier. Majority of the patient suffering from this dystrophy have a normal life span.

LIMB GIRDLE MUSCULAR DYSTROPHY

It is seen in the second or third decade. Lower limb girdle weakness appears first followed by upper limb. Muscular hypertrophy is rare. Winging of the scapula is seen. There is no involvement of cardia.

Treatment for Muscular Dystrophies

This consists of physiotherapy, mental and physical support, speech therapy, and mechanical aids like splints, walking aids, etc.

NEURAL TUBE DEFECTS (DYSTROPHISM)

SPINA BIFIDA

Definition Neural tube defects are due to failure of neuralisation of the primitive neural tube between the 3rd and 4th week *in utero*.

This is due to the failure of the fusion of the two vertebral arches in the embryological stages of development usually during the 17th to 35th day after conception. The failure of fusion could be limited, only to the spinous process resulting in spina bifida occulta, the most common variety or the entire vertebral arch including the neural elements may fail to fuse giving rise to the rare variety of spina bifida aperta.

Note: Spina bifida is a Latin term which means "split or open spine".

SPINA BIFIDA OCCULTA

This is the most common variety and is generaly mild. Lumbosacral spine and the first sacral vertebra are

[1]**Guillaume BA Duchenne** (1806-1875), a French neurologist, described muscular dystrophy.

commonly affected. The overlying skin may be normal or there may be presence of a tuft of hair, pigmentation, lipoma, dimple, etc.

There may be muscle imbalance in the lower limbs resulting in equinovarus or cavus deformity of the foot due to tethering of the cord by a membrane either to the skin or filum terminale. Rarely, there could be a bifid cord.

Treatment

Asymptomatic cases require no treatment except physiotherapy and back exercises. Surgical correction of foot deformities is as discussed in earlier chapters.

SPINA BIFIDA APERTA OF MANIFESTA

A must know facts:

- About 80–90% infants born with NTDs survive
- In India, about 107,814 children are born with NTDs every year.

Causes of Spina Bifida

The actual cause is still unknown. However, the likely causes are:

- Poor economic status
- Alcohol use
- Vitamin A deficiency
- Folic acid deficiency
- Familial
- Maternal use of valproic acid.

Note: Incidence of spina bifida is 1/1000 live births

Here the defect involves the vertebral arches, skin, meninges and cord. The following varieties are described (Figs 43.9A to D):

a. *Meningocoele* in which there is protrusion of the meninges (4%).
b. *Myelomeningocoele* in which there is protrusion of meninges and cord (96%).
c. *Syringomyelocoele* in which the central canal of the cord is dilated and the cord is protruded.
d. *Myelocoele* in which the central cord remains unfused and exposed.

Next to spind bifida occulta, myelocoele is the next common variety. Most of the cases of spina bifida aperta are either still born or die within a few days of birth. The surviving children may suffer from paralysis and complex severe orthopaedic deformities, bladder and bowel incontinence and foot deformities.

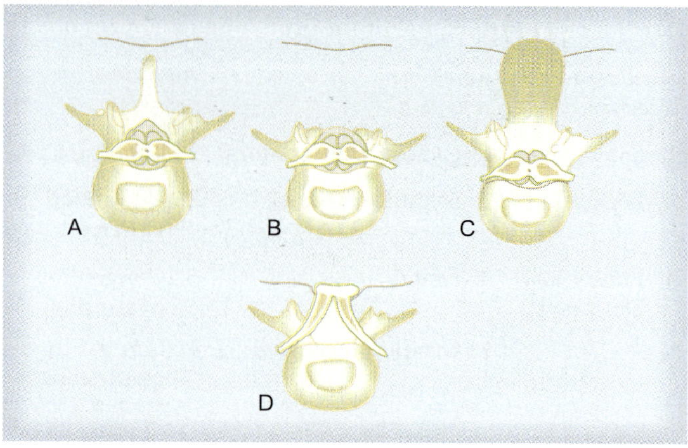

Figs 43.9A to D: Showing different types of spina bifida: (A) Spina bifida occulta, (B) Spina bifida aperta (meningocele), (C) Myelomeningocoele, (D) Myelocoele

Do you know what orthopaedic problems are encountered in myelomeningocele?

- Kyphosis (10–20%)
- Scoliosis (42–90%)
- Hip dislocations
- Congenital club feet.

And what about associated CNS defects:

- Congenital hydrocephalus (most common)
- Acquired hydrocephalus
- Tethered cord syndrome leading to traction injury of the cord and cauda equina
- Syringomyelia (40%).

Early Diagnostic Tools to Detect Neural Tube Defects (Dysraphism)

- *Ultrasound scanning*: Sensitivity is 96–100 per cent Specificity is 30 to 80 per cent
- *Amniotic fluid examinations*: This is to detect the presence of α-fetoprotein (AFP) and acetylcholinesterase levels by 15 to 16 weeks.
- Estimation of AFP in maternal serum.

Other Investigations

- *Radiology:* X-ray of the LS spine (AP/Lat/Oblique) helps to detect this abnormality (Fig. 43.10).
- CT scan and MRI are extremely useful in studying the entire spectrum of this problem.

Treatment

I. ***Preventive measures*** Needles to say that this is the most easiest and effective way of tackling

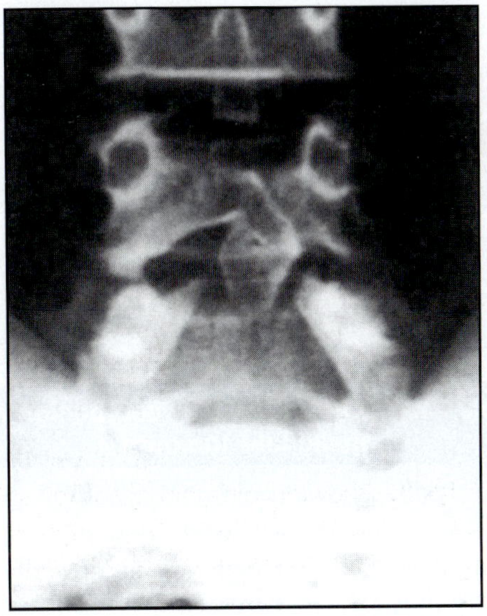

Fig. 43.10: Radiograph showing spina bifida

this menace. Instead of trampling the head of this unkind problem, it is better to see that it does not raise its ugly head in the first place. Some of the recommended measures are:

- All pregnant women should take folic acid or fortified folic acids during the period of pregnancy
- Dose of folic acid:
  a. In all women — About 400 mcg/day
  b. In high risk and those with familial history, previous history of NTD's birth, etc.
     — 4000 mcg/day for 3 to 4 months before conception.

II. ***Curative measures*** Surgery is the treatment of choice to close the neural tube defects or correct the orthopaedic deformities. Surgery to close NTDs should be done within 24 hours after birth to preserve the function of the spinal cord and minimise infection. Shunting operation is performed to tackle the associated hydrocephalus.

Treatment is aimed to surgically correct the spina bifida, foot deformities and other orthopaedic deformities. Bladder incontinence may require urological treatment.

BIBLIOGRAPHY

Cerebral palsy

1. Baker LD. A rationale approach to the surgical needs of the cerebral palsy patient. J Bone Joint Surg 1956;38-A:313.
2. Bax MCO. Terminology and classification of cerebral palsy. Dev Med Child Neurol 1964;6:295.
3. Bleck EE. Orthopaedic Management of Cerebral palsy. Philadelphia: WB Saunders, 1979.
4. Bost FC, Ashley RK, Kelly WJ. Role of the orthopaedic surgeon in the treatment of cerebrla palsy. JAMMA 1956;160-256.
5. Lord J. Cerebral palsy: a clinical approach. Arch Phys Med Rehabil 1984;65:542.
6. Person P, Williams CE. Physical Therapy Services in the Developmental Disabilities. Springfield III, 1980, Charles C Thomas.
7. Steindler A. Orthopaedic operations Springfleld, III, 1940, Charles C Thomas, Publisher.

Poliomyelitis

8. Barr JS. The management of poliomyelitis: The late stage: In poliomyelitis. First International Poliomyelitis Congress, Philadelphia: JB Lippincott Co, 1949.
9. Goldner JL, Irwin CE. Paralytic deformities of the foot. In American Academy of orthopaedic surgeons: Instructional Course lectures, Vol 5, Ann Arbor Mich 1948, JW Edwards.
10. Perry J, Barmes G. The postpolio syndrome. Clin Orthop 1988;233:145.
11. Shar WJ. Muscle recovery in poliomyelitis. J Bone J Surg 1955;37-B:163.
12. Steindler A. Orthopaedic operations: indications, techniques and results. Springfield III, 1940, Charles C Thomas, Publisher.

Spina bifida

13. Allan JH. The challenge of spina bifida cystica. In Adams, JP (Ed), Current Practice in Orthopaedic Surgery. St Louis. CV Mosby Co, Vol II, 1963.
14. Sharard WJW. The orthopaedic management of spina bifida. Acta Orthop Scand 1975;46:356.

44

Bone Neoplasias

INTRODUCTION

Like other systems in the body, musculoskeletal system may also develop tumours, either as a ***primary*** from this system itself or as a ***secondary*** from a distant primary location. The *latter appears to be more common*. Some of the tumours are benign and others are malignant. The accurate diagnosis of a neoplasm is a must before planning the treatment strategy. Diagnosis is best established by history, a proper physical examination and investigations like histological examination, biochemical assays, X-ray, CT scan, MRI, bone scans, arteriography, ultrasound, biopsy (both frozen section and permanent paraffin section), etc.

Primary bone tumours may be benign or malignant. Here is a quick review of the differences between benign and malignant tumours (Table 44.1):

Table 44.1: Differences between benign and malignant tumours

Benign tumours	*Malignant tumours*
• Slow growing	• Rapidly growing
• Well circumscribed	• Not well circumscribed
• Non-invading	• Invading
• No or few symptoms	• Associated with pain and disability
• Does not metastasise	• Metastasises
• X-ray shows lesions confined to the bone	• X-ray shows ill-defined borders, mottled appearance, cortex may be broken
• Does not cause death of the patient	• May cause death of the patient

Since the cells of the skeletal system are derived from the mesoderm, primary malignant bone tumours are called *sarcomas.*

Tumours spreading secondarily to the bone are generally primary carcinomas of breast, kidney, thyroid and lung. These tumours are called *metastatic carcinomas* because the tissue of origin is ectoderm.

Tumour cells may produce either tumour bone or osteoid (e.g. osteogenic sarcoma) or may cause reactive bone formation. Periosteal response may also be seen (e.g. Codman's triangle or onion peel appearance, etc.).

Treatment of benign tumours is usually by excision and if the defect is large, it is packed with bone grafts. Malignant tumours require a multipronged approach in the form of surgery, radiation, chemotherapy, immunotherapy, etc. With a combination of the above modalities of treatment, the recurrence rate has dropped considerably.

Knowledge of the origin, biologic behaviour and treatment of bone tumours is quite incomplete at the present time and much of the information is conflicting and controversial.

GENERAL PRINCIPLES OF TUMOURS

A proper understanding of the general principles of tumours enables one to make a correct diagnosis, choose the correct line of treatment which helps to minimise the recurrence rate and improve the survival rate.

The following are the parameters of general principles of tumours.

HISTORY Salient features are:

1. Pain, mass, disability are the usual presenting symptoms.
2. Anorexia, weight loss and fever are more pronounced in malignant tumours.
3. Onset—it is acute in malignant tumours and insidious in benign tumours.
4. Age—certain tumours have predilection for certain age groups, e.g. Ewing's sarcoma has a predilection for children.

Clinical Examination

General examination for evidence of anaemia, cachexia, lymphadenopathy, etc.

Local examination to know the extent, plane of the tumour, presence of pathological fractures, etc.

Joint examination to know the involvement of the joint, mechanical effects, etc.

Neurological examination to assess the damage to the peripheral nerves due to the spread of tumour.

Assessment of the status of arterial and/or venous circulation.

Investigations

Routine laboratory investigation Hb percentage is decreased, total WBC count and differential count is increased or decreased, ESR is increased, urianalysis. Serum calcium and phosphorous is increased, serum alkaline phosphatase is increased in tumours like osteogenic sarcoma, serum acid phosphatase is increased in metastatic tumours, etc.

Special investigations

Radiological examination of the part is done in two planes anteroposterior and lateral.

Chest radiographs for evidence of secondaries.

CT scan detects pulmonary metastasis at the earliest. It picks up the metastasis of the size of 2 mm compared to X-ray which does so at 2 cm size. It also helps in cross-sectional study of the tumour.

Arteriography This helps to determine the spread of the tumour to the vessel.

Ultrasonography This helps in some situations, though it has a very limited role.

MRI This is the most accurate method of assessing the bone and soft tissue involvement. It also helps in assessing the medullary spread of the tumour.

Bone scans help to detect the extent of spread of bone tumour to other areas of skeletal system and also to detect occult bone metastasis.

Biopsy This is an ultimate diagnostic technique in diagnosing bone tumours.

Usually, closed biopsies are preferred in malignant tumours. Needle biopsy has an accuracy rate of over 90 per cent in malignant tumours. If incisional biopsy is chosen, the incision should be placed longitudinally and should not exceed more than 2 cm.

Types

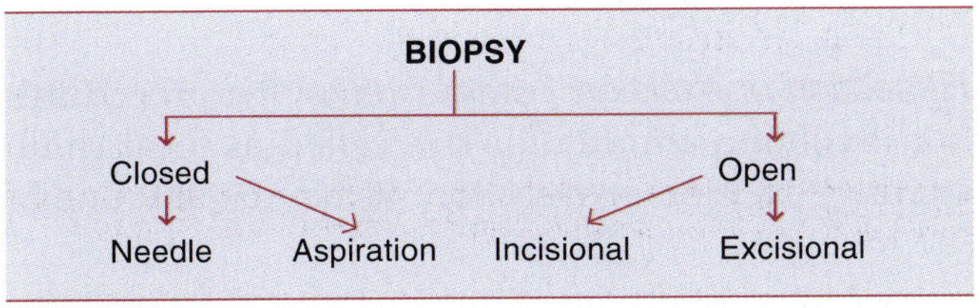

Remember

Tumour biopsy rules

- In malignant tumours, remove the tumour *en bloc*.
- No transverse incisions.
- No important neurovascular structures should be exposed.
- It should traverse only one compartment.
- Collect the sample from periphery of the tumour.
- If bone sample is to be taken, make a small circular or oval hole in the bone to prevent pathological fracture.

All the above investigations help to stage the bone tumour. Staging helps in detecting the type of surgical procedures needed for local control of the tumour.

Enneking's Staging

Enneking's staging is based on three criteria, histological grading, anatomical site, presence or absence of regional or distant metastasis.

I A *Low-grade* Intracompartmental (lesion confined to single anatomical plane)

I B *Low-grade* Extracompartmental (beyond a single compartment)

II A *High-grade* Intracompartmental

II B *High-grade* Extracompartmental.

III *Lesion high- or low-grade* Intra- or extracompartmental with distant or regional metastasis.

The high- or low-grade is a histological grading done on the basis of changes within the cells like pleomorphism, anaplasia, multicellularity, etc. due to malignancy.

0 = benign; 1 = low-grade malignancy; 2 = high-grade malignancy.

Surgical Techniques

Curettage Many benign bone tumours and locally malignant tumours are treated this way, but it leaves microscopic remnants. It gives good results if combined with cryosurgery, bone cement, or allografts, etc. If the lesion is diaphyseal, bone grafting is rarely necessary; but if it is epiphyseal or metaphyseal, allografting is necessary. Since curettage alone is associated with a high rate of recurrence, its role is limited.

Resection or excision Tumour removing procedures not involving amputation are called as local (limb sparing) excision or resection. It may be any one of the following.

Debulking or intralesional excision Here excision is done within the lesion.

Marginal margins Here excision is done through the pseudocapsule which is a thin rim of fibrous tissue formed by the surrounding tissues due to the compression by the tumour mass.

Wide margin Here the excision is carried out through the surrounding normal tissues. It is not useful in high-grade tumours because here the spread is along the fascial planes and this method still leaves some metastasis.

Radical resection Here all normal tissues of one or more compartments involved are removed from the origin to the insertion.

Radical amputation Here amputation is done at a high level.

Extracorporeal irradiated and reimplantation (ECIR) with composite arthroplasty: Here autogenous bone graft is either autoclaved or irradiated and reimplanted back combined with conventional arthroplasty which is fast emerging as an alternative to limb salvage surgery.

Choice of the Surgical Procedures

Surgery is usually advocated for local control of the tumour. Enneking's staging of the tumour decides the choice of surgery as suggested below.

Grade IA	Requires local procedure
Grade IB	Wide excision
Grade IIA	Radical excision
Grade IIB	Radical amputation
Grade III	Multipronged approach like Surgery + Chemotherapy + Radiotherapy

Adjunctive Therapy

Radiotherapy It should not be used for benign tumours (exception, pigmented villonodular synovitis) for the fear of inducing malignant changes within the cells. Its role is mainly *palliative* in non-resectable malignant tumours; but sometimes, it has a *definitive role* in shrinking the size of the tumour making the surgery less traumatic, and it is also known to make the cells *non-viable* and thereby minimise the chances of metastasis elsewhere, when these cells get into the circulation during the surgical procedure.

Chemotherapy This is the treatment of choice for micrometastasis with almost 100 per cent cure rate. If it is given early, it prevents the formation of metastasis. If given late, it shrinks the size of the tumour and thereby facilitates excision. It is highly effective against small tumours when given in combinations. Dosage, sequence, schedule and proper monitoring are matter of extreme importance.

Frequently, a combination of treatment modalities like radiotherapy, chemotherapy, etc. are used along with surgery. In these cases, less radical surgery are used to achieve local control. Limb sparing procedures are preferred over amputations.

Newer Modalities of Treatment

a. *Hyperthermia* This is usually tried in combinations with radiotherapy or chemotherapy.

b. ***Therapeutic embolisation***
c. *Immunotheraphy* Bacille-Calmette-Guérin (BCG) vaccines are found to be of use in control of certain tumours. The above three treatment modalities are at an experimental stage and are outside the scope of discussion here.

CLASSIFICATION OF BONE TUMOURS

Various classifications have been proposed for bone tumours like Dahlin's classification, Mercer's classification, Turek's classification, etc. The ABC classification of *Bristol Bone Tumour Registry* proposed by *Charles Price* is by far the easiest to understand and remember (Table 44.2).

Table 44.2: Classification of bone tumours

Section	*Benign*	*Malignant*
Section A Angioid tumours	• Angioma • Aneurysmal bone cyst • Glomus tumour	• Angiosarcoma
Section B Bone forming tumour	• Osteoma • Osteoblastoma • Osteoid osteoma	• Osteosarcoma • Parosteal osteosarcoma
Section C Cartilage forming tissue	• Chondroma • Osteochondroma • Chondroblastoma	• Chondrosarcoma
Section D Dental and allied structure	• Odontogenic cyst • Amelloblastoma	• Malignant odontoma
Section E Embryonic vestigeal tissue		• Chordoma
Section F Fibroblastic	• Fibroma	• Fibrosarcoma
Section H Heterotropic tissue	• Dermoid	• Adamantinoma of long bones
Section N Non-osseus connective tissue	• Lipoma • Neurofibroma • Neurilemmoma	• Liposarcoma • Reticulum cell sarcoma • Myeloma • Leukaemia • Hodgkin's • Ewing's • Leiomyosarcoma
Section S Synovial tissue	• Synovioma • Chondroma	• Synovial sarcoma
Section U Undifferentiated connective tissue	• Osteoclastoma	• Malignant osteoclastoma
Section X	• Undiagnosed primary bone tumours	• Undiagnosed primary bone tumours

BONE TUMOURS OF CARTILAGINOUS ORIGIN

OSTEOCHONDROMA (EXOSTOSIS)

This is the most common benign bone tumour. It is an offshoot from the spongy bone tissue covered with a cartilaginous cap (size of the cap may vary from 1 to 40 cm).

Age It is common during the growth period.

Sex It has a male preponderance.

Area Location favours the sites of *tendinous attachments* which are usually around the metaphysis of long bones in the region of knee, ankle, hip, shoulder and elbow.

Theory of Histogenesis

1. Though the exact cause is not known various theories have been postulated suggesting the possible mechanism of origin of this tumour. The cambium layer of the periosteum retains throughout life its ability to form cartilage and bone. It may be due to perverted activity of the periosteum, that it reverts to its role as the "perichodrium".
2. At points of tendinous insertion, there are focal accumulation of embryonic connective tissue.

Clinical Features

Symptoms Usually, it is symptomless, but the patient may complain of pain, swelling, etc. once complications like bursitis, malignant change, fracture, etc. have developed (Fig. 44.1A).

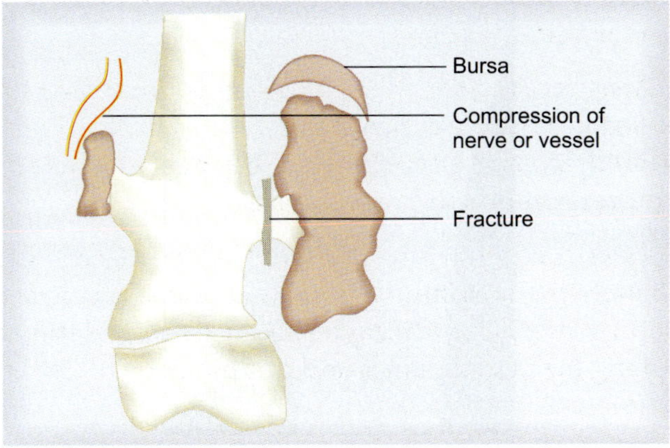

Fig. 44.1A: Showing osteochondroma and some of its complications

Signs A firm non-tender swelling fixed to the bone around the joints is the most common clinical finding. A bursa if inflamed will give rise to tenderness and local warmth. Joint movements may be decreased because of the tumour causing a mechanical block rather than the extension of the tumour into the joint.

Radiographic features This consists of an outgrowth of bone at the metaphysis. This attachment is sessile or pedunculated. The tumour is composed of cortical and medullary portions *which are continuous with the main bone.* The cartilage and capsules are not seen *unless it calcifies* (Fig. 44.1B).

Treatment

Usually, it requires no treatment, but complete surgical excision is indicated in the following situations:

1. *Joint interference* If the tumour is large and obstructing the joint movements, it needs excision of the tumour along with its periosteal cover to prevent recurrence of the tumour.
2. *Painful bursitis* A bursa usually develops because of the constant friction between the tumour and the surrounding soft tissues. If inflammation develops within this bursa, it gives rise to pain necessitating its excision.

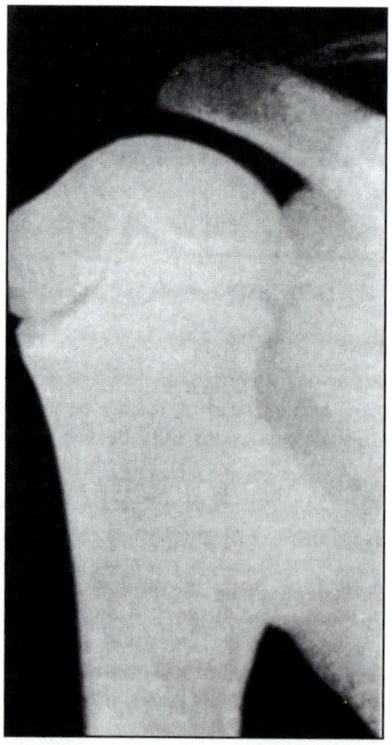

Fig. 44.1B: Radiograph showing osteochondrome upper end of humerus

3. *Fracture* of the bony stalk may occur due to trauma.
4. *Malignant change* (1–2%) Local irradiation may convert this benign tumour into malignant. It grows rapidly and has to be excised.
5. *Pressure on the neighbouring vessels* and nerves may give rise to neurovascular complications.

CHONDROMA (ENCHONDROMA, CHONDROMYXOMA)

This is a benign cartilaginous tumour centrally located when it occurs in phalanges and humerus. It causes destruction of the cancellous bone and has a potential for undergoing malignant change, especially when it is situated in the long bones.

- Age—10 to 50 years.
- Site—metaphysis is usually involved. It is common in the phalanges of hand (little finger common) and feet. Innominate and large long bones may also be involved.
- Symptoms are practically none. There may be slight pain and the phalanx may be enlarged (Fig. 44.2A).
- The course of the tumour is very slow.

Radiology

The tumour appears cystic (loculated or non-loculated), cortex is thin and expanded, it may be

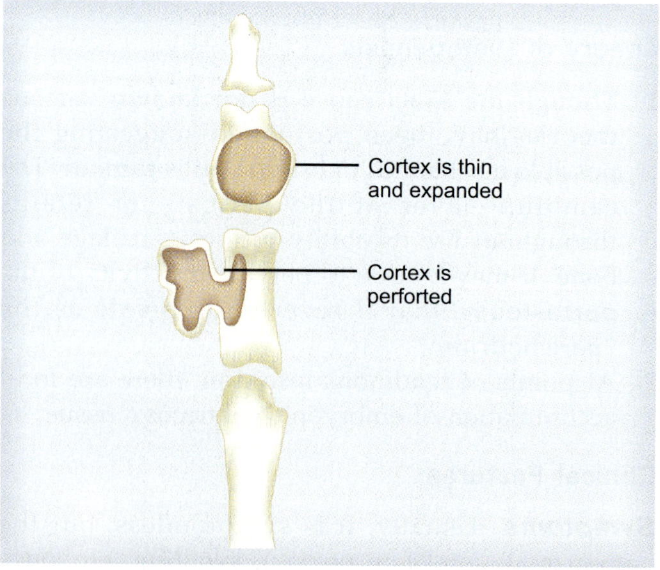

Fig. 44.2A: Showing enchondroma and its features

Section 5

perforated; and at the centre, fibrous septa may be seen interspersing the central cavity (Fig. 44.2B). Stippling or calcification may be present. There is *no reactive bone formation.*

Treatment

Curettage is done and the wall is cauterised if the tumour is small. The surgery done in cases of large tumours is excision and removal of the capsule to prevent recurrence. Radical resection is done for tumours of long bones and pelvis. *Recurrence is common with chondromas of the long bones.*

Prognosis

The incidence of malignant change is 25 per cent, especially in the pelvis.

CHONDROBLASTOMA

This is a highly cellular, vascular, and cartilaginous benign bone tumour of the cancellous bone. Here the cancellous bone is destroyed and multiple calcium deposits are usually found within the tumour.

Age 10 to 20 years.

Sex Male preponderance.

Sites Epiphyseal ends of long bones are commonly affected.

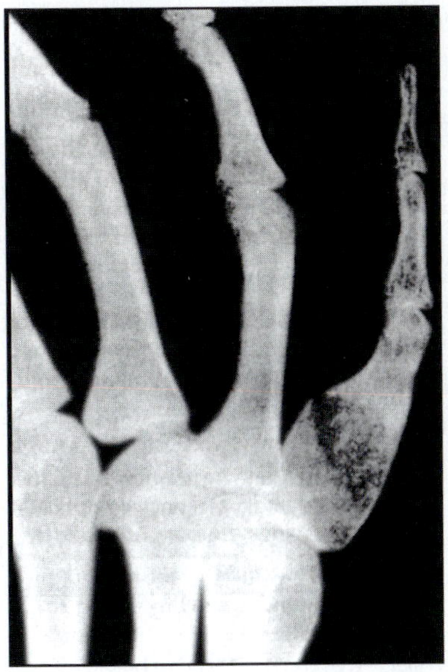

Fig. 44.2B: Radiograph showing enchondroma of the proximal phalanx

Symptoms The patient may present with pain, swelling, joint effusion, etc.

Radiology

Radiographic features of the tumour are areas of rarefaction at epiphysis, eccentric position of the tumour, thin cortex and mottled areas of calcification.

Treatment

This consists of curettage and bone grafting if the lesion is small, excision in bigger tumours. If it is accidentally irradiated, it may turn malignant. Recurrence rate after excision is 25 per cent.

CHONDROSARCOMA

This is *second* in frequency to osteosarcoma. It arises from the cartilage cells. It is a malignant but *slow* growing tumour. It has a long history and a better prognosis. Unlike osteogenic sarcoma, there is *no neoplastic osteoid formation and alkaline phosphatase is usually not raised.* It ranges from being locally aggressive to high-grade malignancy.

Classification

Primary/secondary Secondary tumours develop when benign cartilaginous tumours are irradiated.

Peripheral/central/juxtacortical depending on the situation of the tumour within the bone.

Low, medium and high grade malignancy depending on the cellularity.

Antecedent lesions

1. Multiple enchondroma (Ollier's disease)
2. Osteochondroma, etc.

Location It is common at the sites of proximal femur, humerus, ribs, scapula, innominate bones, rare in hands and feet except in calcaneus, occur in pelvis or upper femora.

Sex Males are more commonly affected than females.

Age Twenty to sixty years, rare below 20 years, peak in the sixth decade.

Symptoms The duration of symptoms are usually less than 2 years in 75 per cent of the cases and less than 5 years in the remaining 25 per cent. Pain is usually not a prominent feature unlike osteogenic sarcoma. The central tumour remains entirely asymptomatic till it has eroded and penetrated the cortex or caused a pathological fracture. A palpable firm mass attached to the bone is the common physical sign. The tumour may assume large proportion (Fig. 44.3A).

Radiology

1. *Central tumours* Central lytic lesion with calcification gives a fluffy, cotton wool, popcorn or breadcrumb appearance (Fig. 44.3B). Metaphysis or diaphysis of the long tubular bone is usually affected. Very rarely epiphysis may be involved. Greater degree of calcification is observed in slow growing tumours. It invades the soft tissue, there is little or no periosteal reaction seen.
2. *Peripheral tumours* These are very large tumors and the central part is heavily calcified.
3. *Juxtacortical tumours* are seen adjacent to the cortex.

Diagnosis

Biopsy is the only criterion to establish a diagnosis with certainty. This tumour is notorious for soft tissue seeding during biopsy. Hence, the biopsy scar should be small and within the area of resection.

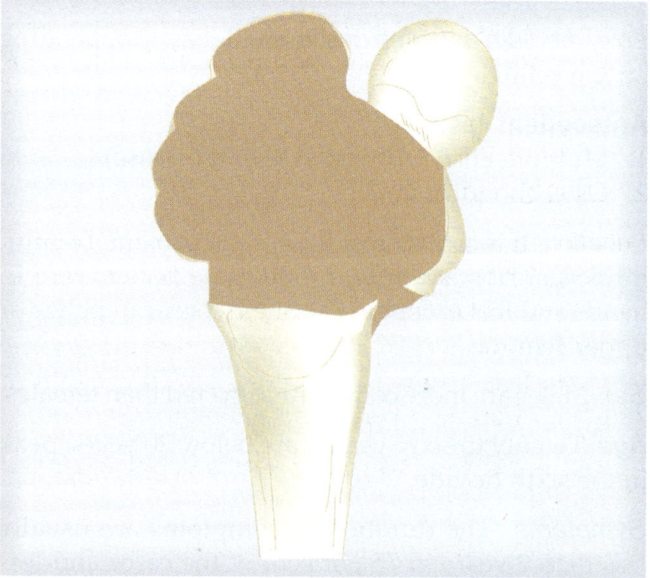

Fig. 44.3A: Showing chondrosarcoma affecting the upper end of the femur

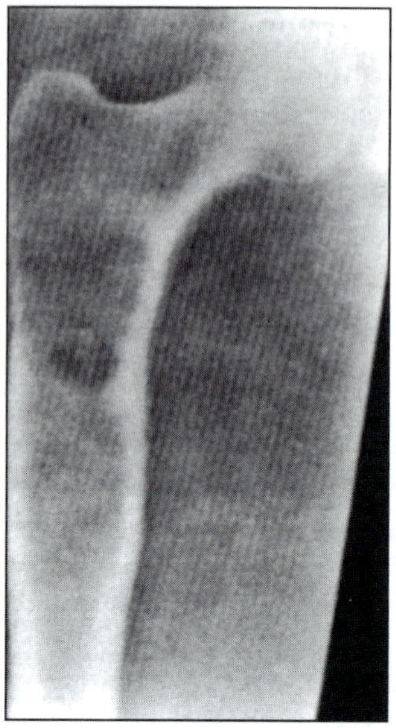

Fig. 44.3B: Radiograph showing chondrosarcoma

Treatment

Surgery is the treatment of choice.

Low and medium grade lesions require wide excision, e.g. Forequarter amputation (Thikor-Linberg) for the shoulder girdle; hindquarter amputation for the pelvic girdle.

High grade lesions require radical marginal excision Role of systemic chemotherapy in chondrosarcoma is controversial.

Palliative radiotherapy is indicated when the tumour cannot be resected because of its enormous size or if the tumour is present in inaccessible region.

Prognostic Factors

The following factors indicate poor prognosis:

1. *Location* Axial skeleton and proximal portions of the long bones.
2. *Age* More aggressive in childhood and young adults.
3. *Cytological features* suggesting high-grade malignancy are:
   - Increased water and calcium (85%).
   - DNA more than 5.5 µg/mg.
   - Excess protein more than 350 µg/mg.
   - Increased Ch-4-SO_4, decreased Ch-6-SO_4 (ratio > 1).
   - Decreased keratin sulphate.
   - Galactosamine/xylose ratio more than 10.
   - Hexosamine concentration less than 75 µg/mg.

4. *Size* larger the tumour, greater is the chance of malignancy.
5. *Secondary chondrosarcomas* are more malignant.
6. Survival time after treatment is 10 years. The comparative statistics are as follows after treatment:
   - Low grade tumours have 70 per cent survival rate.
   - Medium grade tumours have 50 per cent survival rate.
   - High grade tumours have 30 per cent survival rate.

Quick facts in Chondrosarcoma

- Second in frequency to osteosarcoma.
- No neoplastic osteoid.
- Long history.
- Pain is not a prominent feature.
- X-ray—*popcorn* appearance.
- Wide excision is the treatment of choice.
- Better survival rate.

CHONDROMYXOID FIBROMA

This is the least common benign cartilaginous bone tumour.

Age Young adults in the 2nd and 3rd decade are commonly affected.

Sex Equal incidence.

Location Metaphyseal ends of the long bones are commonly involved.

Clinical Features

Usually, the patient does not give a history of pain but complains of increasing swelling. A tender tumour mass may be palpable. Symptoms are more severe if the tumour develops in patients less than 10 years of age. Usually, it does not show sarcomatous change or metastasis.

Radiology

Radiographic features show eccentrically located tumour in the metaphysis. Cortex is expanded, thin and interrupted (Fig. 44.4). Medullary margins are scalloped and sclerosed, the base of the tumour shows triangular periosteal bone formation.

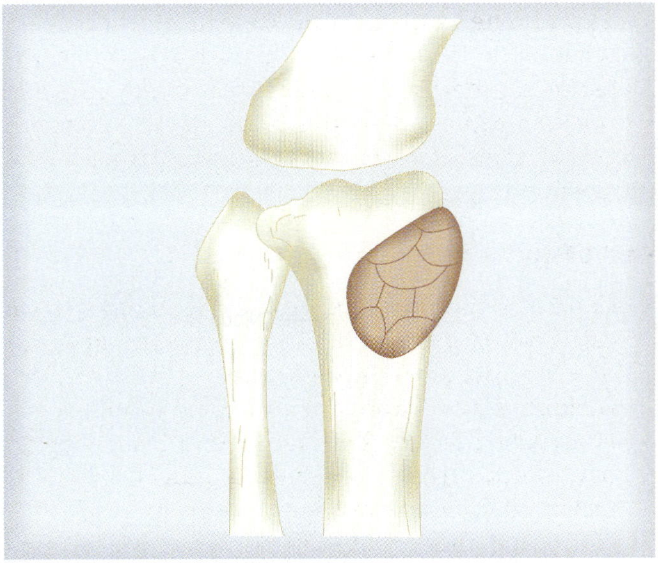

Fig. 44.4: Showing chondromyxoid fibroma, characteristic findings, lytic lesion, trabecular pattern and cortex slightly expanded

Treatment

The treatment of choice is local excision and bone grafting for small tumours, wide *en bloc* excision for large tumours.

OSSEOUS ORIGIN BONE TUMOURS

OSTEOMA

Osteoma is a benign bone tumour, occurs in membranous bones of skull and face. Usually, there are very few complaints, the history is long and the finding is a diffuse bony hard tumour. It rarely requires treatment.

[1]OSTEOID OSTEOMA

This is a benign osteoblastic tumour with a well-demarcated nidus of less than one cm surrounded by a distinct reactive bone (Fig. 44.5).

This tumour presents very interesting clinical features. It is a tumour of young adults, benign in nature and occurs in enchondral bones.

Age It is common in young adults between 10 and 25 years of age.

Sex Male preponderance (M:F = 2:1).

[1]**Osteoid osteoma**. This was described by Jattle H.L. of USA in the year 1935.

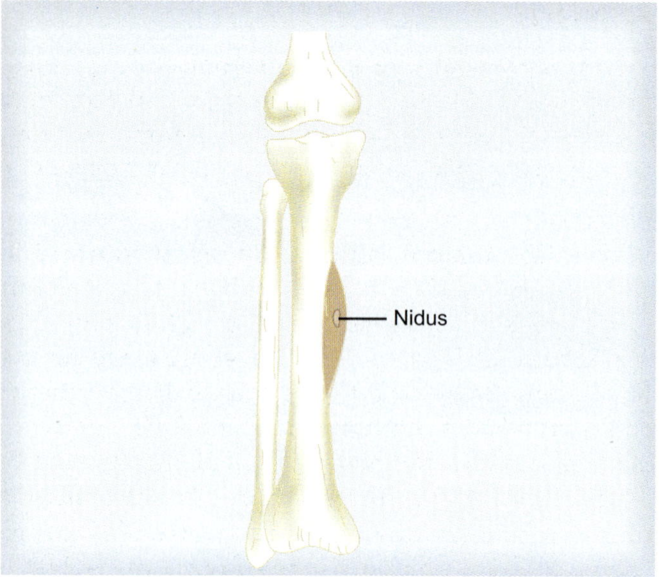

Fig. 44.5: Showing osteoid osteoma in tibia

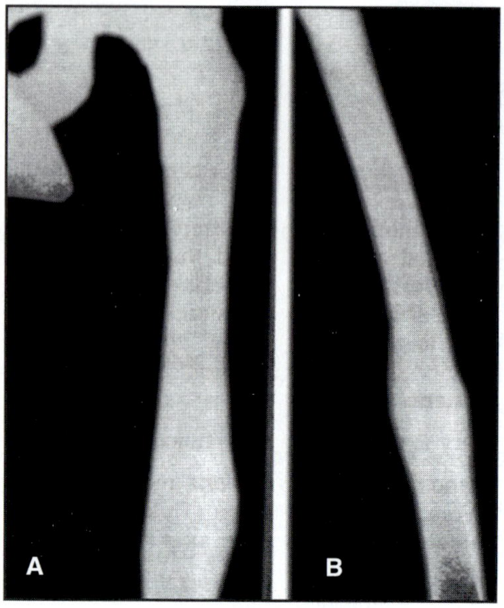

Figs 44.6A and B: Radiographs showing osteoid osteoma of the femur

Sites Long bones usually tibia and femur are more commonly affected.

Clinical Features

The patient complains of vague and intermittent pain which is more at night. The pain dramatically decreases after giving aspirin so much so that this is called the *therapeutic test*. The patient also complains of limp due to pain. There is a mild swelling, the local area may be tender, temperature is not raised, the skin is not stretched, shiny or warm. When the lesion occurs in the spine, the patient presents with acute low backache.

Radiology

It usually shows small rarefied lesion < 2 cm in diameter found in either the cortex, subcortical or subperiosteal regions. It is surrounded by a thick sclerotic bone. A small dense centre of ossification seen in the centre as the *nidus* (Figs 44.6A and B). Five per cent of the cases of sciatica are due to osteoid osteoma.

CT scan and MRI also help in diagnosing this tumour.

Treatment

Conservative line of treatment consists of rest to the part and analgesics. If the tumour is too troublesome, complete excision of the cortex containing the nidus is sufficient.

Do you know what is new in the management of osteoid osteoma?

- For the rare intra-articular situation, arthroscopically assisted excision is done
- CT-guided endoscopic removal
- Percutaneous excision
- MRI-guided cryotreatment
- CT-guided biopsy and thermocoagulation.

OSTEOGENIC SARCOMA

Osteogenic sarcoma is a highly malignant bone tumour (Fig. 44.7). Here tumour cells invariably form a neoplastic osteoid or bone or both. It arises from a common multifactorial mesenchymal tissue; and hence, the tumour could be either *fibroblastic, osteoblastic* or *chondroblastic*.

This is the most frequent primary bone tumour next only to multiple myeloma.

Age It is common in the second decade, rare below 10 years of age, 75 per cent of the cases are seen below the age of 25 years.

Sex Male preponderance. When found in females, it starts at an early age.

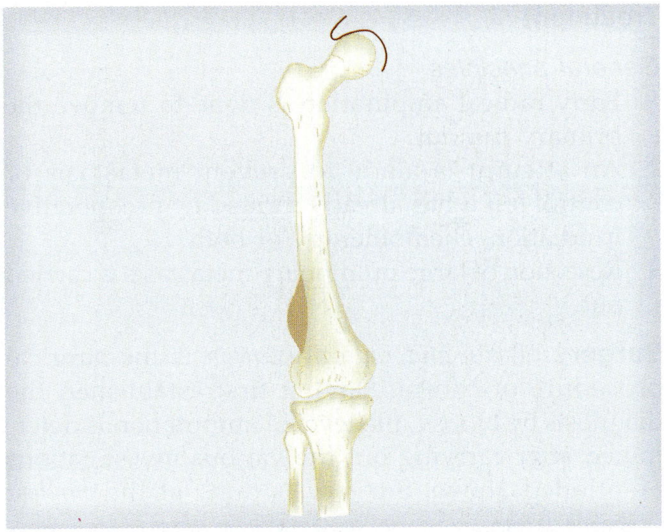

Fig. 44.7: Showing osteogenic sarcoma lower end of femur

Incidence is 1/75,000 population.

Site Ninety per cent of the tumour occurs in the metaphysial region of the ends of long bones. It has a predilection around the knee and upper humerus. It may affect the jaws in the aged.

Location

— Fifty-two per cent of the cases occur in the femur (9% in greater trochanter).
— Twenty per cent of cases are seen in the tibia (90% in upper medial aspect).
— Nine per cent are seen in the humerus. It is common in the upper end but rare below the deltoid tubercle.

Exciting Factors

The predisposing factors of this tumour are:

a. *Virus*
   - DNA virus—Polyoma and SV 40 virus.
   - RNA virus—Harvey and Moloney mouse sarcoma virus. These are known to produce tumours in experimental animals but not known in humans.

b. *Radiation* If a dose of more than 2000 rads are given to osteoprogenitor cells situated in areas of active growth at the metaphysis, malignancy sets in.

c. *Chemicals* Twenty methyl cholanthrene, beryllium compounds are known to induce malignancy changes.

Pathology

The tumour could be either osteoblastic, chondroblastic or fibroblastic. Consequently, the tumour may be osteosclerotic or osteolytic. Most common tumour is both a combination of osteosclerotic and osteolytic variety.

Gross The tumour is more commonly situated in metaphysis of a large long bone. It is a large tumour with areas of destruction (Fig. 44.8) gives an appearance of *leg of mutton.* The consistency ranges from stony hard to soft. The colour of the tumour could be *white* if the tumour is *fibroblastic, yellowish white* if *osteoblastic; bluish white;* if the tumour is *cartilaginous.* At the areas of rapid growth, there is necrotic foci, cavitation and haemorrhage. *Sunray* appearance is seen in the subperiosteal space due to bone deposition along the vessels. *Codman's triangle* is a reactive bone formation parallel to the bone and is triangular in shape.

Histology

Small spindle cells with hyperchromatic nuclei are seen. The shape may be round, cuboidal or columnar. Cells are pleomorphic in nature. Large spindle-shaped cells are rare. Giant cells are often present. Matrix may be either myxomatous, cartilaginous or

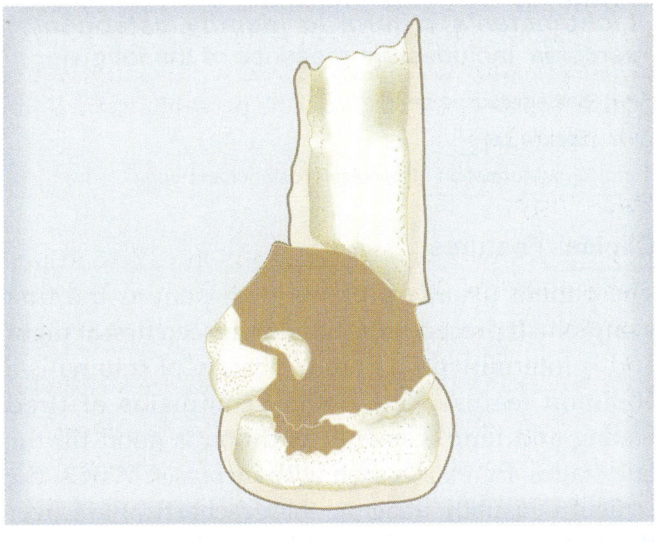

Fig. 44.8: Showing osteogenic sarcoma showing widespread destruction of the metaphysis, extension into the soft tissue and epiphysis. Spread to the joint is limited by the growth plate

osseous. Areas of haemorrhage may be present. Normally, when the bone forms an osteoid tissue, it is preceded by the stage of chondrification. *Neoplastic or tumour osteoid formed from the primitive malignant cells skip the stage of chondrification and form the ossified tissue directly without any intervening stage of chondrification.*

Classification

1. Primary and secondary.
2. Dahlin's (prognostic) classification:
   a. *Osteoblastic* Poor five-year survival rate.
   b. *Chondroblastic* Five-year survival rate is three times more than that of osteoblastic variety.
   c. *Fibroblastic* Five-year survival rate is two times more of osteoblastic variety.
3. *Geschickter and Copeland* classification:
   a. Sclerosing type.
   b. Osteolytic type.
   c. Mixed type of both osteoblastic and osteolytic varieties.
   d. Telangiectatic type.

Secondary osteosarcoma *This is less malignant than the primary, develops in bones affected with Paget's disease, diaphyseal aclasia, enchondromas, irradiation, etc. It is more common in older age groups and is treated on the same lines as the primary.*

***Lichtensten's criteria to identify osteogenic sarcoma* includes the presence of the following:**

a. Sarcomatous stroma
b. Spindle cells
c. Direct formation of neoplastic osteoid and bone.

Clinical Features

The patient usually presents with pain as the first symptom. It precedes the tumour, is seen first at night and is intermittent in nature. History of trauma is a common feature. The patient complains of tired feeling and limp. General condition is good till the late stages. Pyrexia is seen with increased WBCs. the patient is usually anaemic than cachectic. Skin over the tumour is stretched, shiny and mobile. Local temperature is increased, consistency of the tumour is variable, dilated veins are present (and is evident at an early stage).

Treatment

General principles

1. Early radical amputation is done to remove the primary tumour.
2. An attempt is made to prevent metastasis or control it if it has already formed by preoperative irradiation, chemotherapy or both.
3. Resection of large pulmonary metastasis is carried out.

Surgery *Early and radical ablation* is the surgical procedure of choice. Having first established the diagnosis by biopsy, the level of amputation is determined after carrying out the various investigations mentioned above. Surgery is done at the *earliest* possible time.

Quick facts

Osteosarcoma: Levels of amputation

a. Upper end of humerus: Forequarter amputation.
b. Upper end of tibia: Midthigh amputation.
c. Upper end of femur: Hindquarter amputation and hip disarticulation.
d. Lower end of femur: Midthigh amputation and hip disartication.

Newer techniques:

- ***Limb salvage with tumour endoprosthesis*** This is showing a better final clinical outcome in recent times
- In juxta-articular osteogenic sarcoma, intra-epiplyseal excision and biological reconstruction to give excellent functional results.

Megavoltage radiotherapy Megavoltage irradiation is given preoperatively before amputation to decrease the *viability* of the cells that may be disseminated into bloodstream by surgical trauma. It is an useful adjunct in the treatment of resectable tumours. Its efficacy is doubtful in the non-resectable tumours, e.g. vertebra. Irradiation destroys tumour cells with minimal effect on the uninvolved parts.

Preliminaries before irradiation

1. Bone scans are done to detect the skip lesions.
2. Biopsy scar is limited to < 2 cm size to avoid skin necrosis.
3. Chemotherapy is given to increase the susceptibility of tissues to irradiation.
4. Dose—Total dose of irradiation is 6,000–8,000 rads or 230 rads/day or 1000 rads/week.

Chemotherapy (CT) Role of chemotherapy is as follows:

- After ablation of the primary tumour, it produces a disease-free state for many months.
- If given before the metastasis is apparent, it improves the 5-year survival rate by 60 per cent.
- Chemotherapy approach assumes, that at least 80 per cent of the patients have microscopic foci in the lungs at the time of initial diagnosis.
- Chemotherapy started early after the diagnosis destroys the microscopic foci at a stage when they are most susceptible to the action of chemotherapy drugs.
- It prevents metastasis in 60 per cent of the cases. The remaining 40 per cent become disease free due to aggressive attack on the metastasis. After metastasis has occurred, chemotherapy decreases the tumour size and enables easy surgical removal.
- When the patient refuses amputation, but accepts local resection and implant, chemotherapy decreases the size of the tumour.

Earlier osteogenic sarcoma was refractory to chemotherapy. But it has now been found that high doses of methotrexate, citrovorum factor rescue (CFR) and adriamycin are effective. By using the above drugs in short cyclical courses, toxic effects can be held to a minimum. Addition of an alkylating agent, like cyclophosphamide, has increased the interval between the administration of individual drugs. This has markedly reduced the toxicity of the drugs. The treatment triad in order of sequence are shown in Figure 44.9.

In summary, after having established the diagnosis of osteogenic sarcoma with certainty, the patient is initially put on chemotherapy. The role of chemotherapy has already been discussed. Local irradiation of the tumour is done next. Early radical surgical ablation is then carried out at the appropriate time.

Treatment of Pulmonary Metastasis

Pulmonary microemboli are best managed by chemotherapy. Large lesions require removal by wide resection or lobectomy after giving chemotherapy.

Another experimental approach to manage the lethal metastasis is the immunological approach. The immunological status is increased by giving specific antibiotics, BCG vaccine, allogenic sarcoma tumour cell vaccine for two years, interferon therapy, etc.

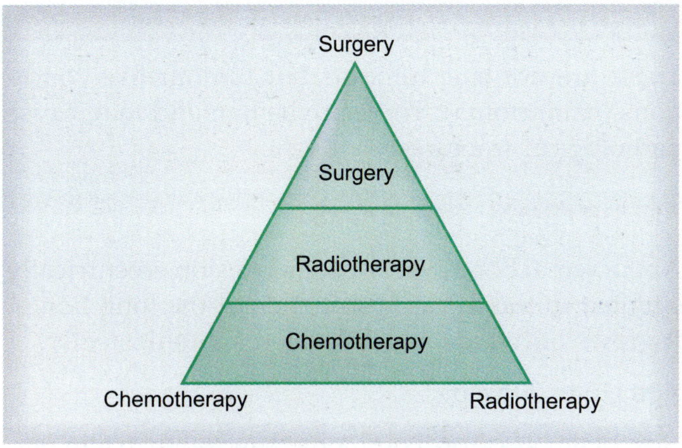

Fig. 44.9: Showing triad of treatment in osteogenic sarcoma

Prognosis

Prognosis of osteogenic sarcoma has dramatically improved by the combined approach of ablation, megavoltage irradiation and chemotherapy.

In untreated cases, survival time after pulmonary metastasis has developed (around 2.9 per cent).

With the combined approach of chemotherapy, radiotherapy and pulmonary resection, the five-year survival rate has increased by 60 per cent.

Osteogenic sarcoma is curable and warrants intensive treatment with chemotherapy and surgical resection.

Remember

Charactreristic facts of osteogenic sarcoma

- Highly malignant bone tumour.
- Arises from multipotent cells.
- Most frequent primary bone tumour next only to multiple myeloma.
- Seventy-five per cent are below 25 years of age.
- Ninety per cent occur in the metaphysis.
- Neoplastic osteoid is always present.
- Both osteosclerotic and osteolytic variety is the most common.
- Leg of mutton appearance.
- Spindle cells.
- No giant cells.
- Pain is the first symptom.
- Skin is stretched shiny, dilated veins are present.
- Pathological fractures are not common.
- Eighty per cent has blood spread.
- Sunray appearance and Codman's triangle are special X-ray features.
- Multipronged approach gives better survival rate.

RESORPTIVE BONE TUMOURS

These are not true tumours but tumour-like conditions (hamartoma). These are benign and may cause pathological fractures.

ANEURYSMAL BONE CYST

Aneurysmal bone cyst is a benign lesion eccentrically situated in the metaphyseal ends of the long bones. It grows outwards and is located subperiosteally.

Age 10 to 30 years.

Sex Males are more commonly affected than females.

Clinical Features

The patient usually gives history of mild trauma. Pain and swelling are the main complaints. Joint movements may be decreased.

Radiology

Radiographic features of the tumour consists of radiolucent area situated at the metaphysis. It extends outwards eccentrically, periosteal new bone formation is seen, and pathological fractures may be present (Figs 44.10A and B).

Pathology

It is a thin shell of bone enclosing cystic blood-filled spaces. Partially organised clots remain in the centre of the tumour. Microscopy shows blood-filled spaces. Giant cells are seen.

Treatment

Surgery is the treatment of choice. Curettage and bone grafting is the procedure commonly followed.

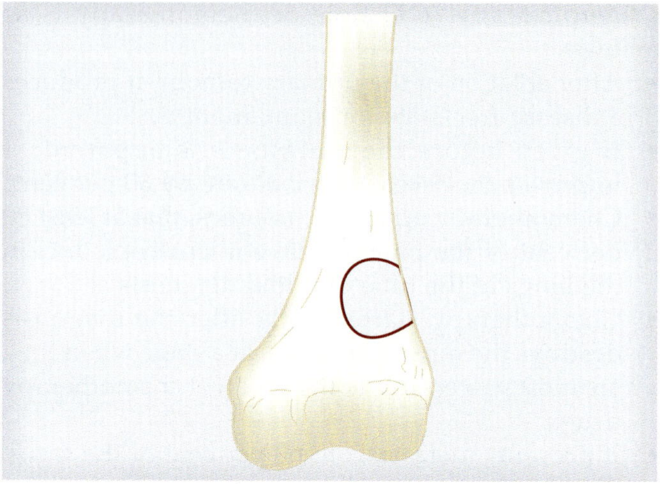

Fig. 44.10A: Aneurysmal bone cyst

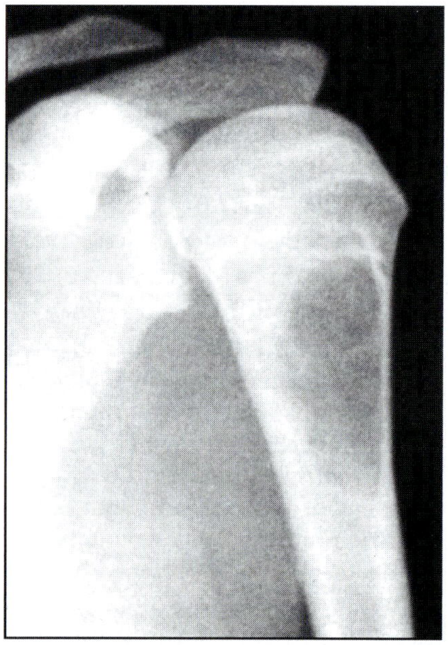

Fig. 44.10B: Radiograph showing aneurysmal bone cyst upper end of humerus

UNICAMERAL BONE CYST

Unicameral bone cyst was first described by Jaffe and Lichtenstein in the year 1942.

It is an uncommon, non-neoplastic lesion commonly seen in the first two decades of life. It is situated in the metaphysis of the long bones and its proximity towards the epiphysis may affect the growth plate. Pathological fracture is a common entity. The cyst will not disappear on its own and remains so unless obliterated by surgery.

Age Fifty per cent lesions are seen in less than 10 years of age, forty per cent between 10 and 20 years.

Sex The male to female ratio is 2:1.

Location Upper end of humerus in 55 per cent, upper end of femur in 26 per cent.

Pathology

Gross It is a fusiform swelling, occupying the metaphyseal region of the bone. The underlying bone is thin with areas of haemorrhage present.

Section 5

Microscopy The cells are flat and vascular tissue is present. It has characteristic *giant cells.*

Types of cyst There are two types of bone cysts:

Active cyst is so called if the cyst is situated close to the epiphyseal plate.

Latent cyst is so called if the cyst moves away from the growth plate.

Clinical Features

The tumour is asymptomatic till fracture occurs through the cyst wall which causes pain and draws the attention of the patient towards the problem. In most cases, the cyst is juxtaepiphyseal. Due to its proximity to the growth plate, the cysts may cause shortening, lengthening, coxa vara or coxa valga deformities. The tumour weakens the bone and the patient is susceptible to pathological fractures. Spontaneous obliteration of the cyst is seen in 15 per cent of the cases and in 30 per cent of the cases, cyst is displaced down the shaft due to continuous bone growth.

Radiology

Radiographic examination of the tumour shows lytic lesion in the juxtaepiphyseal portion of the metaphysis, the lesion is expansive, the regional cortex is attenuated and pathological fractures may be seen (Figs 44.11A and B).

Complications

Since the tumour is situated in the juxtaepiphyseal region, complications like shortening, coxa vara, coxa valga and bone overgrowth may develop.

Treatment

Surgical excision is the treatment of choice. The following are some of the surgical procedures.

Types of Surgery

a. *Curettage and bone grafting* This procedure is associated with high rate of recurrence.
b. *Subtotal resection and bone grafting* Here 1 cm of the normal bone above and below the lesion is excised.
c. *Total resection and bone grafting* is the other method of treatment.

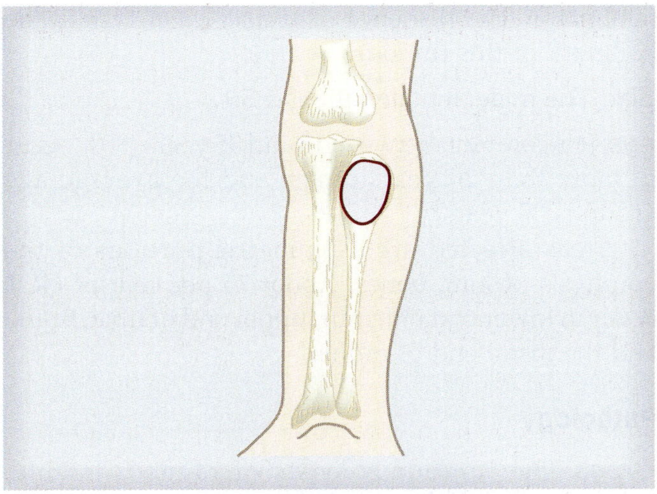

Fig. 44.11A: Showing features of unicameral bone cyst

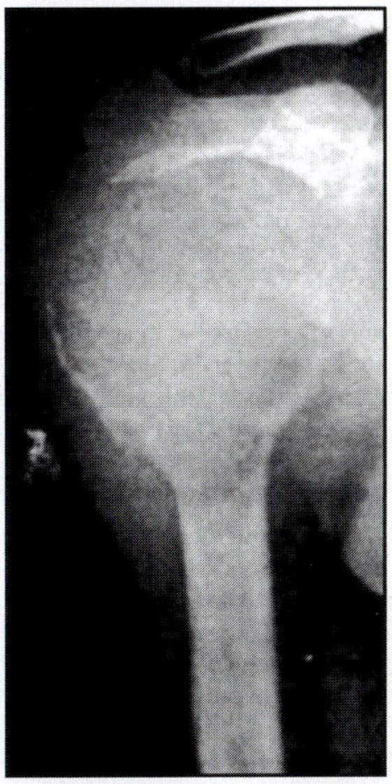

Fig. 44.11B: Radiograph showing unicameral bone cyst of upper end of humerus

d. *Intracystic injection of corticosteroids* Steroids injected into the cysts are known to cause obliteration of the cyst 40 to 80 mg of prednisolone for smaller cysts recommended, larger cysts may require 200 mg of prednisolone.

GIANT CELL TUMOUR (GCT) (SYN: OSTEOCLASTOMA)

BENIGN GIANT CELL TUMOUR

Benign giant cell tumour (GCT) is an osteolytic tumour arising from the *epiphysis* and is common in young adults. Though it is benign, it is *locally* malignant. The presence of *tumour giant cells* is the hallmark of this tumour.

Sex The male: female ratio is 1.5:1.

Age It is common between 15 and 35 years (80% occur in more than 20 years of age and the average age group is 35 years).

Areas affected are asymmetric portions of the epiphysis of long bones. About 75 per cent of GCT occur in lower end of femur, upper end of tibia, fibula and the distal end of radius.

Pathology

Gross The tumour consists of ragged, friable, bleeding tissue filled with old or fresh blood clots with various sized cysts and cavities. Colour varies from red to brown. Epiphyseal end of the bone is distorted. Tumour extension into the joint cavity is usually not seen and also there is no evidence of periosteal reaction.

Microscopy The tumour is encompassed by a fibrous capsule at the periphery. Presence of abundant tumour giant cells are quite characteristic. These cells are characterised by their larger size, multiple nuclei more than 150 in number which are distributed throughout the cell. Appearance of spindle cells indicate *malignant* potential.

Histological Grading (Jaffe's Criterion)

Grade I	• Presence of characteristic stromal cells • Little intercellular collagen • Spindle cells are adjacent to the necrotic tissue
Grade II	• Random distribution of giant cells are seen among the stromal cells
Grade III	• Nuclei of giant cells are identical to those of the stromal cells

Clinical Features

The course of the tumour is chronic. Unlike osteogenic sarcoma, pain is not the presenting feature but trauma is, the patient complains of swelling which is situated on one side of the bone. Skin over the tumour is stretched, but there are no dilated veins. Tenderness is moderate or absent, *egg shell crackling* sensation may be present or absent. Limitation of joint movements is not seen till the late stages. There is no increase in joint fluid and the joint is rarely invaded. Pathological fracture is a late feature.

Radiology

- An osteolytic area is seen near the epiphysis
- The cortex is expanded and thin
- There is no periosteal new bone formation
- Thin septa of bone traverse the interior and produce a *soap-bubble appearance* (Figs 44.12A and B)
- The cortex may be disrupted in late stages
- Joint extension is rare.

Campanacci's radiographic grading

1. *Grade 1* Cystic lesion.
2. *Grade 2* Cortex is thin but not perforated.
3. *Grade 3* Cortex is perforated with extension into soft tissues.

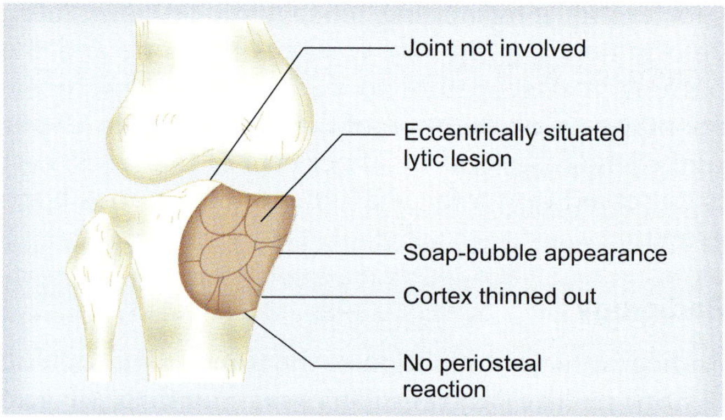

Fig. 44.12A: Radiological features of giant cell tumor

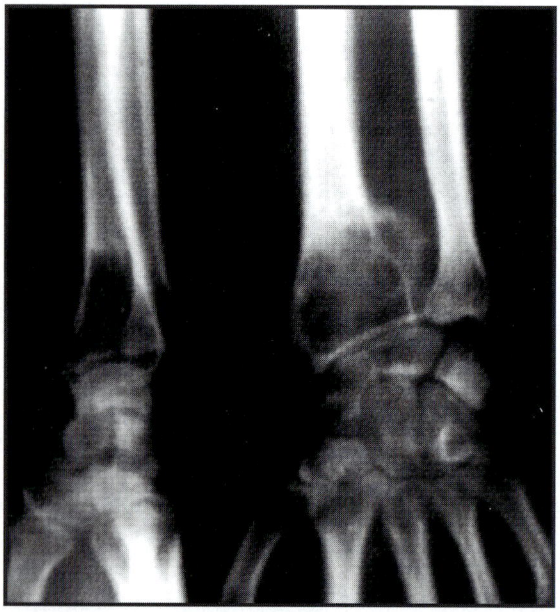

Fig. 44.12B: Radiographs showing the giant cell tumour of the lower end of radius showing the soap bubble appearance

Malignant GCT

Primary This develops as a frank sarcomatous lesion.

Secondary This develops at the site of previously treated GCT.

Enneking's Staging of Benign GCT

Stage I (Latent)	• Incidence is 10 to 15 per cent • Discovered accidentally, no symptoms. • Pathological fracture may be present
Stage II (Active)	• Incidence is 70 per cent • Symptomatic, pathological fracture may be present • Benign
Stage III (Aggressive)	• Incidence is 10 to 15 per cent • Symptomatic, rapidly growing • Benign • Cortex is perforated

Treatment of GCT

Principles of tumour treatment:

- The tumour is invasive and aggressive.
- It commonly recurs, may become malignant after unsuccessful removal.
- Recurrence is treated with *en bloc* excision.
- *En bloc* excision is also indicated if the tumour has eroded the cortex and extended into the soft tissues.

Surgical Methods

More aggressive approach is adopted for more aggressive lesions and the surgical methods described are:

Curettage and bone grafting It is a simple technique but is associated with high recurrence rate (about 30%).

En-bloc excision This is the initial procedure of choice and here 2 cm of normal tissue is also excised. Defects are filled with cancellous bone grafts, freeze dried allografts or prosthesis. This technique has low recurrence rate.

Curettage and arylic bone cementation This has a low rate of recurrence and the heat of polymerisation destroys residual stromal and giant cells (0.5 cm).

Curettage and cryosurgery This destroys the residual tumour at its margin of curettage by repetitive freezing and thawing by liquid nitrogen. Malignancy change rate decreases from 15 to 1.9 per cent.

Excision and reconstruction This procedure can be followed for GCT affecting the lower end of femur or upper end of tibia. After *en bloc* excision, reconstruction can be done by one of the following methods.

a. *Turn-o-plasty technique* Here after excision of the tumour in the lower end of femur, the required length of the proximal tibia is chosen, split into two halves and one-half of it is turned upside down and fixed with the left over stump of the femur. If the lesion is in the tibia, the procedure is done by taking half of the femur.
b. Arthrodesis is done by using the fibula from both the sides to bridge the excised gap.
c. *Arthroplasty* After tumour excision, arthroplasty is done either by using an autograft, allograft or prosthesis.

Irradiation therapy induces malignant change if it is given to the benign lesion. Megavoltage therapy is permissible only for inaccessible lesions located in the spine, sacrum, pelvis, etc. The recommended dosage is 1,500 to 5,000 rads for 5 to 6 weeks.

Other Methods

1. *Marginal resection with curettage* This is done using power burrs with copious irrigation of 5 per cent phenol and 70 per cent alcohol.
2. *Resection of distal radius* and using ipsilateral proximal fibula to reconstruct the wrist joint.
3. *Amputation* is done for widespread aggressive tumour as a last resort.

Treatment facts of GCT

Site	Surgical option
I. Upper limb	
a. Lower end of ulna	Excision
b. Lower end of radius	Excision with reconstruction by ipsilateral fibula
II. Lower limbs	
a. Lower end of femur	Excision with Turn-o-graft
b. Upper end of tibia	Excision with Turn-o-graft

Quick facts of GCT

- Locally malignant.
- Affects young adults.
- Arises from the epiphysis.
- Giant cells are characteristic.
- Egg shell crackling may be present.
- Soap-bubble appearance is characteristic.
- *En bloc* excision and reconstruction is the surgical method of choice.
- One-third are benign, one-third is locally malignant and one-third is malignant.

Note: **Mnemonic BLUNACH denotes lesion with giant cells. (Differential diagnosis of GCT)**

Benign chondroblastoma
Localised osteitis fibrosa
Unicameral bone cyst
Non-ossifying fibroma
Aneurysmal bone cyst
Chondromyxoid fibroma
Hyperparathyroidism

TUMOURS OF NON-OSSEOUS ORIGIN

[2]EWING'S SARCOMA

Ewing's sarcoma was first described by Ewing in the year 1928. This is a rare primary malignant bone tumour (10–14% of all malignant bone tumours) affecting children. It is a lethal tumour with a poor 5-year survival rate.

Clinical Features

Age persons commonly affected are four to twenty five years of age group (about 80%).

Sex More common in males.

Site Long bones affected are femur, tibia, fibula and humerus in that order. About 20 per cent of tumours are seen in flat bones.

Location Diaphysis of the long bones is commonly affected.

Pathology

Gross It is a greyish white tumour encapsulated by fibrous tissue. It may contain haemorrhagic foci and areas of cystic formation. From the medulla, it reaches to the surface through the haversian canals.

Histology

The tumour is very *cellular.* The cells may be small, round or polyhedral in shape and may be arranged as cords or sheets. Intercellular substance is minimal. Necrosis is common. Cells are arranged round the vessels justifying the term *perithelioma.* Many tumours show *Rosette* formation with central fibril. *Pseudorosettes* are more common (no central fibril). Giant cells are not found and there is no new bone formation.

Differential diagnosis is between reticulum cell sarcoma and Ewing's sarcoma:

1. Ewing's stains for *Glycogen positivity* by PAS.
2. In reticulum cell sarcoma *Silver stain* is positive.

Clinical Features

The patient presents with pain which is intermittent in nature. The pain is worse at night. The tumour is diaphyseal and fixed to the bone, skin is red, dilated veins may be present (Fig. 44.13A). Sometimes the tumour may present with constitutional symptoms like fever, sweating, chills, leucocytosis, anaemia. This may create confusion as it mimicks acute osteomyelitis.

Course

- Exacerbation and remission is characteristic.
- Blood and lymphatic spread is common.
- Metastasis to other bones like skull, vertebrae, ribs, lungs, etc. may occur.

Investigations

Radiographic features

- The lesion could be lytic, sclerotic or mixed.
- Diaphysial lesion with irregular destruction (moth-eaten appearance or cracked ice appearance).
- Periosteal new bone formation is in layers giving an *onion peel* appearance (Fig. 44.13B).
- Permeative margin.

Biopsy is necessary for diagnosis.

Other tests

- *Urine* for vanillylmandelic acid (VMA).
- *Tissue* for glycogen stain.
- Immunohistochemical markers.
- *Electron microscopy study.*

N.B. Onion peel appearance is also seen in:

- Osteomyelitis
- Osteosarcoma
- Malignant lymphoma

[2]**James Ewing** (1966-1943), Oncologist (USA). It was first described by Ewing in the year 1928.

Recommended Treatment

This tumour is highly radiosensitive, disappears with radiation only to recur back again (melts like snow). Hence, a combination of local radiotherapy with systemic chemotherapy brings down the recurrence rate dramatically. But even this treatment has a recurrence rate of 20 to 30 per cent and because of the possibility of radiation-induced sarcomas, surgical resection for the control of the primary lesion is being used. The surgery planned is conservative in nature and aims at limb preservation.

Effective chemotherapy is given using newer chemotherapeutic drugs like Ifosfamide, cisplatinum, epipodophyllin toxin for a short period of time.

Radiation is the mainstay of local treatment, especially in axial skeleton. Dose required is high 4,000 rads for the entire limb and 1000 rads as boost to the tumour.

Surgery Conservative surgery like debulking of the tumours, or limb preservation surgery has a role.

Unfavourable prognostic features are

- *Male patients.*
- *Humerus if involved.*
- *Pelvic bones if involved.*
- *Distant metastasis.*

Primary irradiation followed by amputation has a two year survival rate of 15 per cent. A combination of chemotherapy, radiotherapy with surgery improve the survival rate to 50 to 75 per cent for 3 to 5 years.

Quick facts of Ewing's sarcoma

- Rare primary malignant tumour.
- Common between 5 and 15 years.
- Tumour of the diaphysis.
- Clinically may mimick acute osteomyelitis.
- X-ray shows moth-eaten appearance and onion peel appearance.
- Tumour is highly cellular.
- Highly radiosensitive (melts like snow).
- High rate of recurrence.
- Combination of radiotherapy, chemotherapy and surgery has improved 2-year survival rate.

MULTIPLE MYELOMA (Plasmacytoma)

This is the most common bone tumour in adults. It accounts for 50 per cent of all bone tumours. Here plasma cells replace the bone. It affects elderly persons between 40 and 60 years of age.

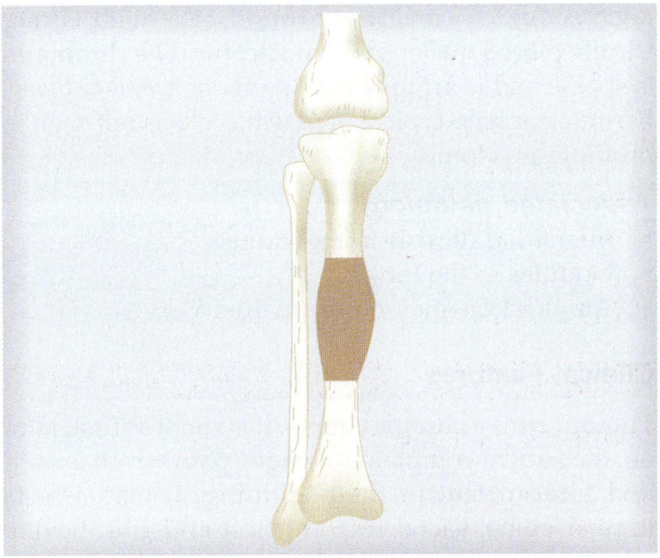

Fig. 44.13A: Showing features of Ewing's sarcoma

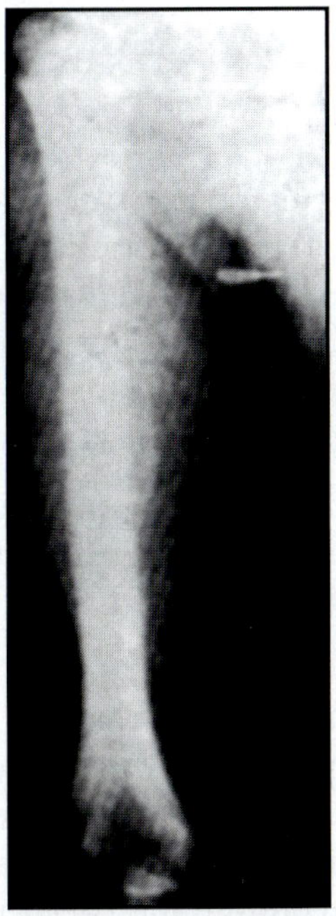

Fig. 44.13B: Radiograph showing Ewing's sarcoma of femur

Sex Males and females are equally affected.

Pathology

Gross The tumour is dark red in colour, soft in consistency and lies within the medulla. The cortex is thin and broken.

Microscopy It consists of round cells with eccentrically placed nucleus with nucleolus. The chromatin is sparse and is arranged in *"spokes of wheel fashion"*. Perinuclear halo typical of plasma cells is not seen in multiple myeloma.

Associated pathology

- Interstitial fibrosis in the kidney.
- Nodules in the lungs.
- Amyloidosis may occur (in 10–15%).

Clinical Features

Tumour runs a chronic course. It is silent at first; later on, the patient complains of vague pain which is mild and intermittent in the beginning. It also affects lumbar spine, sacral region, chest and ribs. Severe attacks of sharp pain, superimpossed at intervals may develop. Often, the patient may complain of a diffuse, persistent, backache.

Findings

In the early stages, there are hardly any clinical findings. Later on, the patient may complain of soft tissue swelling in about 10 per cent of cases. Signs of pathological fracture is present in about 20 per cent of cases. The sternum and ribs may be tender and there may be signs of vertebral collapse.

Course The tumour is chronic, later the marrow replacement causes anaemia, thrombocytopenia and haemorrhages. Renal failure due to tubular block by protein casts may also be seen ***(myeloma kidney).***

Laboratory findings

1. *Bence Jones protein* is found in only 30 per cent of the cases. On boiling, a white precipitate appears at 50°C, dissolves at boiling point after acidifying the urine; on cooling, the precipitate reappears.
2. Serum globulin is increased.
3. Hypercalcemia.
4. ESR is increased (sludged blood).
5. *Low alkaline phosphatase* is seen despite extensive bone destruction or it may be normal.
6. *Marrow biopsy* reveals anaemia, is refractory to iron, B_{12}, folic acid, etc.

Radiology

The affected bones show diffuse osteoporosis or lytic lesions. *Biconcave* vertebral bodies and collapse of vertebra. *Punched-out* lesions in skull and pelvis are the characteristic findings in the X-rays.

Typical lesions

- Osteolytic lesion penetrates the cortex, but there is no periosteal reaction.
- Rarefaction of vertebrae may be extensive *(disappearing vertebrae)*, vertebral pedicle involvement is more common, when involved it is called as the "pedicle sign" (common in secondaries).

Treatment

When the tumour is widespread, it is usually fatal and then treatment is only palliative. The tumour is radiosensitive.

Chemotherapy Agents like steroids, cyclophosphamide, urethane and melphalan *(SCUM)* are found to be effective.

What is new?

High dose VDD (vincristine, doxorubicin, dexamethasone) with stem cell infusion is emerging as a better alternative to the conventional chemotherapy.

Surgery

- Laminectomy is done when there is evidence of compression of spinal nerves.
- Intramedullary fixation is done for pathological fractures of long bones.

Prognosis

- The disease is widespread and fatal.
- Death occurs within three years in majority of cases and in all by five years.

Complications

- Pathological fracture of the ribs.
- Spinal cord or nerve root compression.
- Anaemia, leucopenia, thrombocytopenia.
- Renal failure.
- Severe infection.
- Amyloidosis.

METASTATIC TUMOURS OF BONES

Definition These are cancerous tumours originating in other organs and involving the skeletal structures of the body.

Bones may be involved by:
- Direct invasion.
- Blood-borne metastasis (most common route).
- Very-rarely through the lymphatics.

Blood-borne metastases to the bone greatly outnumber the primary bone tumours.

Incidence is twenty-seven to seventy per cent.

Tendency percentage wise	
Ca Breast	73 per cent
Ca Lungs	32 per cent
Ca Kidneys	24 per cent
Ca Rectum	13 per cent
Ca Stomach	11 per cent

Sites The secondary bone tumours commonly involve vertebrae (Fig. 44.14), ribs, pelvis, sternum, skull and proximal ends of femur and humerus. It is unusual for metastatic neoplasms to involve bones distal to the elbows or knees.

Occurs in Three Clinical Settings

1. Pain in the spine or extremity without a known history of primary tumour *(rare)*.
2. Pathological fracture with or without known primary.
3. The third and most common is a patient with a known primary tumour with a painful lesion in the spine or extremities.

Clinical Features

The patient is usually an adult, in the middle or late life, and may present with pain, pathological fracture or anaemia. The patient complains of headache if the skull is involved. Spine involvement causes girdle pains, spastic paralysis, etc. Pathological fractures are frequent in femur. Collapse of vertebrae may be present.

Laboratory Diagnosis

- Blood picture may be normal or bizarre showing features of anaemia, thrombocytopenia or thrombocytosis, leucocytosis or leucopenia, eosinophilia, etc.
- Sometimes anaemia is associated with leucoerythroblastic reaction.
- Sometimes a syndrome of haemolytic anaemia, thrombocytopenia, fibrinogenopenia can be seen with cancer of stomach and pancreas, etc.
- Alkaline phosphatase is increased normally, but acid phosphatase increases in cancer of prostate.

Other Investigations

Radiology Radiographs fail to detect secondaries in the bone in 20 to 25 per cent of the cases.

Two types are recognised:

1. Osteolytic variety is frequent.
2. Osteoblastic variety shows increased density (cancer prostate).

Periosteal reaction and mottled or marble appearance are the other radiographic features.

Bone scan This is the most sensitive method of investigation.

Fine needle biopsy is accurate in over 90 per cent of the cases.

Treatment

The following are the various modalities of treatment.

Radiotherapy is by ^{60}Co 3000 to 4000 rads for 3 to 4 weeks.

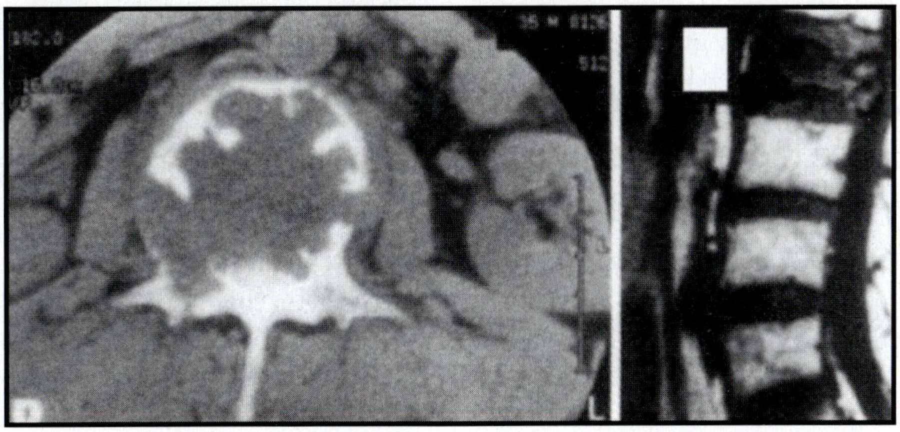

Fig. 44.14: CT scan showing metastasis in a vertebral body

Surgery If the patient has developed pathological fracture, internal fixation with acrylic cement is done. Decompressive laminectomy is done for secondaries in the spine. Endocrine surgery for cancer breast, cancer prostate, etc.

Hormone therapy
- For prostatic cancer, oestrogen.
- For breast cancer, diethylstilboesterol.
- For thyroid cancer, T_3 and ^{131}I.

Radioisotope therapy is by using
- Radioactive phosphorus
- Radioactive ^{131}I

Chemotherapy is by using drugs like alkylating agents, antimetabolites, etc.

Treatment of hypercalcaemia is by using cortisone, mithramycin, etc.

Amputation is indicated for intractable pain and as a last resort.

Prophylactic nailing is considered for those cases with more than 50 per cent destruction of the cortex.

What is new?

Radiofrequency Ablation (RFA)
In failed or poor candidates for conventional radiation or chemotherapy, RFA has emerged as an effective alternative palliative treatment of osteolytic metastatic lesion. However, ablation has to be done right up to the bone and not just in the centre of the tumour.

INCLUSION TUMOURS

SYNOVIOMA (SYNOVIAL SARCOMA)

Definition Synovioma is a slowly growing malignant tumour occurring in juxtaposition to and attached to the synovial tissue but almost invariably lies outside the joint.

Pathology

It is difficult to find the synovial attachment of the tumour. The tumour may be circumscribed, rounded, lobulated, and may be surrounded by a pseudocapsule. The tumour lies closely to the tendons, bursae and joint capsules.

Microscopy Three basic patterns indicate synovial origin (i) formation of tissue spaces, (ii) formation of cell tufts, and (iii) the presence of epithelial cell tufts.

Evidence of malignancy is seen in fibrosarcomatous stroma.

Clinical Features

This is a tumour of young adults, rare in people more than 40 years of age, common in the lower extremity, around the knee. Soft tissue outside the joint is involved, painful swelling, slowly increasing in size, firm or soft and tender. Restriction of joint movements may be seen.

Course The course is very slow, metastasis is eventually into the lungs.

Radiology

Soft tissue shadows are seen. Stippling is observed if the tumour contains small areas of calcification.

Treatment

Synovioma is a slow growing tumour. It metastasises late. Surgery is the treatment of choice and includes local excision. Radical amputation is preferred if the tumour has a widespread involvement.

RECENT TRENDS IN LIMB SALVAGE SURGERY

Mercifully, gone are the days when amputation was an inevitable and inescapable event in the surgical management of bone tumours. Due to improvement in tumour control due to modern chemotherapy, limb salvage operation is gaining prominence.

The principles of limb salvage in bone tumour management is to eradicate the tumor, retain the integrity of the skeletal system and preserve the limb with useful function. After the resection, skeletal reconstruction can be done by bone grafting (auto- or allografts) or by endoprosthesis (modular or custom made) (Figs 44.15A and B). Prosthetic reconstruction is found to be more effective from a functional point of view than other alternatives.

When compared to the radical amputation and external prosthetic fitting or limbsparing surgery with bone grafting, this method of treatment is found to

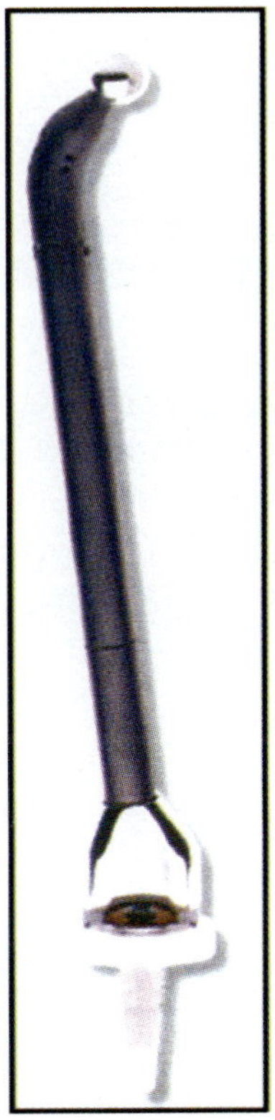

Fig. 44.15A: Showing custom prosthesis

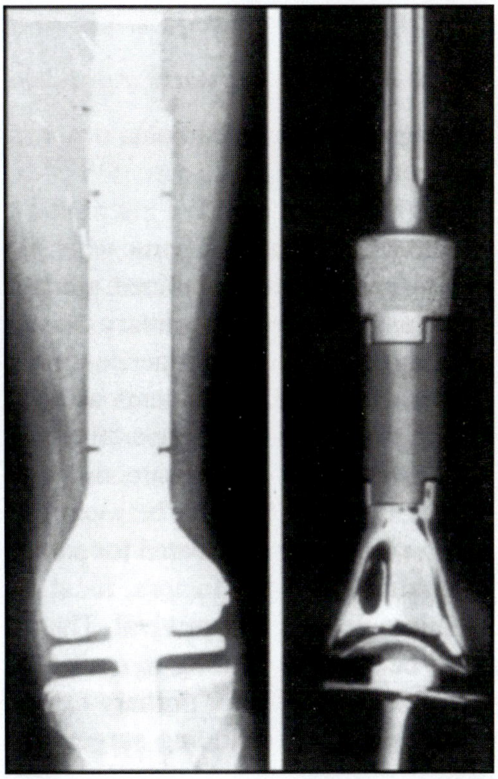

Fig. 44.15B: Showing custom prosthesis

be more effective in early mobilisation of the patient, limb function that is satisfactory and a better emotional acceptance by the patient.

BIBLIOGRAPHY

1. Baker DM. Benign unicameral bone cyst: a study of 45 cases with long-term follow-up. Clin Orthop 1970;71:140.
2. Bhansali SK, Desai PP. Ewing's sarcoma: observations in 107 cases. J Bone and Joint Surg 1963;45-A:541.
3. Bhulla SK. Metastatic disease of the spine. Clin Orthop 1970;73-52.
4. Biesecker JL et al. Aneurysmal bone cysts: a clinicopathologic study of 66 cases. Cancer 1970;26:615.
5. Brostrom LA. On the natural history of osteosarcoma: aspects in diagnosis, prognosis and endocrinology. Acta Orthop Scand Suppl 1984;53(Suppl):183.
6. Campanacci M, Bacci G, Pagani P, Giunti A. Multiple drug chemotherapy for the primary treatment of osteosarcoma of the extremities. J Bone Joint Surg 1980;62-B:93.
7. Campanacci M, Guinti A, Ohm R: Giant cell tumors of bone. a study of 209 cases with long-term follow-up in 130. Ital J Orthop Traumtol 1975;1:249.
8. Coventry MB, Dahlin DC. Osteogenic sarcoma: a critical analysis of 430 cases. J Bone Joint Surg 1957;39-A:741.
9. Craig FS. Metastatic and primary lesions of bone. Clin Orthop 1970;73-33.
10. Dias LS, Frost HM. Osteoid osteoma: osteoblastoma. Cancer 1974;33:1075.
11. Enneking WF, Spanier SS, Goodman MA. A system for the surgical staging of musculoskeletal sarcoma. Clin Orthop 1980;153:106.
12. Erikkson AL, Schiller A, Mankin HJ. The management of chondrosarcoma of bone. Clin Orthop 1980;153:44.
13. Grimmer RJ, Cannon SR et al. Royal Orthopaedic Hospital, London.
14. Jaffe HL, Lichtenstein L, Portis RB. Giant cell tumor of bone: its pathologic appearance, grading supposed variant and treatment. Arch Pathol 1940;30:993.
15. Johnston JO. Local resection in primary malignant bone tumors. Clin Orthop 1980;153:75.
16. Lichtenstein L. Bone tumors, 5th edn. St Louis: CV Mosby Co, 1977.
17. Mizuta H, Yamaski M. Nuclear magnetic resonance studies on human bone and soft tissue tumors. J Jpn. Orthop Assoc 1984;58:97.
18. Murray JA. Multiple myeloma. Curr Pract Orthop Surg 1975;6:145.
19. Onolenghi CE. Diagnosis of orthopaedic lesions by aspiration biopsy: results in 1,063 punctures. J Bone Joint Surg 1955;37-A:443.
20. P Sonneveld et al. Dept. of Clinical Oncology, Leiden, Netherlands.
21. Radiofrequency ablation (RFA). Source Orthonet 2003;63:5.
22. Treatment of osteoid osteoma, recent trends. Source: Orthonet India, April 2002.
23. W Piotz et al. Clinical orthopaedics and related research. Dec 02.

SECTION SIX

MISCELLANEOUS

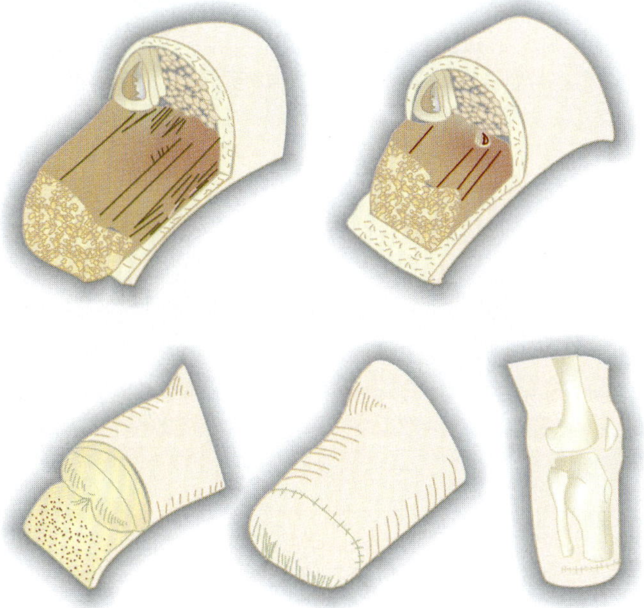

45

Amputations

INTRODUCTION

Definition

Amputation is defined as removal of the limb through a part of the bone.

Disarticulation is the removal of the limb through the joint.

Incidences

Age Common in 50 to 75 years age group.

Sex Seventy-five per cent men, 25 per cent women.

Limbs Eighty-five per cent is through the lower limbs, 15 per cent is through the upper limbs.

Indications: Mercifully, due to recent advances in medicine and technology, the incidences of amputations are showing a downhill trend.

However, there are certain specific indications that require amputations (see the flow chart). But indications are not constant and keep changing according to the age of the patient.

Indications for amputations

- **Common causes**
  - < 50 yr
    - Injury
  - >50 yr
    - Peripheral vascular disease
- **Less common causes**
  - Infection (fulminating gas gangrene)
  - Tumours
  - Nerve injuries
  - Congenital anomalies
  - Miscellaneous

Note: Injury is the most common cause for amputations.

Remember

The only real absolute indication for amputation is irreparable loss of blood supply of a diseased or injured limb.

Quick Facts: Age vs Indications in Amputations

- Children — Congenital anomalies
- Young adults — Injuries
- Elderly — Peripheral vascular diseases like TAO.

TYPES

Closed amputation This is done most of the times as an elective procedure and may be above knee or below knee, above elbow and below elbow, etc.

Open amputation In open amputation, the wound is left open over the amputation stump and is not closed. This is done as an emergency procedure in the face of life-threatening infections. There are two types in this depending upon the skin flaps:

a. Open amputations with inverted skin flap.
b. Circular open amputation in which skin is closed at a later date.

Amputation Levels

Upper limbs (Fig. 45.1)

- Shoulder disarticulation
- Short above elbow
- Standard above elbow
- Elbow disarticulation
- Very short below elbow
- Medium below elbow
- Long below elbow.

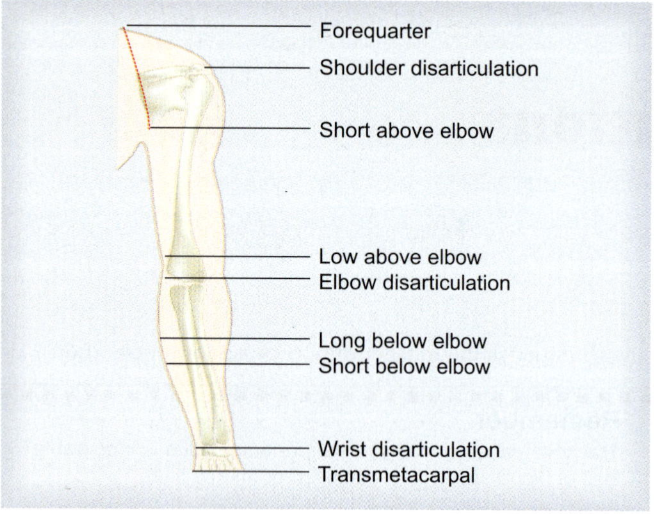

Fig. 45.1: Showing different levels of amputations in the upper limb

Lower limbs (Fig. 45.2)
- Hip disarticulation
- Very short above knee
- Short above knee
- Medium above knee
- Long above knee
- Very long above knee
- Knee disarticulation
- Very short below knee
- Short and below knee.

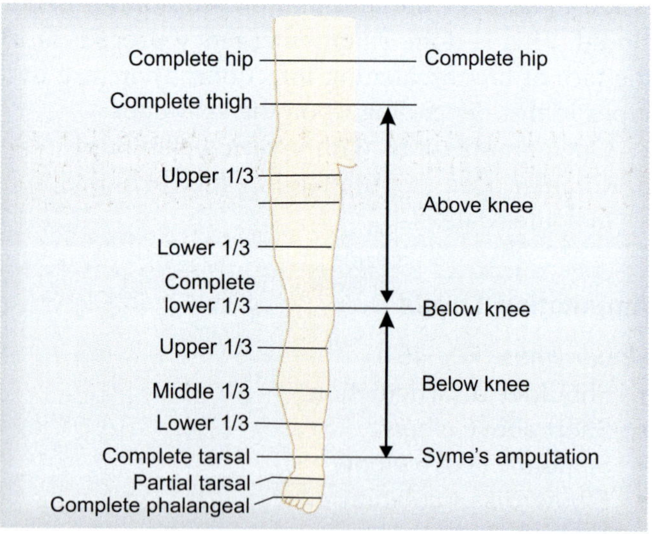

Fig. 45.2: Showing different levels of amputations in the lower limb

Ankle amputation
- *Syme's amputation* Here the level of bone section is 0.6 cm proximal to the ankle joint
- *Sarmiento's amputation* Here the level is 1.3 cm proximal to the joint.
- *Wagner's* is two-stage Syme's amputation.
- *Boyd's* This consists of talectomy and calcaneo-tibial arthrodesis.
- *Pirogoff's amputation* In this only anterior part of the calcaneum is removed.

Foot amputation
- Amputation of great toes and other toes.
- Amputation through the metatarsal bones.
- *Lisfranc's operation* Amputation is at the level of the tarsometatarsal joints.
- *Chopart's operation* Amputation is through the midtarsal joints.

PRINCIPLES

CLOSED AMPUTATIONS

In this, the skin is closed primarily after amputation.
1. *Tourniquets* These are desirable except in ischaemic limbs.
2. *Level of amputation* As in the past, the level of amputation is no longer important, thanks to the modern and sophisticated present-day prosthesis.

Remember: The cardinal rule

Amputate through the tissues that will heal satisfactorily and preserve all possible lengths consistent with good surgical judgement.

- *Skin flaps* Good skin coverage for the amputation site is of vital importance. The skin should be mobile and sensitive. Location of the scar is not important.
- *Muscles* The muscle is divided at least 5 cm distal to the level of intended bone section and sutured.

Remember

Two methods of muscle suture
- *Myodesis* Here muscle is sutured to the bone.
- *Myoplasty* Here muscle is sutured to the opposite muscle group under appropriate tension.

These two techniques of *myodesis* and *myoplasty* help improve the function of the muscles and circulation in the stump and thereby help to prevent phantom pain.

- *Nerves* The nerves are cut proximally and allowed to retract.
- *Blood vessels* are doubly ligated and cut.
- *Bone* The bone is sectioned above the level of muscle section.
- *Drains* are removed after 48 to 72 hours.

OPEN AMPUTATIONS (GUILLOTINE OPERATION)

In this type of amputation, the skin is not closed primarily and later, it is followed by any one of the closure methods like secondary closure, reamputation, revision amputation or plastic repair.

Indications

- Severe infections
- Severe crush injuries.

Types

Open amputations with inverted skin flaps is the method of choice.

Circular open amputation Here the wound is kept open and closed secondarily either by secondary suture after a few days, split thickness skin graft, revision of the stump or by reamputation.

AFTER TREATMENT

Two concepts are widely accepted.

Rigid dressing concept Here, plaster of Paris cast is applied to the stump over the dressing after surgery. This presents the following advantages:

- Prevents oedema.
- Enhances wound healing.
- Decreases postoperative pain.
- Encourages early upright posture which has both physiologic and psychologic benefits.
- Reduces hospital stay.
- Helps in early temporary prosthetic fitting.

Soft dressing concept This is the conventional method wherein the stump is dressed with a sterile dressing and elastocrepe bandages are applied over it. The bed is elevated to facilitate venous drainage and prevent stump oedema (Figs 45.3 and 45.4). The sutures are removed after 10 to 14 days and the muscle exercises are commenced. Prosthetic fitting is taken up as the last step.

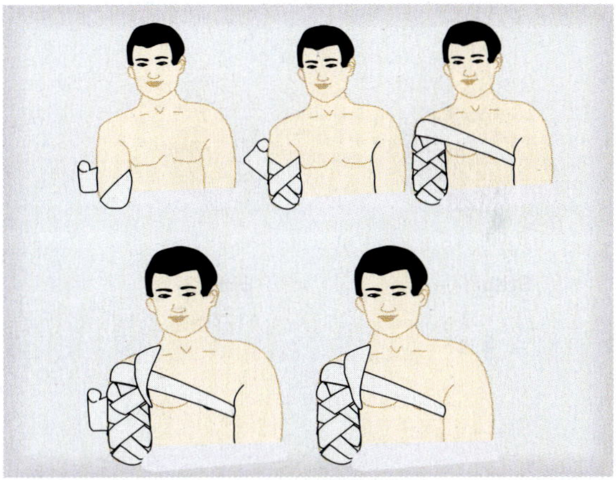

Fig. 45.3: Different steps in the stump bandaging of the above elbow amputation

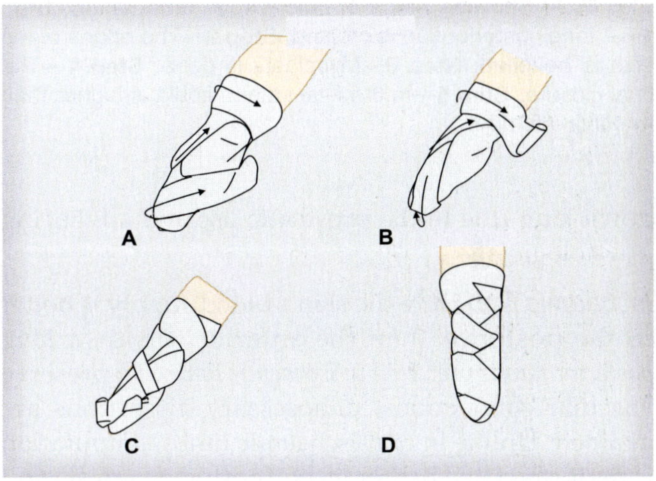

Figs 45.4A to D: Showing bandaging techniques of the below knee stump: anterior views (A and B). Posterior views (C and D)

IMPORTANT AMPUTATIONS OF LOWER EXTREMITY

Amputations of lower extremity accounts for nearly 85 per cent of all amputations. *To succesfully use a prosthesis, it is desirable to perform amputation of the lower limb at the distal most possible level.*

Below knee amputation (Fig. 45.5) This is the most common amputation performed. Techniques vary in non-ischaemic and ischaemic limbs.

Non-ischaemic limbs Here, the ideal level of amputation is at the *musculotendinous junction of the gastrocnemius* because distal to this level the tissues are relatively avascular and soft tissue padding is scanty. Though soft tissue may heal early, it usually breaks

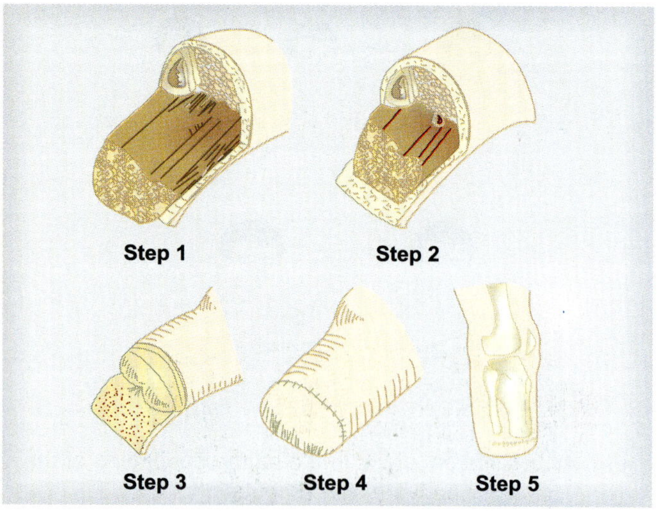

Fig. 45.5: Showing steps of below knee amputation: **Step 1**—A long posterior flap is created. **Step 2**—The edges of the tibia is bevelled. **Step 3**—Myoplasty is done. **Step 4**—The final closure. **Step 5**—In the final stump, fibula is higher than the tibial stump

down later due to the prosthetic use and advancing physiologic age.

Ischaemic limb Here the skin's blood supply is better to the posterior than the anterior. *Hence, a long posterior flap is preferred in ischaemic limbs.* To preserve vascular connections, unnecessary dissections are avoided. Unlike in non-ischaemic limbs, amputation is performed at a higher level. Tension myodesis and myoplasty are contraindicated for fear of damaging the already precarious blood supply.

Knee disarticulation This gives an excellent end bearing stump. Large end bearing surfaces of the distal femur are naturally suited for weight bearing and the prosthesis will be stable.

Amputation through the thigh This is second in frequency to the knee. Because knee joint is lost, it is extremely important that the stumps be as long as possible to provide a strong lever arm for the control of prosthesis.

[1]**Syme's amputation** (Fig. 45.6) It is indicated in severe crush injuries of the forefoot. A healthy heel pad is required for the successful outcome of this surgery.

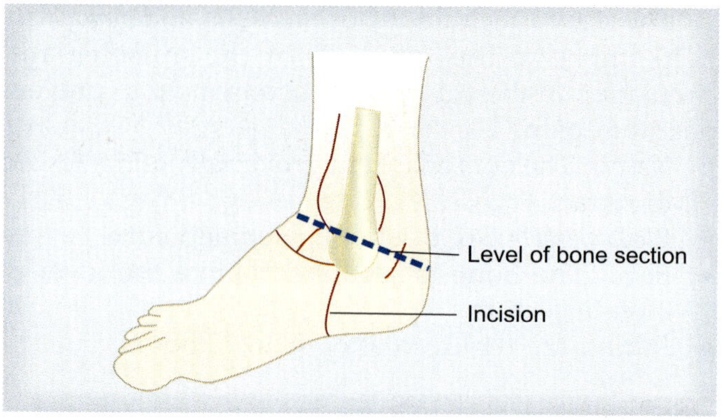

Fig. 45.6: Syme's amputation

COMPLICATIONS

Haematomas This delays the wound healing and acts as a culture media for the growth of the organisms.

Infections This is more common in peripheral vascular disease and diabetics.

Necrosis of the skin flaps are usually due to insufficient circulation and requires revision amputations.

Contractures This is largely preventable by positioning the stump properly.

Neuromas form always on the end of a cutaneous nerve and any pain from a neuroma is usually caused by a traction on a nerve when it is embedded within the scar tissue.

Phantom sensation This is a pseudo feeling of the presence of the amputated limb. It could be of a painless or a painful variety.

Causalgia It is due to division of the peripheral nerves. Even local stimulus stimulates pain.

Remember in amputations

- Eighty-five per cent amputations are through the lower limbs.
- Severe injury forms the most common indication.
- Level of amputation is no longer important as in the past due to efficient prosthesis.
- The latest concept is to preseve as much stump length as possible.
- Guillotine amputations are salvage procedures for life-threatening infections.
- Stump care is very vital to prevent post-amputation problems.

[1]**James Syme** (1799-1870). Edinburgh British Surgeon described it in 1843.

46

Prosthetics and Orthotics

- Prosthetics
  - Classification
  - Types
  - Prosthesis for the lower limbs
  - Prosthesis for below knee amputations
  - Prosthesis for Syme's amputation
  - SACH foot
  - Jaipur foot
- Orthotics
  - Classification of orthotics
  - Varieties of orthoses
  - Types
  - Lower limb orthosis
  - Upper limb orthosis

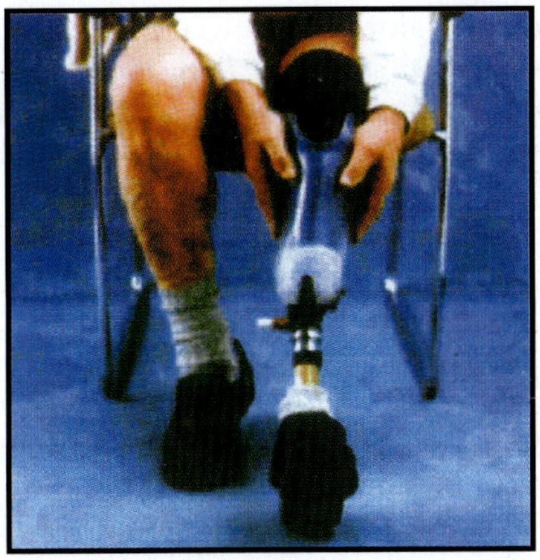

Fig. 46.1: Showing patient wearing an artificial leg

PROSTHETICS

Prosthesis in Greek means "in addition". Thus, a prosthesis is *defined as a replacement or substitution of a missing or a diseased part*.

Prosthetics is the theory and practice of the prescription, fitting, design, assessment and production of prosthesis.

CLASSIFICATION

Endoprostheses These are implants used in orthopaedic surgery to replace joints, e.g. Austin Moore prosthesis.

Exoprostheses These are for replacement externally for a lost part of the limb. They are more extensively used in the lower limbs (Fig. 46.1).

TYPES

1. *Temporary prosthesis* (e.g. Pylon). These are used following an amputation till the patient is fitted with permanent prosthesis (Fig. 46.2).
2. *Permanent prosthesis.* The following are some of the important ones:

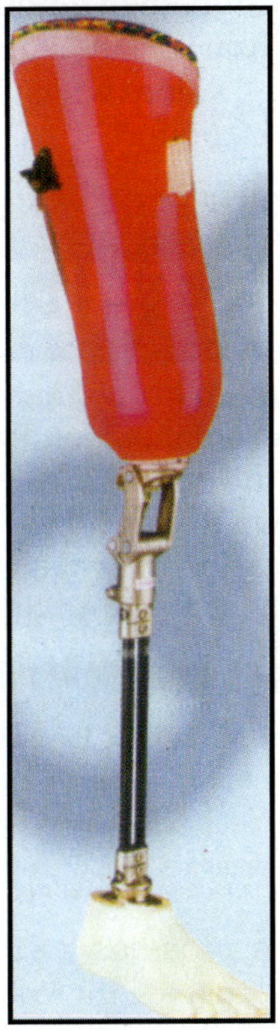

Fig. 46.2: Showing a temporary prosthesis

PROSTHESIS FOR THE LOWER LIMBS

Prosthesis for the lower limbs are required in the following situations:

1. For disarticulation of hip and hemipelvectomy (Fig. 46.3).
2. Following transfemoral amputations: Two types of prostheses are recommended.
   a. *Suction-socketted limb* This is useful in young adults and is best suited for cylindrical stumps. It snuggly fits and has a two-way valve mechanism to maintain negative pressure.
   b. *Non-suction-socketted limb* Here, no negative pressure is employed to hold the prosthesis, but pelvic bands or harness are made use of for holding.

The advantages of suction-socketted limb are that skin infection is less common, there is freedom from harness of any kind, greater feel of close contact of the prosthesis and the patient feels that it belongs to him or her. Stump socks are not necessary in this variety. On the contrary, the advantages of non-suction-socketted limb are, it is easy to wear, there is no perspiration, it provides a comfortable fit, and there is no difficulty in changing the stump circumference.

Prothesis for through knee amputation As already mentioned, knee disarticulation gives a good, stable, long weight bearing stump which enables to operate the prosthesis with comfort.

PROSTHESIS FOR BELOW KNEE AMPUTATIONS (Fig. 46.4)

Two varieties are described:

Patellar tendon bearing (PTB) prosthesis In this, the socket is made in such a way that it fits exactly over the patellar tendon and the sides of the tibial condyles such that when in full extension the weight is transferred to some extent through this to the prosthesis (Fig. 46.5). This has the advantage over the conventional prosthesis which require the knee supports.

Quick facts: About lower limb prosthesis

- Quadrilateral socket prosthesis for above knee amputation.
- PTB prosthesis for below knee amputation.
- Syme's prosthesis for Syme's amputation.
- Shoe fillers for partial foot amputation.

Conventional type prosthesis This consists of the thigh corset, the side steels, the knee joint, shin piece, ankle joint unit and the foot piece. It definitely has

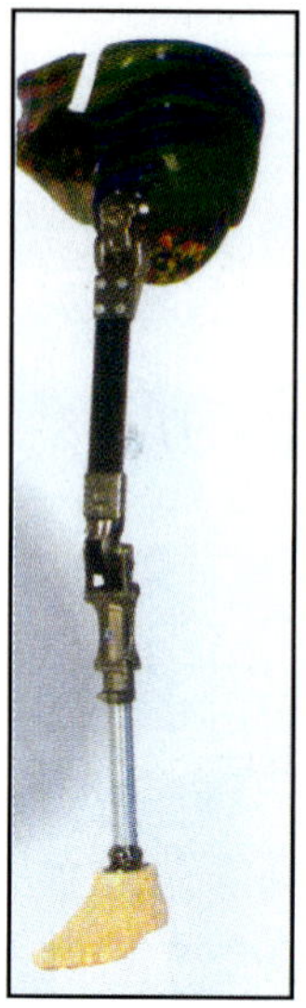

Fig. 46.3: Showing prosthesis for hemipelvectomy and hip disarticulation

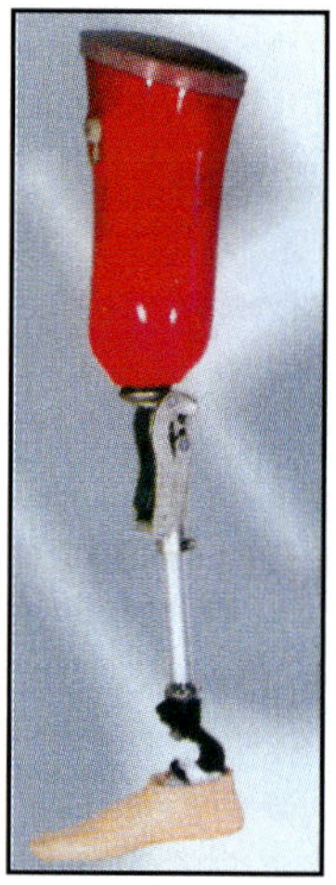

Fig. 46.4: Showing prosthesis for below-knee amputation

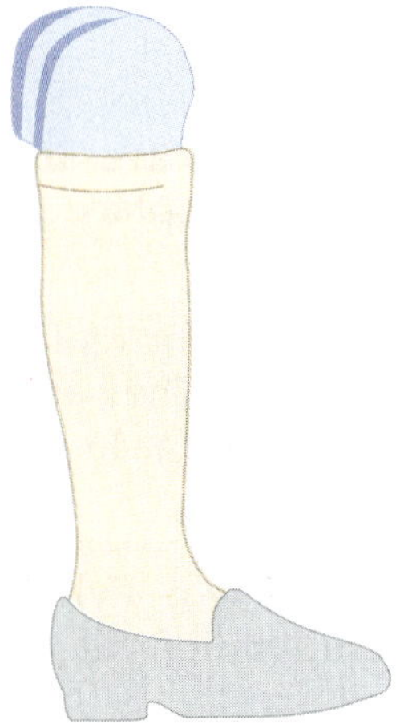

Fig. 46.5: Showing PTB prosthesis

the disadvantage in that it is more cumbersome to put on and use it when compared to the PTB prosthesis.

PROSTHESIS FOR SYME'S AMPUTATION

This is a below knee prosthesis used after Syme's amputation (Fig. 46.6). These prostheses may have closed sockets or open sockets and may be full weight bearing or modified end bearing.

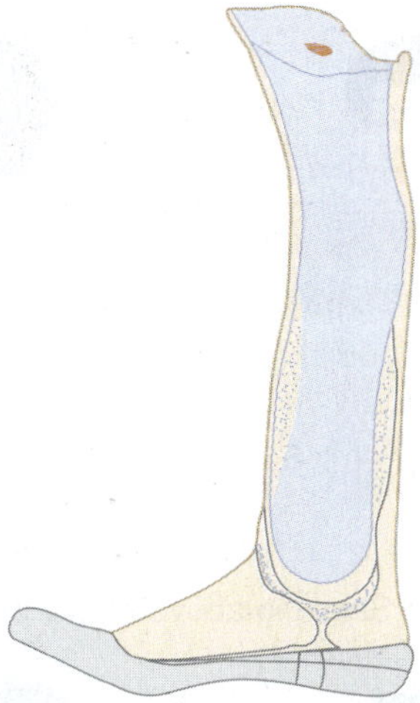

Fig. 46.6: Showing Syme's prosthesis

SACH FOOT

Ankle Units and Artificial Feet

Solid action cushion heel (SACH) (Fig. 46.7A) foot has no ankle joint, but a simulated action is gained by the compression of wedge-shaped rubber heel and the whole foot is incorporated with various layers of rubber with its density varying, all placed over a wooden insert for the heel and wooden side keel. This allows smooth movements of the foot.

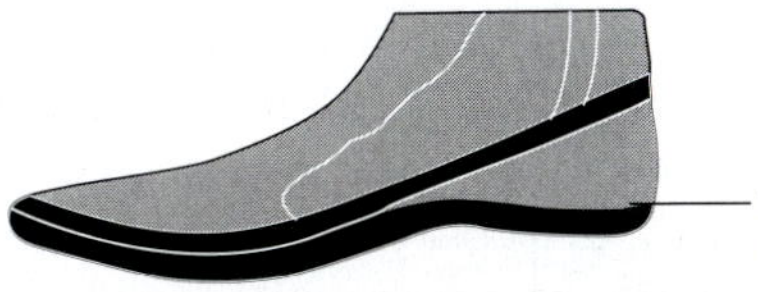

Fig. 46.7A: Showing SACH foot

Remember

Aims of prosthetic fitting

- To substitute for a lost part.
- To restore a lost function.
- In lower limbs it must provide a comfortable ambulation with minimal expenditure of energy.

JAIPUR FOOT (INDIA'S PRIDE)

- This is the brain child of Dr PK Sethi and Masterji Ram Chander Sharma of Jaipur
- Rubber and aluminium are the mainstay. Rubber is waterproof, aluminium is used for the leg piece, because it is cheap, strong and rust proof
- Unlike the Western model, Jaipur foot is best for foot conditions in developing countries as it allows sitting on the floor, squatting and does not require a shoe (Fig. 46.7B).

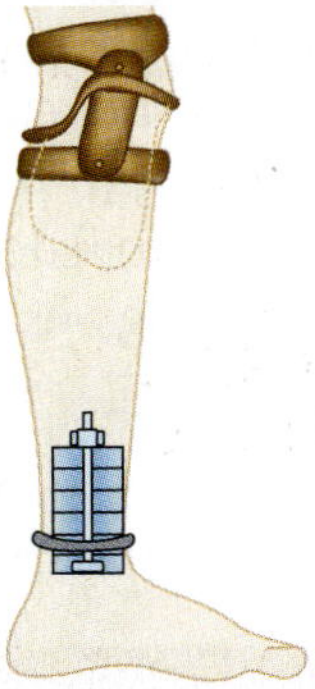

Fig. 46.7B: Showing Jaipur foot

Remember in prosthesis for lower extremities:

Long stump is prosthetically superior to a shorter one because it provides

- Longer lever arm.
- More sensory feedback.
- Greater area for distribution of pressure forces.

Prosthesis for upper limb amputations

Forequarter amputations Here the prosthesis merely serves a cosmetic purpose. A sleeve fitter prosthesis with a plastozoate cap padded inside with foam and retaining straps is used.

Shoulder disarticulation

- *Shoulder piece* extended cap to hold the prosthesis.
- *Elbow piece* It can be flexed by pulling on the flexion cord with the protractors of the shoulder.
- *Handpiece* Either cosmetic or splint hook type.

Above elbow amputation Same as above except that the elbow flexion is more stronger due to the action of the arm muscles along with the protractors of the shoulder (Fig. 46.8).

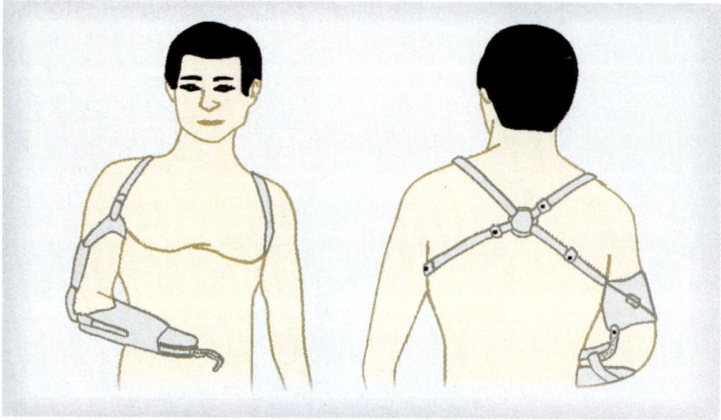

Fig. 46.8: Showing above elbow prosthesis

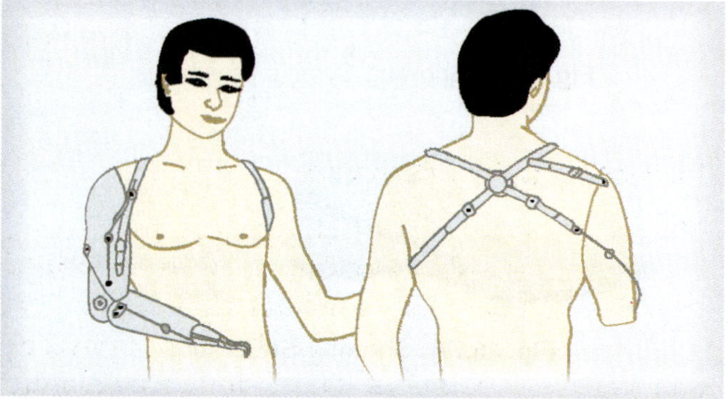

Fig. 46.9: Showing below elbow prosthesis

Below elbow amputation Here there is a cup socket attached to the terminal device through an operational cord. The terminal device can be activated through a loop harness (Fig. 46.9).

For wrist disarticulation In this, a split socket forearm and a wrist rotation device is provided. A device can be provided to lock for supination and pronation.

ORTHOTICS

Orthosis is an appliance which is *added* to the patient to enable better use of that part of the body to which it is fitted.

Prosthesis replaces a missing part of the body, while an orthosis provides support to a weak part of the body.

An orthotist is a person qualified to measure and fit all types of orthoses.

CLASSSIFICATION OF ORTHOTICS

One single classification is very difficult. Hence, GK Rose has grouped them as follows:

- Functional biomechanical
- Functional descriptive
- Nosological (according to disease)
- Regional.

Terminology for orthosis The three major anatomical regions of the body are divided as follows and the initials given are as in Table 46.1.

Table 46.1: Major anatomical regions of the body

Upper limb		*Lower limbs*	*Spine*
S-Shoulder		H-Hip	C-Cervical
E-Elbow		K-Knee	T-Thoracic
W-Wrist		A-Ankle	L-Lumbar
H-Hand		F-Foot	S-Sacroiliac
F-Fingers	MP	Subtalar	
(2–5)	DIP	Midtarsal	
	PIP	Metatarsal	
Thumb	CM		
	MP		
	IP		

Orthotic facts

Nomenclature for orthosis now used has the first letter of the name of each joint which the orthosis crosses in power sequence, and the letter 'O' for orthosis is attached at the end. Accordingly, we have the following types of orthoses:

a. CO—Cervical orthosis
b. CTLSO—Cervico-thoraco-lumbar-sacral orthosis
c. WHO—Wrist hand orthoses
d. HKAFO—Hip-knee-ankle-foot orthoses
e. KAFO—Knee-ankle-foot orthoses
f. KO—Knee orthoses
g. AFO—Ankle foot orthoses

Action of orthosis The action of an orthosis on a joint is indicated by initials which are as follows:

F—Free
A—Assist
R—Resist
S—Stop
H—Hold
V—Variable
L—Lock.

VARIETIES OF ORTHOSES

- Spinal orthosis.
- Cervical orthosis.
- Lower limb orthosis.
- Upper limb orthosis.

Spinal orthoses These fall into two categories:

1. Supportive
2. Corrective.

Functions of spinal orthosis

- To relieve pain.
- To support weakened paralysed muscles.
- To support unstable joints.
- To immobilise joints in functional position.
- To prevent deformity.
- To correct deformity.

TYPES

Supportive Spinal Orthosis

Belts and corsets These are most commonly used for the treatment of low backache. *Belts are prescribed for men and corsets for women.* These orthoses encircle the sacral region and extend a variable distance upwards, the term applied to them depends upon their depth posteriorly (sacroiliac, lumbosacral (Fig. 46.10), thoracolumbar). Anteriorly they have buckles.

Remember

The role of belts

- They do not immobilise the spine but only restrict extremes of forward, lateral flexion and extension.
- They provide subjective support.
- They remind the patients to avoid movements.

Rigid spinal brace All rigid spinal orthoses are constructed on the basis of a metal frame which takes firm support from the pelvis. To this is added the metal uprights which are joined by cross bars and straps, e.g. tailor brace, night tailor brace, etc.

Moulded spinal orthosis of leather, plastic, etc.

Indications for supportive spinal orthosis

- Sacroiliac strain.
- Low backache.
- Prolapsed intervertebral disc.
- Spondylolisthesis, etc.

Remember

The mechanisms of pain relief by spinal orthoses

- Psychological.
- Increases intra-abdominal pressure.
- Decreases lumbar lordosis.
- Causes local inactivity of associated muscle groups and ligaments.

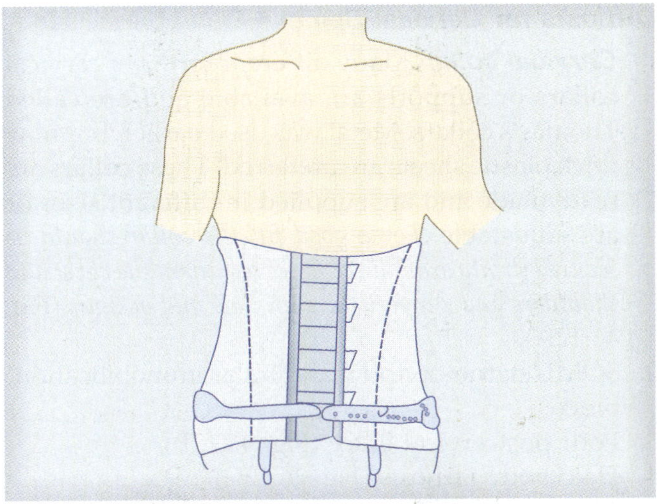

Fig. 46.10: Showing lumbosacral belt

Corrective Spinal Orthosis

Milwaukee brace (Fig. 46.11) This is an active corrective spinal orthosis used almost exclusively in the ambulant treatment of structural scoliosis.

The main aim of Milwaukee brace is to postpone, temporarily or permanently, the need for operation.

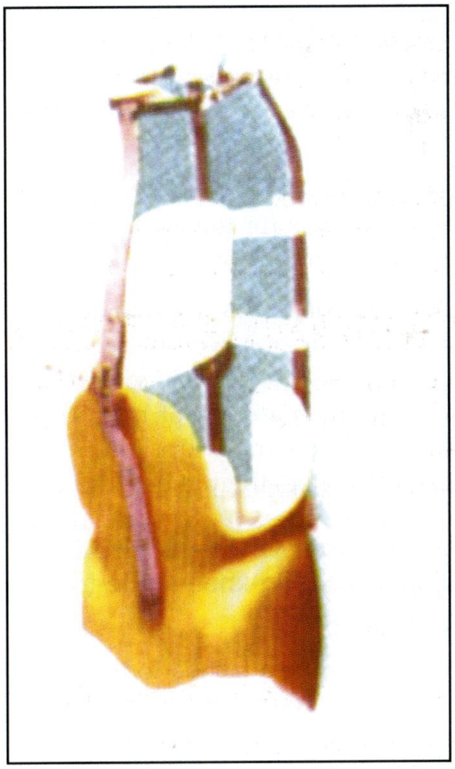

Fig. 46.11: Showing Milwaukee brace

Orthosis for Cervical Spine

1. ***Cervical collar*** Many different forms of cervical collars or supports are available and are called Thomas's collars. Metal was used earlier, but now thick plastic sheets are preferred. These collars are readymade and are supplied in different sizes or are adjustable. *For a good fit, the collar should be secured firmly around the neck, rest upon the chest and shoulders and support the chin, jaw and occiput* (Fig. 46.12A).
2. SOMI (sterno-occipit mandibular immobilisation) brace.
3. Four postcervical brace (Fig. 46.12B)
4. Halo body orthosis (Fig. 46.12C)
5. *Minerva jacket* (Fig. 46.13) In lesions of uppermost part of the cervical spine the forehead must be included in the external support. In such situations, Minerva jacket made from plaster of Paris is used.

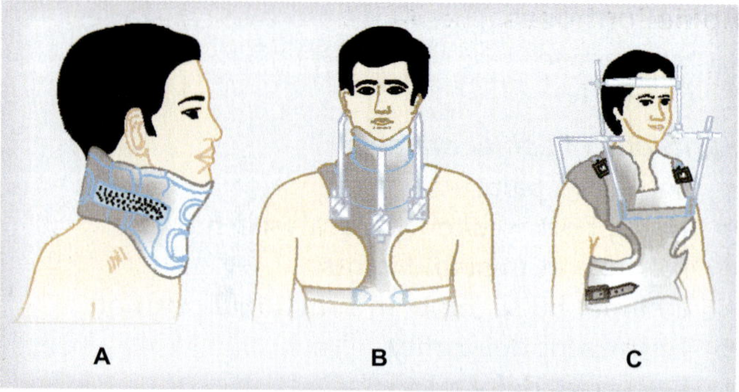

Figs 46.12A to C: Showing different cervical orthosis; (A) Cervical collar, (B) Four postcervical brace, (C) Halo body orthosis

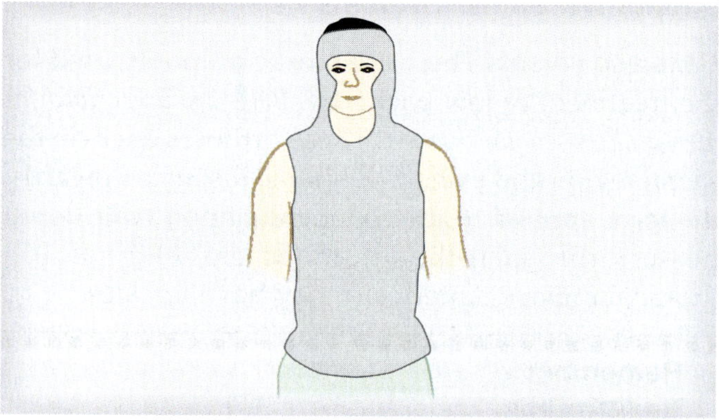

Fig. 46.13: Showing Minerva jacket

Remember

The functions of calipers

- It provides stability
- It relieves weight bearing
- It relieves pain
- It controls deformity
- It restricts movements
- It assists movements
- A combination of the above functions

LOWER LIMB ORTHOSIS

Caliper is an orthosis for the lower limb which may be used permanently or for a very short time only.

Knee-ankle-foot orthosis (KAFO) These are either weight relieving or non-weight relieving calipers (Fig. 46.14). It consists of the following parts, an upper end which may be made up of ring, cuff or bucket top. It has two side bars or upright, the knee joint, the ankle joint, a shoe, thigh, knee and calf bands.

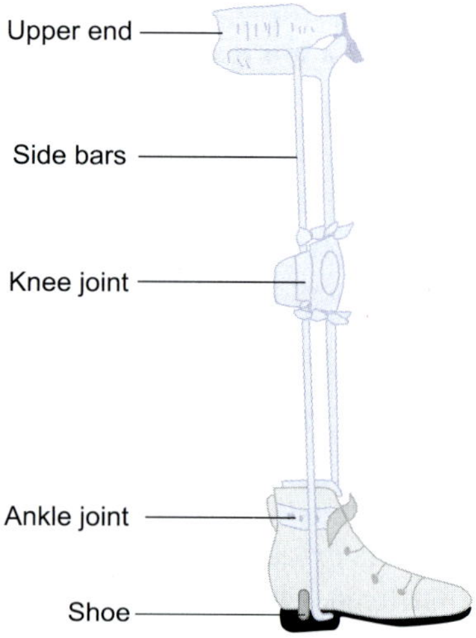

Fig. 46.14: Showing knee-ankle-foot orthosis (KAFO)

Hip-knee-ankle-foot Orthosis (HKAFO) and Lumbosacral Hip-knee-ankle-foot Orthosis (LSHKAFO)

A pelvic band may be attached to the KAFO with or without a hip joint to convert to an HKAFO. And if this is extended upwards, a lumbosacral support is obtained converting it to an LSHKAFO.

The purpose of the pelvic band at the hip joint is to:

1. Prevent development of a flexion deformity in polio, cerebral palsy, etc.
2. To increase the stability of spine.

Ankle-foot Orthosis (AFO)

This is a below-knee orthosis in which the ankle joint can be controlled by mechanical ankle joints or by heel straps (Fig. 46.15).

All the above lower limb orthoses so far mentioned are useful either to prevent or correct deformities due to polio, cerebral palsy, spina bifida, etc. They can be used either temporarily or permanently.

Footwear and its Modifications

The following are some of the modifications of footwear useful in the clinical situations mentioned below:

a. *Rocker bar* For hallux rigidus.
b. *Outside heel float* For lateral ligament injuries of the ankle.
c. *Heel pad* For heel pain (Fig. 46.16A).
d. *Medial longitudinal arch support* To relieve pain, the following supports are used:
   - Valgus insole
   - Thomas heel (extension of medial aspect of the heel)
   - Filling of the medial half of the shank of the shoes (medial shank filler).
e. *Metatarsal arch* is supported by the doom-shaped metatarsal bars (Fig. 46.16B).
f. *More roomy footwear* To accommodate deformed toes.

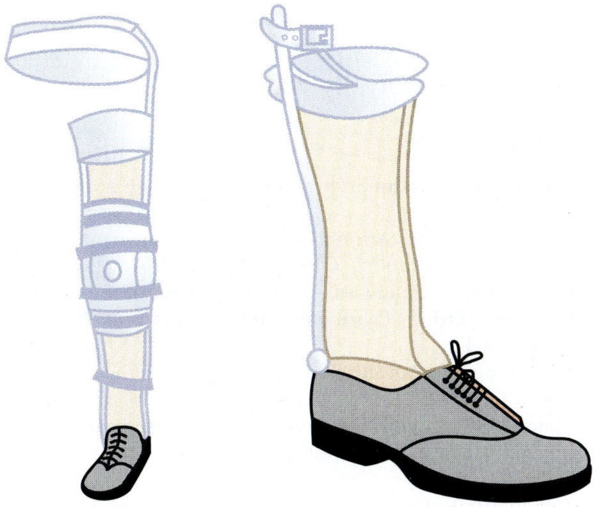

Fig. 46.15: Showing ankle-foot orthosis (AFO)

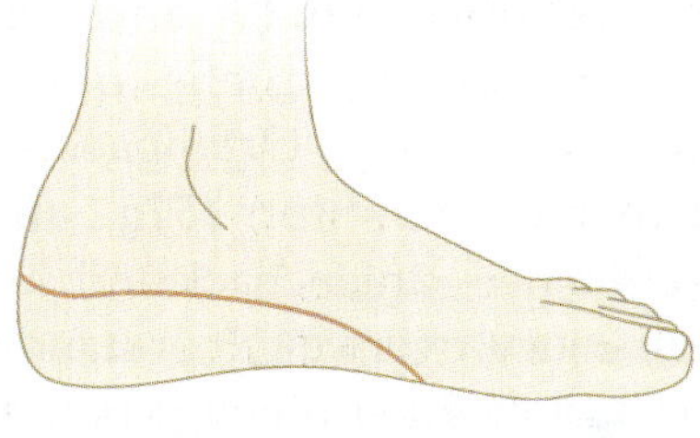

Fig. 46.16A: Showing UC-BL shoe inserts to relieve heel stress in plantar fascitis and calcaneal spur

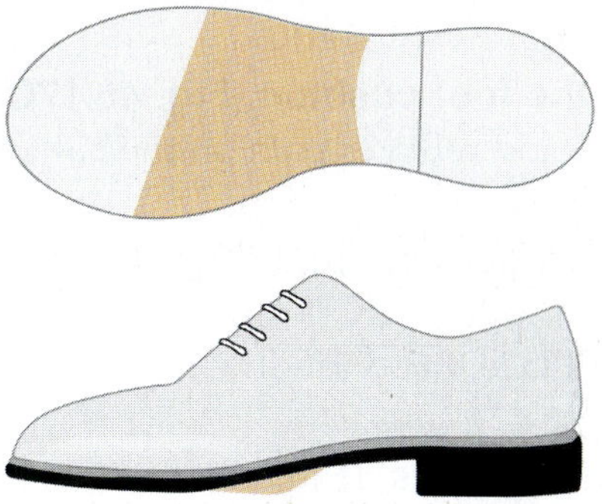

Fig. 46.16B: Showing incorporation of metatarsal bars, under the sole of the footwear

Quick facts: Surgical footwears

Footwear with	Indications
a. Thomas heel	Flat foot
b. Arch support	Flat foot
c. CTEV shoes	For CTEV (Fig. 46.16C)
d. Heel pad	Calcareal spur and plantar fascitis
f. Metatarsal pad	For corns
g. Metatarsal bar	Metatarsalgia
h. Medial raise	Genu valgum
i. Lateral raise	Genu varum
j. Universal	For short leg

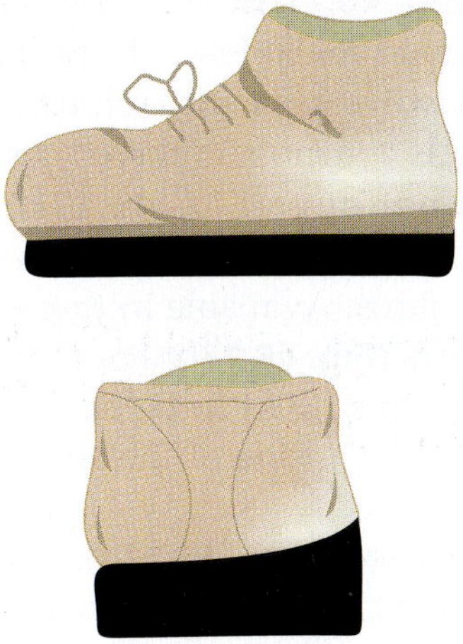

Fig. 46.16C: Showing CTEV shoes

Foot supports (Figs 46.17 and 46.18): The following are the different varieties of heel and foot supports currently in use in Orthopaedic practice.

a. **Podo-tech heel cushion (Fig. 46.17A):** For severe pain in heel, ankle, back and anterior knee pain due to injury, overweight or standing for long time. The heel cushion relieves pain by altering the line of weight bearing. Available in 3 sizes.

b. **Astro-sorb heel seat (Fig. 46.17B):** The cushion protects against stress and relieves pain on the ball of foot from overactivity.

c. **Ball of the foot cushion (Fig. 46.17C):** Reduces pressure and relieves pain on the ball of foot from overactivity.

d. **Stompers gel heel pad (Fig. 46.17D):** For knee and back pain, tibial shin pain, athletes and joggers. Place this under the heel and wear shoes. *Do not use adhesives.*

e. **Duosoft insoles (Fig. 46.17E):** For diabetic patients to reduce pain and burning sensation for uncontrolled diabetic neuropathy. Absorbs shock, reduces friction, and disperses weight and protects the foot from harmful forces. Available in two sizes.

f. **Stompers work and sports insoles universal (Fig. 46.17F):** To relieve tired, achy legs, try one of the shock absorbing insoles which have a wide variety of uses such as for work on hard surfaces and all sports or simply to relieve the day-to-day stress on feet, knees and back, pain relief for a number of conditions and enhanced cushioning with mild anatomical support.

g. **Starflex (Fig. 46.17G):** For use in children above 2 years who have flat foot. The Starflex™ orthotic blank is a polyester resin, reinforced with glass fibre threads available in three sizes.

h. **Globus heel cup (Fig. 46.17H):** For use in children above 18 months who have flat foot with calcaneo valgus. Available in three sizes.

i. **Valgus pads (Fig. 46.17I):** For flat foot and weak medial arch in adults. To be pasted using rubber adhesive on the inside of the shoes. Available in two sizes.

j. **Tri-lam insoles (Fig. 46.17J):** For adults with plantar fascitis, flat foot and transverse arch pain. Available in five sizes.

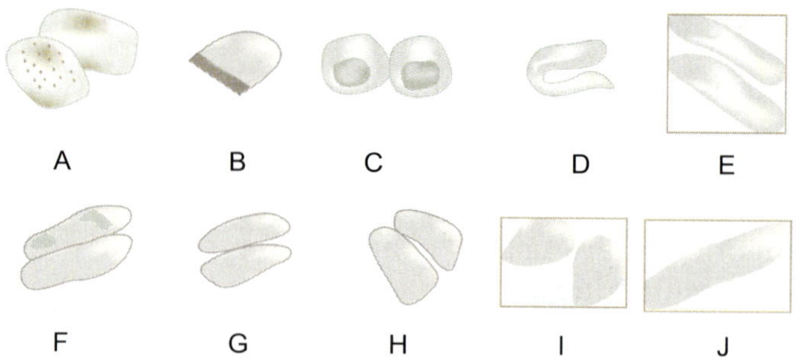

Figs 46.17A to J: Showing various foot supports

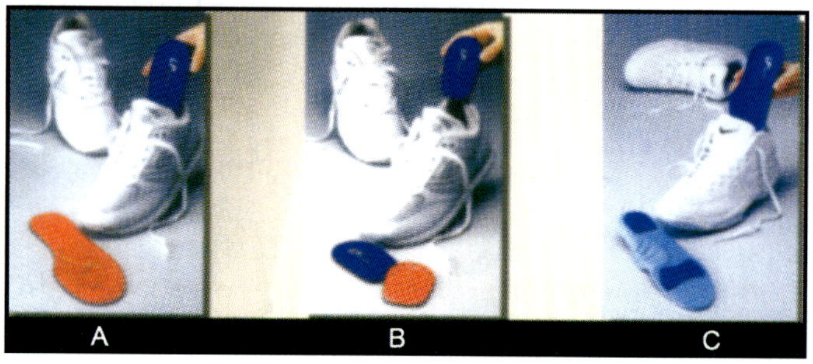

Fig. 46.18A to C: Showing foot inserts

UPPER LIMB ORTHOSIS

Upper limb orthoses ranges from a simple splint to the very complex varieties which are manufactured to the following basic requirements:

1. Limitation of movements could be either total or partial.
2. Exercise of muscles and joint range against energy storing devices such as springs or elastics.
3. Replacement of paralysed muscles using similar devices.
4. Preventive deformity control.

BIBLIOGRAPHY

1. Brittain HA. Hindquarter amputation. J Bone and Joint Surg 1949;31-B:104.
2. Brown PW. The rational selection of treatment for upper extremity amputations. Orthop Clin North Am 1981;12:843.
3. Burges EM, Romano RL, Traub JE. Immediate postsurgical prosthetic fitting. Prosthetic Study Report Bull Prosthet Res 1965;10-4:42.
4. Little Wood H. Amputations of the shoulder and at the hip. Br Med J 1922;381.
5. Malone JW, Moore WS, Goldstone J. Therapeutic and economic impact of a modern amputation program. Am Surg 1979;189:798.
6. Marquardt E, Correll J. Amputations and prosthesis for the lower limb. Int Orthop 1984;8:139.

7. Mccollough NC. The bilateral lower extremity amputee. Orthop Clin North America 1972;3:303.
8. Peizer E, Pirrello T. Principles and practice in upper extremity prosthesis. Orthop Clin North Am 1972;3:197.
9. Phelan JT, Nodular SH. A technique of hemipelvectomy. Surg Gynaecol Obstet 1964;119:311.
10. Pillet J. The aesthetic hand prosthesis. Orthop Clin North Am 1981;12:961.
11. Room AJ, Moore WS, Goldstone J. Below knee amputation: a modern approach. Am J Surg 1977;134:153.
12. Sarmiento A. A modified surgical-prosthetic approach to the Syme's amputation, a follow-up report. Clin Orthop 1972;85:11.
13. Tooms RE. Amputation surgery in the upper extremity. Orthop Clin North Am 1972;3:383.
14. Wagner FW (Jr). Amputations of the foot and ankle: current status. Clin Orthop 1977;122:62.
15. Weiss. The prosthesis on the operating room from the neurological point at view. Report of Workshop panel on lower extremity prosthetics fitting, 1966. Committee on prosthetics. Research and Development, National Academy of Sciences.

47

Sports Injuries

INTRODUCTION

Our cricketing icons; master blaster Sachin Tendulkar, ace spinner Anil Kumble, Nawab of Najafgarh Virender Sehwag, the effervescent VVS Laxman and the rock of Gibraltar Rahul Dravid all were in the news recently for sports injuries. For once, these injuries outfamed and outshone these cricketing demigods and were discussed and talked by everyone than the cricketers themselves. So these injuries fall within the gambit of sports medicine which is in fact a developing science with tremendous potential. With more and more people taking up sports as a career, the sports-related injuries are on the rise.

Sports medicine, like all other branches of medicine, aims at the complete physical, mental and spiritual well being of a sportsperson. A healthy mind in a healthy body is a concept which is more true to a sportsperson than anybody else. Positive thinking, fairplay and sportsmanship should be the hallmark of a true sportsman. We, the doctors and the therapists, aim to keep a sportsperson physically fit so that the rest of the objectives mentioned above are attained automatically.

Like in other branches of medicine so in sports medicine, prevention is better than cure. To prevent sports injuries, the first step is to ascertain whether a person choosing sports is fit to take it. An unfit person taking up sports is a sure prescription for future sports injuries. A fitness testing for those who wish to take up sports as their career should include various relevant parameters (see box).

Quick facts: Sports vs fitness testing

- Muscle power should be adequate.
- Active joint movements.
- Range of passive movements.
- Body balance.
- Coordination skills.
- Symmetrical and coordinated movements between the limbs and the body.
- Elasticity and extensibility of muscles and ligaments.
- Presence of any unwanted or accessory movements.

  These and a lot of other factors determine whether a person is fit enough to take to sports.

But one has to remember that fitness testing is not done only at the initial stages but needs to be done repeatedly at every stage of an athlete or a sportsperson's life. The second stage of prevention of sports-related injuries is assessing whether a sportsman is fit enough to resume the sporting activity after the initial layoff. There is nothing more dangerous than an unfit or a partially fit person resuming the sporting activity. It may spell a doom to his otherwise flourishing career in sports. A sportsperson has to satisfy certain norms before he can finally be sent back to the field (see box).

Quick facts

A sportsperson has to satisfy the following norms before he resumes sports again:

a. Should be able to jump from a height of 1 metre.
b. Full range of painless active movements.
c. Slight pain at extreme movements against resistance.
d. No running limp.
e. Can fully squat with one or both legs.
f. Can do full press up.
g. Can extend the knee with 20 lb × 10 in 45 sec.
h. Persons engaged in contact sports should be able to lift 45 lb × 10 in less than 45 sec.
i. The sportsperson should be independent of any strapping or support.

   If a person satisfies all the above criteria, he can be safely returned back to his passion, i.e. sports.

CLASSIFICATION OF SPORTS INJURIES

Among the various classifications proposed for sports injuries, the one proposed by Williams (1971) is widely used and recommended.

Williams' Classification

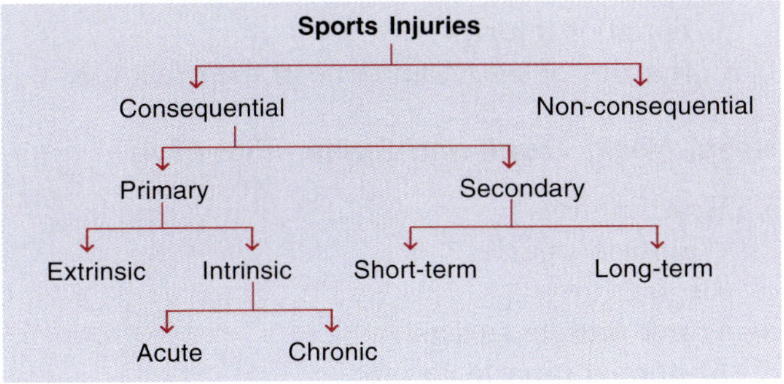

Among the Consequential Injuries

Primary extrinsic This is further subdivided into:

a. *Human:* Black eye due to direct blow.
b. *Implemental:* May be incidental (as in blow from a hard ball) or due to overuse (blisters from oars).
c. *Vehicular:* Clavicle fracture due to fall from cycle, etc.
d. *Environmental:* Injuries in divers.
e. *Occupational:* Jumper's knee in athletes, chondromalacia in cyclists, etc.

Primary intrinsic This could be acute or chronic.

a. *Incidental:* Strains, sprains, etc.
b. *Overuse:*
   - Acute, e.g. acute tenosynovitis of wrist extensors in Canoeists.
   - Chronic, March fracture in soldiers, etc.

Secondary short-term: For example, quadriceps weakness.

Secondary long-term Degenerative arthritis of the hip, knee, ankle, etc.

Nonconsequential Injuries

These are not related to sports but are due to injuries either at home or elsewhere and are totally not connected to any sports (e.g. slip and fall at home).

COMMON SPORTS INJURIES

Sports medicine usually deals with minor orthopaedic problems like soft tissue trauma (Fig. 47.1).

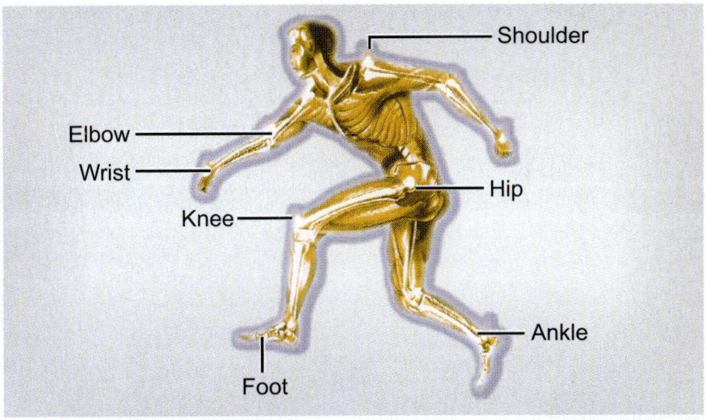

Fig. 47.1: Showing common sites of soft tissue injuries in sports

Very rarely, there may be serious fractures, head injuries or on the field deaths. There is nothing unusual about these injuries except that a sportsperson demands a 100 per cent cure and recovery while an ordinary person is satisfied and happy with a 60 to 80 per cent recovery. The difference is because of the desire of the sportsperson to get back to the sport again which requires total fitness.

Note: The incidence of sports injuries among all orthopaedic injuries is 5 to 10 per cent.

The following are some of the most common sports-related injuries one encounters in clinical practice.

Upper Limbs

1. *Shoulder complex*
   a. Rotator cuff injuries
   b. Shoulder dislocations
   c. Fracture clavicle
   d. Acromioclavicular injuries
   e. Bicipital tendinitis or rupture.
2. *Elbow*
   a. Tennis elbow (Fig. 47.2)
   b. Golfer's elbow
   c. Dislocation of elbow.
3. *Wrist*
   a. Wrist pain
   b. Carpal tunnel syndrome.
4. *Hand*
   a. Mallet injury (Fig. 47.3)
   b. Baseball finger
   c. Jersey thumb
   d. Injuries to the finger joints.

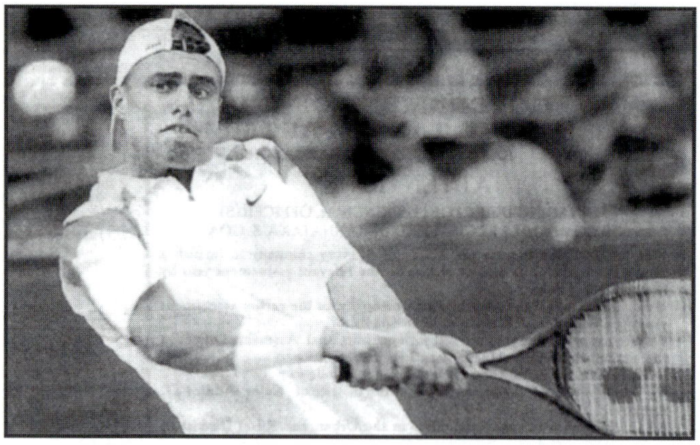

Fig. 47.2: Professional tennis players most commonly suffer from a famous sports disorder tennis elbow

Lower Limbs

1. *Hip*
   a. Iliotibial or tract syndrome
   b. Quadriceps strain
   c. Hip pain
   d. Groin pain due to adductor strain.
2. *Knee joint*
   a. Jumpers knee
   b. Chondromalacia
   c. Fracture patella
   d. Knee ligament injuries
   e. Meniscal injuries.
3. *Legs*
   a. Calf muscle strain
   b. Hamstrings sprain
   c. Stress fracture tibia
   d. Compartmental syndrome of the leg.

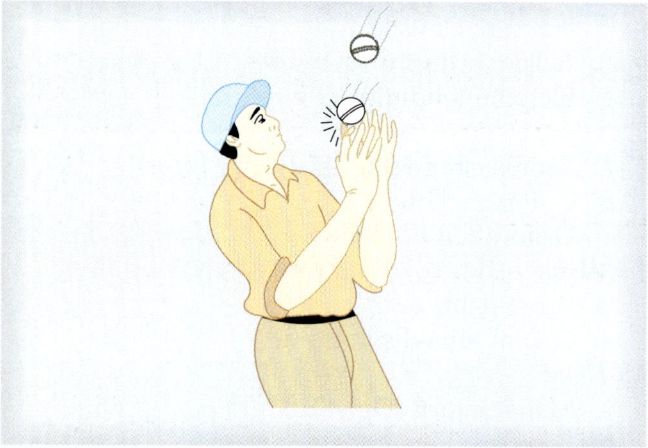

Fig. 47.3: Mechanism of mallet finger injuries in cricketers while trying to catch a ball

4. *Ankle injuries*
   a. Ankle sprain
   b. Injuries to tendo-Achilles
   c. Tenosynovitis.
5. *Foot*
   a. March fracture
   b. Jones fracture
   c. Forefoot injuries
   d. Injuries of sesamoid bone of the great toe.

Head, Neck, Trunk and Spine (Fig. 47.4)

a. Head injuries
b. Whiplash injuries
c. Rib fractures
d. Trunk muscle strains
e. Abdomen muscle strain
f. Low backache.

All these injuries have been discussed in relevant sections.

INVESTIGATIONS

These are the same as for any orthopaedic-related disorders and consists of plain X-ray, CT scan, bone scan, MRI, arthroscopy, arthrography, stress X-rays, etc.

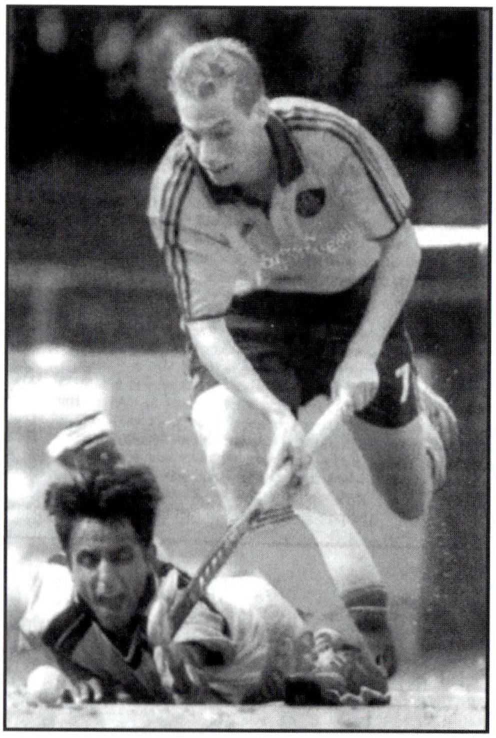

Fig. 47.4: Frequent falls, contact injuries and high speed activities are the common causes of sports injuries

TREATMENT OF SPORTS INJURY

This is discussed under three headings prevention, treatment proper and training.

Preventive Measures

The best way to treat a sports injury is to prevent it from happening. Nothing is better than preventing the injury.

Quick facts

Preventive measures

a. Proper clinical examination to identify any bodily defects.
b. Fitness training.
c. Correcting the wrong body mechanics and posture.
d. Conditioning exercises to overcome particular deficiencies.
e. Cardiopulmonary conditioning exercises to develop endurance.
f. Proper warm up exercises and relaxation techniques before and after the sports.
g. Wearing proper footwears and other protective devices like helmet, gloves, etc.
h. To prevent overuse syndrome, taking adequate breaks in between the vigorous sports is advised.
i. Avoiding sports in very high or low temperature climates.
j. Not allowing to aggravate minor problems like contusion, sprain, etc. by taking adequate rest and treatment.

Treatment

Treatment of individual sports-related disorders are discussed under suitable sections. However, a mention is made here of the general principles of treatment which is applicable to all sports injuries.

General Principles

1. *Concept of RICEMM* This sums up the early treatment methodology of sports injuries and consists of:
   R—Rest to the injured limb
   I—Ice therapy
   C—Compression bandaging
   E—Elevation of the injured part
   M—Medicines like pain killers, etc.
   M—Modalities like heat, straps, supports, etc.
2. After immobilisation and rest, early vigorous exercises should be commenced at the earliest to prevent muscle weakness and atrophy.
3. To prevent joint stiffness, early mobilisation has to be done first by passive movements and later by active movements. To improve the strength, resistive exercises are added.
4. Unlike the conventional once-a-day treatment, a sportsperson needs to be seen at least 2 to 3 times a day.
5. As mentioned earlier, allow resumption of sporting activity only after the sportsperson assumes 100 per cent fitness.
6. Mind training is as important as physical training. By repeated counselling, improve the psychological status of the patient to avoid depression, anxiety and negative attitudes which may develop during the injury.
7. Orthopaedic and surgical treatment to be undertaken at appropriate situations.

Training

The physiotherapist has to train a sportsperson in various exercises to enable him to keep his fitness level very high. After conducting a fitness testing, (mentioned earlier), the therapist has to subject an athlete to various forms of exercises to increase the endurance, strength, running, weight-bearing, etc. The following are the various forms of exercises.

Exercises to Increase the Cardiopulmonary Capacity

These exercises are done to increase the endurance level of an athlete or sportsperson.

Exercises to Increase the Muscle Strength

By carefully planned, graded, progressive resistive exercises (PRE), the therapist aims at improving the strength of the muscles of the upper limbs, lower limbs, trunk and spine.

Quick facts: PRE (Progressive Resistive Exercises)

- For upper limb muscles—bench press
- For lower limb muscles—squatting exercises
- For trunk and muscles of the limbs—power clean.

Exercises for Free Weight Training

Strength training with machines has a disadvantage in training only the prime movers. This anomaly is converted by free weight training which helps to strengthen not only the prime movers but also the synergistic and stabilising groups of muscles (e.g. exercises with dumbbells). They are also known to increase the tensile strength of the muscles, ligaments and tendons.

Measures to Improve the Agility

The measures to improve the agility levels of sportsperson are two-leg hops, one-leg hop, cross over-run turning, bending and backward running. These exercises help to improve balance, co-ordination and movements at a faster rate.

Measures to Improve the Speed-Polymetrics

In this, the neuromuscular system is trained to such an extent that it can react very quickly to sudden increase of speed and power which is so often required in sporting activities.

Measures of Relaxation

After the vigorous workout mentioned above, the sportspersons are taught methods of relaxation and body stretches.

Quick facts: About polymetrics

- Hops
- Speed jumps
- Running drills
- These above exercises must be done very fast with sudden burst of energy.
- The speed strength of a sportsperson depends on how fast the muscle action changes from eccentric to concentric ones.
- This is then followed with graded resistance exercises.

Before an athlete or a sportsperson resumes his sporting activities, a fitness testing is carried out (*ref page 609*) and only then he is allowed to take to the sports provided he is 100 per cent fit.

BIBLIOGRAPHY

1. Bass AL. Rehabilitation after soft tissue injury. Proceedings of the Royal Society of Medicine, 653-6.
2. Fowler JA. Fitness and its components. Physiotherapy 63.
3. Hornor Z, Werpravnik C. Mechanisms, types and treatment of injuries. British Journal of Sports Medicine, 1: 45-6.
4. Williams JGP. Classification of Sports Injuries, 1971.
5. Wright D. Fitness testing after injury. In Reilly T (Ed): Sports Fitness and Sports Injuries. London: Faber and Faber.

APPENDICES

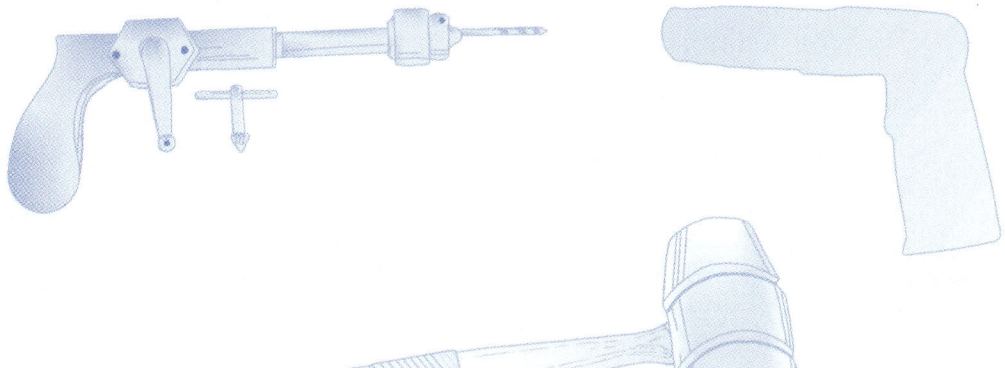

Instruments and Implants in Orthopaedics

For convenience and easy understanding, instruments used in orthopaedic surgery can be categorised into three groups:

1. General surgical instruments
2. Regular orthopaedic instruments
3. Instruments used in special orthopaedic situations.

Now let us try to analyse each one in detail.

GENERAL SURGICAL INSTRUMENTS

a. Surgical knife and blade is used to incise the skin and soft tissues.
b. Artery forceps is used to catch the bleeding vessels.
c. Allis forceps is used to catch the soft tissues.
d. Retractors are used to retract the soft tissues.
e. Scissors are used to cut the soft tissues.
f. Tissue holding forceps, needles, etc.

The general surgical instruments help in the initial stage of surgery, for exposure, to deal with the soft tissue structures, to expose the bones, etc.

REGULAR ORTHOPAEDIC INSTRUMENTS

After reaching the bone, general orthopaedic instruments help to deal with the bone to place implants, etc. The following are the general orthopaedic instruments mentioned in order of priority.

BONE HOLDING, PLATE HOLDING AND ROD HOLDING INSTRUMENTS

Instruments

1.

Bone hook

2.

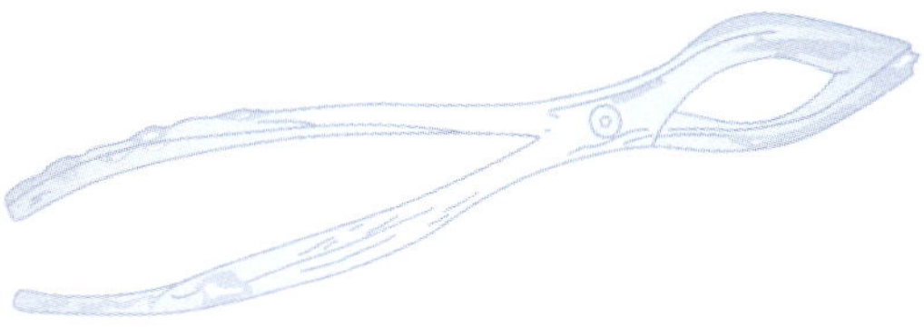

Fergusson's lion-toothed bone holding forceps

3.

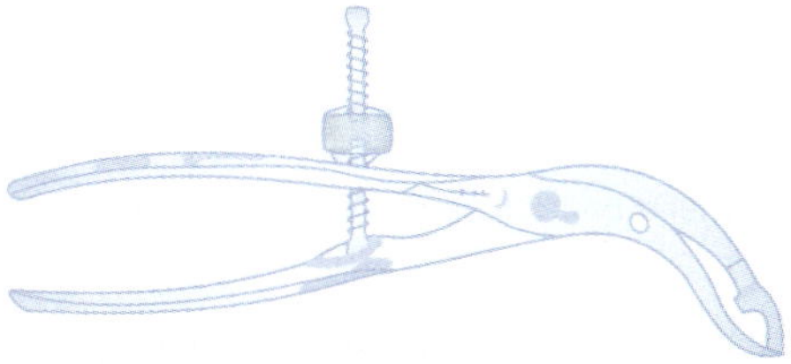

AO forceps

4.

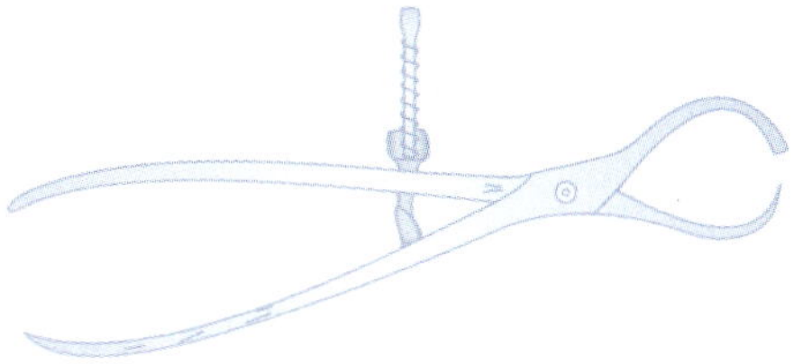

Patella forceps

5

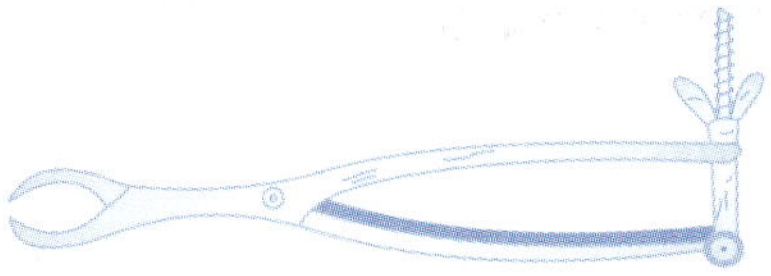

Heygrove's bone holding forceps (sizes 8"/10"/12")

9.

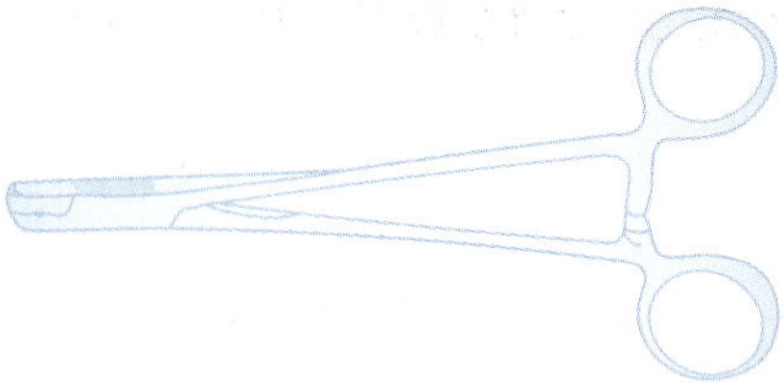

Rod holding forceps

6.

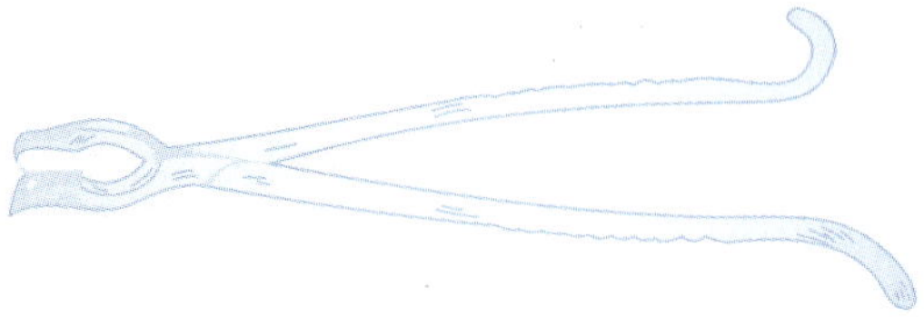

Lane's Fagg's bone holding (sizes 12 ½")

10.

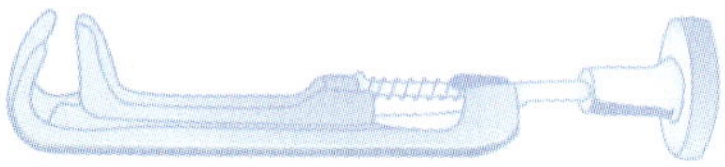

Lowman's bone holding clamp (sizes 4", 5", 8")

7.

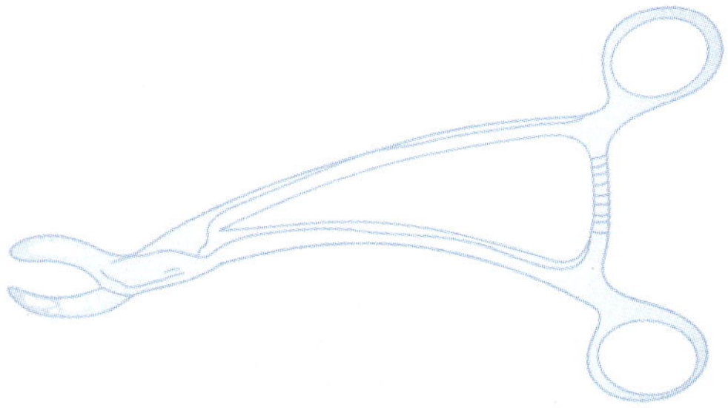

Burn's bone holding forceps

11.

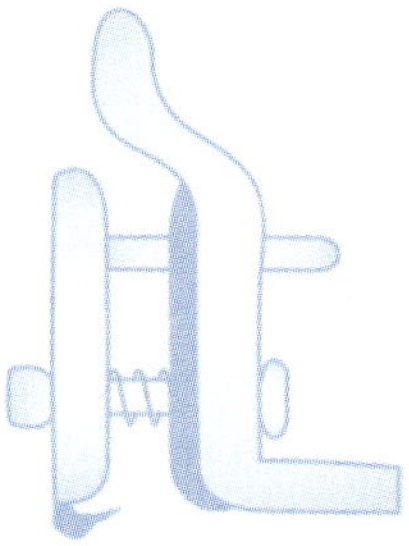

Müller's compression device with handle

8.

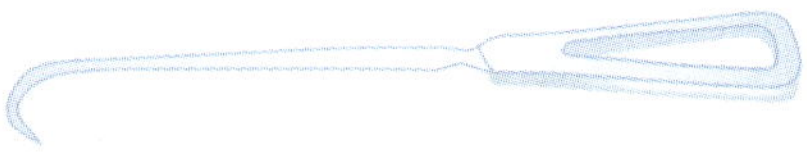

Kocher's bone hook (sizes: small/medium/large)

12.

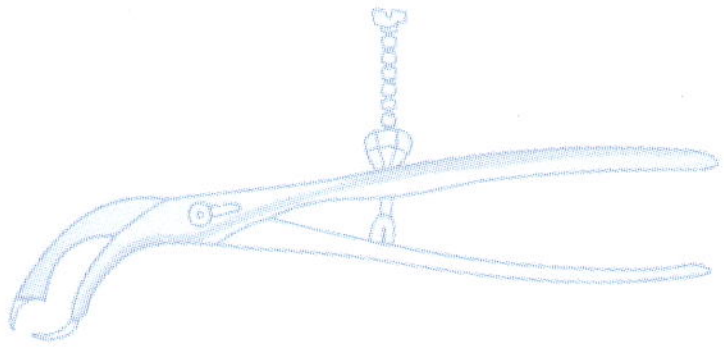

Self-centering bone holding forceps

Instruments from 1 to 8 are used to pick up and hold the bone firmly during surgery, instrument No. 9 is used to hold and steady the intramedullary nails. No. 10 is to hold the plate to the bone for fixation.

INSTRUMENTS USED TO CUT, NIBBLE, CURETTE AND MAKE HOLES IN THE BONES

Instruments

1.

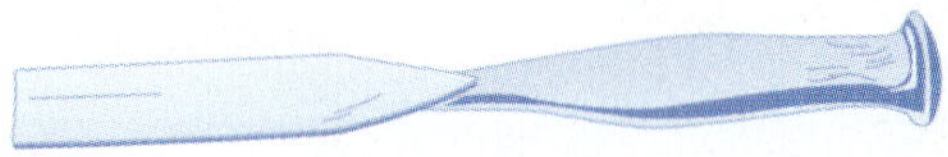

Smith-Peterson osteotome—straight
(sizes—5 to 35 mm with 5 mm variation)

2.

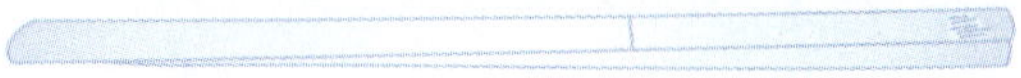

Lambotte osteotomes—9" length (straight ½", ¾", 7/8" width)

3.

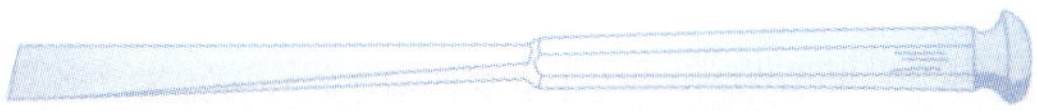

Stille type osteotome (straight—5 to 35 mm
with 5 mm variation)

4.

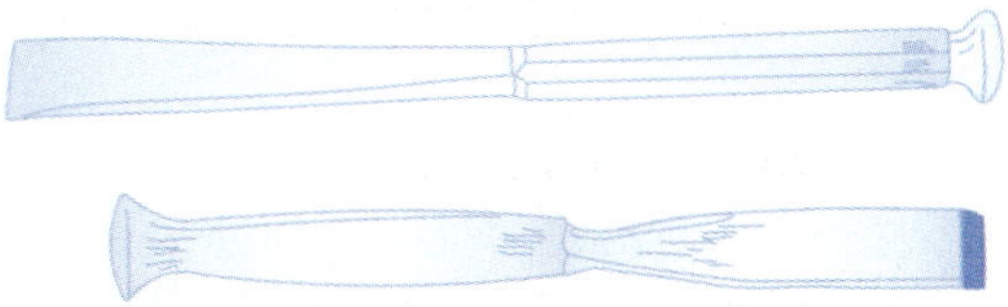

Stille type chisel—straight 7"
(sizes—5 to 30 mm with 5 mm variation)

5.

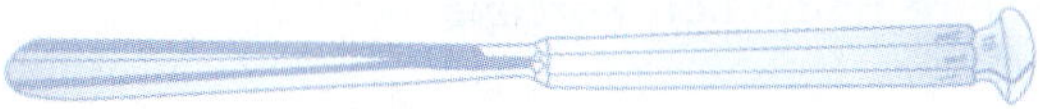

Stille gauge—curved
(sizes—5 to 35 mm with 5 mm variation)

6.

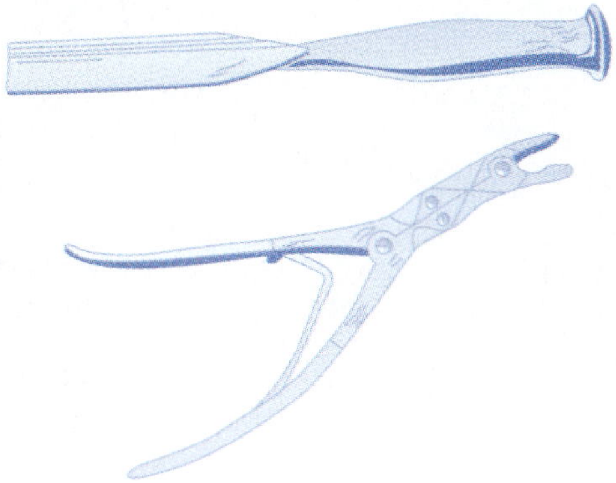

Leksell's rongeur (double action)

7.

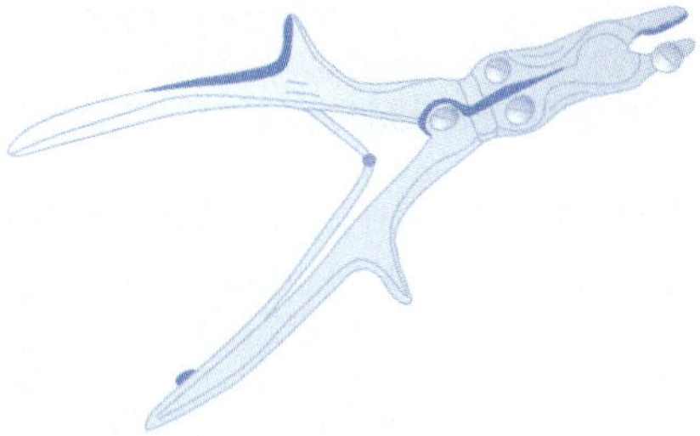

Northfields rongeur (heavy double action)

8.

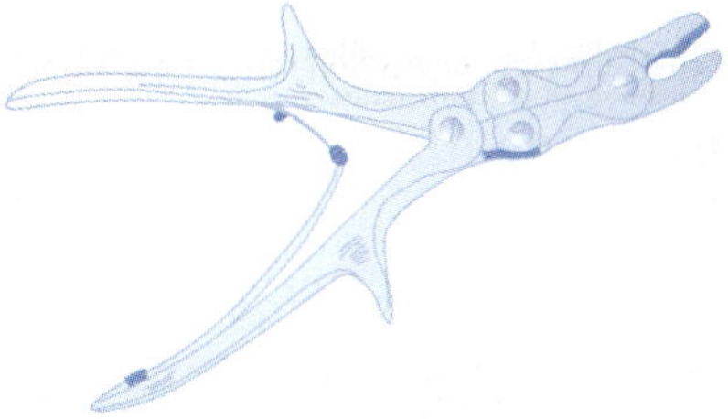

Sargent rongeur (double action)

9.

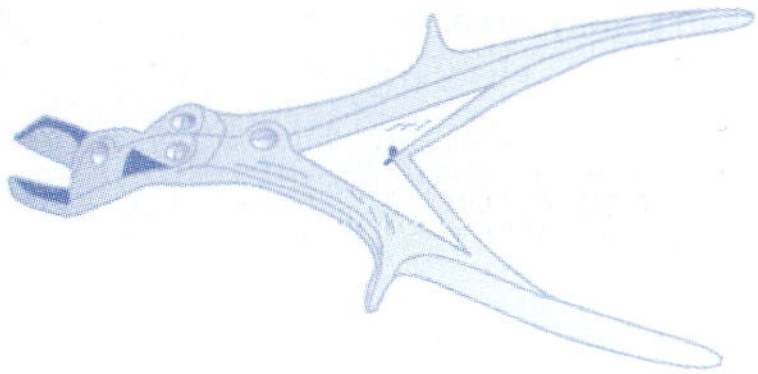

Stille-Horsley bone cutting forceps (10" length)

10.

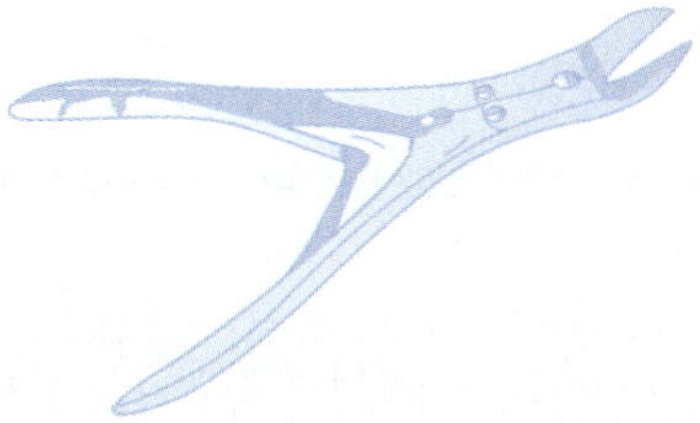

Ruskin bone cutting forceps (double action) 7½"

11.

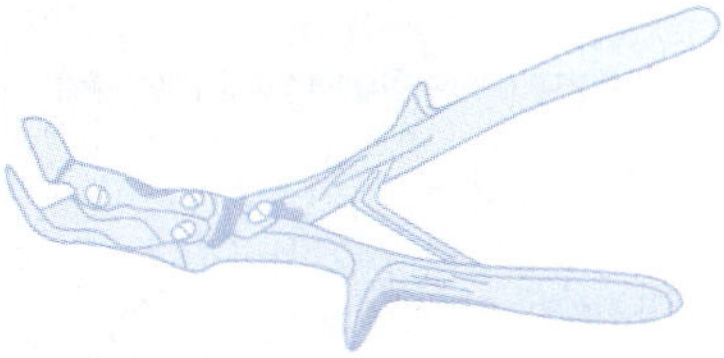

Tudor Edward bone cutting forceps (9½" length)

12.

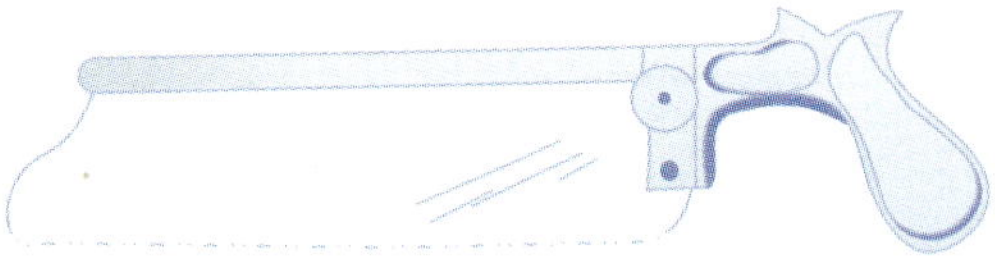

Amputation saw

13.

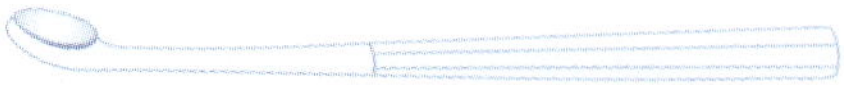

Cup curette (sizes 3 to 10 mm)

14.

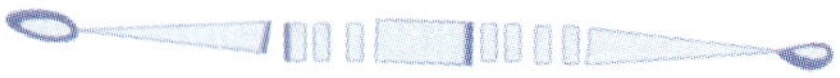

Volkman curette double ended (sizes 4 mm)

15.

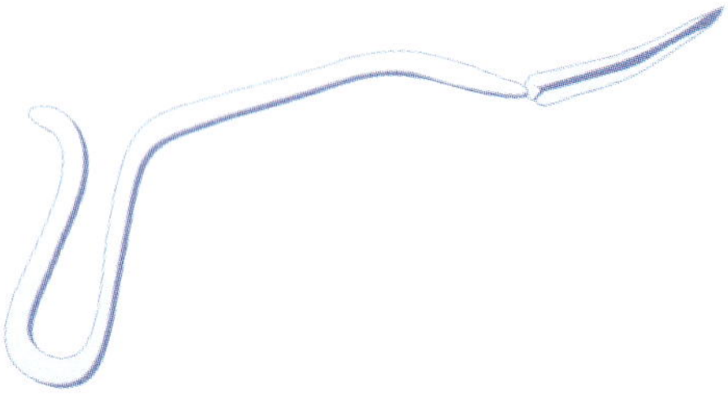

Kuntscher's diamond pointed AWL

MISCELLANEOUS ORTHOPAEDIC INSTRUMENTS

INSTRUMENTS

I. Periosteal Elevators

1.

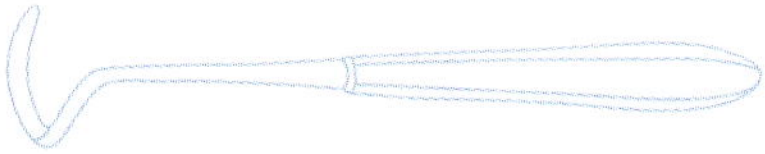

Doyan's periosteal elevator Adult—right/left

2.

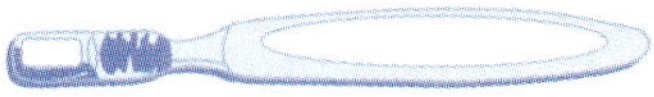

Farabeauf rugine straight/curved

3.

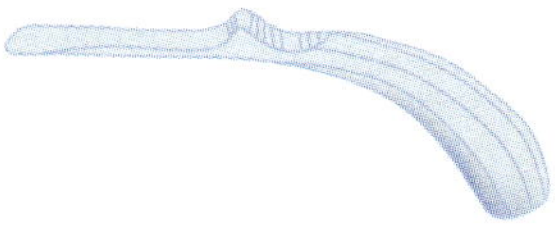

Jone's periosteal elevator (pistol-shaped handle)

4.

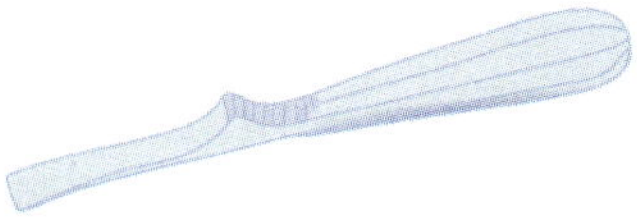

Mitchell elevator—straight 8¼"

5.

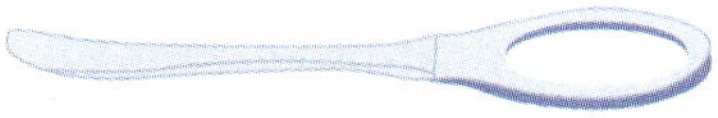

Bristows periosteal elevator

II. Bone Levers

1.

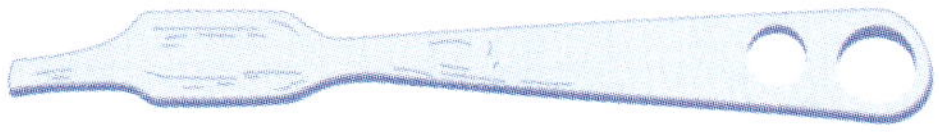

Retractor wide tip—width 22 mm

2.

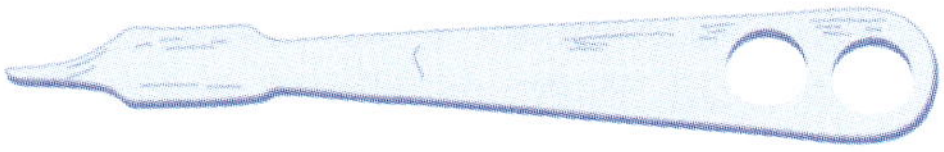

Retractor long narrow tip (for hip surgery)—width 18 mm

III. Fracture Reduction Forceps

1. • Ratchet lock

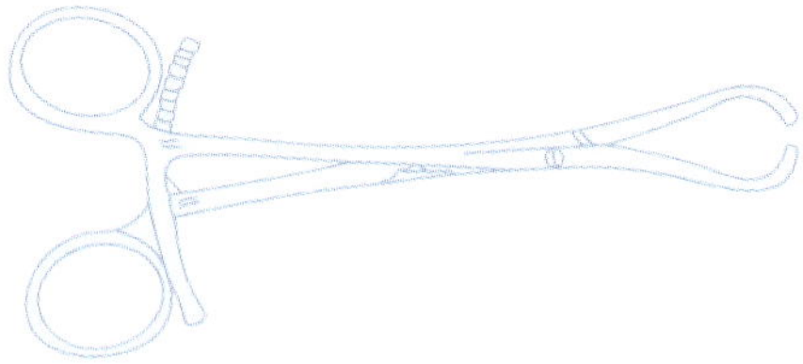

With points

2. • Speed lock

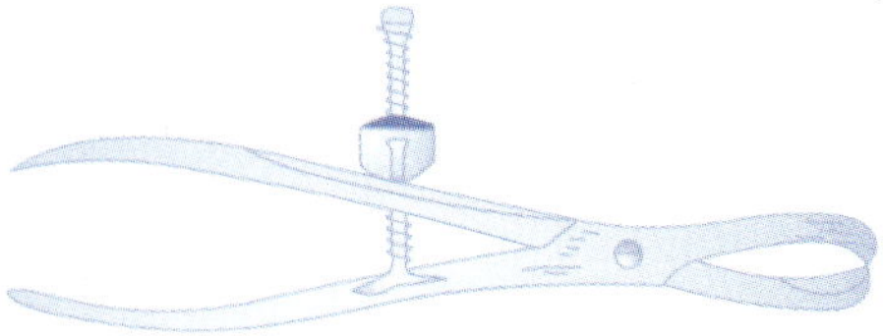

Large forceps

Appendices

3.

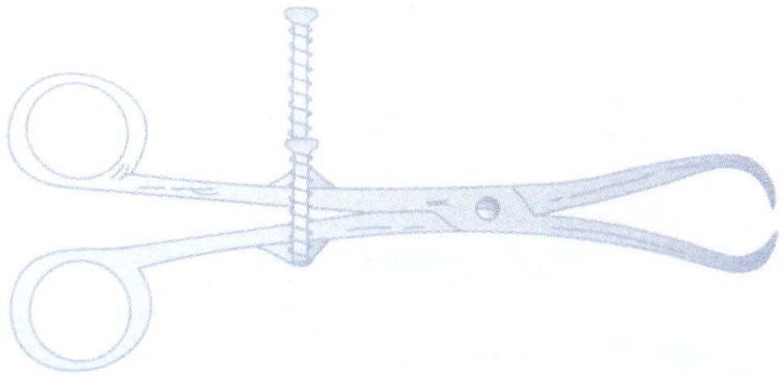

• Speed lock

4.

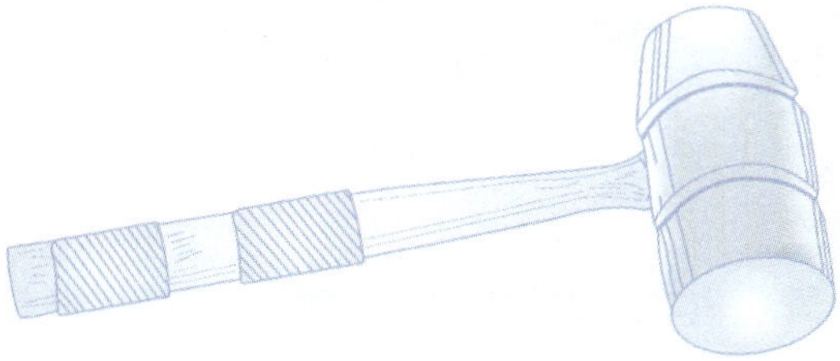

• Mallet

Serrated

INSTRUMENTS USED FOR INSERTION OF PLATE AND SCREWS

Instruments

1.

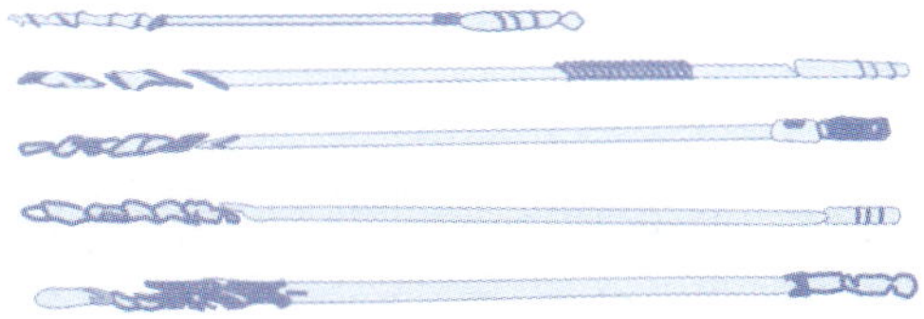

Drill bits

2.

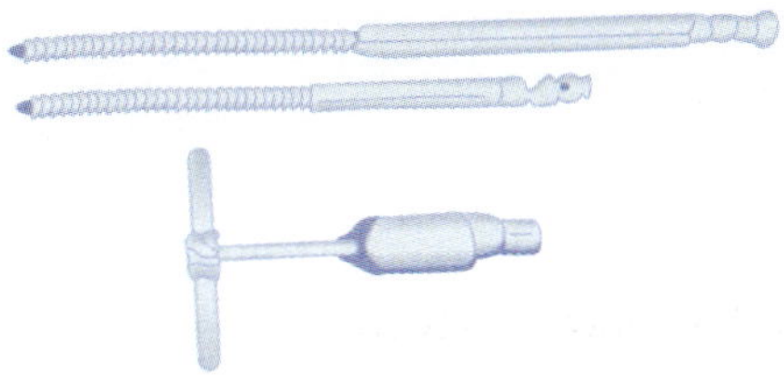

Tap and T-handle

3.

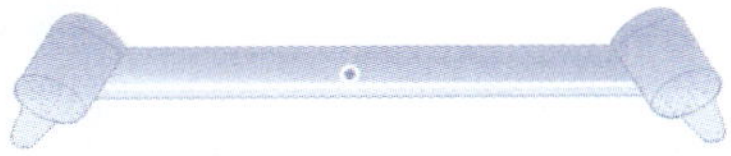

DCP drill guide position

4.

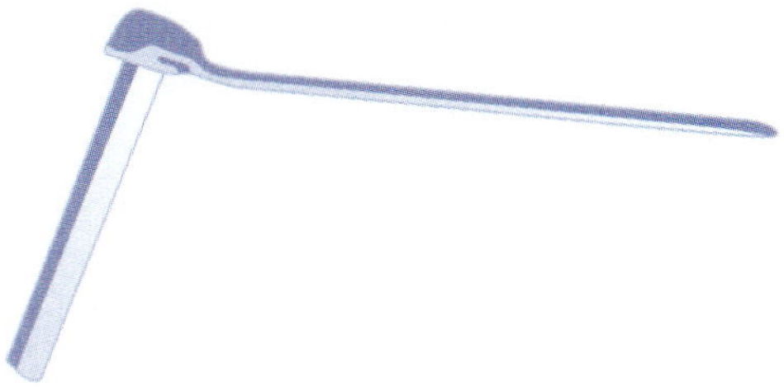

Protection sleeve

5.

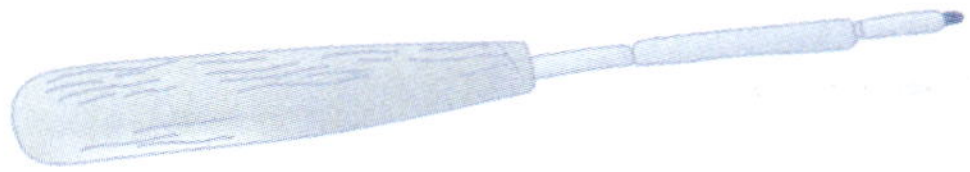

Hexagonal screwdriver

6.

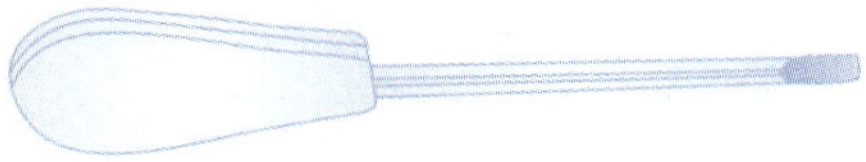

Ordinary screwdriver

7.

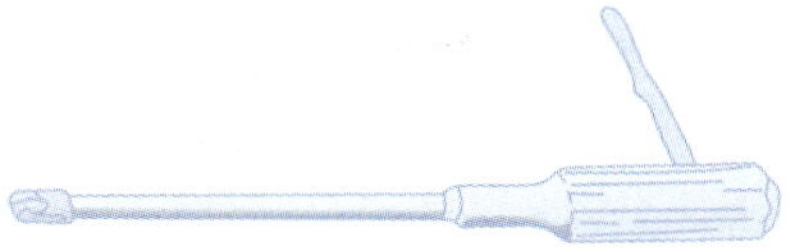

William' screwdriver

8.

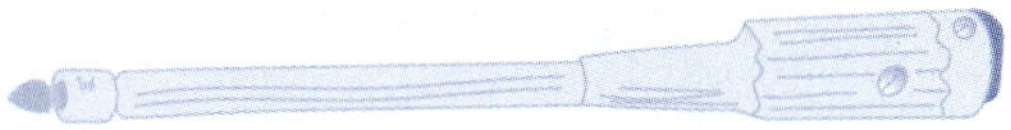

Burn's self-holding screwdriver

9.

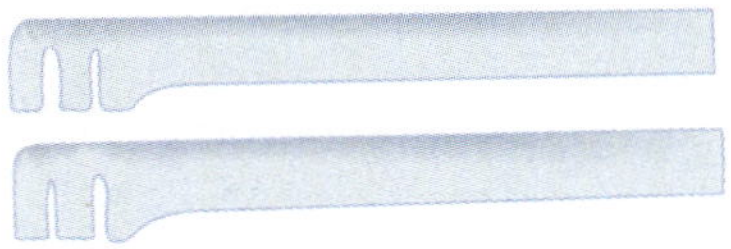

Plate benders

10.

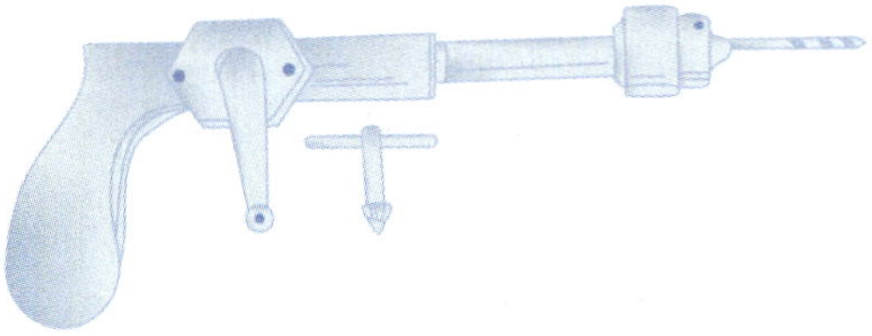

Hand operated drill and Chuck

12.

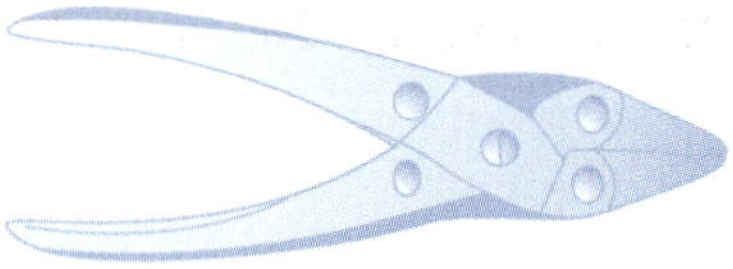

Cutting pliers

13.

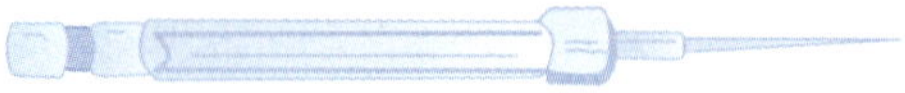

Depth guage

11.

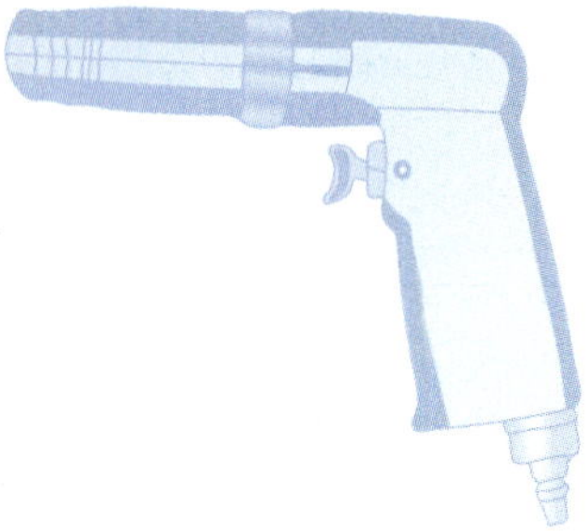

Universal airdrill

14.

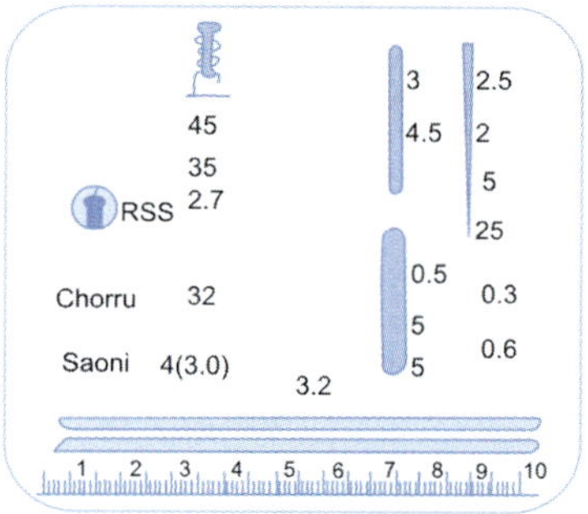

Measuring device

INSTRUMENTS USED FOR CUTTING PLASTER CASTS

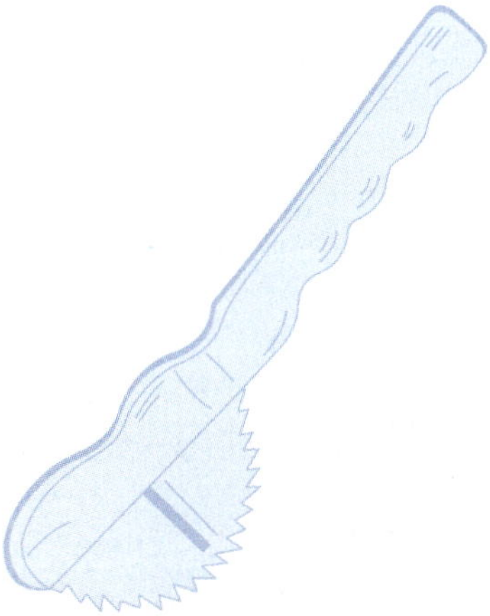

Plaster saw with aluminium handle

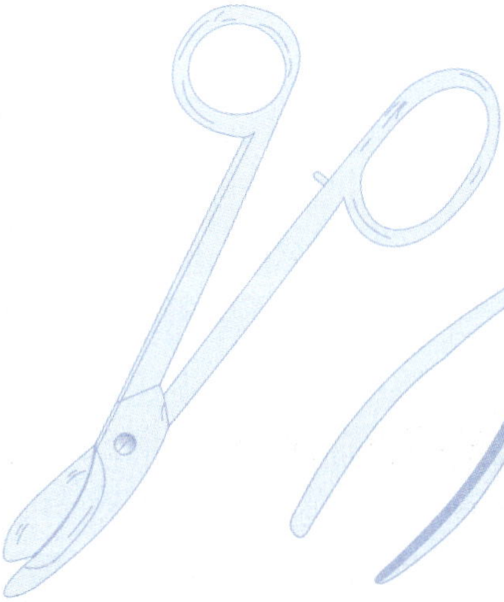

Plaster cutting scissors

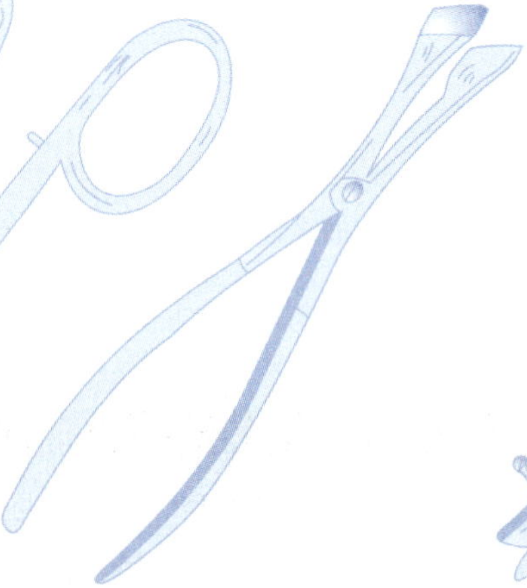

Plaster cast spreader

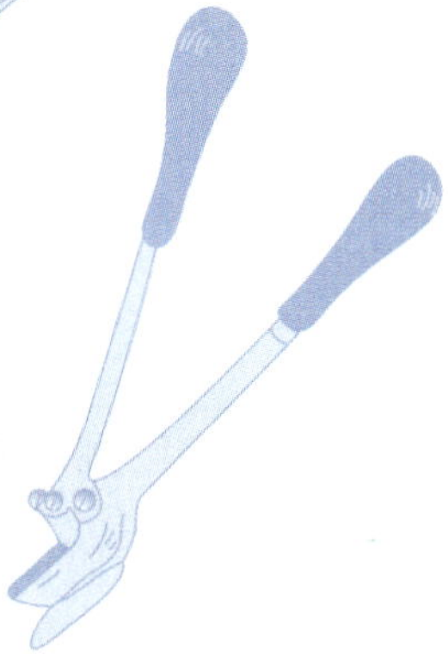

Lorenz plaster shears

INSTRUMENTS USED FOR WIRE INSERTION

Instruments

1.

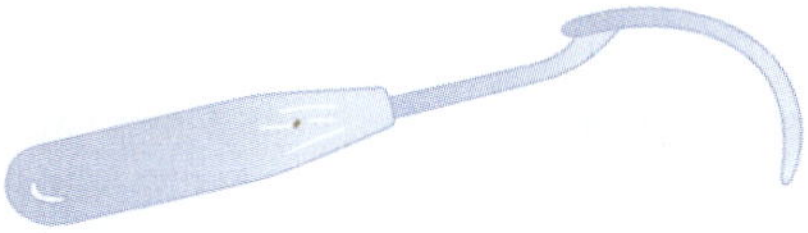

Wire sleeve

2.

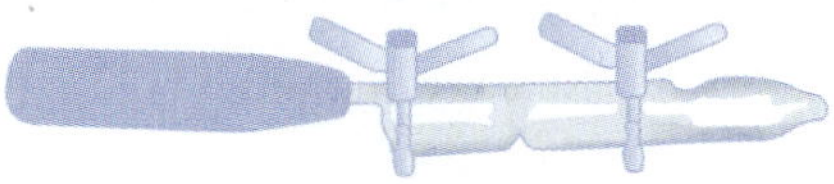

Wire tightener

3.

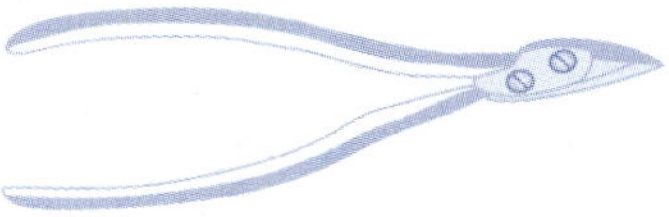

Wire bender

4.

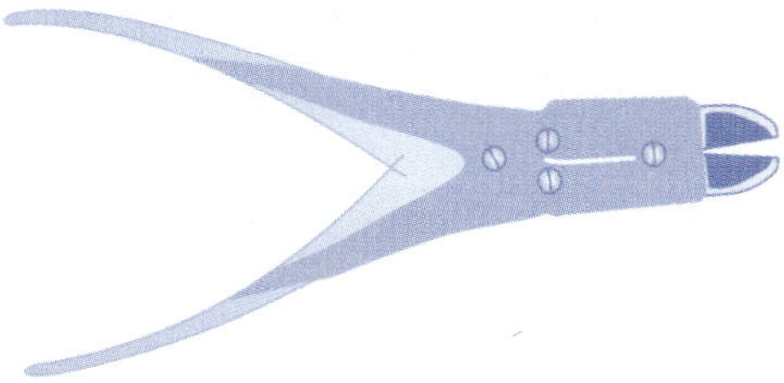

Wire cutter

5.

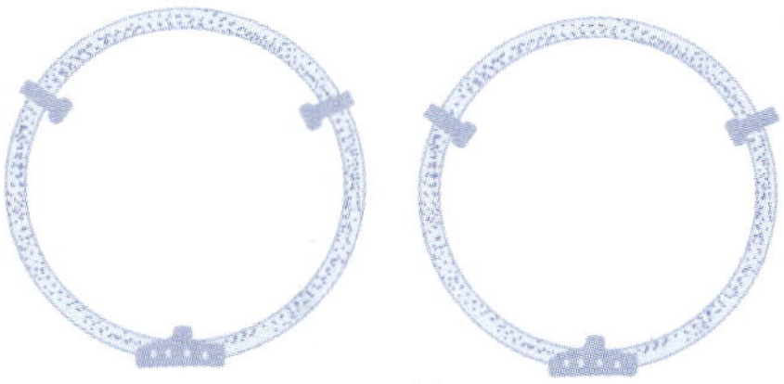

Circlage wire

6.

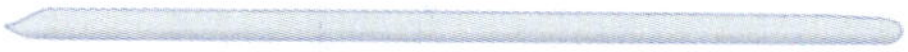

Kirschner wire

IMPLANTS IN ORTHOPAEDICS

Different Types of Plates Used in Orthopaedics

Instruments

1.

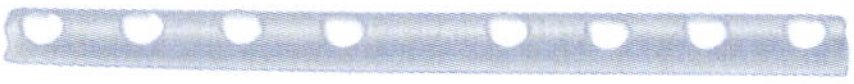

Semitubular plate

2.

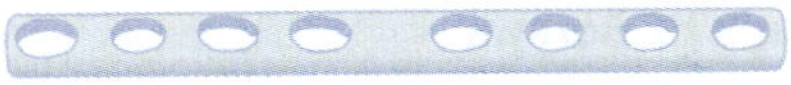

Narrow DCP 4.5

3.

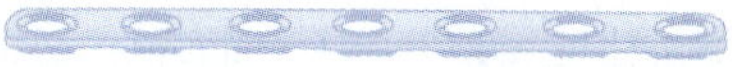

Narrow LC-DCP 4.5

4.

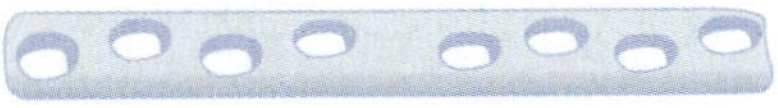

Broad DCP 4.5

5.

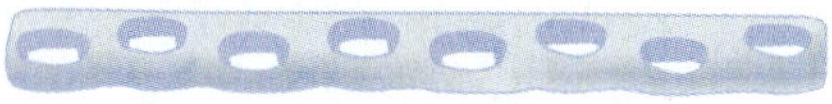

Broad LC-DCP 4.5

6.

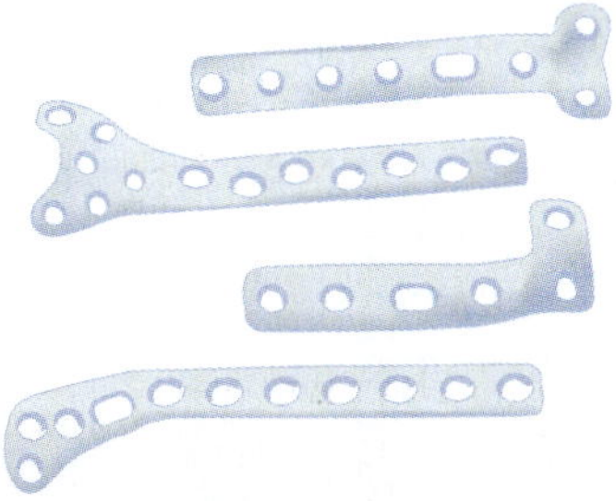

Form plates

7.

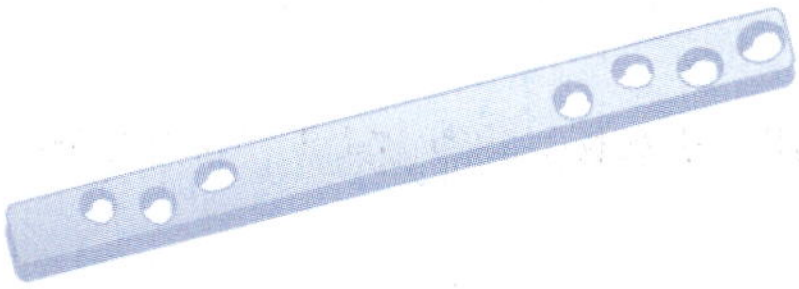

Broad lengthening plate

8.

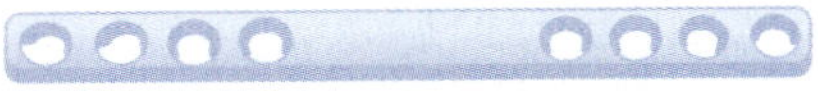

Narrow lengthening plate

9.

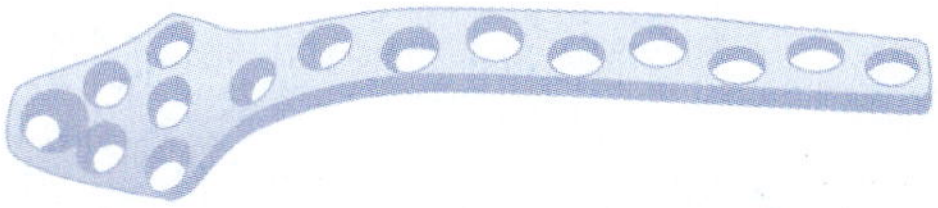

Cobra head plate

Semitubular plate is used for fracture of subcutaneous bones like ulna

Note: Narrow DCP—is used for tibia and is not intended for femur
Broad DCP—is used for femur and humerus and is not intended for tibia
LC-DCP—is a limited contact dynamic compression plate.

Different Sets of Screws

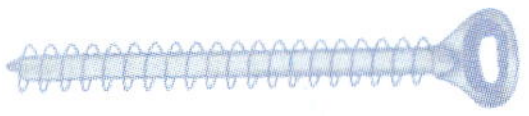

4.5 mm malleolar screw

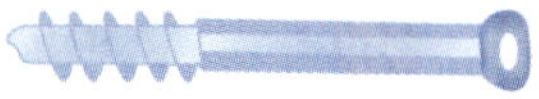

4.5 mm cortex screw

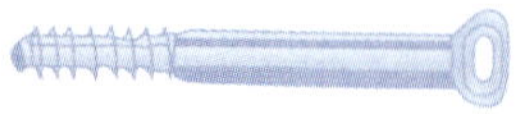

4.5 mm shaft screw

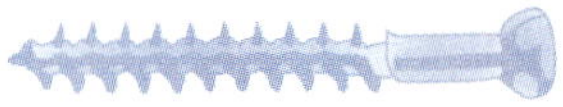

6.5 mm cancellous bone screw/fully threaded

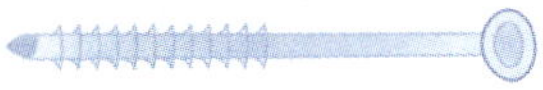

6.5 mm cancellous bone screw/32 mm

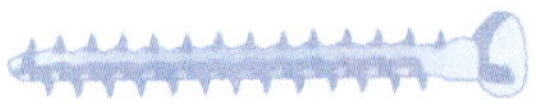

6.5 mm cancellous bone screw/16 mm

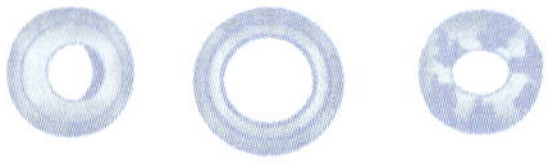

Nuts and washers

DYNAMIC HIP AND ANKLE IMPLANTS

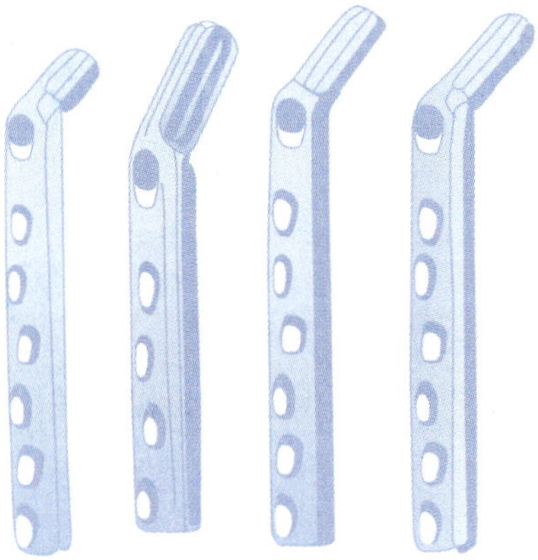

Dynamic hip plate

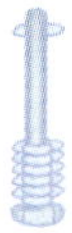

DHS Locking device

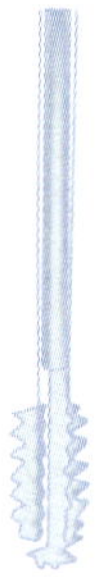

DHS/DCS Screw

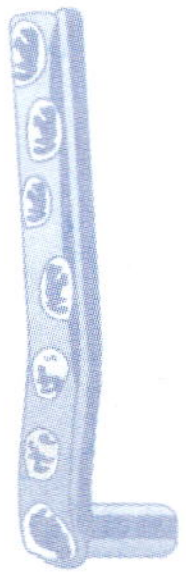

DCS Plate

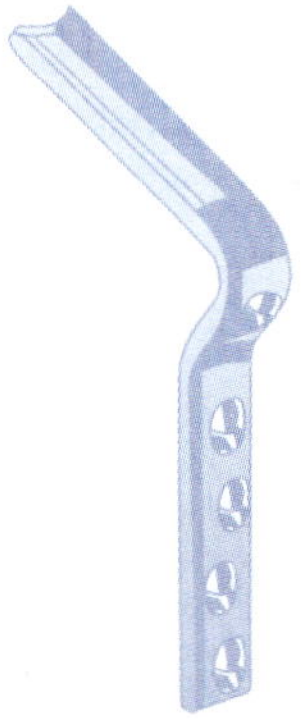

Angled blade plate for intertrochanteric femoral osteotomies in adults

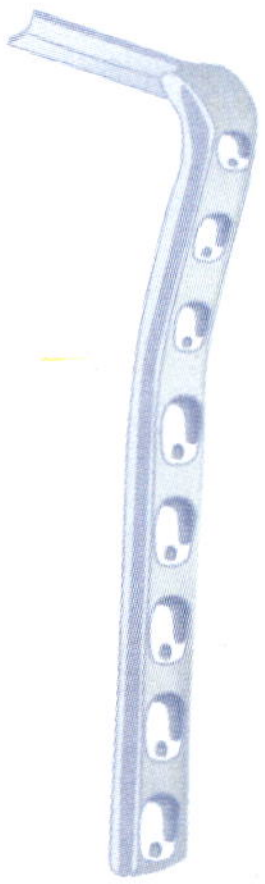

Condylar plates 95° for small adults and adolescents

SOME OF THE SPECIAL PLATES USED IN ORTHOPAEDICS

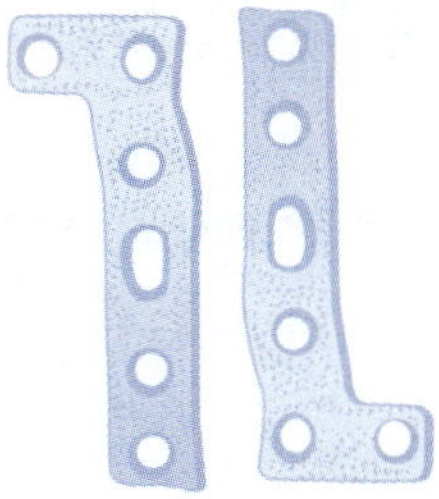

L-Plate

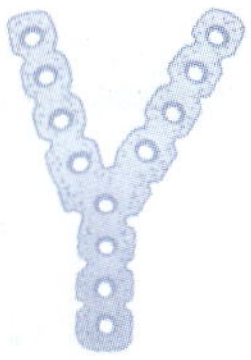

BO805.01 'Y' plate

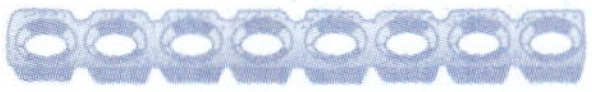

Reconstruction plate for 3.5 mm

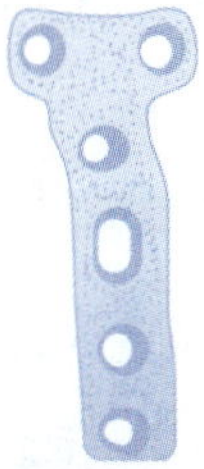

Small 'T'-plate

DIFFERENT CONVENTIONAL INTRAMEDULLARY NAILS

1.

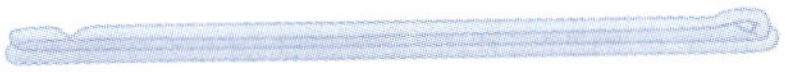

Küntscher's cloverleaf medullary nail with two slots for femur (K-nail)

2.

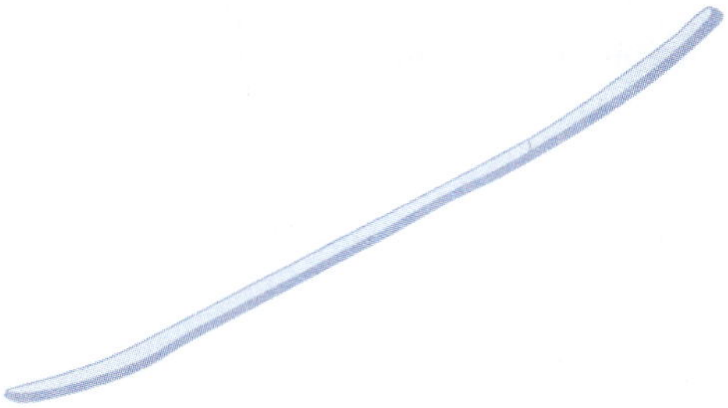

Küntscher's 'V'-shaped medullary nail with curved end—tibia

3.

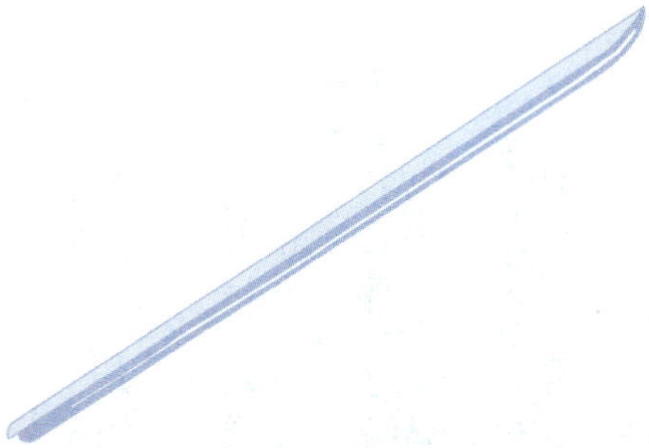

Küntscher's 'V'-shaped medullary nail straight for humerus

4.

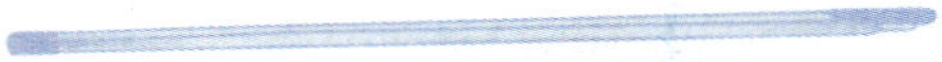

Square nail for radius

5.

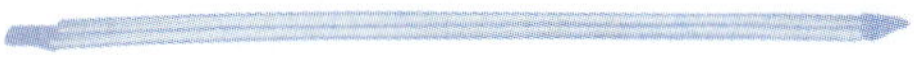

Square nail for ulna

INSTRUMENTS USED FOR K-NAIL INSERTION FOR FEMUR

1.

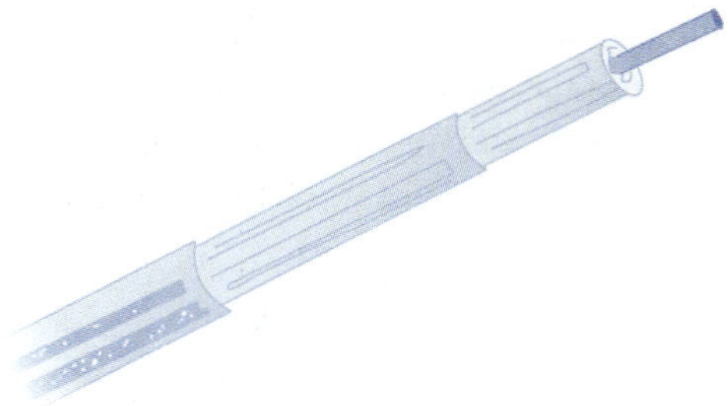

Nail set

2.

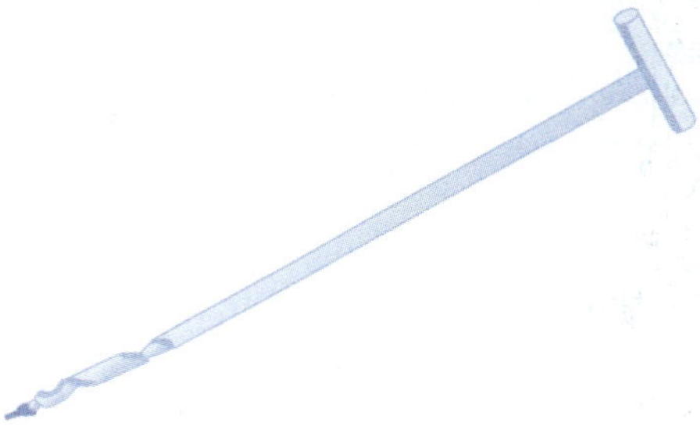

Intramedullary reamer
(Sizes 6 to 15 mm with 1 mm variation)

3.

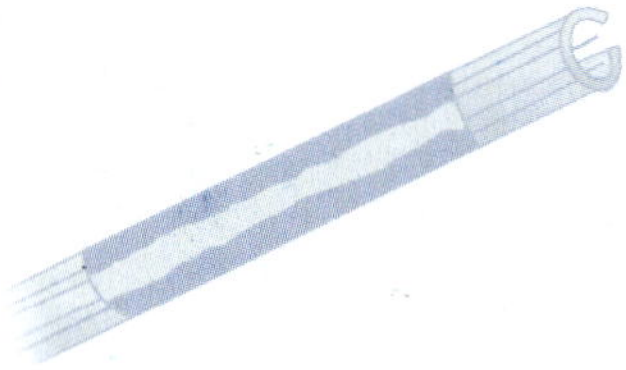

Küntscher's nail driver

4.

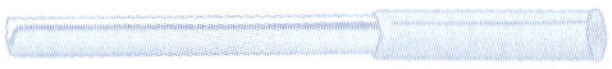

Küntscher's nail punch for final tapping

5.

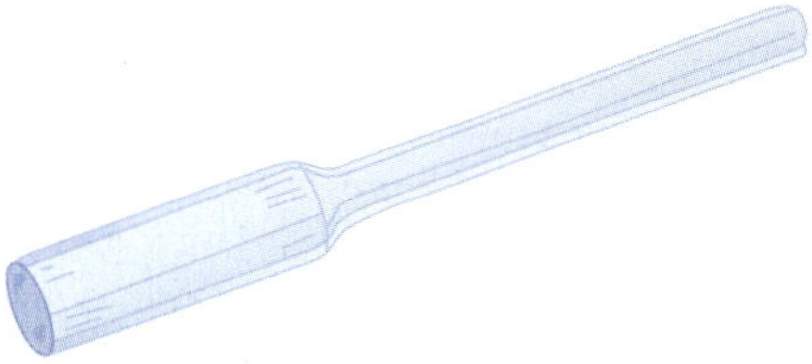

K-nail impactor

6.

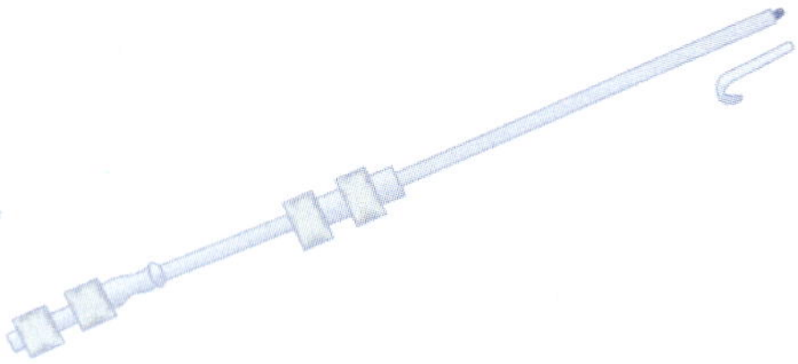

K-nail extractor with two hooks

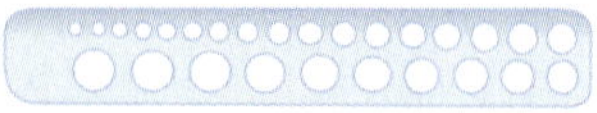

Diameter measuring gauge

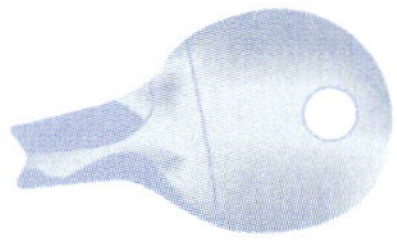

Tissue protector

KÜNTSCHER'S CLOVERLEAF* INTRAMEDULLARY NAIL

For information about intramedullary nail, its requirements, mode of action, and its varieties please refer to page No. 72. The technique of nail insertion is described on page No. 213.

Methods of insertion It could be either open or closed. A comparative study is presented here.

Open technique	Closed technique
Disadvantages	*Disadvantages*
• Infection is more common.	• Technically difficult.
• Exposure time is more.	• Require sophisticated equipment.
• Fat embolism may occur.	• Expensive.
• Blood loss is more.	
• Fracture haematoma is lost.	
• Tissue trauma is more.	
Advantages	*Advantages*
Good anatomic reduction can be obtained.	All the disadvantages of open technique are absent.

PROSTHESIS OF THE HIP

Prostheses are used for replacement of head of femur following nonunion and avascular necrosis due to fracture neck of femur.

Advantages

- It helps to mobilise the patients early.
- It eliminates the complications like avascular necrosis, nonunion, fixation failure, etc.

Disadvantages

- Function after hemireplacement arthroplasty and prosthesis is not equal to patient's own femoral head.
- The surgery is extensive and time consuming.

Indications (9 Ps)

1. **P**oor general health.
2. **P**athological fracture.
3. **P**orosis.
4. **P**auwel's type III fracture.
5. **P**hysiological age 60 years and above.
6. **P**araplegia and paresis.
7. **P**aget's disease.
8. **P**rimary internal fixation failed.
9. **P**oor union (nonunion and delayed union).

Primary prosthesis replacement is required only in 10 per cent of all fracture neck of femur cases.

Types of Prosthesis (Fig. AII.1A and B)

There are two types of hemireplacement prostheses used in orthopaedic practice, the Austin Moore prosthesis and the

*(So called because on cross-section the nail has cloverleaf shape and this gives good rotational stability).

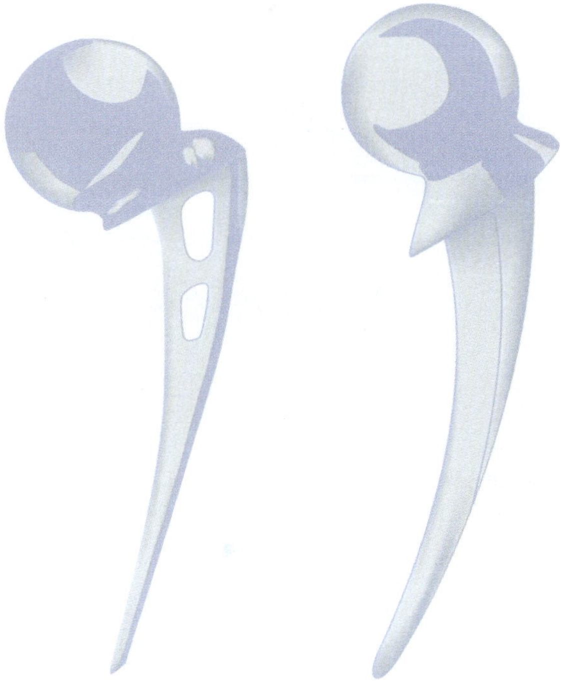

Fig. AII.1A and B: (A) Austin Moore and (B) Thompson's prosthesis

Thompson prosthesis. Table AII.1 shows the differences between the two varieties of prostheses used in hemireplacement arthroplasty.

Approaches

Posterior This is the commonly used approach. In this approach, incidence of posterior dislocation is common due to poor healing of the capsule due to flexion, adduction contractures of the hip and increased incidence of sepsis due to proximity of the perineum.

Anterior This is less commonly employed and is known to cause increased incidence of fracture shaft femur.

Technique of Prosthesis Insertion (Moore's)

The hip can be approached either by the anterior (Watson Jones), lateral (Gibson's) or posterior (Moore's or Southern) approaches. The one commonly preferred is the Moore's approach.

The hip is exposed through the posterior approach and the hip is dislocated posteriorly and the head is removed. The medullary canal of the neck and upper shaft is opened and reshaped with a rasp. A notch is cut in the proximal end of the greater trochanter. Now measure the size of the head removed from the acetabulum and select a prosthesis of the same size. Confirm the size of the prosthesis so chosen by inserting it directly into the acetabulum. Now using a hand saw or a motor saw, prepare the end of the femoral neck leaving about 1.3 cm of the calcar to seat the A-M prosthesis. The prosthesis is now inserted into the canal and reduced back into the acetabulum. A check is made for the stability of the prosthesis. Close the wound needed in layers. No external immobilisation is required. After two weeks, active and passive movements are begun and the patient can begin to walk between parallel bars after 2 to 3 weeks.

Table AII.1: Differences in prostheses

S. No.	*Features*	*Austin Moore's prosthesis*	*Thompson's prosthesis*
1.	Indications	Fracture neck femur with at least 1/4" calcar femoral left intact	For fracture neck femur with no calcar
2.	Neck	Present	Absent
3.	Collar	Present	Absent
4.	Bone cement	Not required	Always required
5.	Holes	Present	Absent
6.	Locking mechanism	Self-locking	Not self-locking

Complications

1. *Infection* This is due to poor aseptic measures and due to close proximity to the perineum. Incidence is 2 to 20 per cent.
2. *Dislocation of prosthesis* This is rare in posterior approach. Incidence is 1 to 10 per cent.
3. *Fracture of femoral shaft* This can occur if the stem of the prosthesis is forced into an improperly reamed medullary canal and while trying to reduce the head into the acetabulum. The incidence is 4 to 5 per cent.
4. *Breakage of prosthesis* This is a rare complication and can be due to undue stress and strains or faulty material.
5. *Pain* This can be due to tightness into the acetabulum due to the large size of the prosthesis. If the size is too small, the joint will be painful and unstable.
6. *Heterotropic calcification* This is seen in some patients in the dissected gluteal muscles and the capsule.
7. *Damage to the acetabular articular cartilage* This is due to excessive and constant pressure of the prosthesis over the acetabular cartilage.

DIFFERENT HIP IMPLANTS

1. Fixed angles nails and plates (sizes 2.5" to 7" with 0.25")

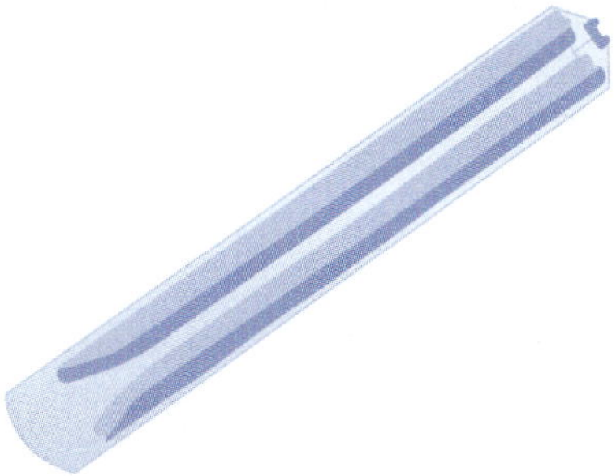

a. Smith-Peterson nail

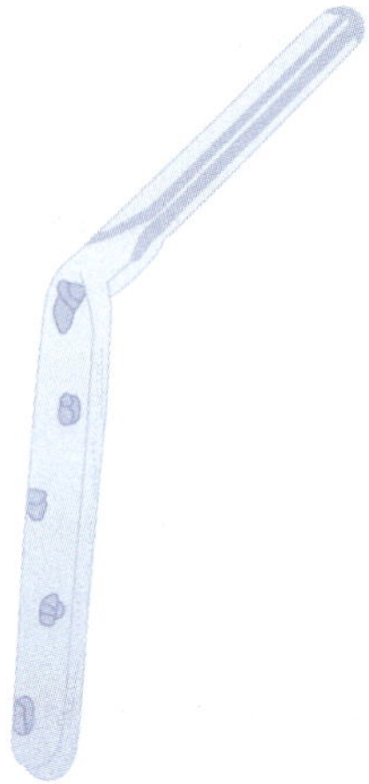

b. Jewett nail 120 DEG, pin length 2.5" to 4" with 0.25" variation (Plate sizes 3 to 6 holes)

2. Hip fixation pins

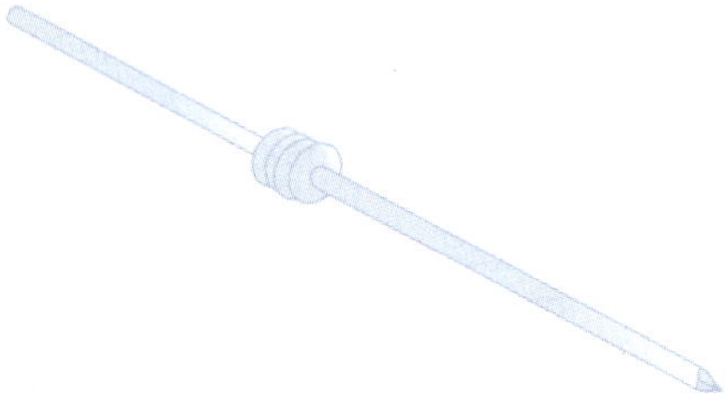

a. Moore pin with two nuts
Sizes 2.5" to 5" with 0.25" variation

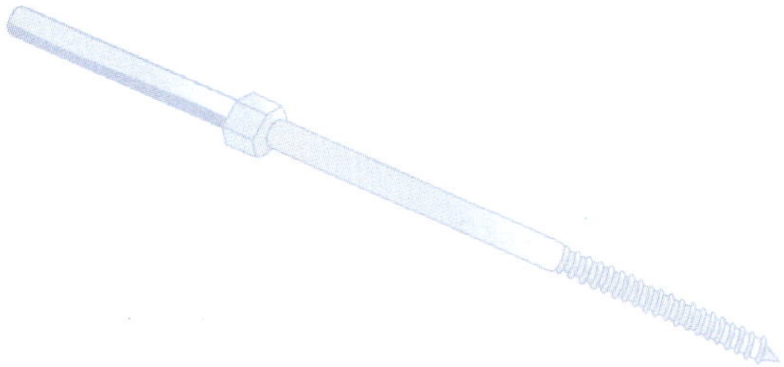

b. Knowles pin 4 mm diameter
Sizes 2.5" to 5" with 0.25" variation

3. Hemi-hip replacement prosthesis

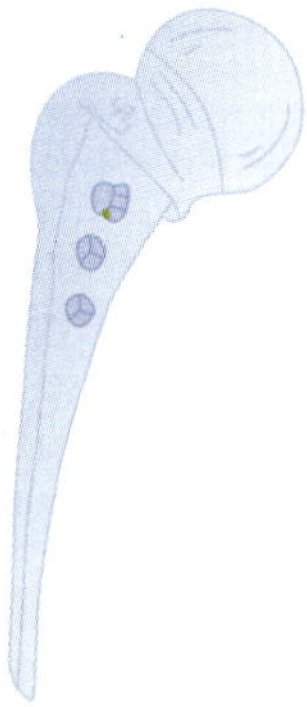

a. Austin moore prosthesis
Sizes 35 mm to 55 mm with 2 mm variation

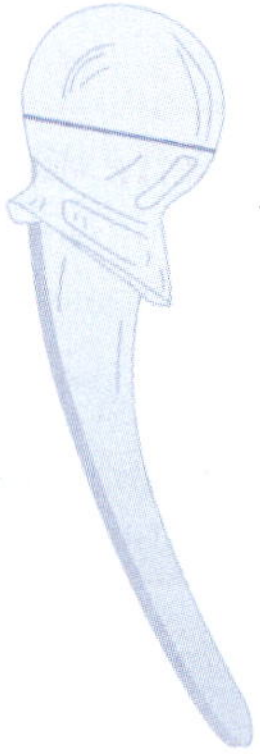

b. Thompson prosthesis
Sizes 35 mm to 55 mm with 2 mm variation

4. Hip screws

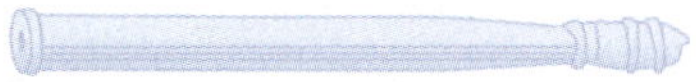

a. Garden screw—short tapping
Sizes 2.25" to 5" with 0.25" variation

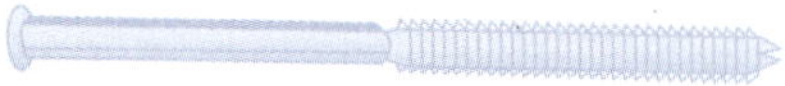

b. Garden screw—extended tapping
Sizes 2.25" to 5" with 0.25" variation

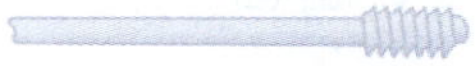

c. Cannulated hip screws (CHS).
Length: 50 mm to 115 mm with 5 mm variation

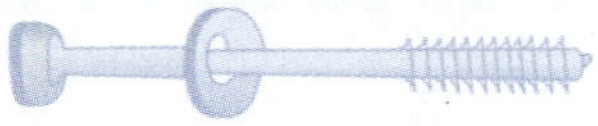

d. Cannulated bolts
Sizes 2.5" to 4.5" with 4.25" variation

5. Osteotomy fixation plates

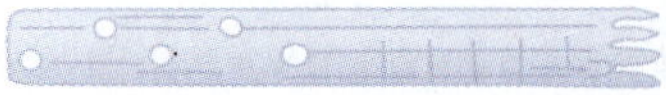

a. Kessel plate 3 or 4.7 mm thick.
Sizes 5 or 6 holes

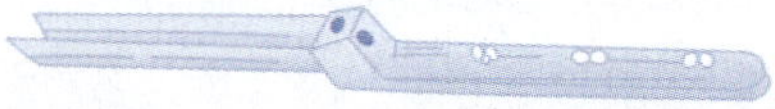

b. Wainwright plate, Blade sizes 2" to 2.5"
plate sizes 3 and 4 holes

INSTRUMENTS USED FOR HIP HEMIREPLACEMENT SURGERY

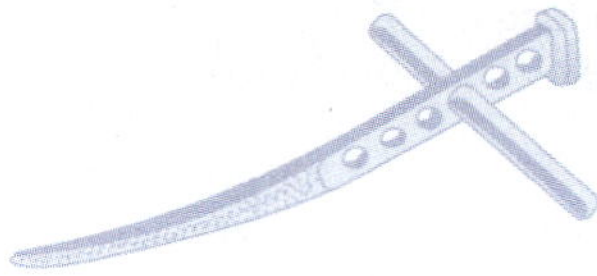

Rasp for intramedullary canal reaming for AM prosthesis

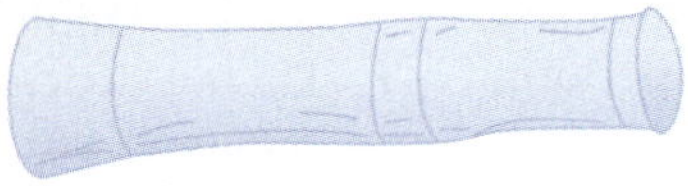

Alluminium impactor for AM prosthesis

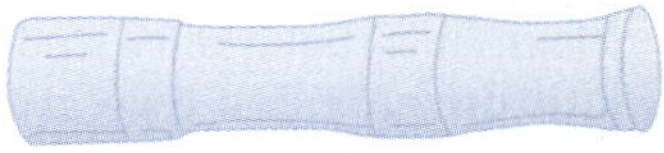

Alluminium impactor with tufnol head for AM prosthesis

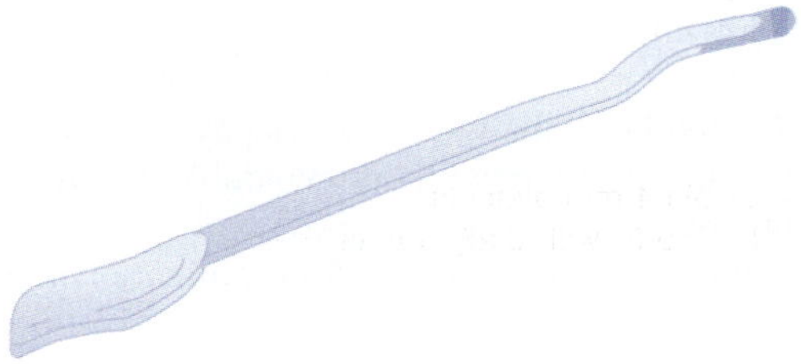

Murphy skid

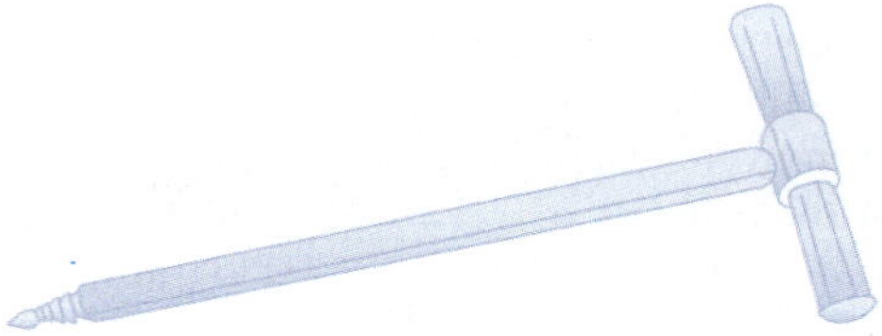

Head extracator—Judet extractor

INSTRUMENTS USED FOR SMITH-PETERSON NAILING

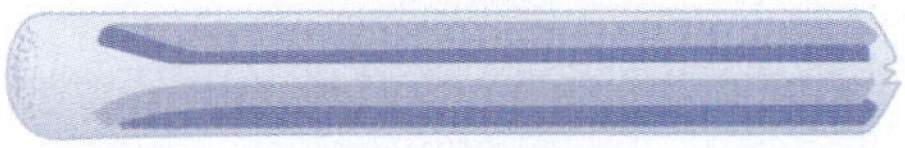

Smith-Peterson nail

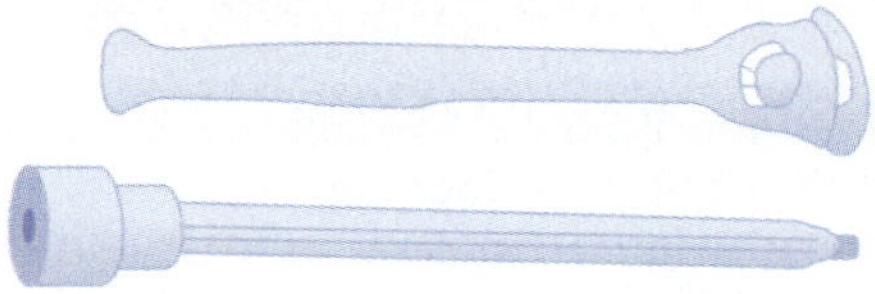

Smith-Peterson impactor for SP nail

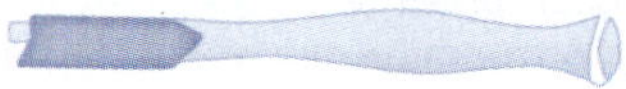

Smith-Peterson trifin nail starter

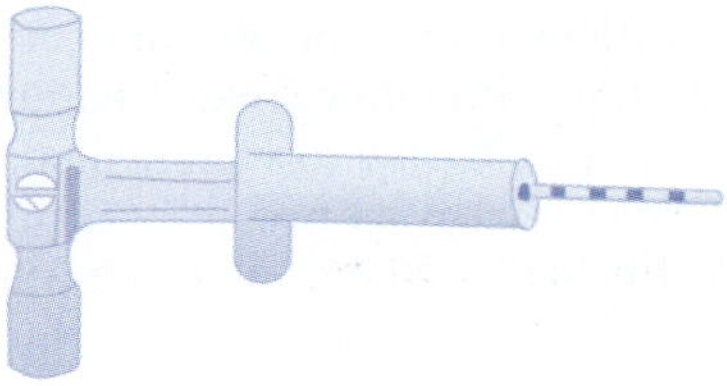

Watson Jones handle for guidewire

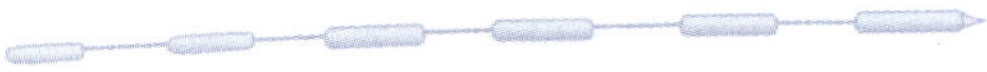

Guidewire—calibrated 9° for SP nail

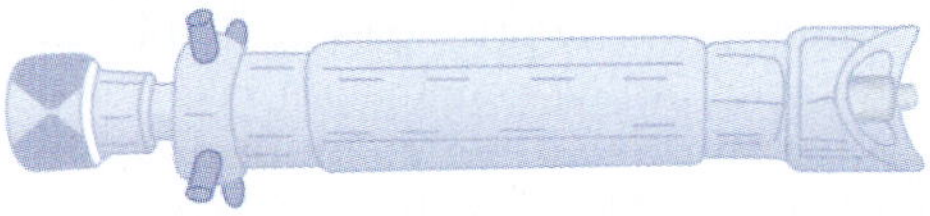

Extractor/impactor for SP nail

Guidelines for Practical Examinations

Time and again students have requested me to give practical suggestions to perform better in clinical examination. This section is intended to give some guidelines to help the students to fare better in the practical examinations. *I would like to remind the students that this is only a guideline and not a passport to success.* I can only give clues, but it is the student who has to perform. One has to develop his own method built upon the information given here.

This section is presented under the following headings:

1. *Guidelines to perform well in the clinical examination.*
2. *Common pitfalls which can be avoided during the examination.*
3. *A list of common short cases, the diagnostic clues and pitfalls in each case.*

(Remember only the common cases are mentioned here. There could be a few others also).

Apart from clinical presentation of short cases, a practical examination consists of viva voce which is mainly oral question and answers identifying radiographs of classical cases, instruments and specimens. The important radiographs have been given at the end of each chapter and the instruments have been clearly displayed on the chapter on implants. One need to read them prior to the examinations.

GUIDELINES TO FARE BETTER IN CLINICAL EXAMINATION IN ORTHOPAEDICS

- Attend the clinical postings regularly.
- See all the examination cases at least once during the postings or later.
- Read standard books on orthopaedics right from the beginning and not at the time of examination.
- Become familiar with clinical examination methods by reading and practicing the correct methods.
- Present as many cases as possible during the clinical postings. This will make you fluent and boost your confidence.
- Inculcate the habit of discussion with the staff, professor and fellow students.
- Try to understand the principles behind treatment, etc.

  Do not read for the examination sake. Read to acquire knowledge, since you are going to practice in future. *Examination should just be a part of the exercise and not your goal.*

- In cases of ambiguity, do not give a very accurate diagnosis even though you are very sure. This creates suspicion and hence always give a differential diagnosis.
- Do not argue even though you feel that the examiner is wrong. Mildly, but firmly, express your opinion.
- Do not depend on luck. Try to do things correctly and minimise the errors. Always put up a brave front, look straight into the examiner's eye. Remember luck always favours the brave.
- Do not cry and try to gain examiner's sympathy. Snatch the result with both your hands rather than spread your hands pleading for results.
- Keep cool, use plenty of common sense and be opportunistic. Remember hard work always pays.
- Certain amount of tension is unavoidable, but do not be overcome by it.
- Keep all the instruments needed for examination in proper shape.
- Remember the examiners were students once and they know all the trials, tribulations and mischiefs. So do not bluff and try to outsmart them.
- Usually clear-cut and straight forward spotters are given in the examination. Diagnosis is not a problem, but discussion is.

AVOID THE FOLLOWING PITFALLS IN THE EXAMINATION HALL

- Make your own diagnosis.
- Do not heed to prompts by examination experts.
- Be cautious with the patients. Fed up with repeated examination by many students and you, they may mislead you.
- Do not look into the case papers, as things may be erroneous in it.
- Follow a methodical and analytical approach.
- Do not stop after making a diagnosis, look beyond for complications and other changes.
- Make a common diagnosis and be skeptical about rare diagnosis.
- Be on your guard if you are the first student or the last student in the examination. *A fresh examiner and a tired examiner both are dangerous.*

- When things are going tough, keep yourself cool, have presence of mind and look for clues. *Never panic even in extremely difficult situations.*
- By making smart, intelligent moves always lead the examiners into areas of your strength and do not get led into areas of your weakness.

INSTRUMENTS REQUIRED FOR CLINICAL EXAMINATION

- Measuring tape
- Skin marker
- Knee hammer
- Goniometer
- Common pin
- Cotton
- Stethoscope.

COMMON EXAMINATION CASES

Case	Relevant clues	Pitfalls	Ref. page
I. UPPER LIMB **1. Cubitus varus**	• H/o old trauma • Gunstock deformity • Loss of carrying angle (compare with opposite elbow) • Movements of elbow full • Arms short	• 95% of cases are due to old supracondylar fracture • 5% other causes • Measurements to be interpreted cautiously The bony measurements are not very useful but are useful in acute cases	140
2. Unreduced posterior dislocation of elbow	• H/o old trauma • Slightly older child • Fixed flexion deformity of elbow movements are definitely restricted • Wasting of muscles and forearm is short	• Likely to confuse with old supracondylar fracture of humerus • See for points above • Look for other complications of posterior dislocation of elbow	145
3. Malunion Colles' fracture	• H/o of old trauma • Usually patient is an elderly female but not necessarily. • *Dinner fork deformity if present helps but if absent does not rule* out diagnosis • If styloid processes are at the same level, it clinches the diagnosis with certainty • Movements of the wrist decreased	• Dinner fork deformity If present, helps in the diagnosis; but if absent, does not rule out.	164
4. Claw hand	• Classical claw hand deformity • Look whether total or ulnar. • H/o trauma ± • Look for features of leprosy • Carry out tests for all three peripheral nerves • Look for wasting of hypothenar and intermetatarsal space • Trophic changes may be present	• If total, lesion could be higher • Leprosy is a common cause • If ulnar, lesion could be low down • Do not confuse with Dupuytren's contracture. Here there is flexion of both MP and IP joints. In clawing there is extension of MP joints and flexion of IP joints of the fingers • VIC is another important differential diagnosis	300
5. Dupuytren's contracture	• Long history • Usually affects little and ring finger • See above • Flexion of both MP and IP joints • Examine the other hand also • Cord-like structure felt on the ulnar aspect of palmar fascia • Peripheral nerve tests are usually normal	• Likely to be confused with claw hand	357

Contd...

Appendices

Contd...

	Case	Relevant clues	Pitfalls	Ref. page
	6. Wrist drop	• Inability of extend wrist, thumbs, and MP joints of the fingers • Extension of IP joints is present. It is brought about by intrinsic muscles of the hand, supplied by ulnar nerve and median nerve	• Tendency to ignore the diagnosis on seeing extension of fingers of IP joints	307
	7. VIC	• Old history of trauma • Old supracondylar fracture in child. • Old both bone fracture in adults • Extensive forearm scarring • Forearm thin, atrophic • Function of elbow and wrist joints are affected • Peripheral nerves affected • Volkmann's sign, if present is characteristic • Claw hand deformity	• Confused with other causes of claw hand • Confused with Dupuytren's contracture	35
	8. Rheumatoid hand	• Chronic history • Bilateral, symmetrical • Other joints involved • Swan neck. Boutonniére deformity ulnar deviation, etc. • Generalised pain, swelling	• Confused with other hand anomalies described above	530
II.	**LOWER LIMBS** **1. Genu valgum**	• If bilateral, could be idiopathic • If unilateral, look for history of trauma or infection • Deformity is the only complaint if idiopathic • Intermalleolar distance is increased • Late onset genu valgum is a feature of renal rickets (11–14 yr) • Movements usually are full range	• In idiopathic variety deformity is the only complaint • Late onset deformity is common with renal rickets • Lock carefully for any general causes, other accompanying deformities, etc.	383
	2. Genu varum	• Spot diagnosis • Deformity is the only complaint in the idiopathic variety • If unilateral, look for infection and trauma • Common deformity in OA knee • Movements are usually normal	• Not to be confused with genu valgum	384
III.	**FOOT** **1. CTEV**	• Present since birth • Classical five deformities • In idiopathic, deformity is the only complaint • Look for other causes • Examine spine and other features of congenital disorders	• If generalised and rigid, suspect AMC • Defect in the spine with a tuft of hair, etc. Suspect spina bifida • Carefully check for muscle imbalance	452
	2. Foot-drop	• Traumatic history • Leprosy is a common cause • If complete, inability to dorsiflex, evert and invert • Look for trophic ulcers • Follow the course of sciatic nerve to detect the cause	• Always check whether foot-drop is complete or incomplete • Common peroneal nerve affection, either due to trauma or leprosy is the most common cause of foot-drop	309

Contd...

Contd...

Case	Relevant clues	Pitfalls	Ref. page
IV. GENERAL 1. **Chronic osteomyelitis** *Any bones not joints*	• Chronic history • H/o acute osteomyelitis • Characteristic point in history is *discharge of bony spicules* • Irregular bone thickening • Multiple scars and sinuses adherent to bone. • Movements of neighbouring joints are decreased • Wasting of the muscles • Sprouting granulation tissue is seen	• Septic arthritis. Here joint movements grossly disturbed unlike chronic osteomyelitis • Ewing's sarcoma	494
2. **TB knee** **TB shoulder** **TB ankle**	• Chronic history • Constitutional symptoms • Monoarticular • Gross wasting of muscles • Movements markedly affected • Lymphadenopathy	• Other joint disorders	515 518
3. **Tumours**	**Diagnostic clues**	**Pitfalls**	**Ref. page**
Exostosis Common sites are: • Lower end of radius • Around knee joints • Around shoulder	• Bony hard swelling at the ends of long bones • Immobile • Chronic • Movements of neighbouring joints may be decreased • No symptom unless associated with complications	• Look for multiple exostosis which is a developmental disorder	571
Osteoclastoma Common sites: • Lower end of radius • Lower end of femur • Upper end of tibia • Upper end of fibula	• General condition of the patient is normal • Slightly longer history • Young adults • Epiphyseal ends of long bones • No dilated veins • Egg shell crackling may be present or absent • Joint movements are usually affected late • Age: slightly middle age group is affected	• Confused with osteomyelitis • Malignant bone tumour • Other bone cysts	581
Chondrosarcoma	• Usually a long history • Metaphyseal ends of long bones • Huge size • Patient usually not very moribund	Confused with osteosarcoma which has: • Short history • Patient is more cachectic • Dilated veins are present • Other features of malignancy • Slightly younger patient	573
Ewing's sarcoma	• 5–15 years of age • Very short history • Diaphysis situation • History of fever present • Features of malignancy present	• Confused with acute osteomyelitis • Look for features of osteomyelitis	584

Contd...

Contd...

Case	Relevant clues	Pitfalls	Ref. page
4. Nonunion of any bone			36
Characteristic sites	**Diagnostic clues**	**Confused with**	
• Lower end of tibia • Patella • Both bones forearm • Neck of femur • Humerus lower 1/3	• H/o trauma • Prolonged history of treatment • *Painless abnormal mobility* • Loss of function • Wasting • In infected nonunion, look for features of chronic osteomyelitis, sinus scars, implants, etc.	• Delayed union • Maluniting fracture • Pseudarthrosis tibia	
5. Malunion of any bone			
Sites	**Diagnostic clues**	**Confused with**	**Ref. page**
• Humerus shaft • Supracondylar fracture of humerus • Both bones forearm • Femur • Tibia • Clavicle	• H/o trauma • H/o long treatment • H/o treatment by quacks • Cosmetic deformity • Shortening • Altered function • Wasting of muscles	• Nonunion • Delayed union • Deformities due to other causes	41

Index

G

H

I

N

O

P

Q

R

S